EMT
PREHOSPITAL
CARE

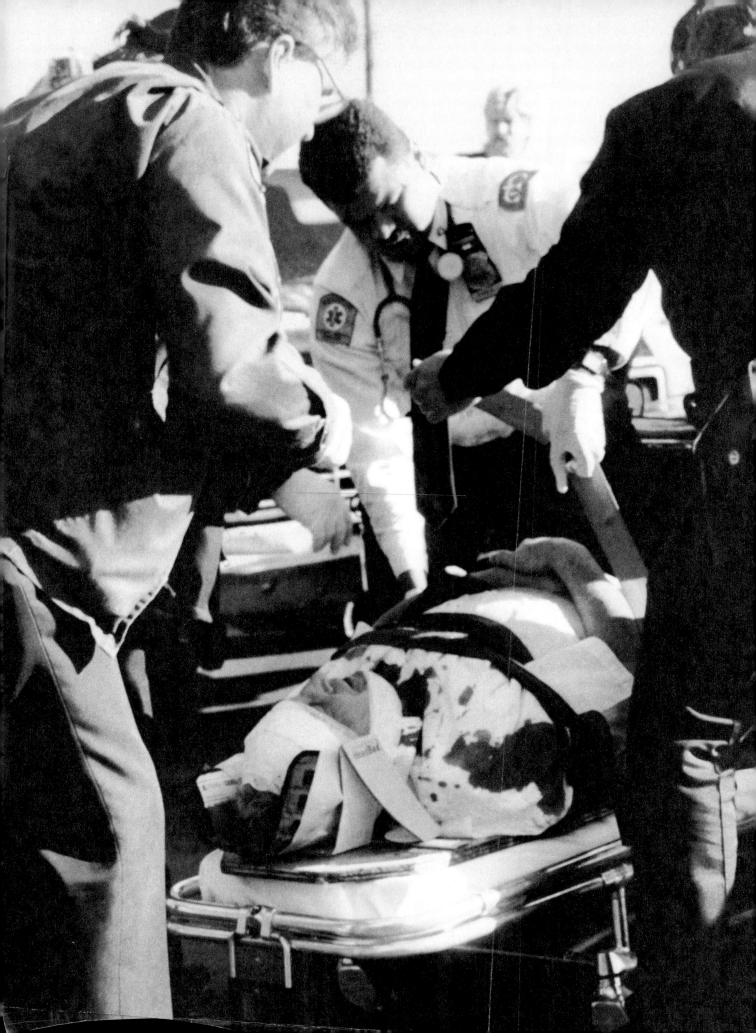

EMT
PREHOSPITAL
CARE

Mark C. Henry, MD
Associate Professor and Chairman
Department of Emergency Medicine
School of Medicine
State University of New York at Stony Brook
Stony Brook, New York

Edward R. Stapleton, EMT-P
Director of Prehospital Care and Education
University Hospital
Instructor
Department of Emergency Medicine
School of Medicine
State University of New York at Stony Brook
Stony Brook, New York

W.B. SAUNDERS COMPANY
A Division of Harcourt Brace & Company
Philadelphia London Toronto Montreal Sydney Tokyo

W.B. SAUNDERS COMPANY
A Division of
Harcourt Brace & Company

The Curtis Center
Independence Square West
Philadelphia, Pennsylvania 19106

Library of Congress Cataloging-in-Publication Data

Henry, Mark C.
    EMT, prehospital care / Mark C. Henry, Edward R. Stapleton.
        p.   cm.
    Includes index.

    ISBN 0-7216-1301-2

    1. Emergency medicine.   2. Emergency medical technicians.
    3. Medical emergencies.   I. Stapleton, Edward R.   II. Title.
    [DNLM: 1. Emergencies.   2. Emergency Medical Services.   WX 215
    H523e]
    RC86.7.H47   1992
    616.02'5—dc20
    DNLM/DLC   91-35156

Editor: Margaret M. Biblis
Developmental Editor: Shirley Kuhn
Designer: Paul Fry
Production Manager: Carolyn Naylor
Manuscript Editor: Tina Rebane
Illustrator: Laurence Ward
Mechanical Illustrator: Risa Clow
Illustration Coordinator: Cecilia Roberts
Page Layout Artist: Holly McLaughlin
Indexer: Norman Duren
Cover photo by: Mark C. Henry, MD

EMT: Prehospital Care   ISBN 0-7216-1301-2

Last digit is the print number: 9   8   7   6   5   4   3   2

To **Diane**,
for her continuous support and encouragement
and to my children
Matthew, **Rachael**, *and* **Adam**

MCH

To **Donna**,
for her love, enthusiasm, and hard work during this project
and to my children
Lara *and* **Edward**

ERS

CONTRIBUTORS

WILLIAM H. BENSKY, PA

Formerly Director of Hyperbaric Medicine, Mount Sinai Medical Center, New York, New York

(Contributed to Diving Emergencies in Chapter 11—ENVIRONMENTAL EMERGENCIES)

JONATHAN BEST, EMT-P

Chief, Fairfield Fire Department, Fairfield, Connecticut

(Coauthored Chapter 17—DISASTERS AND TRIAGE; and Chapter 18—EXTRICATION)

ROBERT ELLING, EMT-P

Associate Director, EMS Program, New York State Department of Health, Albany, New York

(Contributed to Operating an Emergency Vehicle in Chapter 19—AMBULANCE OPERATIONS)

GEORGE FOLTIN, MD

Director, Pediatric Emergency Services, Bellevue Hospital Center; Assistant Professor of Clinical Pediatrics, New York University, School of Medicine, New York, New York

(Coauthored Chapter 14—PEDIATRIC EMERGENCIES)

NEAL FLOMENBAUM, MD

Chairman, Department of Emergency Medicine, Long Island College Hospital; Associate Professor of Clinical Medicine, State University of New York at Brooklyn, Brooklyn, New York

(Contributed to Poisons in Chapter 12—MEDICAL EMERGENCIES)

RICHARD GUERIN, EMT-P

EMS Representative, EMS Program, New York State Department of Health, Albany, New York

(Contributed to Operating an Emergency Vehicle in Chapter 19—AMBULANCE OPERATIONS)

JAMES MARTIN, EMT-P

Captain, New York City Emergency Medical Services, EMS Academy, Bayside, New York

(Contributed to Operating an Emergency Vehicle in Chapter 19—AMBULANCE OPERATIONS)

JONATHAN POLITIS, EMT-P

Director, Town of Colonie, Department of Emergency Medical Services, Colonie, New York

(Contributed to Hazardous Materials in Chapter 11—ENVIRONMENTAL EMERGENCIES)

ANDREW STERN, NREMT-P

Paramedic Supervisor, Town of Colonie, Department of Emergency Medical Services, Colonie, New York

(Contributed to Hazardous Materials in Chapter 11—ENVIRONMENTAL EMERGENCIES)

DONNA STAPLETON, RN

Obstetrics Nurse, Good Samaritan Hospital; Member of the Faculty, Paramedic Training Program, Department of Emergency Medicine, Booth Memorial Medical Center, Flushing, New York

(Chapter 13—OBSTETRICAL AND GYNECOLOGICAL EMERGENCIES)

PETER SHIELDS, MD

Mount Sinai Medical Center, New York, New York

(Contributed to Chapter 8—ABDOMINAL EMERGENCIES)

PETER VICCELLIO, MD

Vice Chairman and Residency Program Director and Assistant Professor, Department of Emergency Medicine, School of Medicine, State University of New York at Stony Brook, Stony Brook, New York

(Chapter 15—PSYCHOLOGICAL ASPECTS OF EMERGENCY CARE and contributed to Communicable Disease in Chapter 12—MEDICAL EMERGENCIES)

FOREWORD

The extension of medical care outside the walls of a hospital illustrates uniquely how real—and how essential—is medical teamwork in the service of patients. Many have long paid lip service to the theory that physicians, nurses, and paramedical personnel must work closely to provide the best care possible in a modern medical system. Prehospital care requires more than lip service to make it work. Emergency medicine is the specialty that perhaps most practically illustrates the need for the team to be close-knit, efficient, and "singing from the same songsheet." Prehospital care depends more on this "team" approach than does any other branch of medicine, but bridging the gulf between hospital and field requires a special approach to both training and clinical practice.

The bridge was more easily built in the early days when prehospital care programs were largely experiments by hospital clinicians and designed to duplicate the care provided in specialized units. The link between physician-EMT, EMT-nurse, and nurse-physician was more readily forged and maintained due to the "pioneering" nature of these programs and the common purpose felt by all involved. As we grew, and as programs became more complex, the ties binding the team together began to weaken and fade.

In *EMT: Prehospital Care*, Dr. Mark Henry and his colleague Ed Stapleton make a major effort to strengthen the link that binds hospital and field teams together. *EMT: Prehospital Care* presents solid medical principles tampered and shaped by long experience in field practice. It is a product of physician/EMT-P collaboration, and the influence of this collaboration is evident throughout the work. It is wonderfully balanced with sound medicine and practical principles. This is no "ivory tower" work but rather is spattered and soiled from the lessons of the streets. It is a welcome addition, and a unique one.

Impressive in this text is the bold, decisive nature of the medical principles presented. The authors do not shy away from the complex physiologic or anatomic facts necessary for a student or veteran to understand and remember important medical facts. Rather, they use the principles to help the learner understand and—perhaps more important—remember "need-to-know" essentials. The presentation of anatomy and physiology is relevant to prehospital clinical practice, and it is done in such a way as to be understandable yet accurate. This text is refreshing in the fact that it is not a "cookbook" and avoids taking a "cookbook" approach to the provision of prehospital care. Though it is easily understood, it is not simplistic. This fact alone makes it stand out. It should, for this reason, set a standard.

The text is wonderfully illustrated, and its organization is excellent. Its use of real patient problems reinforces its clinical base and relevance to field practice.

The philosophy behind this text is evident: that prehospital care is medical care, and that it must be practiced by informed and well-trained team members. The text is a bridge, sound in construction and solid underfoot. But most of all, it is patient-centered. What better could be said of it?

RONALD D. STEWART, MD, FACEP, FRCPC, DSc (Hon)
Professor of Anaesthesia (Emergency Medicine)
Dalhousie University, Halifax, Nova Scotia, Canada

PREFACE

Prehospital and emergency care is an exciting and challenging endeavor. The steps taken in the first minutes after an emergency medical problem has occurred may make the difference between life and death. Emergency medicine is a relatively new field, and emergency medical services systems are still evolving in scope and sophistication. Emergency medical technicians are often the first formally trained medical personnel to encounter the critically ill or injured patient and are the foundation of the prehospital emergency medical response system in a community.

The emergency medical technicians are recognized by the emergency medicine community as a key link in the "chain of survival." Whether the patient has had a heart attack or has suffered a severe injury, the actions of the EMT contribute to the patient's outcome. At the heart of the EMT's knowledge is the ability to conduct an efficient and organized assessment, design a plan of action, institute emergency treatment, and make triage and transport decisions necessary for the patient's survival. The EMT encounters patients of all ages and with multiple conditions in various and unpredictable environments. As knowledge and technology advance, EMTs take on more and more responsibility. The scope of knowledge required of EMTs is broad indeed.

We have taught and practiced emergency medical care for several years. We recognize that the EMT is routinely faced with life and death decisions and must be prepared to act instinctively and with confidence. As with all medical care professionals, EMTs are most effective when they have an understanding of the "why" and "how" of the actions that they undertake in the field.

To lay a foundation of understanding, we have coupled the traditional style of medical education with the pragmatic approach to the patient that the student will use in the field. The medical content is explained by introducing anatomy and physiology, followed by pathophysiology (disease and injury states), assessment, and treatment. This allows the acquisition of knowledge and skills to proceed as "building blocks" that are logically layered one on another and prepares the student for the final "assessment based" approach to the patient. The assessment discussion is divided into trauma and medical (nontraumatic) sections, since the conditions encountered and the approach to the patient vary. This organization—anatomy and physiology, pathophysiology, assessment, and treatment— is followed in most chapters. Most clinical chapters are grouped by organ systems, with respiratory, circulatory, and nervous systems introduced first since the assessment of these systems is the basis for the *primary survey*, a rapid assessment and treatment approach applied to all patients.

Procedures employed in patient treatment are emphasized in separate and distinct layouts. With each skill, there is an attempt to provide the rationale for the prehospital treatment. Protocols or treatment plans are used to summarize the approach to the patient. These are invaluable tools for learning, reinforcement, and retention.

This book is designed to serve as a text for EMT-ambulance, EMT-defibrillation, and EMT-intermediate training. It covers all the current Department of Transportation objectives for EMTs, and includes advanced skills such as defibrillation, intubation, IV fluid therapy, and administration of critical drugs that may be used by EMTs, such as epinephrine for anaphylaxis and glucose and glucagon for patients with low blood sugar.

The study guide is designed to supplement the text, offering the student a chance to reinforce and evaluate acquisition of the knowledge objectives and to prepare for course tests and the certifying examination. Also offered are an instructor's guide and slide package, both of which are keyed to the DOT curriculum.

Writing this text has been a tremendous learning experience for us. We have relied on our own education and practice, feedback from our EMT students, and information and illustrations from textbooks and articles, and we acknowledge the significant influence of our teachers and peers. Whenever possible, we have based our recommendations on the standards and guidelines of nationally recognized organizations such as the National Association of EMS Physicians, the American Heart Association, the American College of Surgeons, the American College of Emergency Physicians, the National Association of EMTs, and the American College of Orthopedic Surgeons. Our greatest reward, however, is to share the students' joy in grasping new concepts that will be part of their basic understanding of the human body and emergency care.

How to Use This Book

Since much of the information in the text is likely to be new to you, it is important to organize yourself to ensure *acquisition* and *retention* of the essential knowledge. This includes learning new terms, recognizing anatomy, grasping concepts of physiology and pathophysiology, and learning the signs and symptoms of various injuries and diseases and prehospital treatments.

A practical study strategy would be use of the "whole–part–whole" approach:

1. **Review the Chapter Objectives.** The objectives at the beginning of each chapter define the important learning points to be covered. Carefully review them and keep the objectives in mind as you read the material.

2. **Skim the Chapter.** Read the introduction on the first page and then quickly browse through the chapter, looking at the main headings to appreciate the basic organization of the subject matter.

3. **Review Questions.** Before reading the chapter in detail, look at the review questions to appreciate the focus of the chapter and reflect on them during your reading.

4. **Read Section by Section.** Begin to read the book carefully, stopping to understand information or vocabulary that is unclear. Write down words that you do not comprehend and return to the text or refer to the glossary for clarification. At the end of each section, attempt to answer the relevant review questions at the end of the chapter. If you have difficulty with a question, briefly review the related material.

5. **Use Tables and Illustrations.** Tables and illustrations are powerful ways to present information. Tables are used to summarize and organize key points. Illustrations include photographs, line drawings, and anatomical drawings that help the reader visualize relevant anatomic and physiologic facts, key clinical signs, and treatment steps.

6. **Review the Procedures and Protocols.** The clinical chapters contain both procedures and protocols. Procedures are step-by-step descriptions of how to perform necessary techniques to assess and treat the patient and are specially highlighted for clarity and emphasis. Protocols summarize actions to take when encountering patients with specific signs, symptoms, or diagnoses. They also provide a method for summarizing and condensing key information. We have included protocols from the New York State EMS Program and the New York City Emergency Medical Services as examples. While these protocols were derived by practicing experts in emergency care and are based in large part on national standards and guidelines, we recognize that there are constant changes and variations from region to region. Therefore we recommend that whenever possible the reader become familiar with local protocols early in the study of this text.

7. **Perform a Self-Test.** At the end of a chapter, conduct a self-test using the review questions or the related workbook or have a fellow student ask you questions directly out of the book.

We hope the readers will find the text interesting and stimulating and will continue to update their education. We have tried to make the text as accurate and as practical as possible. We recommend that EMTs follow the procedures and protocols of their respective EMS system.

We welcome feedback from the readers.

MARK C. HENRY, MD
EDWARD R. STAPLETON, EMT-P

ACKNOWLEDGMENTS

We wish to extend our gratitude to the wide variety of friends, co-workers, and W.B. Saunders Company staff who have contributed their time and expertise in the development of this text. Thanks also to our friends who willingly gave of their time and skills to create the manuscript and illustrations:

Sal Aquilato	Jeff DePrima	Frank Mazzagatti
Joseph Asti	Lisa Epstein	Sunil Nath
Pearl Bartels	Frank Fillaramo	William Powell
Grace Leora Bartolillo	Peter Finamore	Eva Rivera
Joseph Bartolillo	Madeline Fong	Joseph Savasta
George Benedetto	Raymond Gasper	Sandy Shulder
Robert Bentkowski	Howard Gelfman	Yvonne Siegel
Andrew Bonadia	Marianne Gelfman	Bruce Stark
Nicholas Boukas	Linda Gordon	Barbara Tenney
Jane Brandt	Timothy Gray	Carol Timpa
Christopher Cassela	Noreen Groome	Alvin Toro
Allison Cassidy	Matthew Henry	Robert Torres
Michael Cassidy	Lester Kallus	Nancy Whitfield
Mary Ann Citarella	Peter Kwiath	Willard Wright
Michael Corr	Hoon Jae Lin	

We are grateful to the Booth Memorial Medical Center for providing the academic environment that supported our work in EMS education.

The New York State Department of Health EMS Program contributed both important information and materials for this text. We especially thank Michael Gilbertson, Bob Elling, Richard Guerin, and John Clair for their invaluable contributions. We also thank our Colleagues in New York City Emergency Medical Services and the Medical Advisory Committee for their advice and protocols.

We would also like to recognize the Fairfield Connecticut Fire Department for their logistical support and expertise in the development of the rescue illustrations.

A special expression of gratitude is extended to Kathryn Barrett, from Ruttle, Shaw and Wetherill, who helped immeasurably to keep the project moving, and to Marcie Biello for her superb editing skills.

Much of the original artwork in this book can be attributed to the highly skilled professionals assigned to our project. Barbara Proud paid meticulous attention to every detail to ensure exceptional clarity in her photographs. Larry Ward, our illustrator, was able to express both aesthetic beauty and function in his work.

Finally, we thank our editors, Margaret Biblis, who used her outstanding management skills to secure the vital manpower and resources needed to make this project a success; and Baxter Venable, who believed in our abilities and provided inspiration and leadership in the early phases of this effort.

Shirley Kuhn, our developmental editor, provided her extraordinary organizational talents and caring attitude to make a very complex task seem much easier. And thank you to all of the other editorial and production personnel who have contributed to this project, especially Ceil Roberts, Risa Clow, Tina Rebane, and Paul Fry.

MARK C. HENRY, MD
EDWARD R. STAPLETON, EMT-P

REVIEWERS

Thank you to our reviewers for the invaluable feedback:

BRYCE BREITENSTEIN, MD

Medical Director
Occupational Medicine Clinic
Brookhaven National Laboratory
Clinical Associate Professor
Community Medicine
State University of New York at Stony Brook
Stony Brook, New York

FRANK CARIELLO, MD

Department of Obstetrics and Gynecology
Good Samaritan Hospital
West Islip, New York

DENNIS DePASS, RpT

Manager
Respiratory Therapy
Booth Memorial Medical Center
Flushing, New York

SHIRLEY KOTCHER, JD

Legal Council
Booth Memorial Medical Center
Flushing, New York

ERIC NIEGELBERG

EMS Coordinator
University Hospital
Paramedic Training Coordinator
School of Allied Health Professions
State University of New York at Stony Brook
Stony Brook, New York

ARSEN PANKOVICH, MD

Clinical Professor of Orthopaedic Surgery
New York University Medical Center
Attending Physician
Booth Memorial Medical Center
Flushing, New York

GUSTAVE PAPPAS, EMT-P

Director
Emergency Medical Services Academy
New York City EMS
Fort Totten, New York

KENNETH RIFKIND, MD

Associate Chairman of Surgery and
Director of Trauma Services
Booth Memorial Medical Center
Flushing, New York
Assistant Professor of Clinical Surgery
New York University School of Medicine,
New York, New York

CONTENTS

CHAPTER 11

ENVIRONMENTAL EMERGENCIES 487

Mark Henry, Edward Stapleton, Andrew Stern, and Jonathan Politis

CHAPTER 12

MEDICAL EMERGENCIES 537

Mark Henry, Edward Stapleton, and Neal Flomenbaum

CHAPTER 13

OBSTETRIC AND GYNECOLOGIC EMERGENCIES 597

Donna Stapleton

CHAPTER 14

PEDIATRIC EMERGENCIES 643

George Foltin, Mark Henry, and Edward Stapleton

CHAPTER 15

PSYCHOLOGICAL ASPECTS OF EMERGENCY CARE 679

Peter Viccellio

CHAPTER 16

LIFTING AND MOVING PATIENTS 689

Mark Henry and Edward Stapleton

CHAPTER 17

DISASTERS AND TRIAGE 717

Mark Henry, Edward Stapleton, and Jonathan Best

CHAPTER 18

EXTRICATION............................ 735

Mark Henry, Edward Stapleton, and Jonathan Best

CHAPTER 19

AMBULANCE OPERATIONS.......... 755

Mark Henry, Edward Stapleton, James Martin, Robert Elling, and Richard Guerin

CHAPTER 20

APPROACH TO THE MULTIPLE TRAUMA PATIENT.................... 795

Mark Henry and Edward Stapleton

PROCEDURES

CHAPTER 16

EMT
PREHOSPITAL
CARE

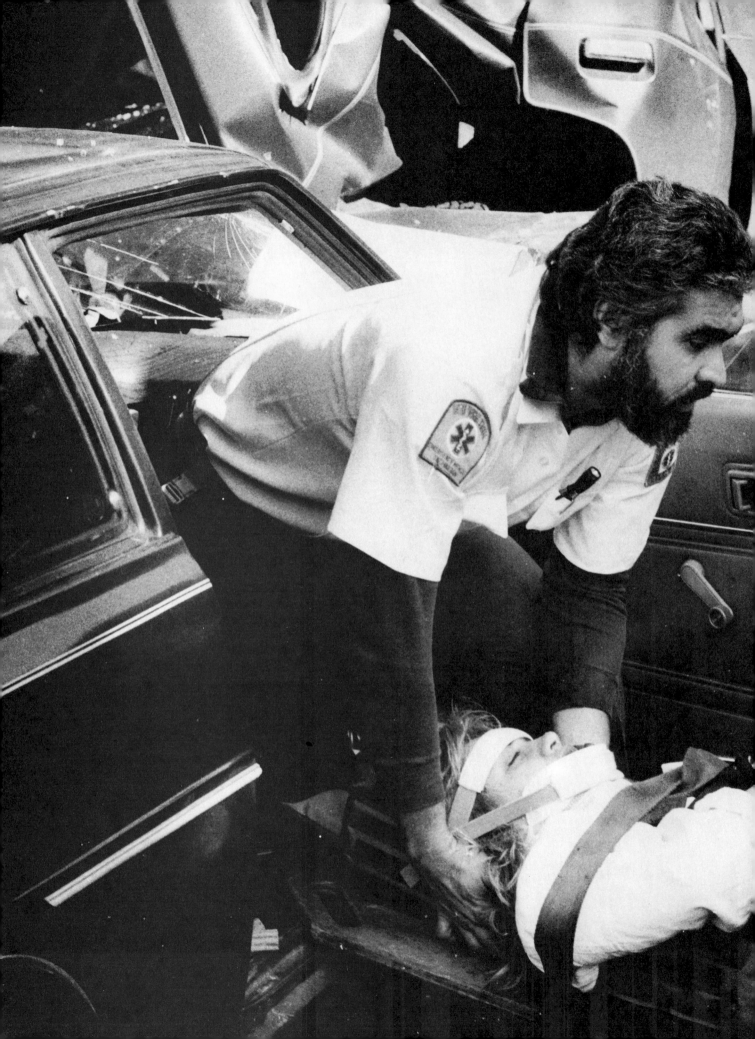

CHAPTER 1

INTRODUCTION TO PREHOSPITAL EMERGENCY CARE

OBJECTIVES

At the conclusion of this chapter the reader will be able to:

1. Define an EMS system.

2. List each component of an EMS system and describe its role.

3. Define medical control.

4. List four primary and three other responsibilities of an EMT.

5. Discuss ethical principles related to prehospital care.

6. List and describe the four elements of medical malpractice.

7. Describe the following types of consent:
   Implied
   Informed

INTRODUCTION

Working as an emergency medical technician (EMT) can be very challenging and rewarding. As an integral part of emergency medical services (EMS), the EMT usually provides the first professional medical aid to victims of an illness or accident. By assessing patients' conditions, treating and transporting them, and communicating with other rescue and medical personnel, EMTs are able to save countless lives.

This chapter explains the evolution and development of the modern EMS system. It also discusses the training, duties, and obligations of the EMT and how he or she works within the EMS system.

EMERGENCY MEDICAL SERVICES SYSTEM

Webster's Dictionary supplies the following definitions:

Emergency—An unforeseen combination of circumstances or the resulting state that calls for immediate action. A pressing need.
Medical—Relating to or concerned with physicians or the practice of medicine.
Service—The occupation or function of serving; a contribution to the welfare of others.
System—A regular interacting or interdependent group of items forming a unified whole.

An emergency medical services system (EMSS) is the planned configuration of community resources and personnel necessary to provide immediate medical care to patients who have suffered sudden or unexpected illness or injury.

Historical Perspective

EMS is a relatively new and exciting field that is still in the process of evolving. The origins of EMS date back to the simple idea of one human being helping another. The altruistic human motivation to respond to someone in need led to the development of the sophisticated EMSS that exists today. The "Good Samaritan" is the model that EMS personnel should emulate when called to the aid of someone in distress.

BATTLEFIELDS AS A LABORATORY

The growth and development of EMS systems were relatively slow and occurred primarily over the past 20 to 30 years. While much of this growth is due to technological advances, the value of a coordinated response to expected injury was ironically first identified on the

battlefields. During the Napoleonic Wars, an army surgeon, Baron Dominique Jean Larrey, introduced his *ambulance volantes*, or flying field hospital (Kennedy, RH). To increase the chances for survival, light carriages were used to remove the wounded from the battlefield, and preliminary care was provided.

In the United States, horse-drawn ambulances were first introduced during the Civil War, under the direction of Dr. Jonathan Letterman (Fig. 1–1). During the Korean War in the 1950s, helicopters were used to rapidly evacuate the wounded to mobile army surgical hospitals (MASH units). Immediate lifesaving surgery was performed there prior to transfer to more permanent definitive care units. The Vietnam War experience reinforced the value of rapid transport and early surgery for trauma victims. The death rates of battle casualties who reached a hospital dropped from 8% in World War I, to 2.5% in Korea, to less than 2% in Vietnam.

CIVILIAN EVOLUTION

The civilian evolution of EMS varied greatly from area to area. One of the first hospital-based ambulance services was initiated by Cincinnati General Hospital in the mid-1860s. The first motorized ambulance is said to have been provided by Michael Reese Hospital of Chicago in 1899 (Fig. 1–2). As automotive technology progressed, the style and capabilities changed accordingly (Fig. 1–3). Prior to World War II, physicians often rode on hospital-based ambulances as part of their clinical training. This model for prehospital emergency care still exists in some countries, including the Soviet Union.

TRAUMA AS AN IMPETUS FOR EMERGENCY MEDICAL SERVICES

Accidental injury is the leading cause of death in persons 1 to 34 years of age. In civilian life the automobile has caused a powerful surge in trauma deaths. In 1900

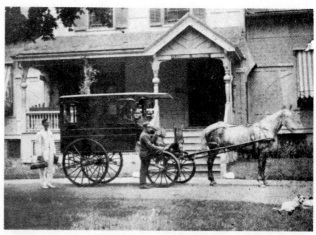

FIGURE 1–1. A horse-drawn ambulance. (Courtesy of Flushing Hospital, Flushing, NY.)

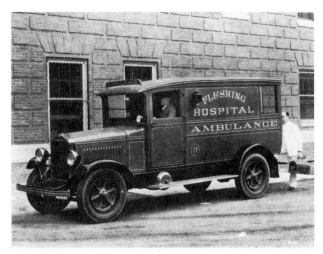

FIGURE 1–2. An early motorized ambulance. (Courtesy of Flushing Hospital, Flushing, NY.)

trauma due to accident was the seventh leading cause of death in the United States. It is now the third leading cause of death, with automobile accidents accounting for about half of these fatalities. Physicians observed the deaths of accident victims who might have been saved had they been treated on the battlefield. These losses brought to national attention the need for the rapid prehospital intervention demonstrated so successfully on battlefields during wartime. The simple steps necessary to intervene in the dying process were recognized. Application of bleeding control at the scene, safe patient handling, and rapid transportation to organized trauma centers were introduced to varying degrees throughout the country.

Since the resuscitation and stabilization of the injured person requires knowledge of the critical body systems (respiratory, circulatory, and nervous), care of the acute medical patient was also improved. The recent success in the resuscitation of victims of cardiac arrest provides the most dramatic evidence of the effects of a modern EMS system.

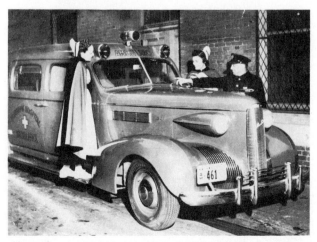

FIGURE 1–3. An ambulance of the 1930s. (Courtesy of Flushing Hospital, Flushing, NY.)

Medical knowledge and related technology were incorporated into EMS as they became available. For example, cardiopulmonary resuscitation (CPR) was not developed until 1960. Portable defibrillators, needed to resuscitate victims of cardiac arrest in the prehospital phase of care, were not available until the mid-1960s. The introduction of biotelemetry in the late 1960s improved prehospital care dramatically by allowing paramedics to perform defibrillation, to do advanced airway procedures, and to administer drugs under the direction of a physician at a base hospital.

THE PHYSICIAN AND EMERGENCY MEDICAL SERVICES

The physician's role in the development of EMS systems was extremely important. Medical societies such as the American Academy of Orthopaedic Surgeons and the American College of Surgeons played a significant role in EMS systems development. For example, the National EMT Training Curriculum that is used today was an outgrowth of work done by these physician groups in the 1960s. Physicians have been involved in EMT training from its beginning, and many still work with the Department of Transportation (DOT) to ensure the medical accuracy of national training curricula. Today the American College of Emergency Physicians and the National Association of EMS Physicians also play an active role in EMS.

Although physicians have functioned as prehospital providers in some areas of the United States, their role as field personnel has been limited. For many reasons, including resource allocation and costs, most ambulances are staffed by nonphysicians. In France and West Germany, however, physicians still respond in ambulances or helicopters.

THE LANDMARK PAPER

The National Academy of Sciences published a landmark paper in 1966 entitled "Accidental Death and Disability: The Neglected Disease of Modern Society." This document prompted federal initiatives to provide the original grants for the safe transportation and handling of ill or injured people. In 1973, after demonstrations of effective trauma systems in Illinois and Maryland, these grants accounted for the rapid proliferation of EMS systems across the country. Money was allocated for the development of training programs, communication systems, hospital designations, and other essential system components.

In 1973 federal legislation provided funding for the development of EMS systems throughout the country. The goal of this act was coast-to-coast proliferation of regional EMS systems. This legislation defined 15 components of an EMS system: manpower, training, communications, transportation, facility categorization, critical care units, use of public safety agencies, consumer participation, access to care, transfer of patients, record keeping, consumer education, review and evaluation, disaster linkage, and mutual aid agreements. Many systems have developed rapidly as a direct result of this legislation and funding.

Since there has not been time to finish this considerable task in most areas, EMS is still developing. Owing to widespread acceptance of the DOT National Curriculum, broad-based standardization exists in some areas of EMS, such as training. However, there are different methods that have been developed to provide the various components within an EMS system. There have not been sufficient evaluation and validation of the various models to determine which is best. Some variation may always exist because of differences in geography, distances between hospitals, number of hospitals in the area, population density, and other resources. These variables still affect the local strategy for the provision of emergency medical care.

THE EMERGENCE OF THE EMERGENCY MEDICAL TECHNICIAN

The EMT represents a major and relatively recent advance in emergency care. Prior to the late 1960s, ambulance personnel ranged from totally untrained individuals to physicians. The personnel utilized in any given area depended upon its economic base, the vehicles available for suitable patient transport, and local resources. For example, in communities with existing volunteer fire departments, the provision of EMS often became a secondary function, with the firefighters serving as EMTs. In large cities, hospitals frequently assumed the responsibility for providing ambulance services because of the availability of individuals trained in medical care.

Components of an Emergency Medical Services System

There is a wide range of illnesses and injuries that require immediate intervention by an EMS system. The leading cause of death in the United States is heart disease. Every year there are approximately 512,000 deaths due to myocardial infarctions, commonly referred to as heart attacks. More than half of these deaths occur outside the hospital. An additional 110,000 deaths each year are caused by trauma. Those undergoing unexpected and imminent childbirth, suffering from poisoning, or experiencing shortness of breath are just a few more examples of the types of medical emergencies that require immediate attention. For each category of patient there

are distinct interventions that are needed to improve the chances for survival.

Patients themselves should know the signs and symptoms of illnesses that require immediate intervention and how to access the EMS system. They should also know some basic self-help measures, in the event that immediate help from bystanders is not available.

LAY RESCUERS AND FIRST RESPONDERS

Often the first person to recognize an emergency condition is another member of the community. For certain conditions that render the victim helpless, actions by bystanders and those "first to respond" can make the critical difference. These members of the community need to know the same information as do prospective patients. Knowledge of a simple measure, such as how to control bleeding, may be all that is necessary to save a life.

CPR, when performed in a timely fashion, may save thousands of lives each year (Fig. 1–4). CPR and other basic skills, when taught as a body of knowledge to lay people, may result in first-aid or first-responder certification. Groups such as the American Heart Association and the American Red Cross are leaders in this type of training.

Community education programs that provide the public with more basic skills are also taught and advocated by these and other groups. Programs taught in public schools and to community groups are used to educate a significant cross section of the community. First-responder and first-aid training take time. Basic actions such as recognizing the signs of a heart attack, accessing the system, establishing an airway, providing relief to the choking victim, administering CPR, and establishing bleeding control are often taught in shorter courses so that they reach more people.

Sometimes a community will plan for a formal

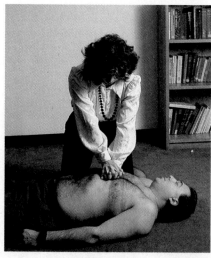

FIGURE 1–4. A lay rescuer performing one-rescuer CPR.

4-26-94

response to the call for help by training police or fire-fighters to administer first aid. These individuals are often trained in a first-responder program that provides them with the necessary skills to save a life, using a minimum of equipment.

EMERGENCY MEDICAL TECHNICIANS

There are more than 400,000 trained EMTs in the United States today, and they provide the foundation for prehospital care (Fig. 1–5). An EMT, by national definition, is someone who has successfully completed an EMT-Ambulance (EMT-A) training program according to the DOT's national curriculum. This involves attending lectures as well as receiving practical and clinical instruction in the assessment and management of the acutely ill or injured patient.

Originally, the EMT was primarily trained to provide safe handling and transportation of the ill or injured patient. This is reflected in the fact that the first EMT courses were only 24 hours long. However, the scope of prehospital care is in a dynamic state of change. As medical knowledge and technology progress, more treatments become available that are applicable in the prehospital setting. They are then incorporated into the EMT curriculum. This trend toward continually upgrading prehospital patient care has resulted in several revisions of the national curriculum.

Today, with additional training, EMTs may function at the "advanced level" as an *EMT-Paramedic (EMT-P)* or as an *EMT-Intermediate (EMT-I)*. An EMT-P is someone who has completed the standardized national curriculum as prescribed by the DOT. This individual performs advanced techniques, such as electrocardiogram (ECG) interpretation, drug therapy, invasive airway techniques, and defibrillation. Paramedic training is available throughout the country through programs sponsored by hospitals, community colleges, and other agencies.

An EMT-I is an individual who is trained in a limited number of advanced techniques, such as endotracheal intubation or IV therapy. The training programs for EMT-Is are generally shorter than paramedic programs. This gives a higher level of prehospital care to communities that rely upon volunteer ambulance services.

The specific therapeutic interventions taught and practiced by EMTs at different levels may vary somewhat from state to state.

Ambulance design has also changed to accommodate room for treatment while en route to the hospital. At one time the hearse was used in many communities that had little to offer in the way of prehospital care. The present-day vehicles allow two personnel members to attend to an individual, using specialized adjunctive equipment such as spine boards and airway devices.

EMERGENCY DEPARTMENTS

The emergency department is the location where the next phase of care is provided within an EMS system. Today's emergency departments are vital centers of acute medical and trauma care that serve as the "intersection" of the EMS system for the emergency patient (Fig. 1–6). In the emergency department the patient may receive stabilizing drug therapy or surgical procedures prior to transfer to a specialized critical care unit within the hospital. Many emergency departments have specialized cardiac arrest or trauma teams that respond in the event of a patient in a serious unstable condition. It is essential that the EMT on the scene notify the emergency department by radio or telephone.

Emergency medicine is a very young specialty of medical practice. It was only in the 1970s that a need to formalize this area of patient care was identified. Prior to that time, physicians of varied specialties and often physicians in training served as the primary staff for the emergency department. Modern day emergency physicians are trained in specialized programs that prepare them to respond to both medical and surgical emergen-

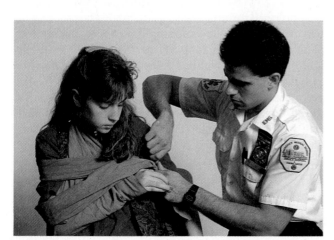

FIGURE 1–5. An EMT administering to an injured patient.

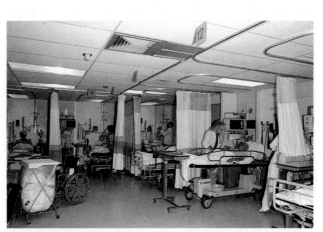

FIGURE 1–6. A modern emergency department.

cies. The emergency physician serves as the team leader for both inhospital and prehospital personnel.

The standards for emergency departments have also advanced over the last 20 years. Many communities have developed minimum standards for staff, space, equipment, and the availability of specialists (i.e., neurosurgeons, orthopedists, and so forth). Much of this progress can be attributed to the national EMS grants of the 1970s.

CRITICAL CARE UNITS AND OPERATING ROOMS

After being stabilized, the acutely ill or injured patient is usually transferred to the operating room or critical care unit for additional lifesaving treatments or close monitoring to avoid subsequent problems (Fig. 1–7). There are various types of these critical care or intensive care units, such as cardiac, respiratory, and neonatal (newborn) (Fig. 1–8).

Many medical centers specialize in a particular area of acute care. For example, some facilities specialize in care of the burn patient, employing expensive and unique equipment needed to effect the survival of the severely burned patient. The staff consists of physician and nurse specialists who deal exclusively with this type of patient. This kind of care, because of its restrictive cost, could not be available in every hospital and is usually offered on a regional basis. Protocols are often developed that allow EMTs to bypass the closest hospital in order to transport the patient directly to the specialized center. Patients who are unstable may be brought to the closest hospital and later transferred to the specialty center. There are also special trauma, poison, neurosurgical, cardiac, neonatal, and hyperbaric centers.

REHABILITATION

The ultimate goal of an EMS system is to return the patient to the community. For many patients, specialized, long-term care is needed to rehabilitate and restore the function of body systems. A severely injured patient may have musculoskeletal or central nervous

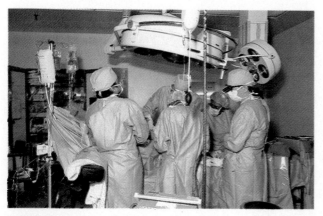

FIGURE 1–7. A modern operating room.

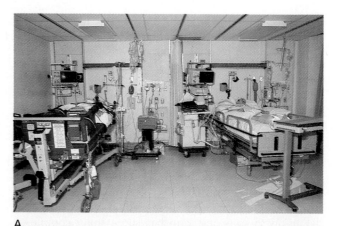

A

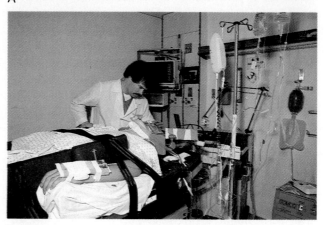

B

FIGURE 1–8. A modern critical care unit.

system problems that require long-term care to maximize function. Treatments may be provided during the hospital stay or on an outpatient basis.

COMMUNICATIONS

Since an EMS system involves a large number of resources, some method of coordination and communication is essential. In many cities and towns this is accomplished through the 911 emergency telephone system. This system allows for rapid access to all elements of medical care and support services. The 911 system utilizes a single telephone number for the dispatch of ambulances and other emergency vehicles. A central dispatch center coordinates resources and personnel within the system. Prior to the introduction of the 911 system, many communities had several different numbers dedicated to ambulance access. This resulted in an inefficient utilization of the emergency resources and needless delay for victims of illness and injury.

ELEMENTS OF A COMMUNICATION SYSTEM. A modern day EMS system may contain several components. A *dispatch system* receives the call for help and sends the appropriate response vehicles to the scene. An *ambulance-to-hospital communication system* allows the physician at the hospital to communicate with the EMT or paramedic in the field.

The Dispatch System. The dispatch center is the "central nervous system" of EMS resources. The center receives calls, categorizes them according to priority, and dispatches the appropriate ambulance. It serves as a communication point through which an EMT at an accident scene can call for additional resources, such as police, fire, and rescue personnel and equipment. The dispatch center also relays information from the accident scene to the receiving facilities and advises the EMT on facility selection and the availability of other rescue personnel (Fig. 1–9).

A formal national training program has been developed to train dispatch personnel to deal with the complexities of their job. Dispatchers often make critical decisions regarding the type of unit required for any given call. In dual response systems where both EMT and paramedic units are utilized, the dispatch person must ensure the appropriate use of advanced life support vehicles.

Ambulance-to-Hospital Communication Systems. Many EMS systems provide communication from the field personnel to the physician at a base hospital. These systems may include both voice and biotelemetric components. Biotelemetry permits the transmission of ECG data from the patient in the field to the physician at the base hospital (Fig. 1–10). These systems also allow the EMT to notify the hospital that an acutely ill or injured patient is being transported (Fig. 1–11). The few extra minutes provided by this advance warning allows the hospital to set up an operating team or have specialized equipment and personnel standing by.

MEDICAL CONTROL

Since the conception of an EMS system in the 1960s, advocates of the "systems approach" have stressed the need for coordination between the prehospital and hospital components of EMS. A major aspect

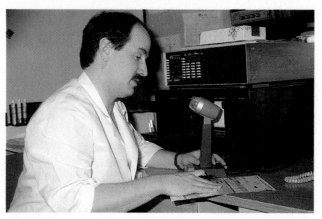

FIGURE 1–10. A physician monitoring a patient's status at a hospital communication base station.

of this approach was the establishment of medical direction and involvement by physicians in both the prehospital and hospital phases of care: *medical control.* This became crucial as advanced life support systems were developed, since the use of drugs and other invasive techniques required physician direction and orders.

Today, most systems that provide an advanced level of care have some form of medical control. In many systems, however, EMTs may not have a formal relationship with a physician at the local hospital. Fortunately, this is changing as more and more physicians are getting involved with prehospital care and providing medical leadership for prehospital personnel. This benefits both the EMT and the patients being treated.

MEDICAL RESPONSIBILITY. For EMS systems to be effective, the medical care rendered by all providers should be coordinated to achieve maximal benefit to the patient. Medical control of prehospital emergency care

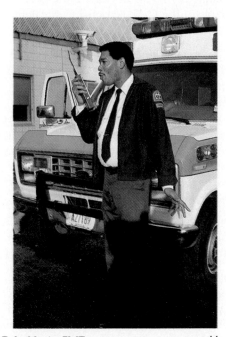

FIGURE 1–11. An EMT communicating via a portable radio.

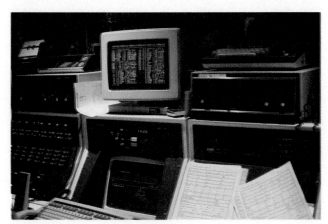

FIGURE 1–9. A dispatch communications center.

implies that there is accountability at the physician level for the medical conduct of EMS field personnel.

The type of care provided in the field should be carefully considered and judged to be medically prudent by physicians who are experts in emergency medicine. Depending on the size of the service, more than one physician may accept this responsibility.

Medical responsibility for the system may be shared through common protocols and mechanisms for on-line (i.e., direct radio communication) and off-line (i.e., education, call review, and evaluation) physician control as appropriate. However, the foundation of medical control is the premise that an individual physician will accept responsibility for a limited number of EMTs.

ELEMENTS OF MEDICAL CONTROL.   The involvement of physicians varies from system to system but usually includes assessment of patient needs and analysis of local resources, training and certification, continuing education and call review, protocol development, and evaluation to determine the effectiveness of the EMS system.

Needs Assessment and System Design.   The first aspect of medical control is assessment of the community's needs to determine the best design for the system. This may involve analysis of the patient population and regional resources, including examination of hospital records, response times, transport times, availability of facilities and manpower, geography, and financial resources. Physician involvement in this process is essential in determining the most efficient medical response to the emergency care needs of the community.

Training and Certification.   Physicians have played an important role in the development of the National EMT Training Program through the DOT. The DOT recommends in the EMT National Curriculum, 3rd Edition, 1984, that:

- A physician should serve as the course medical director with responsibility of ensuring the medical accuracy of the course.
- The inhospital phase of training must be planned in conjunction with the course medical director and representatives of an emergency medical facility.
- All EMT training should be arranged under the sponsorship of the local medical society or medical advisor to ensure medical accuracy and compliance with local treatment protocols.

These recommendations from the EMT National Curriculum illustrate the national intent regarding the physician's role in course organization and presentation.

Continuing Education and Call Review.   The development of knowledge and skills should not end with the initial EMT course. The medical control physician plays an important role in the process of continuing education. This includes lectures on various clinical topics, training in new skills, and reinforcement of old skills. Continuing education should also include follow up after specific calls. The physician can be an invaluable resource for the EMT in clarifying confusing cases. Questioning about these patients is often best done upon arrival at the emergency department.

Call review is another aspect of continuing education. It is a formal session where calls of a particular unit are presented by the responding EMTs for discussion. The physician can provide the inhospital evaluation of each case and how it was handled.

Protocol Development.   A *protocol* is a standardized approach to emergency care that reflects regional and national guidelines. Protocols provide the basis for prehospital practice within a given community. Because variations in regional resources and operating conditions can influence treatment and transport decisions, protocols are best developed on a local or regional level rather than at the national level. Protocols identify conditions that require either therapeutic intervention in the field or rapid transport. Their guidelines for selecting an appropriate receiving facility are based on a community's resources and its EMTs' ability to assess patients according to pre-established criteria. Because these protocols have such a far-reaching impact, it is essential that they be written by physicians actively involved with prehospital care and education (Fig. 1–12).

There have been many changes in the level of care provided by basic EMTs. These changes involve the care of the most critically ill patients, including those who formerly would have died before reaching a hospital. For example, defibrillation is performed by many EMTs who have completed a short additional training module.

Evaluation and Quality Assurance.   The final aspect of medical control is evaluation. The medical director and EMS team evaluate the effectiveness of aspects of the system or the system as a whole. This may include audits of charts, studies of past performance, or controlled studies of future performance. This measurement of success or failure allows for improvement of the existing system and for designing future systems for the optimal benefit of the patient.

The Roles and Responsibilities of the Emergency Medical Technician

The work of an EMT is extremely diversified and provides both challenge and gratification. As an EMT you will function in several roles that require medical, technical, clerical, and social interaction skills. Many of

BASIC LIFE SUPPORT PROTOCOL: OBSTRUCTED AIRWAY—ADULT

A. IF THE PATIENT IS *CONSCIOUS* AND CAN BREATHE, COUGH, OR SPEAK:
1. **DO NOT INTERFERE!** Encourage coughing.
  IF THE FOREIGN BODY CANNOT BE DISLODGED BY THE PATIENT COUGHING:
2. Administer high-concentration oxygen.
3. Transport in a sitting position, keeping the patient warm.
4. Obtain and record the vital signs, and repeat en route as often as the situation indicates.
5. Record all patient care information, including the patient's medical history and all treatment provided, on a prehospital care report.

B. IF THE PATIENT IS *CONSCIOUS* BUT CANNOT BREATHE, COUGH, OR SPEAK:
OR

IF THE PATIENT IS OR BECOMES UNCONSCIOUS:
1. Perform obstructed airway maneuvers according to AHA/ARC standards.

> **C A U T I O N !**
> **IF OBSTRUCTED AIRWAY IS TRAUMATIC, MANUALLY IMMOBILIZE THE HEAD AND CERVICAL SPINE IN A NEUTRAL POSITION WHILE OPENING THE PATIENT'S AIRWAY USING THE JAW-THRUST MANEUVER AND TRANSPORT THE PATIENT WITHOUT DELAY!**

IF AIRWAY OBSTRUCTION PERSISTS AFTER TWO SEQUENCES OF OBSTRUCTED AIRWAY MANEUVERS:
2. Transport, keeping the patient warm.
3. Repeat the sequences of obstructed airway maneuvers en route until the foreign body is forced out.
4. Obtain and record the vital signs, and repeat en route as often as the situation indicates.
5. Record all patient care information, including the patient's medical history and all treatment provided, on a prehospital care report.

IF AIRWAY OBSTRUCTION IS REVERSED AND THE PATIENT RESUMES BREATHING:
2. Administer high-concentration oxygen.
3. Transport, keeping the patient warm.
4. Obtain and record the vital signs, and repeat en route as often as the situation indicates.
5. Record all patient care information, including the patient's medical history and all treatment provided, on a prehospital care report.

FIGURE 1–12. EMT protocol. (New York State Department of Health, EMS Program, 1990.)

these skills will be acquired during your classroom training sessions, others will develop during your clinical field work under the supervision of senior EMTs or instructors.

PRIMARY RESPONSIBILITIES

PATIENT ASSESSMENT. Assessment is one of your primary responsibilities as an EMT. It involves the systematic collection of information through a patient history, an analysis of vital signs, and a careful physical examination to arrive at a working diagnosis or impression (Fig. 1–13). You must become a skilled observer who can recognize problems quickly and respond accordingly. This may be difficult when, for example, there are distraught family members or severely injured victims at the scene of a serious motor vehicle accident.

Patient assessment is probably the most difficult skill to master as an EMT because it involves so many different areas of knowledge. You will learn to take a concise history from a patient who may be hysterical. For this you will need patience and a great deal of

practice. You will learn which facts are relevant to each type of chief complaint and how to avoid unnecessary questioning that wastes time.

Continued monitoring of the vital signs and an ongoing evaluation of the effectiveness of the treatments you have instituted are also vital to the welfare of the patient.

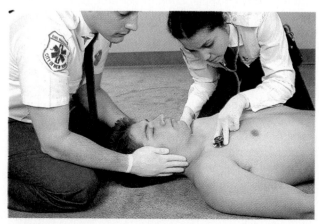

FIGURE 1–13. An EMT performing patient assessment.

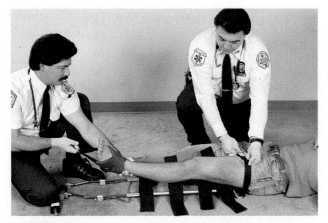

FIGURE 1–14. An EMT splinting a fractured extremity.

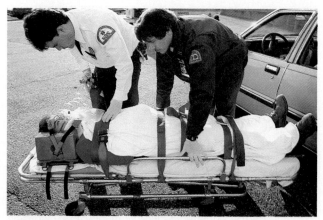

FIGURE 1–15. An EMT applying an immobilization device to prevent spinal cord injury.

PROMPT AND EFFECTIVE TREATMENT. Your training will prepare you to handle a variety of critical problems, ranging from resuscitation of a cardiac arrest victim to the immobilization of a fractured leg (Fig. 1–14). In some cases there may not be time for a thorough analysis, since many true emergencies may result in death if not treated immediately. A severe hemorrhage or a complete airway blockage requires a reflex reaction that you can develop only with intensive classroom and clinical practice. Other treatments you will learn include CPR, oxygen therapy, assisting at childbirth, management of poisoning and overdose, treatment of shock states, and psychological first aid. Knowing when to transport and when to choose a special institution (e.g., burn center) is a component of treatment that is not emphasized sufficiently.

PATIENT HANDLING. A large portion of the patients you encounter will be injured and require immobilization and careful handling. The movement of a suspected spinal injury victim must be done with extreme caution and consideration for the underlying injuries (Fig. 1–15). Rough and careless handling of the patient could result in paralysis. As an EMT, you will become familiar with a variety of spinal immobilization methods, splinting, different types of stretchers, and rapid removal techniques.

SAFE AND EFFICIENT TRANSPORT. If your rapid response to a call results in injury to yourself, your partner, or a patient, you have defeated your purpose. When you get behind the wheel of an emergency vehicle, you take on a great responsibility. Although the law permits you certain exemptions while operating an ambulance, you are still responsible for maintaining control of that vehicle at all times.

Familiarity with the best possible routes in your area is essential. You should know things such as traffic patterns at certain times of the day and alternate routes to take in the event that your original route is obstructed.

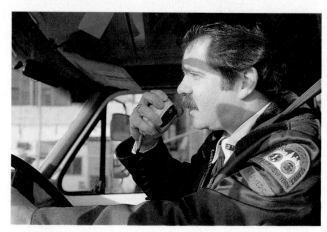

FIGURE 1–16. An EMT driving an ambulance.

The safe and appropriate transport of your patient is another aspect of emergency vehicle operation. Contrary to popular belief, most patients do not benefit from a frantic ride to the hospital with lights flashing and siren blaring (Fig. 1–16).

TRANSFER OF RESPONSIBILITY TO THE HOSPITAL STAFF. When you arrive at the emergency department with your patient you should be ready to transfer care of the patient to the emergency room staff. You may have to continue certain aspects of care, such as resuscitation, until the nurse, physician, or other health care professional assumes responsibility. You should have a brief history prepared that highlights key aspects of the assessment and treatment performed in the field (Fig. 1–17).

OTHER RESPONSIBILITIES

EXTRICATION. Although not a primary responsibility, you may sometimes be called upon to gain access

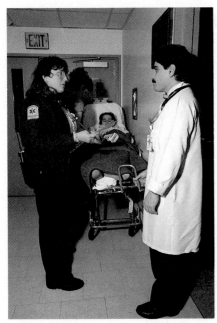

FIGURE 1–17. An EMT presenting a patient history to the emergency department physician.

to and extricate people trapped in automobiles (Fig. 1–18). This is usually the function of specialized rescue personnel within EMS, the police department, or fire department. However, when these units are not immediately available, or when regional systems incorporate these functions into the EMT's protocols, you must be prepared to effect a safe and efficient rescue. In most instances you will perform "light extrication," or extrication with the use of basic tools, such as screwdrivers, crowbars, and hacksaws.

If heavy extrication is assigned through regional protocols, specialized programs are usually conducted to teach you proper use of the larger and more powerful devices typically used by rescue personnel.

Before extrication occurs, you may have to gain

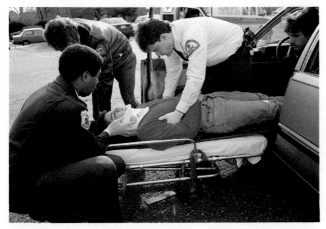

FIGURE 1–18. EMTs extricating an accident victim from an automobile.

control of the accident scene. This may mean having visual warning devices set up on a highway or choosing a person to direct traffic or effect crowd control.

COMMUNICATIONS. The use of radio codes and proper utilization of the radio itself will be part of your training. Communications over the radio should be short and clear, since long conversations tie up the airwaves and may obstruct other critical messages. The radio is a useful tool to mobilize essential resources, notify hospital personnel of the imminent arrival of an acutely ill patient, and document unusual circumstances that may have medicolegal implications at a later time. For example, a patient who leaves the scene against your advice and without a proper signature on a release form can be documented by radioing the information to the dispatcher. Many systems record all conversations to provide another form of documentation.

Obviously, communication is not limited to radio conversations. You must learn to be an effective communicator in person with patients, family members, and hospital personnel. In this function you will be required to use medical terminology, which is the language of health care systems.

RECORD KEEPING. Accurate records play an important role in the management of the patient because they become the reference point for information after your departure from the hospital (Fig. 1–19). The prehospital assessment findings and the chronology of prehospital events and treatments play an important role in the definitive care of the patient and must be recorded properly. These records are an essential aspect of protection against lawsuits. You must develop good habits in recording all pertinent data collected from the time of the initial patient encounter until arrival at the hospital. A call report must be thorough, chronological, and clear. It should be written with the concept in mind that someone may want to retrieve this information at a later time. Accuracy is another necessary ingredient in effective documentation. Times, vital sign values, and other diagnostic findings should be recorded carefully, to aid in the physician's assessment of the patient.

VEHICLE AND EQUIPMENT MAINTENANCE. Vehicles and equipment that are well cared for last longer and perform better for you and the patient. It is very frustrating and dangerous to attempt a resuscitation or other task only to discover that essential equipment is not serviceable or is missing. Proper inspection and maintenance of the vehicle and equipment is an essential role of every EMT (Fig. 1–20). The aesthetic value of a clean ambulance and equipment cannot be stressed too highly, not to mention that dirt and debris promote an infectious environment for both you and the patient. Additionally, medical providers have a responsibility to ensure that equipment is functional and effective. Ambulance failure

Prehospital Care Report

USE BALL POINT PEN ONLY.

Press Down Firmly. You're Making 4 Copies.

2—1128038

M   D   Y   DATE   RUN NO   AGENCY CODE   VEH. ID

Name	Agency Name		MILEAGE		USE MILITARY TIMES
Address	Call Location		END	CALL REC'D	
	CHECK ONE ☐ Residence ☐ Health Facility ☐ Farm ☐ Indus. Facility ☐ Other Work Loc. ☐ Roadway ☐ Recreational ☐ Other		BEGIN	ENROUTE	
Ph #	Call Origin		TOTAL	AT SCENE	
AGE ☐☐☐ DOB M ☐ D ☐ Y ☐ SEX M☐ F☐	Dispatch Information			FROM SCENE	
Physician	CALL TYPE AS REC'D. ☐ Emergency ☐ Non-Emergency ☐ Stand-by	INTERFACILITY TRANSFER ☐ Yes TYPE OF TRANSFER ☐ BLS ☐ ALS	HOSPITAL COMMUNICATIONS ☐ Yes ☐ Directly ☐ Thru Dispatch ☐ VHF ☐ UHF ☐ Phone ☐ No ☐ Communications Difficulties	AT DESTIN IN SERVICE IN QUARTERS	
Next of Kin					

MECHANISM OF INJURY
☐ MVA (complete seat belt section) ☐ Fall of ___ feet ☐ GSW ☐ Other ___
☐ Struck by vehicle ☐ Unarmed assault ☐ Knife
☐ Extrication required ___ minutes Seat belt used? ☐ Yes ☐ No ☐ Unknown Seat Belt Use Reported By ☐ Crew ☐ Patient ☐ Police ☐ Other

CHIEF COMPLAINT   SUBJECTIVE ASSESSMENT

PRESENTING PROBLEM

☐ Airway Obstruction
☐ Respiratory Arrest
☐ Respiratory Distress
☐ Cardiac Related (Potential)
☐ Cardiac Arrest

☐ Allergic Reaction
☐ Syncope
☐ Stroke/CVA
☐ General Illness/Malaise
☐ Gastro-Intestinal Distress
☐ Diabetic Related (Potential)
☐ Pain

☐ Unconscious/Unresp.
☐ Seizure
☐ Behavioral Disorder
☐ Substance Abuse (Potential)
☐ Poisoning (Accidental)

☐ Shock
☐ Head Injury
☐ Spinal Injury
☐ Fracture/Dislocation
☐ Amputation

☐ Other ___

☐ Multiple Trauma
☐ Trauma-Blunt
☐ Trauma-Penetrating
☐ Soft Tissue Injury
☐ Bleeding/Hemorrhage

☐ OB/GYN
☐ Burns
Environmental
☐ Heat
☐ Cold
☐ Hazardous Materials
☐ Obvious Death

PAST MEDICAL HISTORY

☐ Hypertension ☐ Stroke
☐ Seizures ☐ Diabetes
☐ COPD ☐ Cardiac
☐ Allergy ☐ Other (List)
☐ Medication

VITAL SIGNS

TIME	RESP	PULSE	B.P.	LEVEL OF CONSCIOUSNESS	GCS	TS	R PUPILS L	SKIN
	Rate: ☐ Regular ☐ Shallow ☐ Labored	Rate: ☐ Regular ☐ Irregular		☐ Alert ☐ Voice ☐ Pain ☐ Unresp.			☐ Normal ☐ Dilated ☐ Constricted ☐ Sluggish ☐ No-Reaction ☐	☐ Unremarkable ☐ Cool ☐ Pale ☐ Warm ☐ Cyanotic ☐ Moist ☐ Flushed ☐ Dry ☐ Jaundiced
	Rate: ☐ Regular ☐ Shallow ☐ Labored	Rate: ☐ Regular ☐ Irregular		☐ Alert ☐ Voice ☐ Pain ☐ Unresp.			☐ Normal ☐ Dilated ☐ Constricted ☐ Sluggish ☐ No-Reaction ☐	☐ Unremarkable ☐ Cool ☐ Pale ☐ Warm ☐ Cyanotic ☐ Moist ☐ Flushed ☐ Dry ☐ Jaundiced
	Rate: ☐ Regular ☐ Shallow ☐ Labored	Rate: ☐ Regular ☐ Irregular		☐ Alert ☐ Voice ☐ Pain ☐ Unresp.			☐ Normal ☐ Dilated ☐ Constricted ☐ Sluggish ☐ No-Reaction ☐	☐ Unremarkable ☐ Cool ☐ Pale ☐ Warm ☐ Cyanotic ☐ Moist ☐ Flushed ☐ Dry ☐ Jaundiced

OBJECTIVE PHYSICAL ASSESSMENT   COMMENTS

☐ Physical Findings Unremarkable

Head/Neck, Upper Extr., Chest/Back, Abd/Pelvic, Lower Extr.

1) Pain
2) Wound
3) Fracture/Disloc. Open
4) Fracture/Disloc. Closed
5) Bleeding/Hemorrhage
6) Loss of Motion/Sensation
7) Sprain/Strain
8) Burn ___ Deg ___ %
9) Internal

TREATMENT GIVEN   MEDICAL CONTROL INFORMATION   Insurance Data

☐ Airway Cleared
☐ Oral Airway
☐ Esophageal Obturator Airway/Esophageal Gastric Tube Airway (EOA/EGTA)
☐ EndoTracheal Tube (E/T)
☐ Oxygen Administered @ ___ L.P.M., Method ___
☐ Suction Used
☐ Artificial Ventilation Method ___
☐ C.P.R. in progress on arrival by: ☐ Citizen ☐ Firefighter ☐ Police Officer
☐ C.P.R. Started @ Time ▶ ___   Time from Arrest Until C.P.R. ▶ ___ Minutes
☐ EKG Monitored (Attach Tracing) [Rhythm(s) ___]
☐ Defibrillation/Cardioversion No. Times ___ With ___ Watt/Sec.

☐ Medication Administered (Use Continuation Form)
☐ IV Fluid ___ No. Established ___ No. of Attempts ___
☐ Mast Inflated (Time Inflated: ___)
☐ Bleeding/Hemorrhage Controlled (Method Used: ___)
☐ Spinal Immobilization ☐ Neck ☐ Back
☐ Limb Immobilized by ☐ Fixation ☐ Traction
☐ (Heat) or (Cold) Applied
☐ Vomiting Induced @ Time ___ Method ___
☐ Restraints Applied, Type ___
☐ Baby Delivered @ Time ___ In County ___
   ☐ Alive ☐ Stillborn ☐ Male ☐ Female
☐ Other ___

DISPOSITION   (See list)   DISP. CODE   CONTINUATION FORM USED   YES ←

CREW

IN CHARGE	DRIVER'S NAME	NAME	NAME
☐ EMT ☐ AEMT #	☐ EMS-FR ☐ EMT ☐ AEMT #	☐ EMS-FR ☐ EMT ☐ AEMT #	☐ EMS-FR ☐ EMT ☐ AEMT #

*COPYRIGHT 1986 NEW YORK STATE DEPARTMENT OF HEALTH   EMS 100 (11/86) provided by NYS-EMS PROGRAM

AGENCY COPY/**WHITE**   HOSPITAL PATIENT RECORD COPY/**PINK**   RESEARCH COPY/**BLUE**   EXTRA SERVICE COPY/**GREEN**

FIGURE 1–19. An ambulance call report. (From New York State Department of Health, EMS Program, 1990.)

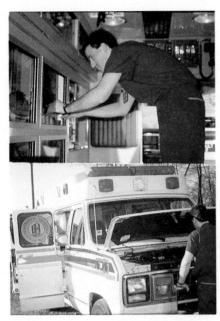

FIGURE 1-20. An EMT inspecting the ambulance prior to the first run.

or equipment malfunction provides fertile ground for litigation.

CERTIFICATION

Each state establishes license or certification requirements for the practicing EMT, that may include written, practical, and clinical requirements. Although there are variations, the DOT EMT-A curriculum usually provides the framework for programs throughout the country. States may also add various specialty training modules that enhance the local or regional provision of prehospital care, such as, EMT-defibrillation, specialized trauma programs, emergency vehicle operation, extrication training, and other specialty programs.

Recertification is usually required every 2 to 3 years and may involve ongoing continuing education requirements, challenge testing, or attendance of a formalized refresher program.

NATIONAL REGISTRY OF EMERGENCY MEDICAL TECHNICIANS. The National Registry was developed to establish a high quality and standardized competency level for basic and advanced EMTs. It provides written and practical testing and a continuing education program at the basic and advanced levels. The National Registry of EMTs is used by many states to provide reciprocity to EMTs and paramedics. It also maintains continuing education requirements that encourage the professional development of EMTs nationwide. EMTs can be registered at either the basic or the advanced level.

NATIONAL ASSOCIATION OF EMERGENCY MEDICAL TECHNICIANS. The National Association of Emergency Medical Technicians (NAEMT) is an organization that represents EMTs throughout the United States. It was founded in 1975 with the support of the National Registry and other national leaders to serve as a national voice for EMTs and paramedics. It maintains three societies that serve other subdivisions of prehospital care—the National Society of EMS Administrators, the National Society of Instructor Coordinators, and the National Society of EMT-paramedics.

The NAEMT serves several functions, including working for legislative change in EMS, providing continuing education, representing EMTs in other national organizations, providing job placement for EMTS, and in general working for the development and recognition of EMTs nationwide. Among the continuing education efforts offered by NAEMT are a national educational conference and prehospital trauma life support (a continuing education trauma program).

THE AMERICAN HEART ASSOCIATION. The American Heart Association (AHA) establishes standards and guidelines for emergency cardiac care for both hospital and prehospital providers. Approximately every 4 to 5 years AHA publishes the *Standards and Guidelines for Emergency Cardiac Care* in cooperation with other health care organizations that provide the basis for CPR performance and advanced protocols used in prehospital care.

ETHICS AND MEDICOLEGAL ISSUES

Ethics
THE "GOLDEN RULE"

"Do unto others as you would have them do unto you." This time-tested philosophy provides a sound basis for defining ethical practices within all aspects of medical care. It implies that the individual is acting in a manner that he or she believes to be in the best interest of the patient. There are many instances where personal convenience, comfort, and self-interest may potentially stand in the way of providing the best possible care for the patient.

For example, it may be easier to walk a patient from the scene rather than provide the appropriate stretcher transport, or it may be more expedient to deliver a patient to a nearby but less suitable emergency department at the end of a shift. These are examples of clearly unethical practices. Practices such as these destroy the essence and intent of quality prehospital care and often provide a basis for lawsuits.

COMPETENCE

The golden rule implies an intent by an individual to provide adequate care. However, this intent is only effective when combined with the knowledge and ability to properly recognize and treat critical conditions. In other words, the EMT has an additional ethical responsibility to maintain competence in the practice of prehospital care. This includes a serious effort to acquire the requisite skills taught in the initial training program, as well as a continued effort to polish those skills and reinforce knowledge.

Remaining skillful in the administration of prehospital care requires diligence and careful self-evaluation on the part of the EMT. Many states require attendance at refresher courses every few years in order to qualify for recertification. These courses are especially valuable to the "part-time" EMT or volunteer who practices the profession only a few hours a week and is therefore not exposed to a large volume of calls. Reading journals, attending lectures, participating in call review sessions, and other types of educational endeavors are essential ingredients to personal development and optimal patient care.

PROFESSIONALISM

The term that probably best embodies these basic values is *professionalism*. Webster describes professionalism as *"acting requisite to the body of knowledge which defines the service and abilities of the professional... according to the oath of the profession."* While the term professional is used more loosely now, the expectations of behavior can easily be understood by reading a traditional medical oath.

A professional appearance and attitude evoke a sense of confidence in the patient and family members (Fig. 1–21). Since emergency care providers have little

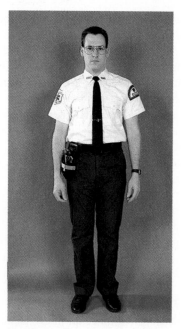

FIGURE 1–21. A properly attired EMT.

time to establish a rapport with their patients, the sight of an EMT in a clean and appropriate uniform helps establish a sense of authority and trust. Conversely, an EMT who arrives at the scene wearing jeans and sneakers appears unprofessional. To the already anxious patient, this attire creates a heightened sense of concern that he or she is not yet in able hands.

The attitude of the EMT is as important as his or her outer appearance. You should show an interest in your job and possess a sensitive awareness of your environment and the needs of others around you. The provision of medical care is a giving profession and should not be taken lightly.

CONFIDENTIALITY

By the nature of the work, the EMT enters into some very private situations and circumstances. Every patient has the right to feel that the information he gives in order to be treated will be kept confidential. Many individuals have genuine concerns regarding the effect of public knowledge of their illness or injury. For example, patients with a seizure disorder may be worried about the status of their jobs if their employers become aware that they have epilepsy. You have a responsibility to regard all information provided in a patient's history, by observation, and in physical assessment as confidential. However, there are cases such as those involving child abuse and other crimes where the EMT is required to report information to the appropriate authorities.

You may be thrust into a situation where you must deal with reporters or requests for information from family members or friends. Personal information regarding the diagnosis or care of the patient should be left for the physician to discuss. Some instances arise where the EMT may provide the press with general facts regarding an accident. When possible, you should consult with your supervisor, administrator, or medical control physician to confirm the appropriateness of releasing any given information to the press.

Medicolegal Considerations

Aside from moral responsibilities, you will also be bound by law to provide timely and effective care to your patient. This includes a rapid response, proper assessment and treatment, and careful documentation of the care rendered in the field.

THE STANDARD OF CARE

The guiding standard of effective medical practice is referred to as the "standard of care." This term is used to describe the body of knowledge, laws, policies, standards, and guidelines set forth by various standard-setting organizations that provide the basis of prehospital and other medical care. For example, the American Heart Association and National Research Council establish standards and guidelines for CPR performance. These standards are reevaluated and published every few years. The changes that are recommended are based upon the collective research data that have been developed since the previous standards were established. The standard of care is also defined by protocols.

You will find that your practice as an EMT is governed by laws, rules, and regulations. The extent of regulation varies from region to region. State or local statutes may specifically define the practice of prehospital care. This may include limitations on your role as well as the requirement to perform specific skills for a specific situation. For example, EMTs in New York State are legally required to attempt resuscitation of every cardiac arrest victim with only a few exceptions in specific circumstances.

Another way an EMT is evaluated relative to the standard of care is in comparison to others functioning at a similar level. In a lawsuit situation, EMTs are often brought in as expert witnesses to establish how they would have acted in similar circumstances in a similar region.

Further definition of the standard of care is established by state or local certification. This certification attests to the attainment of a measured level of performance. A state agency, usually the state health department, may develop training and testing standards for EMT level work. This is accomplished with the use of standardized written and practical examinations.

LAWS PERTAINING TO PREHOSPITAL CARE

Many states enact laws that define the practice of prehospital care. These laws may address issues such as minimum training standards, medical control, vehicle and equipment specifications, and licensure or certification. These laws and regulations vary from state to state according to the level or scope of practice performed by the EMT. In New York State, prehospital care is governed by Public Health Law, Article 30 (Emergency Medical Services). The current Article 30 was developed to promote "The public health, safety, and welfare" by requiring registration or certification of all ambulance services and by creating regional EMS councils as well as the New York State EMS Council. The latter were created to develop minimum training, equipment, and communication standards. Other states, such as Indiana, have very detailed legislation that clearly states specific requirements regarding medical control and other essential components of the system.

SCOPE OF PRACTICE. The scope of practice refers to the parameters and limitations of a given medical provider. For example, an EMT's certification may not permit the performance of certain invasive skills practiced by paramedics or EMT-Is. If you were to perform one of these skills while working as an EMT, you would be functioning beyond your designated scope of practice. For instance, an EMT who performs a surgical invasion of the airway, such as a tracheostomy, to allow a patient with a blocked airway to breathe may believe there is justification in trying to save the patient's life. However, whether the EMT is familiar with the procedure or not, undertaking this action goes beyond the limits of the EMT's scope of practice and may result in severe consequences. Even if no injury occurs to the patient, going beyond the defined scope of practice may result in revocation of your certification.

LEGAL PRINCIPLES

There are four major ingredients involved in successful litigation against EMTs: duty to act, breach of duty, damage, and causal connection. In order for medical malpractice to be established, all four ingredients must be present.

DUTY. For litigation to be successful, the complainant's attorney must first establish that the EMT had a duty to the patient. An EMT has a duty to act when responding to a critical illness or accident while working on the ambulance, whether as a volunteer or a professional. On the other hand, an *off-duty EMT* has no *initial* duty to act when encountering an emergency situation. He or she may have ethical or moral reasons to intervene, but there is usually no legal mandate. However, an off-duty EMT can establish a duty to act by becoming involved with the patient. But, the standard of care required of such a samaritan is far less than that which is required of the same EMT in the course of his work. As a matter of fact, an EMT not on duty and acting as a samaritan is only held liable for gross negligence.

For our purposes, here we shall deal strictly with the more common situation where EMTs on duty become involved in accusations of negligence. The minute you take part in the care of a sick or injured individual, you lose bystander status by having established a patient-provider relationship.

BREACH OF DUTY. A breach of duty refers to a negligent act or omission that violated the standards of care expected from an EMT under the circumstances. Every medical provider is expected to act with reasonable care so as to prevent injury to the patient. EMTs may breach their duty by performing a procedure incorrectly, by lack of timely and appropriate action, by failure to act in the circumstances required, and by other acts deemed negligent.

INJURY. In order to initiate a medical lawsuit

based on malpractice, the plaintiff must first demonstrate damage. If the patient suffered no damage following an omission of treatment or the alleged use of improper methods or following an alleged omission by an EMT, there would be no basis for a lawsuit.

CAUSAL CONNECTION.   The final ingredient necessary to initiate a successful lawsuit is a clear connection between the patient's injury and actions taken or omitted by the EMT. It is not enough to demonstrate injury; the plaintiff must prove that the injury was caused by the actions of the EMT. For example, if a patient who was paralyzed following an accident sued the care provider (EMT), the patient would be required to prove that the paralysis was related to an action or inaction on the part of the EMT and not the result of his accident.

CONSENT

Before treating a patient you must obtain the consent of the patient, parent, or guardian. Patients have a right to consent to treatment. EMTs should only enter into a care-giving role with the consent of the patient. In a hospital, patients may be asked to sign a statement of consent. In emergency prehospital care, this is not usually done. Because of the emergency situation, a verbal approval or other indication of agreement (such as a nod) may be the form of consent. An unconscious patient may receive emergency treatment by implied consent. The EMT should understand basic concepts of consent and seek to obtain consent for care in all cases. However, consent is not always possible. For example, you will encounter patients who are disoriented, minors with no parent or guardian immediately available, and individuals who are mentally handicapped and incapable of providing consent. Remember that consent may take several forms.

INFORMED CONSENT.   Consent for any invasive procedure must be an informed consent. In order for consent to be informed, the patient must be made aware of the risks, benefits, and consequences of the care provided and alternatives to the care. In prehospital care, fully informing the patient is especially important when a patient wants to withhold consent. If a patient or patient's family refuses medical treatment, it is necessary for you to inform them of the potential consequences of delayed treatment prior to having the patient or patient's family sign a release form.

IMPLIED CONSENT.   Implied consent refers to circumstances where verbal or written consent is not possible. For example, when you encounter an unconscious person, treatment should be provided since a reasonable person would want such actions to be taken under these circumstances. This concept also applies to persons unable to legally give consent such as children or mentally handicapped individuals. As previously mentioned, a par-

ent or guardian should provide consent in these circumstances. However, if the delay caused by seeking such consent would affect the health or life of the patient, the EMT should pursue treatment.

PERSONS CAPABLE OF CONSENTING TO TREATMENT.   An individual is capable of consenting when he or she is a mentally competent adult or an emancipated minor. An *emancipated minor* refers to an individual who is under the legal adult age but who is living independently of the parents, is financially self-supporting or is or was married, or is or was a parent.

A difficult aspect of establishing legally valid consent is the issue of mental competence. For example, an individual who is oxygen deprived may have impaired judgment and may not be capable of giving an informed consent. When a patient who is exhibiting signs of an altered mental state refuses medical treatment, you should attempt to secure the consent of a family member or engage the assistance of a police officer prior to removing a patient against that person's will.

REFUSAL OF TREATMENT.   You will encounter many instances where a patient refuses medical treatment. Again, only a competent adult has the right to refuse medical care that is deemed essential by the EMT. However, a person may refuse care if he or she is mentally competent and therefore capable of making a clear judgment. You run the risk of a charge of "false imprisonment" should you forcibly remove this patient against his or her expressed wishes. When the patient appears in need of medical care, every attempt should be made to convince the patient to go to the hospital. Family members, friends, and physicians provide an excellent source of motivation in these trying situations.

REFUSAL OF TREATMENT/TRANSPORTATION
NEGATIVA A RECIBIR TRATAMIENTO/SER TRASLADADO

RELEASE
EXONERACION DE RESPONSABILIDADES

COMPLETE ON WHITE (AGENCY) COPY ONLY
LLENE UNICAMENTE LA COPIA BLANCA (DE LA AGENCIA)

I hereby refuse (treatment/transport to a hospital) and I acknowledge that such treatment/transportation was advised by the ambulance crew or physician. I hereby release such persons from liability for respecting and following my express wishes.

Mediante la presente declaro que me niego a aceptar el tratamiento/traslado a un hospital y reconozco asimismo que el medico o el personal de la ambulancia recomendaron ese tratamiento/traslado. Consiguientemente, eximo a dichas personas de toda responsabilidad por haber respetado y cumplido mis deseos expresos.

Signed:
Firma: _____

Witness:
Testigo: _____

FIGURE 1–22. Refusal of care form. (From New York State Department of Health, EMS Program, 1990.)

If, after reasonable attempts to convince the patient, medical care is still refused, a "refusal of aid" release form should be signed by the patient. Again, it is essential that the patient appreciate the potential consequences of refusing medical care prior to signing the release form (Fig. 1—22).

IMMUNITIES

Federal and state laws often provide legal immunities for institutions, medical professionals, and lay people, which provide an extra degree of protection from lawsuits. These laws are designed to protect people who come to the aid of an ill or injured person in a "volunteer" capacity. They also serve to protect government agencies, such as the military, from costly lawsuits.

"GOOD SAMARITAN LAWS." Specific laws designed to protect the private citizen who is functioning in a nonprofessional capacity and without an expectation of remuneration are often referred to as "Good Samaritan laws." These laws were developed to encourage medical professionals and lay persons to provide aid without undue fear of litigation. Some states have limited statutes that protect only medical professionals such as physicians, nurses, and volunteer EMTs. Other states provide comprehensive protection for any citizen who may render care to an ill or injured patient.

ABANDONMENT

As an EMT who is part of an EMS system, you assume the responsibility of providing care to an ill or injured patient from the time you arrive on the scene until you transfer the patient to the care of hospital personnel. A special form of litigation that EMTs and other health professionals are subject to is "abandonment." Abandonment occurs when an EMT or other health professional discontinues a patient—provider relationship without giving the patient time or opportunity to obtain substitute treatment. This would include circumstances in which an EMT leaves the patient on the scene in need of emergency care and transportation to a hospital, or in which care is prematurely discontinued.

For a case of abandonment to hold up in court the complainant must first establish that he was owed a duty and that the duty was breached.

Charges of abandonment are also possible in cases in which a patient who refused care was incompetent, such as a child or an adult with an altered mental state. If the EMT suspects that a patient who is refusing care is not capable of making a reasonable judgment, every attempt should be made to transport that patient to the hospital. If the patient adamantly refuses, the EMT should secure the aid of family or police officers. In some instances, it may be appropriate and necessary to take the patient against his or her will. If administrative or legal advice is available in such circumstances, you should avail yourself of this help.

EQUIPMENT-RELATED INJURIES

Upon responding to an emergency call you are expected to provide reasonable care according to your level of training and certification. This includes having available the equipment essential to the treatment of common emergencies. Malfunctioning or missing equipment invites lawsuits. It is important to check all equipment, including the vehicle, at the beginning of each tour of duty and to replace or repair missing or malfunctioning items before responding to your first call. Equipment failure that occurs during the treatment of a patient should be carefully documented and reported to administrative personnel. When practical, replacement items should be available in the vehicle's storage compartment.

PSYCHIATRIC PATIENTS

The management of emotionally or mentally disturbed patients represents an area of high legal risk for both inhospital and prehospital personnel. Since these patients are often held against their expressed wishes, charges of "false imprisonment" and "battery" are sometimes brought in relation to an injury sustained during the restraining process.

You should exercise due caution when removing psychiatric patients against their will. Generally, such actions are taken to prevent the patients from injuring themselves or others around them. In such circumstances, many state and local governments permit the police to remove the patient under the concept of "protective custody." If conditions permit, the patient's family or doctor should be contacted to encourage the patient to submit to care. However, with violent or suicidal patients this is sometimes not possible.

When forcible removal is necessary, care should be taken to not harm the patient. Soft restraints should be available and utilized in these circumstances. The use of handcuffs should be discouraged owing to the injury that is likely to occur during the patient's struggle. After removal to the hospital, precise documentation is essential to record the circumstances that warranted the use of force. Extreme care should be taken not to use subjective words or phrases to describe the patient's behavior; instead, the patient's behavior should be documented specifically, for example, "The patient attempted to strike the EMTs and police during the patient interview," or "The patient stated that he was going to kill himself." In most states patients may also be removed forcibly under a court order or multiple-physician order. You should consult with your administrative staff about the policy within your organization.

WITHHOLDING CARDIOPULMONARY RESUSCITATION

Many EMS systems permit EMTs either to leave patients at the scene who are "obviously dead" and who will be removed later by the medical examiner, or to transport them directly to the morgue. This means that the EMT has a serious responsibility and must exercise good judgment. In general, CPR should always be instituted if there is any hope for the patient's, survival or any doubt that death has occurred.

CRITERIA. Legally, CPR is withheld when there is evidence of obvious death that can be well documented. Such signs may include *rigor mortis*, a state of body stiffness caused by changes of proteins in the muscles following a prolonged period of cardiac arrest. *Extreme dependent lividity* is the discoloration of body tissues in the lower or dependent areas of the body, which is caused by the collection of coagulated blood. This also occurs after a prolonged period of cardiac arrest. Death may also be documented if obvious evidence such as decapitation, decomposition of the body, or similar signs are present.

TERMINAL ILLNESS. A more controversial area regarding the withholding of CPR is in cases of terminally ill patients who have expressed their desire that extraordinary measures of life support be avoided. With the growing trend toward homecare of dying patients such circumstances will probably be on the rise. Some cases may be well defined, such as calls where a doctor is present and indicates that no resuscitation should be attempted. In these cases the doctor should be requested to sign the call report to document his or her actions. In a situation that is not as clear-cut, where the patient's wishes are expressed by bystanders, you should probably attempt a resuscitation until there is more definitive evidence for withholding resuscitation.

Many states have developed Do Not Resuscitate legislation or policies that clarify the actions to be taken by emergency personnel in complying with the wishes of the terminal patient or his or her family.

CARDIOVASCULAR UNRESPONSIVENESS. Once CPR is started it should be continued until the patient is transferred to hospital personnel or other resuscitation teams, such as paramedics. Again, premature discontinuation of treatment may constitute abandonment. In prehospital care CPR may be discontinued only when no reasonable means of transport exists and the rescuer is totally exhausted, or when "cardiovascular unresponsiveness" is established following advanced life support measures. Such measures can be done only by paramedics or other advanced EMTs following comprehensive resuscitation measures, including defibrillation, drug therapy, and application of advanced airway skills. In other words, after every attempt has been made to resuscitate the heart, the patient may sometimes be pronounced dead because of cardiovascular unresponsiveness. However, some systems do not permit paramedics to work under this concept and require the transport of all patients.

REPORTING REQUIREMENTS

There are laws in various states that require EMTs and other emergency personnel to report certain conditions to the police, health department, and other authorities. Child abuse, infectious diseases, and violent crimes such as rape and assault are examples of potentially reportable cases. You should familiarize yourself with local protocols to determine your responsibility in this area.

RISK MANAGEMENT

The saying "An ounce of prevention is worth a pound of cure" very much applies to the medicolegal aspects of prehospital care. This is not to say that as an EMT you should approach every patient with an apprehension about lawsuits, since this may impair your judgment and interfere with the application of timely and effective management. However, you can incorporate certain principles into your day-to-day approach to patient care that will minimize the potential for litigation.

ACT ACCORDING TO THE STANDARD OF CARE. First and foremost, you should act according to the current standard of care prescribed by curricula, textbooks, protocols, and local and state policies and laws. This again illustrates the importance of solid continuing education for every EMT. Admittedly, there are controversial areas of EMT practice, but these are often clarified by local protocols or through consultation with your medical control physician. When in doubt, you should be guided by your best judgment and act in the best interest of the patient.

DOCUMENT ACTIONS CAREFULLY. Essentially, the patient record is the backbone of a defense in any lawsuit against an EMT. Most lawsuits come to the attention of the EMT months or sometimes years following an incident. Your individual recollection of circumstances and actions is likely to be extremely vague and blurry. The patient record will be your primary reference point in these instances. Effective record keeping ensures continuity of patient care and protection to all care providers. All assessment steps, treatments, times, and other significant events should be meticulously documented for retrieval at a later time.

ACT IN THE BEST INTEREST OF THE PATIENT. Although interaction with the patient and family members is usually brief, the nature of the circumstances is likely to generate strong and sometimes turbulent emotions. The patient and family view you as the individual charged with lifesaving responsibilities. Your attitude and demeanor should reflect an appropriate sense of the significance of the circumstances. EMTs who present an immature or careless attitude are likely to provoke both concern and anger from the patient and family. This kind of negative experience often provides the "breeding ground" for lawsuits. Patients and families may often manifest anger or impatience during the care of themselves or their loved one. An understanding and tolerant attitude is essential to avoid destructive and often unnecessary confrontation. It helps to imagine how you might behave under similar circumstances. An EMT with an empathetic and caring manner is one of the best preventions against lawsuits.

REVIEW EXERCISES

1. Define an EMS system.

2. Give two examples of how war, technology, and physicians contributed to the evolution of EMS.

3. List the number of deaths per year caused by coronary heart disease and accidents.

4. List each component of an EMS system and describe its role.

5. Describe the differences between an EMT-A, EMT-I, and EMT-P.

6. List five functions of a dispatch communication system.

7. Provide the definition of medical control.

8. List five elements of medical control.

9. List four primary and three other responsibilities of an EMT.

10. Write a paragraph discussing the significance of the following issues related to ethics:
    Competence
    Professionalism
    Confidentiality

11. List three elements that comprise the standard of care.

12. List the four ingredients of medical malpractice and describe how each ingredient is established.

13. State the difference between informed and implied consent.

14. State the purpose of a "Good Samaritan law" and list two reasons why such laws are necessary.

15. Define *abandonment*.

16. List three criteria for withholding CPR.

17. List three ways to reduce the chances of a lawsuit while practicing prehospital emergency care.

REFERENCES

Accidental Death and Disability: The Neglected Disease of Modern Society. Washington, DC, National Academy of Sciences/National Research Council, 1966.

Boyd DR: Trauma—A controllable disease in the 1980's. J Trauma 20:14–24, 1980.

Community-wide emergency medical services. JAMA 204(7), May 13, 1968.

Consumer Health Perspectives: Emergency Medical Care in the United States: A New Frontier. Consumer Commission in the Accreditation of Health Services, January 1981.

Essential equipment for ambulances. Bulletin of the American College of Surgeons, May 1970.

Farrington JD, Hampton OP: A curriculum for training emergency medical technicians. Bulletin of the American College of Surgeons, September–October 1969.

Hampton OP: The systematic approach to emergency medical services. Bulletin of the American College of Surgeons, September–October 1968.

Henry M, Stapleton E: EMTs and medical control. Journal of Emergency Medical Services 1(I):32–34, 1985.

Kennedy RH, et al: Emergency care. The Committee on Trauma, American College of Surgeons. Philadelphia, WB Saunders, 1966.

Kennedy RH: Community responsibility in the care of emergency patients. Journal of Oral Surgery 27, July, 1969.

Kimball KF: The importance of ambulance design to emergency care. Journal of the Ambulance Association of America, August 1970.

Medical Control of Emergency Medical Services: An Overview for Emergency Physicians. Dallas, American College of Emergency Physicians, 1984, p.1.

Subcommittee on Medical Control, Committee on Emergency Medical Services, Assembly of Life Sciences: Medical control in emergency medical service systems. Washington, DC, National Research Council, National Academy Press, 1981.

Morrissey JM, Hoffmann AD, Thrope JC: Consent and Confidentiality in the Health Care of Children and Adolescents: A Legal Guide. New York, The Free Press, 1986.

Nagel EL, Hirschman JC, Nussenfeld SR, et al: Telemetry—medical command in coronary and other mobile emergency care systems. JAMA, 214(2), 1970.

NASA-developed system transmits electrocardiograph by RF and telephone links in emergency situations AID. Journal of the Ambulance Association of America 3(11), November 1968.

Peisert M: The Hospital's Role in Emergency Medical Services Systems. Chicago, American Hospital Publishing, 1984.

Roush WR (ed): Principles of EMS Systems: A Comprehensive Text for Physicians. Dallas, American College of Emergency Physicians, 1989.

Safer P, Esposito G, Benson DM: Ambulance design and equipment for mobile intensive care. Arch Surg 102, March 1971.

Standards for emergency ambulance services. Bulletin of the American College of Surgeons, June 1971.

Stapleton E, Best J: Developing a hospital based ambulance service. In Pascarelli E: Hospital based ambulatory care. Norwalk, CT, Appleton-Century-Crofts, 1982.

Taubenhaus LJ, Kirkpatrick JR: Analysis of a hospital ambulance service. Public Health Rep 82(9), September 1967.

Textbook of Advanced Cardiac Life Support, 2nd ed. American Heart Association, 1987. US Bureau of the Census: Statistical abstract of the United States: 1990 (110th Edition). Washington, DC, 1990.

US Department of Health, Education and Welfare: Medical requirements for ambulance design and equipment. Emergency Health Series C-3.

US Department of Health, Education and Welfare: Training of ambulance personnel and others responsible for emergency care of the sick and injured at the scene and during transport. Emergency Health Series C-4.

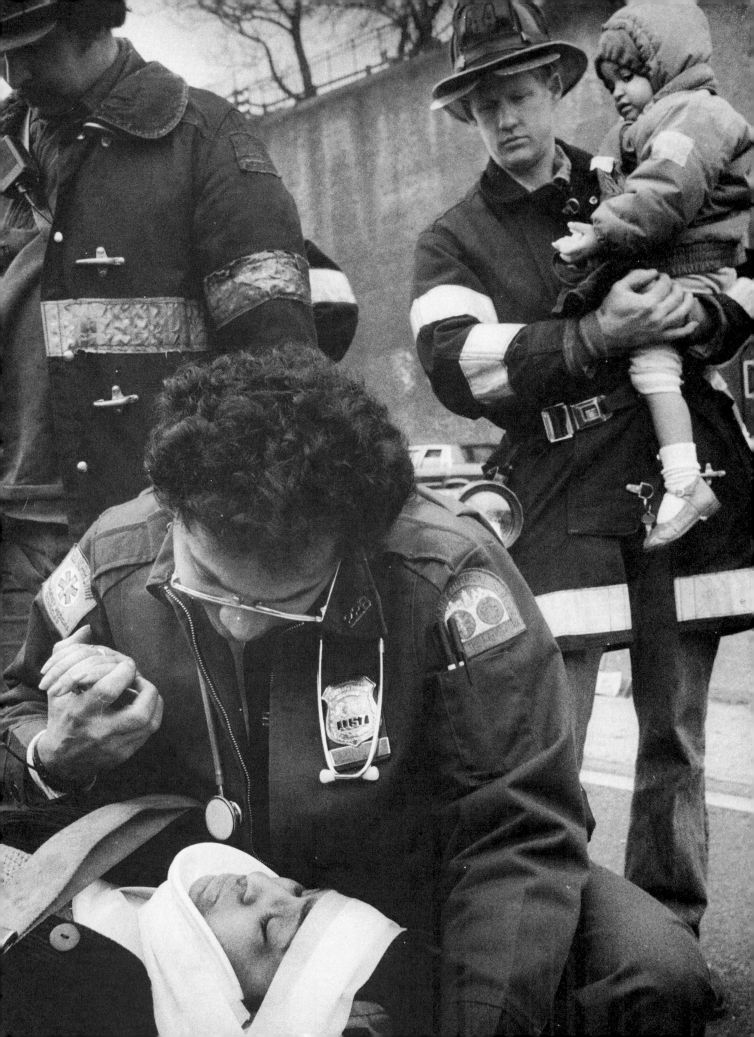

CHAPTER 2

ANATOMY, PHYSIOLOGY, AND PATIENT ASSESSMENT

OBJECTIVES

At the conclusion of this chapter the reader will be able to:

1. Define the following anatomical terms:

Medial	Anterior	Posterior
Lateral	Proximal	Midline
Distal	Right	Left
Superior	Inferior	

2. Describe the general function of the following major body systems:

Respiratory	Nervous	Circulatory
Digestive	Muscular	Genitourinary
Skeletal	Reproductive	

3. List four vital signs.

4. List five diagnostic signs in addition to vital signs.

5. Demonstrate on a role-playing "patient" the technique for completing a total patient assessment. Identify and record diagnostic signs and describe normal and abnormal findings.

ANATOMY AND PHYSIOLOGY

The study of anatomy and physiology is the study of the body's structure and function. Anatomy is the study of the structure of body parts, and physiology is the study of processes and activities of living organisms.

A knowledge of anatomy and physiology is essential for all practitioners of medical care, and it is the starting point for understanding the significance of disease and injury. Understanding how the body works provides a rational basis for recognizing abnormal conditions and their treatment.

Structural Organization of the Human Body

ATOMS AND MOLECULES

Atoms are the smallest units of matter. Atoms can bind together chemically to form elements and molecules. Molecules are small particles made up of more than one atom that form a chemical substance. When a substance is made of identical atoms, it is called an *element.* Oxygen gas is an example of an element. It is composed of two atoms of oxygen and is written symbolically as O_2. The main molecules that make up the body are water and *proteins.* A water molecule is made from two atoms of hydrogen (H) and one atom of oxygen (O) and is written as H_2O (see Fig. 2–1*A*). Water makes up approximately 60 to 70% of the body by weight. Proteins are the building blocks from which many body substances are formed. Proteins are molecules composed of various combinations of carbon, hydrogen, oxygen, and nitrogen atoms. Other important molecules and atoms found in the body include fats, carbohydrates, minerals, and electrolytes (atoms with an electric charge when in solution). Examples of electrolytes include calcium (an important mineral that hardens bone), sodium, potassium, magnesium, and phosphorus.

Water is vitally important because it dissolves or surrounds other molecules within the body. When water disperses, or separates, other molecules by surrounding the individual molecules with water molecules, it is said to act as a *solvent.* The substance that is dissolved is called a *solute* and is said to be in solution (see Fig. 2–1*B*). Sugar and salt are common examples of solutes that can be dissolved (dispersed) in water. The concentration of a solute in solution depends on the amount of the solute and volume of water. The concentration of a salt solution depends on the amount of salt in proportion to the volume of water. For example, a teaspoon of salt in a quart of water is not as concentrated as three teaspoons of salt in a quart of water. The first example would be considered a more dilute solution.

THE CELL

The cell is the fundamental unit of all living things. There are one-celled animals, as well as large animals made up of billions of cells. While cells can have different and distinct functions, all cells have some characteristics in common. The *cell membrane* contains the contents of a cell and separates it from other cells and the outside environment. This allows the cell to have an internal environment that is regulated by the flow of substances across the membrane. The control center of the cell is the *nucleus,* which is also contained in its own membrane. The nucleus contains the genetic material, or genes. When cells grow by cell division, the genes are reproduced so that each new cell has the same genetic material as the original cell.

The cell, being a living structure, does work. To do work, it requires nutrients and energy. Specialized structures called *mitochondria* convert food into a form of energy that can be used by the cell for synthesis of proteins and other substances. *Ribosomes* are special structures in which large molecules called proteins are assembled or synthesized from smaller molecules. These proteins may be needed for cell growth, reproduction, or production of proteins to be secreted out of the cell membrane and used by other cells. The special structures inside the cell membrane are bathed in a fluid called *cytoplasm.* The membrane serves to keep this cytoplasm distinct from the external environment that surrounds the cell (Fig. 2–2).

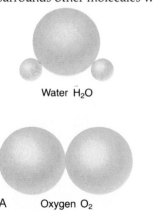

Water H_2O

A   Oxygen O_2

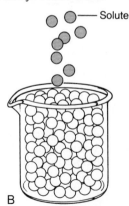

— Solute

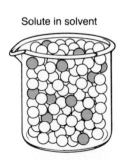

Solute in solvent

B

FIGURE 2–1. (*A*) Water and oxygen molecules. (*B*) A solute in a solvent.

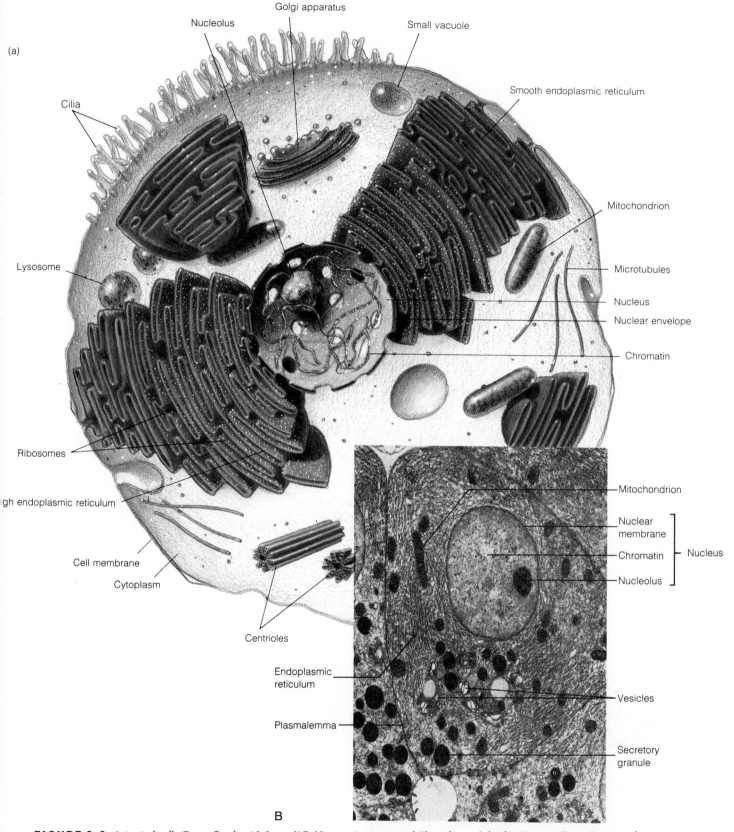

FIGURE 2–2. A typical cell. (From Gaudin AJ, Jones KC: Human Anatomy and Physiology. Orlando, Harcourt Brace Jovanovich, 1989, p. 48.)

TISSUES

Although cells have some basic components in common, they also may have unique characteristics that enable them to serve a specific function. When many specialized cells are grouped together, they compose a *tissue*. A tissue is a group of cells working together to serve a given function. There are four basic types of tissues (Fig. 2–3). For example, *muscle tissue* is made up of many cells that can contract to allow motion. *Nerve tissue* conducts impulses that are used to direct body functions and for communication. The other types of tissues in the body are *epithelial tissue*, a protective covering that can selectively allow certain substances to pass across while prohibiting passage of others, and *connective tissue*, which provides structure, attaches, and protects.

However, each basic tissue type can have specialized functions as well. For example, muscle tissue can

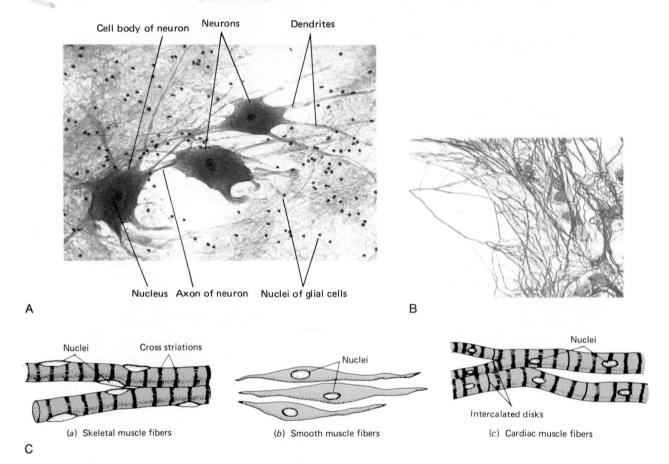

A

B

(a) Skeletal muscle fibers   (b) Smooth muscle fibers   (c) Cardiac muscle fibers

C

Simple Columnar Epithelium

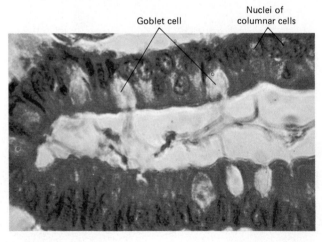

Approximately × 450

D

FIGURE 2–3. (*A*) Nerve tissue. (*B*) Connective tissue. (*C*) Muscle tissue. (*D*) Epithelial tissue. (From Solomon EP, Phillips GA: Understanding Human Anatomy and Physiology. Philadelphia, WB Saunders, 1987, pp. 48, 51, and 53.)

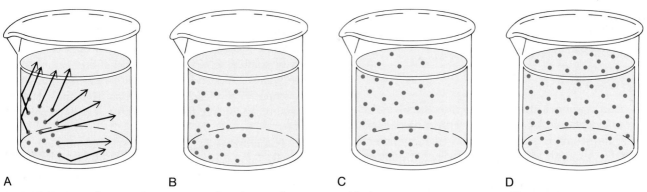

A   B   C   D

FIGURE 2–4. Diffusion is the movement of a substance from an area of higher concentration to an area of lower concentration. In this experiment, when a lump of sugar is dropped into a beaker of water, its molecules dissolve (*A*) and begin to diffuse (*B* and *C*). Eventually, diffusion results in an even distribution of sugar molecules throughout the water (*D*). (From Davis WP, Solomon EP: The World of Biology, 4th ed. Philadelphia, Saunders College Publishing, 1990.)

be classified as *voluntary* or skeletal muscle, used for willful movement as in walking; *involuntary* or smooth muscle, used for processes such as movement of food through the digestive tract; and *cardiac* muscle, a specialized form of involuntary muscle found in the walls of the heart, which pumps blood throughout the body.

INTERSTITIAL OR TISSUE FLUID

The cells within a tissue are surrounded by fluid called *interstitial fluid*, or tissue fluid. Nutrients from the blood vessels pass through the interstitial fluid as they move to the cells. Waste products produced by the cells pass through the interstitial fluid as they move to the vascular space to be excreted from the body. The cell membrane regulates the passage of substances between the interstitial or extracellular fluid and the cytoplasm or intercellular contents.

The passage of substances may occur in different ways. Examples include *diffusion*, where a substance crosses a membrane freely and flows from an area of higher concentration to an area of lower concentration (Fig. 2–4), and *osmosis*, in which a solvent flows across a membrane from an area of lower concentration to an area of higher concentration (Fig. 2–5). Diffusion and osmosis are methods whereby substances move across cell membranes without expenditure of energy. (Diffusion and osmosis are concepts used in understanding functions within the respiratory system, discussed in Chapter 3, and the circulatory system, discussed in Chapter 4.) Active transport is an example of solute transport across a membrane that does require the cell to use

FIGURE 2–5. Osmosis and the living cell. (*A*) The concentration of solutes is the same in the solution as in the cell. No net movement of water occurs across the cell membrane. Below are seen normal-appearing red blood cells. (*B*) The concentration of solutes is greater in the solution than in the cell. Water moves from the cell (across the cell membrane) into the solution in an attempt to reach equilibrium. As a result, the cell is left with less water (dehydrated), shrinks, and can die. (*C*) The concentration of solutes is lower in the solution than in the cell. Water moves from the solution across the cell membrane into the cell. The cells swell and perhaps even burst. (Micrographs of human red blood cells courtesy of Dr. R.F. Baker, University of Southern California Medical School; from Davis WP, Solomon EP: The World of Biology, 4th ed. Philadelphia, Saunders College Publishing, 1990.)

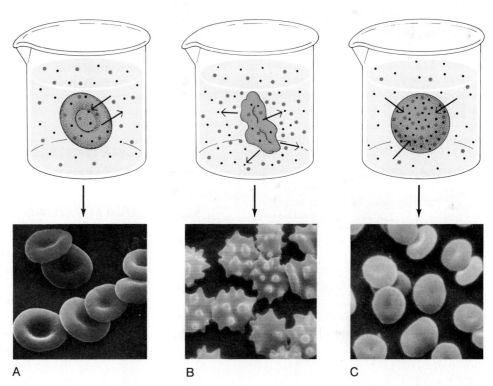

A   B   C

energy. Through the expenditure of metabolic energy, materials move across cell membranes. Active transport is utilized by muscle and nerve cells.

ORGANS

An *organ* is a structure composed of several types of tissues that work together to serve a particular function. The stomach is an organ that contains several tissues. For example, epithelial tissue lines the inside and outside of the stomach, muscular tissue mechanically churns the food, and nerve tissue regulates the body's activities. Collectively, these tissues work together to give the stomach its specialized ability to contribute to the digestion and transport of food.

ORGAN SYSTEMS

An organ system is a group of organs that work together to perform a complex function. For example, the stomach and several other organs, including the mouth, esophagus, gallbladder, liver, pancreas, intestines, and rectum, form the digestive system. Other major organ systems include the skeletal, muscular, respiratory, circulatory, nervous, endocrine, urinary, reproductive, and integumentary (or skin).

ESSENTIAL PROCESSES

Nutrition, growth, reproduction, and elimination of waste products are essential processes that are part of life. Nutrients must be taken into the body for manufacture of the proteins and other molecules necessary for cell maintenance and cellular division. The sum of all chemical processes in the body is referred to as *metabolism*. Heat is given off during metabolic processes. Since metabolism is continuously occurring, the internal production of heat given off during metabolism is used to maintain body temperature. Waste products are formed during metabolic processes and must be eliminated from the body.

NUTRIENTS

The essential nutrients are oxygen, water, and sources of nitrogen and carbon (protein, carbohydrates, fats). Minerals and trace elements are required as well. All nutrients except oxygen are taken in through the digestive system. Oxygen is acquired through the respiratory system.

How often these essential nutrients are taken in varies and depends on how fast they are used and how they can be stored.

Oxygen is used continuously and, although vitally important, cannot be stored. If one stops breathing, life stops within minutes.

Water is acquired from liquids and foods and as a byproduct of metabolism. Water is not stored for future use. Rather, to keep and maintain the proper concentration of solutes within cells, interstitial fluid, and blood, both water intake and excretion are carefully regulated. The importance of water is obvious from the fact that a person cannot live for more than a few days without water.

Food brings in the other essential nutrients and minerals. Food is broken down and stored for future use. Furthermore, the body can convert one type of food substance to another. Because food can be stored, a person may live for weeks without food intake, provided there is limited activity and access to water.

HOMEOSTASIS

While conditions in the environment can change significantly, body processes tend to work best under relatively constant conditions. *Homeostasis* is the word used to describe the tendency of the body functions to maintain this constant internal environment. Examples of conditions that must be carefully regulated in order for the body to function include temperature, water balance, and the acid content of body fluids.

For example, the normal temperature for the human body is 98.6 degrees (°) Fahrenheit (F) or 37 degrees Celsius (C). While outside temperatures can range from below 0° to over 100° F, body processes work to maintain the internal temperature at a relatively constant 98.6° F. Many different processes may be employed to achieve homeostasis. For example, when exposed to cold temperatures the body increases heat production by changing its metabolism and by shivering (forced muscular activity) and reduces heat loss by reducing blood flow to the skin so less heat will be radiated to the outside environment. To maintain homeostasis when a person exercises, the blood vessels in the skin dilate so more body heat is given off to the outside; the person perspires heavily and loses heat through the evaporation of sweat.

Anatomical Terms and Relationships

ANATOMICAL POSITION

The relationship of each of the body's parts to one another is described by use of anatomical terms. These terms are applied to a body in the anatomical position. Regardless of the actual position a body may assume, the terms remain fixed when describing the relationship of one body part to another.

The *anatomical position* refers to a body standing erect with the feet together and parallel, the arms at the sides, and palms and the head facing forward (Fig. 2–6).

From this position any part further from the ground or closer to the head is referred to as *superior*. Any part closer to the ground or the feet is referred to as *inferior*. For example, the knee is superior to the ankle. The heart is inferior to the head. At times you may see the word *cephalad* (head) used instead of "superior," and *caudal* (tail) used instead of "inferior" (see Fig. 2–6).

Structures toward the front of the body are said to be *anterior*. Structures toward the rear of the body are *posterior*. In the anatomical position, the *sternum* (breast bone) is anterior to the heart; the spine is posterior.

Reference to the midline of the body is facilitated by imagining a plane through the nose, sternum, and *umbilicus* or navel, separating the body into right and left halves. If a structure is further away from the midline, it is said to be *lateral*. Conversely, if a structure is closer to the midline, it is said to be *medial*. For example, the arm is lateral to the torso; the nose is medial to the eyes.

On the extremities, additional terms are sometimes used to describe location. The term *proximal* means closer to the trunk, and *distal* means further away from the trunk. For example, the elbow is proximal to the hand, and the foot is distal to the knee.

Other useful terms include *superficial* and *deep*, used to describe relative distance from the surface of the body. For example, a wound might be described as superficial if it scrapes the upper level of skin and deep if it punctures through the skin and underlying tissues. *Central* and *peripheral* are terms used to describe the relative distance from the center of the body. For example, arteries and nerves in the extremities are referred to as peripheral vessels. The major arteries and veins that leave and enter the heart would be appropriately referred to as central vessels.

Confusing relationships for some students are those of the arms and hands. Confusion is avoided by always referring to the picture of the anatomical position where the arms are at the sides and the palms are facing forward (see Fig. 2–6). In this position, the thumb is lateral and the little finger is medial. Actually, all structures on the

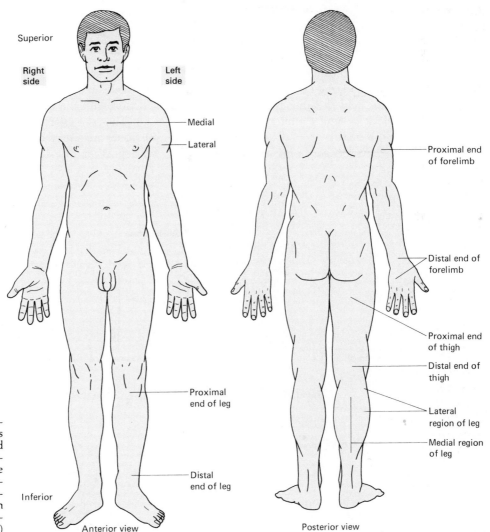

Know this Direction

FIGURE 2–6. The standard anatomical position: body erect, palms forward. This allows for a standard reference when communicating anatomical relationships. Relate the terms found in the text to the drawing above. (From Solomon EP, Phillips GA: Understanding Human Anatomy and Physiology. Philadelphia, WB Saunders, 1987, p. 11.)

thumb side of the arm in this position would be considered lateral, and those on the side of the little finger, medial. Also confusing when dealing with the extremities are the anatomical meanings of the words "arm" and "leg." In anatomy, the arm refers to the upper arm only, from the shoulder to the elbow. The leg refers to the lower leg, from the knee to the ankle.

TERMS RELATING TO POSITION AND MOVEMENT

Special terms are used to describe body position and movement. The body standing upright is called *erect*, and lying on its back, *supine*. If the body is lying face down it is said to be *prone*. A body lying on its side is said to be in the *lateral recumbent* position. The lateral recumbent position is further described by the inferior side, or side on the ground. For example, a patient lying on the right side would be said to be in the right lateral recumbent position.

Movement away from the midline is referred to as *abduction* (ab = away); movement toward the midline is called *adduction* (ad = toward). For example, raising the arm from the side upward would be abduction. Returning the arm to the side would be adduction. In the hand, abduction and adduction refer to movement with respect to an arbitrary line drawn through the third finger. When the fingers are spread apart, they are said to be abducted; when the fingers are held together they are adducted (Fig. 2–7). In the foot, a similar arbitrary line is drawn through the second toe.

Flexion and extension are terms used to describe motion about a joint. When a joint is bent and the two parts are brought closer together they are in *flexion*, or flexed. When the joint is apart they are said to be in *extension*, or extended (Fig. 2–8). The head is flexed when it is bent forward toward the chest and extended when it is brought back to anatomical position or slightly beyond. When the head is further extended toward the back it is said to be *hyperextended*.

Medial rotation is used to describe motion of a limb when the anterior surface of the limb is rotated to face medially; the term *lateral rotation* is used when the anterior surface rotates to face laterally (Fig. 2–9). For example, medial rotation describes rotation of the arm from the anatomical position to a position where the anterior surface faces the trunk instead of forward.

Specific Organ Systems

Each organ system has a specific role in the body's activities and functions. Understanding the contributions of each organ system helps one appreciate the body as a whole.

SKELETAL SYSTEM

The skeletal system gives structure and support to the body and serves to protect vital organs. In conjunction with the muscles, it allows for movement.

There are 206 bones in the body (Fig. 2–10A and B). Bones are a form of connective tissue that is hardened by deposition of calcium. Bone is a living substance and

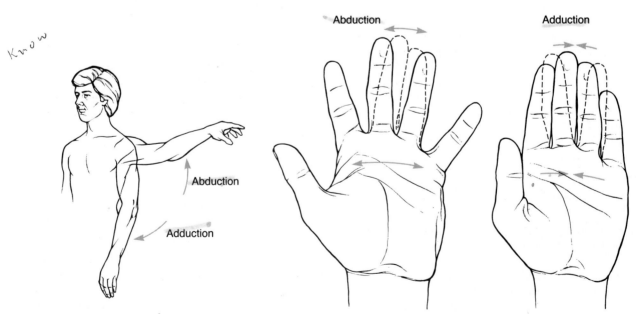

FIGURE 2–7. Abduction versus adduction.

Know

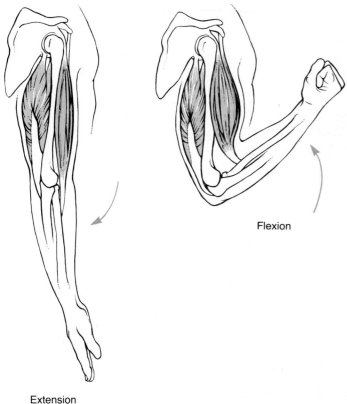

Flexion

Extension

FIGURE 2–8. Flexion versus extension.

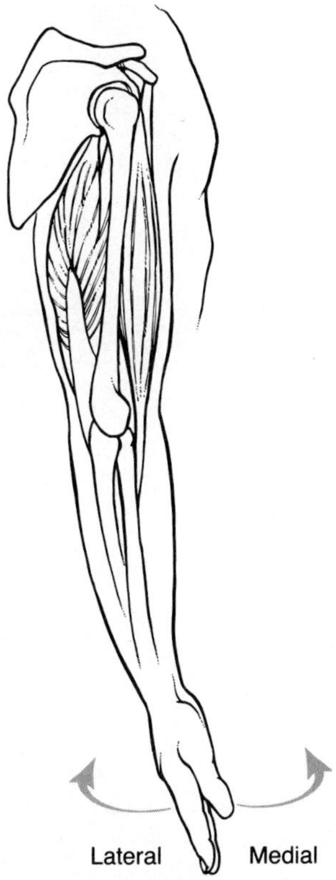

Lateral   Medial

FIGURE 2–9. Medial and lateral rotation.

capable of growth and repair. Other forms of connective tissue that compose the skeletal system include *cartilage*, a softer, more flexible support substance, and *ligaments*, which attach bone to bone, and *tendons*, which attach muscle to bone.

SKULL.   The skull is made up of the bones of the *cranium* and the face. The cranium encases the brain and, in the adult, has about a 1-liter internal capacity that is fully occupied by brain, cerebrospinal fluid, and blood vessels. The cranium serves mainly to protect the delicate brain tissue within (see Fig. 2–10*A* and *B*). The cranial and vertebral cavities enclose the central nervous system (Fig. 2–11).

SPINAL COLUMN.   The spinal column consists of 33 bones called *vertebrae*, which give support to the neck, thorax, abdomen, and pelvis. The spinal column can be divided into five sections.

- Cervical—the seven vertebral bones that form the neck
- Thoracic—the twelve vertebrae to which the ribs are attached
- Lumbar—the five vertebrae forming the lower back
- Sacral—the five fused vertebrae that form the *sacrum*, or back of the pelvis
- Coccygeal—the four fused vertebrae that form the *coccyx*, or tailbone

The cervical, thoracic, and lumbar vertebrae are separated by cartilaginous discs that allow for varying degrees of mobility in addition to support. The fused sacral vertebrae offer support and protection to the pelvis. In the center of the spinal column is a hollow opening called the *spinal canal*. As the spinal cord extends downward from the brain through a hole in the base of the skull, it is protected within the spinal canal.

The *cranial vault* (inside of the cranium) and the spinal canal are sometimes referred to as body cavities.

THORACIC CAVITY.   The *thoracic cavity* begins just below the neck and extends down to the *diaphragm* (a respiratory muscle that separates the *thorax* [chest] and abdomen). The rib cage surrounds the thoracic cavity and is attached to the sternum on the anterior side and to the thoracic spine on the posterior side. The upper 10 pairs of ribs are attached to the sternum on the anterior side and to the thoracic spine on the posterior side. These ribs are attached to the sternum by cartilage that is called *costal cartilages*. The 11th and 12th pairs of ribs are not attached to the sternum. They are attached only to the 11th and 12th thoracic vertebrae and are referred to as "floating" ribs. The sternum is composed of three separate bones: the upper *manubrium*, the *middle body*, and the lower *xiphoid*.

The *clavicles*, or collarbones, lie over the anterior

Text continued on page 34

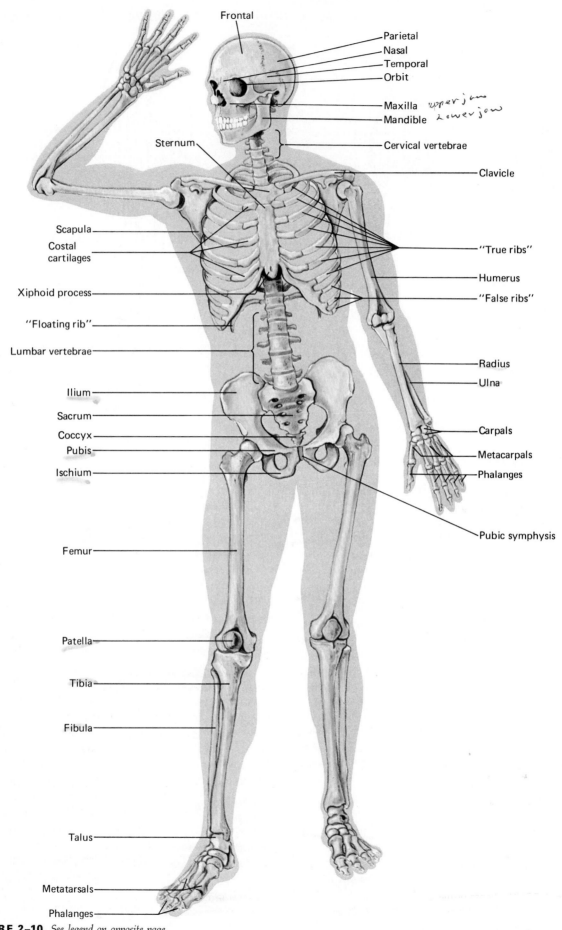

Frontal

Parietal
Nasal
Temporal
Orbit

Maxilla *upper jaw*
Mandible *lower jaw*

Cervical vertebrae

Clavicle

Sternum

Scapula

Costal
cartilages

Xiphoid process

"Floating rib"

Lumbar vertebrae

Ilium

Sacrum

Coccyx

Pubis

Ischium

Femur

Patella

Tibia

Fibula

Talus

Metatarsals

Phalanges

"True ribs"

Humerus

"False ribs"

Radius

Ulna

Carpals

Metacarpals

Phalanges

Pubic symphysis

A

FIGURE 2–10. *See legend on opposite page*

32

Know

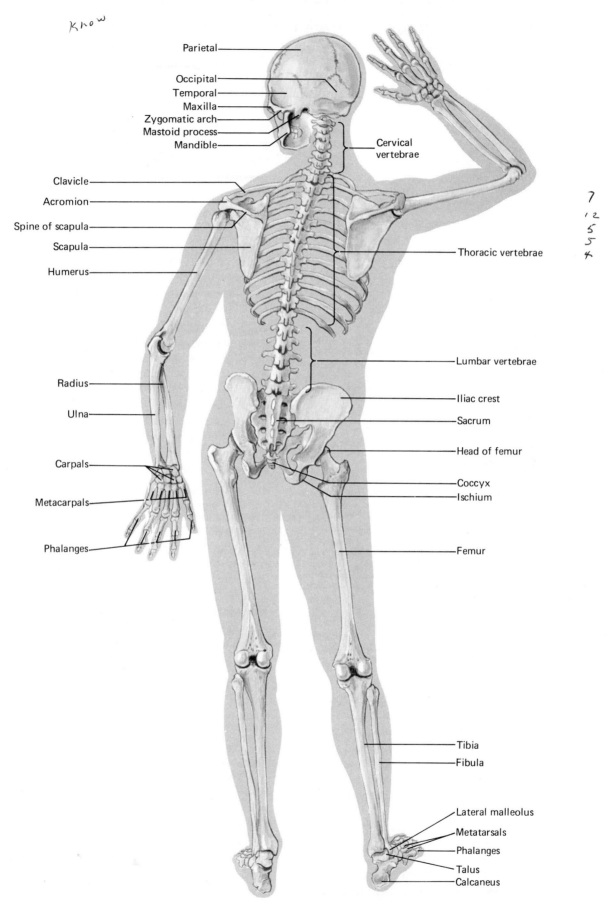

7
12
5
5
4

Parietal

Occipital
Temporal
Maxilla
Zygomatic arch
Mastoid process
Mandible

Cervical
vertebrae

Clavicle
Acromion
Spine of scapula
Scapula
Humerus

Thoracic vertebrae

Radius

Ulna

Lumbar vertebrae

Iliac crest
Sacrum
Head of femur

Carpals

Coccyx
Ischium

Metacarpals

Phalanges

Femur

Tibia
Fibula

Lateral malleolus
Metatarsals
Phalanges
Talus
Calcaneus

B

FIGURE 2–10. The bones of the skeletal system. (A) Anterior view. (B) Posterior view. (From Solomon EP, Phillips GA: Understanding Human Anatomy and Physiology. Philadelphia, WB Saunders, 1987, pp. 75 and 76.)

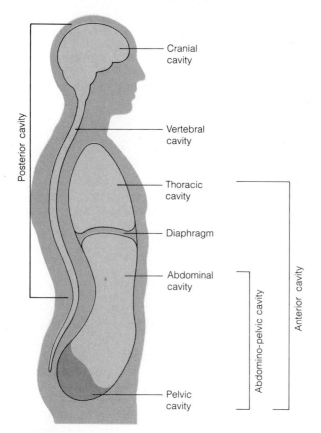

FIGURE 2–11. The cranial vault is composed of several bones, including the frontal, two parietal, occipital, and two temporal bones, which encase the brain and spinal cord. The spinal cord exits the base of the brain and is surrounded by vertebrae as it travels through the spinal canal. The thoracic cavity extends from the base of the neck down to the diaphragm (the primary muscle of breathing). The abdominal cavity begins at the diaphragm and extends down to the pelvic cavity, which is surrounded by the pelvic bones and sacrum of the spine. (From Gaudin AJ, Jones KC: Human Anatomy and Physiology. Orlando, Harcourt Brace Jovanovich, 1989, p. 10.)

upper ribs and extend from the sternum to the shoulders. The *scapulas*, or shoulder blades, lie over the upper posterior ribs and attach to the clavicles and humerus to form the shoulder (see Fig. 2–10*A* and *B*).

The *diaphragm* is a dome-shaped muscle that forms the base of the thoracic cavity. It contracts and pushes downward into the abdomen to allow air to enter the lungs during *inspiration* (breathing in). The diaphragm relaxes and rises within the thoracic cavity during *expiration* (breathing out). As mentioned, the diaphragm forms the division between the thoracic and abdominal cavities. Since it moves with breathing, the boundary between these two cavities may move as well, which is something to consider when evaluating penetrating injuries.

The attachments of the diaphragm are the xiphoid process of the sternum, the lower six ribs, and the upper lumbar vertebrae. There are openings in the diaphragm for the *aorta* (major artery), *vena cava* (major vein), and *esophagus* (food pipe).

Contained within the thoracic cavity are the heart, lungs, and great vessels. The esophagus travels through the middle of the thoracic cavity posterior to the airway.

The thoracic cavity is subdivided into two smaller spaces, the *mediastinum* (in the center) and the *pleural spaces* on either side. The mediastinum is occupied by the heart, great vessels, esophagus, *trachea* (windpipe), and mainstem bronchi. The lungs occupy the pleural spaces.

ABDOMINAL-PELVIC CAVITY. The abdominal cavity is bounded by the diaphragm superiorly and the bony pelvic cavity inferiorly (see Fig. 2–11). Posteriorly it is protected by the spine. The sides and anterior portions are protected by layers of muscle. Additional protection over the superior portion is provided by the lower ribs.

The abdominal cavity contains several organs of digestion and excretion, including the stomach, the small and large intestine, the liver, the gallbladder, the pancreas, the kidneys, and the ureters. Also, the spleen is contained within the abdominal cavity.

The abdominal cavity is lined with a membrane called the *peritoneum*. This membrane separates the organs from the abdominal wall and surrounds most surfaces of the organs within the abdominal cavity. Portions of the small intestines, the pancreas, the kidneys, and the great vessels lie behind the peritoneum and are said to be *retroperitoneal*.

The pelvic cavity is the lowermost portion of the abdominal cavity (see Fig. 2–11). The pelvic girdle is a ring of bones formed by the sacrum, the ilium (two, left and right), the ischium (two) and the pubis (two). They provide protection to the pelvic organs within, including parts of the lower intestine and the rectum and the urinary bladder, as well as the reproductive organs in the female. The superior boundary of the pelvic cavity is formed by an imaginary plane extending between the pubic bone anteriorly to the top of the sacrum posteriorly. The floor of the pelvis is made up of muscles and connective tissue.

QUADRANTS. The abdominal-pelvic cavity can be divided in various ways to describe the location of pain, tenderness, or other physical findings. A common system is to divide the abdomen into quadrants by two imaginary lines that intersect at the *umbilicus*, or navel. Horizontal and vertical lines through the umbilicus form right and left upper quadrants and right and left lower quadrants. See Figure 2–12 for examples of the quadrants and organs that lie beneath. Some organs are contained within a single quadrant and others lie in more than one.

Other terms used to describe specific locations in the abdomen are *epigastric*, *umbilical*, and *suprapubic* (see Fig. 2–12). These terms are helpful in localizing findings near the midline. The term *epigastric* includes the area below the xiphoid and costal margins. The term *periumbilical* describes the area immediately surrounding the umbilicus. The term *suprapubic* (also *hypogastric*) is used

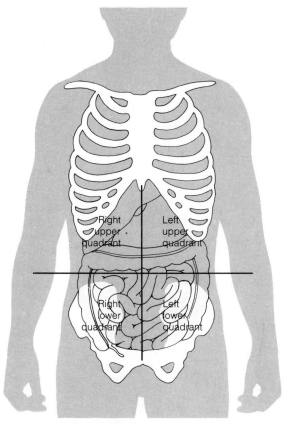 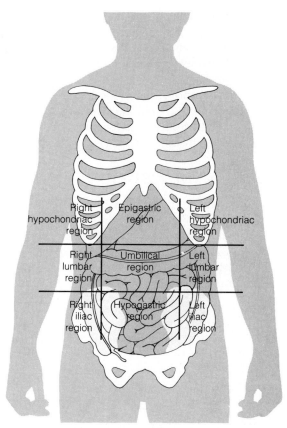

FIGURE 2–12. Quadrants of the abdomen and the location of major organs. (From Gaudin AJ, Jones KC: Human Anatomy and Physiology. Orlando, Harcourt Brace Jovanovich, 1989, p. 11.)

to describe the area just above the symphysis pubis. The term *flank* describes the posterior portion of the abdomen between the ribs and the ilium of the pelvis.

UPPER EXTREMITIES. The upper extremities consist of the shoulder, the arm, the elbow, the forearm, the wrist, and the hand.

The only bone in the upper arm is the *humerus.* The shoulder is formed by the *articulation* (joining) of the humerus with the scapula. The head of the humerus fits against the glenoid process of the scapula to form a ball-and-socket joint. The shoulder receives support from attachments between the scapula and the clavicle. The muscles of the shoulder give this joint added stability.

Bones in the forearm are the *radius* and *ulna.* The radius is on the lateral side (thumb side) of the arm in the anatomical position. The ulna is on the medial side. The elbow is the joint formed by the articulation of the humerus, radius, and ulna. The wrist is made up of eight bones called *carpal* bones. The hand is made up of *metacarpal* bones and *phalanges* (see Fig. 2–10A and B).

LOWER EXTREMITIES. The lower extremities are made up of the hip, the thigh, the knee, the leg, the ankle, and the foot. The *femur* is the bone of the thigh and is the largest bone in the body. The hip joint is the

articulation of the head of the femur and the *acetabulum*, or socket, of the pelvis. It is a ball-and-socket joint.

The bones of the lower leg are the *tibia* and the *fibula.* The tibia, the major weight-bearing bone, is larger and located medially. It is covered by a thin layer of skin and soft tissue anteriorly and is easily palpable. The fibula is a thinner bone that lies lateral to the tibia.

The knee is a hinge joint formed by the articulation of the femur and the tibia and the femur and the *patella* (kneecap). The patella is a triangular-shaped bone that is situated in the tendon of the *quadriceps* muscle (which extends the knee) at the anterior aspect of the knee. The patella is felt subcutaneously on its anterior surface. Its posterior surface articulates with the femur. The patella aids in extension of the knee.

The ankle is made up of seven bones called *tarsal* bones. The foot is composed of *metatarsal* bones and *phalanges* (see Fig. 2–10A and B).

MUSCULAR SYSTEM

The muscles are tissue capable of contraction, or shortening. They are attached and designed in such a way that the power of their contraction results in movement. There are three types of muscles (Fig. 2–13):

voluntary, or skeletal, muscle (Fig. 2–14*A* and *B*); involuntary, or smooth, muscle; and cardiac muscle. Skeletal muscles (voluntary) are any muscles that are normally controlled by a person's will. Contraction of the smooth (involuntary) muscles results in automatic functions such as *peristalsis*, or movement of food through the digestive tract. Cardiac muscle, although similar in structure to skeletal muscle, functions automatically to pump blood with each heartbeat (see Figs. 2–13 and 2–14*A* and *B*).

RESPIRATORY SYSTEM

The respiratory system brings oxygen into the body and rids the body of *carbon dioxide*, the waste product. It is composed of the nose and mouth, the *nasopharynx* and *oropharynx*, the *larynx*, the *trachea*, the *bronchi*, and the *lungs* (Fig. 2–15). The respiratory system allows an exchange of gases with the outside environ-

ment. The nose, nasopharynx, and oropharynx are designed to filter, moisten, and warm or cool the air, as needed, before it reaches the delicate *alveoli*, or air sacs, in the lungs. The larynx (which also contains the vocal cords), the trachea, and the bronchi conduct air to the lungs. The diaphragm and the muscles of the chest cause the thoracic cavity to expand and contract like a bellows to create air flow during ventilations.

CIRCULATORY SYSTEM

The blood is the medium through which oxygen and nutrients are transported to the cells and waste products are returned to the organs of elimination. The blood vessels are the conduits through which blood travels, and the heart is the pump that provides the driving force to move blood through the circulatory system (Fig. 2–16).

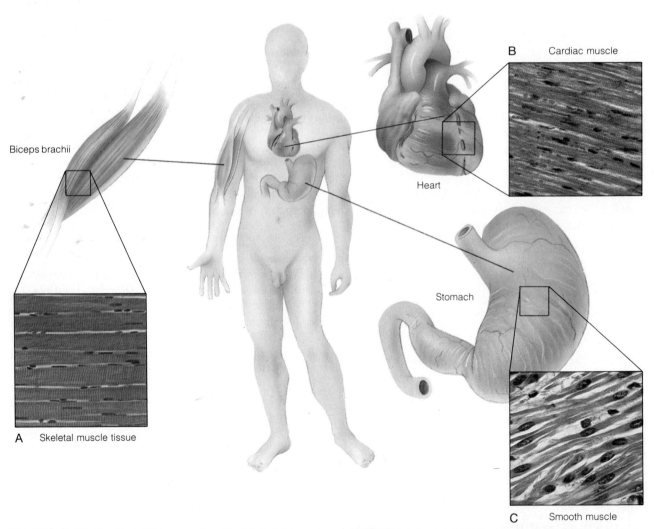

FIGURE 2–13. There are three types of muscle. (*A*) Skeletal muscle provides the force for voluntary motor activity throughout the body. (*B*) Cardiac muscle found in the heart provides the force for contraction and blood flow. (*C*) Smooth muscle is found in the blood vessels and in the linings of the gastrointestinal and respiratory tracts. (From Gaudin AJ, Jones KC: Human Anatomy and Physiology. Orlando, Harcourt Brace Jovanovich, 1989, p. 181.)

The blood has both cellular and liquid components. The liquid portion of blood is called the *plasma*, which makes up over half the volume of blood. The principal cellular component is the red blood cells, whose main job is the transportation of oxygen. Additional cellular components of blood are the white blood cells, used to fight infection, and *platelets*, which are essential for blood clotting.

There are three major types of blood vessels: *arteries*, *capillaries*, and *veins*. The arteries carry oxygen-rich blood away from the heart to the body, forming smaller and smaller blood vessels until finally they are thin-walled capillaries. The capillaries are microscopic vessels in which red blood cells come in close contact with the individual cells throughout the body. It is at the capillary level that oxygen and other nutrients pass from the blood cells and plasma through the walls of the blood vessel to the tissue cells. At the same time, carbon dioxide and other waste products of metabolism pass through the capillary walls in the opposite direction, from the tissue cells to the blood, to be taken away. The veins return the blood to the heart. From there it is delivered to the lungs to obtain more oxygen. There are also lymphatic vessels that return tissue fluid to the blood stream.

The heart is actually two separate parallel pumps, referred to as the left heart and the right heart. Each side of the heart is further divided into collecting and pumping chambers. The right heart collects blood returning from the body and pumps it into the lungs, where it eliminates carbon dioxide and is enriched with oxygen. The left heart receives the oxygen-enriched blood returning from the lungs and pumps it throughout the entire body, to deliver more oxygen to the cells. Blood that is rich in oxygen is bright red in color. When it has given up its oxygen, it is dark bluish red.

Actually, there are two different circulatory systems operating simultaneously, the *pulmonary* and the *systemic*. The pulmonary circulation is the right circulation, since the right side of the heart pumps blood through the lungs. Blood flow through the systemic, or left, circulation is pumped by the left side of the heart.

NERVOUS SYSTEM

The nervous system is the controlling and regulating organ system for all parts of the body. It is both the decision maker and the communicator. The decision-making takes place in the *central nervous system*, which consists of the brain, the brain stem, and the spinal cord. Communication to distal body parts takes place through nerves that compose the *peripheral nervous system* (see Fig. 2–17). The peripheral nervous system has two components, *sensory nerves*, which bring information to the central nervous system, and *motor nerves*, which transmit messages from the central nervous system to all parts of the body.

Some decisions of the central nervous system are conscious; others are made without our awareness. The nervous system can be divided into *voluntary* and *involuntary* parts on the basis of whether we have conscious control of the action. For example, the voluntary system controls body movement, speech, and other activities of daily life. The involuntary nervous system, known as the *autonomic nervous system*, is concerned with vegetative processes such as control of respiration, circulation, and digestion. The autonomic nervous system is further divided into two parts called the *parasympathetic* and *sympathetic* divisions, which have opposing influences on organs. For example, with the heart, the parasympathetic division slows the pulse rate, whereas the sympathetic division speeds it up. The balanced influence of these two divisions regulates the heart rate.

ENDOCRINE SYSTEM

The endocrine system is also a regulatory system. Endocrine tissue is gland tissue that secretes special chemicals within the body or into the blood. These special chemicals, called *hormones*, can influence body functions distant from the site where they are produced. The hormones help regulate metabolism and maintain homeostasis, as well as influence reproduction, growth, and response to stress.

The major hormones that are helpful for the emergency medical technician (EMT) to understand are *epinephrine*, or adrenaline, and *insulin*. Epinephrine is secreted by the adrenal glands, located above the kidneys. This hormone is released in times of stress and is part of a survival mechanism that enhances the activity of the sympathetic nervous system. Insulin is secreted by the pancreas and regulates metabolism of glucose.

Other hormones include growth hormone (from the pituitary gland), *thyroxine* (from the thyroid gland), *testosterone* (from the testes), and *estrogen* (from the ovaries). See Figure 2–18 to review the organs of the endocrine system.

DIGESTIVE SYSTEM

The digestive system is the source of all nutritional intake except for oxygen. Throughout the digestive system food is processed both mechanically and chemically to allow its absorption into the blood. Water is absorbed by the digestive tract as well. Foodstuffs that cannot be used by the body are eliminated through the rectum and anus as feces.

Food first enters through the *mouth* where it is broken down mechanically by the *teeth* and *tongue* and is mixed with *saliva* to begin chemical processing (Fig. 2–19). As food is swallowed, it is moved from the *oropharynx* into the *esophagus*. The epiglottis closes to

Text continued on page 40

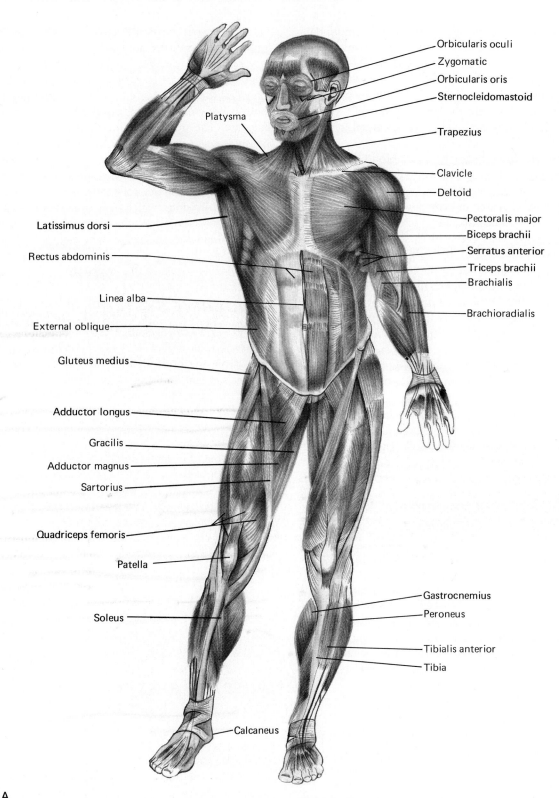

Orbicularis oculi
Zygomatic
Orbicularis oris
Sternocleidomastoid
Trapezius
Clavicle
Deltoid
Pectoralis major
Biceps brachii
Serratus anterior
Triceps brachii
Brachialis
Brachioradialis

Platysma
Latissimus dorsi
Rectus abdominis
Linea alba
External oblique
Gluteus medius
Adductor longus
Gracilis
Adductor magnus
Sartorius
Quadriceps femoris
Patella

Gastrocnemius
Peroneus
Tibialis anterior
Tibia

Soleus

Calcaneus

A

FIGURE 2–14. Major muscles of the body. (*A*) Anterior view. (*B*) Posterior view. Illustrated here are some of the major muscles of the body. As an EMT, you need not commit all of these muscles to memory, but rather be familiar with the major muscles in the upper and lower extremities. These will be discussed in Chapter 10. (*A*, from Solomon EP, Phillips GA: Understanding Human Anatomy and Physiology. Philadelphia, WB Saunders, 1987; *B*, from Villee CA, Solomon EP, Martin C, Martin D: Biology, 2nd ed. Philadelphia, Saunders College Publishing, 1989.)

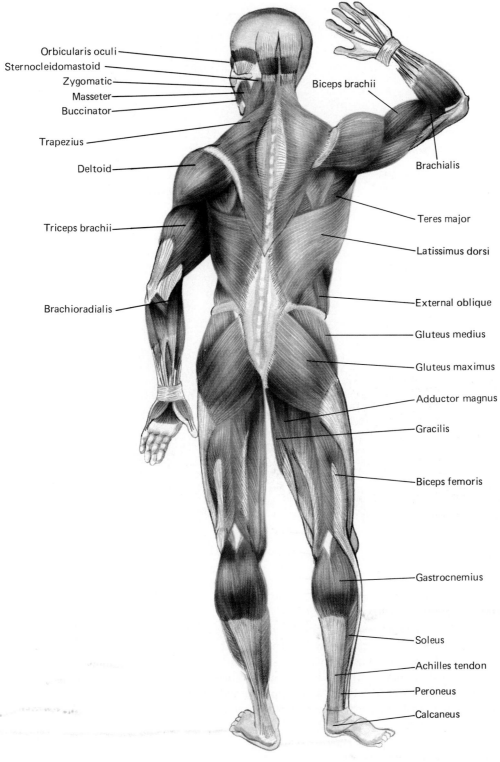

Orbicularis oculi

Sternocleidomastoid

Zygomatic

Masseter

Buccinator

Trapezius

Deltoid

Triceps brachii

Brachioradialis

Biceps brachii

Brachialis

Teres major

Latissimus dorsi

External oblique

Gluteus medius

Gluteus maximus

Adductor magnus

Gracilis

Biceps femoris

Gastrocnemius

Soleus

Achilles tendon

Peroneus

Calcaneus

B

FIGURE 2–14. *Continued*

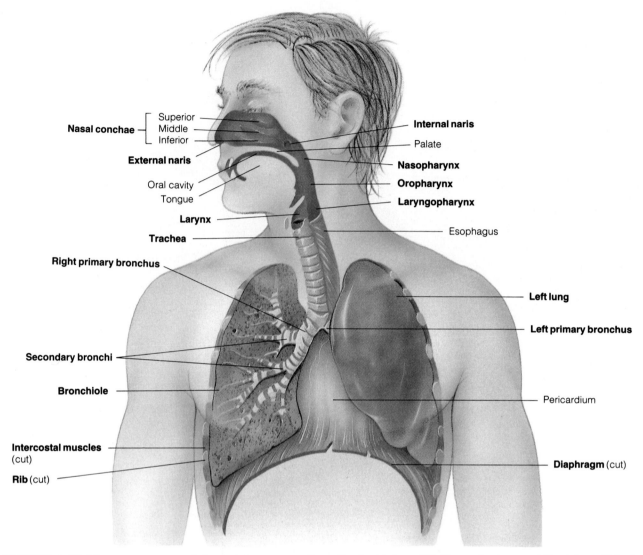

FIGURE 2–15. The major structures of the respiratory system. (From Gaudin AJ, Jones KC: Human Anatomy and Physiology. Orlando, Harcourt Brace Jovanovich, 1989, p. 505.)

protect the trachea during swallowing. Food moves along the esophagus via *peristaltic* contractions of the smooth muscle that lines the esophageal walls. This wave-like contraction of smooth muscle that propels substances forward, called *peristalsis*, is found throughout the digestive tract from the esophagus to the anus. Food passes from the esophagus into the *stomach*, where it is churned and mixed with stomach acid and other secretions to continue chemical processing. Food leaves the stomach as *chyme* (partially digested food) through the *pylorus*, a sphincter-type muscle at the end of the stomach. It enters the *duodenum*, or the first part of the small intestine. Here alkaline and enzyme-rich *pancreatic secretions* neutralize the stomach acids and break down the chyme into smaller units, and the *liver* secretes bile to aid in fat absorption. The *gallbladder* stores bile until it is needed.

The small intestine is the main site for absorption. The small intestine begins with the duodenum at the outlet of the stomach, then continues as a long tube that is initially called the *jejunum* and later, as the nature of the intestinal walls changes, the *ileum*. After the chemical and mechanical processing has broken the chyme into small enough components, these small fragments can enter the blood vessels within the intestinal walls. The blood from the intestines passes through a capillary bed within the liver on its return to the general circulation. The liver serves to filter blood and is concerned with the storage, breakdown, and synthesis of the proteins, carbohydrates, and fats that are the basic constituents of food. *Interconversion* of proteins, fats, and carbohydrates, or the changing of one form of food constituent to another (i.e., fat to carbohydrate, etc.), also takes place in the liver.

Text continued on page 42

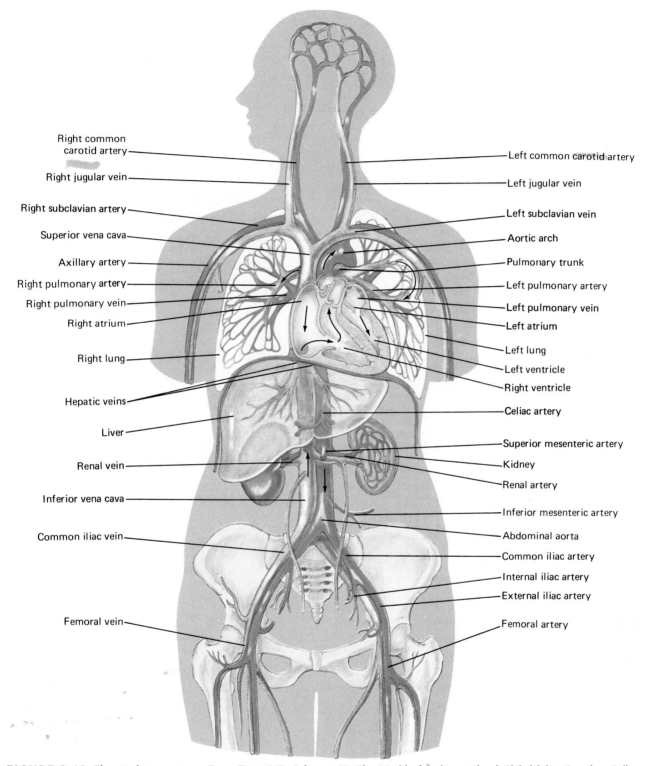

FIGURE 2–16. The circulatory system. (From Davis WP, Solomon EP: The World of Biology, 4th ed. Philadelphia, Saunders College Publishing, 1990.)

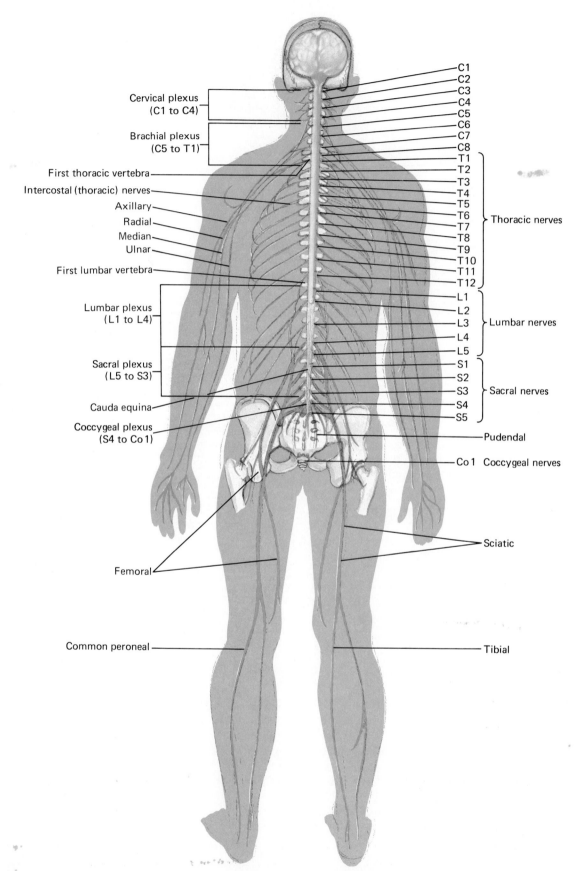

FIGURE 2–17. The central and peripheral nervous systems. (From Solomon EP, Phillips GA: Understanding Human Anatomy and Physiology. Philadelphia, WB Saunders, 1987, p. 153.)

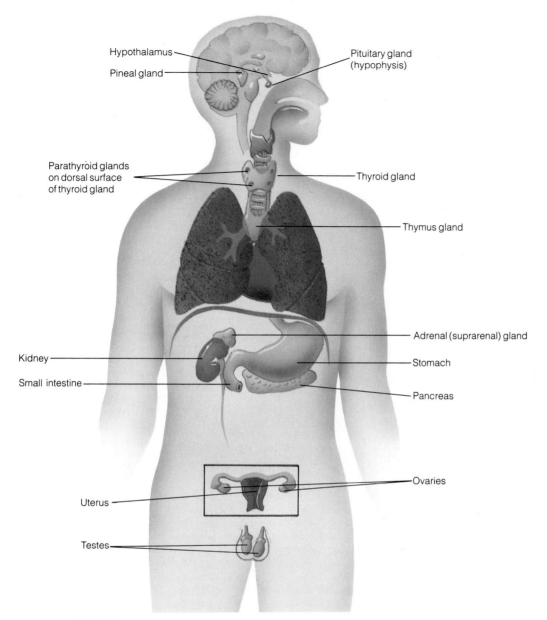

FIGURE 2–18. The endocrine system. (From Gaudin AJ, Jones KC: Human Anatomy and Physiology. Orlando, Harcourt Brace Jovanovich, 1989, p. 409.)

The *large intestine* absorbs excess water as the unused foods are converted to feces, which are excreted through the anus. The large intestine begins in the right lower quadrant at the *cecum*. Off the cecum is the *appendix*. The large intestine continues as the ascending colon as it passes upward to the right upper quadrant, travels across the abdomen as the transverse colon, then descends along the left side as the descending colon, where it changes to the sigmoid colon in the left lower quadrant. The feces are stored in the descending and sigmoid colon until it passes into the *rectum* and through the *anus* during defecation. The sigmoid colon and the rectum lie within the pelvis.

While the digestive system functions automatically, contractions and sensations within the intestines and stomach stimulate us to eat food and to eliminate feces. Although involuntary muscle is found from the esophagus to the rectum, there is voluntary muscle in the mouth and pharynx for chewing and swallowing and at the anal canal for control of defecation.

URINARY SYSTEM *Know*

The urinary system, which is composed of the kidneys, the ureters, the urinary bladder, and the urethra, filters the blood and excretes water and waste products

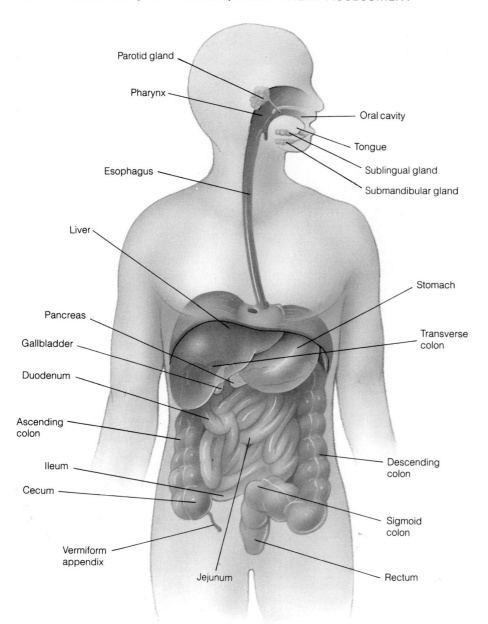

FIGURE 2–19. The digestive system. (From Gaudin AJ, Jones KC: Human Anatomy and Physiology. Orlando, Harcourt Brace Jovanovich, 1989, p. 441.)

Parotid gland
Pharynx
Oral cavity
Tongue
Sublingual gland
Submandibular gland
Esophagus
Liver
Stomach
Pancreas
Transverse colon
Gallbladder
Duodenum
Ascending colon
Descending colon
Ileum
Cecum
Sigmoid colon
Vermiform appendix
Jejunum
Rectum

(Fig. 2–20). To maintain homeostasis, excesses of water, salts, and other constituents of the body fluids, as well as waste products, must be eliminated from the body. For example, if we drink more water than we need, we must eliminate the excess or we will *dilute* the concentration of the blood and body fluids.

The *kidneys* filter the blood and reabsorb essential ingredients while selectively excreting excesses and waste products. The urine thus formed is transferred via peristalsis through the *ureters* to the *bladder*, where it is stored. The bladder is emptied during urination when urine is released through the *urethra*.

REPRODUCTIVE SYSTEM

The female reproductive organs, located within the pelvis, are the *ovaries*, the *fallopian tubes*, the *uterus*, and the *vagina* (Fig. 2–21A). In the male, the *testes* are located

in the *scrotum*. *Sperm* manufactured by each testis travels through the *vas deferens* and then the *prostate*, where it is mixed with secretions to form *semen* and ejaculated through the urethra in the penis (Fig. 2–21B).

INTEGUMENTARY SYSTEM

The skin and its associated structures make up the largest organ of the body. The skin protects the internal environment from the external. It serves as a barrier to bacteria, prevents water loss, insulates, regulates heat, and allows for sensation. The skin has two main layers. The outer *epidermis* has no blood vessels and rests on the *dermis*, which contains the vessels, nerves, and other specialized structures such as sweat glands, sebaceous glands, hair follicles, and specialized nerve endings. The dermis rests on a subcutaneous layer of fat and connective tissue (Fig. 2–22).

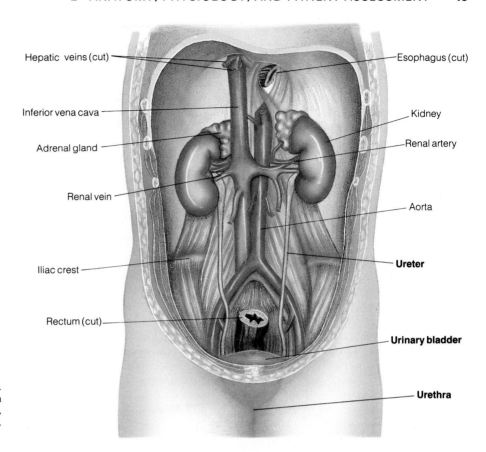

Hepatic veins (cut)
Inferior vena cava
Adrenal gland
Renal vein
Iliac crest
Rectum (cut)

Esophagus (cut)
Kidney
Renal artery
Aorta
Ureter
Urinary bladder
Urethra

FIGURE 2–20. The urinary system. (From Gaudin AJ, Jones KC: Human Anatomy and Physiology. Orlando, Harcourt Brace Jovanovich, 1989, p. 647.)

HEART, LUNGS, AND BRAIN RELATIONSHIP

The vital organ systems are the nervous, the respiratory, and the circulatory. These three systems are intimately interrelated. Failure of any one system may rapidly lead to collapse of the other two. For this reason, primary emphasis in emergency assessment and treatment in the prehospital phase of care is directed to these three organ systems.

HEART. Tracing the need for oxygen demonstrates the most dramatic example of the organ systems' interdependence. The brain can only function for 10 seconds or less if deprived of all oxygen. If the heart stops and circulation of blood to the brain ceases (cardiac arrest), consciousness is lost within 10 seconds, and shortly thereafter all respiratory effort ceases. Lack of oxygen flow to the brain, as evidenced by no pulse and respirations, causes the condition known as *clinical death*. If the brain is deprived of oxygen for 4 to 6 minutes, *biological death* begins. Biological death defines a state of sustained oxygen deprivation after which recovery without brain damage is unlikely.

The time to biological death is modified by certain factors or conditions. For example, children have greater tolerance for sustained pulselessness than do adults. A cool body temperature lowers the body's metabolism and improves the chances of recovery. Drowning often

arouses reflexes (e.g., the mammalian diving reflex—a reaction to cold water that shuts off major blood flow throughout the body, except to the brain, heart, and lungs) that improve the chances of recovery as well.

LUNGS. When breathing stops, the level of oxygen in the blood begins to fall. After a few minutes, the brain will no longer have enough oxygen delivered to maintain consciousness. *The brain is the organ most sensitive to oxygen deprivation.* The heart, being a muscle, requires oxygen to sustain contractions. The heart and the other tissues have been extracting the oxygen that remains in the lungs and the blood, causing the oxygen content to drop lower and lower. Eventually, in from 5 to 12 minutes, there will be inadequate oxygen to power heart contractions and circulation will stop.

BRAIN. The brain regulates respiration. A brain injury may cause failure of ventilation, which in turn can lead to cardiac arrest.

It should be noted that failure of any one of these three vital organ systems can lead to clinical death in seconds or minutes. Carefully review Table 2–1 to appreciate the relationship among these three essential organs.

SUDDEN AND UNEXPECTED DEATH. The common causes of sudden and unexpected death are cardiovascular disease, cerebrovascular disease, and accidental in-

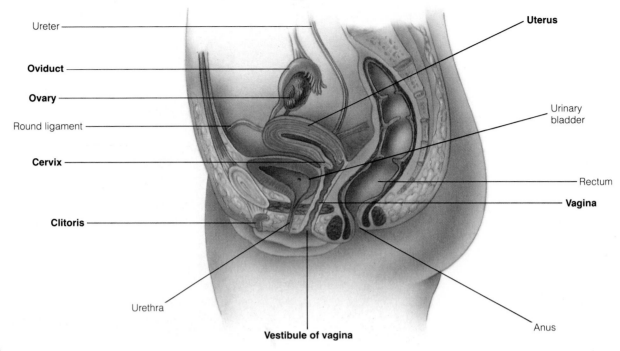

A

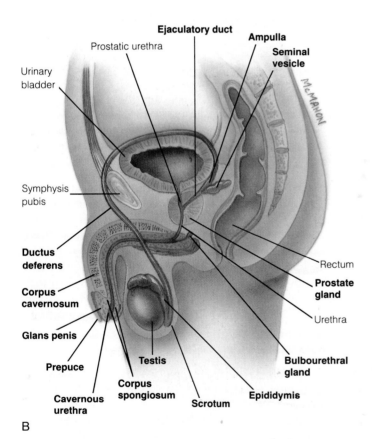

B

FIGURE 2–21. (*A*) Female reproductive system. (*B*). Male reproductive system. (From Gaudin AJ, Jones KC: Human Anatomy and Physiology. Orlando, Harcourt Brace Jovanovich, 1989, pp. 699 and 709.)

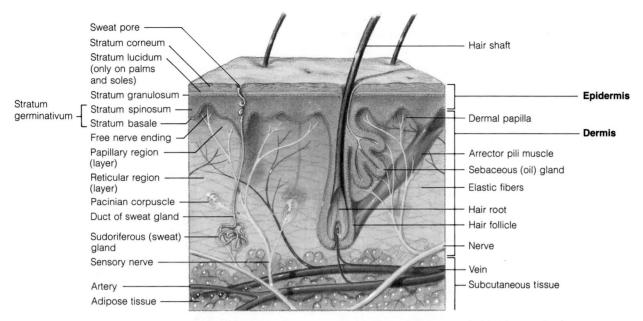

FIGURE 2–22. The major structures of the skin. (From Gaudin AJ, Jones KC: Human Anatomy and Physiology. Orlando, Harcourt Brace Jovanovich, 1989, p. 101.)

TABLE 2–1. Interrelationships of Vital Organs

Organ	Function	Some Causes of Organ Failure	Signs of Failure	Response of Rescuer
Brain	Maintains consciousness Controls breathing	Stroke Injury Electric shock Drug overdose	Unresponsive to stimuli	Check for breathing
Lungs	Oxygenate blood Remove carbon dioxide	Drowning Airway obstruction Chest injury Suffocation Asphyxiation	No breathing or inadequate breathing	Provide ventilation by mouth-to-mouth breathing
Heart	Circulates blood	Myocardial infarction Electric shock	No pulse	Provide circulation by external chest compression

juries. Understanding how these conditions lead to clinical death and the time intervals involved in the dying process is useful for many reasons. First, it helps focus the EMT on the very conditions that he or she will be facing in the community. Second, it helps in understanding the priorities built into standardized approaches to assessment and treatment, as in the primary survey; and third, it helps in recognizing the importance of rapid delivery of definitive medical care for critical patients.

PATIENT ASSESSMENT

Overview

The foundation of emergency care is patient assessment. Treatment, transportation, and triage are all dependent upon the collection of the *signs* and *symptoms*

of disease or injury. Clues from the environment, visualization of the mechanism of injury, a solicitation of facts from patients and bystanders, and findings on the physical examination are all part of this process. Symptoms are subjective complaints or descriptions of how a patient feels and are obtained through patient interview (history). Examples of symptoms include pain, difficulty breathing, chills, and nausea. Signs are clues confirmed and elicited by the EMT through physical examination, including visual observation, touching (palpation), listening (auscultation), and smell. Examples of signs include bruises, swelling, gurgling breath sounds, and odor of alcohol on the breath. The EMT combines this information with his or her knowledge of those illnesses and diseases that require emergency care—helping to formulate a prehospital impression, or "working diagnosis." At times, a therapeutic response immediately follows clues that are apparent upon arrival at the scene. For example, stabilization of the cervical spine is routinely performed when the mechanism of injury suggests injury to the cervical spine. Recognition of *cyanosis* (a bluish color from oxygen deprivation) would lead to immediate oxygen therapy and support of breathing. Sometimes, brief periods of assessment are followed by intervention, and then the survey is continued. Obvious external bleeding would call for immediate intervention to control bleeding. In other instances, the condition requiring emergency care may not be clear until a number of diagnostic clues pointing to that condition are obtained.

To be effective, the EMT must maintain a consistently systematic approach. The most life-threatening conditions are assessed first, with treatment instituted as the need is encountered. Assessment then proceeds in an orderly fashion to be sure that less obvious conditions requiring emergency treatment are not overlooked. Furthermore, in order to identify some conditions, it is necessary to collect many facts about them.

The key to effective patient assessment is to proceed in an organized manner that is "goal oriented." There are two primary goals: (1) develop enough information to provide immediate and necessary prehospital care, and (2) accumulate additional useful information to help guide subsequent care.

Prehospital assessment is divided into four distinct areas: *the dispatch review, the scene survey, the primary survey,* and *the secondary survey.* This organization is structured so that the most life-threatening conditions are evaluated first. Following this sequence makes sure that data are searched for in phases that are logically ordered to provide for diagnostic and treatment decisions. This sequence is usually maintained except where history (due to an unconscious patient) is not available. Some components are performed concurrently when a sufficient number of EMTs are available. For example, one EMT collects a history while another conducts a secondary survey.

The importance of structure during assessment cannot be overstated. The price of a random, haphazard approach is usually failure to arrive at the correct conclusion.

The Dispatch Review

Initial information about the patient's condition may be available from the dispatcher before you arrive at the scene. This first phase of assessment gives you valuable time to anticipate the worst possible events and review a plan of action with your partner. A careful review of dispatch data such as location and type of call will allow the EMT time to contemplate likely possibilities. For example, a dispatched call "Pedestrian struck on a main thoroughfare" should initiate a mental rehearsal, including anticipating the most critical injuries likely to be encountered. It would be useful to expect respiratory problems, cervical spine injury, chest trauma,

shock states, etc.; to consider the immediate needs of a patient; to plan equipment needs; and to discuss the roles that each EMT will assume. This will result in more of a "reflex" response upon arrival at the scene, thus saving valuable time.

During the dispatch review, the route of response is also planned to ensure the fastest possible arrival. Factors such as traffic conditions, construction obstacles, and weather should be considered in planning the best route.

The Scene Survey

Upon arrival at the scene, the EMT should make a series of rapid observations that will frequently result in immediate action:

- Assess the need for additional units.
- Identify hazards
- Determine the mechanism of injury or illness.

When arriving at a scene where there are multiple casualties, it is important for the EMT to quickly assess the need for additional units. A timely call may result in the saving of many lives rather than delaying response to the other patients while the EMT becomes involved in treating just one victim. For the safety of rescuers and others, it is also critical to quickly identify hazards such as traffic or fire prior to initiating care. An area should be secure as a first measure to reduce the chance of further injuries to both patients and EMTs.

Another component of the scene survey is determining the mechanism of injury or illness. While approaching the patient, the EMT should observe the patient's environment, since it may provide valuable clues to the underlying problem. For example, a broken windshield or steering wheel would lead one to suspect certain types of injuries such as head *trauma,* cervical spine injury, and chest trauma. On a medical call for an unconscious patient, a medication vial might give information about past medical conditions or suggest a possibility of overdose. The mechanism of injury and other clues obtained from the patient's immediate environment should always be conveyed to the emergency department staff. Failure to do so might result in a delay in diagnosis and essential treatment.

The Primary Survey

The primary survey is the first step upon physical encounter with the patient. As the name implies, the primary survey is directed toward the most life-threatening conditions by quickly assessing the three most critical organ systems: the nervous system, the respiratory system, and the circulatory system. The mnemonic "ABCDE" is used to provide a reminder of the recommended sequence of evaluation and treatment. This rapid review includes:

Airway
1. Establish responsiveness.
2. Ensure a clear airway.

Breathing
3. Check for breathing.
4. Evaluate the adequacy of breathing.

Circulation
5. Check for a pulse.
6. Look for obvious chest wounds and external bleeding.
7. Evaluate the adequacy of circulation.

Disability
8. Determine the level of consciousness.
9. Evaluate the neurologic (central nervous system) function.

Expose
10. Expose the head and trunk to identify signs of major trauma.

During the primary survey, the EMT performs each component of assessment and then, if needed, reacts quickly with an intervention. For example, once identified, a respiratory or cardiac arrest is treated immediately. Likewise, respiratory or circulatory distress is recognized and treated during the first moments of care. Positive findings in the primary survey may also lead to a rapid transport decision.

A—AIRWAY

ESTABLISH RESPONSIVENESS. Each step in the primary survey should be performed quickly and carefully. When *checking for responsiveness*, the EMT should provide verbal and, if necessary, *tactile* (pinch, tap, or rub) stimuli. There should be enough stimuli applied to get a response in a patient with a depressed mental status. When approaching unresponsive patients with a possible head or neck injury, care must be taken not to aggravate existing injuries. Establish responsiveness by using the procedure that follows.

PROCEDURE 2–1   ESTABLISHING RESPONSIVENESS

1. If it is suspected that the patient suffered trauma, one EMT should maintain in-line cervical immobilization while the other performs the primary assessment.
2. Tap on the patient's chest or vigorously rub the *sternum* (breast bone) while shouting "Are you OK?" (Fig. 2–23). This can be done with the patient in the same position as when you arrived.

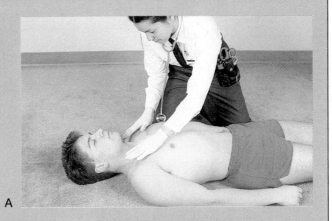

A

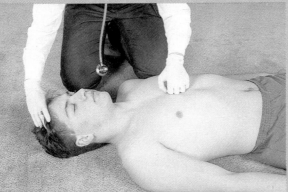

B

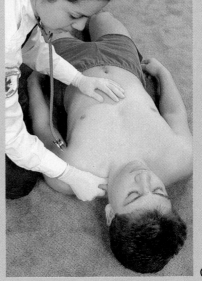

C

FIGURE 2–23. There are three methods used to check for responsiveness: (*A*) Tap the patient's shoulder region with both hands. (*B*) Firmly rub the breast bone with the knuckle of one hand (be careful not to be too vigorous). (*C*) Apply a firm pinch to the muscles of the neck. Regardless of the technique, you should shout, "Are you okay?" while providing physical stimuli.

Continued

3. A patient who is unresponsive and found in a position other than supine should be rolled into the supine position. In suspected trauma patients, this can be done while maintaining alignment of the spine (Fig. 2–24).

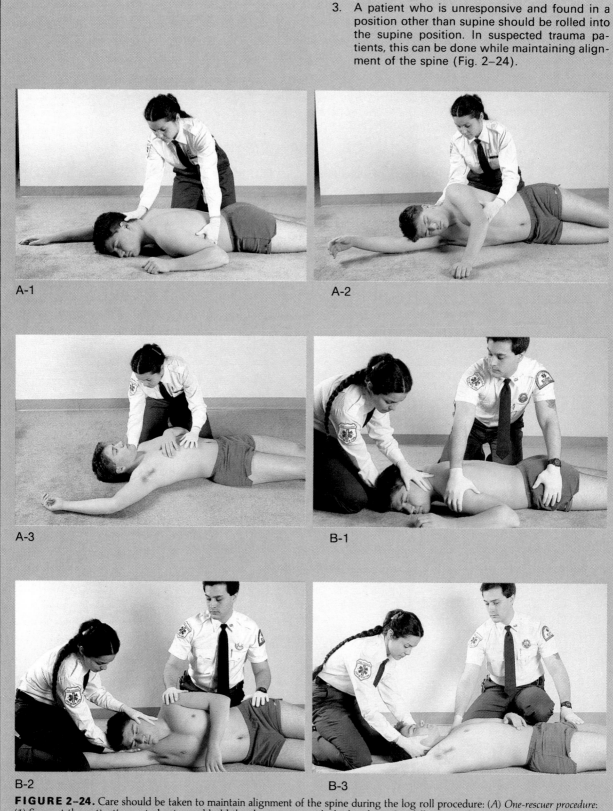

FIGURE 2–24. Care should be taken to maintain alignment of the spine during the log roll procedure: (*A*) *One-rescuer procedure*: (1) Support the patient's cervical spine and hold the chest region with the hand. (2) Carefully rotate the patient while maintaining alignment of the spine. (3) Place the patient in the supine position. (*B*) *Two-rescuer procedure*: (1) Rescuer number 1 maintains alignment of the cervical spine while rescuer number 2 supports the shoulder and hip region. (2) The patient is rotated smoothly to the lateral position on the command of rescuer number 1. (3) The patient is then carefully rotated to the supine position.

ENSURE A CLEAR AIRWAY. The next priority is to ensure an open airway and adequate ventilations. If the patient is unresponsive, you may need to open the airway to check for breathing. There are two basic methods used to open the airway. The names of the methods are descriptive of the technique employed. The *head tilt–chin lift* procedure uses hyperextension of the neck and forward displacement of the jaw to lift the tongue away from the back of the pharynx. The *jaw thrust—without* *head tilt* is used in patients with suspected cervical spine injuries. This maneuver displaces the jaw forward and lifts the tongue away from the pharynx without extension of the cervical spine. An alternate maneuver for cervical-spine-injury patients is the *tongue–jaw lift*. This may be the method of choice when there is a fracture of the *mandible* (jaw), which might make the jaw thrust maneuver less effective.

PROCEDURE 2–2 HEAD TILT–CHIN LIFT

1. Place one hand on the forehead and the fingers of the hand closest to the feet along the patient's jawbone.
2. Apply a gentle, rotating force to the forehead while lifting the jaw upward, taking care not to close the mouth. The thumb may be used to distract the lower lip away from the upper lip if necessary (Fig. 2–25).

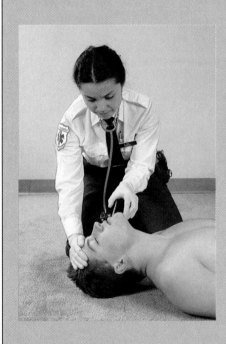

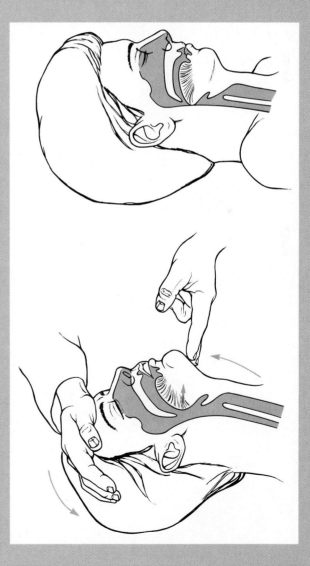

FIGURE 2–25. Head tilt–chin lift. Place the hand closest to the patient's head on the patient's forehead and the index and middle fingers of the hand closest to the patient's feet on the bony margin of the chin. Carefully rotate the head at the same time you lift the chin upward until the teeth are touching but the mouth is not completely closed.

In cases where injury to the neck is suspected, the airway maneuver of choice is the jaw thrust-without head tilt. A description of this follows.

P R O C E D U R E   2 – 3   JAW THRUST–WITHOUT HEAD TILT

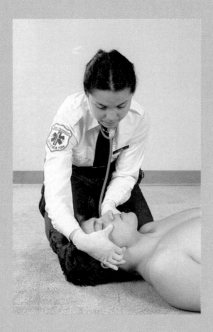

1. Place both thumbs on the patient's *maxilla* (cheekbones) and your index and middle fingers on both sides of the *mandible* (lower jaw) where it angles toward the ear.
2. Apply upward pressure with your fingers to displace the jaw forward WITHOUT TILTING THE HEAD (Fig. 2–26)!

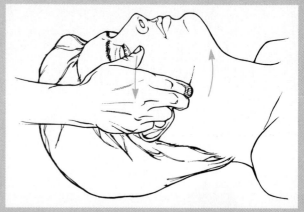

FIGURE 2–26. Jaw thrust—without head tilt. Place your thumbs on the patient's cheekbones just below the eyes and your index and middle fingers at the angles of the patient's jaw just below the ears. While using the cheekbones to stabilize the head, lift the jaw upward, *without tilting the head or flexing the cervical spine.*

P R O C E D U R E   2 – 4   TONGUE–JAW LIFT

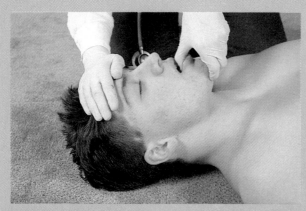

1. Grasp the lower jaw with your thumb and index and middle fingers, placing your thumb inside the lower teeth and your fingers along the margin of the mandible inferiorly.
2. While stabilizing the head with your other hand, pull the jaw forward (Fig. 2–27).

FIGURE 2–27. Tongue—jaw lift. Grasp the patient's lower jaw with a gloved hand closest to the patient's feet. While stabilizing the forehead with the hand closest to the patient's head, lift the jaw upward.

All three of these maneuvers achieve the same result. They move the lower jaw forward and carry the tongue (which is attached to the lower jaw) away from the back of the throat (Fig. 2–28). This will open the airway and allow for easy passage of air if the patient is breathing. Sometimes this maneuver is all that is necessary to activate normal breathing in the unconscious patient.

B—BREATHING

Once the airway is opened, the adequacy of ventilation and oxygenation must be evaluated.

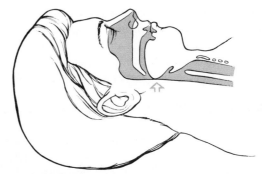

FIGURE 2–28. The airway may be obstructed by the tongue in unconscious patients. The purpose of airway maneuvers is to lift the tongue away from the pharynx.

PROCEDURE 2–5 CHECKING FOR BREATHING

1. During the check for breathing, utilize the following three of your senses. Once the airway is opened, you should place your ear directly over the patient's mouth and nose and *LOOK*, *LISTEN*, and *FEEL* for breathing.
2. With your eyes in visual contact with the patient's chest and abdomen, observe for movement, listen for air exchange, and feel for warm breath against your cheek (Fig. 2–29*A*).

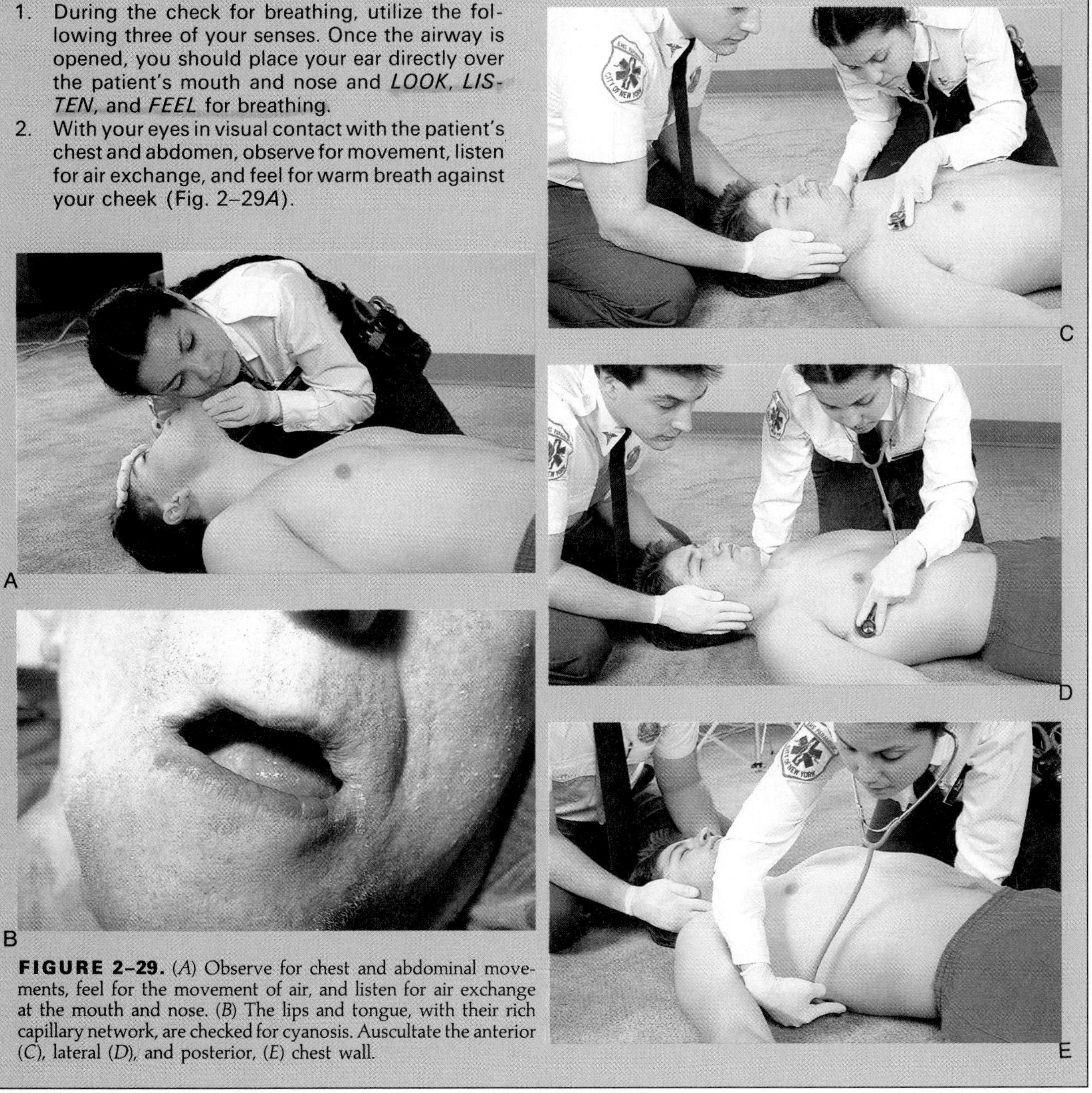

FIGURE 2–29. (*A*) Observe for chest and abdominal movements, feel for the movement of air, and listen for air exchange at the mouth and nose. (*B*) The lips and tongue, with their rich capillary network, are checked for cyanosis. Auscultate the anterior (*C*), lateral (*D*), and posterior, (*E*) chest wall.

Quiet breathing may be difficult to detect especially in environments that are noisy or distracting, such as in the street or during transport in an ambulance. Using all three senses maximizes the information that can be gathered to establish the presence and help gauge the adequacy of ventilations.

Absent breathing requires positive-pressure ventilations (i.e., mouth-to-mouth or mouth-to-mask). Inadequate breathing is evidenced by infrequent or shallow breaths accompanied by other signs of respiratory ineffectiveness. Alterations in consciousness are another sign. The neck and chest are carefully inspected for signs of respiratory compromise, including:

- Difficulty breathing
- Respiratory rate less than 12 and over 28
- Altered mental state
- Cyanosis (bluish mucous membranes or skin) (Fig. 2–29B).
- Absent or diminished breath sounds (sounds heard through a stethoscope) (Fig. 2–29C, D, and E). This will be discussed in Chapter 3.

- Use of the neck muscles (accessory muscles) to breathe
- Wound or other injury to the chest wall

EVALUATE THE ADEQUACY OF BREATHING. If breathing appears to be inadequate, the need for positive-pressure ventilation or supplemental oxygen is determined. The decision to ventilate and the specific techniques of positive-pressure ventilation will be addressed in Chapter 3.

C—CIRCULATION

CHECK FOR A PULSE. After checking for responsiveness and breathing, the next priority is to establish the presence of a pulse. The *carotid pulse* should be felt on any patient who is unconscious or where pulselessness may be suspected. The carotid pulse is an excellent pulse to assess the adequacy of circulation due to its accessibility to the rescuer. For example, the rescuer can remain in position to provide positive-pressure ventilation and be ready to perform cardiac compressions in the event that they are needed.

PROCEDURE 2-6   ESTABLISHING A PULSE

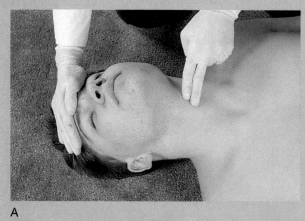

1. Use the hand closest to the patient's feet to gently palpate the carotid artery on the side of the neck closest to the rescuer.
2. Locate the larynx (voicebox) with your index and middle fingers and gently slide them down into the groove between the trachea and the neck muscles (Fig. 2–30A and B).
3. Gently palpate the carotid artery while maintaining a head tilt (if no trauma) for 5 to 10 seconds.

The carotid pulse is felt in unresponsive patients. Pulses in the arm or other regions may be more difficult to palpate, particularly in severe shock states. It is essential to palpate for 5 to 10 seconds to detect weak or slow pulses. Failure to carefully assess the carotid pulse may result in application of chest compressions when they are not indicated. The technique of chest compressions will be covered in Chapter 4.

FIGURE 2–30. Taking the carotid pulse. (A) Locate the larynx and (B) slide your index and middle fingers in the groove between the larynx and the sternocleidomastoid muscle.

LOOK FOR LIFE-THREATENING BLEEDING AND OPEN CHEST WOUNDS. The next phase of the primary survey is the identification of life-threatening bleeding or obvious open chest injuries. Either of these conditions can result in rapid death if not treated immediately. Rapid external blood loss must be controlled with appropriate techniques.

Holes in the chest wall must be sealed with an airtight dressing, since they can lead to rapid ventilatory failure (see Chapter 3).

CHECK FOR SIGNS OF CIRCULATORY COMPROMISE. Other signs of circulatory compromise are sought in order to determine if there is internal bleeding and also to identify other causes of shock. Some general signs associated with poor circulation include:

- Altered mental status
- Thready or nonpalpable radial or brachial pulses
- Rapid or very slow pulse rate
- Pale, cool, and sweaty skin (Fig. 2–31)
- Delayed capillary refill (this will be discussed later in this chapter)

When circulatory compromise is noted, essential life support is provided along with immediate transport. This is particularly important when the condition (i.e., internal bleeding) may require a surgical intervention.

D—DISABILITY

DETERMINE THE LEVEL OF CONSCIOUSNESS. During the primary survey the central nervous system is quickly evaluated to identify signs of life-threatening conditions and neurologic impairment. Bleeding within the brain, stroke, diabetic states, and respiratory and circulatory compromise are examples of causes of neurologic impairment.

The most sensitive indicator of neurologic function is "level of consciousness." The level of consciousness is evaluated quickly by administering verbal and painful stimuli and noting the specific degree of response from the patient in relation to the stimulus provided. For example, a patient may be alert and capable of normal conversation, or the patient may require verbal or painful "prodding" to respond or may not respond regardless of the stimuli provided.

A mnemonic that is used to categorize the stimulus and response is "AVPU":

A—Alert (the patient is alert and capable of normal communication)
V—Verbal (the patient responds to verbal stimuli)
P—Painful (the patient does not respond to voice but responds to painful stimuli)
U—Unresponsive (the patient does not respond to either verbal or painful stimuli)

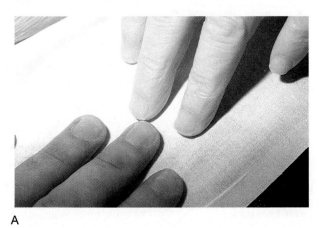

A

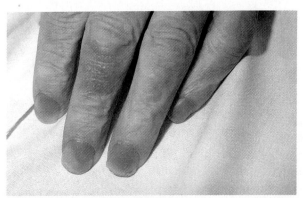

B

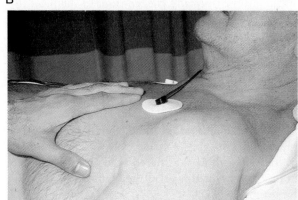

C

FIGURE 2–31. Note color of skin and nailbeds for important clues. (*A*) Normal skin and nails are contrasted with pale color seen with severe deficiency of red blood cells (anemia; see Chapter 5). (*B*) Cyanosis of nailbeds is due to poorly oxygenated red blood cells. It is always an indication for supplemental oxygen and often positive pressure ventilation. (*C*) Jaundice or yellow coloring of skin may indicate severe liver disease.

EVALUATE NEUROLOGIC FUNCTION: PUPIL AND MOTOR AND SENSORY EXAMINATION. The patient's pupils are evaluated to determine the diameter, reactivity to light, and the relative equality of one pupil to the other. The patient's ability to move his or her extremities can be briefly assessed. The specific techniques for these evaluation components are discussed in the secondary survey in this chapter.

E—EXPOSE

The final element of the primary survey is to expose the patient's head, trunk, and extremities to inspect for significant wounds or hemorrhage. Obviously, this may already have been done during the breathing and circulation components of the survey. However, with trauma patients a more complete observation of the torso and extremities may be necessary.

TREATMENT AND TRANSPORTATION DECISION

As the need is encountered during the primary survey, lifesaving treatments are provided such as positive-pressure ventilation (rescue breathing), oxygen therapy, and immobilization of the spine. Additionally, a decision is made whether to further evaluate the patient or to transport the patient immediately. Patients who are unstable and have conditions that may lead to cardiac arrest or require immediate hospital care should be rapidly transported to the appropriate medical facility. Other patients will be further evaluated prior to transport (secondary survey).

The Secondary Survey

The secondary survey continues the examination for signs or symptoms that will identify a need for subsequent emergency care. The secondary survey is the period of assessment during which a history is developed and further examination of the patient is performed. It includes the history, vital signs, the head-to-toe survey, and the neurologic examination.

The history is usually elicited prior to the head-to-toe examination in conscious medical patients. On the other hand, in unresponsive patients and in trauma patients the history may be limited, and the physical examination may play a larger role in the decision-making process.

The scope of the secondary survey may vary according to the patient's problem and be altered or modified by the identification of immediate life-threatening conditions. For example, if evidence of internal bleeding exists, rapid transport is required while the rest of the secondary survey continues in the ambulance en route to the hospital.

THE PATIENT HISTORY

The *history* is frequently the most significant part of patient assessment. The history is the patient's story of significant events related to and surrounding the present problem that has necessitated seeking medical attention. The patient usually begins the history with words describing the main problem, which is called the *chief complaint*. This may be "Chest pain," "I can't breathe," or "It's the worst headache I've ever had." You should then go about a systematic and chronological gathering of relevant information associated with the chief complaint. This also includes pertinent past medical history.

Many serious diseases or conditions are often diagnosed primarily on the basis of history. For example, a heart attack victim is usually diagnosed in the prehospital setting based on information in his or her history.

The history is obtained by following a set sequence during the interview. This is done by all medical professionals to ensure collection of relevant data in an efficient manner. Properly taken, a history proceeds in an orderly fashion that allows information gathered to be processed together with physical signs to achieve a working diagnosis. Knowledge of signs and symptoms of diseases and injuries is essential. Throughout the following chapters, diseases and injuries are described by their clinical presentation.

The components of the history include *the chief complaint, the history of present illness, the past medical history, and medications and allergies.*

The history is the most subjective aspect of the diagnostic process. It relies upon the patient's description and interpretation rather than on objective findings directly observed, heard, or felt by the evaluator. Therefore, one should follow certain principles to maximize the validity and reliability of information gathered.

1. *Use open-ended questions.* As much as possible patients should express all complaints and facts in their own words. For example, if a patient complains of chest pain, the EMT should ask, "Can you describe the pain?" When the interviewer offers adjectives such as "Was this a sharp pain?" or "Did it feel like a burning sensation?" the interviewer runs the risk of "putting words in the patient's mouth." This would make the information far less reliable.

2. *Direct the interview.* Maintain the order of chief complaint, history of present illness, past medical history, and medications and allergies. This will ensure that relevant information is not overlooked. One component should lead to the next. Do not allow the patient to drift off the topic. Failure to maintain control can waste valuable time. Maintain the focus of the interview within relevant boundaries.

3. *Do not delay urgent treatments.* Although you should try to collect the most comprehensive history, it

should not delay any therapy if an indication for such is evident. For example, oxygen therapy for a heart attack patient may be started as soon as the need has been determined. Other conditions may result in immediate transport. In any case, the history should be continued in the ambulance while en route to the hospital. This technique will achieve both important goals: RAPID INTERVENTION and MAXIMUM DATA COLLECTION.

4. *The patient is the best source for the history*. Keeping in mind that there are exceptions to this rule (an unconscious patient or small child), it is generally important to allow the patient to express the problem. Bystanders may interpret and misrepresent facts and, again, may put words in the patient's mouth. A bystander's history, while it may be important, should supplement rather than replace the patient's own history.

The direction that a history takes is very much determined by each developing fact. As you gain knowledge of signs, symptoms, and presentations of various disease states, this will become more evident to you. Like any investigative process, a single fact may alter your impression and your subsequent questioning. However, there are questions that are common to most complaints. These will be addressed as we discuss the various categories.

CHIEF COMPLAINT. After learning basic facts about a patient (age and sex), you should ask the patient to describe the problem. The patient's single-sentence response becomes the chief complaint. Examples are "I woke up this morning with chest pain," "I have difficulty breathing," "I have a severe pain in my lower back." These statements will determine to some extent your follow-up questions.

If the patient's initial statement is too vague, such as "I feel sick," or "I hurt myself," you should request more specifics from the patient about the reason for calling for medical aid.

HISTORY OF PRESENT ILLNESS. After the chief complaint is obtained, a series of questions are asked to expand and identify the cause of the chief complaint. The patient's activity at the time of the problem, a description of other associated symptoms, the sequence of events leading up to the incident, factors that aggravate or alleviate the problem, and similar past experiences are elicited at this time.

Throughout this text, these questions will be presented in the context of each critical condition. However, there are facts to be ascertained that are common to all complaints. The purpose of these questions is to identify the pattern of events that led up to, and is associated with, the immediate problem. These include:

1. *Sequence of events*. Have the patient express the order in which each sign or symptom occurred.

2. *Activity at the onset or immediately preceding the event*. Ask the patient to describe the activity involved when the problem first presented itself, e.g., running, sitting, walking up stairs, eating, and so forth.

3. *Aggravating and relieving factors*. Have the patient relate any behavior that makes the symptoms worse or alleviates them. For example, "Walking increases the pain" or "Sitting makes the pain go away."

4. *Similar past experiences*. Ask the patient if a similar problem has occurred before. If so, was a doctor consulted? Was there a hospital admission? What was the diagnosis? This line of questioning frequently identifies the cause.

5. *Associated symptoms*. Ask the patient if there are other complaints or abnormal sensations associated with the chief complaint. If there are no associated symptoms, you may ask about specific symptoms commonly associated with the chief complaint. For example, a person with severe abdominal pain who denies any associated symptoms might be questioned specifically about nausea and vomiting.

6. *Describing pain*. Questions about the complaint of "pain" should address several descriptive variables including location, duration, quality, severity, radiation (flow from one area to another), and aggravating and relieving factors.

During the *history of present illness*, you should start formulating a mental list of the possible causes of the patient's condition. The amount of information gathered during this phase will be determined by the effectiveness of your interview technique, as well as by the ability of the patient to respond. For example, brain hypoxia (poor oxygen delivery to the brain), drugs, disease states, and other factors may diminish thought processes and hamper the interview.

PAST MEDICAL HISTORY. One should always ask certain questions about a patient's past medical history for many reasons. It frequently clarifies or reinforces the diagnosis suspected from the history of the present illness. A variety of medical conditions are either progressive in nature (worsen over time) or are often associated with, or may aggravate, other conditions. A patient who has high blood pressure is at increased risk for a heart attack. Likewise, a history of *hemophilia* (a bleeding disorder) is of considerable importance when treating trauma patients.

When collecting the past medical history, the interviewer must use the time efficiently. Major illnesses requiring prior hospitalizations, illnesses presently under treatment, and illnesses similar to, or associated with, the present illness should be elicited. You may start this phase of the interview with open-ended questions such as "What major illnesses or injuries have you had in the past?" or "Are you undergoing treatment at this time?" This can be followed by more specific inquiries about diseases or injuries that may be related to the immediate condition.

In adult patients always inquire specifically about four conditions. These conditions can be remembered as "the big four" and include heart disease, hypertension (high blood pressure), diabetes, and chronic obstructive pulmonary disease (emphysema and bronchitis). These conditions can be progressive in nature, are risk factors for emergency conditions, and can alter treatment.

MEDICATIONS AND ALLERGIES. Be sure to inquire specifically about an allergy history and whether the patient is taking any medications. Bring the medications to the hospital if they are readily available. An elderly person may not be able to describe the name of a specific disease that may be suspected by the need for a certain drug.

An allergy history may be useful for both prehospital diagnosis and as information to guide the choice of drug therapy in the hospital.

MEDIC ALERT TAGS. Some patients with a known disease such as diabetes or with severe allergies may wear or carry a Medic Alert tag or card. This bracelet, necklace, or wallet card may contain the only history available for an unconscious or disoriented patient. They may indicate specific conditions, medications, allergies, or other personal information needed to institute care.

Confidentiality

Information given to a medical practitioner is confidential and privileged information. You are entrusted to keep confidential both personal and medical information elicited during your patient interviews. Whenever possible, care should be taken to conduct the interview in a private setting. For example, in the workplace you should clear bystanders and co-workers from the immediate area before asking medical questions. While this may be modified by the patient's condition and the surroundings, it should still be a fundamental rule of practice. Conduct the interview with the same respect you would want shown to yourself or your family.

SUMMARY

Becoming a skillful interviewer requires adherence to the structure outlined above and a great deal of practice. The latter can be achieved by clinical experience in an emergency department or on an ambulance with a veteran EMT, physician, or nurse observing your technique. It is best to practice under supervision to learn proper techniques and avoid repeating mistakes. You may also team up with a fellow student and take turns "role playing" patients, attempting to extract information from each other, followed by discussion of your effectiveness.

EXAMINATION

During the secondary survey, the EMT uses his or her senses to elicit *visual*, *auditory*, and *tactile* findings or signs that may be encountered while examining the patient. You observe, palpate (feel with the fingertips), listen, and auscultate (listen with a stethoscope), noting any variations from the norm (see Fig. 2–31). Unlike the primary survey, you will usually perform the entire examination prior to initiating interventions. There are exceptions when life-threatening conditions are encountered, such as massive internal bleeding, which call for immediate treatment or transport once identified.

Certain principles should be followed when performing a secondary survey:

- *Utilize personnel.* When two or more EMTs are present on the scene, work as a team. One may check vital signs while the other conducts a head-to-toe survey and neurologic examination. Or, one may initiate therapy, such as supplemental oxygen, while the other performs the examination.

- *Do not lose your focus.* A grossly angulated fracture or a grotesque avulsion may capture the attention of the best observers. This will sometimes lead to the EMT's becoming preoccupied with the more obvious problems, causing delay in identification of life-threatening conditions.

- *Perform gentle palpations.* Excessive or forceful manipulation may cause pain and aggravate injuries. Particular care should be exercised when spinal injury is suspected or when palpating the skull, so as not to cause neurologic injury (brain and spinal cord damage).

- *Do not forget the dependent areas.* When patients are found in the prone and supine positions, it is essential to examine the dependent areas of the body. Failure to do so can result in overlooking potentially fatal wounds or missing important physical signs.

- *Consider the mechanisms of injury.* When assessing the significance of physical findings, the mechanism of injury must be considered. A small contusion of the chest may appear harmless. However, with a driver involved in a high speed accident, it may suggest a severe chest injury caused by impact with the steering wheel. Each sign should be considered in the context of the situation, and each situation should cause you to search for specific signs. As we discuss the various types of trauma within the text, common mechanisms of injury will be addressed.

As in all aspects of assessment, you must avoid "too much or too little" evaluation. The time spent on the scene should be the amount necessary to establish the need to initiate essential prehospital treatment. The head-to-toe approach helps ensure that no appreciable findings are overlooked. Remember, not everything must be done at the scene. Examination components can be performed in the ambulance if the circumstances dictate early transport.

Vital Signs

Vital signs are measurements of the functions of vital body systems and are good indicators of abnormal conditions. They include respirations, pulse, blood pressure, and temperature.

The interpretation of vital signs plays a central role in determining prehospital management. They may serve as a basis for initiating specific treatments, such as oxygen therapy, ventilation, application of a pneumatic antishock garment (PASG), and general shock therapy, and provide a baseline by which the effectiveness of therapy can be measured. When evaluating the significance of vital signs we do so in the context of *norms*.

What Are Norms?

Norms are the general range of vital signs that are considered normal. For example, the normal pulse rate for adults should fall somewhere between 60 and 80 beats per minute. These values were developed by considering typical ranges among healthy individuals. However, athletes may have pulse rates well below 60 and still be considered normal.

Vital signs should always be considered in the context of the entire situation. Factors such as stress, anxiety, age, and medications are variables that may alter the expected norms. One may ask certain patients, such as those with a history of hypertension or athletes, what is "normal" for them.

Respirations

The process of breathing is evaluated in four ways: rate, depth, pattern, and sound of respirations. The EMT should be stationed at the side of the patient, with a clear view of the chest and abdominal regions. The patient's breathing should be observed without the patient's being aware of it.

RATE. Observing the margin of the chest and abdomen, you should count the number of breaths occurring in a 15-second period and multiply by four. The normal respiratory rate in adults is approximately 12 to 20 breaths per minute. The rate in children tends to be fastest during infancy and gradually decreases to adult rates with age.

DEPTH AND PATTERN. While observing the chest and abdomen, you should also note the depth and pattern of respirations. Depth will be categorized as either normal, deep, or shallow in character. The pattern will either be regular, evenly spaced breaths or one of the abnormal

sequences that are indicative of either brain trauma or metabolic disturbances. (The specific abnormal patterns are presented in Chapter 7, Central Nervous System Emergencies.)

SOUNDS. While observing respirations, sounds emitted during breathing might also be noted. Sounds heard externally, without the use of a stethoscope, are usually an indication of some obstructive process that exists in the upper or lower airways. Sounds that may sometimes be heard include:

- *Gurgling*—A sound created by air moving through fluid. It sounds similar to blowing through a straw beneath water. This usually indicates the presence of fluid in the upper airway.
- *Wheezing*—High-pitched whistling sounds created by narrowed bronchioles (the small divisions of the airway). This is usually a result of asthma, allergic reactions, or bronchitis.
- *Stridor*—A harsh, high-pitched sound heard usually on inspiration. It is indicative of upper airway obstruction involving the vocal cords or epiglottis.
- *Snoring*—A harsh, low-pitched sound usually caused by the tongue partially blocking the upper airway. An unconscious patient may suffer from this type of obstruction.

Pulse

The pulse is the alternating expansion and contraction of the artery due to the rhythmic propulsion of blood with each heartbeat. It is perceived by palpating an artery close to the skin.

A pulse is evaluated according to the following criteria: rate, rhythm, and quality. All three in some way reflect function within the cardiovascular system. The pulse point most frequently utilized to monitor these functions is the radial pulse, which is located in the distal end of the forearm, on the anterior side, at the base of the thumb (Fig. 2–32). It is important to compress gently with your index and middle fingers so as not to obliterate the pulse.

RATE. Pulse rate can be determined by counting the number of impulses, or beats, in a 15-second period and multiplying by four. The normal pulse range in an adult is approximately 60 to 80 impulses per minute. The generally accepted average is about 72 beats per minute.

QUALITY. The quality of a pulse may be either normal, bounding (a well-defined thumping sensation), or thready (a barely detectable impulse). In some instances, such as shock states, pulses in the extremities may not be palpable. In these circumstances, you should monitor more central arteries such as the carotids or femorals.

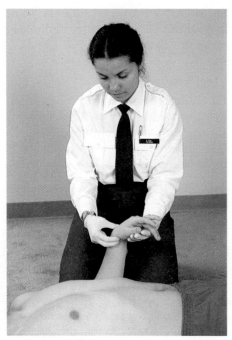

FIGURE 2–32. Locate the radial pulse at the base of the thumb on the anterolateral aspect of the wrist.

RHYTHM. The palpated rhythm will be described as either regular or irregular and directly reflects the function of the pacemaker and electrical conduction system of the heart. Obviously, a regular rhythm reflects optimal function. However, certain individuals may chronically maintain an irregular heartbeat that produces sufficient blood flow. The rhythm should always be reported when communicating the status of the pulse.

Blood Pressure

The blood pressure is a measure of the force that blood exerts on the walls of the arteries. It is determined by two factors: the amount of blood ejected from the heart each minute and the space within the arteries that the blood can occupy. Changes in heart function, blood vessel diameter, and total blood volume may alter the blood pressure.

Blood pressure is measured with a sphygmomanometer (blood pressure machine). The cuff of the sphygmomanometer is placed around the arm above the elbow.

There are two techniques that the EMT may use to measure the blood pressure—auscultation and palpation. *Auscultation* is the preferred method of measuring blood pressure and involves listening to sounds emitted from an artery while changing its diameter from a collapsed state to a fully opened state (Figs. 2–33 to 2–35)

The method of *palpation* is used when you are unable to ascertain blood pressure by auscultation. This may be due to environmental noise or very low blood pressures such as in shock states. This method utilizes the monitoring of a distal pulse (usually the radial or brachial) to determine the point at which blood first flows through the artery (Fig. 2–36).

PROCEDURE 2-7   MEASURING BLOOD PRESSURE BY AUSCULTATION

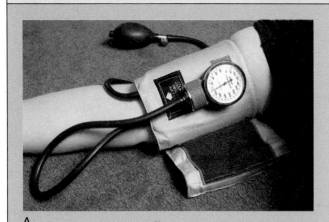

A

1. The cuff of the sphygmomanometer is placed on the arm just above the elbow, with the bladder portion of the cuff over the brachial artery (Fig. 2–33*A*). Most cuffs provide markings that aid in the correct placement. The cuff should be snug enough so as not to move freely but not so tight as to cause discomfort to the patient.

FIGURE 2–33. Auscultation of the blood pressure. (*A*) Place the bladder portion of the cuff around the upper arm just above the crease in the elbow. (*B*) A simple rule for quickly measuring a cuff in prehospital care is that the cuff's bladder width should be approximately 40% of the circumference of the patient's arm.

There are various types and sizes of blood pressure cuffs that range from newborn through obese adult. To select the appropriate size, you should compare the width and length of the bladder within the cuff to the patient's arm. The *width* of the bladder should be *approximately* 40% of the circumference of the patient's arm. The *length of the bladder should be approximately* 80% of the circumference of the patient's arm (Bates, 1991) (Fig. 2–33*B*).

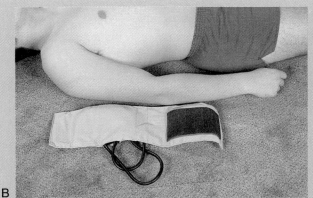

B

FIGURE 2–33. *Continued*

2. Locate the brachial pulse point that is found in the crease of the anterior side of the elbow in a straight line up from the little finger (see Fig. 2–34*B*). Your stethoscope is placed over the pulse point (see Fig. 2–34*A*). Close the valve located above the bulb of the sphygmomanometer and pump air into the cuff until the mercury (Hg) or dial on the gauge stops undulating as it moves upward. In most cases, this occurs between 150 and 200 mm Hg. Listen for pulse sounds with the stethoscope over the brachial artery. If sounds are heard at this point, continue pumping until sounds disappear; then pump 20 mm Hg further.

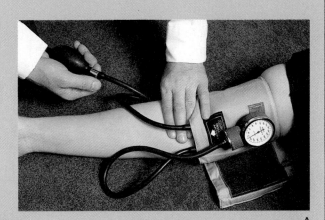

A

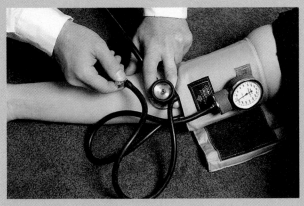

B

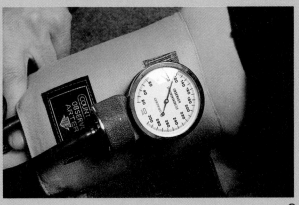

C

FIGURE 2–34. (*A*) Palpate a brachial pulse. (*B*) Place the diaphragm portion of the stethoscope over the pulse point and inflate the cuff until no sounds are heard through the stethoscope. (*C*) Begin releasing air slowly (no faster than 3 mm/second), and note the first sound (systolic). (*D*) Continue releasing air and note a decrease or cessation of sounds (diastolic).

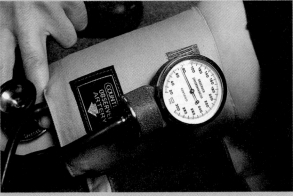

D

Continued

3. At this point, you will have totally occluded the flow of blood past the site of the cuff (Fig. 2–35). When the pressure in the cuff exceeds the pressure of the blood within the artery, no blood can flow through, and you will hear no pulse sounds. Release the valve slowly (about 3 mm/second) and listen for the soft sounds created by blood beginning to flow as the pressure in the cuff goes below the highest pressure within the blood vessel (see Figs. 2–34C and 2–35). Because the artery remains partially occluded, the blood flow that occurs is *turbulent*. This turbulence creates the sounds heard over the brachial artery distal to the occlusion. The first sound will reflect flow during the *systolic phase* (the contracting phase) of the heart. Therefore, we refer to the first sound as the *systolic blood pressure*.
4. Continue to release pressure and listen until the sounds disappear or suddenly diminish in volume. This point will be reached when the pres-

sure in the cuff is less than the blood pressure during the heart's *diastole*, or relaxation phase, allowing blood to flow without turbulence (see Figs. 2–34D and 2–35). The point where the sounds disappear or significantly diminish in volume is recorded as the *diastolic blood pressure*.

Note: The normal values for adult blood pressure vary with age. A generally accepted rule for the systolic pressure is 100 plus the patient's age, up to 140 to 150. The diastolic range is from 65 to 90 mm Hg. Women tend to have blood pressures approximately 8 to 10 mm Hg lower than men of the same age. Children and young adults normally have lower pressures and will be addressed in the pediatric section of this text (see Chapter 14).

5. Record the measured values by placing the systolic reading over the diastolic reading, using a diagonal line to divide the two values, e.g., 120/80.

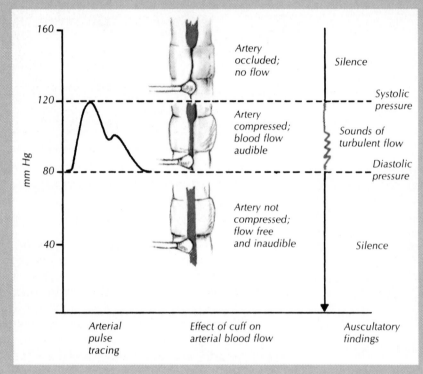

FIGURE 2–35. The artery is totally occluded when the systolic pressure is exceeded (*top*); no sounds are heard. As the artery opens during cuff deflation, the first blood flows, creating turbulent sounds (systolic). When the diameter of the artery allows free, nonturbulent blood flow, no sounds are heard (diastolic). (From Bates B: A Guide to Physical Examination, 5th ed. Philadelphia, JB Lippincott, 1991, p. 284.)

There are many factors and disease states that will affect a patient's blood pressure. Stress, anxiety, drugs, metabolic disturbances, and central nervous system diseases and injuries are among the common causes of increased pressure. Shock states, drugs, heart rhythm disturbances, and simple fainting are associated with decreased pressures. Again, the significance of variations must be evaluated in the framework of the entire clinical situation. It is important to question patients about their "normal" blood pressure when considering its significance.

Temperature

The final vital sign gathered by the EMT in most cases is retrieved simply by touching the patient and subjectively interpreting the patient's body *temperature*. Measuring the temperature with a thermometer in the field is rarely done due to time constraints and the fact that detection of gross variations is usually adequate. However, with the advent of electronic thermometers that enable rapid measurement, some EMT units are collecting specific readings.

P R O C E D U R E   2 – 8   *Measuring Blood Pressure by Palpation*

1. After applying the cuff, monitor the radial pulse and pump up the pressure until the pulse disappears.
2. Slowly release the pressure until the pulse first reappears. This point establishes the systolic blood pressure.

   Note: When taking the pressure by this method, one is unable to determine the diastolic measurement because the changes that occurred in auscultation are audible but not detectable by palpating.

3. Record your findings as the systolic value over "palpation," e.g., 120/palpation or 120/p. This method is also of value in confirming the systolic reading of the auscultated blood pressure (Fig. 2–36).

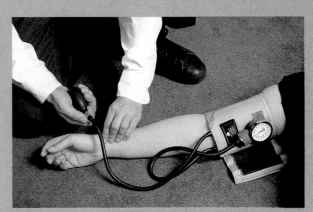

FIGURE 2–36. Palpate the distal pulse while releasing the pressure within the cuff. The first pulse wave is recorded as the systolic reading.

To obtain a temperature, place the posterior surface of your hand against the side of the patient's face. Besides determining the temperature, you should also note the relative moisture of the skin at this time. You will then record your findings: warm and moist, warm and dry, cool and dry, and so forth. For example, the changes in the temperature of the skin range from *hypothermia* (general body cooling) through *heat stroke* (excessive heat retention due to failure of the heat-regulating system).

SUMMARY

When the components of assessment are processed to make diagnosis and treatment decisions, vital signs are always given significant weight. They are the most objective measurements available in the prehospital setting. The EMT must therefore maintain a consistently accurate approach to gathering these data. Particularly in blood pressure monitoring, you must perfect your technique through practice to ensure validity and reliability in your measurements.

Vital signs should be taken early in the secondary survey to aid in establishing the seriousness of the underlying disease. As frequently as possible, additional readings should be obtained to monitor progress or deterioration during therapy. Upon arrival at the hospital, a chronological summary of these measurements should be communicated to the nurse and physician in the context of the history and treatment rendered.

THE HEAD-TO-TOE SURVEY

The remainder of the secondary survey is devoted to a comprehensive body examination to identify significant trauma or diagnostic signs. Certain observations and tests included in this examination will be performed in most cases regardless of the chief complaint. Other aspects are performed selectively in specific instances. Effectiveness during this evaluation is dependent upon a good working knowledge of topographic anatomy and recognition of a variety of diagnostic signs.

As the heading implies, the observations are performed in a set order, starting from the head and finishing at the toes. The EMT records mental notes of all significant findings and initiates treatment upon completion of the examination, unless life-threatening conditions are found that need immediate attention. Four techniques are utilized during the evaluation:

- *Observe*—Look for visual clues, such as cyanosis, contusions, abrasions, deformities, and the status of anatomical structures, including veins, respiratory muscles, chest movements, abdominal shape, and any other pertinent findings.
- *Listen*—Listen for grossly audible sounds, as well as those auscultated through a stethoscope. Stridor,

TABLE 2–2. Examples of Smells and Their Medical Significance

Smell	Possible Significance
Alcohol	Overdose: intoxication
Toxic chemicals	Poisoning
Gasoline (hydrocarbons)	Kerosene, gasoline
Garlic	Organophosphates
Acetone—fruity	Diabetic ketoacidosis
(like nailpolish remover)	
Bitter almonds	Cyanide poisoning
Urine	Kidney failure
Fecal vomitus	Low-bowel obstruction

snoring, and air moving through a sucking chest wound are examples of sounds heard with the ears alone. Lung sounds are auscultated with the aid of a stethoscope.

- *Palpate*—Depressions in bone, swelling, grating of broken bone ends, and air beneath the skin may be felt with your fingers during the survey. You should also note any tenderness experienced by the patient while you are palpating the various regions.
- *Smell*—Many diseases and poisonings will result in odors that are useful in diagnosis. You should routinely check the breath of the patient for such information (Table 2–2).

It is helpful during initial practice sessions to mentally recite these four techniques as you scan the various body regions. It will decrease the possibility of overlooking valuable information.

Mental Status

While responsiveness is checked during the primary survey, a patient's mental status may require further evaluation. Level of consciousness, orientation, eye opening, verbal behavior, and ability to move body parts are all significant indicators of *neurologic* (brain) function.

Level of Consciousness

This is defined in many ways. Again, the type of response to verbal or painful stimuli is the best way to express this concept. For example, a patient may not respond to verbal inquiries but when a pain stimulus is applied, such as rubbing over the sternum (breast bone) or pinching the shoulder, the patient may moan or speak. This patient would be described as being "responsive to painful stimuli." Other terms utilized to describe the level of consciousness are:

Alert—Able to express concepts clearly and maintain normal conversation.
Confused—Capable of some sustained conversation but gives incorrect answers or appears disoriented.
Lethargic—Pertaining to a sleepy, depressed state in

which the patient may still be aroused with painful and verbal stimuli.
Coma—Totally unresponsive to verbal and painful stimuli.

Orientation

Orientation refers to one's awareness of person, place, and time. In conditions such as head trauma, patients may become disoriented. The degree of orientation can be more specifically established by asking patients their name, the location, and the day and approximate time. An individual who fails to answer all three questions correctly is said to be "disoriented times three." If one or two of these components are missed, the individual is categorized as "oriented to person and place" or "oriented to person." Rarely will an individual be disoriented to self or person.

The Glasgow Coma Scale

A standardized approach to evaluating brain or neurologic function is the Glasgow Coma Scale (GCS). It utilizes eye opening, verbal response, and motor (ability to move) functions to define a patient's neurologic status.

EYE OPENING. Eye opening is noted when initiating verbal or painful stimuli. Types of possible responses include *open without stimuli, open with verbal stimuli, open with painful stimuli,* or *do not open.*

A numerical grade is given to each level of eye opening ability on a scale of *1* to *4* (Table 2–3).

VERBAL RESPONSE. Verbal response is also scored, but on a scale of *1* to *5*. If an individual is alert and oriented, a score of *5* is given. If the patient is *confused* (gives incorrect answers) but is able to maintain a conversation, a score of *4* is given. If the patient speaks words clearly but is not only confused but also unable to maintain a conversation without repeated prodding by the examiner, the words are said to be *inappropriate* and the patient receives a *3.* The examiner has a difficult time maintaining the attention of the inappropriate patient. A patient who is moaning incomprehensively receives a *2*, and a patient who emits *no sounds* is given a *1.* A summary of grades for verbal response is provided in Table 2–4.

TABLE 2–3. Glasgow Coma Scale—Eyes

Sign	Score
Eyes are open	*4*
Verbal stimuli—opens eyes	*3*
Pain stimuli—opens eyes	*2*
Eyes do not open	*1*

TABLE 2-4. Glasgow Coma Scale—Verbal

Sign	Score
Alert and oriented	5
Confused	4
Inappropriate words (unable to maintain conversation)	3
Incomprehensible sounds	2
No sounds	1

TABLE 2-5. Glasgow Coma Scale—Motor

Sign	Score
Obeys commands	6
Localizes (pain)	5
Withdraws (pain)	4
Abnormal flexing (pain)	3
Abnormal extension (pain)	2
No response (pain)	1

MOTOR RESPONSE. Motor functions receive scores ranging from *1* to *6*. A patient who is able to *move upon verbal command* receives a *6*. If painful stimuli cause the patient to *localize* (reach for the source of pain), a score of *5* is given. When pain is applied and the patient *withdraws* from the source of pain, a score of *4* is given. A patient who *flexes* the upper extremities upon application of pain receives a *3*. This posturing is also referred to as *decorticate posturing* (Fig. 2–37A). If the patient *extends* both arms in response to painful stimuli, a score of *2* is given. This extension is called *decerebrate posturing* (Fig. 2–37B). Finally, a patient who *does not respond to pain* receives a *1* (Table 2–5).

The GCS should be noted for each patient and repeated at frequent intervals on those with head trauma and impaired mental status. This will provide a baseline measurement of central nervous system function and will chart improvement or regression following treatment or during transport.

When expressing the GCS to the nurse or physician, you should note the total score (*3* to *15*) *and* the individual scores for each category if the total score is less than *15*. (See Chapter 7 for a fuller discussion of the GCS.) Table 2–6 summarizes the Glasgow Coma Scale.

Examination of the Head

Examine the head for evidence of soft tissue injuries, fractures, central nervous system function, and the status of the eyes, ears, nose, and oral cavity.

OBSERVATION AND PALPATION. When examining the head of a suspected trauma victim, you should always assume the presence of a neck injury (Figs. 2–38 and 2–39A and B). You should observe and palpate the skull and face carefully; cuts, bruises, and deformities should be noted. Palpation should be gentle to avoid compressing bone fragments into the brain should a skull fracture exist.

PUPILS. An important diagnostic sign found when examining the head is the status of the pupils. The pupil is the center, black portion of the eye that normally changes diameter in relation to light. When exposed to bright light, the pupil should *constrict*, or become smaller. Conversely, pupils should be *dilated*, or wide, in a dark environment. Furthermore, the two pupils should be equal in size. We measure the function of the pupils according to three parameters: *diameter*, *reactivity to light*, and *equality*.

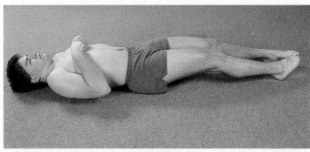

A

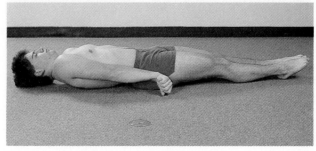

B

FIGURE 2–37. (*A*) Decorticate posturing (abnormal flexion). (*B*) Decerebrate posturing (abnormal extension).

TABLE 2–6. Glasgow Coma Scale—Total

Eye Opening	Spontaneous	4	
	To Voice	3	
	To Pain	2	
	None	1	
Verbal Response	Oriented	5	
	Confused	4	**Patient's Best Verbal Response**
	Inappropriate Words	3	Arouse patient with voice or painful stimulus.
	Incomprehensible Sounds	2	
	None	1	
Motor Response	Obeys Command	6	
	Localizes Pain	5	
	Withdraw (pain)	4	**Patient's Best Motor Response**
	Flexion (pain)	3	Response to command or painful stimulus.
	Extension (pain)	2	
	None	1	
Total GCS Score		:3-15	

From Champion HR, Sacco WJ, Carnazzo AJ, et al: Trauma score. Crit Care Med 9(9): 672–676, 1981.

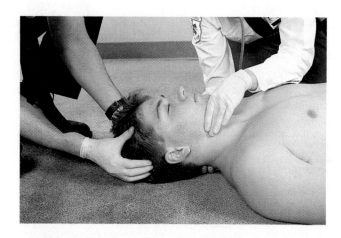

FIGURE 2–38. Carefully palpate the head, using gentle flat-hand pressure. Note any crepitus, deformities, or depressions. In-line immobilization of the head should be maintained during this procedure.

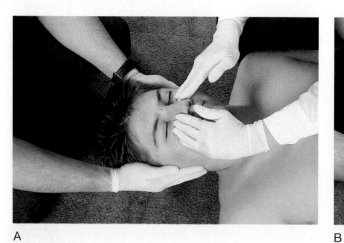

A

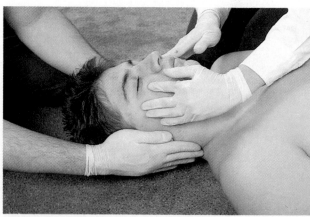

B

FIGURE 2–39. Palpate the bones below the eyes and anterior to the ears and the lower jaw, and note any crepitus, deformity, tenderness, or loose segments.

P R O C E D U R E   2 - 9   EXAMINING PUPILS

1. Face the patient and turn on your light before shining it into the patient's pupil.
2. Observe the diameter of the pupil while holding the lid open.
3. Then quickly shine the light beam into the pupil and observe the reaction and the diameter following exposure to light (Fig. 2–40).

    Note: This should be done on both sides, noting whether the pupils react identically to light.

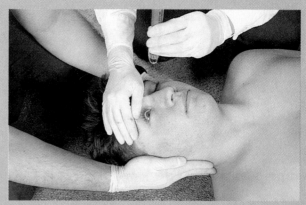

FIGURE 2–40. Observe the pupil while shining the light from the lateral corner of the eye.

4. Record the findings according to the diameter, equality, and reactivity. For example, "The patient's pupils are mid-positional, equal, and reactive to light," or "The pupils were dilated, equal, and nonreactive." Some EMTs record the specific diameter by using a pupil chart (Fig. 2–41) that is frequently found on ambulance call reports. Many factors will alter pupillary function including hypoxia, drugs, brain damage, eye injuries, and eye diseases. Look at the sclera (white portion of the eye) for changes in color.

    Also note whether the conjunctival or covering membrane on the inner eyelids is pink or pale (Fig. 2–42).

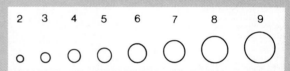

FIGURE 2–41. This chart provides an accurate measurement of pupil diameter in millimeters.

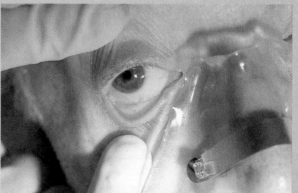

B

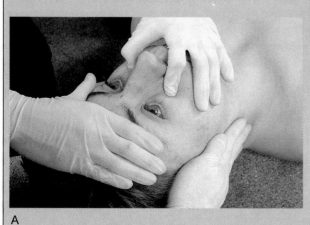

A

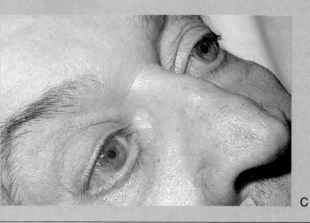

C

FIGURE 2–42. (*A*) Inspect the sclerae and conjunctivae for appearance. (*B*) Note the pale conjunctivae due to a deficiency of red blood cells (anemia). (*C*) Note the jaundice (yellow) of the sclerae (white portion of the eye) due to liver disease.

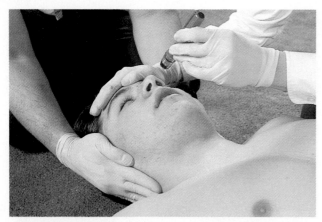

FIGURE 2–43. Inspect the nose for bleeding or fluid leakage.

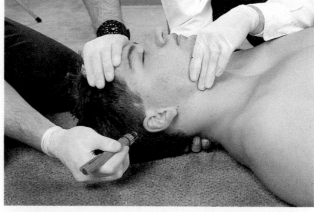

FIGURE 2–44. Inspect the ear for evidence of fluid or blood.

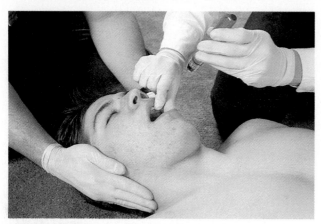

FIGURE 2–45. Inspect the mouth for broken teeth, bleeding, or foreign bodies.

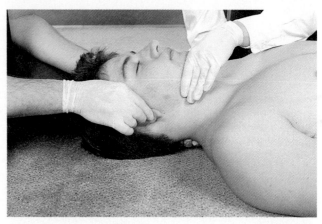

FIGURE 2–46. Battle's sign. Inspect behind the ears for ecchymosis (black and blue marks). The presence of Battle's sign suggests a basilar skull fracture.

NOSE AND EARS. The nose and ears should be inspected for the presence of cerebrospinal fluid that will appear clear or upon mixing with blood will have a pink-tinged color. Either finding is suggestive of a skull fracture (Figs. 2–43 and 2–44).

Inspect the mouth for broken teeth, bleeding, or foreign bodies (Fig. 2–45).

The soft tissue around the eyes and behind the ears on the mastoid process should be examined for *ecchymosis* (black and blue marks). Positive findings are referred to as "raccoon eyes" (around the eyes) and "Battle's sign" (over the mastoid process), respectively (see Fig. 2–46). They are both indicators of a *basilar* skull fracture (base of the skull).

The Neck

The neck offers valuable information about the status of the respiratory and cardiovascular systems, as well as signs of soft-tissue and possible cervical-spine injury (Figs. 2–47 and 2–48). The neck should be observed and palpated circumferentially for signs of wounds, contusions, and deformity.

Active neck muscles during respiratory efforts suggest impairment or obstruction of respiratory function requiring increased work of breathing. The larynx and trachea, which are located midline just above the suprasternal notch, should be palpated (Fig. 2–49). Tracheal deviation to either side and the development of *subcutaneous emphysema* (air beneath the skin) are both signs of *tracheobronchial injury* or chest trauma. Subcutaneous emphysema is characterized by a crackling sensation (similar to squeezing cellophane wrapping) beneath the skin's surface.

THE NECK VEINS. The external jugular veins, which extend from the mastoid process down to the clavicle on both sides of the neck, should be examined for distention. The neck veins are valuable indicators of obstructive shock and heart failure and will be discussed in detail in Chapter 5, Cardiovascular Emergencies. As an exercise, observe the neck veins of a friend or classmate in the erect and supine positions. They should distend in the supine position and disapppear while standing erect.

FIGURE 2–47. Major structures in the neck.

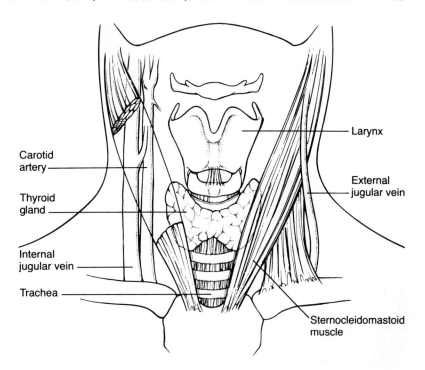

Carotid artery

Thyroid gland

Internal jugular vein

Trachea

Larynx

External jugular vein

Sternocleidomastoid muscle

The Chest

The thorax should be observed and palpated on the anterior, posterior, and lateral planes (Figs. 2–50 and 2–51). Open wounds should be identified and promptly sealed with an airtight dressing. Areas of suspected fractures should be closely observed for signs of *paradoxical breathing.* This is characterized by sections of the chest wall moving in the opposite direction from the rest of the thorax. These types of injuries will be discussed more specifically in Chapter 3. Subcutaneous emphysema may also be observed and may be associated with an underlying lung injury.

The chest should be observed for symmetrical expansion. Decreased movement on one side of the chest is suggestive of underlying chest injury. This is called "splinting."

AUSCULTATION. The chest should be auscultated with the *diaphragm* (flat) end of the stethoscope at several locations. At each location you should listen to at least one complete respiratory cycle. When abnormal breath sounds are discovered you should note their relationship to inspiration and expiration, as well as the nature of the sound. Specific techniques and clarification on the issue of breath sounds will be provided in Chapter 3.

The Abdomen

Examination of the abdomen should begin with observation for distention and, in cases of trauma, evidence of wounds on all areas of the abdomen and lower back (Fig. 2–52). Distention may be characterized by a bloated appearance, which can be caused by air or fluid collecting within the abdomen.

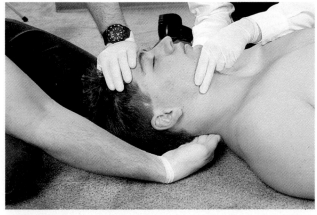

FIGURE 2–48. While maintaining in-line immobilization, carefully palpate the posterior cervical spine and note any crepitus, tenderness, or deformity.

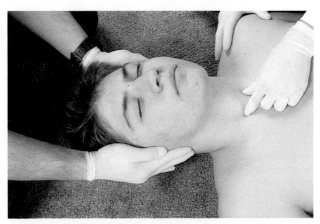

FIGURE 2–49. Observe the muscles in the neck and palpate the trachea and note if it is midline. Also note any wounds, ecchymosis, crepitus, or swelling in the neck region.

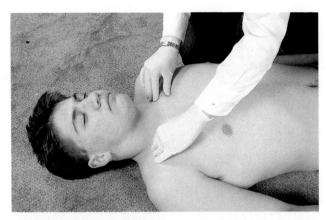

FIGURE 2–50. Carefully and gently palpate the clavicles and note any tenderness, deformity, crepitus, or ecchymosis.

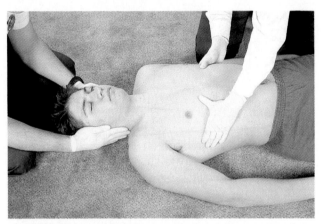

FIGURE 2–51. Palpate the chest by compressing gently on the anterior and lateral wall, noting any ecchymosis, tenderness, crepitus, or deformity.

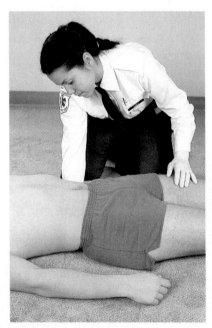

FIGURE 2–52. Observe the abdomen for any swelling, ecchymosis, or wounds.

The abdomen may then be palpated for masses, rigidity, or tenderness (Fig. 2–53). Palpation should be gentle to avoid causing undue pain or aggravation of organ injury. (See Chapter 8 for a more detailed discussion.)

The Pelvic Girdle

The pelvis and hip region are evaluated by palpating the pelvis circumferentially while observing for evidence of wounds or contusions. The integrity of the pelvis is checked by applying gentle pressure medially, posteriorly, and over the pubic symphysis (Fig. 2–54A, B, and C). If the patient complains of pain or if there is movement of these normally fixed bones, a pelvic fracture should be assumed. Great care and gentleness are essential during this examination to avoid complicating underlying fractures. If the circumstances permit, the genitalia should be observed for bloody discharge, which suggests underlying trauma to the genitourinary structures. Obviously, patient privacy and concern for individual needs should be respected.

The buttocks can be evaluated by palpation and, if possible, by log rolling the patient, particularly if trauma to the back is suspected or, in the case of gunshot wounds, to identify possible exit wounds (Fig. 2–55).

Lower Extremities

When examining the lower extremities, you should observe and palpate "bilaterally" while moving downward to compare one leg with the other. Subtle evidence of swelling and deformity can only be noted when you recognize the relative difference between the two legs. The importance of this is reinforced by the fact that when a liter of blood is lost into the thigh, the circumference increases by only 1 to 2 cm. (Fig. 2–56).

When palpating the lower extremities, start at the top and work your way down. The entire extremity should be palpated completely around. Certain bones including the patella, tibia, metatarsus, and phalanges are palpable on the surface (Fig. 2–57). Feel for deformity

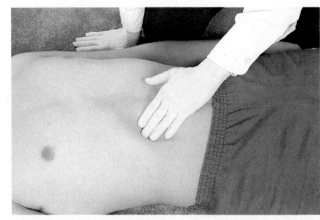

FIGURE 2–53. Carefully palpate the abdominal wall, starting away from the area of pain, and note tenderness, rigidity, or pulsatile masses.

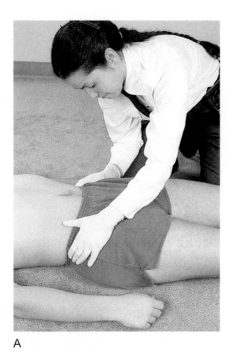

A

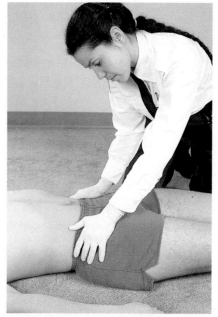

B

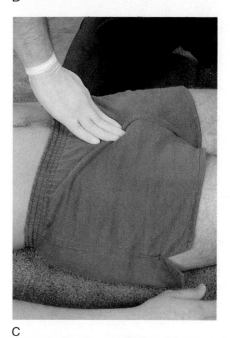

C

FIGURE 2–54. Gently compress the iliac crests (*A*) toward the midline and then (*B*) posteriorly. (*C*) Palpate the pubic bone. Be very careful and gentle, and stop compression when movement is noted in the normally rigid pelvic bone.

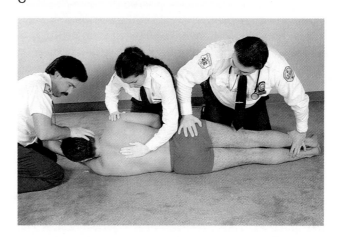

FIGURE 2–55. If circumstances permit, rotate the patient as a unit and inspect and palpate the back region. This is particularly important when dealing with a gunshot wound victim.

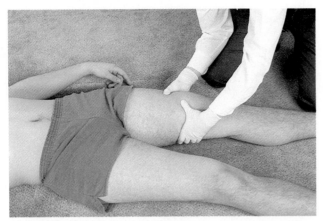

FIGURE 2–56. Palpate both thighs, comparing the size to identify swelling. Also note any crepitus, ecchymosis, tenderness, or deformity.

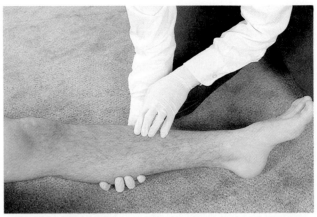

FIGURE 2–57. Inspect and palpate the lower leg, noting any crepitus, ecchymosis, tenderness, or deformity. Run your fingers along the tibia, which can be felt on the anterior surface of the lower leg. Note any deformity.

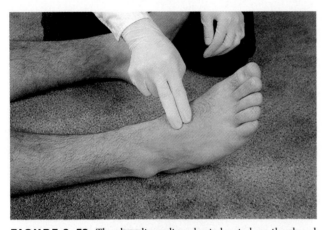

FIGURE 2–58. The dorsalis pedis pulse is located on the dorsal *(top)* surface of the foot by drawing an imaginary line up from the junction of the great and second toe.

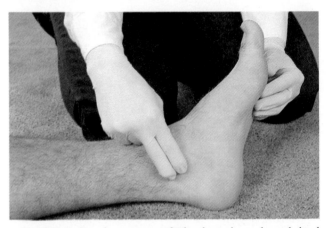

FIGURE 2–59. The posterior tibial pulse is located just behind the medial ankle bone (medial malleolus).

and evidence of *crepitus,* a crackling or grating sensation or sound that may be elicited during palpation. Crepitus can be caused by broken bone ends rubbing together or a collection of air beneath the skin.

Certain types of fractures in the lower extremity may cause the leg to assume a specific posture. For example, a fracture of the hip bone (head and neck of the femur) causes the leg to externally rotate and shorten. An anterior dislocation of the hip causes a similar presentation. A posterior hip dislocation results in internal rotation, adduction (upper leg bent toward midline), and flexion at the knee. These are classic findings and will be discussed in greater detail in Chapter 10.

The final aspect of the lower extremity examination is the neurocirculatory evaluation. Circulation and nerve function are always of great priority when evaluating injured extremities. Should an injury cause a laceration to, or pressure on, nerves or vessels, total loss of function is possible. For this reason, the distal pulses are palpated and, when possible, the patient is asked to move both feet and toes to determine neurocirculatory function. The pulses that can be utilized are the *dorsalis pedis* (Fig.

2–58), located on the dorsal surface of the foot, and the *posterior tibial,* which is behind the *medial malleolus* (Fig. 2–59). Absence of pulses should always be reported to the emergency department staff so that restoration of blood flow can be attempted early in the patient's treatment.

To evaluate the nervous supply, you should ask the patient to flex and extend the foot and press the foot against the examiner's hand (Fig. 2–60A, B, and C). This will evaluate function of the main motor nerves innervating the lower extremity. Ask the patient if he or she can feel you touching the bottom of the feet (Fig. 2–61). When a patient does not feel a light touch, you can apply mildly painful stimuli such as a pinch to the skin to check further for sensory function. If no sensation is felt distally, check for sensation higher up on the leg. You might ask the patient to close both eyes and to tell you when the sensation is felt, while you provide the stimulus in several locations on the anterior, posterior, medial, and lateral areas of the lower extremities. Be careful not to cue the patient while performing this examination. A verbal cue may result in a "false positive

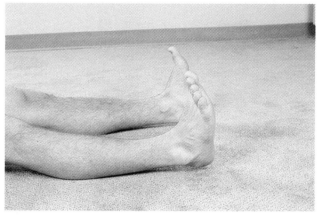

A

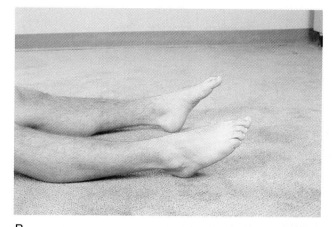

B

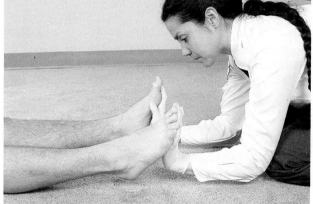

C

FIGURE 2–60. Motor examination of the lower extremity. Have the patient tilt both feet up (A) and down (B), and ask the patient to press both feet against your hands (C) and note comparative strength.

response." Again, all findings should be communicated to the emergency department staff when you give the patient's history.

Upper Extremities

The upper extremities should be palpated and observed starting at the clavicles and shoulders and working down toward the hands (see Fig. 2–62). As with the lower extremities, you should compare the two extremities during your examination to elicit variances in diameter or deformity. Like the lower extremities, there are bones in the upper extremity that reach the surface in certain areas. These areas include the proximal and distal ends of the humerus, the radius and ulna, and the metacarpals and phalanges.

Check for sensation on the fingers and then higher up if there is no feeling distally (see Fig. 2–63). To evaluate motor nerves, the patient is asked to move the hands, spread the fingers, and to squeeze your fingers and then push and pull against your resistance to gauge strength (see Fig. 2–64).

The distal pulses utilized to evaluate circulation to the upper extremities include the radial pulse, located on the anterior, lateral surface of the wrist just proximal to the thumb, and the ulnar pulse, which is located on the anterior, medial surface of the wrist proximal to the little finger.

A final important evaluation to be performed in the

upper extremity is to check for capillary refill. This test is a measurement of cardiovascular function that is used to identify shock states or so-called circulatory collapse, and is also evaluated during the primary survey. The test is performed by compressing the patient's nail surface with your finger, then releasing the pressure and observing the color changes before and after (Fig. 2–65). Normally the nail bed should be pink before compressing,

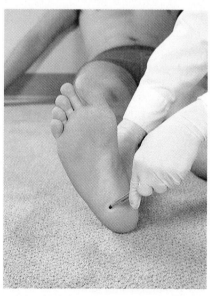

FIGURE 2–61. Check for sensation on the bottom of each foot.

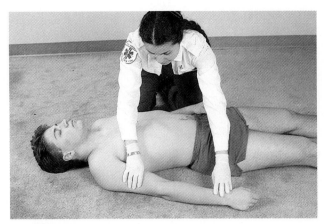

FIGURE 2–62. Inspect and palpate the lower arm, noting any crepitus, ecchymosis, tenderness, or deformity.

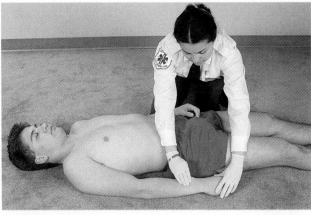

FIGURE 2–63. Sensory examination of the upper extremities. Start with the fingers and then move up. Ask the patient to indicate when your touch is felt.

pale immediately after, and then return to a pink color within 2 seconds. Delay in capillary refill of more than 2 seconds is consistent with *hypovolemia* (or low blood volume, as from bleeding). This test will be discussed in more detail in Chapter 5.

The Neurologic Examination

The conclusion of the secondary survey is devoted to the neurologic examination. The neurologic exami-

nation evaluates the function of the central and peripheral nervous system, in other words, the brain and spinal cord (central) and the nerves that travel to and from the various regions of the body (peripheral). Furthermore, much of the neurologic examination has already been performed in the primary and secondary surveys, including establishing unresponsiveness, mental status evaluation, orientation, the Glasgow Coma Scale, the pupil check, and the motor and sensory examination in

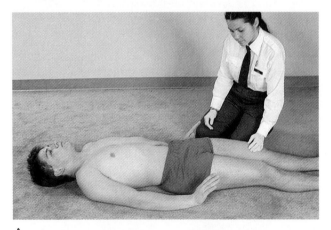

A

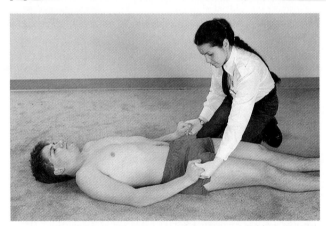

B

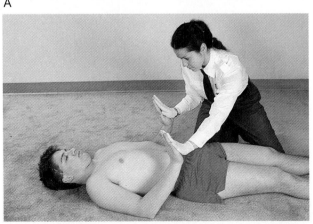

C

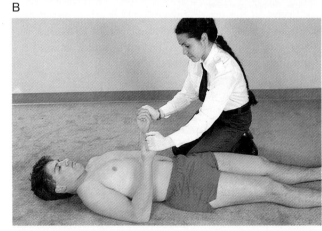

D

FIGURE 2–64. Motor examination of the upper extremities. Have the patient (*A*) tilt both hands up, (*B*) squeeze your hands, (*C*) push you away with both hands, and (*D*) pull you forward with both hands.

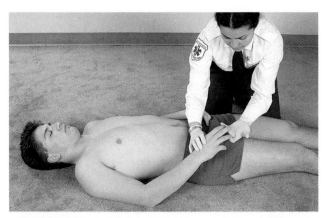

FIGURE 2–65. Capillary refill test: squeeze the fingernail bed and note the time for a pink color to return.

the extremities. The remainder of the examination will cover evaluation of the spinal cord, identification of specific diseases, and locating lateralizing signs (paralysis, weakness, sensory loss, or dysfunction of one side of the body). These lateralizing signs are very important in identifying many neurologic diseases and injuries.

Motor and Sensory Evaluation

The evaluation of motor and sensory function has already been discussed in the section on the extremity examination. However, in instances of medical illness or where extremity injury is not suspected, this examination should be performed to identify brain or nerve abnormalities. The evaluation is performed in exactly the same way as discussed in the extremity examination, with the addition of some other tests.

Facial muscles can be checked by asking the patient to smile and frown. In some neurologic problems, a characteristic droop on one side of the face may be quite noticeable. All findings should be carefully recorded.

SENSORY EXAMINATION. A very important neurologic examination is used when spinal injury is suspected. This test determines the "level" of injury to the spine. As the spinal cord descends from the brain, nerves depart and return at each level. These nerves innervate muscles and other organs and bring back sensory information from the various structures, including the skin.

When the spinal cord is damaged, a disruption of these functions may occur, causing a loss of movement and/or sensation. When you perform the motor and sensory check of the extremities, you are also evaluating the level of function. For example, if the spinal cord was damaged in the upper neck region, paralysis and sensory loss may occur bilaterally in both the upper and lower extremities. If the spinal cord was damaged in the back, the patient might develop loss of function in only the lower extremities. Paralysis of all extremities is called *quadraplegia*, and lower extremity paralysis is referred to as *paraplegia*.

To identify the level of injury more specifically, you can check at several locations for sensation and correlate it to its relationship to the spinal cord. There are five locations you should remember (see Fig. 2–66):

● The skin just above the clavicle is innervated by the nerve arising from the fourth cervical vertebra interspace (C4).
● The level of the breast nipple is supplied by the nerve arising from the fourth thoracic vertebra interspace (T4).

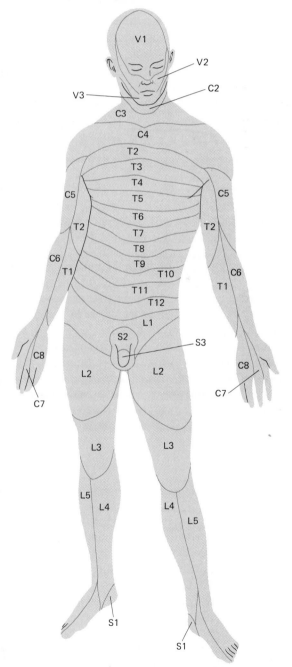

FIGURE 2–66. Dermatome chart. (Solomon EP, Phillips GA: Understanding Human Anatomy and Physiology. Philadelphia, WB Saunders, 1987, p. 155.)

- The umbilical level receives and sends messages through the tenth thoracic interspace (T10).
- The groin region is supplied by lumbar interspace one (L1).

This information has a practical application. If a person were to fall and damage or *transect* (cut through) the spinal cord at the level of thoracic vertebra one, during the sensory examination a *stimulus* (a pinch or needle prick) applied to the shoulder just behind the clavicle should reveal normal sensation. However, a stimulus to the thoracic region at nipple line should reveal an absence of sensation. The level of injury would then be suspected to be between C4 and T4.

This evaluation process should be performed on all suspected spinal victims who are responsive to pain. Ask them to note pain with their eyes closed while you provide stimuli in the respective regions. Again, be careful not to provide verbal cues.

MENINGEAL EXAMINATION. A specialized test that is a useful diagnostic tool for unconsciousness in nontraumatic patients is a test for meningeal irritation. IT SHOULD ONLY BE UTILIZED WHEN THERE IS NO POTENTIAL FOR SPINAL INJURY because it involves flexion of the neck. It is called the meningeal examination because it evaluates the presence of irritation to the meninges (the brain covering). When bleeding occurs between the brain coverings or when the meningeal layers become infected, an irritation develops. To identify the presence of this irritation, a simple neck flexion test is used. By flexing the patient's neck the meningeal tissues are stretched, resulting in pain or stiffness in the neck region. In some instances, the neck will become totally rigid and will be unable to bend. Either response constitutes a positive test and suggests the presence of meningeal irritation. It is important to note that the absence of these findings does not eliminate the possibility of meningitis or meningeal hemorrhage. In the early phase of both problems or when a patient is in deep coma, the test may be negative. (See Chapter 7 for further discussion.)

SUMMARY

At the completion of the neurologic examination, you should review all of the information gathered in the secondary survey and quickly develop a priority treatment plan. Those wounds, fractures, and other soft tissue injuries that remain untreated are cared for in order of their importance. The issue of treatment priorities will be discussed in the various chapters, with special attention in Chapter 17, Disasters and Triage.

Obviously, the survey described in this chapter constitutes a broad overview of patient assessment. Some aspects of the scene survey, as well as the primary and secondary evaluation, will be irrelevant in many instances. The essential aspects of assessment for each disease or traumatic condition are highlighted as each

TABLE 2–7. Equipment Carried to the Scene for Initial Patient Assessment, Resuscitation, and Immobilization

1. Patient Assessment/Trauma Kit
   The package should be clearly marked for easy location of items.

1	small flashlight
1	blood pressure cuff (preferably single gauge/multi-cuff sizes)
1	stethoscope
1	bandage scissors (preferably heavy duty clothes cutting)
3	disposable surgical masks
3	sets of disposable gloves
4	triangular bandages
3–5	rolls of 4″ unsterile Kling
3	rolls of 6″ unsterile Kling or Kerlex
1	roll 3″ plastic adhesive tape
1	roll 2″ plastic adhesive tape
12	topper 4 × 4 sterile sponges
20	4 × 4 unsterile gauze
1	multi-trauma 10 × 30 dressing
1	full size sterile burn sheet
1	500 ml plastic bottle of sterile water or saline
6–8	5 × 9 sterile dressings
2	3″ Ace bandages
3	Vaseline gauze of various sizes
1	hypothermic thermometer
1	turkey baster for emergency suction
1	a few large band aids
1	note pad and pen
1	set of extrication collars (three 10-foot 2-inch web straps with D-rings and a second blanket, which can be used in place of the head immobilizer)

2. Portable oxygen
3. Bag valve mask
4. Suction unit
5. Patient carrying device
6. Other appropriate equipment (PASG, backboard, etc.) deemed appropriate from dispatch information
7. Watch with "second" hand

Adapted from Critical Trauma Care Manual, New York State Emergency Medical Services.

system is covered. Furthermore, practicing during your EMT course in patient assessment will help you become organized and focused in your approach to the patient. Finally, as you work in prehospital care, the repetitive use of a systematic method will fine tune your evaluation skills. During your actual clinical experience, it is essential that you follow up on the inhospital course of your patients in order to correlate your impressions with those of the physicians. This exercise is the most specific and valuable way to improve upon your ability to recognize key diagnostic signs and symptoms and to integrate them to achieve a working prehospital diagnosis.

See Protocol: Approach to the Prehospital Patient for a summary of guidelines. Table 2–7 lists essential equipment for initial assessment and treatment.

Presenting Your History in the Emergency Department

Upon arrival at the emergency department, it will be necessary to present the information gathered in a systematic and concise manner. It should include all of the pertinent historical facts about the patient, such as mechanisms of injury as well as signs and symptoms relative to the condition or conditions being treated. Also included are important "negatives." For example, in someone complaining of chest pain, the denial of a previous heart attack history or high blood pressure is worth noting. Furthermore, normal physical findings such as good capillary refill during a hemorrhage condition will provide an important perspective.

When presenting your history, you should follow the same pattern utilized during your assessment: scene survey, primary survey, patient history, secondary survey, the prehospital treatment, and any changes in the patient's condition following treatment or during transport. Presenting the information in this format achieves the most comprehensive transfer of a patient history. The sequence is important because physicians and nurses routinely anticipate this pattern of presentation. A more haphazard approach can be confusing. Read the following example and relate it to the patient assessment format presented in this chapter. Note the flow of information and connecting phrases that link the various components:

• CASE HISTORY •

Dr. Viccellio, this patient is a 25-year-old male who was struck on the left side of his body by an auto traveling approximately 20 mph. He was thrown about 10 feet and landed on his left side. According to bystanders, he was conscious and oriented immediately following the accident. Upon our arrival approximately 4 minutes after the accident, we found him supine and responsive to verbal stimuli. The primary survey revealed that he had rapid and shallow breathing and a rapid, weak pulse with no evidence of open chest or external hemorrhage. During the secondary survey, vital signs were: respirations 30 and shallow, pulse 130 and thready and regular, blood pressure 80/60, and skin pale, cool, and clammy. With verbal stimuli, he showed eye opening and confusion, and he obeyed commands for a Glasgow Coma Score of 13. The head-to-toe survey revealed a con-

tusion just above the left eye and that his pupils were equal, dilated, and sluggishly reactive. Upon chest examination, we discovered abrasions and tenderness over the left lower lateral ribs. The breath sounds were normal. His abdomen showed a contusion and tenderness over the left upper quadrant. Examination of his lower extremities revealed deformity, tenderness, and crepitus in the mid-lower leg region. His pulses were bilaterally present, and his upper extremities showed no evidence of trauma. He also had delayed capillary refill. Neurologic examination indicated normal motor and sensory findings in the upper and lower extremities. He denies any significant past medical history but states he is allergic to penicillin. Our working diagnosis is hypovolemic shock secondary to internal bleeding, head injury, and possible fractures of the left lower legs and left ribs. The prehospital treatment included spinal immobilization, oxygen via a nonrebreather mask, and application of the pneumatic antishock garment (PASG) with all three sections inflated. Ten minutes after application of the PASG, his vital signs were respirations 24 and shallow, pulse 100 weak and thready, and blood pressure 100/80. His mental state improved and he remained slightly lethargic but oriented times three with a Glasgow of 15. Time from injury to our arrival at the hospital was approximately 22 minutes.

This scenario demonstrates a clear development of information. The flow proceeded from arrival on the scene through the current status of the patient. Each component of the assessment was presented with inclusion of the important positive findings and some key negative ones (e.g., chest examination). This provides the emergency staff with a good starting point for in-hospital management, as well as important facts about the status of the patient from the accident through arrival.

As you first present your history in your early clinical experience, you may find it difficult to be thorough and organized. However, constant use of the same evaluation and presentation format will ultimately refine your technique.

PROTOCOL

APPROACH TO THE PREHOSPITAL PATIENT

1. INITIAL SCENE ASSESSMENT

   A. Assess the scene for safety.

   B. Note the number of patients, the mechanism(s) of injury, environmental hazards, etc.

   C. Call for additional personnel (i.e., A-EMTs, police, firefighters, etc., as appropriate) and/or additional equipment if needed.

2. EXPANDED PRIMARY ASSESSMENT/RESUSCITATION

   A. AIRWAY—Is the airway open?
      —Will it stay open?
      —Use jaw thrust/manually stabilize the head/neck for cervical spine precautions.
      —Suction the patient's pharynx if necessary.
      —Insert oral/nasal airway if indicated.

   Identify and correct any existing or potential airway obstruction, while protecting the cervical spine, if indicated.

Continued

B. BREATHING—Is breathing present?
—Is it adequate?
—Does anything endanger the patient's breathing? Is the patient talking?
—Can the patient take a deep breath?
—Check the respiratory rate.
—Any pain during breathing?
—Assess the chest.
    Inspect
    Palpate
    Auscultate
    Cover wounds with occlusive dressings.
    Stabilize flail segments.
—Administer high-concentration oxygen.
—Ventilate as necessary.

Identify and correct any existing or potentially compromising factors.

C. CIRCULATION—Is a pulse present?
—Is obvious, serious internal/external bleeding present?
—Check capillary nail bed refill.
—Is the patient in shock?
—Note skin color.
—Check pulses:
    If radial pulse is present = 80 systolic BP
    If femoral pulse is present = 70 systolic BP
    If carotid pulse is present = 60 systolic BP
—Obtain baseline set of vital signs.
—Support circulation as necessary.
—Leg elevation (beware of fractures), if indicated.
—PASG (beware of contraindications), if indicated.

Identify and correct any existing or potentially compromising factors.

D. DISABILITY—What is the patient's level of consciousness?
—Assess the patient's level of consciousness as follows:

Alert—Adult patient knows:
    1. his/her name
    2. where he/she is
    3. day of the week

—Infant or child patient:
    1. recognizes parents
    2. responds to presence of rescuers

Verbal—Patient responds to verbal stimuli but does not respond appropriately.

Painful—Patient responds only to pain.

Unresponsive—The patient does not respond verbally or react to pain.

—Assess the pupils.
—Quick assessment of ability to move extremities.
—Apply a rigid collar and stabilize the head/neck.

E. EXPOSE the patient as appropriate to locate life-threatening problems.

IMMEDIATE TRANSPORT DECISION

THE VITAL SIGNS, SECONDARY SURVEY, AND TREATMENT MAY BE DONE AT THE SCENE ONLY IF THE PATIENT IS STABLE!

---

3. VITAL SIGNS: Obtain and record the following on every patient initially, and repeat as indicated.

A. Pulse: rate and quality.
B. Respirations: rate and quality.
C. Blood pressure: systolic and diastolic BP.
D. Skin: color, temperature, and moisture.

4. SECONDARY SURVEY: Complete as indicated by the patient's condition.

A. Reassure and inform the patient about the treatment.
B. Obtain and record chief complaint, subjective information, any pertinent history of present illness, and any pertinent medical information from the patient, family, and bystanders. Check for medical identification.
C. Perform a head-to-toe assessment as indicated.

5. FIELD TREATMENT: Administer appropriate treatment in order of priority.

6. COMMUNICATIONS: If there is a need to notify the hospital of the arrival of a seriously ill or injured patient, the following information should be relayed to the dispatcher:

A. Patient information:

   1. Age and sex.
   2. Chief complaint.
   3. Subjective and objective patient assessment findings.
   4. Level of consciousness and vital signs.
   5. Pertinent history as needed to clarify the problem (mechanism of injury, previous illness, allergies, medications).
   6. Treatment given and patient's response, if any.
   7. Other pertinent information as necessary.

B. Notification of any delay in transport or any unusual circumstances.

C. Estimated time of arrival (ETA).

7. ARRIVAL AT THE HOSPITAL: Upon arrival at the hospital emergency department submit a verbal report summarizing the above information to responsible medical personnel. Submit the hospital copy of the Ambulance Call Report to the responsible emergency department personnel after all crew members have had the opportunity to review it.

From Manual for Emergency Medical Technicians. Emergency Medical Services Program. Albany, New York State Department of Health, 1990.

REVIEW EXERCISES

1. Define the following topographic and anatomic terms:

Medial	Anterior	Posterior
Lateral	Proximal	Midline
Distal	Inferior	Abduction
Superior	Lateral recumbent	Adduction

2. Write a list of the major anatomic structures and describe the general functions of the following major body systems:

Respiratory	Nervous	Circulatory
Digestive	Muscular	Genitourinary
Skeletal	Reproductive	

3. Explain the concept of the heart–lung–brain relationship.

4. List four vital signs and their normal range.

5. Make a detailed list of the steps of patient assessment starting with the dispatch review and ending with the secondary survey.

6. List in the correct order the questions that should be asked when collecting a patient history.

REFERENCES

American Heart Association: Standards and guidelines for cardiopulmonary resuscitation and emergency cardiac care. JAMA 255:2905–2989, 1986.

Bates B: A Guide to Physical Examination, 5th ed. Philadelphia, JB Lippincott, 1991.

Guyton AC: Textbook of Medical Physiology, 7th ed. Philadelphia, WB Saunders, 1990.

Passmore R, Robson JS (eds): A Companion to Medical Studies, Vol 1. Oxford, Blackwell Scientific Publications, 1969.

Prehospital Trauma Life Support Committee of The National Association of EMTs: Prehospital Trauma Life Support, 2nd ed. Akron, OH, Emergency Training, 1990.

Raynor J: Anatomy and Physiology. New York, Harper & Row, 1977.

Safer P, Bircher N: Cardiopulmonary Cerebral Resuscitation, 3rd ed. Philadelphia, WB Saunders, 1988.

Solomon EP, Gloria GA: Understanding Human Anatomy and Physiology. Philadelphia, WB Saunders, 1987.

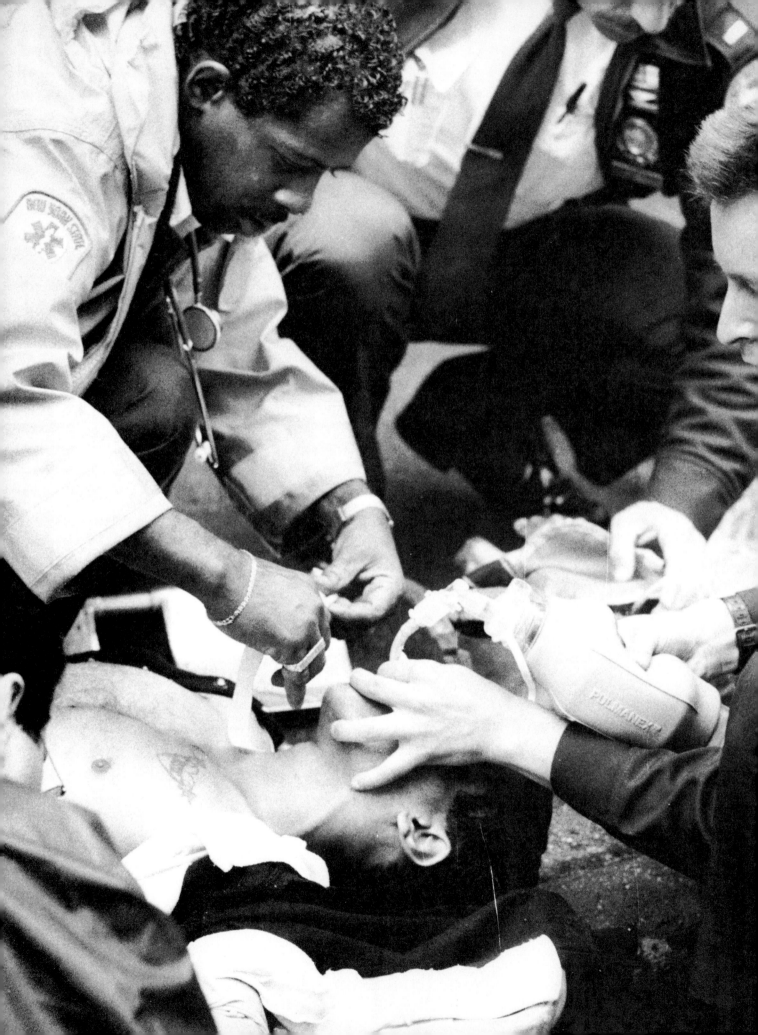

CHAPTER 3

RESPIRATORY EMERGENCIES

O B J E C T I V E S

At the conclusion of this chapter the reader will be able to:

---

1. Describe the significance of oxygen to body tissues, particularly to the brain.

---

2. List five components of the respiratory system and the function of each.

---

3. List three signs of adequate air exchange.

---

4. Define dyspnea.

---

5. List the signs and symptoms of COPD.

---

6. Define hyperventilation.

---

7. List the boundaries of the thoracic (chest) cavity.

---

8. Describe the emergency care treatment for:
   Traumatic pneumothorax   Chronic obstructive
   Tension pneumothorax   pulmonary disease
   Hemothorax   Asthma
   Flail chest   Respiratory arrest
   Airway obstruction

---

9. List the indications, purpose, and functions of the following airway devices:
   Oropharyngeal airway
   Nasopharyngeal airway
   Endotracheal intubation
   Esophageal gastric tube airway (EGTA)

INTRODUCTION

Humans Are Oxygen-Dependent Organisms

Humans are oxygen-dependent organisms. When living cells are deprived of oxygen, they begin to die. Brain cells are the most sensitive to oxygen deprivation and begin to die within 4 to 6 minutes.

HEART, LUNGS, AND BRAIN RELATIONSHIP

The three body systems most involved in ensuring oxygen delivery are the *respiratory system*, the *cardiovascular system*, and the *central nervous system*. The respiratory system retrieves oxygen from the environment and delivers it to the blood. The cardiovascular system transports the oxygen molecules to the cells, where they produce energy and sustain life. The central nervous system monitors the body's needs and regulates the delivery of oxygen to the cells throughout the body.

Because of the interdependency of these systems, failure of any one can result in damage to the others. Consider the following three examples:

• CASE HISTORY 1 •

—Mr. Jones is a 48-year-old male whose airway became completely blocked by a piece of meat while he was eating. He is unable to take in any air and becomes totally *anoxic* (without oxygen). Initially, his heart continues beating, but as the body cells use up the available oxygen his brain begins to die. Ten minutes later he goes into *cardiac arrest* (heart stoppage) due to hypoxia (low oxygen) to the heart muscle.

• CASE HISTORY 2 •

—Ms. Smith, a 65-year-old woman, suffers a heart attack, and shortly after, cardiac arrest. Blood ceases to circulate and the brain is instantly without oxygen. About 10 seconds later she becomes unconscious. Within 30 seconds her brain is unable to send impulses to the respiratory muscles, and she suffers a *respiratory arrest* (breathing stoppage).

• CASE HISTORY 3 •

—Mr. Long, a 24-year-old male, takes an overdose of heroin. The drug suppresses central nervous system respiratory controls, and Mr. Long stops breathing. Ten minutes later he is in cardiac arrest due to heart hypoxia and suffers irreversible brain damage.

Each of these examples illustrates the dramatic relationship of the heart, lungs, and brain. Their functions are by no means separate. For this reason, priority management in any emergency is directed toward ensuring stability of respiratory and cardiovascular function and brain viability.

Components of Respiration

Respiration means the uptake and delivery of oxygen from the atmosphere to the cells of the body, where it is utilized to provide energy for all life functions. Humans cannot store oxygen for future use. This becomes quite apparent when people hold their breath and are rapidly forced by the central nervous system to take another breath and replenish their oxygen supply. Respiration is a delicate and complex process that can be thought of in terms of the following four distinct components.

Ventilation—The inflow and outflow of air from the atmosphere to the *alveoli* (air sacs) in the terminal end of the pulmonary tree.

Diffusion—The exchange of gases between the alveoli and the blood, which takes place at the junction of the *capillaries* (the smallest blood vessels) and the alveoli (tiny air sacs), and again between the capillaries and the body cells.

Transport—The movement of gases in the blood to the site of exchange between the blood and body tissues. Oxygen is delivered to cells for energy production, and carbon dioxide (the waste product of cell activity) is returned to the lungs for excretion into the atmosphere.

Regulation—The needs of the tissues to use oxygen and excrete carbon dioxide are carefully monitored by the central nervous system. The nervous system regulates respiratory and cardiovascular function to maintain a correct balance.

ANATOMY AND PHYSIOLOGY OF THE RESPIRATORY SYSTEM

Overview

The *respiratory system* serves three main functions: the delivery of oxygen from the atmosphere to the blood, the removal of carbon dioxide (the waste product of the body's metabolism) from the blood to the atmosphere, and the creation of voice by the movement of air past the vocal cords.

To meet the above goals requires the cooperative,

effective function of several parts of this system. First, the air passage must be clear of obstructions. The "air sacs" where oxygen and carbon dioxide are exchanged must be functional. The nerves and muscles of respiration must be working effectively, and the portion of the brain that controls these muscles and nerves must be operational and send impulses at the appropriate time. Should any one of these areas fail to perform its required function, respiratory function would be impaired and result in the deprivation of oxygen to the body's cells.

The Airway and Alveoli

The airway is a series of tubes that extend from the mouth and nose down into the lungs. In order for oxygen to be delivered to the blood, the airways must be clear of obstructions and must maintain a sufficient diameter to move an adequate supply of air.

THE NOSE

The first portion of the airway is the *nasal passage*. The nasal passage consists of external and internal sections (Fig. 3–1). The external section includes the nose, which is formed by cartilage and skin and opens at the *nares*, or nostrils. The upper portion contains the nasal bone, and the entire nose is divided into two compartments by the *nasal septum*, which is made of cartilage and bone. Three functions of the airway that begin at the nose are filtering, moisturizing, and warming the air that is breathed in. The nose also provides the function of smell. Injuries to the nose are of great concern to the EMT. First, fractures of nasal or facial bones can compress the *patency* (openness) of the airway. Also, bleeding from the nose in unconscious patients may lead to aspiration of blood into the lungs.

THE PHARYNX

The passage extending from the back of the nasal cavity down to the esophagus and larynx is called the *pharynx*. Each part of the pharynx is further classified according to its relationship to other structures: the *nasal pharynx*, the *oral pharynx*, and the *laryngopharynx* (see Fig. 3–1A). This portion of the airway anatomy may become obstructed when the tongue falls back against it in an unconscious patient or when swelling of pharyngeal tissues develops due to allergic reactions or trauma (see Fig. 3–1).

THE LARYNX

Most anterior in the laryngopharynx is the *larynx* or "voice box." This structure is formed by cartilage, bone, and ligaments, and contains the *vocal cords* (Figs. 3–2A and 3–21G). The vocal cords serve two primary functions: they create voice, and they prevent foreign objects that have slipped past the epiglottis from entering the lungs. When foreign material attempts to enter the airway, the vocal cords, which are muscular bands within the larynx, go into spasms and close shut. This accounts for the so-called "dry drowning," where some persons who drown are found to have little or no water in the lungs due to closure of this structure. The opening of the larynx is commonly called the *glottis* or *glottic opening*.

The two main cartilages forming the larynx are the *thyroid* and *cricoid* cartilages. The thyroid cartilage is superior and is commonly referred to as the "Adam's apple." The cricoid cartilage is inferior and forms a circle just above the trachea. A membrane lies just between these two structures and is called the *cricothyroid membrane*. The cricothyroid membrane is surgically opened to gain access to the airway when an obstruction exists above the larynx. This procedure is called a *cricothyroidotomy* (Fig. 3–2B).

THE EPIGLOTTIS

The vocal cords provide backup protection from *aspiration* (inhaling foreign material). The primary job belongs to the *epiglottis* (see Fig. 3–1). The epiglottis is a flap of cartilage that covers the larynx during swallowing to prevent food from entering the lungs. The epiglottis obviously plays an important role in protecting the airway. However, a disease of the epiglottis that can cause rapid swelling of this structure can result in progressive obstruction of the airway. This is called *epiglottitis* and most commonly affects small children. This is a problem that EMTs may encounter because of the rapid onset of swelling.

THE TRACHEA

Extending down from the larynx is the *trachea* or "windpipe" (Fig. 3–3). It is a hollow tube with several horseshoe-shaped rings of cartilage on the anterior surface that support this portion of the airway. Posteriorly, the trachea is composed of a muscular wall that permits food to move freely down the esophagus, which is located directly behind the trachea. In infants, the trachea is so pliable that great care must be taken not to hyperextend the neck to open the airway. Much like a hose when bent, the infant's trachea may kink and cause an obstruction. The trachea, like the cricothyroid membrane, is often used in emergencies to gain access to the airway. The process of surgically making an entrance into the trachea to provide an airway is called a *tracheostomy*. Take a moment to feel the tracheal rings just above your sternum in the anterior portion of your neck.

THE BRONCHI

At approximately the second intercostal space, the trachea subdivides into two tubes made of cartilage

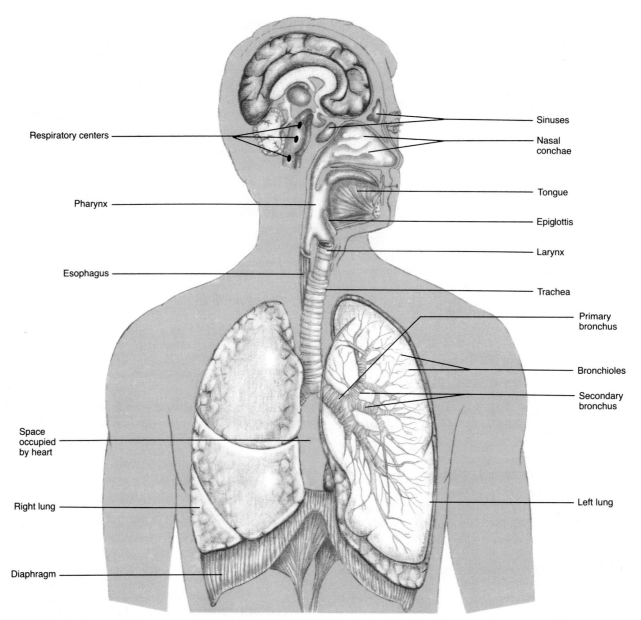

FIGURE 3–1. Anatomy of the respiratory system. (From Davis WP, Solomon EP: The World of Biology, 4th ed. Philadelphia, Saunders College Publishing, 1990.)

which are called *bronchi*. This first division of the "bronchial tree" is referred to as the *main stem bronchi*. Each main stem bronchus (singular term) extends into the left and right lung, respectively. Because of the location of the heart, the left main stem bronchus is at a sharper angle to the trachea than is the right. Small particles that manage to enter the airway tend to fall along the more direct path, into the right main stem bronchus. (see Figs. 3–1 and 3–3).

THE BRONCHIOLES

Much like a tree, the bronchi in turn subdivide to form smaller and smaller bronchi. As they become smaller, they contain less cartilage and more muscle. At about the fifteenth generation of division these tubes

lose their connective tissue sheath and are then referred to as *bronchioles*. Bronchioles are the smallest type of airway tube and have a muscular quality, which permits changes in the diameter of the tubes. A major factor in the disease of asthma is *bronchial constriction*, which increases the work of breathing by narrowing and increasing the resistance within the airways. Reversal of this condition is achieved by drugs that dilate the smooth muscle of the bronchioles.

THE ALVEOLI

The final results of all the subdivisions of the tracheobronchial tree are the *alveoli* (see Fig. 3–4A and B). These microscopic air sacs are the portion of the lungs where gas exchange takes place. Alveoli arise in grape-

FIGURE 3–1. *Continued.*

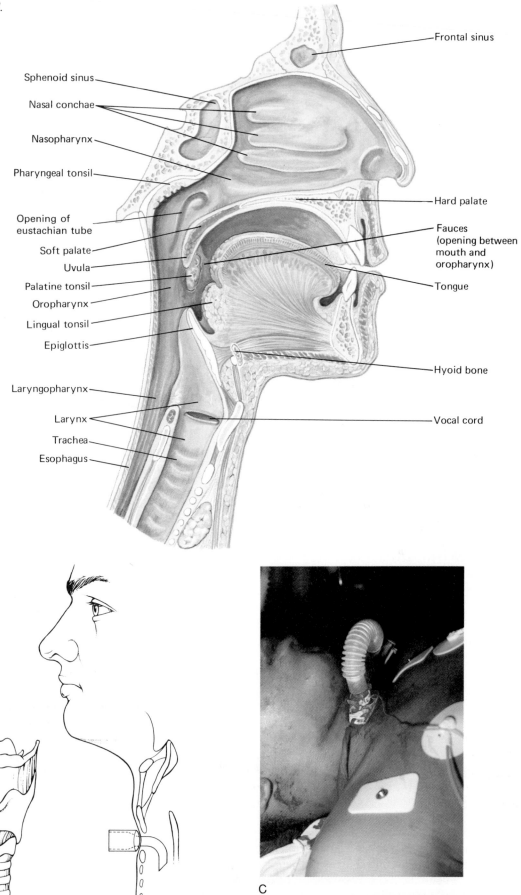

Frontal sinus

Sphenoid sinus

Nasal conchae

Nasopharynx

Pharyngeal tonsil

Hard palate

Opening of
eustachian tube

Fauces
(opening between
mouth and
oropharynx)

Soft palate

Uvula

Tongue

Palatine tonsil

Oropharynx

Lingual tonsil

Epiglottis

Hyoid bone

Laryngopharynx

Larynx

Vocal cord

Trachea

Esophagus

Thyroid
(Adam's
apple)

Cricoid

A

B

C

FIGURE 3–2. *(A)* The major structures of the larynx. *(B and C)*
A surgical cricothyroidotomy is an artificial airway opening made to
ventilate patients with obstructions at or above the larynx.

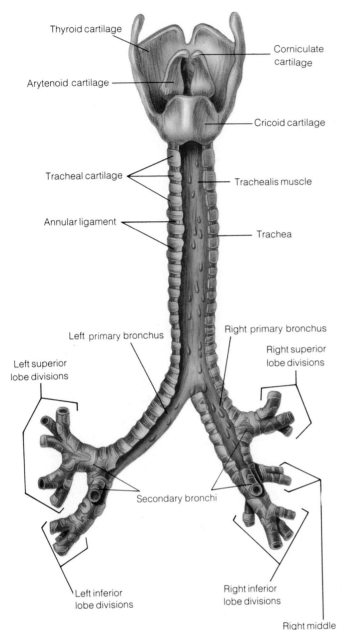

FIGURE 3–3. The trachea (shown from posterior) is formed by rings of horseshoe-shaped cartilage on the anterolateral walls. The posterior wall consists of a muscular band that is located directly anterior to the esophagus. The trachea subdivides into left and right bronchi. (From Gaudin AJ, Jones KC: Human Anatomy and Physiology. Orlando, Harcourt Brace Jovanovich, 1989, p. 511.)

like clusters at the end of the bronchioles. The wall of an alveolus (singular term) is *one cell thick*. The walls must be thin to permit the exchange of gas with blood in the adjoining capillaries (the smallest units of a blood vessel). The ability of the lung to exchange oxygen with the blood is also dependent on the total number of functional alveoli in contact with capillaries. If spread out, the alveoli in a normal adult would cover an area greater than 50 square meters. In diseases such as emphysema where the alveoli are damaged or destroyed,

patients have less ability to take up oxygen from the lungs.

SURFACTANT

The alveoli and bronchioles have an elastic quality. During movement of the lungs, the elastic quality allows the lungs to expand during inspiration and recoil during expiration. A significant factor that contributes to this elastic property is *surfactant*. Surfactant is a special filmy fluid that lines the alveoli and keeps them open through both inspiration and expiration. The surfactant has a property known as surface tension. Surface tension can be seen in soap bubbles. The larger bubbles have a tendency to break down into smaller bubbles, or to diminish in size. The uniqueness of surface tension is also seen in the fact that the bubbles have greater strength as they diminish in size. Remember how when a child blows bubbles the larger ones break first, while the smaller ones float in the air for a longer period. Such is also the case with the surfactant in the alveoli. As the alveoli reach their smallest size during expiration, the surfactant inside them helps keep them open and prevents their total collapse.

The need for surfactant is most dramatic in prematurely born infants. Their lungs are deficient in surfactant into the seventh month of gestation. Without an adequate amount of surfactant, their alveoli tend to collapse easily, and they must be ventilated with a ventilator.

Another condition that affects surfactant is drowning. The drowning victim who aspirates water may wash away the surfactant, resulting in collapse of the alveoli.

THE MUCOUS BLANKET

Alveoli are also sensitive to dry air and irritants that may enter the airway. As explained above, the job of filtering, warming, and moistening the air begins in the nasal passages and continues through the conducting portion of the airway. The lining of the airway has a rich blood supply and specialized mucus-secreting cells and is called a *mucous membrane*. Particles are filtered by hairs called *cilia* and trapped by the sticky mucous secretions. The cilia continually beat particles upward from the lower airway to the pharynx, where they are swallowed. Coughing is a vigorous expiration that also rids the airway of foreign material. If there is excessive mucous because of an infection or a heavy concentration of irritating particles, as in smoke inhalation, the patient may expel thick, viscous *sputum*. We have all noted sputum production during chest colds.

The rich blood supply of the mucous membrane also serves to humidify the air, or saturate it with water vapor before it reaches the delicate alveoli. Likewise, the surface blood vessels exchange their warmth with the air to bring the air temperature close to that of the body's

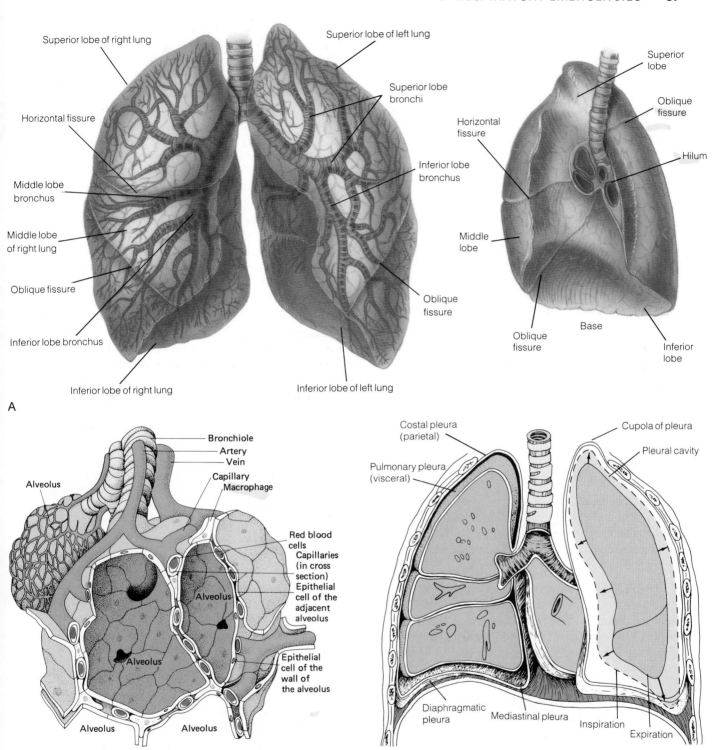

FIGURE 3–4. (*A*) The bronchioles subdivide several times and become less cartilaginous and more muscular with each subsequent division. (*B*) At the lowest division, the respiratory bronchioles terminate as alveolar ducts and alveolar sacs. Alveoli are the tiny air sacs at the end of the bronchiole tree where diffusion of gases takes place. (*C*) The pleura consists of a parietal pleura that covers the lining of the chest wall and a visceral pleura that lines the lung. The space between these two layers is called the pleural space. Each side of the chest cavity has a separate and distinct pleural space. (*A* and *C*, from Gaudin AJ, Jones KC: Human Anatomy and Physiology. Orlando, Harcourt Brace Jovanovich, 1989, pp. 512 and 513; *B*, from Davis WP, Solomon EP: The World of Biology, 4th ed. Philadelphia, Saunders College Publishing, 1990.)

core. We are reminded that the air reaching our lungs is warm and saturated with water when we see our exhaled air as "fog" on a cold day.

Lungs, Thorax, and Muscles

THE LUNGS

The bronchi, bronchioles, and alveoli together form two cone-shaped organs we call *lungs* (see Fig. 3–4*A*). Each lung is divided into lobes, which are separate sections of lung tissue. The left lung has two lobes and the right lung has three lobes. Patients with lung cancer may have lobes or even an entire lung removed to prevent the spread of the disease. The vast surface area of our alveoli permits us to survive with a relatively small portion of our lung tissue intact.

Both lungs are suspended within the chest cavity and attached only at the *hilum*, where the main stem bronchus enters each lung. The lungs are separated by the *mediastinum*, which is a space occupied by the heart, great vessels, trachea, main stem bronchi, esophagus, and nerves.

BORDERS OF THE THORACIC CAVITY

The borders of the thoracic cavity include the sternum, muscle, and ribs anteriorly; the thoracic spine, the scapula, muscle, and ribs posteriorly; the clavicle and neck as superior border; and the diaphragm, which is the primary muscle of respiration, inferiorly.

THE PLEURA. The inner surface of the chest cavity is lined with a thin, membranous sheath called the *parietal pleura* (see Fig. 3–4*C*). The lung also has a similar covering on its outer surface, called the *visceral pleura*. The parietal and visceral pleura are in direct contact and slide against each other during breathing. This is a smooth process because of a lubricating film between the two pleura. When inflammation occurs between the pleura, or scarring results from a disease or injury, the normal smooth process is interrupted and pain results during ventilatory movements. This condition is commonly called *pleurisy*. This term is more generally used in establishing possible causes of chest pain. Pain resulting from, or made worse by, the process of ventilation is called *pleuritic chest pain*.

MUSCLES OF RESPIRATION

The chest movement that results in air exchange between the atmosphere and the alveoli occurs by actions of the muscles of respiration. These muscles change the

diameter of the chest cavity by contracting and relaxing, and therefore create a *bellows effect,* much like the device used by blacksmiths to fan a fire. In normal, quiet breathing, the principal muscle of respiration is the *diaphragm,* aided by the *external intercostals* (Fig. 3–5*A*). The diaphragm, which is a dome-shaped muscle at rest, separates the chest and abdomen in the inferior portion of the thoracic cavity. Quiet inspiration occurs when the diaphragm contracts downward and "flattens" out while the external intercostals pull the ribs upward and outward, thereby increasing the anterior-posterior, superior-inferior, and lateral-lateral dimensions of the chest cavity.

When the chest cavity increases in size, the pressure within the chest cavity becomes lower than the pressure in the atmosphere, and air rushes into the tracheobronchial tree (Fig. 3–5*B*). Air continues to rush in until the pressure within the lungs becomes equal to the atmospheric pressure. This is the end of inspiration. Quiet expiration occurs as a result of (1) the *relaxation of the muscles of respiration* and (2) *the elastic recoil of lung tissue.* It is essentially a passive process. As the chest cavity becomes smaller, the pressure increases, causing the gas to be expelled (Fig. 3–5*C*). The end of expiration occurs when the pressure inside the lung is again equal to atmospheric pressure (Fig. 3–5*D*).

NEGATIVE PRESSURE CONCEPT

How do the lungs stay expanded in the chest? As was previously mentioned, lung tissue has an elastic quality. This quality creates a natural tendency of the lungs to collapse. Furthermore, when the chest cavity becomes larger there is an increase in this potential. The ability of the lungs to remain expanded within the chest cavity is due to a relatively "negative" pressure (subambient or less than atmospheric pressure) within the pleural space. To better understand this concept of negative pressure, consider the experiment (Fig. 3–6).

A balloon is placed in a bottle with the edges of the balloon folded around the opening (see Fig. 3–6*A*). A hole is then made in the bottle, and air is sucked out through the hole. This will result in the balloon conforming to the shape of the bottle and contacting its inner wall (see Fig. 3–6*B* and *C*).

The lungs are maintained in a state of expansion by this principle of negative pressure. At rest, the pressure within the pleural space is about 4 mm of mercury *less* than atmospheric pressure, therefore causing the lung to stay expanded. This difference in pressure is critical to lung function. A condition that can interfere with this relationship is called *pneumothorax* (air within the pleural space). When the chest wall or lung is penetrated by a knife or missile, the difference between atmospheric and pleural pressure causes air to rush into the pleural space, separating the lung from the chest wall. The elastic property of lung tissue then causes the lungs to collapse. A

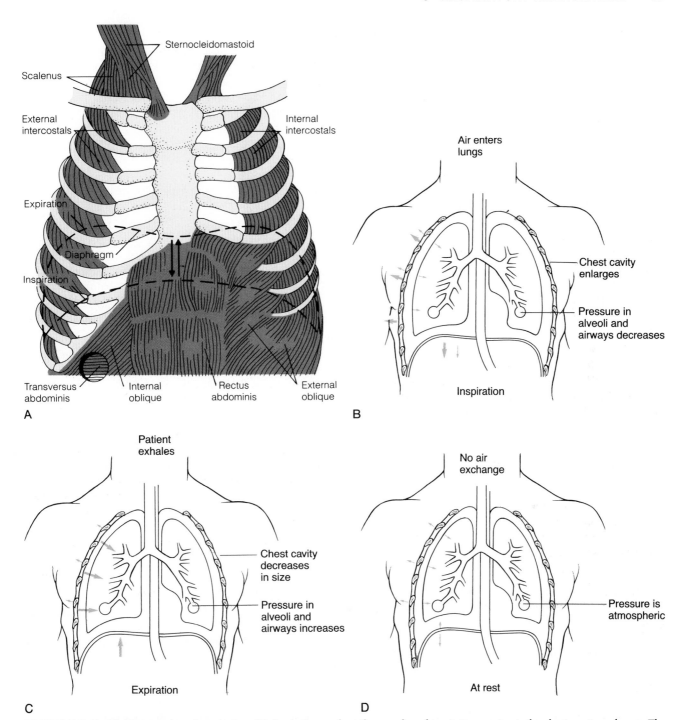

FIGURE 3–5. (*A*) The muscles of respiration. (*B*) *Inspiration*—when the muscles of inspiration contract, the chest cavity enlarges. The pressure of the air within the airway and alveoli falls below atmospheric pressure. Air rushes into the lungs. (*C*) *Expiration*—when the muscles of inspiration relax, the elastic recoil of the lungs and chest wall decreases the size of the chest cavity. This increases the pressure within the airway and alveoli in relation to the atmosphere. Air will then rush out through the airway until the pressure within the lungs and that of the atmosphere equalize. (*D*) *At rest*—the air pressure within the lungs is equal to atmospheric pressure. (*A*, from Gaudin AJ, Jones KC: Human Anatomy and Physiology. Orlando, Harcourt Brace Jovanovich, 1989, p. 516.)

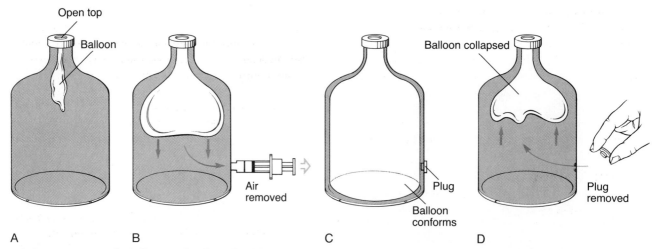

FIGURE 3–6. (A) The balloon is placed in a bottle with its edges around the opening. (B) Air is then sucked out of the bottle using a syringe, and the balloon conforms to the inner wall of the bottle. (C) The bottle wall is closed with an airtight seal and the balloon stays expanded because of lower pressure between the balloon and the inner wall of the bottle. (D) When the seal is removed, the air rushes into the bottle due to the differences in pressure, and the balloon collapses.

similar comparison can be made to the balloon in the bottle. If you puncture the bottle or remove the plug, the balloon collapses as outside air rushes into the bottle (see Fig. 3–6D). Try this experiment at home. This concept of "negative pressure" is essential to understanding certain types of chest trauma and diseases of the lung.

ACCESSORY MUSCLES OF RESPIRATION

During quiet breathing, the diaphragm and external intercostals are more than capable of providing the appropriate volumes of air needed to sustain effective oxygen levels. However, during strenuous exercise or in instances of respiratory disease or trauma, the *accessory muscles* come into play. There are two types of accessory muscles: muscles of inspiration and muscles of expiration. The accessory muscles of inspiration primarily increase the size of the thoracic cavity by pulling the ribs further in the upward direction and increasing intrathoracic diameters. They include the *scalene muscles* in the neck, which elevate the upper ribs; the *sternocleidomastoids*, which pull and elevate the sternum; and the *parasternals*, which pull up on the cartilaginous portion of the ribs adjacent to the sternum. These accessory muscles add to the efforts of the external intercostals and diaphragm to increase tidal volume or respiratory effort. This can occur during exercise, with respiratory compromise from disease or injury, or when destruction of the airway creates greater resistance to airflow.

Accessory muscles of expiration are used when more rapid forceful breathing is needed and when obstructive processes exist. The muscles are the *internal intercostals*, which pull the ribs down and inward, and the *abdominal muscles*, which pull the lower ribs down-ward and compress the abdominal contents, pushing the diaphragm upward to decrease the size of the thorax. Figure 3–5A illustrates these muscles.

During patient assessment, active accessory muscle use provides a key warning signal of respiratory distress. Bulging of the neck muscles, retraction of the spaces between the ribs, and active abdominal muscle use collectively comprise these warning signals.

Physiology of Respiration

RESPIRATORY VOLUMES

There are several parameters that quantify the amount of air contained within the lungs and that measure breathing potential. Some of these values are obtained with a special instrument called a spirometer. These important measurements include the minute volume, tidal volume, vital capacity, residual volume, and total lung capacity.

MINUTE VOLUME. The adequacy of breathing is determined by evaluating two parameters: the *tidal volume* and the *respiratory rate*. The tidal volume times the respiratory rate is called the *minute volume*. The normal respiratory rate is approximately from 12 to 20 breaths per minute, and the normal tidal volume (at rest) is approximately 500 ml. Thus, the normal minute volume is approximately 6,000 to 10,000 ml of air per minute. As an emergency medical technician (EMT), you will not be able to record a specific tidal volume, but generally, well-defined visible chest expansion indicates a tidal volume of about 700 ml in the average adult. This is used as a guide during *assisted ventilation* that an adequate volume has been delivered.

RESIDUAL VOLUME. The amount of air that remains in the lungs after a forceful expiration is the *residual volume*. The residual volume is an important concept to the EMT, as it relates specifically to obstructive disease. A primary component of chronic obstructive pulmonary disease (COPD) is "air trapping." In patients with COPD, the residual volume is increased when excessive air remains in the lungs. This increases the work of breathing and leads to the characteristic barrel-shaped chest found in these patients.

VITAL CAPACITY. The *vital capacity* is defined as the maximum amount of air that can be exhaled after a maximum inspiration. The average vital capacity for a healthy adult is about 4,500 to 5,500 ml. This potential for the movement of large quantities of air is what allows patients to compensate in the face of respiratory compromise. It also allows rescuers to provide effective ventilation with mouth-to-mouth or mouth-to-mask resuscitation.

TOTAL LUNG CAPACITY. The *total lung capacity* represents the total amount of air that the lung can contain after a maximum inspiration. It therefore includes the vital capacity and the residual volume. The average total lung capacity for an adult is about 6,000 ml. Figure 3–7 reviews these various volumes. Think about your own tidal volume and vital capacity.

NERVOUS SYSTEM REGULATION OF BREATHING

Much like a home heating system, the body has a "thermostat" that monitors respiratory function. As certain changes take place, it turns breathing "on" or "off." Messages from this system are sent to the muscles of breathing and cause them to contract and relax. This mechanism of control is the function of the central nervous system and the peripheral nerves that stimulate these muscles. There are essentially two methods of nervous control, *unconscious* and *conscious*. Our unconscious controls regulate our breathing most of the time. Our conscious controls permit us to slow down, speed up, increase, and decrease our volume of breathing at will. As you sit reading this section, your unconscious controls dominate, unless, of course, you "override" these mechanisms and consciously alter your pattern of respiration.

Unconscious controls consist of regulators, connecting sensors with a feedback mechanism. The respiratory centers in the brain stem communicate with receptors in the *carotid arteries* in the neck and the *aorta*, the main artery leading out of the heart. There are other receptors located within the brain itself. These receptors monitor three parameters in the blood to determine the body's respiratory and cardiovascular needs; These parameters are *oxygen (O_2), carbon dioxide (CO_2), and the pH (the relative acidity or alkalinity of fluid)*. The receptors in the aorta and carotid arteries monitor oxygen and carbon dioxide levels. The brain receptors monitor the pH of the fluid surrounding the brain.

The conscious stimulus of breathing arises from the higher brain centers, which communicate through the unconscious control centers via nerve pathways extending into the brain stem.

As we take each breath, we change the levels of oxygen, carbon dioxide, and the pH in our blood. When we increase the rate and depth of breathing, blood oxygen levels tend to increase, while carbon dioxide levels decrease as we "blow off" CO_2. Conversely, as we decrease our respiratory rate and depth, blood oxygen

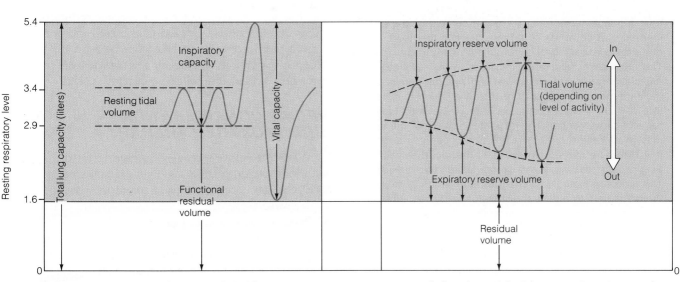

FIGURE 3–7. Respiratory volumes. (From Gaudin AJ, Jones KC: Human Anatomy and Physiology. Orlando, Harcourt Brace Jovanovich, 1989, p. 518.)

levels will decrease, while carbon dioxide will increase as we "retain" CO_2. The pH will change because some carbon dioxide in the blood takes the form of acid called *carbonic acid*. Thus, more CO_2 equals more carbonic acid; less CO_2 equals less carbonic acid. Carbon dioxide changes the pH of the blood. In a normal person, CO_2 *plays the most dominant role in altering ventilation.*

Metabolism also changes the values of O_2, CO_2, and pH. Metabolism represents the sum of cellular activity. As cells become more active, they consume more oxygen and produce more carbon dioxide or waste. As carbon dioxide increases, the pH also changes due to an increase in carbonic acid.

The respiratory centers are constantly monitoring these parameters. When O_2 levels decrease or CO_2 levels increase, messages are sent to the pons and medulla (respiratory centers of the brain) to increase the respiratory rate and depth. These brain centers in turn send messages to the muscles of respiration through nerve fibers. The *intercostal nerves*, which arise from the spinal cord in the thorax, travel along the respective ribs and stimulate the *intercostal muscles* to contract. The *phrenic nerve*, which arises from the spinal cord in the neck, stimulates the *diaphragm* to contract. These messages from receptor to brain and from brain to muscle are continually adjusted to balance supply and demand (Fig. 3–8). Consider the following example:

• CASE HISTORY •

Kelly wakes up from sleep and is about to go jogging. At this moment her respiratory rate is 12 breaths per minute and her depth of breathing is relatively shallow, which more than meets her oxygen requirements at rest. As she starts to jog, the muscles in her legs begin to consume more oxygen and give off more carbon dioxide into the blood. A few seconds later, her receptors detect these changes and notify the brain centers of the increased oxygen needs of the muscles and the need for more rapid excretion of accumulating carbon dioxide. The brain stem then sends impulses to the respiratory muscles through the intercostal and phrenic nerves to increase the rate and depth of breathing. Two minutes into the jog, Kelly's respiratory rate is 24, with more forceful movement of her respiratory muscles. Immediately after the run, Kelly is breathing deeply at a rate of 40 times per minute. However, the muscles then begin to consume less oxygen and excrete less carbon dioxide. The receptors note these changes and gradually cause the brain stem to reduce the stimulus to the respiratory muscles. Five minutes following the run, Kelly's respiratory efforts return to their resting level.

In addition to the respiratory changes, the circulatory status would experience a similar stimulation to transport the needed O_2 and CO_2. To review the func-

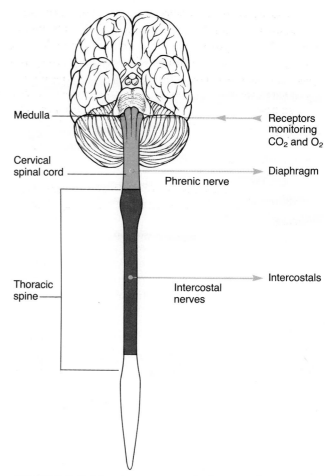

FIGURE 3–8. Messages are sent to the brainstem from receptors in the carotid artery and aorta, which monitor oxygen and carbon dioxide levels in the blood. This and other information is used by the brain to regulate breathing. Messages are sent along the phrenic nerve and intercostal nerves to cause the diaphragm and intercostal muscles to contract or relax.

tions described above, monitor your own respiratory patterns during exercise, or hold your breath and notice the drive that forces you to take your next breath. As we discuss the various respiratory emergencies, the concept of neuro-regulation will be constantly useful.

SPECIAL CONSIDERATIONS DURING OXYGEN THERAPY

When patients are exposed to high levels of CO_2 over a long period of time, as occurs in some cases of COPD, changes occur in the neuro-receptors. They gradually become insensitive to increases in carbon dioxide and switch over to *hypoxic drive*. Therefore, less O_2 will become the dominant force to increase ventilation, and more O_2 will cause a decrease in ventilation. The danger of this alteration in the monitoring mechanism is that excessive oxygen administration may result in *hypoventilation* or even *respiratory arrest*. Thus, when treating COPD patients, oxygen must be administered with caution, usually at levels of about 24% to avoid depressing the respiratory drive. However, when COPD patients are severely hypoxic, in shock, or are having *ischemic chest* pain (i.e., pain resulting from coronary artery disease), oxygen concentrations should be increased and the patient should be monitored for respiratory depression or arrest. If the patient should start to hypoventilate, positive pressure ventilation should be administered.

DIFFUSION

Diffusion is the tendency of molecules to move from an area of higher concentration to an area of lower concentration. The movement of oxygen and carbon dioxide across the alveolar-capillary membranes occurs

as a result of this principle. Capillary blood moving past the alveolar surface is lower in oxygen content and higher in carbon dioxide than the gas within the alveoli. This imbalance permits oxygen to move into circulating blood and attach to the hemoglobin molecule. The hemoglobin molecule is a pigment found in the red blood cell, which is responsible for carrying oxygen. It gives oxygen-rich blood its red color. Carbon dioxide, which is in a higher concentration in the blood than in the alveoli, in turn leaves the blood and enters the alveoli (Fig. 3–9).

During ventilation, the concentrations of gas within the alveoli reflect the environmental air that we breathe. The gas within our environment accounts for the 760 mm Hg of pressure in the atmosphere (at sea level). Atmospheric air contains 21% oxygen, less than 1%

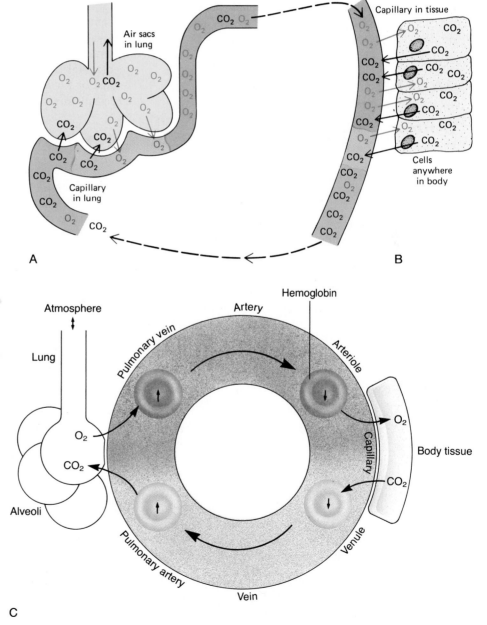

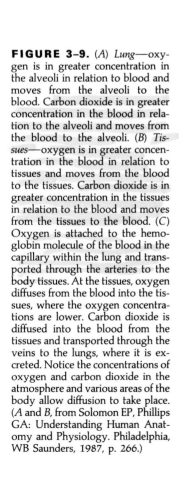

FIGURE 3–9. (*A*) *Lung*—oxygen is in greater concentration in the alveoli in relation to blood and moves from the alveoli to the blood. Carbon dioxide is in greater concentration in the blood in relation to the alveoli and moves from the blood to the alveoli. (*B*) *Tissues*—oxygen is in greater concentration in the blood in relation to tissues and moves from the blood to the tissues. Carbon dioxide is in greater concentration in the tissues in relation to the blood and moves from the tissues to the blood. (*C*) Oxygen is attached to the hemoglobin molecule of the blood in the capillary within the lung and transported through the arteries to the body tissues. At the tissues, oxygen diffuses from the blood into the tissues, where the oxygen concentrations are lower. Carbon dioxide is diffused into the blood from the tissues and transported through the veins to the lungs, where it is excreted. Notice the concentrations of oxygen and carbon dioxide in the atmosphere and various areas of the body allow diffusion to take place. (*A* and *B*, from Solomon EP, Phillips GA: Understanding Human Anatomy and Physiology. Philadelphia, WB Saunders, 1987, p. 266.)

carbon dioxide, and 79% nitrogen. Each of these gases exerts a partial pressure that collectively accounts for the atmospheric pressure (760 mm Hg). Oxygen accounts for 159 mm Hg of pressure, and nitrogen accounts for 601 mm Hg.

As atmospheric air is pulled into our lungs, the percentages and pressures change. Water vapor is added by the airway, and the gases mix with air already in the tracheobronchial tree. The partial pressure of oxygen is referred to as the pO_2, and the partial pressure of carbon dioxide is referred to as the pCO_2. The normal partial pressure of oxygen (pO_2) in the alveoli is about 100 mm Hg, while the normal partial pressure of carbon dioxide (pCO_2) is approximately 40 mm Hg. These pressures are important to diffusion because the difference between alveolar and capillary partial pressures determines the driving force of the gases. If we increase the percentage of oxygen delivered to a patient, we also increase the partial pressure of oxygen within the alveoli, and therefore the driving force of oxygen into the blood.

PATIENT ASSESSMENT

General Signs and Symptoms

There are some relatively universal complaints and physical signs that are common to most respiratory problems. Familiarity with these indicators will allow you to suspect and investigate the causes with greater ease. These signs and symptoms are discussed below.

DYSPNEA

Dyspnea (difficulty breathing) is a subjective feeling of shortness of breath. It cannot be accurately quantified, but you may note relative degrees of dyspnea and interpret this information with other data. It is by far the most common chief complaint among most respiratory problems. Questions to ask in developing the history of present illness in dyspneic patients include the following:

"Did anything cause or worsen the shortness of breath, e.g., increased activity; walking up stairs, position, for instance, lying down?"
"Does anything decrease the sensation, e.g., reducing activity, sitting in an upright position, resting, etc.?"
"Did this ever happen before? If so, what was the diagnosis?"
"Have you recently had cold, cough, or fever?"
"Do you have associated pain or dizziness?"

Record positive and negative responses to these questions and include them when presenting your history to the physician or nurse.

PLEURITIC CHEST PAIN

Many respiratory diseases and trauma cause chest pain. This kind of pain, which is aggravated by breathing, is called *pleuritic pain*. *Pleurisy* (inflammation of the pleura), pneumothorax, and chest trauma are likely to precipitate pleuritic chest pain. Therefore, it is important to ask your patient with chest pain if the character of the pain changes on inspiration or expiration to differentiate this type of pain from other causes of chest pain, such as cardiac chest pain. Cardiac chest pain does not vary with ventilations or chest wall movement.

MENTAL STATUS

A variety of alterations in mental status may be observed as a result of hypoxia. Variances range from agitation, restlessness, and *lethargy* (sleepy appearance), to coma. The type of response is frequently dictated by the degree of oxygen deprivation or the perception of dyspnea on the part of the patient. Any alteration in mental status should dictate the need for a careful examination for respiratory problems and for supplemental O_2 treatment.

CYANOSIS

Cyanosis, which is a bluish discoloration of the mucous membranes or skin, results from oxygen-depleted hemoglobin. Oxygen-rich hemoglobin is a red color; oxygen-poor hemoglobin is more blue or a darker red. The presence of cyanosis indicates poor oxygen content of the blood. It is important to note that the absence of cyanosis does not guarantee that there is good oxygenation (Fig. 3–10).

PUPILS

The pupils are relatively good indicators of brain oxygenation in the prehospital phase. Dilated and sluggishly reactive or non-reactive (to light) pupils may be the result of hypoxia or anoxia. However, since other factors affect pupillary response, you should consider the possible causes of pupil variations prior to interpreting this data. All clinical findings should be considered collectively.

HEMOPTYSIS

Many respiratory conditions, including pulmonary edema, pulmonary lacerations, tracheobronchial tree injuries, and pulmonary embolism, cause hemoptysis. Hemoptysis (coughing up blood) can appear in two ways. The patient may either cough up blood-stained sputum or expel frank, red blood.

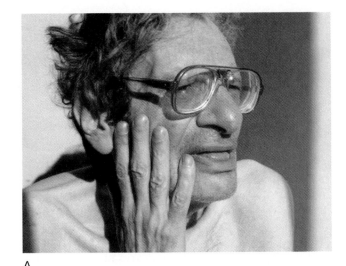

A

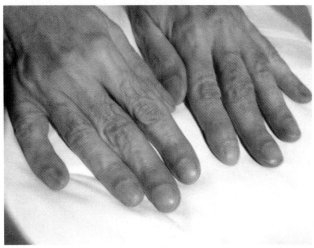

B

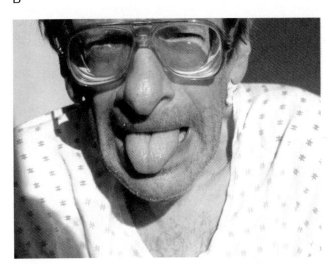

C

FIGURE 3-10. Cyanosis can be noted in the lips, nail-beds, and skin. (*A* and *B*) Patient with a longstanding congenital heart condition and hypoxia. Note cyanosis of the nail-beds and lips. (*C*) Cyanosis of the tongue. In prehospital care, patients with cyanosis should always receive supplemental oxygen and possibly positive-pressure ventilations.

ACCESSORY MUSCLE USE

Remember that the muscle groups used during normal resting breathing are the diaphragm and the intercostals. When a person is experiencing dyspnea or when the diaphragm and intercostals must work against an obstruction, the accessory muscles are used. Bulging of the neck muscles, retraction of the rib spaces, and hypercontouring of the abdominal muscles are strong indicators of increased work of breathing. This may indicate respiratory distress.

VENTILATION

Previously we discussed the normal range of respiratory rates and volumes. Most respiratory problems have an impact on the rate, depth, and sometimes the pattern of breathing. You should be familiar with these variations to recognize the underlying conditions with which they are associated.

HYPOVENTILATION. A decreased minute volume is referred to as *hypoventilation*. Remember that the min-

ute volume is the product of the tidal volume times the respiratory rate. Therefore, one may hypoventilate by decreasing either or both parameters. In the prehospital phase, tidal volume is evaluated by observing chest and abdominal movements. If respiratory movements are barely visible or "shallow," or if the respiratory rate is below 10 breaths per minute or above 30 breaths per minute (with shallow breathing), then hypoventilation should be suspected. The most common cause of hypoventilation is depression of the neuro-stimulation mechanisms. Hypoxia, drug overdose, brain injury, stroke, or any other problems that affect brain function can result in hypoventilation.

HYPERVENTILATION. An increase in the minute volume is known as *hyperventilation*. Again, an increase in either the tidal volume or the respiratory rate may result in hyperventilation. This can be caused by several underlying conditions. It is a normal compensatory response to most causes of hypoxia. Trauma to the respiratory system, obstructive disease, anxiety, and hypoxia may cause hyperventilation. It may also be caused by damage to the neuro-regulation systems in the brain, disease, or trauma. Hyperventilation may also occur as an attempt to rid the body of carbon dioxide (or acid) to compensate for metabolic acidosis (which can be caused by kidney failure, diabetes, or other problems).

TACHYPNEA. Rapid breathing is known as *tachypnea*. It simply means an increase in the respiratory rate. Tachypnea may occur without causing hyperventilation. Frequently, in circulatory failure or so-called shock states, respirations are rapid and shallow. The net result is tachypnea with hypoventilation. This is due to a significant decrease in the tidal volume that is not compensated for by the increased respiratory rate.

SPECIFIC RESPIRATORY PATTERNS. Many neurologic problems alter the basic pattern of breathing. These patterns are defined in Chapter 7 and should be reviewed for further clarification of these signs.

Auscultation of Breath Sounds

To perform *auscultation* of breath sounds properly requires patience, good technique, reasonably good hearing, and, of course, knowledge of the various sounds. In order to retrieve reliable and valid information you should listen over several locations, listen to both inspiratory and expiratory sounds, control for extraneous noises as much as possible, and be familiar with the variants in breath sounds.

TECHNIQUE FOR AUSCULTATION

Ideally, the patient should be sitting upright when the chest is auscultated. This will allow for auscultation of all aspects of the chest wall. You should apply the diaphragm portion of your stethoscope firmly to the patient's chest wall. Optimally, the chest is auscultated on both the anterior, posterior, and lateral chest wall (Fig. 3–11). This may not always be possible, since trauma patients often cannot be moved, and other patients may not tolerate the sitting position. Furthermore, a prolonged examination of the chest may not be necessary to establish a "working impression" and may contribute negatively to the seriously ill or injured patient by delaying time to definitive care.

Have the patient open his or her mouth and take slow, deep breaths following placement of the diaphragm in each location. In confused patients or patients who are unable to communicate, it may be helpful to demonstrate the desired breathing pattern. Listen carefully at each of the locations, noting any abnormalities. Usually, one breath cycle is all that is required in each location. However, should you encounter a vague ab-

normality in any given location, you should listen longer to clarify your findings. While performing this technique, you must be careful not to allow your patient to hyperventilate. If dizziness, tingling sensations, or a feeling of faintness occurs, the patient should rest before further auscultation.

TYPES OF BREATH SOUNDS

There are two primary findings that you are concerned with when auscultating for breath sounds: the character of the basic sounds (length of inspiration and expiration, the pitch of sounds, and the amplitude) and sounds that are superimposed over the basic sounds, such as rales (or crackles), wheezing, rhonchi (rattling sounds), and friction rubs. The character of breath sounds varies with the location on the chest wall and relates to air flow through the different anatomical structures of the airway, from large, windy pipes with turbulent flow to softer sounds in the terminal airways. With your stethoscope, listen to the variations of chest sounds described in the following paragraphs as you move the stethoscope to the locations pictured in Figure 3–12A.

TRACHEAL. Heard directly over the trachea, these are loud, very high-pitched, windy sounds that have a relatively equal inspiratory and expiratory phase. There is also a break between the inspiratory and expiratory phases (Fig. 3–12A and B).

BRONCHIAL. Sounds normally found at the top of the sternum and between the scapulae (posteriorly) are *bronchial*. Sounds here are also loud and high-pitched, but have a somewhat longer expiratory phase. Again, there is also a break between the phases (see Fig. 3–12A and C).

BRONCHOVESICULAR. Sounds heard over the upper/middle sternum and to its left and right are referred to as *bronchovesicular*. These sounds have a lower pitch, are somewhat softer than tracheal and bronchial sounds, and have equal inspiratory and expiratory phases (combination of air through bronchioles and alveoli). There is no break between inspiration and expiration (Fig. 3–12A and D).

VESICULAR. Sounds found in all other areas of the chest are called *vesicular*. They are lower pitched, softer sounds that normally have a longer inspiratory phase (Fig. 3–12A and E).

When routinely auscultating the chest, you will usually limit your examination to the *bronchovesicular* and *vesicular* areas.

ABNORMAL BREATH SOUNDS

Changes in the character of breath sounds and superimposed sounds may occur independently or simul-

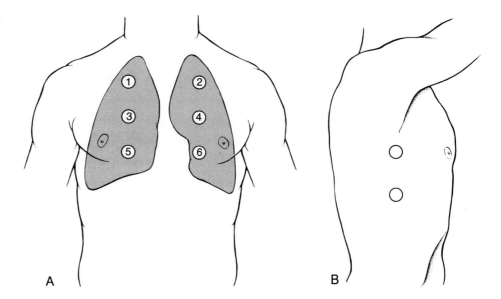

FIGURE 3–11. Locations for auscultating breath sounds on the (*A*) anterior and posterior and (*B*) lateral chest wall.

taneously. These may include any of the following sounds.

ABSENT OR DIMINISHED SOUNDS. A decrease or absence of breath sounds may occur following pneumothorax (collapse of a lung) or when there is blood in the chest cavity, as from trauma. Comparisons can sometimes be noted by comparing equivalent regions on each side of the chest wall. Other diseases such as COPD or even obesity can cause diminished breath sounds on both sides.

STRIDOR. This high-pitched sound arises from the upper airway and usually occurs on inspiration. It commonly occurs in children suffering from croup or epiglottitis, both of which cause narrowing of the upper airway. This sound may be accompanied by a "barking" cough.

RALES (CRACKLES). Crackling sounds, *rales* are usually caused by the presence of fluid in the lungs and sound similar to rubbing hair together near your ear. The intensity and the presence of rales in the inspiratory

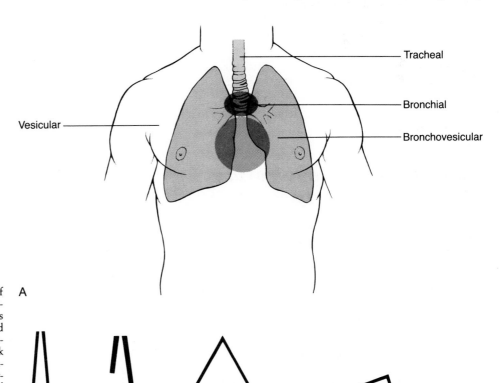

FIGURE 3–12. (*A*) Location of various breath sounds. (*B*) *Tracheal*—high-pitched, loud sounds with break between inspiration and expiration. (*C*) *Bronchial*—high-pitched, loud sounds with break between inspiration and expiration. (*D*) *Bronchovesicular*—lower-pitched, softer, and relatively equal inspiratory and expiratory phases. (*E*) *Vesicular*—lowest-pitched, softer sounds, with a longer inspiratory phase.

and expiratory phase are very much determined by the degree of fluid buildup in the lungs. Generally, excessive fluid buildup results in more coarse, loud rales. Typically, rales first appear at the base of the lungs and evolve to the upper lobe, due to the effects of gravity (Fig. 3–13).

RHONCHI.   Low-pitched continuous sounds, *rhonchi* are created by obstruction in the larger airways. Mucous plugs, tumors, and other sources of obstruction may cause rhonchi. They may occur in the inspiratory or expiratory phase (Fig. 3–13).

WHEEZES.   A *wheeze* is a sound that usually occurs on expiration and is the result of narrowed bronchioles. It is a high-pitched, whistling-type noise that lengthens the expiratory phase. More severe episodes can involve the inspiratory phase and tend to be of a greater intensity. Wheezing is commonly associated with asthma and chronic lung disease, although pulmonary edema may occasionally present with wheezing instead of rales. The expiratory phase in pulmonary edema is usually not lengthened as it is in asthma (see Fig. 3–13).

FRICTION RUB.   A *friction rub* is a coarse, grating sound created by inflamed pleura rubbing against the opposite pleural surface. It is usually found in painful local areas on the chest and is accompanied by pleuritic pain (Fig. 3–13).

SOUNDS IN COMBINATION.   It is important to realize that many conditions can result in changes of sound character and the creation of superimposed findings.

To become effective at auscultation of breath sounds, you should listen frequently in the presence of a physician, nurse, or clinical EMT instructor. There are also tapes available through medical libraries, which are an excellent source of learning. As an exercise, listen to the breath sounds of friends and family members to refine your listening skill.

Overview of Respiratory Pathophysiology

The essence of emergency respiratory care is to ensure oxygen delivery to the blood. There are several

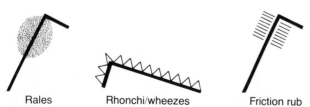

Rales   Rhonchi/wheezes   Friction rub

FIGURE 3–13. Adventitious sounds. *Rales*—moist crackles heard during inspiration or expiration. *Rhonchi and wheezes*—continuous sounds heard during inspiration and expiration. *Friction rub*—coarse, grating sounds heard over local areas of the lung, caused by rubbing of the pleural surfaces.

problems that may need to be addressed to achieve this goal.

AIRWAY BLOCKAGE

For air to reach the alveolar capillary membrane, the airway must be clear of obstruction. Because mechanisms of obstruction are different, obstructions are divided into two types, upper and lower.

UPPER AIRWAY OBSTRUCTION.   The upper airway can become obstructed by the tongue falling back against the oropharynx; food blocking the passage; or swelling occurring in the larynx, pharynx, or epiglottis.

LOWER AIRWAY OBSTRUCTION.   The lower airway can become blocked by *bronchospasm* (constriction of the bronchi or bronchioles) or when secretions such as mucus or foreign bodies become lodged in the tracheobronchial tree. Often, some bronchi or bronchioles become totally obstructed with secretions. This results in the alveoli supplied by these bronchi not participating in air exchange. Thus, when blood passes by the affected alveoli, no oxygen will be available to diffuse into the bloodstream. This is called a *shunt*.

A shunt is a condition in which some blood circulates through nonventilated alveoli and returns to the heart unoxygenated. Consider the following example carefully to better understand the significance of this problem:

Alveolus A is completely without air exchange due to a mucus plug in the bronchiole. No oxygen is being delivered to the alveolus, and no carbon dioxide is being removed. Blood passing this alveolus cannot gain oxygen or rid itself of carbon dioxide.

Alveolus B is normally ventilated and diffusion occurs across the alveolar-capillary membrane. Blood passing by this alveolus gains oxygen and releases carbon dioxide. Blood from both alveoli mixes together in the veins returning to the heart, and the *net* result is that there will be less oxygen and more carbon dioxide in the bloodstream than is normal (Fig. 3–14).

Shunts can result from many different causes, including fluid in the alveoli, collapsed alveoli, and airway obstruction. Regardless of the cause, the treatment that is usually beneficial is oxygen therapy. By increasing the concentration of oxygen breathed by the patient, the working alveoli will increase the pO_2 of the blood.

Consider the following example with the addition of oxygen therapy:

By administering oxygen-enriched air we increase the pO_2 in Alveolus B. This increases the pO_2 in the blood. Blood passing by this alveolus will leave with an increased quantity of oxygen. Alveolus A remains unaffected due to mucus plug and subsequent absence of air exchange. However, when the blood mixes in the veins returning to the heart, the net result will be a partial compensation for the nonfunctional alveolus (Fig. 3–15).

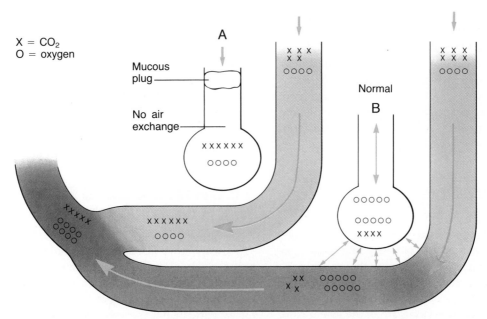

FIGURE 3–14. Effects of a shunt. Alveolus A has no ability to exchange oxygen with the atmosphere, due to a mucous plug in the bronchiole. Blood passing alveolus A has no net gain of oxygen or loss of carbon dioxide. Alveolus B has normal exchange of gases with the atmosphere. When blood passes by alveolus B, oxygen diffuses into the blood, where it is in lower concentration, and carbon dioxide diffuses to the alveolus. When the blood returning to the left side of the heart mixes, there is decreased oxygen concentration and increased carbon dioxide compared with normal.

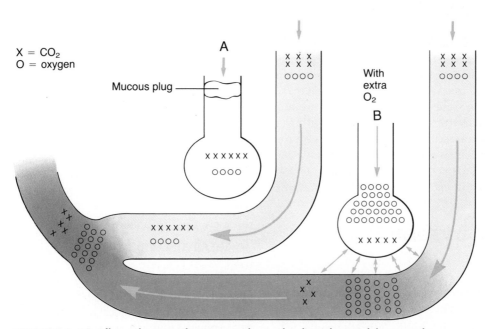

FIGURE 3–15. Effects of oxygen therapy on a shunt. Alveolus A has no ability to exchange oxygen with the atmosphere, due to a mucous plug in the bronchiole. Blood passing alveolus A has no net gain of oxygen or loss of carbon dioxide. Alveolus B has a normal exchange of gases with the atmosphere. Additionally, the patient is receiving supplemental oxygen, and the partial pressure of oxygen is much higher within the alveolus. When blood passes by alveolus B, a greater amount of oxygen diffuses into the blood. When the blood returning to the left side of the heart mixes, the increased oxygen concentration from alveolus B helps compensate for the shunt.

This demonstrates the significance of oxygen therapy when dealing with obstructions of the lower airway. Your ability to reverse conditions causing lower airway blockage is very limited. The administration of *humidified oxygen* helps by loosening dried secretions and improving alveolar oxygen levels. Another very simple treatment is decreasing the oxygen needs of the patient. By calming and reassuring the patient, you can reduce oxygen consumption and thereby help to balance supply and demand.

RESPIRATORY DEPRESSION OR ARREST

In patients who overdose with central nervous system depressants such as heroin, or when trauma damages the respiratory centers of the brain, the stimulus to breathe can be depressed. Patients may hypoventilate (slow, shallow breathing) or suffer a respiratory arrest. Respiratory arrest may also occur when the spinal cord, which contains the nerves of respiration (phrenic and intercostals) is cut due to trauma. This separates the muscles of breathing from the respiratory brain centers. Regardless of the cause of respiratory depression or arrest, management is the same: institute positive-pressure breathing and give supplemental O_2 (increase delivery of oxygen). Positive-pressure breathing is a mechanism for forcing air down to the alveoli. It achieves this goal by reversing the normal breathing process. In normal breathing, our chest cavity is enlarged and air is pulled into the lungs due to a decrease in pressure within the thorax. This was referred to earlier as the "bellows" effect. In positive-pressure breathing, air is forced into the airway by mouth-to-mouth breathing or with the aid of a mechanical resuscitator. Either mechanism provides the same benefit: alveolar ventilation. When a patient is hypoventilating or is in respiratory arrest, positive-pressure breathing must be instituted immediately.

DECREASED ALVEOLAR SURFACE

Oxygen can only enter the blood through the wall of the alveoli. When the alveolar surface is decreased or obstructed with fluid, diffusion of oxygen is impaired. This can occur in pneumothorax (when the lung collapses), when individual alveoli collapse due to surfactant insufficiency (near-drowning), from emphysema, and from other causes. When this happens, you can compensate by increasing the concentration of oxygen delivered to the normal alveoli.

DAMAGE TO MUSCLES OF RESPIRATION OR CHEST WALL

When the muscles of respiration are damaged or ribs are broken, the mechanics of air movement are neg-atively affected. The bellows effect within the chest cavity is less. Less air will be pulled in during inspiration and exhaled during exhalation. You must learn to assess the effectiveness of your patient's ventilatory efforts and, if necessary, be prepared to institute positive-pressure breathing. In certain cases, splinting of the chest wall may be indicated. When any compromise to ventilation is encountered, supplemental O_2 is recommended.

TECHNIQUES OF MANAGEMENT

Respiratory management techniques have three essential goals: (1) establish and maintain a patent airway, (2) ensure adequate ventilation, and (3) ensure adequate oxygenation. The techniques are not limited to respiratory patients but represent primary management of all emergency conditions.

Airway Management

The first step in any emergency is to ensure a patent (open) airway. Once established, it must be maintained. Methods of airway control include manual techniques, mechanical airway devices, and suctioning.

MANUAL AIRWAY TECHNIQUES

Immediate opening of the airway is the first and most basic skill of cardiopulmonary resuscitation (CPR). The most common cause of airway obstruction occurs when the tongue falls to the back of the throat as the muscles of an unconscious victim relax. Since the tongue is attached to the lower jaw, bringing the jaw forward lifts the tongue away from the back of the throat, and the airway opens. There are two techniques that are routinely used to open the airway:

HEAD TILT–CHIN LIFT. Place the fingers of one hand under the bony part of the lower jaw. Place the other hand on the victim's forehead. Lift the lower jaw upward, without completely closing the mouth, while you tilt the forehead back with your other hand. The neck should be hyperextended (see Fig. 2–25 in Chapter 2).

JAW THRUST WITHOUT HEAD TILT (MODIFIED JAW THRUST). The modified jaw thrust maneuver is performed by placing your elbows on the surface surrounding the victim. WITHOUT TILTING THE HEAD, place your index and middle fingers beneath the angle of the jaw (just below the ears). Then displace the jaw upward with your fingers. This technique should be used on patients with suspected cervical spine injury, as it opens the airway without extension of the neck. If ventilations are ineffective in the neutral position, it might be necessary to slightly extend the neck.

Manual airway techniques are used as the first step in opening the airway. Either of these methods is recognized to be effective, and they are interchangeable. When the airway must be maintained for an extended period of time, mechanical airway devices are usually used (see Fig. 2–26 in Chapter 2).

MECHANICAL AIRWAY DEVICES

The purpose of mechanical airway devices is to maintain a clear route to the tracheobronchial tree by keeping the tongue away from the pharyngeal wall. Certain devices will prevent air escape into the esophagus and the risk of aspiration. The principal methods include the oropharyngeal airway, nasopharyngeal airway, esophageal airway, and endotracheal intubation. All of these techniques involve the application of certain principles that ensure the correct insertion of these devices and minimize any complications.

OROPHARYNGEAL AIRWAY. The *oropharyngeal airway* is the most basic airway device and is designed to elevate the tongue away from the oropharynx in unconscious states. Although there are a variety of types, the basic design is essentially the same. They consist of a curved plastic device that extends from just anterior to the lips down the base of the tongue in the oropharynx. The outer portion has a flange that extends over the mouth's opening to help prevent the device from slipping into the airway.

P R O C E D U R E   3 – 1   INSERTING AN OROPHARYNGEAL AIRWAY

1. Measure the airway to ensure proper placement (Fig. 3–16A).
2. Place the index finger of one hand on the top teeth and the thumb on the lower teeth and apply pressure in opposite directions (Fig. 3–16B).
3. Insert the device into the mouth with the tip pointing toward the roof of the mouth.
4. Be careful not to push the tongue into the oropharynx, and rotate the device into place just behind the tongue.
5. *If the patient begins to gag, remove the airway immediately* and do not attempt reinsertion. This could result in vomiting and aspiration of vomitus.
6. Once the airway is in place, test the patency of the airway by ventilating the patient (Fig. 3–16C). If you are unable to ventilate, remove the airway, maintain manual maneuvers, and reinsert, when possible (Fig. 3–16A).

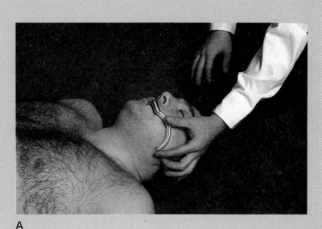

A

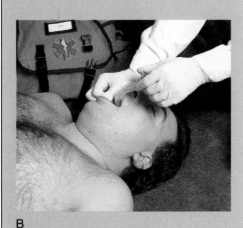

B

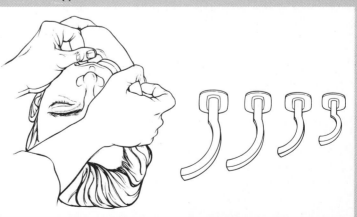

FIGURE 3–16. (A) Measure the airway from the center of the patient's mouth to the angle of the jaw. (B) To open the mouth, place your index finger on the top teeth and the thumb on the lower teeth and apply pressure in opposite directions. Insert the oropharyngeal airway in the mouth with the tip pointing toward the roof of the mouth.

Continued

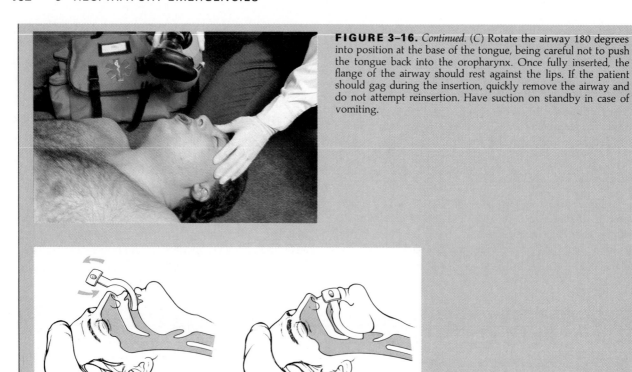

FIGURE 3–16. *Continued.* (C) Rotate the airway 180 degrees into position at the base of the tongue, being careful not to push the tongue back into the oropharynx. Once fully inserted, the flange of the airway should rest against the lips. If the patient should gag during the insertion, quickly remove the airway and do not attempt reinsertion. Have suction on standby in case of vomiting.

The oropharyngeal airway can also be inserted using a tongue blade:

- The tongue is retained in the lower area of the mouth with the tongue blade (Fig. 3–17A, B, and C).
- The airway is then inserted with the tip pointing toward the tongue and is directed into the pharynx.

Insertion of the oropharyngeal airway should be done without undue interruption in ventilation. As a rule, ventilations should not be interrupted for more than 10 seconds.

NASOPHARYNGEAL AIRWAY.   The *nasopharyngeal airway* has the same purpose as the oropharyngeal airway—to maintain the tongue away from the pharynx. It is used in instances where an oropharyngeal airway cannot be tolerated by the patient or when the mouth cannot be accessed due to trauma or clenching of the teeth. The nasopharyngeal airway consists of a soft rubber tube that, when properly positioned, extends from the nares down into the oropharynx. It also has a lip that extends around the outside of the nose to prevent slippage into the airway. The nasopharyngeal airway is measured from the nares to the tip of the ear.

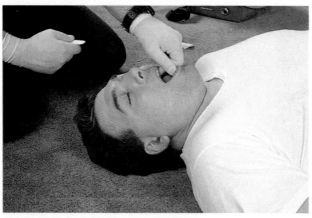

A

FIGURE 3–17. Measure the airway as described in Figure 3–16. (A) Open the mouth using the crossed-finger technique and retain the tongue in the lower jaw with the tongue blade.

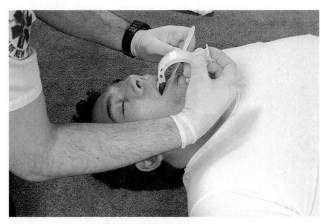

B

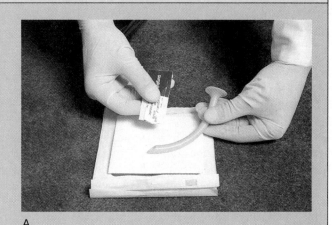

B

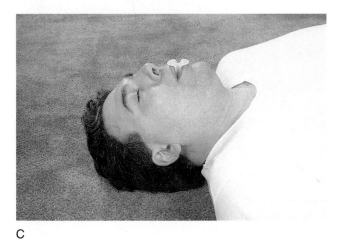

C

FIGURE 3–17. *Continued.* (B) Insert the oropharyngeal airway into the mouth with the tip pointing toward the floor of the mouth until the tip is at the base of the tongue. If gagging should occur, proceed as described in Figure 3–16. (C) Fully inserted airway.

PROCEDURE 3–2   INSERTING A NASOPHARYNGEAL AIRWAY

1. Lubricate the outside of the tube with a water-soluble gel to decrease irritation to the nasal passage (Fig. 3–18A).
2. Slowly insert the tube into either nasal passage. Do not force it in or nasal bleeding may occur, resulting in potential aspiration. Gentle, firm pressure sometimes results in dilation of one nasal passage and facilitates insertion (Fig. 3–18B and C).
3. If you are unable to successfully insert the tube in one nostril, you may try the opposite one.
4. Once inserted, test patency by initiating a ventilation and observing the chest rise while listening and feeling for air exchange.

A

FIGURE 3–18. (A) Lubricate the airway, using a water-soluble gel.

Continued

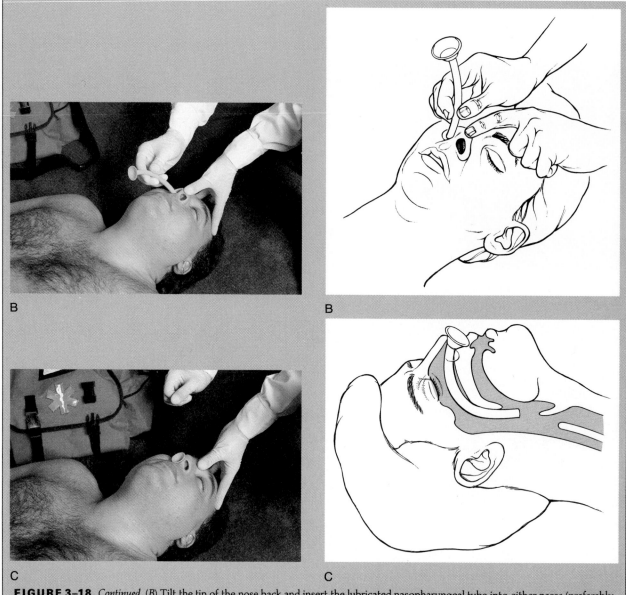

FIGURE 3–18. *Continued.* (B) Tilt the tip of the nose back and insert the lubricated nasopharyngeal tube into either nares (preferably the right). (C) Gently advance the tube. If you feel resistance; do not force it; rather, try the other nostril. Continue insertion until the flange of the airway rests against the opening of the nares. Insertion of the airway between the tongue and posterior pharynx ensures an open upper air passage.

ESOPHAGEAL GASTRIC TUBE AIRWAY. The esophageal gastric tube airway (EGTA) is a device designed to obstruct the esophagus with a gastric tube while permitting positive-pressure ventilation through a mask device. The main objective of the device is to prevent air from entering the stomach during mask ventilation and therefore avoid gastric distention. The insertion technique is relatively simple. However, failure to adhere to proper technique can result in severe complications, including anoxia, esophageal or tracheobronchial trauma, tracheal obstruction, and *necrosis* (tissue death) to the wall of the esophagus. The esophageal airway should be utilized only for patients who are totally unresponsive and in need of positive-pressure ventilation.

The EGTA consists of an esophageal tube, mask, and gastric lavage tube. The esophageal tube, which is inserted in the esophagus, has a distal inflatable cuff. Once inserted, the cuff is inflated by a syringe through a one-way valve with about 35 ml of air and obliterates the esophageal opening. The inflated cuff serves to prevent air from entering the stomach and vomitus from entering the airway and should be checked for leaks before the device is inserted. The mask snaps over the esophageal tube and the patient is ventilated through one opening while a gastric tube can be inserted through a second hole into the stomach to relieve distention (Fig. 3–19).

FIGURE 3–19. The esophageal gastric tube airway consists of a gastric tube that is inserted into the esophagus. This tube has a central lumen that allows the insertion of a gastric lavage tube to relieve distention. The mask has two ports: one for the gastric tube and the other for ventilation to the upper airway. The tube has a cuffed end that is inflated with approximately 35 ml of air to close off the esophagus and prevent air from entering the stomach and gastric regurgitation.

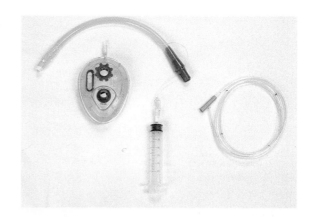

PROCEDURE 3–3   INSERTING THE ESOPHAGEAL GASTRIC TUBE AIRWAY

1. Place the patient in the supine position, with the head in a neutral or slightly flexed position. Grasp the lower jaw between your thumb and index finger and pull the jaw up away from the pharynx (Fig. 3–20A).
2. While maintaining this position, insert the tube against the posterior wall of the pharynx and down into the esophagus until the mask comes in contact with the face (Fig. 3–20B and C). If you encounter resistance, remove the tube and attempt to reinsert.
3. Seal the mask against the face and ventilate through the mask while observing for chest excursions (Fig. 3–20D).
4. Once you observe the chest rise, auscultate both lung fields with your stethoscope to confirm placement. Then inflate the cuff with 35 ml of air and continue ventilation (Fig. 3–20E and F).

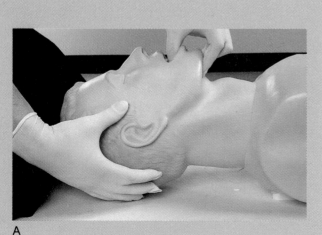
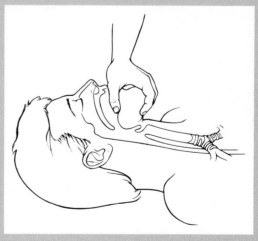

A

FIGURE 3–20. (A) Place the patient in the supine position, keeping the head in the neutral or slightly flexed position, and grasp the lower jaw between your thumb and index finger.

Continued

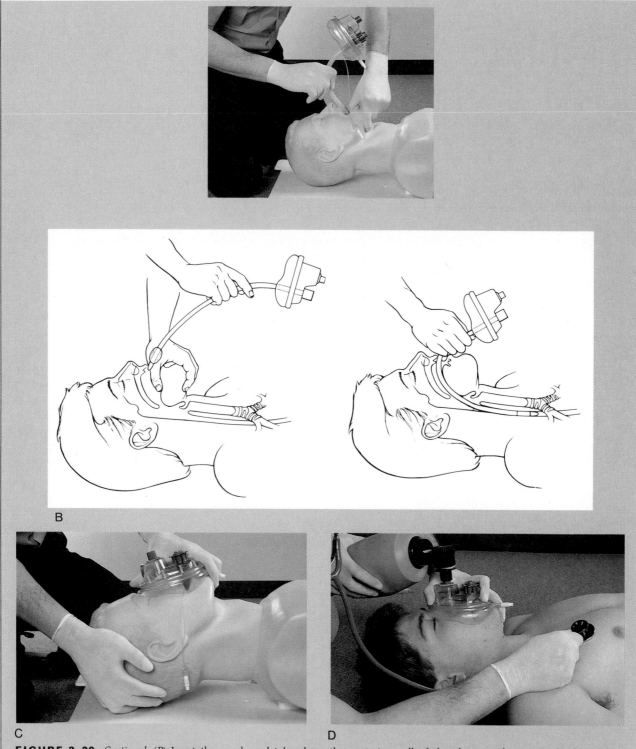

FIGURE 3–20. *Continued.* (*B*) Insert the esophageal tube along the posterior wall of the pharynx. If gagging should occur, discontinue the procedure and do not attempt reinsertion. (*C*) Continue inserting the tube until the face mask comes in contact with the face. (*D*) Seal the mask against the face with the nose portion of the mask aligned with the bridge of the nose, and ventilate the patient while observing chest rise. Confirm placement by auscultating the lungs and stomach with a stethoscope.

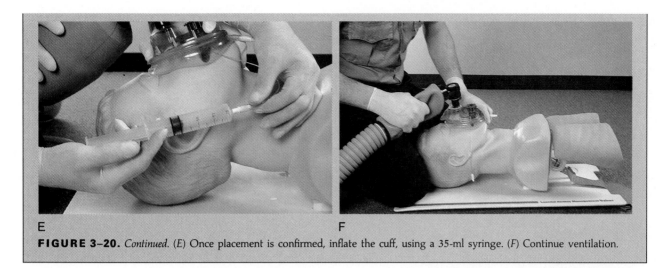

FIGURE 3–20. *Continued.* (E) Once placement is confirmed, inflate the cuff, using a 35-ml syringe. (F) Continue ventilation.

If difficulty is encountered during insertion, ventilation should be resumed with mouth-to-mouth, mouth-to-nose, or other quickly applied positive-pressure techniques. As a rule, the insertion process should not exceed 15 to 30 seconds from the last ventilation to the post-insertion ventilation. A "trick of the trade" that might help you to remember this is to hold your breath at the point of the patient's last ventilation. When you feel the need for your next breath, you should immediately resume ventilation of the patient as well.

Contraindications. There are some instances in which the EGTA must not be used. They include the following:

- In children under 16 years of age or less than 5 feet tall. The tube is too long for these individuals.
- Persons over 7 feet tall, since the cuff would rest directly behind the trachea and result in a posterior collapse of the trachea.
- In persons with known esophageal disease or who have ingested caustic poisons. Here the integrity of the esophageal wall may be compromised, resulting in rupture.
- When there are facial injuries that prevent a tight seal with the mask.
- In conscious or breathing patients and patients who gag upon insertion of the device.

Removal of the EGTA. When removing the EGTA, you should exercise great concern for aspiration. There is a high incidence of vomiting following removal of this device. Unless there is a need for immediate removal, the patient should have an endotracheal tube inserted prior to removal of the EGTA. However, if the patient becomes responsive and develops a gag reflex, then the device should be removed immediately while turning the head to one side (see Figure 3–20G). Have a suction machine ready in case vomiting should occur.

ENDOTRACHEAL INTUBATION. The most effective form of airway management is *endotracheal intubation.* It

requires skill and practice to be performed properly. Most EMTs are not trained to perform endotracheal intubation. However, as an EMT you may assist an advanced EMT during intubation, and some emergency medical services systems may include the skill in future protocols.

Endotracheal intubation is performed with the aid of an instrument called a *laryngoscope.* A laryngoscope is a plastic or metal device used to see the vocal cords in order to insert the endotracheal tube. It consists of a handle that contains batteries and a detachable blade with a light at the distal end. There are two types of blades that may be used——*straight or curved.* The choice of blades depends on which technique is preferred, since the technique varies with each type. To light the bulb, the blade is attached to a bar at the end of the handle and then brought to a 90-degree angle to the handle, causing it to light.

The tube that is inserted into the trachea is called an *endotracheal tube.* One end extends out of the mouth and has a "universal" adapter that can connect to various free-flow and positive-pressure devices. The other end, which is inserted into the trachea has an inflatable cuff around its outer surface. This cuff can be inflated and deflated via a pilot tube with a one-way valve.

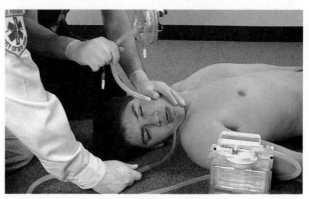

G

FIGURE 3–20. *Continued.* (G) If the patient should begin to gag or become responsive, turn the head and remove the airway, keeping suction on standby.

PROCEDURE 3-4   INSERTING AN ENDOTRACHEAL TUBE

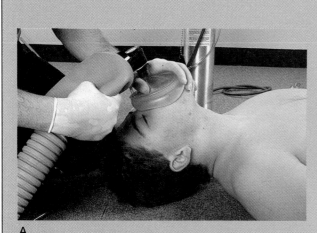

A

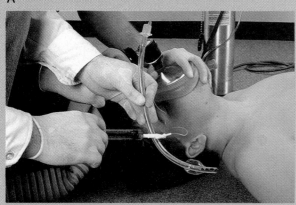

B

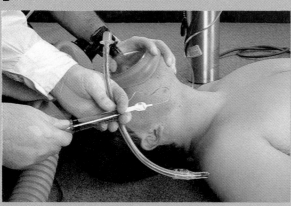

C

1. Ventilate with a mask device (Fig. 3–21*A*).
2. Test the cuff on the endotracheal tube for leaks (Fig. 3–21*B* and *C*).
3. Always have suction ready. Stimulation of the oropharynx during intubation attempts may induce vomiting in patients with no gag reflex.
4. Open the mouth, using the cross finger technique, and place the head in the sniffing position (Fig. 3–21*D* and *E*).
5. Holding the laryngoscope handle in your left hand, place the blade into the mouth, being careful not to strike the teeth (Fig. 3–21*E*). Do not use the blade to open the mouth. (Broken teeth are one of the most common complications of endotracheal intubation and result from leverage, not insertion.)
6. Under direct visualization, when you reach the uvula, move the tip of the blade forward toward the epiglottis. With a curved blade, the tip of the blade should rest just above the epiglottis in the space called the vallecula (Fig. 3–21*F*). You should see the epiglottis at the tip of your blade. When using a straight blade, lift the edge of the epiglottis directly with the tip of the blade.
7. Lift the laryngoscope anteriorly and superiorly until you visualize the glottic opening (Fig. 3–21*G*). Do not use the teeth for leverage during intubation, as this may result in broken teeth.
8. Once the vocal cords are visualized, the endotracheal tube should be inserted between the cords so that the cuff lies just distal to them. It is crucial that you observe the insertion of the tube (Fig. 3–21*H*).
9. Inflate the cuff using the syringe and attempt ventilation while observing the chest rise while your partner auscultates the lungs and stomach with a stethoscope to confirm proper placement (Fig. 3–21*I*).
10. If breath sounds are heard on only one side (usually the right), you should deflate the cuff and pull it out slowly (about an inch at a time) and recheck placement after each repositioning until breath sounds can be heard on both sides.
11. Once inserted properly, an oropharyngeal airway should be placed alongside the endotracheal tube so that the patient will not occlude it by biting down with his or her teeth. Tape or tie the tube in place (Fig. 3–21*J*).

FIGURE 3–21. (*A*) Prior to endotracheal intubation, the patient is ventilated with a mask device (pocket mask, bag-valve-mask, etc.). (*B*) The syringe is attached to the one-way valve connected to the bladder of the endotracheal tube. Air is introduced and the bladder is checked for tears. (*C*) Then the air is withdrawn. (*D*) Upon command, ventilation is interrupted and the head is placed in the hyperextended position (a folded sheet can be placed below the occipital region to displace the head forward into the sniffing position). This technique aligns the mouth and glottic opening. (*E*) Using the crossed-finger technique described previously, open the mouth and advance the laryngoscope blade toward the pharynx, while sweeping the tongue to the left side of the oral cavity. Use special care not to strike the teeth. (*F*) When using a curved blade, slide the tip of the blade into the *vallecula* (the space between the epiglottis and the base of the tongue). You will be able to visualize the epiglottis at the tip of the blade. When using a straight blade, place the tip of the blade directly beneath the epiglottis. Once the tip of the blade is in place, lift the laryngoscope handle up at a 45-degree plane to the floor. *Do not rotate the blade back on the teeth.* Using the teeth as a fulcrum will often result in breaking the upper teeth. While maintaining visualization of the glottic opening, slide the endotracheal tube into the right side of the mouth and through the glottic opening so that the cuffed end of the tube lies just beyond the vocal cords.

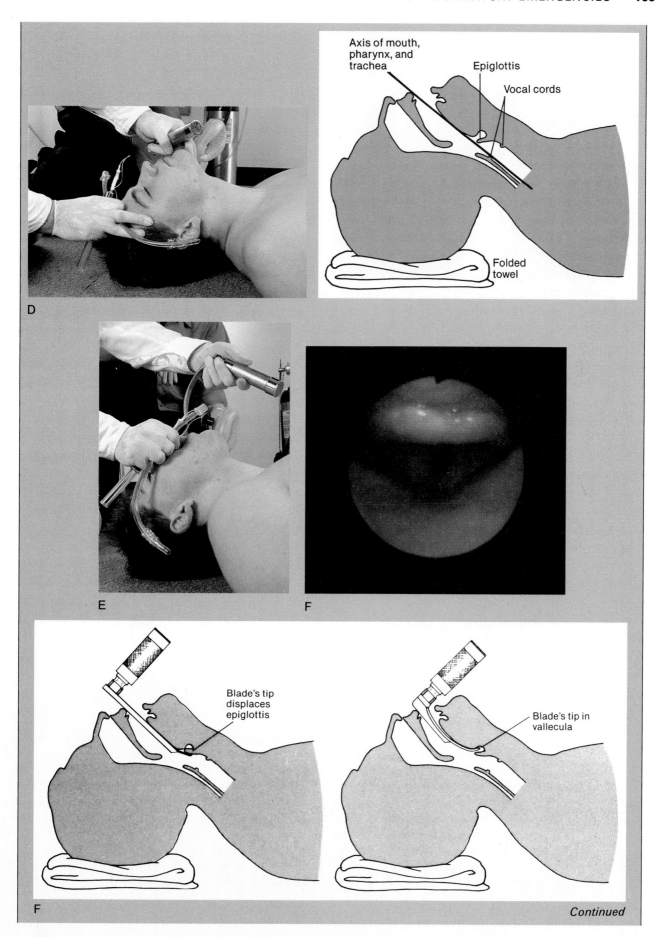

Axis of mouth, pharynx, and trachea

Epiglottis

Vocal cords

Folded towel

D

E

F

Blade's tip displaces epiglottis

Blade's tip in vallecula

F

Continued

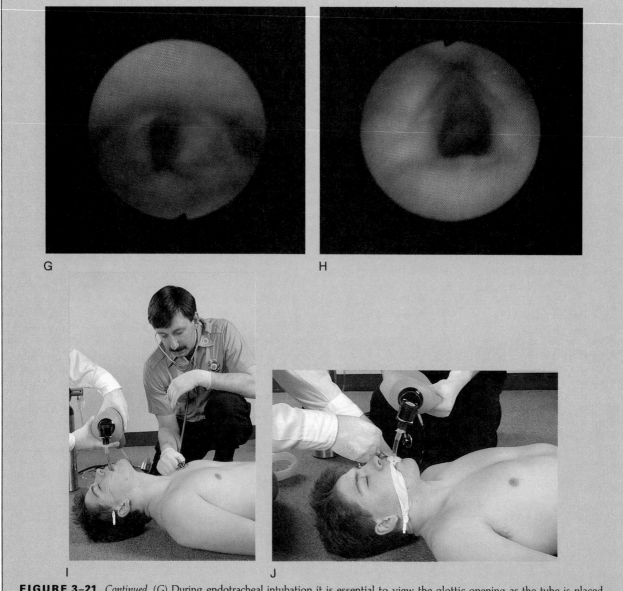

FIGURE 3–21. *Continued.* (G) During endotracheal intubation it is essential to view the glottic opening as the tube is placed in the trachea. It appears as a dark opening with the vocal cords on either side. (H) If the patient is breathing, time the tube insertion with inspiration, when the vocal cords move to the side. (I) Inflate the cuff using the syringe. Attempt ventilation while observing chest rise. Auscultate the lungs and stomach with a stethoscope to confirm proper placement. If ventilation is heard only on one side, deflate the cuff and pull the tube out an inch at a time until both lungs are ventilated. (J) Place an oropharyngeal airway adjacent to the tube and secure the tube in place with tape, umbilical tape, or specific device used for this purpose. (Drawing in *D*, from Kersten LD: Comprehensive Respiratory Nursing: A Decision Making Approach. Philadelphia, WB Saunders, 1989, p. 642; *F*, *G*, and *H*, from Sunil Nath, MD.)

The entire procedure of intubation should take no more than 15 to 30 seconds from the last ventilation to the postinsertion ventilation. Again, the breath-holding technique may be tried to ensure adequate ventilation of the patient. Hypoxia due to delay in the technique is a serious complication that may result in brain damage or death. Other potential complications include broken teeth, intubation of the esophagus or mainstem bronchus, direct injury to the structures of the airway, and aspiration of teeth, blood, or vomitus into the lungs.

TUBE SIZE SELECTION. Tubes for adults range in size from 7.0 mm (internal diameter) to 10.0 mm. The average adult will usually accommodate an 8.0-mm tube, but small females may require a 7.0-mm tube and large males may need a 9.0-mm tube. A good rule for small children is the diameter of their little finger, which should approximate the tube diameter. The volume of air in the cuff varies according to the type of tube and size of the patient. Tubes without a cuff are used for infants and small children. Consult your senior instructor to discuss local equipment. Table 3–1 lists the tracheal tube sizes for patients according to age and sex.

MAGILL FORCEPS. The Magill forceps is an adjunct device used in combination with a laryngoscope to

TABLE 3–1. Endotracheal Tube Sizes

Age of Patient	Endotracheal Tube Size (mm)
Newborn	2.5–3.0
1 year	4.5
2 years	5.0
4 years	5.5
6 years	6.0
8 years	6.5
10 years	7.0
12 years	7.5
Adult male	8.0–9.5
Adult female	7.5–8.5

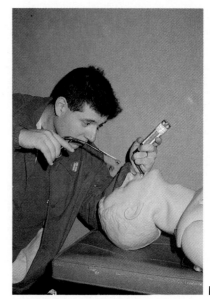

FIGURE 3–21. *Continued*

remove foreign bodies of the upper airway. The device is used when basic life support maneuvers (abdominal thrusts, finger sweeps, etc.) have failed to remove the obstruction. The forceps comes in both adult and pediatric sizes and consists of a "scissor" style handle with forceps that extend at a 90-degree angle, with a rounded tip used to grasp the foreign body (Fig. 3–21*J*).

To remove a foreign body, the airway and foreign body are visualized by using the laryngoscope in the same manner described previously. The Magill forceps is inserted in the airway with the handle pointing downward (Fig. 3–21*K*). The foreign body is then grasped with the tips of the forceps and carefully removed from the airway. If upon removal the patient does not begin to ventilate spontaneously, positive-pressure ventilation is provided.

Positive-Pressure Ventilation

Once an airway has been established, the need for ventilation must be determined. If a patient's own respiratory efforts are inadequate, a variety of techniques are available to positively force air into the lungs. They include mouth-to-mouth and mouth-to-nose breathing, the pocket mask, the bag valve mask, and the manually triggered resuscitator. Each technique requires a conscientious approach by the EMT to ensure adequate ventilation. Adequate ventilation is assessed on the basis of chest excursion and other indicators of oxygenation such as skin color and pupils.

MOUTH-TO-MOUTH AND MOUTH-TO-NOSE BREATHING

Mouth-to-mouth and mouth-to-nose breathing is the most basic form of positive-pressure breathing. It is a reliable method of positive-procedure ventilation, since the EMT actively feels lung expansion and is in a good position to closely observe chest excursion.

When a good seal cannot be made due to injury to the mouth or with edentulous patients (patients without teeth), the alternative procedure for delivering air, mouth-to-nose breathing, may be applied.

P R O C E D U R E   3 – 5   *MOUTH-TO-MOUTH BREATHING*

1. Open the airway with the head tilt–chin lift or modified jaw thrust (Fig. 3–22*A* and *B*).
2. Once the need for mouth-to-mouth breathing has been established, seal your mouth completely around the victim's mouth while pinching the nose and maintaining an airway (Fig. 3–23).
3. When using the modified jaw thrust, seal the nose with your cheek during ventilation.
4. Give two smooth breaths while observing for chest rise out of the corner of your eye. Take your mouth away from the patient's mouth after each breath so that you can take another breath and avoid breathing the exhaled air from the patient.
5. Assuming that the pulse is present (cardiac arrest is covered in the next chapter), administer one breath every 5 seconds until the patient begins to breathe adequately (determined by minute volume).
6. If the patient is breathing at an adequate rate but inadequate depth, assist ventilations by providing a breath each time the patient attempts to breathe, thereby synchronizing your efforts with the patient's.

Continued

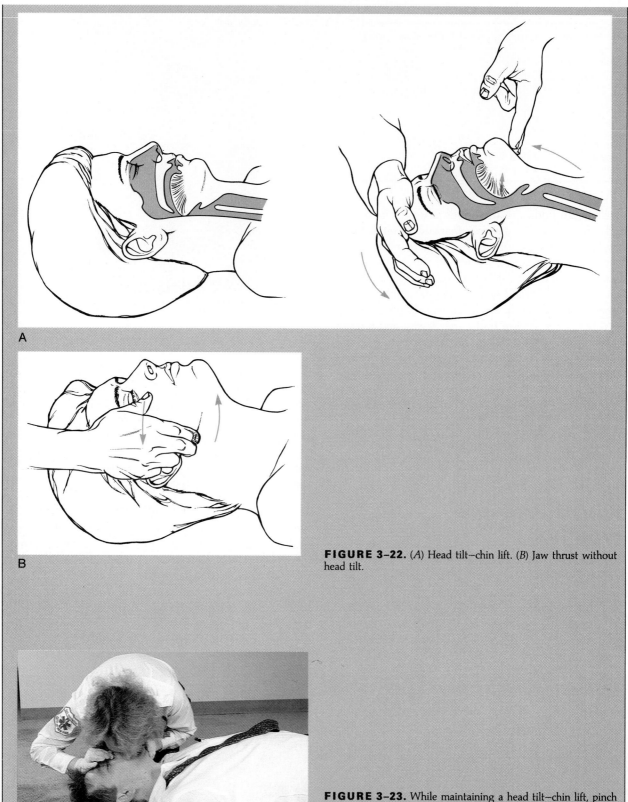

A

B

FIGURE 3–22. (*A*) Head tilt–chin lift. (*B*) Jaw thrust without head tilt.

FIGURE 3–23. While maintaining a head tilt–chin lift, pinch the nose. Seal your mouth around the victim's mouth and administer a smooth breath while observing for chest to rise. The breath should be given slowly over 1 to 1.5 seconds to avoid gastric distention. Remove your mouth from the victim's mouth to take the next breath, and allow the victim to exhale.

PROCEDURE 3-6   MOUTH-TO-NOSE BREATHING

1. Place your hand over the victim's mouth to seal it.
2. Place your mouth over the victim's nose, providing an effective seal with your lips.
3. Blow air forcefully through the patient's nose (Fig. 3–24).
4. The mouth should be opened during exhalation to permit the outflow of air.

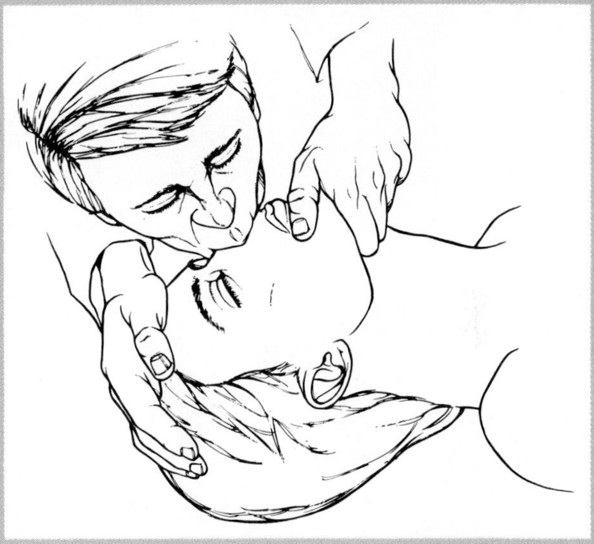

FIGURE 3–24. Maintaining a head tilt–chin lift, seal your mouth around the patient's nose while closing the patient's mouth to prevent air leakage during ventilation. Administer a smooth breath while observing chest rise as described in Figure 3–23. At the end of each breath, remove your mouth from the patient's nose and allow the patient to exhale while you take your next breath.

THE POCKET MASK

The *pocket mask* is a transparent, semirigid mask that, when properly placed, seals around the patient's mouth and nose with an air-filled bladder. The great advantage is that supplemental O_2 can be given and it eliminates the need for you to make direct contact with the patient's mouth or nose. It does not, however, guarantee that there will be no contamination risks from the patient to the EMT (Fig. 3–25).

Like mouth-to-mouth resuscitation, it is an extremely reliable form of ventilation due to the use of two hands in creating a seal with the mask, and because of the sense of lung compliance the EMT can feel. Having two hands available for creating a seal is an advantage over using the bag-valve-mask.

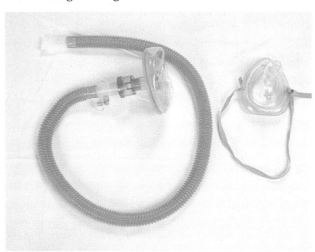

FIGURE 3–25. Two examples of pocket masks. Pocket masks consist of a mask, one-way valve, and, on some units, an oxygen inlet to provide enriched concentrations of oxygen.

PROCEDURE 3-7   USING THE POCKET MASK FOR RESUSCITATION

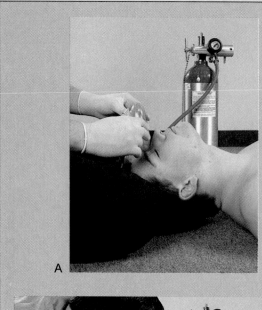

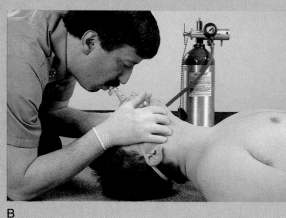

1. Place the mask about the patient's mouth and nose, using the bridge of the nose as a guide for correct placement (Fig. 3–26*A*).

   Note: Positioning of the mask is critical, as gaps between the mask and face will result in leakage.

2. The mask is sealed by placing the heel of each hand on the border of the mask's edge and hyperextending the head and neck.

3. Ventilations are then administered (in the same sequence and at the same rate as mouth-to-mouth) while observing chest excursion (Fig. 3–26*B*).

FIGURE 3–26. (*A*) Position the mask on the patient's face with the nose portion aligned with the bridge of the nose to ensure an airtight fit. (*B*) Place both thumbs and the fatty portion of your palm below the thumb along the outer edge of the mask. Place your index, middle, and ring fingers at the angle of the jaw and perform a jaw lift while squeezing the mask onto the patient's face. Provide a breath through the one-way valve in the same manner described in Figure 3–23, while observing chest rise. Supplemental oxygen can be provided at a flow rate of 15 liters per minute to achieve an oxygen delivery of 50%.

Oxygen can be adapted to some pocket masks through a port on top of the mask. Flow rates of 10 to 12 liters of oxygen per minute will result in oxygen concentrations of approximately 50%.

THE BAG-VALVE-MASK

The *bag-valve-mask* is the most common mechanical aid used in emergency care to initially administer positive-pressure breathing. It can also be the most *unreliable* unless it is used properly. The typical unit consists of a bag that has a capacity of approximately 1200 to 1500 ml of air and a one-way valve that ensures a unidirectional flow of air to the patient. Exhaled air escapes through an exit port on the valve into the environment. A mask is attached to a universal opening adjacent to

the valve. The mask should be transparent (so you can observe for possible vomiting) and capable of achieving an adequate seal. As a rule, air-filled masks tend to be superior in sealing tightly around the patient's mouth and nose. Some units are equipped with a pressure "pop-off" valve to avoid excessive airway pressure during ventilation. In patients with bronchial constriction or other sources of increased resistance, it may be necessary to disable this valve to ensure delivery of adequate volumes of air to the patient.

The unit also has an oxygen inlet that provides increased oxygen concentrations to the patient (Fig. 3–27). A bag-valve-mask with an oxygen-collecting reservoir is capable of delivering 90 to 100% oxygen (Fig. 3–28). Be sure to familiarize yourself with the unit on your ambulance.

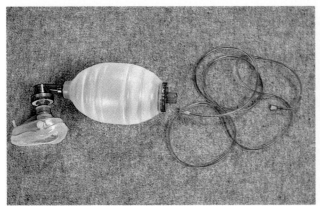

FIGURE 3–27. A bag-valve-mask with oxygen tubing can deliver approximately 50% oxygen (assuming a ventilation rate of 1 breath every 5 seconds).

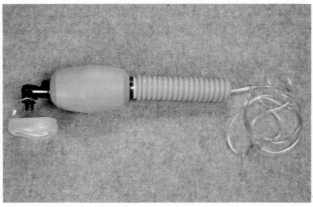

FIGURE 3–28. A bag-valve-mask with an oxygen reservoir can deliver approximately 90% oxygen. The reservoir can consist of long tubes or plastic bags that collect oxygen between breaths.

PROCEDURE 3 – 8   APPLYING A BAG-VALVE-MASK

1. Carefully place the mask about the patient's mouth and nose (Fig. 3–29*A*) in the same way as the pocket mask and seal the mask by grasping it with your index finger and thumb like a "C" clamp. Your remaining fingers should maintain an open airway by lifting the bone edge of the jaw.
2. Squeeze the bag while observing for chest rise (Fig. 3–29*B*). Sometimes it is helpful to squeeze the mask against your abdomen or thigh to maximize deflation of the bag.
3. Oxygen is added to the bag or its reservoir if so adapted.

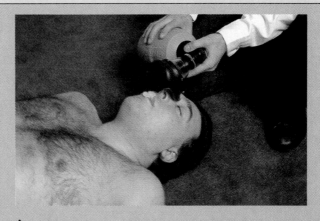

A

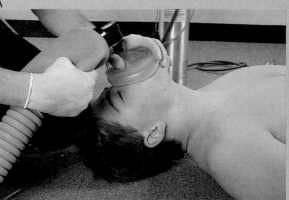

B

FIGURE 3–29. (*A*) Position the mask on the face with the nose portion of the mask aligned with the bridge of the nose. (*B*) The mask is held in place using a "C" clamp technique with the index finger and thumb. The remaining fingers grasp the jaw and execute a chin-lift procedure. While maintaining a head tilt–chin lift, squeeze the bag smoothly with the other hand and observe for chest rise. The bag can be squeezed against the side of the patient's head or your thigh to assist in collapse of the bag.

Continued

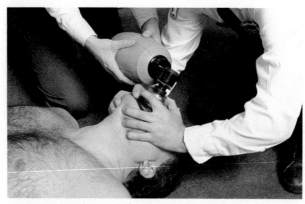

FIGURE 3–29. *Continued.* (C) *Two-handed technique*—when there are enough personnel, one rescuer can achieve a two-handed seal while the other squeezes the bag with two hands. This facilitates more effective ventilation.

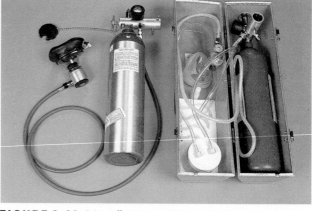

FIGURE 3–30. Manually triggered demand-valve resuscitator.

It is essential to closely monitor chest excursion when using this device, as low tidal volumes are likely when poor technique is used. Figure 3–29C illustrates the two-handed technique for sealing the mask while another EMT squeezes the bag.

MANUALLY TRIGGERED, DEMAND-VALVE RESUSCITATOR

The manually triggered resuscitator can achieve the highest delivered oxygen concentrations of any positive-pressure device (Fig. 3–30). It is an oxygen-powered apparatus and delivers 100% oxygen to the patient's airway. It is activated by a push button or lever located on the valve, or by the negative pressure (demand) created by a breathing patient's inspiratory effort. The valve and regulator reduce the delivered pressure to about 40 to 60 pounds per square inch (PSI) and flow rates to 40 liters/minute, which is a safe level for the adult patient. This device should not be used in infants and small children. Application of the device does tend to cause gastric distention, due to the rapid increase in airway pressure. The patient's abdomen should be observed closely to avoid vomiting secondary to excessive pressure within the stomach. If distention is noted, it may be wise to switch over to a bag-valve-mask or pocket mask.

PROCEDURE 3–9   MANUALLY TRIGGERED RESUSCITATOR

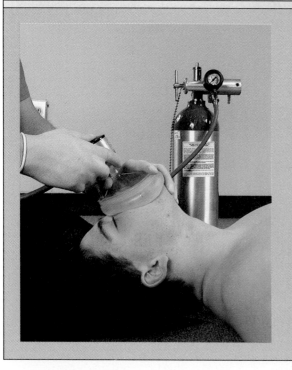

1. Correctly place the mask on the face in the same manner as previously described for the bag-valve-mask.
2. Compress the button or lever until visible chest excursion can be seen and then immediately release to avoid gastric distention (Fig. 3–31).
3. If the patient is breathing and activating the unit, it may be necessary to deliver additional volume by compressing the button or lever.

FIGURE 3–31. Place the mask in the same manner described in Figure 3–29A. While maintaining an airtight seal and lifting the jaw, squeeze the lever (or press the button on top of the device) and observe for chest rise. A breathing patient may trigger the device with the negative pressure generated by his or her inhalation (demand valve).

TABLE 3–2. Positive-Pressure Ventilation Methods and Disadvantages

Method	Advantages	Disadvantages
Mouth-to-mouth	Reliable volume delivery	Fear of disease Low oxygen percentages
Pocket mask	Reliable volume delivery Feel lung expansion	Fatigue of rescuer Lower oxygen percentages
Bag-valve-mask	Higher oxygen delivery Feel lung expansion	Unreliable volume delivery
Demand valve	Higher oxygen delivery	Gastric distention

Note: Pressure in the oxygen cylinder should be monitored closely during operation to ensure an adequate driving force for ventilation. As a rule, when tank pressures fall below 500 Ib, the cylinder should be changed. Review Table 3–2, which summarizes the advantages and disadvantages of the different methods of delivering positive-pressure ventilations.

Oxygen Therapy

Oxygen is a colorless, odorless gas that is plentiful in our environment. Normal atmospheric air contains approximately 21% oxygen. When patients become hypoxic, one method of improving oxygenation of tissues is to increase the oxygen content of their inspired air: *oxygen therapy*. This is achieved by administration of *cylinder oxygen* through a delivery system that includes a regulator that reduces the pressure of the gas and controls its rate of flow, plus oxygen tubing through which the gas is delivered to the final component, the delivery device.

OXYGEN CYLINDERS

Oxygen is carried by the EMT in a steel or aluminum cylinder. This cylinder is extremely strong and contains a proportionately large quantity of gas that is stored at very high pressure (usually 2000 PSI). These cylinders are color coded green, which identifies them as containing oxygen. Other gases are identified with various colors. This reduces the chance of inadvertently administering the wrong gas. Another safeguard is called the *pin index safety system*. This method varies the openings at the top of the cylinder valve so that the tank only accepts a special regulator designed for oxygen (Fig. 3–32A and B). The holes include one opening through which air flows out of the cylinder and two other openings that receive stabilizing pins that extend out of the regulators. Larger oxygen cylinders do not have this pin index system and use a thread system.

CYLINDER SIZES. Oxygen cylinders are available in several sizes. The smaller sizes are referred to as *D* or *E* cylinders. These tanks are portable and designed to bring oxygen to the patient's side. Larger cylinders are identified as *M* or *H* and are used to store large quantities of gas in the vehicle. Obviously, as the size

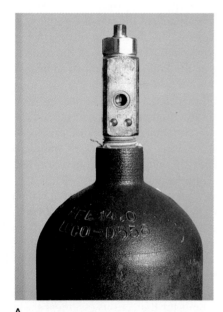
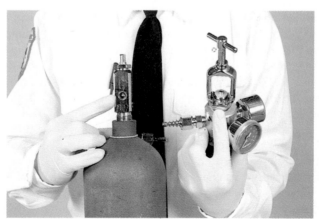

A   B

FIGURE 3–32. (*A*) An oxygen pin index system consists of two small holes below an opening on the cylinder valve (where gas exits the cylinder). (*B*) These holes interface with the pins on a regulator that prevents the misplacement of an oxygen regulator on a cylinder containing a different gas (i.e., nitrous oxide).

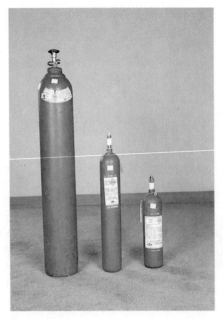 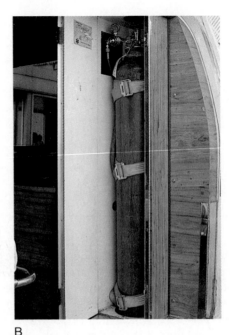

A   B

FIGURE 3–33. (*A*) Oxygen D, E, and M cylinders. (*B*) An M cylinder stored in an ambulance cabinet.

of the cylinder increases, so does the volume of gas it can contain (Fig. 3–33*A* and *B*).

REGULATORS. The regulator is a device that reduces the very high pressure of gas within the cylinder to a level that will not injure the patient. There are essentially two types of regulators: single-staged or double-staged. The single-staged regulators have only one phase of pressure reduction and usually result in an exiting pressure of approximately 40 to 70 PSI. This is the most common type of regulator used in emergency medical services.

A double-staged regulator reduces gas pressure in a two step process. First the pressure is reduced as the gas enters the regulator to approximately 700 PSI and is further reduced at the interface with the liter flow gauge to 40 to 70 PSI. This two-staged reduction has the advantage of saving wear and tear on the reducing valve and serves as an additional safety measure.

All regulators have a *pressure gauge* that informs you of the tank pressure (Fig. 3–34*A*). A fresh tank should measure approximately 2000 PSI.

Some regulators also have a *flowmeter* that records the flow rate of gas leaving the cylinder. These flowmeters usually range from 0 to 15 liters per minute. There are three types of flowmeters used in emergency medical services (EMS). A *Bourdon gauge flowmeter* utilizes the pressure gauge to measure flow rates to the delivery

device (Fig. 3–34*A*). A *pressure-compensated flowmeter* (Thorpe tube flowmeter) uses a gravity-regulated ball on a vertical meter to record flow (see Fig. 3–34*B*). The liter flow is read at the center of the ball as it rises. The pressure-compensated flowmeter has the advantage of being more accurate, since it measures actual flow. If the tubing on a device is clogged or kinked the flow rate will accurately reflect the actual amount of gas delivered to the patient. The third type of flowmeter is a *constant flow selector valve*. This type of flowmeter uses a flow marking at the adjustment dial to indicate flow rates.

With the use of the cylinder size, pressure gauge, and the flowmeter, we can predict the time of gas consumption when administering oxygen. For example, an *E* cylinder containing *1200 lb* of pressure and opened to deliver *8 liters* of oxygen per minute will last approximately *35 minutes*. This conclusion was reached by applying the formula in Table 3–3.

The tank pressure is obtained by observing the pressure gauge. The figure 200 is subtracted from this pressure to ensure an adequate residual amount of gas at which point the cylinder should be changed. This value is then multiplied times a constant, which is a figure that controls for the variance in cylinder size. The product of this multiplication is then divided by the liter flow. The constants for the various cylinders are listed in Table 3–3.

In theory, this formula allows you to predict the

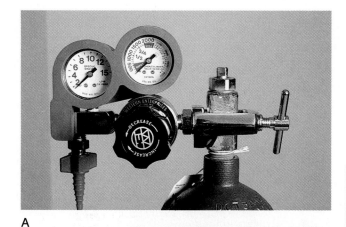

A

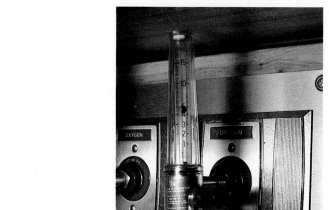

B

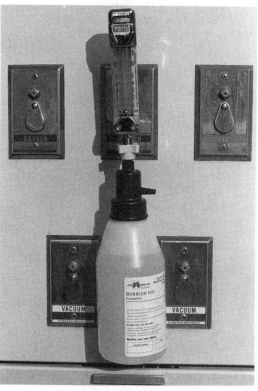

C

FIGURE 3–34. (*A*) Bourdon gauge regulator. (*B*) Pressure compensated regulator. (*C*) Humidifier. (*C*, from Kersten LD: Comprehensive Respiratory Nursing: A Decision Making Approach. Philadelphia, WB Saunders, 1989, p. 602.)

point at which the cylinder must be changed. However, in instances where you use large quantities of oxygen, such as positive-pressure ventilation with a demand

TABLE 3–3. Formula for Computing Amount of Time Remaining in an Oxygen Cylinder in Relation to Flow Rates

$$\text{Time (min)} = \frac{\text{Tank pressure (lb)} - 200\ \text{lb} \times \text{constant}}{\text{Flow rate (liters/min)}}$$

Constant by Tank Size

D Cylinder —0.16
E Cylinder —0.28
M Cylinder—1.56
H Cylinder —3.14

valve, keeping a close eye on the pressure gauge is the safest and most convenient method.

HUMIDIFICATION. A *humidifier* is a water-filled bottle that moisturizes the inspired oxygen. It is useful to loosen secretions and prevent drying of the airway. In the prehospital phase it is especially useful for the treatment of children and for conditions such as inhalation of smoke and irritant gases. However, short periods of oxygen administration without humidification are not harmful, and most patients benefit just as much from administration of oxygen alone in the prehospital phase of care. When humidification is used, care must be taken to prevent contamination of the humidification device, and the device should be changed after each use (Fig. 3–34C).

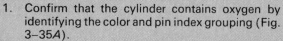

PROCEDURE 3-10   **SETTING UP AN OXYGEN SYSTEM**

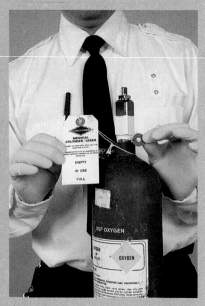

A

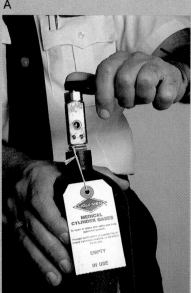

B

1. Confirm that the cylinder contains oxygen by identifying the color and pin index grouping (Fig. 3–35*A*).
2. Check to see that a rubber washer (the O-ring) is in place at either the cylinder opening or the regulator opening (Fig. 3–35*A*).
3. Open the main valve at the top of the cylinder slowly until gas starts to come out, to clear dust from the opening. Then immediately close the valve (Fig. 3–35*B*).
4. Attach the regulator by carefully aligning the pin index from the regulator into the cylinder holes (Fig. 3–35*C*).
5. Tighten the clamp with firm hand pressure to ensure an adequate seal and then open the main valve two full turns (Fig. 3–35*C* and 3–35*D*).
6. Check the pressure gauge, which should record approximately 2000 pounds. If the cylinder leaks, you should turn off the main valve and check the connection and firmness of the attachment.
7. Once the regulator is attached, you should check the flowmeter to ensure that the dial or ball device rises as the valve opens (Fig. 3–35*E*).
8. Attach the tubing or delivery device to the regulator (Fig. 3–35*F*).
9. Attach the delivery device to the patient (Fig. 3–35*G* and *H*).

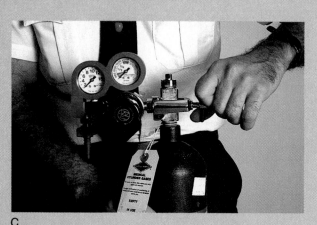

C

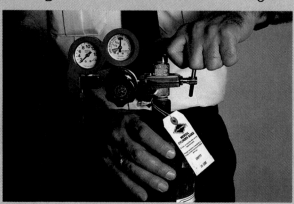

D

FIGURE 3–35. (*A*) Identify the cylinder by the color and pin index safety system. Also note the status of the tank (full vs. empty) from the attached tag. Check to see if a new washer is needed on the regulator. (Most cylinders have a new washer attached.) (*B*) Remove the seal that covers the opening on the cylinder valve. "Crack" the cylinder by opening the main valve to clear dust or other particles from the opening in the valve; then quickly close it. (*C*) Place the yoke of the regulator over the main valve and align the opening and pin index system. Hand tighten the regulator in place. (*D*) Open the main valve and observe the pressure gauge on the regulator. (A full cylinder should register 2000 psi.)

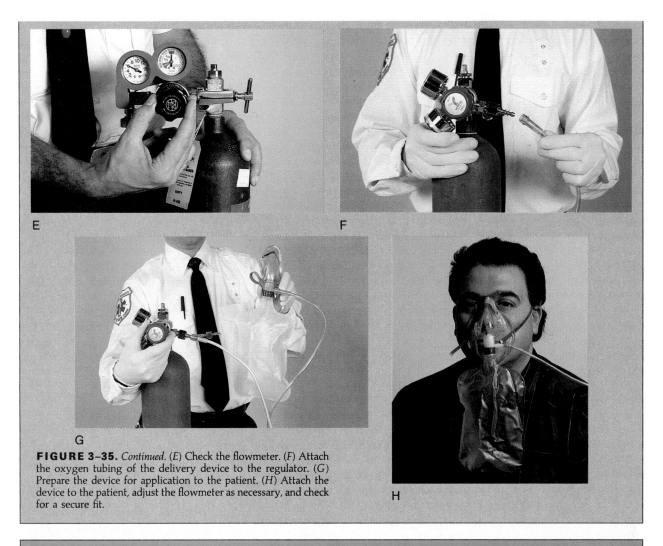

FIGURE 3–35. *Continued.* (*E*) Check the flowmeter. (*F*) Attach the oxygen tubing of the delivery device to the regulator. (*G*) Prepare the device for application to the patient. (*H*) Attach the device to the patient, adjust the flowmeter as necessary, and check for a secure fit.

P R O C E D U R E   3 – 11   *DETACHING THE REGULATOR*

1. Turn off the main valve at the top of the cylinder (Fig. 3–36*A*).
2. Open the flowmeter valve to bleed oxygen out of the system (Fig. 3–36*B*).
3. Detach the regulator by loosening the clamp, mark the cylinder as empty, and store in the appropriate area (Fig. 3–36*C* and *D*).

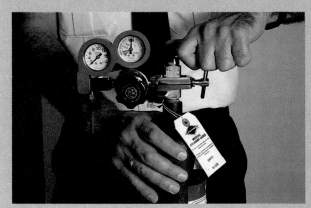

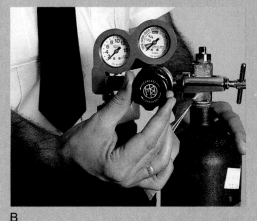

FIGURE 3–36. (*A*) Remove the oxygen administration device from the patient and the regulator, and turn off the main valve. (*B*) Bleed the oxygen from the regulator, and observe the pressure gauge, which should return to zero.

Continued

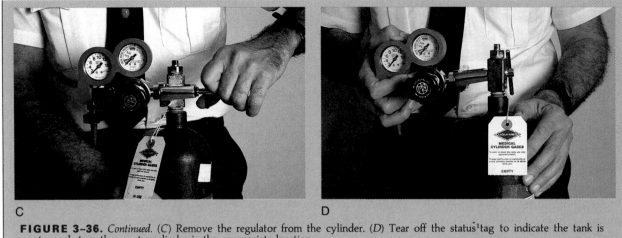

C   D

FIGURE 3–36. *Continued.* (C) Remove the regulator from the cylinder. (D) Tear off the status tag to indicate the tank is empty, and store the empty cylinder in the appropriate location.

At the beginning of each tour of duty, every oxygen device on the ambulance should be checked for function. The discovery of an empty oxygen cylinder during a resuscitation is life threatening to the patient. Table 3–3A reviews key safety issues related to oxygen use.

OXYGEN ADMINISTRATION DEVICES

When patients are ventilating adequately but are in need of supplemental oxygen, free-flow oxygen devices are used. Essentially four devices are most commonly used: a nasal cannula, a Venturi device, a simple face mask, and a non-rebreather device. Each system has advantages and disadvantages and should be selected accordingly. Do not become too comfortable with any single system to the exclusion of others or you may fail to provide your patient with the optimal therapy.

NASAL CANNULA. A *nasal cannula* is a low-flow oxygen delivery system. This means that the device does not deliver the total quantity of gas consumed by the patient. The patient breathes oxygen from the cannula along with room air. A nasal cannula can also be a medium oxygen delivery system. It is capable of delivering 24 to 40% of oxygen at flow rates of 2 to 6 liters of oxygen per minute. As a rule, you should not administer more than 6 liters per minute of oxygen through

a nasal cannula, as it will not increase the delivery concentrations but will dry the nasal mucosa.

Nasal cannulas are useful in treating any condition where low to medium oxygen concentrations are needed, such as COPD, asthma, and uncomplicated heart attacks. It is also valuable when patients cannot tolerate the restrictive feeling of a mask, which is common among dyspneic and hypoxia patients (Fig. 3–37).

VENTURI MASK. A *Venturi mask* is a high-flow oxygen system that allows more precise measurement of the concentration of inspired oxygen. The device can alter either oxygen or air entry from openings in the adapters to vary the ultimate concentration of inspired oxygen. A variety of types of Venturi systems are available. The percentage of oxygen can be controlled by either changing adapters that attach to the base of the mask or sometimes an adjustable, rotating opening alters

TABLE 3–3A. Safety Issues Related to Oxygen Use

1. Monitor the tank pressure frequently.
2. Do not smoke or use an open flame near (within 10 feet) oxygen equipment.
3. Do not use near electrical equipment that gives off sparks.
4. Do not use oils or other flammable substances around oxygen equipment.
5. Store cylinders in a cool, well-ventilated area and secure them in place at all times.
6. Close all valves when oxygen is not in use.
7. Never attempt repair of cylinders or regulators.
8. Never position yourself or the patient above the valve of the cylinder.

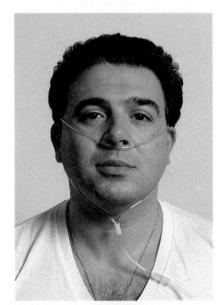

FIGURE 3–37. Place the nasal prongs through the nares and guide the tubing around the ears and under the chin. Adjust the fit of the device under the chin.

the amount of air mixing with oxygen. The final percentages of delivered oxygen are usually found on the adapters or on a marking system at the Venturi opening. Most systems are capable of delivering an oxygen concentration range from 24 to 40% at 4 to 8 liters per minute.

Venturi masks are most useful when treating COPD patients (who are not severely hypoxic, ischemic, or in shock) due to the precise nature of the device. An oxygen delivery component of about 24 to 28% is usually desirable for COPD patients (Fig. 3–38A, B, and C).

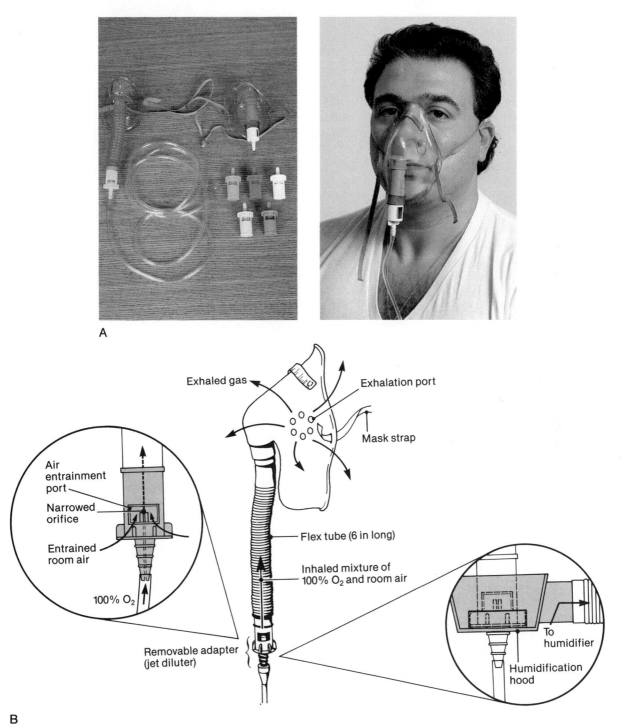

FIGURE 3–38. (A) A Venturi mask is a high-flow, low- to medium-concentration delivery device. It may come with several color-coded adapters that vary the rate of oxygen flow past the air entrainment port. (B) The mix of air and oxygen is adjusted by changing either the flow of oxygen or the size of the air entrainment port. The arrows illustrate the flow of exhaled air. This device is used in prehospital care primarily to administer low concentrations of supplemental oxygen to patients with chronic obstructive pulmonary disease (COPD). The mask should be applied snugly in place to ensure accurate oxygen concentrations. (B, from Kersten LD: Comprehensive Respiratory Nursing: A Decision Making Approach. Philadelphia, WB Saunders, 1989, p. 611.)

SIMPLE FACE MASK. A *simple face mask* is a low-flow oxygen device. It can provide oxygen concentrations ranging from 50 to 60% at liter flow rates of 8 to 12 liters per minute. It has ports on both sides of the mask that provide an environmental air mix with the delivery of oxygen. It is useful in instances where a moderate concentration of oxygen is desired (Fig. 3–39).

PARTIAL AND NONREBREATHER MASKS. A partial rebreather mask uses a reservoir bag to collect oxygen and enrich delivered oxygen concentrations. Figure 3–40A reviews the mechanism of this device. A *nonrebreather mask* is a low-flow, high-oxygen concentration device. It is the best device when high concentrations of oxygen are needed and can achieve concentrations of up to 90% at flow rates on 10 to 12 liters per minute. It consists of a reservoir bag beneath a one-way valve that prevents the patient from exhaling into the bag. Thus the name *nonrebreather*. It is administered by first attaching the oxygen tubing and providing a flow rate of about 8 liters per minute while keeping your finger over the valve. This causes the bag to inflate fully. Then place the mask around the patient's face and pull the elastic straps to properly secure the mask. Leakage around the mask decreases the delivery of oxygen. When the patient inhales, THE BAG SHOULD NOT COLLAPSE. If this occurs, you should increase the delivered oxygen by 2-liter increments until the bag remains inflated.

This device is excellent for severely hypoxic but well-ventilated patients. The nonrebreather mask is used for the treatment of respiratory failure, shock states, and any other cause of poor tissue oxygenation (Fig. 3–40B). Review Table 3–4 for the various administration devices and their oxygen delivery capabilities.

Suctioning the Patient

Suctioning is the act of introducing a tube or rigid cannula into the airway in order to vacuum out liquid and small solid secretions. Vomiting, drowning, and lung secretions are all sources of airway obstruction in unconscious or lethargic patients. Timely removal of these substances ensures a patent airway and more adequate ventilation and oxygenation.

Suction equipment consists of a suction machine that may be portable (Fig. 3–41A) or an inboard wall model (Fig. 3–41B) within the ambulance. It should be capable of removing thick secretions and provide negative pressures of at least 300 mm Hg. A catheter or rigid device is attached to the machine via connecting tubing and is placed in the patient's mouth prior to initiating suction. Some catheters have an opening at the base that activates suctioning, or, in some cases, suc-

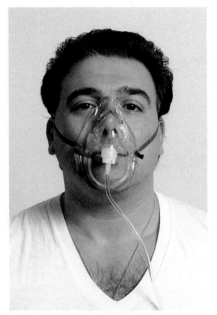

FIGURE 3–39. A simple face mask.

tioning is initiated by pushing a button on the machine itself. To suction, the catheter or rigid tonsil device should be placed into the oropharynx with the suction not activated. Once the device is in place, suction should be applied while spinning the tip of the catheter to avoid plugging by pharyngeal tissue. Suction should not be performed for more than 10 seconds to avoid hypoxia (Fig. 3–42A and B). Review the techniques for using a rigid and soft suction catheter.

When performing procedures related to management of airway, ventilation, and suctioning, standard infection-control practices should be used, including the wearing of goggles, gloves, and a face mask. For further information, see Chapter 12.

TABLE 3–4. Oxygen Percentage Delivery by Device

Device	Approximate Percentage	Liter Flow (liters/min)
Nasal cannula	24–40	2–6
Venturi mask	24–40	4–8
Simple face mask	50	8–12
Partial rebreather	35–60	6–10
Nonrebreather	90	10–12

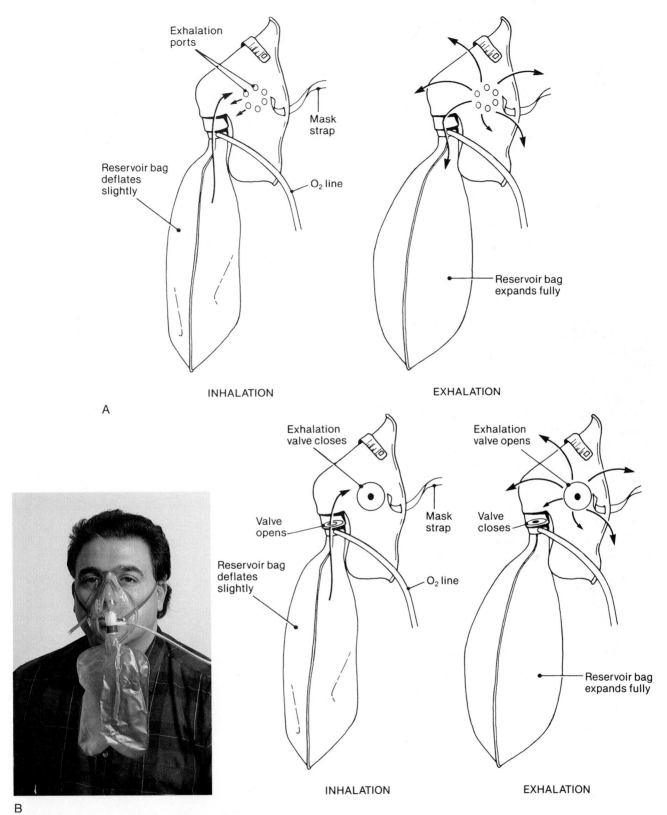

Exhalation ports

Mask strap

Reservoir bag deflates slightly

O₂ line

Reservoir bag expands fully

INHALATION

EXHALATION

A

Exhalation valve closes

Exhalation valve opens

Valve opens

Mask strap

Valve closes

Reservoir bag deflates slightly

O₂ line

Reservoir bag expands fully

INHALATION

EXHALATION

B

FIGURE 3–40. (*A*) A partial rebreather mask provides medium concentrations of oxygen. It consists of a reservoir bag that permits the patient to breathe enriched oxygen concentrations during inhalation. The first third of the patient's exhaled air enters the reservoir bag, while the remainder is directed to the atmosphere through the ports on the side of the mask. A slight amount of carbon dioxide is inhaled on subsequent breaths. This can be reduced by increasing the oxygen being delivered to the reservoir bag. (*B*) *A nonrebreather mask* works in the same manner as a partial rebreather by using an oxygen collection device below the mask, where oxygen collects prior to inhalation. However, a one-way valve separates the reservoir from the mask and directs exhalation out through the sides of the mask. With a tight-fitting mask this device results in approximately 90% oxygen delivery to the patient. The arrows illustrate the flow of air when using this device. This is the delivery device of choice when high-concentration oxygen is needed. A tight-fitting mask will increase the delivered oxygen concentrations. (*A* and drawing in *B*, from Kersten LD: Comprehensive Respiratory Nursing: A Decision Making Approach. Philadelphia, WB Saunders, 1989, pp. 610 and 611.)

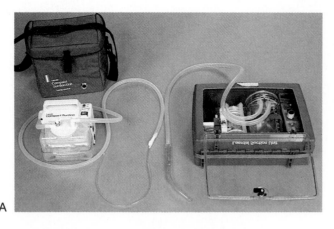

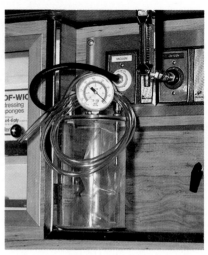

FIGURE 3–41. (A) Two battery-operated suction devices. (B) An inboard suction device with a large collecting chamber.

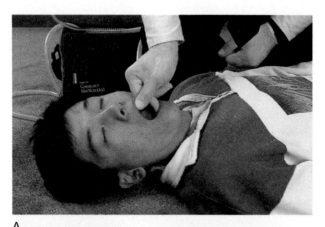

A

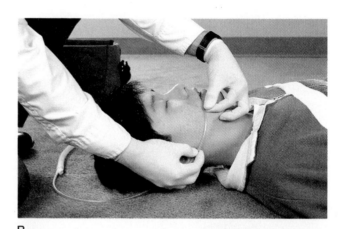

B

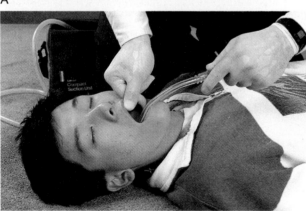

A

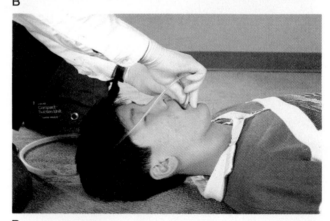

B

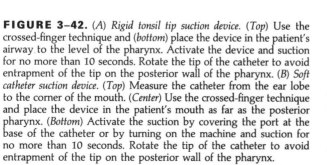

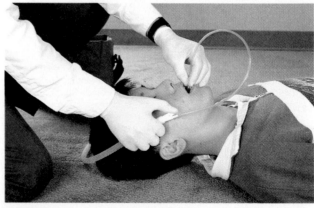

B

FIGURE 3–42. (A) *Rigid tonsil tip suction device.* (*Top*) Use the crossed-finger technique and (*bottom*) place the device in the patient's airway to the level of the pharynx. Activate the device and suction for no more than 10 seconds. Rotate the tip of the catheter to avoid entrapment of the tip on the posterior wall of the pharynx. (B) *Soft catheter suction device.* (*Top*) Measure the catheter from the ear lobe to the corner of the mouth. (*Center*) Use the crossed-finger technique and place the device in the patient's mouth as far as the posterior pharynx. (*Bottom*) Activate the suction by covering the port at the base of the catheter or by turning on the machine and suction for no more than 10 seconds. Rotate the tip of the catheter to avoid entrapment of the tip on the posterior wall of the pharynx.

PROTOCOL

OXYGEN ADMINISTRATION

> #### NOTE!
> 1. OXYGEN SHOULD NEVER BE WITHHELD FROM PATIENTS REQUIRING IT, EVEN THOUGH THEY MAY HAVE COPD!
> 2. WHEN ADMINISTERING OXYGEN, WATCH THE PATIENT CAREFULLY FOR ANY SLOWING OF RESPIRATIONS. BE PREPARED TO VENTILATE THE PATIENT AS NECESSARY!
> 3. IN PATIENTS WHO ARE BEING CHRONICALLY MAINTAINED ON OXYGEN AND WHO ARE BEING TRANSPORTED FOR A CONDITION OTHER THAN ONE REQUIRING HIGH-CONCENTRATION OXYGEN BY THESE PROTOCOLS, CONTINUE ADMINISTERING OXYGEN AT THE PREVIOUSLY PRESCRIBED RATE OF FLOW.

IF THE PATIENT REQUIRES OXYGEN THERAPY:

1. Assure that the patient's airway is open and that breathing and circulation are adequate. IF THE AIRWAY IS OBSTRUCTED, perform obstructed airway maneuvers according to AHA/ARC standards.

2. Administer HIGH-CONCENTRATION OXYGEN.

> #### NOTE!
> There is no contraindication to high-concentration oxygen in pediatric patients in the prehospital setting. Administration of oxygen is best accomplished by ALLOWING the parent to hold the face mask, if tolerated, about 6 to 8 inches from the child's face. Humidified oxygen is preferred, but dry oxygen is better than no oxygen.

  a. First choice—nonrebreathing mask.

    (1) Fill the bag to its capacity initially.

    (2) Adjust the flow of oxygen (usually greater than 10 LPM) so that the bag remains 1/3 full after an inspiration.

  b. Second choice—nasal cannula at 6 LPM (used only if a mask is not tolerated).

IF THE PATIENT DEMONSTRATES INADEQUATE VENTILATION (I.E., THE RESPIRATORY RATE IS LESS THAN 10 PER MINUTE OR GREATER THAN 29 PER MINUTE IN AN ADULT, OR LESS THAN 15 PER MINUTE IN A CHILD, AND THE PATIENT IS CONFUSED, RESTLESS, OR CYANOTIC):

1. Assist the patient's ventilations with 100% oxygen, using a positive-pressure adjunctive device.

  a. First choice—bag-valve-mask (BVM) with reservoir.

> ADEQUATE VENTILATION MAY REQUIRE DISABLING THE POP-OFF VALVE IF THE BAG-VALVE-MASK UNIT IS SO EQUIPPED!

From Manual for Emergency Medical Technicians. Emergency Medical Services Program. Albany, New York State Department of Health, 1990.

SPECIFIC RESPIRATORY PROBLEMS

Upper Airway Obstruction

Blockage of the airway may occur as a result of many causes. It can be partial (allow some flow) or complete (totally prevent flow into the lungs). Functionally, obstructions can be divided into three categories: anatomical, mechanical (foreign body), and pathological. Although all types of airway obstructions may exhibit the same signs and symptoms, the treatment for each type is quite different. For this reason, you must be prepared to rapidly identify the cause of the obstruction and react appropriately.

ANATOMICAL OBSTRUCTION

The most common cause of airway obstruction is an anatomical obstruction by the tongue. In any unconscious state the tongue, which is attached to the jaw, may fall against the oropharynx. This is due to total relaxation of the muscles of the *mandible* (lower jaw) in combination with flexion of the neck (Fig. 3–43). The result is the impairment of air flow through the upper airway. Depending on the degree of relaxation, the flow of air may decrease or be totally obstructed. For example, a person who is sleeping may partially obstruct the airway with the tongue. This will be characterized by snoring. However, in deep states of coma, the tongue may totally block air flow. Obstructions of this type are suspected in all unconscious patients.

The treatment of anatomical obstruction is to displace the tongue away from the pharynx and OPEN THE AIRWAY. These techniques are outlined in Chapter 2 and include the head tilt–chin lift and the jaw thrust without head tilt (utilized in cases of suspected spinal injury).

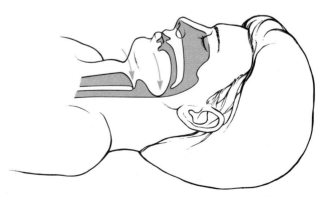

FIGURE 3–43. In the relaxed or unconscious state the tongue may fall against the posterior wall of the pharynx and block the upper airway.

MECHANICAL OBSTRUCTION OF THE AIRWAY

RECOGNIZING THE CAUSES OF AIRWAY OBSTRUCTION.
Obstruction of the airway by a foreign body blocks the passage of air. According to the United States Bureau of the Census, airway obstruction resulted in more than 3,600 deaths in 1986 in the United States.

The principal cause of foreign body airway obstruction is food. Although a variety of foods may be responsible, meat is the most common foreign body to cause obstruction. Other factors associated with airway obstruction, in addition to meat, are excessive alcohol in the blood, false teeth, and large, poorly chewed pieces of food. The symptoms of airway obstruction are sometimes mistaken by lay people for those of a heart attack. For this reason it is often called a "café coronary."

PREVENTING OBSTRUCTION OF THE AIRWAY.
Common sense is probably the best precaution against foreign body airway obstruction. The precautions are quite simple:

- Cut food into small pieces, and chew slowly and thoroughly, especially if you wear false teeth.
- Do not talk or laugh while chewing and swallowing.
- Avoid excessive alcohol before and during meals.
- Do not permit small children to walk, run, or play while food is in their mouths.
- Keep small objects such as marbles, beads, thumbtacks, and buttons away from infants and small children.

WHAT ARE THE SIGNS OF AN OBSTRUCTED AIRWAY?
A foreign body may completely obstruct the airway. If this happens, no air movement is possible at all. The victim will not be able to breathe, cough, or speak. In other cases, a victim may have partial obstruction of the airway. A patient with *partial obstruction may have good air exchange* and may not require any treatment at all. Or a patient may have *partial obstruction and very poor air exchange* and should be treated the same way as the patient with complete obstruction.

Therefore, it is important to recognize the characteristics of complete airway obstruction, partial obstruction with good air exchange, and partial obstruction with poor air exchange.

Partial Obstruction with Good Air Exchange

- The victim can cough forcefully with frequent wheezing sounds between coughs.
- The victim should be encouraged to cough spontaneously and to continue breathing efforts.
- The rescuer should not interfere with the victim's efforts to expel the foreign object.

Partial Obstruction with Poor Air Exchange

- Poor air exchange may occur initially, or good air exchange may become poor air exchange.

- The victim's cough is weak and ineffective.
- Inhaling produces high-pitched noises, such as stridor.
- Breathing is difficult and the patient becomes cyanotic.
- Partial obstruction with poor air exchange should be managed as if it were a complete airway obstruction!

When the airway has been completely obstructed, the victim may at first be conscious. However, as the supply of oxygen is used up the victim will become unconscious.

Complete Obstruction (Victim Is Conscious)

- The victim who is eating or has just finished eating cannot breathe or cough.
- The victim cannot speak even when asked, "Are you choking?"
- The victim shows exaggerated breathing effort without air exchange.
- The victim may give the "UNIVERSAL DISTRESS SIGNAL" by clutching his or her neck between thumb and forefinger (Fig. 3–44).

Complete Obstruction (Victim Is Unconscious)

- In the unconscious victim, complete airway obstruction is recognized by the inability of the rescuer to ventilate the victim.

MANEUVERS FOR RELIEVING AIRWAY OBSTRUCTION.
There are two principal techniques for relieving foreign body airway obstruction: *manual thrusts* and *finger sweeps*. Both of these maneuvers are described below.

Manual thrusts consist of a series of forceful compressions to the upper abdomen or lower chest. Air is expelled from the lungs, creating an artificial cough that may force out the foreign body. Manual thrusts can be given to a victim who is standing, sitting, or lying down. Each thrust should be delivered with sufficient force to remove the obstruction.

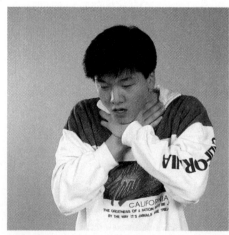

FIGURE 3–44. The universal distress signal.

PROCEDURE 3-12 **PERFORMING ABDOMINAL THRUST WHEN VICTIM IS CONSCIOUS AND STANDING OR SITTING**

1. Stand behind the victim and wrap your arms around the victim's waist (Fig. 3–45).
2. Grasp one fist with your other hand, and place the thumb of that fist against the victim's abdomen, slightly above the navel and below the xiphoid process (Fig. 3–46A, B, and C).
3. Press your fist into the victim's abdomen with a quick upward thrust.
4. Repeat until the obstruction is relieved or until the victim becomes unconscious.

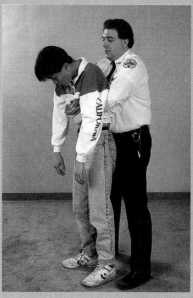

FIGURE 3–45. The rescuer should stand directly behind the victim and with an open stance. This provides a secure position for support should the victim become unconscious.

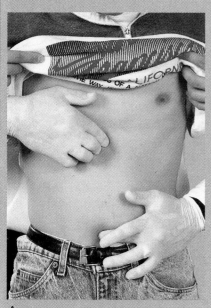

A

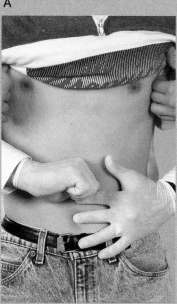

B

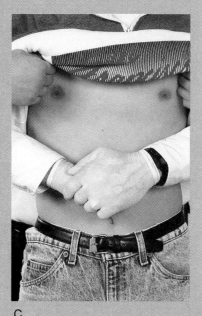

C

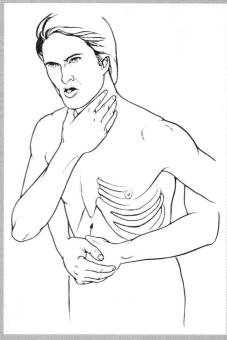

C

FIGURE 3–46. (A) Locate the victim's xiphoid and umbilicus. (B) Place your fist with the thumb side in, just above the umbilicus. (C) Grab the fist with the other hand and apply an inward and upward thrust to the abdominal wall.

Continued

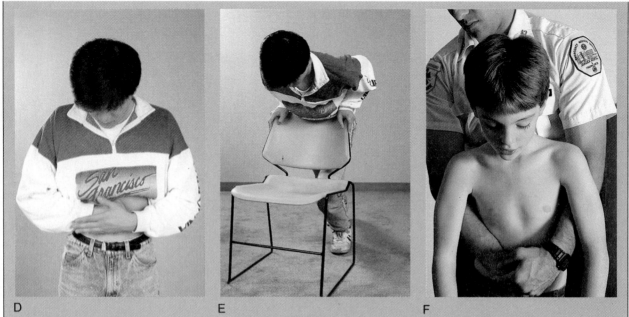

D   E   F

FIGURE 3–46. *Continued.* (*D*) The abdominal thrust can be self-administered in the manner described above, if the victim is alone. (*E*) Self-administration can also be done by thrusting your abdomen against a blunt object, e.g., a chair. (*F*) Abdominal thrust in a child.

It is possible to perform the abdominal thrust maneuver on yourself if you are choking and there is no other person around to provide assistance. Press your fist into the upper abdomen with quick upward thrusts. An alternate procedure is to lean forward and press the abdomen quickly against any firm object such as the back of a chair or table or the edge of a sink or porch railing (Fig. 3–46D and E). Figure 3–46F illustrates the abdominal thrust in a child.

PROCEDURE 3-13   ***PERFORMING ABDOMINAL THRUST WHEN VICTIM IS LYING UNCONSCIOUS***

1. Position the victim on his or her back.
2. Straddle the victim over the thigh area.
3. Place the heel of one hand against the victim's abdomen, between the navel and the xiphoid process. Place the second hand on top of the first (Fig. 3–47A and B). Technique for a child is illustrated in Figure 3–47C.
4. Deliver from 6 to 10 quick upward thrusts.

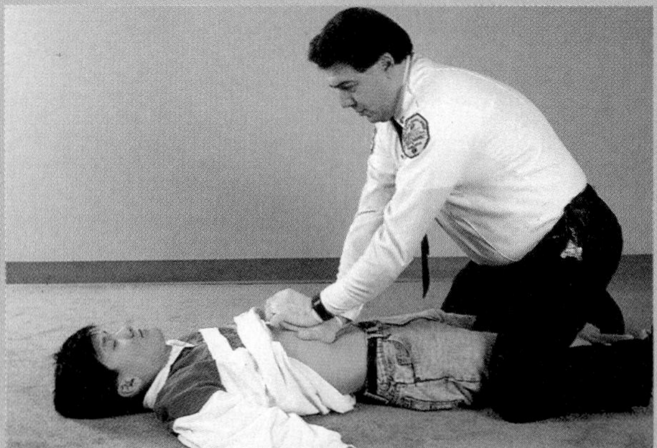

A

FIGURE 3–47. (*A*) Straddle the victim at the level of the thighs and place the heel of one hand just above the umbilicus as described in Figure 3–46.

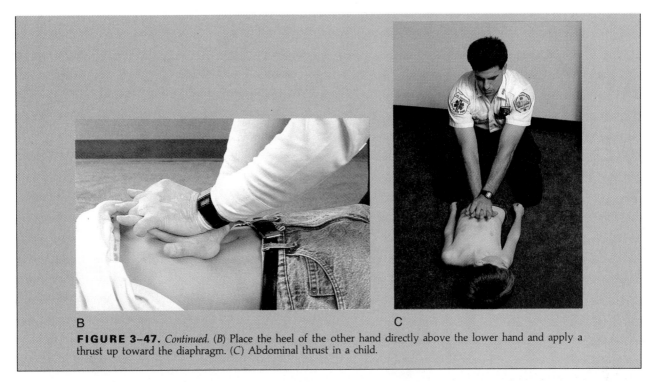

B   C

FIGURE 3–47. *Continued.* (*B*) Place the heel of the other hand directly above the lower hand and apply a thrust up toward the diaphragm. (*C*) Abdominal thrust in a child.

The chest thrust is an alternate technique to the abdominal thrust. It is used for the treatment of a pregnant or obese person, when the rescuer's arms cannot encircle the victim's abdomen. If the victim is obviously pregnant, the chest thrust must be used to avoid injury to the baby.

PROCEDURE 3–14   PERFORMING CHEST THRUST WHEN VICTIM IS STANDING OR SITTING

1. Stand behind the victim: Place your arms under the victim's armpits and encircle the chest.
2. Place the thumb side of your fist on the victim's breastbone above the xiphoid process (the lower tip of the breastbone) (Fig. 3–48*A* and *B*).
3. Grasp your fist with your other hand and deliver forceful backward thrusts (Fig. 3–48*C*).
4. Repeat, if necessary.

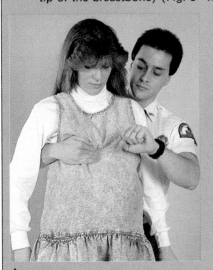
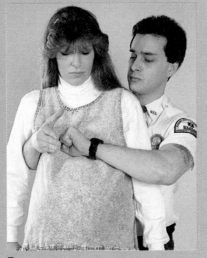
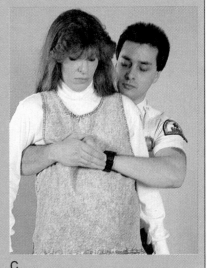

A   B   C

FIGURE 3–48. A chest thrust is applied when encountering a pregnant or extremely obese patient. (*A*) Locate the margin of the rib with your index and middle fingers of one hand and follow it to the base of the sternum. (*B*) Make a fist with the other hand and place the thumb side of the fist just above the fingers of the first hand. (*C*) Grasp the fist with the other hand and apply a quick backward thrust to the sternum. Be careful not to apply pressure to the rib cage, since that may result in fractures.

PROCEDURE 3-15   PERFORMING CHEST THRUST WHEN VICTIM IS LYING UNCONSCIOUS

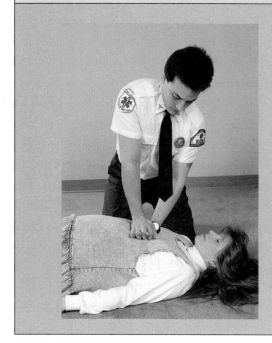

1. Place the victim on his back and kneel beside his chest.
2. Place your hands on the victim's chest as if you were performing external chest compression (Fig. 3–49).
3. Deliver from 6 to 10 chest thrusts in rapid succession.

FIGURE 3–49. Locate the margin of the rib with the index and middle fingers of the hand closest to the patient's feet, and follow it to the base of the sternum. Place the heel of the other hand next to your index finger, keeping your fingers off the chest wall. Place the heel of the hand used for the landmark check directly over the lower hand and apply straight downward pressure on the sternum.

The second technique for removing an airway obstruction is the finger sweep. The finger sweep is not performed on a conscious victim. As the victim is deprived of oxygen and becomes unconscious, however, the muscles of the jaw relax, and the finger sweep can be employed.

PROCEDURE 3-16   FINGER SWEEP WHEN VICTIM IS UNCONSCIOUS

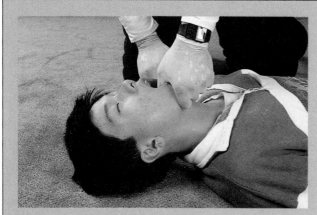

1. Place the victim's head up.
2. Open the victim's mouth by grasping both the tongue and lower jaw between the thumb and fingers and lifting (Fig. 3–50A).

A

FIGURE 3–50. (A) Open the mouth with the tongue-jaw lift procedure.

3. Insert the index finger of the other hand down alongside the inside of the cheek, deeply into the mouth to the base of the tongue.
4. Use a hooking action to dislodge the foreign body and move it into the mouth from which it can be removed (Fig. 3–50*B*).

Note: Be careful not to force the object deeper into the airway.

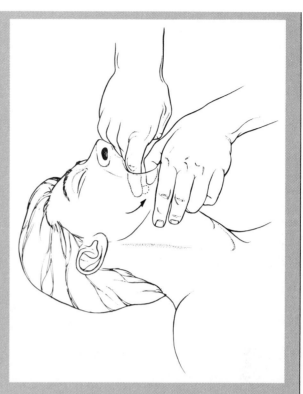

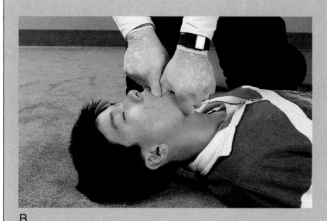

B

FIGURE 3–50. *Continued.* (*B*) Place your index finger along the side of the mouth to the base of the tongue; sweep across with the finger and pull the foreign material up and out of the oral cavity.

If it is not possible to insert your thumb into the victim's mouth for the tongue-jaw lift, use the crossed-finger technique to open the mouth. Cross the thumb over the index finger. Place the crossed fingers firmly against the victim's mouth and forcefully uncross the fingers to pry open the mouth. While doing so, turn the victim's head away from you to provide greater stability. Proceed with the finger sweep.

SEQUENCE OF SKILLS FOR OBSTRUCTED AIRWAY MANAGEMENT

Do the following if the choking victim is conscious:

- Identify complete airway obstruction by asking the victim, "Are you choking?" If the victim cannot speak:
- Apply manual abdominal thrusts (chest thrusts if the victim is pregnant or very obese).
- Repeat delivery of manual thrusts until they are effective or until the victim becomes unconscious.

Do the following if the choking victim becomes unconscious:

- Perform the finger sweep (in a child or infant the finger sweep is performed only if the object is visible).
- Open the airway and attempt to ventilate. If the victim cannot be ventilated:
- Apply from 6 to 10 manual abdominal thrusts (chest thrusts if the victim is pregnant or very obese).
- Perform the finger sweep.
- Open the airway and attempt to ventilate. If the victim cannot be ventilated:
- Repeat the procedure—thrusts, finger sweep, ventilation.

If the victim is found unconscious, and the cause is unknown, the rescuer must determine if the cause of the unconsciousness is cardiac arrest or airway obstruction. The rescuer must:

- Establish unresponsiveness.
- Open the airway.
- Attempt to ventilate.

If the rescuer cannot ventilate successfully, the following sequence of activities must be performed quickly:

- Reposition the head and try to ventilate again. If unsuccessful, and another person is present:
- Activate the EMS system.
- Apply from 6 to 10 manual abdominal thrusts (chest thrusts if the victim is pregnant or very obese).
- Perform the finger sweep.
- Open the airway and attempt to ventilate. If the victim cannot be ventilated:
- Repeat the procedure—thrusts, finger sweep, ventilation—until effective results.

JUDGING THE EFFECTIVENESS OF THE PROCEDURES. When the airway is opened as a result of the procedures that have been described, the victim may develop spontaneous ventilation. It may also be possible to observe the removal of the foreign object from the mouth.

In some victims, after the obstruction has been removed it may be necessary to perform positive-pressure ventilation or complete cardiopulmonary resuscitation. When positive-pressure ventilation is required, deliver one breath every 5 seconds. Even if the victim begins to breathe spontaneously, the victim should be delivered to the emergency department for further evaluation.

FOREIGN BODY AIRWAY OBSTRUCTION IN INFANTS AND CHILDREN

The child or infant with a foreign body obstruction in his or her airway is usually a previously healthy child with a sudden history of choking and signs of upper airway obstruction, i.e., stridor, tachypnea, and difficulty moving air. For the purposes of treatment, an infant is defined as someone less than one year of age and a child as someone between one and eight years of age. These age parameters relate to average size at these ages. In other words, a small 13-month-old may be treated as an infant, and a large 11-month-old may be treated as a child.

In children and infants, one must consider the possibility of obstruction caused by an infectious process such as epiglottitis or croup (see Chapter 14).

To form a working diagnosis, it is important to perform a primary survey and gather the key facts about the patient's history. To determine whether the obstruction is partial or complete, you should assess the patient for level of consciousness, air exchange, and ability to speak or cry. A brief history regarding recent upper respiratory infections, fever, and barking cough, or a history of choking after eating or playing with objects in the mouth helps point to the cause of obstruction.

Treat all cases of suspected infection as if they are epiglottitis, and therefore do not manipulate or attempt to examine the airway. See the discussion of croup, epiglottitis, and foreign body obstruction in Chapter 14 to understand the major differences.

PROTOCOL

OBSTRUCTED AIRWAY—ADULT

A. IF THE PATIENT IS *CONSCIOUS* AND CAN BREATHE, COUGH, OR SPEAK:

1. DO NOT INTERFERE! Encourage coughing.

IF THE FOREIGN BODY CANNOT BE DISLODGED BY THE PATIENT COUGHING:

2. Administer high-concentration oxygen.

3. Transport in a sitting position, keeping the patient warm.

4. Obtain and record the vital signs, and repeat en route as often as the situation indicates.

5. Record all patient care information, including the patient's medical history and all treatment provided, on a Prehospital Care Report.

B. IF THE PATIENT IS *CONSCIOUS* BUT CANNOT BREATHE, COUGH, OR SPEAK:
OR
IF THE PATIENT *IS OR BECOMES UNCONSCIOUS*:

1. Perform obstructed airway maneuvers according to AHA/ARC standards.

> IF OBSTRUCTED AIRWAY IS TRAUMATIC, MANUALLY IMMOBILIZE THE HEAD AND CERVICAL SPINE IN A NEUTRAL POSITION WHILE OPENING THE PATIENT'S AIRWAY USING THE JAW-THRUST MANEUVER, AND TRANSPORT THE PATIENT WITHOUT DELAY!

IF AIRWAY OBSTRUCTION PERSISTS AFTER TWO SEQUENCES OF OBSTRUCTED AIRWAY MANEUVERS:

2. Transport, keeping the patient warm.

3. Repeat the sequences of obstructed airway maneuvers en route until the foreign body is forced out.

4. Obtain and record the vital signs, and repeat en route as often as the situation indicates.

5. Record all patient care information, including the patient's medical history and all treatment provided, on a Prehospital Care Report.

IF AIRWAY OBSTRUCTION IS REVERSED AND THE PATIENT RESUMES BREATHING:

2. Administer high-concentration oxygen.

3. Transport, keeping the patient warm.

4. Obtain and record the vital signs, and repeat en route as often as the situation indicates.

5. Record all patient care information, including the patient's medical history and all treatment provided, on a Prehospital Care Report.

From Manual for Emergency Medical Technicians. Emergency Medical Services Program. Albany, New York State Department of Health, 1990.

THE ALERT CHILD OR INFANT WITH PARTIAL AIRWAY OBSTRUCTION AND GOOD AIR EXCHANGE. If the child is alert, even with severe stridor and a rapid respiratory rate, do not interfere with the child's efforts to cough or breathe. Keep the child and parents as calm as possible and allow the child to remain in the parent's arms in the position of comfort that the child chooses. Supply humidified oxygen without agitating the child (from face mask, nasal cannula, or by holding the mask near the nose and mouth), and transport the child quickly. This holds true regardless of whether you suspect croup, epiglottitis, or a foreign body. *Even if you suspect a foreign body, if the child or infant is alert and moving air, do not intervene.*

THE NONBREATHING COMPLETE OBSTRUCTION OR PARTIAL OBSTRUCTION WITH POOR AIR EXCHANGE. If an infant or child begins to deteriorate with decreasing mental status, severe retractions without air movement, and a rapid respiratory rate and pulse, or especially if the infant or child develops a very slow pulse (a late finding indicating severe hypoxia), intervention becomes necessary.

If the child cannot speak or cry or is exhibiting a weak, ineffective cough, stridor, and cyanosis (partial obstruction with poor air exchange), the child should be treated as having a complete airway obstruction. If you suspect an *infectious cause,* assist breathing with positive-pressure ventilation. If you suspect a foreign body, proceed with the foreign body airway obstruction protocol.

Management of the child with a complete airway obstruction is the same as the management of an adult, with one exception. *The finger sweep procedure is done only when the object is visualized.* Management of the infant with a foreign body airway obstruction differs from that of a child or adult.

THE COMPLETE OBSTRUCTION WITH A FOREIGN BODY IN A CONSCIOUS INFANT. The infant should be supported on your arm and thigh, face down with the head toward your palm and slightly dependent. Four back blows should be administered between the scapula, using the heel of your hand, each blow given with the intent of removing the object (Fig. 3–51). The combination of back blows and gravity often removes the obstruction.

If the obstruction is not removed by back blows, administer 4 chest thrusts. Hold the baby between both arms along the long axis of the body and turn the infant to a supine position. Administer 4 chest thrusts by placing your middle and ring fingers on the sternum 1 finger breadth below the nipple line (Fig. 3–52). Each thrust should depress the sternum $\frac{1}{2}$ to 1 inch.

Repeat 4 back blows followed by 4 chest thrusts until the obstruction is removed or the infant becomes unconscious.

THE INFANT WHO BECOMES UNCONSCIOUS WITH COMPLETE OBSTRUCTION. If the infant becomes un-

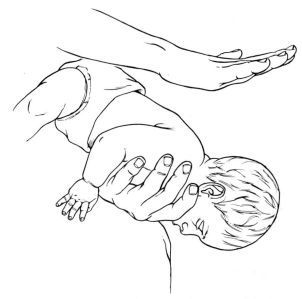

FIGURE 3–51. When administering back blows, to an infant, the infant should be supported on your arm and thigh. The infant's head can rest across your palm to give further support to the head. Strike the infant's back between the shoulder blades with the heel of your hand.

conscious, perform a tongue-jaw lift (Fig. 3–53), visualize the airway, and perform a finger sweep *only if you can see the foreign body.* If you cannot see the obstruction, do not perform a blind finger sweep. After the finger sweep, attempt to ventilate (Fig. 3–54). If you cannot ventilate, repeat the series of back blows and chest thrusts, followed by a finger sweep (when visualized), and then re-attempt ventilations.

The sequence is:

1. Give 4 back blows.
2. Give 4 chest thrusts.

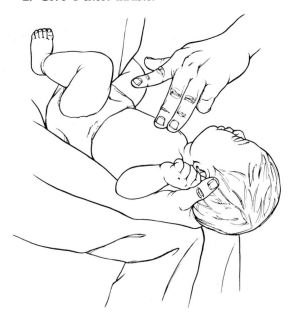

FIGURE 3–52. Chest thrusts for the infant are administered 1 finger breadth below the nipple line. Place 3 fingers on the sternum, with the index finger along the nipple line. Lift the index finger and provide the chest thrusts, using your middle and ring fingers.

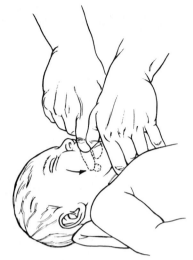

FIGURE 3–53. The finger sweep in the infant should be done while maintaining a tongue-jaw lift. The finger sweep is performed only after you can view the foreign body.

3. Open airway with tongue-jaw lift and perform finger sweep if the foreign body is visible.

4. Attempt to ventilate.

5. If unable to ventilate, repeat Steps 1 through 4.

If you are unable to ventilate after a few cycles, initiate rapid transport while continuing the sequence en route to the hospital.

AN INFANT FOUND UNCONSCIOUS WITH A COMPLETE AIRWAY OBSTRUCTION. If the infant is found unconscious, the presence of a complete airway obstruction is usually established by an inability to ventilate. As with the adult and child, you should first try to reopen the airway and attempt a second ventilation. If you are still unable to ventilate, administer 4 back blows, 4 chest thrusts, and a finger sweep in the same manner described previously. Attempt to ventilate at the end of each sequence. If you are unable to clear the airway after several attempts, rapid transport is essential for surgical intervention.

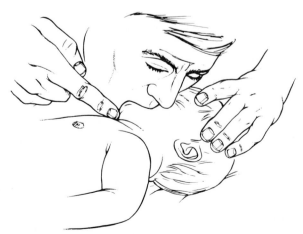

FIGURE 3–54. Keep the airway open with head tilt–chin lift and attempt to ventilate, covering the mouth and nose of the infant.

If the airway is cleared, check the pulse and respirations and proceed accordingly. If there is a pulse with no respirations, provide positive-pressure ventilation at the recommended rate of 1 every 3 seconds. If the infant has no pulse, perform CPR (see Chapter 6 for infant CPR).

PATHOLOGIC OBSTRUCTION

The final type of airway obstruction is a pathologic obstruction. This blockage results from swelling of the tissues of the upper airway. The most common cause of this type of obstruction in adults is anaphylaxis, a severe allergic reaction. (Epiglottitis occurs in adults but is rare.) The release of a substance called *histamine* allows fluid to enter tissue. This fluid may cause swelling throughout the body, but swelling of the tissues of the airway, namely the pharynx, tongue, vocal cords, or epiglottis, is especially dangerous. The swelling narrows, restricts, and sometimes totally obstructs air movement.

There may be other signs and symptoms that precede the obstructive event. Signs and symptoms of an allergic reaction are *hives, blotching of the skin, itching, edema, shortness of breath, wheezing, stridor, and cyanosis.*

The emergency management of anaphylaxis requires medications (e.g., epinephrine) that reverse this process. If this is unsuccessful, a *cricothyroidotomy* or *tracheostomy* (surgical incision of the windpipe) may be necessary to restore breathing (Fig. 3–55). Since most EMTs do not perform such procedures, it is essential to recognize the early signs of an allergic reaction and transport the patient quickly.

When a patient is found in a state of total airway obstruction due to an allergic reaction, you should attempt to provide positive-pressure ventilation during transport in the hope of delivering some oxygen to the alveoli.

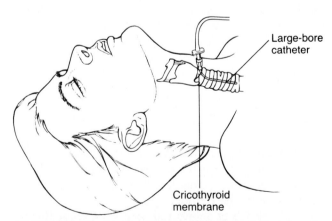

Large-bore catheter

Cricothyroid membrane

FIGURE 3–55. Cricothyroidotomy using the insertion of a catheter into the cricothyroidotomy membrane is a rapid surgical approach to establishing an airway. This technique is a temporary measure that allows for oxygenation until more definitive steps are taken, i.e., tracheostomy. This technique is used by paramedics in some EMS systems.

PROTOCOL

OBSTRUCTED AIRWAY—PEDIATRIC

A. IF THE CHILD IS CONSCIOUS AND CAN BREATHE, COUGH, CRY, OR SPEAK:

1. DO NOT INTERFERE, AND DO NOT PERFORM BLS AIRWAY MANEUVERS! *ALLOW THE CHILD TO ASSUME AND MAINTAIN A POSITION OF COMFORT OR TO BE HELD BY THE PARENT, PREFERABLY IN AN UPRIGHT POSITION.*

2. Administer high-concentration oxygen (preferably humidified) by a face mask IF TOLERATED. *AVOID AGITATING THE CHILD!* Administration of oxygen may best be accomplished by allowing the parent to hold the face mask about 6 to 8 inches from the child's face.

3. Transport immediately, keeping the child warm.

4. Obtain and record the initial vital signs IF TOLERATED, and repeat en route as often as the situation indicates without agitating the child.

5. Record all child care information, including the patient's medical history and all treatment provided, on a Prehospital Care Report.

> REMEMBER: AGITATING A CHILD WITH PARTIAL AIRWAY BLOCKAGE COULD CAUSE COMPLETE OBSTRUCTION! AS LONG AS THE CHILD CAN BREATHE, COUGH, CRY, OR SPEAK, *DO NOT UPSET THE CHILD WITH UNNECESSARY PROCEDURES (E.G., BLOOD PRESSURE DETERMINATION)!* USE A CALM, REASSURING APPROACH, TRANSPORTING THE PARENT AND CHILD AS A UNIT

B. IF THE CHILD IS UNCONSCIOUS AND NOT BREATHING

AND

IF FOREIGN BODY ASPIRATION WAS *NOT* WITNESSED:

> IF FOREIGN BODY ASPIRATION WAS WITNESSED, GO DIRECTLY TO BACK BLOWS OR CHEST THRUSTS AND ATTEMPT TO CLEAR AIRWAY OBSTRUCTION.

1. Attempt to establish airway control using BLS techniques. Open the child's mouth, and remove any VISIBLE foreign body.

2. Administer two breaths using mouth-to-mouth/nose or pocket mask, observing the child for adequate chest rise.

3. IF THE CHILD'S *CHEST DOES NOT RISE*:

   a. Check BLS airway techniques. Reopen the child's airway using the head tilt–chin lift or jaw-thrust maneuver. (Grasping the child's tongue during the chin-lift maneuver may improve the success of opening the airway.)

   b. Reattempt ventilations using mouth-to-mouth/nose or pocket mask.

   c. IF THE CHILD IS YOUNGER THAN 1 YEAR OF AGE (INFANT) AND THE CHEST *STILL DOES NOT RISE*:

      (1) Position the infant in a head-down position.

      (2) Administer back blows and chest thrusts according to AHA/ARC standards.

      (3) Open the infant's mouth, and remove any VISIBLE foreign body.

      > *CAUTION!*
      >
      > DO NOT PROBE FOR SUSPECTED FOREIGN BODY WITH BLIND FINGER SWEEPS. THIS TECHNIQUE COULD INADVERTENTLY FORCE THE OBSTRUCTION FURTHER DOWN THE INFANT'S AIRWAY.

   d. Reattempt ventilations, using mouth-to-mouth/nose or pocket mask.

   e. IF THE INFANT'S CHEST STILL DOES NOT RISE, repeat the sequence of reopening the airway, attempting ventilations, delivering back blows and chest thrusts, removing any VISIBLE foreign body, and reattempting ventilations ONLY ONCE!

   f. TRANSPORT IMMEDIATELY IF UNSUCCESSFUL, repeating step e throughout transport if needed, and keeping the infant warm.

   g. Record all patient care information, including the patient's medical history and all treatment provided, on a Prehospital Care Report.

OR

C. IF THE CHILD IS 1 YEAR OF AGE OR OLDER AND THE CHEST STILL DOES NOT RISE:

   (1) Kneel at the child's feet or straddle the larger child.

   (2) Perform abdominal thrusts according to AHA/ARC standards.

   > *CAUTION!*
   >
   > DIRECT THE THRUSTS UPWARD IN THE MIDLINE. AVOID DIRECTING THE THRUSTS TO EITHER SIDE OF MIDLINE.

   (3) Open the child's mouth, and remove any VISIBLE foreign body.

Continued

CAUTION!

DO NOT PROBE FOR SUSPECTED FOREIGN BODY WITH BLIND FINGER SWEEPS. THIS TECHNIQUE COULD INADVERTENTLY FORCE THE OBSTRUCTION FURTHER DOWN THE CHILD'S AIRWAY.

D. Reattempt ventilations, using mouth-to-mouth/nose or pocket mask.

From Manual for Emergency Medical Technicians. Emergency Medical Services Program. Albany, New York State Department of Health, 1990.
See Epiglottitis in Chapter 14.

Lower Airway Obstruction

CHRONIC OBSTRUCTIVE PULMONARY DISEASE

Chronic obstructive pulmonary disease (COPD) is a common respiratory emergency. This category of disease includes two major diseases: *chronic bronchitis* and *emphysema*. Both diseases are commonly caused by long-term cigarette smoking. Shortness of breath is the primary symptom of both these diseases. Furthermore, although described separately, for an individual patient, the symptoms often overlap.

CHRONIC BRONCHITIS (BLUE BLOATER). Chronic bronchitis is a disease caused by smoking or exposure to environmental pollutants. Long-term irritation results in a number of changes within the lung. Mucus-secreting glands become enlarged and excessive mucus production causes plugging of the bronchi and bronchioles (Fig. 3–56). The retained secretions also cause the characteristic productive cough. This harsh, phlegm-producing cough is especially active on waking in the morning.

The obstructed bronchi result in poorly ventilated alveoli and the *shunting of blood*. This in turn causes poorly oxygenated hemoglobin and cyanosis. Due to the typical cyanotic appearance of these patients, the term "blue bloater" was coined to describe their skin color and puffy, edematous appearance. The edema that accumulates in the ankles, hips, or abdomen is the result of right-sided heart failure, which is a complication of COPD. Heart failure will also cause distention of neck veins. This disease will be discussed in greater detail in Chapter 5.

Auscultation of breath sounds may reveal wheezing, rhonchi, and sometimes rales due to mucous secretions throughout the airway and fluid buildup, which also results from heart failure (Fig. 3–57).

EMPHYSEMA (PINK PUFFER). Emphysema is a disease that is caused by a destruction of alveoli and the

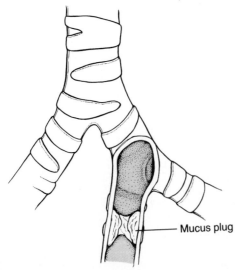

FIGURE 3–56. A mucus plug in the bronchi can obstruct air flow in the airways. Total obstruction can result in non-ventilated alveoli (shunt).

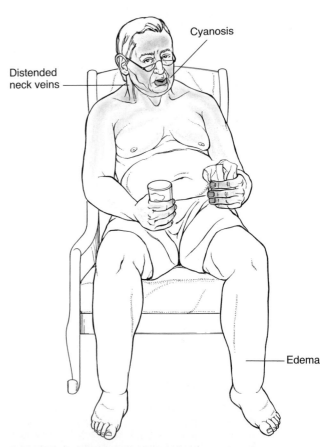

Cyanosis

Distended neck veins

Edema

FIGURE 3–57. The "blue bloater" (chronic bronchitis): cyanosis, edema, and distended neck veins.

loss of elastic recoil within the lung. Patients with this disease are left with less surface area through which oxygen can diffuse into the bloodstream. Emphysema patients also have damage to the muscular portion of the small bronchioles within the lung. These muscular structures, in their normal condition, resist the collapse of the small bronchioles during the increase in pressure within the chest during exhalation. However, the airways of emphysema patients collapse during forced exhalation (Fig. 3–58). They are left with a *higher residual volume* (the amount of air remaining in the lung after a forceful exhalation). This phenomenon is called "air trapping" and is the explanation for the characteristic "barrel chest" appearance of the COPD patient. The chest wall is gradually reshaped as the patient "breathes around" the trapped air. To better appreciate the sensation of air trapping, take a full breath and release only a small amount of air. Now take another few breaths, never releasing beyond this point.

Because their airways tend to collapse during exhalation, emphysema patients find they breathe better when they exhale against a resistance. They make their own resistance to exhalation by pursing their lips, thus narrowing the airway opening.

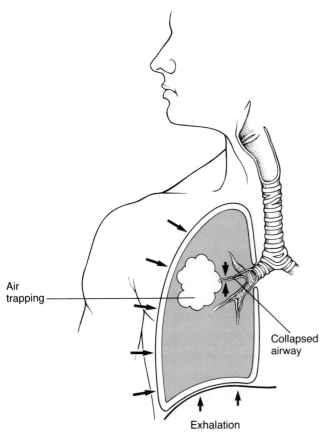

Air trapping

Collapsed airway

Exhalation

FIGURE 3–58. The loss of muscular tissue support in the lower airways can lead to collapse and obstruction of the airways during exhalation when the intrathoracic pressure is increased. This results in "air trapping." The emphysema patient sometimes breathes through "pursed" lips to maintain the pressures within the airway in order to maintain patency (being wide open) during exhalation.

To compensate for chronic lung disease, the body may increase the amount of red blood cells and hemoglobin in the blood. This may result in a characteristic pink appearance. The combination of the pursed-lip breathing and the pink appearance has resulted in the label "pink puffer" being used when describing emphysema patients (Fig. 3–59). Both emphysema and bronchitis patients may have a characteristic "clubbing" of the distal ends of their fingers.

Again, most patients have a combination of both emphysema and chronic bronchitis. The disease is chronic and very disabling and often requires the use of oxygen at home. The patient's daily activity is limited.

COPD PATIENTS IN RESPIRATORY FAILURE. Both emphysema patients and individuals suffering from chronic bronchitis are subject to respiratory infections that can aggravate their condition. During these episodes they are subject to severe hypoxic states. This is caused by the further obstruction of the tracheobronchial tree by inflammation and swelling. In individuals who already have a decreased number of functional airways, this can be life threatening. When their respiratory systems become so ineffective that they can no longer support life, these patients are said to be in a state of *respiratory failure*. Aggressive action by the EMT at this point is essential.

Recognition and Management. COPD patients in respiratory failure initially present with severe dyspnea, while positioned in a bolt upright posture. Their accessory muscles are active, and breath sounds may reveal diffuse wheezing throughout their lung fields. They can be cyanotic and their mental status may be agitated, confused, or depressed, depending on the degree of hypoxia.

If patients exhibit forceful and effective ventilation, they should receive 24% oxygen through a Venturi mask or 2 to 3 liters of oxygen through a nasal cannula if they cannot tolerate a face mask. If patients do not respond, higher oxygen concentration should be used with close monitoring for signs of respiratory depression. Reassurance may decrease their oxygen needs, and they should be transported in the *Fowler's position* (sitting upright). This will allow patients full use of their diaphragms during ventilations. If the patient develops ventilatory depression and shows signs of hypoventilation or respiratory arrest, positive-pressure ventilation should be started. If the patient is still ventilating, positive pressure should be synchronized with the patient's efforts (assisted ventilation) and supplemental O_2 should be added to the positive-pressure device.

ASTHMA

Asthma is an acute and intermittent obstructive respiratory disease that is often precipitated by stress, infection, or an allergic response. The obstruction is the

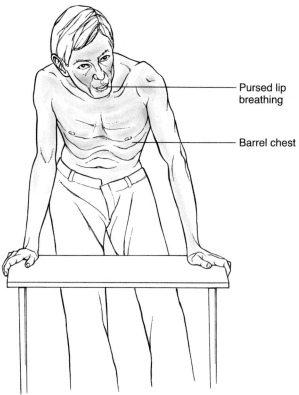

Pursed lip
breathing

Barrel chest

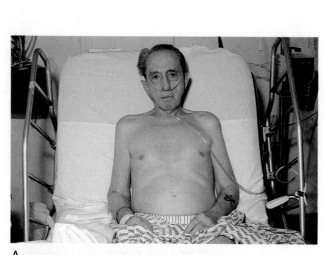

A

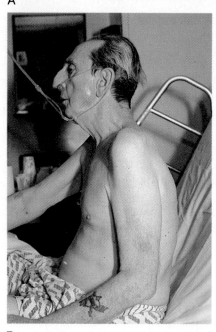

B

FIGURE 3–59. (*A*) The "pink puffer" (emphysema): pink, flushed color; pursed-lip breathing; and (*B*) barrel chest appearance are characteristics of emphysema patients.

result of a spasm of the bronchioles that can be complicated by secretions in the bronchial tree. This reduces air flow to the alveoli and causes the patient to experience dyspnea. Most asthmatic patients are able to compensate for the narrowed airways by hyperventilation and can usually maintain adequate blood oxygen levels. However, if the attack cannot be broken by the medications, which might include oral inhalations of bronchial sprays, they may become exhausted and be unable to maintain

their compensated state. Like the COPD patient, they may experience respiratory failure. Common medications taken by asthmatic patients include epinephrine, isoproterenol, isoetharine, metaproterenol, terbutaline, theophylline, and steroids.

RECOGNITION AND MANAGEMENT. An acute asthmatic attack is characterized by shortness of breath, with the patient assuming the upright posture and using accessory muscles to increase ventilation. The patient may be flushed and breathing forcefully. Wheezing and prolonged expirations may be audible even without the stethoscope. However, as the work of breathing continues, the patient may become fatigued, causing respiratory failure. He or she may become progressively lethargic or sleepy, and cyanosis may develop. Breath sounds, as with the COPD patient, are likely to reveal diffused wheezing and prolonged expiration, and the patient may complain of a "binding" chest pain. When patients have a severe asthmatic attack and become exhausted, they may produce little air flow, have difficulty in speaking, and have decreased breath sounds.

If the patient is ventilating effectively, oxygen via nasal cannula at 6 liters per minute may be administered. If there are signs of hypoxia, high-concentration oxygen should be given. If hypoventilation, cyanosis, and a depressed mental state develop, assistance with positive-pressure breathing should be initiated.

Conditions Affecting the Alveoli and Diffusion of Oxygen

PNEUMONIA

Pneumonia is an inflammation of alveolar spaces caused by various types of infecting organisms or by aspiration of gastric contents into the tracheobronchial tree. The major component of the disease is the collection of fluid in the alveolar space. This reduces the number of functional alveoli, reduces the diffusion surface area, and may lead to respiratory distress. The accumulating fluid is usually the result of the normal body defenses directed against the invading organism. Fluid and white blood cells from the pulmonary capillaries enter the alveolar space to attack the organisms.

ASSESSMENT. Pneumonia may present in many ways, depending on the underlying cause, but there are signs and symptoms that are common to most pneumonias. The disease usually follows a pattern of prior respiratory infection, fever, and cough, often with the production of thick, colored sputum (containing pus). In other cases there may be a sudden onset of cough, fever, and chills in either previously healthy or debilitated people. Pneumonia from aspiration follows unconscious states, including drug and alcohol overdoses.

Patients may complain of dyspnea, chills, headache, and a productive rusty or bloody sputum that may be thick and purulent. They may also complain of local pleuritic chest pain on the affected side. The physical examination may reveal a fever as high as 40.5°C, profuse sweating, and, in the more severe episodes, cyanosis. The mental state may be lethargic and, in some cases,

confused. The vital signs might include a rapid pulse and increased respiratory rate. Breath sounds typically reveal rales and diminished sounds in local areas of pneumonia, with normal sounds in the remainder of the lung field. On examination, the patient is likely to be coughing vigorously and again producing a purulent or bloody sputum.

MANAGEMENT. Emergency care of the pneumonia victim is determined by the degree of distress. If the patient appears hypoxic but is ventilating adequately, then high concentrations of oxygen should be administered through a nonrebreather mask. Usually the patient will prefer to sit in the upright position to improve his or her ventilatory efforts during transport. If the patient develops signs of respiratory failure, including lethargy, hypoventilation, or cyanosis, positive-pressure ventilation with high concentrations of oxygen should be started.

NEAR-DROWNING

Approximately 4,700 people died from drowning in 1986 in the United States. The typical drowning victim has either overestimated his or her endurance, is intoxicated, or has fallen into the water and is unable to swim. The sequence of events often follows a pattern that includes panic, water swallowing, and aspiration of water into the lungs. Sometimes, when water comes into contact with the vocal cords, the resultant "laryngospasm" closes the *glottic opening* (the entrance of the larynx) and prevents water from entering the tracheobronchial tree. This is referred to as a dry drowning and may occur in as many as 10 to 20% of drowning victims. The effects of water that enters the lungs vary according to the type of drowning—salt water or fresh water.

SALT-WATER DROWNING. Aspiration of salt water usually results in massive pulmonary edema due to the salt pulling water from the pulmonary circulation. This results in a massive shunt of blood passing the affected alveoli, resulting in severe hypoxia. The patient eventually becomes unconscious due to poor brain oxygenation.

FRESH-WATER DROWNING. In fresh-water drowning, more water is absorbed into the pulmonary circulation. This results in an increase in the volume of the fluid portion of the blood. The excessive water may also destroy red blood cells and the oxygen-carrying capacity of the blood. Fresh-water drowning also washes away *surfactant*. This results in the collapse of alveoli and again massive shunting of blood passed through the lungs. Hypoxia results in unconsciousness and, ultimately, cardiac arrest.

The time to cardiac arrest may vary, particularly in cold water. Patients have responded with what is called a "mammalian diving reflex." This mechanism slows down metabolism, resulting in decreased oxygen consumption and redistribution of blood to more vital organs: brain, heart, and lungs. This factor has enabled many people to be resuscitated following submersion for long periods of time. Therefore, resuscitation measures should always be initiated on drowning victims.

MANAGEMENT OF NEAR-DROWNING.   Regardless of the type of water in which the victim is drowning, treatment is the same. Priority is given to the ABCs, outlined earlier in this text. An airway should be established as soon as possible—even in the water if conditions permit (a shallow water drowning)—with administration of positive-pressure ventilation. Mouth-to-mouth resuscitation can be initiated until a mechanical aid is either available or feasible. Once a mechanical method is utilized, high-concentration oxygen should be administered (100% if possible). Clearing the lungs of water need not be attempted because the effects of ventilation and oxygenation will drive out the water from the airway. Suctioning of the upper airway may be needed as fluids are expelled. However, suctioning should not last more than 5 seconds because additional oxygen may be removed from the airway. Many drownings occur in shallow water as a result of diving accidents. If spinal injury is suspected, the patient should be removed from the water with alignment of the spine maintained. A backboard or other floatable surface (e.g., surfboard) can be utilized to ensure proper immobilization during the rescue. The jaw thrust–without head tilt maneuver should be utilized for these patients.

Occasionally, the water that is aspirated into the stomach interferes with ventilation efforts. This is characterized by difficulty in delivery of positive pressure. Only in these instances should an abdominal thrust be applied to relieve the obstruction or gastric distention. Suction should be on standby to clear fluid from the upper airway. Obviously, if no pulse is felt, cardiac compressions should be initiated. This is covered in Chapter 6.

Respiratory Depression and Arrest

CAUSES.   A variety of conditions can potentially depress or eliminate respiratory drive: electric shock, head trauma, overdose of depressant drugs, stroke, and any other disease or traumatic condition that causes hypoxia or brain damage. Regardless of the precipitating factor, the central goal is always the same—establish an adequate airway and initiate positive-pressure ventilation.

The mechanisms that cause loss of central nervous system control over ventilations vary. If the cause is one of a depressant nature, such as drug overdose or gradual

---

✠ P R O T O C O L ✠

APPROACH TO THE NEAR-DROWNING PATIENT

1. SPECIAL ASSESSMENT CONSIDERATIONS

   a. Determine if the near-drowning occurred in fresh or salt water. Determine how long the victim was submerged and the temperature of the surrounding water.

   b. Consider possible spinal injuries. Use the appropriate precautions when removing the patient from the water.

   c. If the victim is submerged upon your arrival, request the response of the SCUBA Search and Rescue Unit. Anticipate any necessary medical treatment and *prepare all equipment accordingly.*

   > RESCUES SHOULD NOT BE ATTEMPTED BY THOSE NOT PROPERLY TRAINED IN WATER RESCUE TECHNIQUES!

2. TREATMENT

   a. After access to the victim is gained:

   (1) Perform expanded primary survey.

   (2) Begin artificial respirations as needed.

   (3) Remove the patient from the water. Use spinal precautions as indicated.

   (4) Continue intervention as required.

   > *NOTE!*
   >
   > IN CASES OF COLD WATER DROWNING (WATER TEMPERATURE BELOW 70°F), TREAT FOR HYPOTHERMIA.

   (5) Transport, keeping the patient warm.

   > IN COLD WATER NEAR-DROWNING, CEREBRAL OXYGEN REQUIREMENTS ARE GREATLY REDUCED. THESE PATIENTS CAN WITHSTAND CARDIAC ARREST (EVEN THOUGH SUBMERGED) FOR LONG PERIODS OF TIME WITHOUT SUBSEQUENT BRAIN DAMAGE. THEREFORE, *ALWAYS INITIATE AND MAINTAIN RESUSCITATION PROCEDURES WHEN INDICATED.*

From New York City Emergency Medical Services, Basic Life Support Protocols, New York, NY, 1990.

---

hypoxia, then the evolution from adequate ventilation to depressed ventilation to respiratory arrest tends to be gradual. Acute episodes of breathing stoppage are more likely to be the result of trauma, loss of circulation to the brain such as a stroke, or other sudden factors such as electric shock.

ASSESSMENT. Evaluating the adequacy of ventilation is not a totally objective process. Certainly, when a total respiratory arrest exists, management is obvious. However, patients may be found with various degrees of respiratory depression that cause decision-making to be somewhat ambiguous. Again, adequate ventilation is evaluated grossly by observing chest rise and respiratory rate. Should chest excursion not be visible or barely detectable, or if the patient is exhibiting an altered mental status, inadequate ventilation should be assumed. Other physical findings suggestive of respiratory failure would include a respiratory rate below 12 or greater than 30 per minute, cyanosis, and dilated pupils. If you are unsure about the need for positive-pressure ventilation, it is better to err on the side of treatment.

MANAGEMENT. The emergency care of respiratory depression or arrest is primarily directed toward establishing an airway and initiating positive-pressure ventilation. Supplemental 100% oxygen should be used as soon as possible. Initially, the patient should be given 2 smooth breaths, followed by 1 breath every 5 seconds (in the adult patient). Breaths should be administered no faster than 1 to 1.5 seconds per breath. Otherwise, the pressure created within the upper airway will open the esophagus and cause gastric distention. The abdomen should be closely observed for signs of gastric distention. If it develops, attempts should be made to decrease airway pressures by adjusting the rate and volume of breaths. As with the drowning victim, gastric distention should be relieved only if it interferes with positive-pressure ventilation. When necessary, gastric distention is relieved by applying gentle pressure to the *epigastric region* (just below the xiphoid process), while turning the victim to the side (Fig. 3–60). Again, suction should be available to avoid aspiration of secretions.

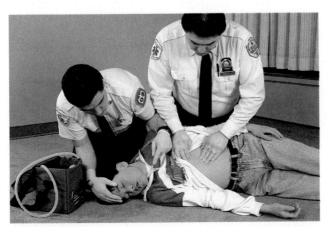

FIGURE 3–60. Rotate the patient on one side and have suction on standby. Gently compress the epigastric region (over the swollen stomach) and be ready to clear vomitus and secretions. *Gastric distention should be relieved only when it interferes with breathing.*

PROTOCOL

RESPIRATORY ARREST—ADULT/CARDIAC ARREST (NONTRAUMATIC)—ADULT AND PEDIATRIC

1. Provide BLS according to AHA/ARC standards.

   IF VENTILATIONS ARE UNSUCCESSFUL, REFER IMMEDIATELY TO THE OBSTRUCTED *AIRWAY* PROTOCOL.

2. Insert an oropharyngeal or nasopharyngeal airway if the gag reflex is absent.

3. Ventilate with an adjunctive device and high-concentration oxygen.

   MINIMUM RATE OF VENTILATION:

   ADULTS—12 TIMES A MINUTE.
   CHILDREN 2 YEARS OF AGE OR OLDER—15 TIMES A MINUTE.
   CHILDREN UNDER 2 YEARS OF AGE—20 TIMES A MINUTE.
   ASSURE THAT THE CHEST RISES WITH EACH VENTILATION!

   > ADEQUATE VENTILATION MAY REQUIRE DISABLING THE POP-OFF VALVE IF THE BAG-VALVE-MASK UNIT IS SO EQUIPPED!

4. Evaluate the effectiveness of the ventilations/compressions.

5. Transport IMMEDIATELY, keeping the patient warm.

6. Record all patient care information, including the patient's medical history and all treatment provided, on a Prehospital Care Report.

From Manual of Emergency Medical Technicians. Emergency Medical Services Program. Albany, New York State Department of Health, 1990.

Hyperventilation Syndrome

An extremely common respiratory problem is *hyperventilation syndrome.* This anxiety-provoked condition is usually precipitated by some emotional event that caused the patient to hyperventilate. The patient overrides the normal stimulus for respiratory rate and volume and begins to breathe more rapidly and forcefully. This will ultimately cause a depletion of carbon dioxide in the blood and result in a more alkaline blood pH.

ASSESSMENT. Patients experiencing hyperventilation syndrome usually have shortness of breath as their chief complaint. Frequently, the history of present illness reveals no other significant respiratory or cardiovascular complaints. Patients commonly complain of tingling about the mouth or fingers, nausea, and a feeling of dizziness. Questioning about a precipitating emotional event should be done whenever hyperventilation syndrome is suspected. The patient's medical history, medication history, or allergies are unlikely to reveal any information specific to diagnosing this problem. A history of similar past episodes or sedative prescriptions for anxiety would reinforce this diagnosis.

PHYSICAL EXAMINATION. These patients typically present with a pronounced appearance of tachypnea and are using accessory muscles, as well as having a rapid pulse rate and possibly an elevated blood pressure due to the anxiety component. A unique sign to look for is *carpopedal spasm* (fingers and toes in a rigid flexed state), which is a reaction to the decreased carbon dioxide levels in the blood.

TREATMENT. When treating hyperventilation syndrome, you must *first be sure that a more serious res-* *piratory or cardiovascular problem does not exist.* Assuming that the diagnosis is correct, the main treatment is to have the patient take slower breaths, thereby allowing carbon dioxide levels in the blood to return to normal. Calm reassurance is needed. Supplemental oxygen will not hurt the hyperventilating patient and should be given if there is any question of the diagnosis or if it helps reassure the patient.

Hyperventilating patients are sometimes asked to breathe into a paper bag. When they rebreath their expired air, the blood carbon dioxide concentration returns to normal more quickly. However, one investigator found that rebreathing from a paper bag caused some people to become hypoxic. Having a patient breathe more slowly through calm direction and reassurance accomplishes the same result without the risk of breathing the lower oxygen levels in expired air.

P R O T O C O L

APPROACH TO THE PATIENT COMPLAINING OF DYSPNEA

1. SPECIAL ASSESSMENT CONSIDERATIONS

    a. Determine scenario of onset.

    b. Determine history of previous episodes.

    c. Note use of accessory breathing muscles and/or obvious respiratory compromise.

    d. Evaluate need for ALS assistance.

2. TREATMENT

    a. Maintain ABCs.

    b. Administer oxygen:
    High concentration should be administered.

    c. Reassure the patient.

> *NOTE!*
>
> IF THE PATIENT IS A CHILD, MAINTAIN A CALM APPROACH TO THE PARENT AND CHILD. ALLOW THE CHILD TO ASSUME AND MAINTAIN A POSITION OF COMFORT OR TO BE HELD BY THE PARENT, PREFERABLY IN AN UPRIGHT POSITION.

> *NOTE!*
>
> AVOID AGITATING A CHILD. ADMINISTRATION OF OXYGEN, PREFERABLY HUMIDIFIED, IS BEST ACCOMPLISHED BY ALLOWING THE PARENT TO HOLD THE FACE MASK, IF TOLERATED, ABOUT 6 TO 8 INCHES FROM THE CHILD'S FACE.

    d. Do not permit physical exertion.

    e. Monitor the patient's condition and document vital signs at least every 5 minutes.

    f. Allow the patient to assume a position of comfort.

    g. Transport the patient to the appropriate hospital.

    h. Record all patient care information, including the patient's medical history and all treatment provided, on the ambulance call report (ACR).

> *NOTE!*
>
> BE PREPARED TO DEAL WITH RESPIRATORY AND CARDIAC ARREST! MONITOR THE RESPIRATORY STATUS CONTINUOUSLY. IN CHILDREN, BE ALERT FOR SIGNS OF INCREASING RESPIRATORY DISTRESS. THESE MAY INCLUDE DECREASED RESPIRATORY RATE AND/OR DEPTH, DECREASED BREATH SOUNDS, CYANOSIS, VISIBLE SOFT TISSUE RETRACTIONS, AND DECREASED LEVEL OF CONSCIOUSNESS. BE PREPARED TO VENTILATE A SLEEPY, ASTHMATIC CHILD WHO HAS A SILENT CHEST!

> *NOTE!*
>
> IF THE PATIENT DEMONSTRATES INADEQUATE VENTILATIONS (THE RESPIRATORY RATE IS LESS THAN 10 PER MINUTE OR GREATER THAN 29 PER MINUTE IN AN ADULT, OR LESS THAN 15 PER MINUTE IN A CHILD, AND THE PATIENT IS CONFUSED, RESTLESS, OR CYANOTIC): USE THE BAG-VALVE-MASK WITH RESERVOIR OR POSITIVE-PRESSURE ADJUNCTIVE DEVICE.

From New York City Emergency Medical Services, Basic Life Support Protocols. New York, NY, 1990.

Trauma to the Respiratory System

PNEUMOTHORAX

Pneumothorax is a condition in which air enters the normally closed space between the visceral and parietal pleura, causing the collapse of lung tissue. As was discussed in the anatomy and physiology section, the lung is dependent on a "relative negative pressure" within the pleural space to stay expanded. This negative pressure keeps the visceral and parietal pleura tightly adherent to each other. When air enters this space, it can dissect along the two pleura, resulting in loss of adherence and lung collapse (Fig. 3–61).

There are essentially two ways in which this condition may occur: first, blunt or penetrating trauma may puncture the chest wall or the lung; or second, the lung wall may spontaneously rupture due to a *bleb* or blister-like defect in the lung tissue.

TRAUMATIC PNEUMOTHORAX

Traumatic pneumothorax occurs when a missile (e.g., a bullet or piece of shrapnel), sharp object, or a broken rib penetrates the chest wall or lung. When the chest wall is perforated, air is drawn into the pleural space during inspiration. This can create a "sucking" sound, and this type of injury is frequently referred to as a "sucking chest wound."

A pneumothorax may also occur when a blunt force is applied to the thoracic cavity, causing the lung to rupture. This happens when a person takes a deep breath and holds it just prior to an automobile collision. As the person's chest cavity strikes the steering wheel, the trapped air causes the lungs to rupture. This is commonly called the "paper bag effect."

When the lung or part of the lung collapses, less alveolar space is available for diffusion of oxygen, and hypoxia can result. The condition can be more serious when the hole in the chest wall is larger than the trachea. In this instance air will preferentially enter through the chest wall over the trachea (air will take the path of least resistance). This will reduce functional air exchange and aggravate the hypoxia.

The pneumothorax patient may present with dyspnea and chest pain that tends to be pleuritic in nature. Breath sounds on the affected side may be diminished or absent. Subcutaneous emphysema may be present (Fig. 3–62). If the chest wall has been penetrated, a sucking wound may be visible. In cases of blunt trauma you may see a contusion or rib fractures, or you may suspect a pneumothorax based on the mechanism of injury when there are diminished or absent breath sounds.

SPONTANEOUS PNEUMOTHORAX

A *spontaneous pneumothorax* occurs in patients who have pulmonary disease that weakens the lung wall or in individuals who have *congenital blebs* (blisters on the

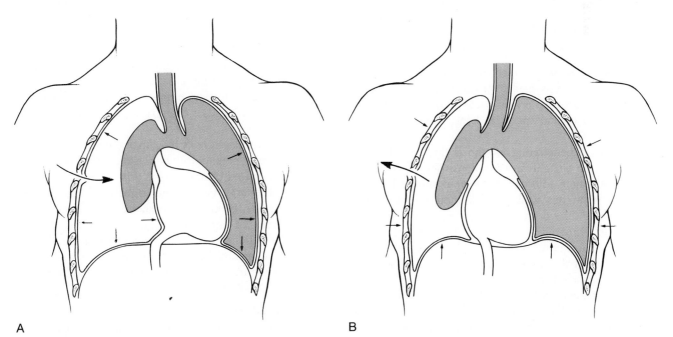

A B

FIGURE 3–61. There are several factors that cause decreased respiratory function in open pneumothorax: (*A*) When the chest cavity is penetrated, the pleural space loses its relative "negative" pressure, causing the lung to collapse (see Fig. 3–6). The hole in the chest wall interferes with the normal air movement of breathing. When the chest cavity expands, air rushes through the hole in the chest wall, as well as the trachea. If the hole in the chest wall is extremely large, air will preferentially enter through the hole, rather than through the airway, resulting in severe hypoventilation and hypoxia. Note the tracheal shift away from the injured side. (*B*) During exhalation, as air leaves through the hole in the chest cavity, the structures in the mediastinum will shift toward the affected side.

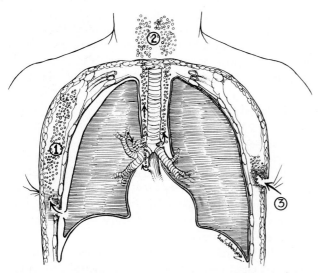

FIGURE 3–62. Subcutaneous emphysema, or air under the skin, may feel like "crepitus" and there may be obvious swelling. It can be felt (1) along the chest wall over a tear in the pleura and intercostal muscles (as from a pneumothorax with rib fractures); (2) in the neck when air dissects along deep tissue planes from tears in the esophagus, bronchus, or mediastinal surface of a lung; and (3) in the area of an external wound. (From Zuidema GD, Rutherford RB, Ballinger WF (eds): The Management of Trauma, 4th ed. Philadelphia, WB Saunders, 1985, p.400.)

lung wall) present since birth. When the lung ruptures and air enters the pleural space, the patient experiences a sudden onset of dyspnea and pleuritic chest pain. The lung may partially or totally collapse following this event. For some reason, this frequently occurs in young, thin, muscular males and therefore should be considered in patients complaining of dyspnea who fit this description. Again, breath sounds may be diminished or absent, depending on the degree of collapse.

MANAGEMENT.   Once the presumptive diagnosis of pneumothorax is made, management is directed at ensuring an adequate airway, preventing further air from entering the pleural space, and increasing delivery of oxygen.

When a penetrating wound is discovered on the chest wall, an airtight dressing consisting of petroleum gauze, aluminum foil, or plastic wrap should be taped securely to the chest wall. The tape should be overlapped around three sides of the dressing to prevent any further air from entering the chest wall but allowing air to escape when the intrathoracic pressure rises (Fig. 3–63). The patient should always be checked for other wounds and for exit wounds in the case of missile injuries.

The patient should then be placed on the *injured* side (unless spinal injury is suspected), to allow maximum expansion and function of the good lung. High-concentration oxygen should be administered through a nonrebreather mask. If the patient is hypoventilating or is in respiratory arrest, great care should be exercised dur-

ing positive-pressure breathing to avoid forcing excess air into the pleural space. Low-pressure methods of ventilation such as the pocket mask or bag-valve mask should be used. High-pressure systems such as oxygen-powered resuscitators may increase and complicate the pneumothorax by forcing more air into the pleural space.

TENSION PNEUMOTHORAX

Occasionally, a simple pneumothorax can be complicated by increased entry of air into the pleural space and thus develop into a *tension pneumothorax*. A tension pneumothorax is a condition in which more air entering the chest cavity becomes trapped within the pleural space. This can occur when a flap of tissue on the lung wall functionally becomes a one-way valve. It permits air to enter through the lung tear, but as air attempts to escape, it applies pressure on the flap and closes the opening. With each breath, as the chest expands, more and more air becomes trapped in the pleural space and the pressure increases. This pressure is exerted on all of the structures within the chest cavity. Initially, the lung collapses further and the diaphragm is displaced downward. Continued pressure will then cause the diaphragm to be displaced downward and the structures of the mediastinum to be pushed away from the affected side. One of the first problems to develop is collapse of the great veins, which have the lowest pressures of the thoracic structures (Fig. 3–64). This will ultimately prevent blood return to the heart, and the patient will go into a profound shock state. Early recognition of tension pneumothorax in the prehospital phase is critical, since transport to definitive treatment is of the highest priority.

Sucking chest wounds may also function as one-way valves, causing tension pneumothorax. Air enters the pleural space during inhalation but closes the flap of tissue during exhalation, trapping the air within. Closing sucking chest wounds is essential to preventing this from occurring.

The cardinal signs of tension pneumothorax include all the signs of pneumothorax plus distended neck veins, which are caused by the obstruction of blood returning through the large veins; other signs of shock (see also the discussion of obstructive shock in Chapter 5); and the shifting of the trachea away from the affected side. The patient becomes progressively more short of breath, the mental status deteriorates, and the patient may become cyanotic. Breath sounds should be noticeably absent on the affected side.

MANAGEMENT.   If these signs and symptoms develop following the application of an airtight dressing to a sucking wound, you should immediately remove the dressing. This may permit trapped air to escape from the chest cavity and release the tension. Immediately

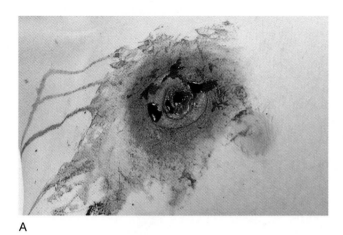

A

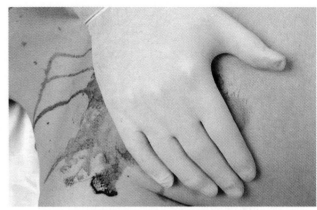

B

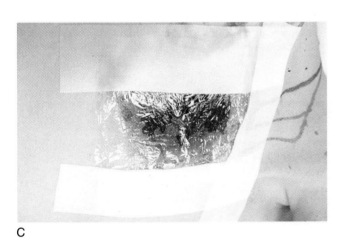

C

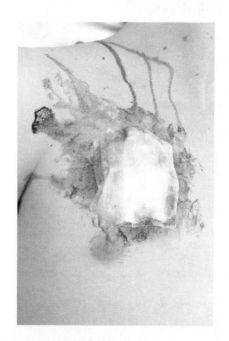

D

FIGURE 3–63. (*A*) A sucking wound may be noted on the chest wall. (*B*) If an airtight dressing is not immediately available, cover the hole with a gloved hand. (*C*) *Airtight dressing using plastic wrap*— ask the patient to forcefully exhale, and place an occlusive dressing over the wound. Tape the dressing on three sides. This will prevent air from entering the wound during inspiration (due to the dressing being sucked against the wound) but will allow air to exit during expiration. (*D*) *Airtight dressing using petrolatum gauze*—Place petrolatum gauze over the wound (do not stuff the dressing into the wound opening). (*E*) Place the sterile side of the aluminum wrapping over the gauze, and tape on three sides. Some protocols advocate taping all four sides. In either case, the patient with a "sealed" open pneumothorax must be watched carefully for signs of a tension pneumothorax. If such signs occur, loosen the seal during expiration to allow release of built-up air pressure.

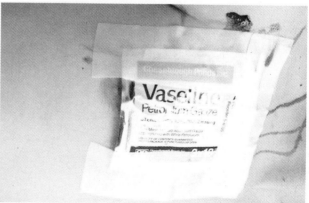

E

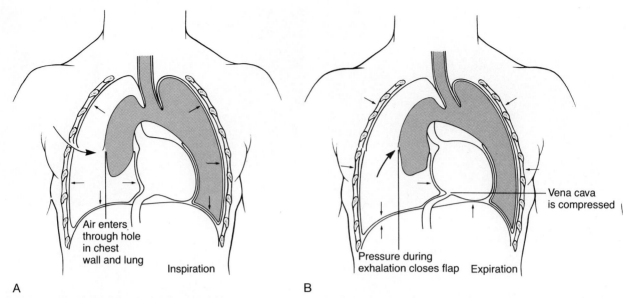

A   B

FIGURE 3–64. There are several factors that cause decreased respiratory and cardiovascular function in tension pneumothorax. (*A*) A flap of tissue on the lung or chest wall acts as a one-way valve. Air enters the chest cavity during inspiration as the flap opens. (*B*) During expiration, pressure within the thorax closes the flap, preventing air in the pleural space from exiting through the airways. If the opening in the chest wall is sealed by an airtight dressing or if the lung is torn without penetration of the chest wall, air cannot escape. Air begins to collect in the pleural space, gradually increasing in pressure. Because of the increased pressure, the diaphragm is pushed downward and the mediastinum is pushed away from the affected side (tracheal shift) and the vessels (veins) collapse within the mediastinum. As the pressure increases, the veins (low-pressure) collapse, obstructing venous return to the heart.

reseal the dressing following the release of tension. You may replace the dressing but observe closely for indications of further tension.

In a pneumothorax resulting from blunt trauma or with a spontaneous pneumothorax that develops tension, you should transport immediately. These patients require a needle to be placed into the chest cavity to relieve the

tension (Fig. 3–65). Some EMS systems permit paramedics to perform this procedure.

HEMOTHORAX

Hemothorax occurs when a blood vessel in the chest cavity is severed and blood begins to accumulate in the

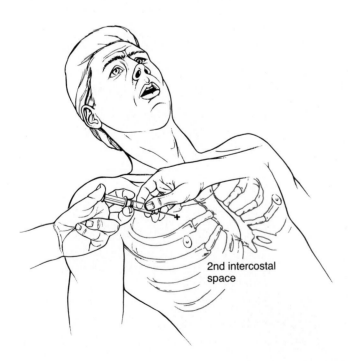

2nd intercostal space

FIGURE 3–65. Needle decompression of the chest is a simple surgical method for relieving tension pneumothorax. This technique is used by paramedics in some EMS systems.

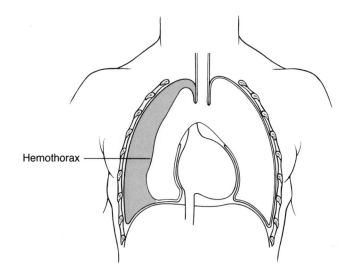

FIGURE 3–66. Hemothorax. Bleeding within the thoracic cavity can be extensive. In fact, the thoracic cavity is capable of storing the entire blood volume. Recognition of hemothorax often rests with recognition of the signs of hypovolemic shock.

pleural space (Fig. 3–66). It can be the result of penetrating or blunt trauma and can cause severe shock. Both hemothorax and pneumothorax can occur independently or in combination. A penetrating wound is likely to result in both.

Recognition of hemothorax in the prehospital phase is extremely difficult. In circumstances where it occurs as a result of penetrating chest injuries, it will be almost impossible to differentiate from pneumothorax. The EMT will primarily identify hemothorax by recognizing signs of hypovolemic shock (rapid pulse; pale, cool, sweaty skin; hypotension; etc.). This is discussed in detail in Chapter 5. In both pneumothorax and hemothorax, breath sounds will be diminished or absent.

MANAGEMENT. The management of hemothorax is the same as that of pneumothorax, with the addition of treatment for hypovolemic shock. Essentially, it includes airway control, oxygen therapy, control of external bleeding, and the application of *pneumatic antishock garment* (PASG). Rapid transport is essential when a shock state exists. This is a surgical emergency that requires surgical intervention.

Conditions Affecting Respiratory Muscle and Chest Wall Function

RIB FRACTURES

Generally speaking, a rib fracture is not a serious emergency. However, complications such as pneumothorax, hemothorax, and flail chest, which are often the result of a rib fracture, should be suspected when a fractured rib is discovered. Rib fractures are most often the result of blunt trauma (steering wheel injuries, falls,

and assault involving blows to the chest are typical examples of mechanisms of injuries). However, penetrating wounds may also result in injury to the ribs.

ASSESSMENT AND MANAGEMENT. Local pleuritic chest pain following a thoracic injury, contusions, crepitus, deformity, tenderness, and "splinting" of the affected side are common signs and symptoms of rib fractures. Splinting refers to the tendency to reduce movement of the injured area on the chest wall. Patients who have rib fractures are likely to display an unequal chest wall movement.

Rib fractures are treated in the prehospital phase by applying a sling and swathe to the affected side of the chest. This will aid in pain relief by splinting the chest wall (Fig. 3–67). Care should be taken not to restrict breathing efforts by applying the swathe too tightly.

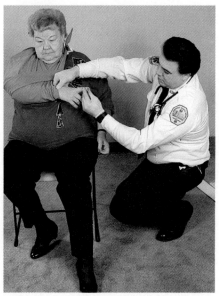

FIGURE 3–67. Treatment for rib fractures—sling and swathe.

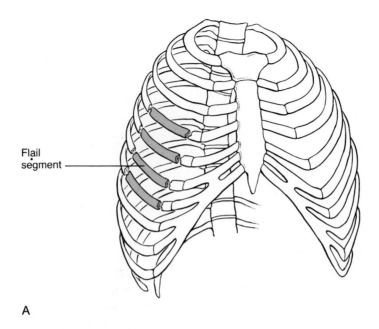

A

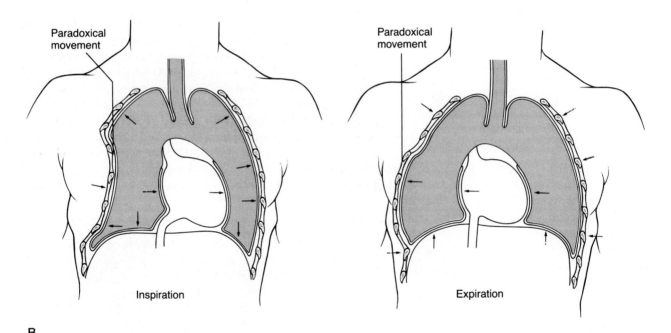

B

FIGURE 3–68. (*A*) *Flail chest*—when two or more ribs are fractured in two or more places, the affected rib segment becomes dissociated from the remaining chest wall. This interferes with the "bellows" mechanism of ventilation. This type of injury often results in severe pulmonary contusions. (*B*) *Paradoxical breathing*—the flail segment moves in an opposite direction to the intact chest wall during breathing. This compromises the normal bellows effect of ventilation.

FLAIL CHEST

Flail chest is strictly defined as *two or more ribs fractured in two or more places* (Fig. 3–68A and B). This results in a portion of the chest wall being dissociated from the remainining chest wall structure. The severity of this condition is determined by the area of the flail segment and the underlying problems such as pneumothorax, hemothorax, or pulmonary contusions (bruising of lung tissue). The typical mechanism of injury causing a flail chest is a high-energy blunt force applied to the chest wall. Steering wheel injuries in automobile collisions are a common cause of flail chest.

When the segment of ribs dissociates from the remaining thoracic cage, a number of problems concerning the mechanics of breathing develop. During inspiration, as the chest cavity enlarges, the pressure within the chest cavity becomes lower than the atmospheric pressure. This causes the flail segment to be pulled in during inhalation. During exhalation, when the pressure within the chest cavity increases, the flail segment is pushed out. In essence, the flail segment is moving in the direction opposite from the remaining chest wall. This is called *paradoxical breathing*. It is the cardinal sign of a flail chest.

ASSESSMENT. Recognition of a flail chest is made first and foremost by considering the mechanism of injury and examining the chest wall for evidence of flail segments. They may be identified during palpation of the thoracic wall. The affected area feels flaccid and easily moves inward. *Great care should be exercised when examining the chest wall.* Observe for paradoxical breathing, although this may not be very obvious in small flail segments. Other signs and symptoms may include chest pain and pale or cyanotic skin, depending on associated injuries. Breath sounds tend to be slightly diminished in the affected area, and signs of pneumothorax or hemothorax should be sought, as there is a good potential for both problems in chest trauma. Flail segments range from relatively small areas of the chest to separation of the entire sternum from the anterior thorax. Obviously, the extent of the flail area affects function.

MANAGEMENT. Management of a flail chest has essentially two objectives: restore the normal mechanics of chest wall movement to improve alveolar ventilation and oxygenation. Two principal methods are used to restore chest wall mechanics. First, the affected flail segment can be splinted to the remaining thoracic cage by placing a pillow or blanket over the flail area (Fig. 3–69A and B). This will prevent outward movement of the flail area during expiration. The second method for treating a flail chest is through the administration of positive-pressure ventilation. During positive-pressure breathing, the forces of lung expansion are reversed. This allows for air to enter all the alveoli simultaneously. However, if the patient is breathing adequately and forcefully without assistance, it is difficult to administer positive-pressure breathing. In these instances, high concentrations of oxygen can be given through a nonrebreather mask. If the patient becomes lethargic, hypoventilates, or exhibits gross cyanosis, positive pressure should be attempted. If the patient is still breathing, breaths can be synchronized with the patient's own efforts.

TRAUMATIC ASPHYXIA

Traumatic asphyxia is an emergency resulting from high velocity compression of the thorax. When the thorax is compressed by the steering wheel of a car or

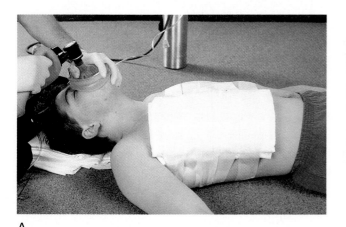

A

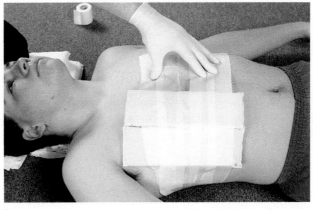

B

FIGURE 3–69. A flail chest can be splinted by several methods. (*A*) Place a towel, folded sheet, or multitrauma dressing over the segment and tape it to the intact chest. Positive pressure is an effective method of restoring adequate ventilation if the patient can tolerate mask ventilation. (*B*) Position padded board splints over the affected area and tape them in place. Either method helps prevent outward (paradoxical) movement of the flail segment during exhalation. Then position the patient on the affected side, if possible.

by another force, the heart is compressed and the blood within the veins is driven into the upper thorax, neck, and brain, causing severe swelling and ecchymosis of the patient's neck and face. The ecchymosis and swelling (traumatic asphyxia) is not of itself life threatening. How-

ever, the critical problems often associated with this condition include pulmonary and cardiac contusion, pneumothorax, hemothorax, rib fractures, and flail chest. These injuries must be diagnosed and treated.

P R O T O C O L

APPROACH TO THE PATIENT WITH CHEST INJURIES

1. SPECIAL ASSESSMENT CONSIDERATIONS

   a. Note any deformities of the chest wall, including abnormalities of the chest wall, i.e., puncture wounds, sucking chest wounds, flail chest, and paradoxical or asymmetrical chest movement.

   b. Note and correct any respiratory distress.

   c. Note if the patient is coughing up bright red blood or pink froth.

   d. Check for the presence of subcutaneous emphysema in the skin overlying the chest or in the neck.

   e. Check for neck vein distention or tracheal deviation.

   f. Note if the systolic and diastolic blood pressures are approximating each other (pericardial tamponade).

   g. Check for presence and equality of lung sounds (pneumothorax or hemothorax).

   h. The patient should be considered as having a developing tension pneumothorax if there exists:

      (1) Increasing difficulty in breathing.

      (2) Absent or greatly diminished breath sounds on one side.

      (3) Neck vein distention.

      (4) Movement of the trachea away from the pneumothorax (to the unaffected side).

      (5) Progressive development of shock.

2. GENERAL TREATMENT

   a. Maintain ABCs.

   b. Administer high-concentration oxygen.

   c. Assist respirations as necessary. DO NOT USE A DEMAND-VALVE RESUSCITATOR.

   d. Control external bleeding, including placement of occlusive dressings as necessary.

   e. Initiate appropriate subprotocols.

   f. Treat for shock.

   g. Monitor vital signs.

   h. Position the patient appropriately.

   i. Transport as soon as possible.

3. OPEN (SUCKING) CHEST WOUND

   a. Control external bleeding.

   b. Seal wound with occlusive dressing (aseptic aluminum foil) and tape on all four sides.

   c. Seal should be made on exhalation.

   d. If tension pneumothorax develops, unseal one side of the dressing to relieve pressure and then reseal it during exhalation.

   e. Position the patient on the affected side.

4. FLAIL CHEST

   a. Place bulky dressings over the flail segment and tape or bind in place.

   b. Position the patient on the affected side.

5. POSSIBLE SIMPLE RIB FRACTURES

   a. Bind the arm to the affected side with a sling and swathe.

   OR

   b. Place bulky dressings over the injury site and bind with sling and swathe.

   c. Allow patient to assume a position of comfort.

   d. Continue to assess for development of complications after chest trauma.

6. SUSPECTED TENSION PNEUMOTHORAX

   a. Maintain ABCs.

   b. Transport is immediately initiated upon determination of a suspected tension pneumothorax.

   c. En route to the appropriate hospital:

      (1) Administer high-concentration oxygen.

      (2) Treat other life-threatening injuries as necessary.

      (3) Position patient on the affected side unless contraindicated.

      (4) Treat for shock.

      (5) If ventilatory assistance is required:

         (a) Place patient in the supine position.

         (b) Assist ventilations by bag-valve-mask with supplemental oxygen.

(c) DO NOT USE A DEMAND-VALVE RE-SUSCITATOR!

7. SUSPECTED PERICARDIAL TAMPONADE

 a. Maintain ABCs.

 b. Transport is immediately initiated upon determination of a suspected pericardial tamponade.

 c. En route to the appropriate hospital:

   (1) Administer high-concentration oxygen.

   (2) Treat other life-threatening injuries as necessary.

   (3) Treat for shock.

   (4) If ventilation assistance is required:

     (a) Place patient in the supine position.

     (b) Assist ventilations by bag-valve-mask with supplemental oxygen.

     (c) DO NOT USE A DEMAND-VALVE RE-SUSCITATOR!

8. TRAUMATIC ASPHYXIA

 a. Maintain ABCs.

 b. Control major external bleeding.

 c. Administer high-concentration of oxygen.

 d. Immobilize the patient's spine and stabilize the flail sternum.

 e. Treat for shock.

 f. If the ventilation assistance is required:

   (1) Use modified jaw thrust and oropharyngeal airway to open the airway.

   (2) Assist ventilations by bag-valve-mask with supplemental oxygen.

   (3) DO NOT USE A DEMAND-VALVE RESUSCITATOR!

From New York City Emergency Medical Services: Basic Life Support Protocols, New York, NY, 1990.

Summary

Respiratory emergencies are among the most life-threatening conditions that the EMT encounters. You must work quickly to provide an airway and ventilation and give supplemental oxygen as required. Certain conditions need rapid transport to the hospital to effect survival. The following protocols summarize the approach to the patients with respiratory problems. These protocols are from New York City EMS and the New York State Department of Health Statewide Basic Life Support Patient Treatment Protocols. Know and follow the protocols in your region.

The EMT should be fully familiar with ventilation and oxygen equipment. A list of essential equipment is presented in Table 3–5. Perfect the skills of oxygen administration, airway control, and positive-pressure ventilation. They are vital in the management of all patients but particularly those who are in critical condition, in whose cases immediate action can seriously affect the outcome.

TABLE 3–5. Ventilation/Oxygen Kit*

The equipment should be in a case that is either hard or soft that protects the oxygen regulator and allows the EMT to secure the oxygen at the foot end of the background so it can be strapped in for transport.

1—complete set of oral airways (#1 to #5)
1—complete set of latex nasal airways (28, 30, 32, 34 French) and water-soluble lubricant
1—adult bag-valve-mask with reservoir system and oxygen tubing attached (NO PEDIATRIC POP-OFF VALVE)
1—pediatric bag-valve-mask with reservoir system and oxygen tubing attached (NO PEDIATRIC POP-OFF VALVE)
1—pocket mask with oxygen inlet and one-way valve
1—adult nonrebreather mask
1—adult multivent mask

1—adult nasal cannula
1—pediatric nonrebreather mask
1—bulb syringe
1—prewrapped disposable bite stick
1—full oxygen D cylinder with a key or wheel attached
1—oxygen regulator capable of liter flow adjustment up to 14 liters per minute, or a multifunction regulator with a positive-pressure ventilator with a trigger, liter flow as described above, and a demand valve.

Note: If you choose to not routinely carry a suction unit as a separate kit, then the ventilation kit should include a small suction unit, i.e., foot pump.

Suction Unit

Whatever brand you choose to use, it is imperative that it be ready to go at all times.

1—portable suction unit (numerous units available)
2—Yankauer rigid tip disposable plastic instruments

*Adapted from The New York State Health Department Critical Trauma Care Manual. Albany, New York State Health Department.

REVIEW EXERCISES

1. State the significance of oxygen to body tissues, particularly to the brain.

2. Make a list of the major anatomic structures of the respiratory system and list their functions.

3. Define diffusion.

4. Define the following respiratory volumes:
   Tidal volume   Vital capacity
   Minute volume   Total lung capacity
   Residual volume

5. List four signs of respiratory distress.

6. State three mental state changes that may occur with hypoxia.

7. Define the following signs and symptoms:
   Hemoptysis   Retractions
   Cyanosis   Paradoxical breathing
   Hypoventilation   Subcutaneous emphysema
   Hyperventilation   Tracheal shift
   Tachypnea

8. Describe the normal character and locations of the following breath sounds:
   Tracheal   Bronchovesicular
   Vesicular   Bronchial

9. Describe the following breath sounds and list one condition in which they might be found:
   Crackles (rales)   Friction rubs
   Rhonchi   Stridor
   Wheezes

10. Describe two infection control measures that should be used during the establishment of airway and ventilation.

11. Write the steps for performing the following airway maneuvers, and if possible, demonstrate them on a family member or friend:
    Head tilt–chin lift
    Jaw thrust without head tilt
    Chin pull

12. Write the steps for performing the following airway techniques:
    Oropharyngeal airway
    Nasopharyngeal airway
    Esophageal gastric tube airway (optional)
    Endotracheal intubation (optional)

13. Write the steps for performing the following ventilation techniques and list one advantage and one disadvantage for each technique:
    Mouth-to-mouth
    Pocket mask
    Bag-valve-mask
    Manually triggered demand valve resuscitator

14. Write the steps for assembly and disassembly of an oxygen cylinder regulator.

15. List the delivered oxygen percentages for the following administration devices:
    Nasal cannula
    Non-rebreather
    Simple face mask
    Venturi mask

16. List three categories of airway obstruction and provide one example of each.

17. Describe the management techniques for the following types of airway obstruction:
    Partial with good air exchange
    Partial with poor air exchange
    Complete

18. List the steps of management for a complete foreign body airway obstruction under each of the following circumstances for an adult, child, and infant:
    Conscious
    Unconscious
    Conscious to unconscious adult

19. List three signs and symptoms and describe the prehospital treatment for pneumonia.

20. List the sequence of a typical near-drowning and discuss the differences between salt- and fresh-water drowning.

21. Describe the management of a patient in respiratory arrest.

22. List three signs and symptoms and describe the prehospital treatment for hyperventilation syndrome.

23. Provide one condition each that may result from blunt, compression, and penetrating (knife vs. missile) injury to the thoracic cage.

24. List two signs and symptoms and describe the appropriate treatment for the following types of chest trauma:
    Rib fracture   Pneumothorax
    Flail chest   Tension pneumothorax
    Hemothorax

REFERENCES

American Heart Association: Standards and guidelines for cardiopulmonary resuscitation and emergency cardiac care. JAMA 244(5):453–509 August 1981.

Bates B: A guide to physical examination, 4th ed. Philadelphia, JB Lippincott, 1987.

Guyton AC: Textbook of medical physiology, 8th ed. Philadelphia, WB Saunders, 1990.

Passmore R, Robson JS (eds): A companion to medical studies, Vol 1. Oxford, Blackwell Scientific Publications, 1969.

Prehospital Trauma Life Support Committee of The National Association of EMTs: Pre-hospital trauma life support. Emergency Training. Akron, OH, 1986.

Raynor J: Anatomy and physiology. New York, Harper & Row, 1977.

Roberts JR, Hedges JR: Clinical procedures in emergency medicine 2nd ed. Philadelphia, WB Saunders, 1990.

Safar P, Bircher N: Cardiopulmonary cerebral resuscitation, 3rd ed. Philadelphia, WB Saunders, 1988.

Schwartz GR, Safar P, Stone JH, et al: Principles and practices of emergency medicine, 2nd ed. Philadelphia, WB Saunders, 1986.

Solomon EP, Schmidt RR, Adragna PJ: Human anatomy and physiology. Philadelphia, WB Saunders, 1990.

United States Bureau of the Census: Statistical Abstract of the United States: 1990, 110th ed. Washington, DC, Bureau of the Census, 1990.

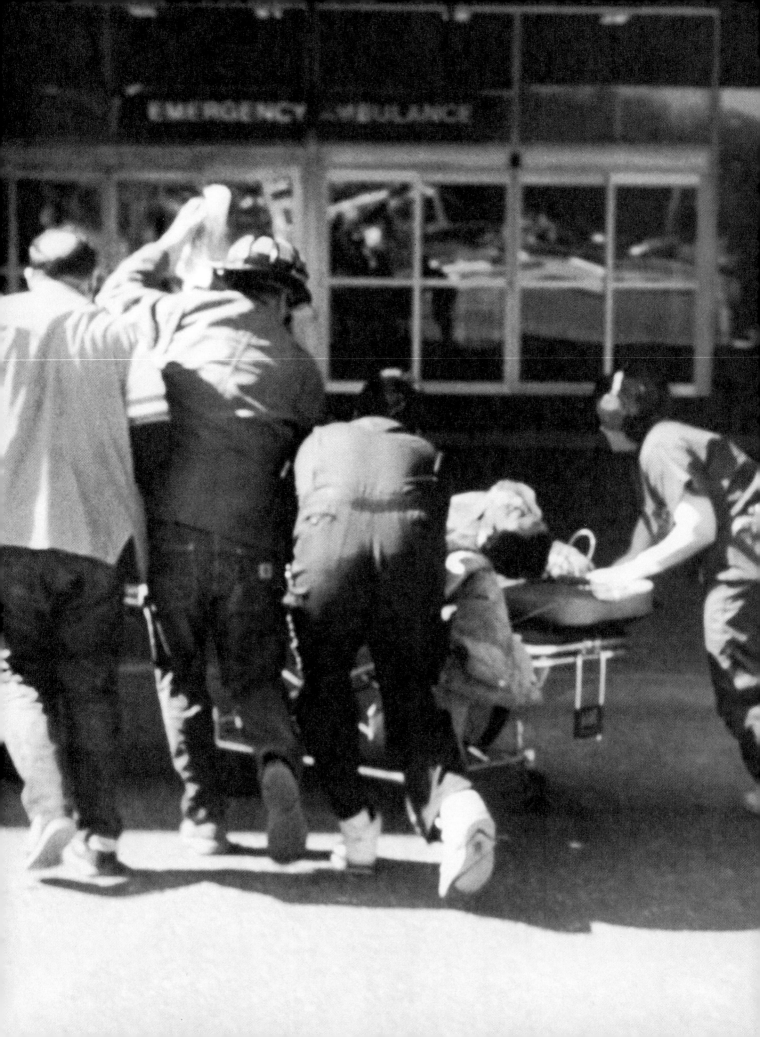

CHAPTER 4

THE CARDIOVASCULAR SYSTEM

OBJECTIVES

At the conclusion of this chapter the reader will be able to:

1. List three functions of the circulatory system.

2. List the three components of the circulatory system.

3. Describe the components of blood and explain their functions.

4. Given an anatomical chart, identify the major parts of the circulatory system.

5. Explain how valves control blood flow within the circulatory system.

6. Describe the function of the conduction system within the heart.

7. Explain the following concepts relating to circulatory physiology:
   Cardiac output
   Starling's law
   Autonomic control
   Pulse pressure
   Blood pressure
   Diffusion
   Osmosis

INTRODUCTION

The circulatory system is the transport system of the body. It has many functions. It delivers oxygen and nutrients to the tissues and returns the waste products of metabolism (carbon dioxide and cellular wastes) to the lungs and kidneys for excretion from the body. It also transports specialized cells to areas of the body where they are needed to repair injured tissues, combat foreign bacteria, and control bleeding. By reducing or increasing the amount of blood in contact with the skin, the circulatory system helps regulate body temperature as well.

Because the tissues are most dependent on an adequate supply of oxygen for survival, any compromise in circulatory function can lead to tissue damage or death. Because the most oxygen-dependent tissues are the central nervous system and the heart, the signs of inadequate oxygenation are looked for when examining these organ systems. Although all organ systems are affected by lack of oxygen, rapid assessment of brain and circulatory function must be given priority in the early part of every examination. The EMT must be able to recognize the indicators of cardiovascular failure quickly and to administer prompt emergency treatment.

COMPONENTS OF THE CIRCULATORY SYSTEM

Proper functioning of the circulatory system depends on three components: the *heart, blood,* and *blood vessels.* These components are *interdependent.*

The blood is the fluid in which oxygen and nutrients are transported. The vessels are the pathways that direct blood to the various cells of the body. The heart is the pump that provides the driving force necessary to keep the blood circulating.

ANATOMY AND PHYSIOLOGY

Blood

The average adult's body contains 5 to 6 liters of blood. The amount of blood volume is proportionate to the size of the patient. For the adult, an estimate of 70 ml of blood/kg of body weight is used. Infants and small children have about 80 ml of blood/kg of body weight. Blood consists of both liquid and cellular components.

PLASMA—THE LIQUID COMPONENT

The liquid portion of blood is called the plasma; it constitutes 55 to 65% of the blood volume. The plasma consists mostly of water in which other elements and particles are dissolved. The dissolved particles include certain nutrients (glucose, fats, and so forth); waste products; small ions such as sodium, potassium, and chloride that are used in the maintenance of cellular function; and proteins. The proteins are used in bleeding control, as hormone carriers, and to help maintain the plasma volume within the blood vessels.

BLOOD CELLS

The cellular component of blood consists of red blood cells, white blood cells, and platelets. The cellular component makes up 35 to 45% of the total blood volume.

RED BLOOD CELLS. The red blood cells constitute the largest portion of the cellular component. They are the carriers of oxygen and carbon dioxide. They contain a large protein called *hemoglobin,* which binds oxygen at the alveoli to form oxyhemoglobin. Oxyhemoglobin is bright red in color and accounts for the pink appearance of the lips and nail beds. Hemoglobin binds oxygen in the lungs and then releases it to the tissues of the body that are oxygen depleted. Hemoglobin that is not bound to oxygen is more blue or purple in appearance. This explains why patients who are oxygen deprived may appear *cyanotic,* especially in the nail beds or the lips, where many small vessels are visible at the skin's surface.

HEMOGLOBIN AND OXYGEN TRANSPORT. Ordinarily, 98% of the oxygen carried in the blood is bound to hemoglobin. The other 2% is dissolved in the plasma. Without hemoglobin, the blood could not carry enough oxygen to meet the body's needs. The body usually requires only one-fourth of the supply of oxygen bound to hemoglobin; the rest is held in reserve. Some patients who have a low supply of hemoglobin and red blood cells are said to be *anemic.* If the hemoglobin supply reaches too low a level, these patients require a transfusion of red blood cells. In cases of severe blood loss, transfusion of red blood cells may be required to restore the blood's oxygen-carrying ability.

The amount of oxygen dissolved in the plasma alone is not adequate to support the body's needs. If a higher concentration of oxygen is inspired, then more oxygen is dissolved in the plasma. However, even with 100% oxygen this *dissolved oxygen cannot meet the body's needs by itself;* rather, it supplements the oxygen carried by the hemoglobin. The *main role of oxygen therapy is to ensure full saturation of the hemoglobin with oxygen.*

The red blood cells have an average life expectancy of 120 days. As individual cells reach the end of their life span, they are replaced by new cells that are produced in the bone marrow.

WHITE BLOOD CELLS. The principal role of the white blood cells is to combat and eliminate infecting organisms and foreign materials. They are fewer in number than the red blood cells and have a much shorter life span. The white blood cells pass through the walls of microscopic vessels and accumulate at the site of an infection. Once there, they break down and attack the offending organism or foreign substance, consume some of the breakdown products, and help direct the remaining *pus* (wastes) out of the body. By following the process that occurs when a splinter is left embedded in a finger, it is possible to understand how this works. Initially, an *erythema* (a redness) and warmth are noted around the puncture site as the white cells begin to assemble at the wound. Later, one may observe a pus formation around the splinter. The pus consists of fluid, dead bacteria, dead tissue cells, and white blood cells.

In other infections such as pneumonia, the number of white blood cells in the blood increases as the body combats the infecting organisms. Physicians look for an increase in the white blood cell count as one indication of an infection.

PLATELETS.   Platelets are fragments of cells that circulate in the blood and are necessary for clotting to begin. Together with proteins in the plasma, the platelets form a *thrombus* (blood clot) when exposed to any surface other than the normal lining of a blood vessel. The clotting process is called *thrombosis* and usually takes 5 to 6 minutes. Without healthy platelets, an individual will bleed excessively after sustaining even a small laceration and will have a tendency to bruise easily. Platelet function may be altered by many drugs, including common ones such as aspirin. Individuals whose platelets are particularly sensitive to these drugs will note a tendency to bruise easily after seemingly slight injuries.

The plasma proteins involved in clotting are equally important for bleeding control. Some patients, such as those with hemophilia, have a deficiency of the proteins used for clotting and can bleed excessively. Patients with severe liver disease may also have a deficiency of clotting proteins and so suffer prolonged bleeding.

The Heart

The heart is a muscular pump that generates the driving force for blood to flow to all parts of the body. The force must be sufficient to *open the vessels* so that blood can pass through and thereby *perfuse* the body's organs and tissues.

LOCATION

The heart is located in the chest cavity between the sternum and the thoracic spine, just left of center. It is positioned between the two lungs in a space known as the mediastinum and occupies an area about the size of a fist. The superior and inferior areas of the heart are commonly referred to as the base and the apex, respec-

tively. The base is located toward the right, at the level of the second rib. The apex of the heart is located to the left and rests on the left diaphragm. Its impulse can be felt anteriorly at the level of the fifth or sixth rib. We sometimes refer to taking an *apical pulse* by palpating over the apex of the heart at the level of the fifth and sixth rib interspace at the mid-clavicular line (Fig. 4–1).

PERICARDIUM

The heart is surrounded by a two-layered sac called the *pericardium*. The pericardium is a protective covering that separates the heart from the other organs in the mediastinum. The inner layer adheres to the heart wall and is separated from the loosely adherent outer layer by a small amount of fluid. This fluid serves as a lubricant between the pericardial layers as the heart beats. It is similar to the pleural linings of the lungs, which, as described earlier, are made up of a visceral layer (attached to the lung) and a parietal layer (the outer covering), also separated by a thin layer of fluid. Like the pleura, the pericardium contains a potential space between its two layers. If this space becomes filled with air or an excess of fluid, the heart will not function properly (Fig. 4–2).

LAYERS OF THE HEART

The heart muscle itself is made up of three layers. The outer layer of the heart is called the *epicardium* and is actually the inner or visceral layer of the pericardium. The middle layer is called the *myocardium* and is the muscular portion that performs the work of contraction. The *endocardium*, or smooth inner layer, lines the chambers of the heart (Fig. 4–3). This inner layer continues on into the blood vessels that enter and leave the heart. The function of the endocardium is to provide a surface lining within the heart and vessels that prevents the clotting of blood. When this layer is disrupted and diseased, clotting is likely to occur.

CHAMBERS AND SEPTUM

The inner portion of the heart is divided into four chambers. The upper chambers, the *right atrium* and *left atrium*, are the receiving chambers for blood returning to the heart from the lungs and the rest of the body.

Since these chambers serve primarily as collecting areas in which blood returning to the heart accumulates, they have relatively thin walls. The two lower chambers, the *right ventricle* and *left ventricle*, are the pumping chambers and have thicker walls. The left atrium is located above the left ventricle, and the right atrium is located above the right ventricle.

The right and left sides of the heart are separated from each other by a wall called a *septum*. The respective atrial and ventricular chambers are thereby arranged par-

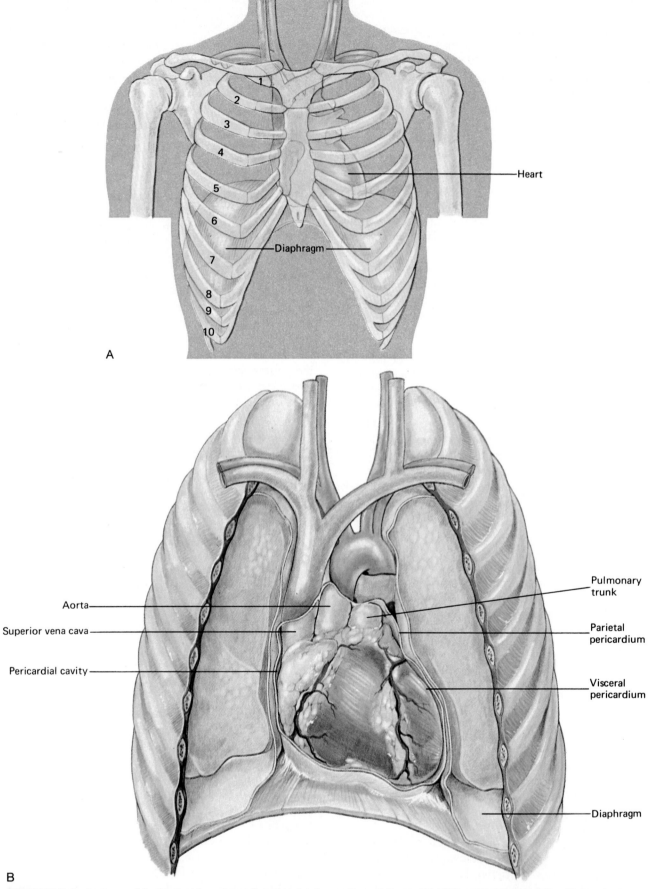

FIGURE 4–1. Anatomy of the heart and great vessels within the thorax. (From Solomon EP, Phillips GA: Understanding Human Anatomy and Physiology. Philadelphia, WB Saunders, 1987, p. 210.)

FIGURE 4–2. The pericardium has two layers. The visceral pericardium (epicardium), or inner layer, closely adheres to the surface of the heart. The parietal pericardium, or outer layer, consists of a more loosely attached, thin, membranous covering.

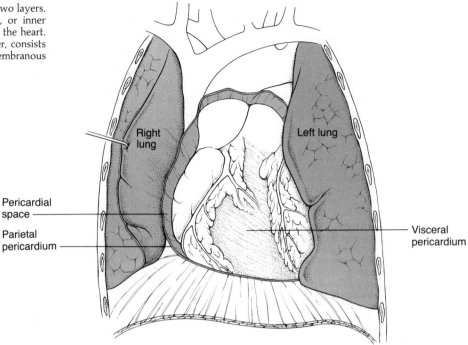

allel to each other. The dividing septum is named for its location as either the *interatrial septum* or the *interventricular septum* (Fig. 4–4).

The two atria beat simultaneously, followed by simultaneous contraction of the two ventricles. However, the septum serves to actually divide the heart into a right and left circulation.

RIGHT AND LEFT CIRCULATIONS—PULMONARY AND SYSTEMIC

Functionally, the circulatory system can be thought of as two distinct systems: the *pulmonary circulation* and the *systemic circulation*.

PULMONARY CIRCULATION—RIGHT. The pulmonary circulation pumps blood through the lungs, where it picks up oxygen and releases carbon dioxide

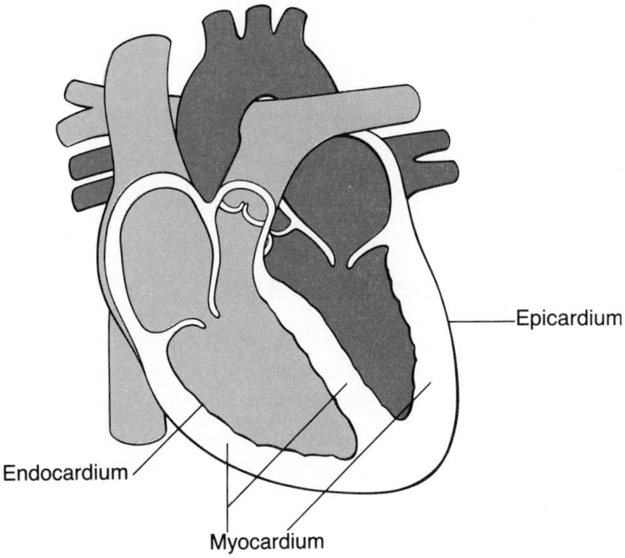

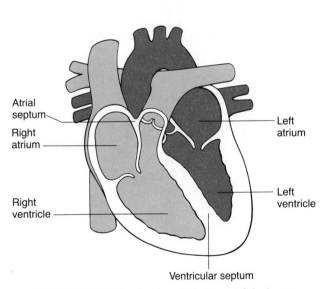

FIGURE 4–3. The layers of the heart: the endocardium (smooth inner lining), myocardium (thick muscular layer), and epicardium (thin outer covering).

FIGURE 4–4. The chambers and septum of the heart.

for excretion from the body. The pump for the pulmonary circulation is the right ventricle. Blood returning to the heart from the pulmonary circulation is now saturated with oxygen, and it collects in the left atrium.

SYSTEMIC CIRCULATION—LEFT. The systemic circulation transports and delivers the oxygen-rich blood (and other nutrients) to the rest of the body, where it is needed for energy. At the same time, it picks up carbon dioxide and other waste products of metabolism. The pump for the systemic circulation is the left ventricle. Blood returning to the heart from the systemic circulation collects in the right atrium. Thus, blood is returned to the pulmonary circulation to begin the cycle once again. Follow the blood flow in Figure 4–5 to understand how blood flows through both the pulmonary and systemic circulations.

VALVES—ONE-WAY FLOW

While the atria and ventricles are contracting, a one-way flow of blood is maintained by the presence of valves. During *systole* (ventricular contraction), the blood in the ventricles is pumped OUT of the heart through

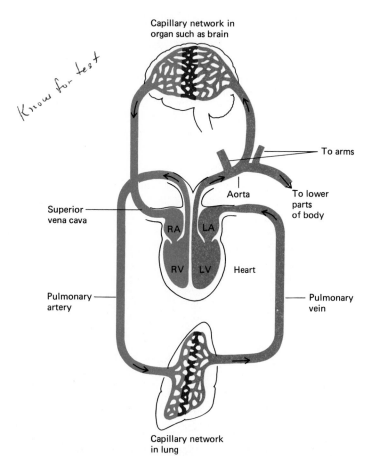

FIGURE 4–5. Pulmonary and systemic circulations. (From Davis WP, Solomon EP: The World of Biology, 4th ed. Philadelphia, Saunders College Publishing, 1990.)

the arteries. During *diastole* (ventricular relaxation), blood flows INTO the empty ventricles from the atria, where it has been collecting. There is a valve at both the INLET and OUTLET of each ventricle to maintain the direction of blood flow from the atrium to the ventricle to the artery.

The valves are composed of flaps of tissue that are cupped in one direction. If pressure is exerted on one side of a valve, it opens. If pressure is exerted on the other side, it closes (Fig. 4–6).

ATRIOVENTRICULAR VALVES—THE INLET VALVES. The valves that separate the atria from the ventricles (at the inlet of the ventricle) are called the *atrioventricular* (AV) valves. Between the right atrium and the right ventricle is the *tricuspid* valve. It is so named because of the three *cusps* or flaps that compose it. Between the left atrium and the left ventricle is the *mitral* valve, which is composed of two cusps.

When the ventricle is relaxed (diastole), the AV valves will open, permitting blood to flow from the atria into the ventricles. During ventricular contraction (systole), the pressure of the blood in the ventricles pushes the AV valves closed, preventing the blood from flowing back into the atria.

SEMILUNAR VALVES—THE OUTLET VALVES. The valves that separate the ventricles from the outlet arteries are called *semilunar valves*. Between the right ventricle and its outlet artery (the pulmonary artery) leading to the lungs is the *pulmonary valve*. Between the left ventricle and the *aorta* (its outlet artery) leading to the rest of the body lies the *aortic valve*. These two valves are composed of three flaps shaped somewhat like a half moon and hence are referred to as the *semilunar valves* (Fig. 4–7). They allow blood to flow freely from the heart through the arteries during ventricular systole but close during diastole to prevent a backflow of blood into the ventricles.

Closure of the valves signals the beginning and end of ventricular contraction. The main heart sounds heard through a stethoscope are caused by the closing of these two sets of valves.

CONDUCTION SYSTEM

The *conduction system* is composed of a series of specialized tissues that order the rhythmic relaxation and contraction of the myocardial cells. The heart must have an ordered relaxation and contraction in order to serve as a pump. The conduction system is anatomically designed to reach all of the myocardium in such a fashion that the atria contract first, followed by the ventricles. During ventricular relaxation, the atria contract and help fill the ventricles with blood. During ventricular contraction, the ventricles pump blood out through the arteries.

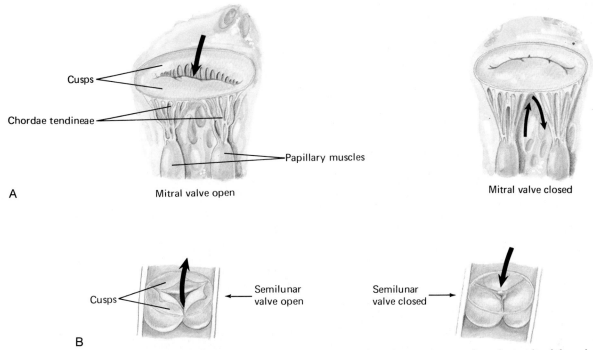

A   Mitral valve open   Mitral valve closed

Cusps

Chordae tendineae

Papillary muscles

Cusps   Semilunar   Semilunar
                     valve open   valve closed

B

FIGURE 4–6. The functions of the (A) mitral and (B) semilunar valves are shown. Pressure exerted on the inside of the valve pushes the flaps open. When the pressure on the outside of the valve increases, the valve is pushed shut. The closing of the AV (i.e., mitral) valves is aided by the contraction of the chordae tendineae and the papillary muscles, which prevent the valves from collapsing backward into the atria. (From Solomon EP, Phillips GA: Understanding Human Anatomy and Physiology. Philadelphia, WB Saunders, 1987, p. 213.)

The conduction system starts with the *sinoatrial (SA) node*, which is the *pacemaker* of the heart and located in the right atrium. The SA node discharges, or fires, about 60 to 80 times a minute in an adult at rest, and begins an electrical impulse that ultimately spreads through the atria and then down through the ventricles.

SEQUENCE OF ELECTRICAL EVENTS.   When the SA node fires, the impulse travels through the atria to a relay station between the atria and the ventricles called the *AV node*. During this time, atrial contraction occurs.

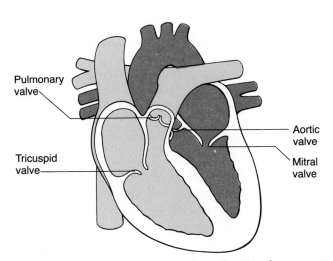

Pulmonary valve

Tricuspid valve

Aortic valve

Mitral valve

FIGURE 4–7. AV and semilunar valves. The AV valves consist of the mitral and tricuspid. The semilunar valves consist of the pulmonary and aortic.

At the AV node the impulse is slowed to allow the atria to finish filling the ventricles. The impulse then travels within specialized conduction tissue between the ventricles, and this tissue divides into right and left bundle branches. These branches deliver the impulse to the respective ventricles and further subdivide into *Purkinje fibers* (specialized fibers) reaching into the myocardium (Fig. 4–8). Finally, the impulse stimulates the myocardial cells within the ventricles, causing a synchronized contraction that results in the ejection of blood into the two outlet arteries.

When considering the sequence of electrical conduction within the heart, the importance of electrical control over mechanical function becomes evident. The pacemaker, or SA node, fires and the atria contract. The impulse is held at the AV junction to allow completion of atrial contraction. The ventricles are filled by the time the impulse reaches them, and they pump the blood to the lungs and the body during ventricular contraction (Fig. 4–9).

Disturbances in the conduction system result in various abnormalities. These include too slow a heart beat, too fast a heart beat, an irregular heart beat, or in the most extreme case, no heart beat at all (cardiac arrest).

THE ELECTROCARDIOGRAM.   The electrical activity of the heart is commonly measured by an instrument that detects and amplifies the electrical signals. The resulting tracing is called an *electrocardiogram*. For further discussion of the heart's electrical activity and the elec-

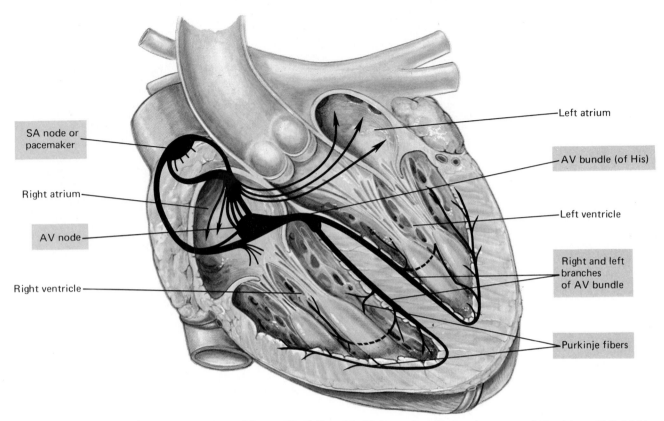

FIGURE 4–8. The conduction system. (From Solomon EP, Phillips GA: Understanding Human Anatomy and Physiology. Philadelphia, WB Saunders, 1987, p. 214.)

trocardiogram, see the section on EMT defibrillation in Chapter 6.

CARDIAC OUTPUT

The volume of blood pumped by the heart in 1 minute is referred to as *cardiac output*. It is calculated by multiplying the number of heart beats per minute times the amount of blood pumped with each beat. The amount of blood ejected with each contraction is referred to as the *stroke volume.*

Heart rate	×	stroke volume	=	cardiac output
(beats/min)		(ml/beat)		(ml/min)

Normally, the stroke volume is about 70 milliliters (ml) of blood. If we take the average heart rate to be 70 beats/minute, we would calculate the cardiac output as follows:

Beats/min	×	ml/beat	=	cardiac output (ml/min)
70	×	70	=	4900 ml/min

or approximately 5 liters (5000 ml) of blood per minute.

The amount of blood pumped out of the heart varies from minute to minute, depending on the changing needs of the individual. One's muscles require more oxygen during exercise and less during rest.

CONTROL OF HEART RATE AND FORCE OF CONTRACTION

Both the rate and the force of the heart's contractions will determine the amount of blood ejected. There are properties peculiar to the heart that will adjust both its rate and force of contraction. Through manipulation of both the heart rate and force of contraction by the *autonomic nervous system*, the cardiac output changes in response to external controls.

HEART RATE. The heart's rate is determined primarily by its pacemaker, which has a normal rate of discharge of from 60 to 80 beats per minute. This rate is altered by the effects of the autonomic nervous system, according to the needs of the body.

FORCE OF CONTRACTION. The myocardial cells are designed in such a way as to allow for *stretching of the chambers* in proportion to the amount of blood entering the ventricles. Not only does this allow for expansion of the chamber to accommodate varying amounts of blood, but the stretching of the ventricles also directly influences the power of contraction as well.

As blood enters the ventricles, it stretches the muscle cells in such a way that the power of the subsequent contraction is proportionate to the degree of stretch. This matches the power of each contraction with the

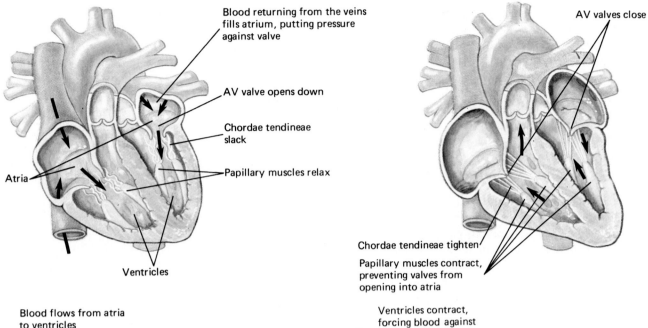

Blood returning from the veins
fills atrium, putting pressure
against valve

AV valve opens down

Chordae tendineae
slack

Papillary muscles relax

Atria

Ventricles

Blood flows from atria
to ventricles

Atria contract
forcing additional
A   blood into ventricles

AV valves close

Chordae tendineae tighten

Papillary muscles contract,
preventing valves from
opening into atria

Ventricles contract,
forcing blood against
B   valve cusps

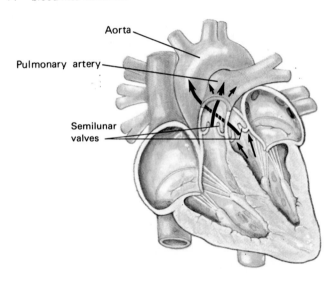

Aorta

Pulmonary artery

Semilunar
valves

When ventricles
contract, blood is
pushed up against
semilunar valves,
C   forcing them open

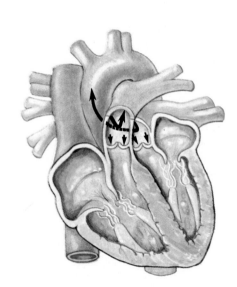

As ventricles relax,
blood starts to flow
back from arteries

Blood fills cusps of
semilunar valves,
D   forcing them to close

FIGURE 4–9. As the pacemaker fires, the atria contract, forcing blood into the ventricles below. The impulse conducts slowly through the AV node (the delay station) to allow the ventricle to fill. The impulse then reaches the Purkinje fibers in the ventricle, causing ventricular contraction. (From Solomon EP, Phillips GA: Understanding Human Anatomy and Physiology. Philadelphia, WB Saunders, 1987, p. 216.)

volume in the chamber. The greater the volume, the greater the stretch, and the greater the power of contraction, the greater the stroke volume. It is an efficient mechanism. Not only will the ventricle expand to accommodate changes in blood volume, but it also adjusts its force of contraction to empty the chamber. It does no more work than is necessary. This physiologic principle is referred to as *Starling's law*.

AUTONOMIC NERVOUS SYSTEM AND EPINEPHRINE

The autonomic nervous system and the hormone epinephrine (adrenaline) alter both heart rate and force of contraction. These alterations are done automatically (without conscious effort) in response to the body's changing needs. The body's needs are monitored by receptors, such as in the aorta and carotid arteries.

EFFECT ON HEART RATE. The autonomic nervous system is composed of sympathetic and parasympathetic components. Both components send fibers to the pacemaker, or SA node (Fig. 4–10). The parasympathetic signal travels down the vagus nerve and slows down the heart rate. The signal from the sympathetic nervous system travels down nerves that branch off the upper thoracic spinal cord and speeds up the heart rate.

The heart's rhythm is also influenced by the circulating hormone epinephrine, or adrenaline. Epinephrine, which is released from the adrenal gland when stimulated by sympathetic nerves, speeds up the heart (Table 4–1). The balance of forces from the autonomic nervous system allows for fine tuning of the heart's rate of contraction to meet the various needs of daily living.

FORCE OF CONTRACTION. Both the sympathetic nervous system and epinephrine increase the force of ventricular contraction. Fibers from the sympathetic nervous system extend into the ventricles, where their stimulation increases the force of contraction. Circulating epinephrine has a similar effect. Fibers from the para-

sympathetic nervous system do not extend into the ventricles and thus have no effect on the force of contraction (Table 4–2).

SEVERANCE OF SYMPATHETIC TONE

The sympathetic fibers to the heart travel from bundles of nerves that branch off the thoracic spinal cord. To communicate with the heart, the nerve impulses must travel from the brain down the spinal cord and through these sympathetic nerves (see Fig. 4–10). Therefore, if

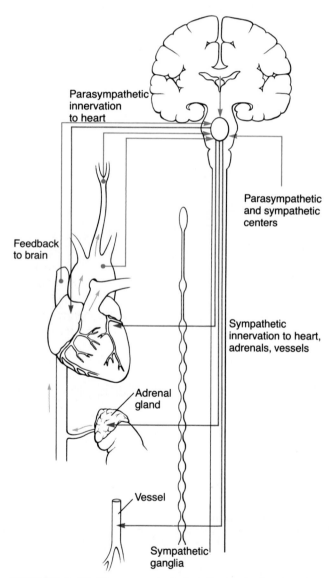

FIGURE 4–10. Nervous control of cardiovascular function. Receptors in the major vessels (i.e., carotid and aorta) send information (blood pressure, oxygen/carbon dioxide content) through nerves (*blue lines*) to the cardiovascular center in the brain. The brain analyzes the information and sends back signals to organs (*black lines*). Parasympathetic signals go through the vagus nerve to the heart. Sympathetic signals travel through the spinal cord and sympathetic ganglia to the heart, blood vessels, and adrenal glands. Destruction of the cervical spinal cord can result in loss of sympathetic nervous control.

TABLE 4–1. Effects of Autonomic Nervous System on Heart Rate

Cause	Effect
Parasympathetic signal	Slows heart rate
Sympathetic signal	Speeds heart rate
Epinephrine	Speeds heart rate

TABLE 4–2. Effects of Autonomic Nervous System on Force of Contraction

Cause	Effect
Sympathetic nerves	Increased power
Epinephrine	Increased power
Parasympathetic nerves	No effect

a patient suffers a fracture of the cervical spine that destroys the spinal cord, the sympathetic nerves cannot communicate with the heart, making it impossible for the heart to speed up.

CHANGES IN CARDIAC OUTPUT

During exercise, the cardiac output can increase several times. We know that the heart rate increases with exercise. Let us say, for example, that a 20-year-old patient reaches a pulse of 180 during exercise. If the stroke volume was still 70 ml/beat, the cardiac output would be

Beats/min	×	ml/beat	=	cardiac output in ml/min
180	×	70	=	12,600

Actually, during exercise the heart beats stronger and faster and can pump more blood out of the ventricles. Assume this young patient's stroke volume is 100 ml/beat.

Beats/min	×	ml/beat	=	cardiac output in ml/min
180	×	100	=	18,000

The heart beats stronger (ejects more blood) as well as faster during exercise because of the increased activity of the sympathetic nervous system as well as Starling's law. As more blood returns to the heart during exercise, the ventricle stretches to accommodate it and, because of Starling's law, has increased contractile strength to empty it as well. The sympathetic nervous discharge that accompanies exercise will increase the contractile strength of the heart and the heart rate as well.

The cardiac output increases during exercise to meet the increased needs of the muscles for oxygen. Both the pulmonary and systemic circulations circulate more blood each minute, picking up extra oxygen from the lungs and delivering it, in turn, to the tissues. Conversely, when one sleeps, there is less need for oxygen because the body is at rest. The cardiac output is reduced accordingly. For example, the patient discussed above may have a heart rate of 60 when sleeping. If the stroke volume remains the same as it was at rest, we can see that the cardiac output will be

Beats/min	×	ml/beat	=	cardiac output in ml/min
60	×	70	=	4,200

CLINICAL APPLICATION

The cardiac output can be estimated, for example, for a patient who has a damaged pacemaker due to heart disease and who cannot increase his or her heart rate to greater than 36 beats a minute. Assuming the stroke volume is 70 ml/beat

Beats/min	×	ml/beat	=	cardiac output in ml/min
36	×	70	=	2,520

If this patient required a cardiac output of 5000 ml/min to meet his or her needs at rest, it would not be surprising to hear the patient complain of weakness when the heart rate is 36. See Table 4–3 for review of factors that affect cardiac output.

The Blood Vessels

There are three major types of blood vessels: *arteries, capillaries, and veins.* Together they form a branching network that directs the blood through every part of the body. The arteries direct blood flowing away from the heart. The veins direct blood returning to the heart. Capillaries are located between the arteries and veins. The capillaries are thin-walled vessels that come in close contact with the cells so that the exchange of oxygen, nutrients, and waste products between the blood and cells can occur.

The vasculature system has often been compared to a tree because of the continuous branching. The arterial system subdivides while branching until it reaches the size of the *arterioles,* whose diameter is approximately that of a hair. The capillary network begins beyond the arterioles and further subdivides to ensure close contact with the cells. The capillaries then start to reconnect, thereby forming the smallest veins, called the *venules.* The venules begin to unite and form larger and still larger tubes called veins, which ultimately connect with the inferior or superior vena cava or the pulmonary veins.

BLOOD VOLUME AND SIZE OF THE VASCULAR SPACE

There is not sufficient blood to completely fill the body's vasculature tree. Blood is directed to those tissues that have the greatest need at a given time. This is

TABLE 4–3. Factors Affecting Cardiac Output

Factor	Examples or Causes	Effect on Cardiac Output
Decreased heart rate	Damage to pacemaker Increased parasympathetic activity Rest or sleep	Decreased
Increased heart rate	Increased sympathetic activity Epinephrine Exercise Fever Fear, anxiety	Increased
Decreased stroke volume	Damage to heart muscle Rest or sleep Blood loss	Decreased
Increased stroke volume	Exercise Pregnancy (late)	Increased

accomplished primarily via the constriction and relaxation of the arterioles, which is regulated by the autonomic nervous system.

The vessels have the ability to vary their diameter by dilatation or constriction. If all vessels were in a state of dilatation, the normal blood volume could not fill the vascular space. Therefore, at any given time, some vessels are dilated while others are constricted, depending on the relative needs throughout the body.

For example, when a person is running, the blood vessels in the skeletal muscles are dilated while the vessels within the gastrointestinal tract are constricted. When one does heavy physical exercise, blood is directed toward the muscles doing the greatest work. The weight-lifter, after curling weights, speaks of the "pump" felt in the biceps, which become engorged with additional oxygen-bearing blood. Likewise, after a heavy meal, one might feel a bit sluggish or tired, as the blood is directed preferentially to the digestive system to pick up nutrients from the food. People are warned not to swim after eating because there may not be sufficient blood to perfuse both the digestive system and the skeletal muscles at the same time. Also, the warning that a cramp could develop in a muscle is based on the fact that insufficient oxygen is being delivered to meet the demands of the muscles used for swimming.

ARTERIES

The arteries are composed of three layers. There is a smooth inner lining called the endothelium, a tough protective outer layer of connective tissue, and a middle layer that is quite elastic in the aorta but which becomes more and more muscular as the arteries decrease in size. The elastic middle layer in the aorta and larger arteries allows them to withstand the high pressure of blood pumped from the left ventricle. They are able to initially expand as blood enters during systole and then contract during diastole. This contraction also serves to propel the blood forward (Figs. 4–11 and 4–13).

ARTERIOLES

The terminal branches of the arteries, the arterioles, are the smallest tubes in the arterial network. Their middle wall consists primarily of circular smooth muscle, which constricts or relaxes at the direction of the autonomic nervous system. The tone of the muscles in the arterioles (constricted or relaxed) regulates the amount of blood permitted to flow into the capillaries beyond.

Vasoconstriction occurs when the muscular wall of the vessel contracts, decreasing its inner diameter. Vasodilation occurs when the muscular wall relaxes, thereby increasing its inner diameter. These changes in the arterioles' diameter are important in controlling the body's blood pressure.

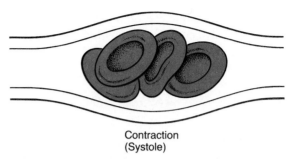

Contraction
(Systole)

FIGURE 4–11. The contraction of the ventricle propels blood into the arteries, causing a wave of blood flow through the vessel. This wave can be felt in the form of a pulse.

CAPILLARIES

The capillaries extend out from the finer branches of the arterioles. The capillary walls are only one cell thick and therefore permit the passage of water, gases, small molecules, and other substances carried in the blood. The diffusion of oxygen and nutrients and the exchange of waste products between the blood and the body cells can occur only at the capillary level. The capillaries are in close contact with all the body's tissues. They are so extensive that if placed end to end, they would extend for 60,000 miles (Fig. 4–12).

Because the capillary walls are so thin, they cannot be subjected to much pressure. The arterioles serve to reduce the pressure of blood before it enters the capillaries. Also, the extensive size of the capillary network presents a greater space for the blood to fill, which also helps to reduce pressure.

VEINS

The basic structure of the walls of the veins is similar to that of the arteries. There is a smooth lining internally, a tougher protective outer lining, and a middle layer that is elastic and muscular in nature. This middle layer is not as thick as that found in the arteries, since there is much less pressure in the veins (Fig. 4–13). However, the veins can expand and contract to accommodate changes in blood volume and normally contain greater than half the circulating blood volume.

THE VENOUS RESERVOIR. Of the total blood volume, approximately 25% is in the heart and pulmonary circulation, 15% in the arterial circulation, and 4% in the capillary bed. The remaining approximately 56% lies within the veins (Table 4–4).

Because the veins contain more than half the blood volume, they serve as a *reservoir* of blood within the vascular tree. The muscular and elastic middle wall allows the veins to contract or expand to accommodate changes in blood volume. For example, should a sudden loss of blood volume occur, the nervous system can tell the muscles in the veins to constrict. Blood from the venous reservoir is then redistributed within the vascular tree.

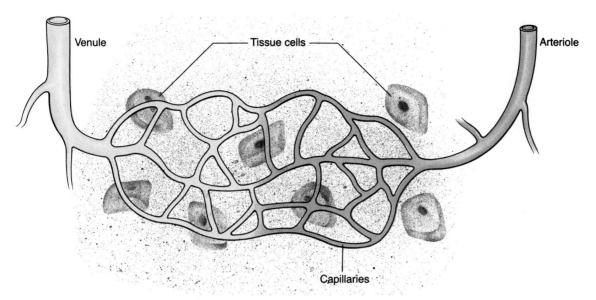

FIGURE 4–12. The capillaries are microscopic vessels that consist of single-celled walls that permit the movement of gases, fluid, and small particles to alveoli and tissue cells.

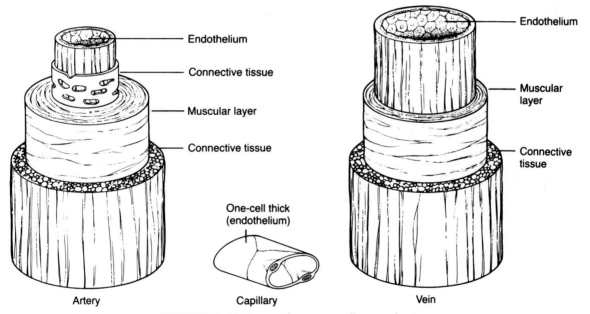

FIGURE 4–13. Layers of arteries, capillaries, and veins.

TABLE 4–4. Blood Distribution in the Circulatory System

Vessel	Percentage of Total Blood Volume
Heart and pulmonary circulation	25
Arteries and arterioles	15
Capillaries	4
Veins and venules	56
	100

Adapted from Rutherford RB, Buerk CA: The patho-physiology of trauma and shock. In Zuidema GD, Rutherford RB, Ballinger WF (eds): The Management of Trauma, 3rd ed. Philadelphia, WB Saunders, 1979.

By decreasing the size of the venous intravascular space and shunting blood to the rest of the circulatory system, blood pressure can be maintained. In fact, this is the first response to blood loss and serves as an important compensatory mechanism.

Conversely, when the blood volume is too great for the circulatory system to handle, the venous system can dilate and enlarge the vascular space. This can occur in common conditions, such as heart failure. In such conditions, distended neck veins may provide an important diagnostic sign.

Clinical application of these concepts will be covered in Chapter 5.

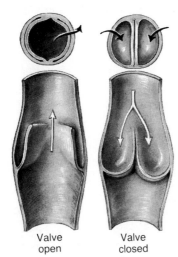

Valve   Valve
open   closed

FIGURE 4–14. Larger veins contain valves that prevent the backflow of blood that could occur owing to the effects of gravity. (From Jacob SW, Francone CA, Lossow WJ: Structure and Function in Man, 5th ed. Philadelphia, WB Saunders, 1982, p. 385.)

VENOUS FLOW AND PRESSURE. Blood moves slowly in the veins as compared with the arteries, owing to the lower pressure. Veins in the lower extremities are particularly aided by the massaging effect of the nearby muscles in promoting blood flow back to the heart. The presence of cup-like valves in some of the larger veins helps prevent backflow (Fig. 4–14).

Blood Pressure

Blood pressure is the force exerted by the blood volume on the walls of the vessels. *Blood pressure is dependent on the volume of blood within the vessels and the size of the vascular space.*

VOLUME OF BLOOD

The amount of blood ejected into the vessels is a function of the cardiac output. It is directly related to the heart rate times the stroke volume. If the size of the vascular space remains the same, an increase in cardiac output will lead to an increase in blood pressure. Conversely, a decrease in cardiac output will lead to a decrease in blood pressure.

INTRAVASCULAR SPACE

The size of the vascular system can vary. The intravascular space is determined by both the internal diameter of the vessels and the number of vessels that are open at any one time. If the cardiac output remains the same, a decrease in the size of the vascular space (vasoconstriction) will lead to an increase in the blood pressure. There is less space for the blood to occupy and the pressure rises. Conversely, an increase in the size of

the vascular space (vasodilation) will lead to a decrease in the blood pressure.

The diameter of the vessels that the blood flows through determines the resistance to flow. The smaller the vessel, the greater the resistance and therefore the greater the pressure. Both the number of vessels that are open and their size constitute the total resistance to blood flow. This is referred to as the *peripheral vascular resistance* or PVR. It is related to blood pressure by the formula

Cardiac output × peripheral vascular resistance = blood pressure				
CO	×	PVR	=	BP

This formula illustrates that blood pressure is elevated by increasing either the cardiac output or the peripheral vascular resistance. On the other hand, blood pressure falls if either the cardiac output or the peripheral vascular resistance is decreased. Being aware of this relationship is basic to understanding how changes in blood pressure occur and what compensatory mechanisms the body uses to maintain blood pressure.

BLOOD PRESSURE AND BLOOD FLOW

Pressure inside the blood vessels exerts a force in all directions. The one-way valves and the containing walls of the vessels enable the pressure to force blood forward through the circulatory system.

SYSTOLIC AND DIASTOLIC BLOOD PRESSURE

When blood is pumped into the arteries during ventricular contraction (systole), the amount of blood in the arteries increases, and the pressure rises. The pressure measured during systole is the *systolic blood pressure.* As the heart relaxes (diastole) and the aortic valve closes, blood continues to move forward through vessels of lower pressure. The contraction of the elastic walls of the arteries aids blood flow during diastole. The amount of blood volume remaining in the arteries decreases and thus the blood pressure falls. The pressure measured during diastole is called the *diastolic blood pressure.*

The normal systolic blood pressure is estimated by calculating 100 mm Hg plus the patient's age (up to 140 or 150 mm Hg for adult men). The diastolic blood pressure is from 65 to 90 mm Hg in normal individuals. In general, the blood pressure is from 8 to 10 mm Hg lower in women.

SUMMARY OF BLOOD PRESSURE DETERMINANTS

Generally, if the cardiac output remains the same, the blood pressure will increase when the blood vessels constrict and decrease when they dilate. Likewise, if the resistance of the vessels remains the same, the blood pressure will increase when the cardiac output rises and decrease when the cardiac output falls. *Cardiac output and the diameter of the vessels are the determinants of blood pressure.* *Baroreceptors* (pressure receptors) in the major blood vessels monitor the blood pressure and provide feedback to the central nervous system. Through the autonomic nervous system, the brain regulates both the cardiac output and the tone or resistance of the vessels to keep the blood pressure within a normal range.

PULSE PRESSURE

Blood flow through the arteries is characterized by a rhythmic pulse or beat. It reflects the rhythmic pumping of the ventricle and can be palpated when taking an arterial pulse. The difference between the systolic and the diastolic pressure is referred to as the *pulse pressure*. The normal pulse pressure is about 40 mm Hg. If the pulse pressure is greater than 50 mm Hg or lower than 30 mm Hg, it is abnormal.

RELATION OF PULSE PRESSURE AND QUALITY OF THE PULSE

If the pulse pressure is large, as can occur when the systolic pressure is 140 and the diastolic is 70, the pulse feels full or bounding. If the pulse pressure is low, as can occur if the systolic pressure is 90 and the diastolic is 70, the pulse feels weak or thready.

DETERMINANTS AIDING INTERPRETATION OF PULSE PRESSURE

The two major determinants of pulse pressure are the stroke volume and the tone of the larger arteries.

If the stroke volume increases, the volume of blood ejected into the arteries is greater, leading to increased stretching and contraction of the elastic walls. If there is no change in the size of the vessel, this leads to an increase in the pulse pressure. Conversely, if the stroke volume is reduced, the pulse pressure is decreased (Table 4–5).

In an elderly person, the vessels can lose their ability to stretch and distend and contract. This often occurs in patients with hardening of the arteries (arteriosclerosis)

TABLE 4–5. Effects of Stroke Volume on Pulse Pressure and Quality*

Stroke Volume	Pulse Pressure	Pulse Quality	Examples
Increased	Increased	Bounding	Exercise
Decreased	Decreased	Thready, weak	Blood loss

* *Assumes constant size and elasticity of vessels.*

when the elastic and muscular properties of the vessels are altered. In individuals with this condition, the arteries do not stretch during systole because they "harden," hence the systolic pressure is greater, resulting in an increased pulse pressure. You will encounter many patients with arteriosclerosis who have an increased pulse pressure.

Conversely, if the vessels are in a state of intense vasoconstriction, this reduces the pulse pressure.

REDUCTION OF BLOOD PRESSURE AND BLOOD FLOW

Blood pressure is highest at the point where the blood leaves the left ventricle. The pressure is successively lowered as blood leaves the pump and travels through the aorta, arteries, arterioles, capillaries, and veins (Fig. 4–15). Blood pressure is significantly reduced as blood flows through the arterioles.

Furthermore, the blood *flow* becomes more continuous than pulsating after it leaves the arterioles and enters the capillaries. This slower and continuous flow persists throughout the capillaries and venous system.

Major Arteries

Blood leaves the heart through either the pulmonary artery or the aorta (Fig. 4–16).

PULMONARY ARTERY

The artery that leaves the right ventricle and branches into the right and left pulmonary arteries that carry blood to the two lungs is called the *pulmonary artery*. These pulmonary arteries in turn subdivide until they become the capillaries that surround the alveoli in

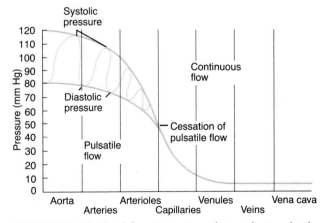

FIGURE 4–15. Blood flow in arteries and arterioles is pulsatile. The maximum pressure is created during ventricular contraction (systole); the lowest pressure occurs just prior to the next pulse wave (diastole). Blood flow in the capillaries, venules, and veins is not under the direct influence of ventricular contraction and is not pulsatile. (Adapted from Solomon EP, Phillips GA: Understanding Human Anatomy and Physiology. Philadelphia, WB Saunders, 1987, p. 236.)

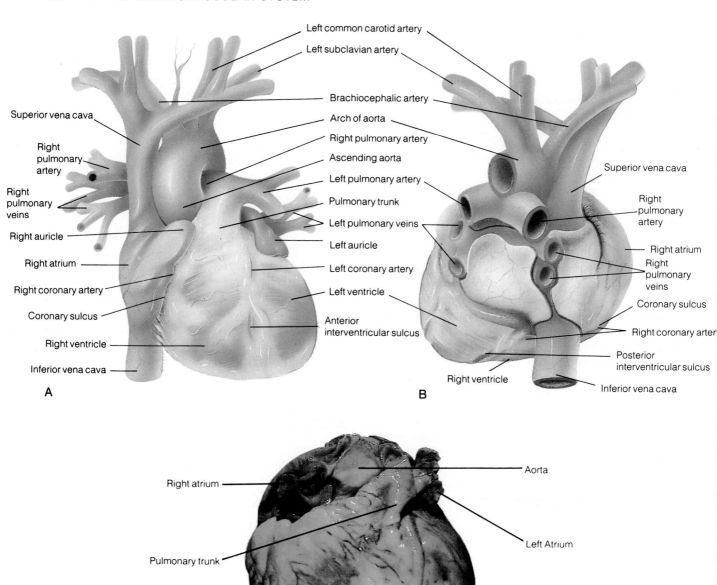

FIGURE 4–16. Pulmonary artery, aorta, and coronary arteries. (*A* and *C*) Anterior and (*B*) posterior views of the human heart. (From Gaudin AJ, Jones KC: Human Anatomy and Physiology. Orlando, Harcourt Brace Jovanovich, 1989, p. 562.)

the lungs. At this site, diffusion of oxygen and carbon dioxide takes place. *In contrast to all other arteries in the body, the pulmonary artery carries blood that is low in oxygen.*

AORTA

The left ventricle pumps out oxygenated blood through the *aorta*. This is a very elastic vessel that is

about 1 inch in diameter where it leaves the heart. Initially, it is directed upward and called the ascending aorta. It then curves backward and to the left at the aortic arch. At the level of the fourth thoracic vertebra it begins to descend downward along the spine where it is named the thoracic aorta, and is then called the abdominal aorta as it traverses the thorax and abdomen. It continues in the abdomen to the level of the fourth lumbar vertebra where it divides into the right and left common iliac arteries.

CORONARY ARTERIES

The first arteries to branch off the aorta are the *coronary arteries*, which exit just above the aortic valve and form a network around the heart. The heart is the first to receive the oxygenated blood. It is estimated that 5% of the blood in the systematic circulation is devoted to the coronary circulation. The pressure in the aorta is the driving force for the blood that flows through the coronary arteries.

The coronary arteries enter the myocardium and branch into capillaries, which give off nutrients and oxygen to the heart and pick up waste products. The capillaries then form into veins that meet at the coronary sinus and return the now oxygen-poor blood to the right atrium.

Blood flow through the coronary vessels to the deeper parts of the left ventricle occurs during rest periods. Therefore, the heart needs diastole so that the deeper parts of the left ventricle can receive oxygen.

HEAD AND UPPER EXTREMITIES

The next group of arteries to branch off the aorta is directed to the head and upper extremities. They arise from the aortic arch and are the brachiocephalic, which becomes the right common carotid and right subclavian; the left common carotid; and the left subclavian (Fig. 4–17A).

The *common carotids* bring blood to the head and neck (Fig. 4–17B). They divide to form the internal and external carotids. The internal carotids provide the main source of blood supply to the head (Fig. 4–17C). The carotid pulse is checked in an unresponsive patient. It passes through the neck along the trachea. To palpate it, slide the tips of your fingers from the Adam's apple (the thyroid cartilage) laterally toward the sternocleidomastoid muscles of the neck. Never compress both carotid arteries at one time; you may obstruct most of the blood flow to the brain if you do.

The external carotids branch further into the superficial temporal and internal maxillary arteries (Fig. 4–17B). The *superficial temporal artery* pulse can be felt by placing two fingers just anterior to the ear. The *facial artery* branches off the internal maxillary artery and can be palpated at the angle of the jaw.

The subclavian and brachiocephalic arteries give rise to branches feeding the thorax, the brain, and the spinal cord and then continue to the upper limbs. The name changes as each artery continues, from *axillary* in the axillary region to *brachial* in the upper arm and then dividing into the *radial* and *ulnar* arteries in the forearm that extend down into the hand (Fig. 4–17D). The brachial and radial arteries are used to check for blood pressure and pulse rate and quality. The brachial artery can be palpated medially, just proximal to the crease of the elbow. The radial artery is palpated on the anterior and radial (thumb) side of the wrist. The ulnar artery can also be palpated on the anterior but ulnar (little finger) side of the wrist.

THORAX, ABDOMEN, AND LOWER EXTREMITIES

The thoracic and abdominal aortas divide into multiple branches along their course to the tissues and organs in the thorax and abdomen. Many of these are labeled in Figure 4–17E. The common iliac arteries are formed by the division of the abdominal aorta. Their branches, the internal and external iliac arteries, branch off to some structures in the lower abdomen. The external *iliac arteries* extend to the inguinal ligament (the crease where the thigh joins the pelvis at the groin), where they enter the thighs and are named the *femoral arteries*. The *femoral artery* is easily palpable at the level of the inguinal ligament, halfway between the superior iliac crest and the symphysis pubis.

The femoral artery gives rise to the *popliteal artery*, beginning in the lower thigh (Fig. 4–17F). The popliteal artery passes behind the knee, where it may be palpated, and then divides to form the *anterior* and *posterior tibial arteries*. The anterior tibial passes between the tibia and fibula and is palpable on the anterior surface of the tarsal bones in the foot, where it is called the *dorsalis pedis*. The posterior tibial artery passes down the calf and is palpable just posterior to the medial malleolus of the ankle. Table 4–6 provides a summary of key arteries and their locations.

Major Veins

The major veins tend to run beside the major arteries. Many of the veins share the names of the arteries that lie parallel to them (Fig. 4–18A). In this section, emphasis will be given to the veins that are used in physical assessment or in the administration of intravenous therapy.

HEAD, NECK, AND UPPER EXTREMITIES

Figure 4–18B and C illustrates the positions of veins in the head and neck. In the cranium, *venous sinuses* are formed under the dura mater lining. Veins from this region empty into the *internal jugular vein*, which travels down through the neck just lateral to the carotid arteries. The *external jugular vein* drains blood from the external portion of the cranium and from the face and neck and is visible over the lateral neck. Both the internal and

Text continued on page 177

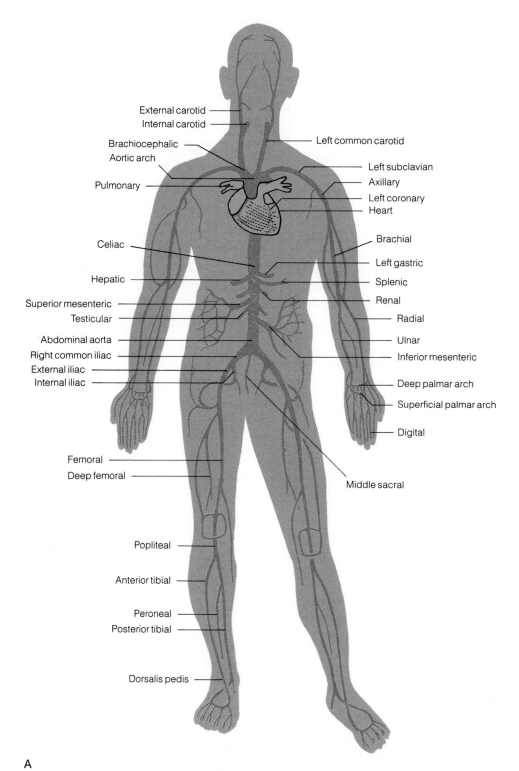

A

FIGURE 4–17. (*A*) Major arteries. (*B*) Arteries of the head and neck. (*C*) Arteries of the brain.

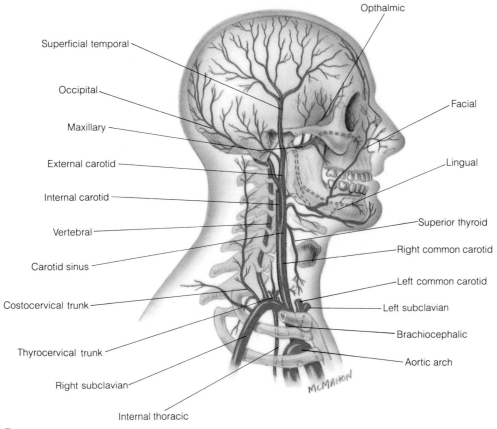

B

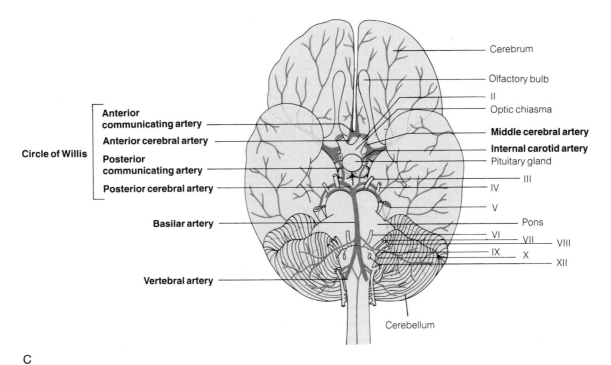

C

FIGURE 4–17. *Continued. Illustration continued on following page*

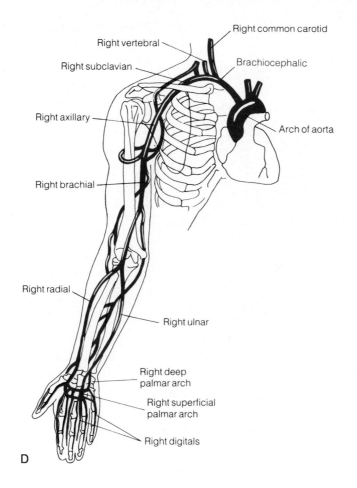

Right common carotid
Right vertebral
Right subclavian
Brachiocephalic

Right axillary

Arch of aorta

Right brachial

Right radial

Right ulnar

Right deep
palmar arch

Right superficial
palmar arch

Right digitals

D

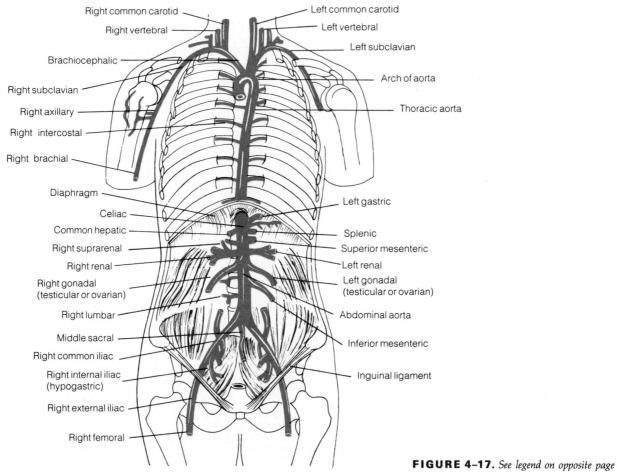

Right common carotid
Right vertebral
Brachiocephalic
Right subclavian
Right axillary
Right intercostal
Right brachial
Diaphragm
Celiac
Common hepatic
Right suprarenal
Right renal
Right gonadal
(testicular or ovarian)
Right lumbar
Middle sacral
Right common iliac
Right internal iliac
(hypogastric)
Right external iliac
Right femoral

Left common carotid
Left vertebral
Left subclavian
Arch of aorta
Thoracic aorta

Left gastric
Splenic
Superior mesenteric
Left renal
Left gonadal
(testicular or ovarian)
Abdominal aorta
Inferior mesenteric

Inguinal ligament

FIGURE 4–17. *See legend on opposite page*

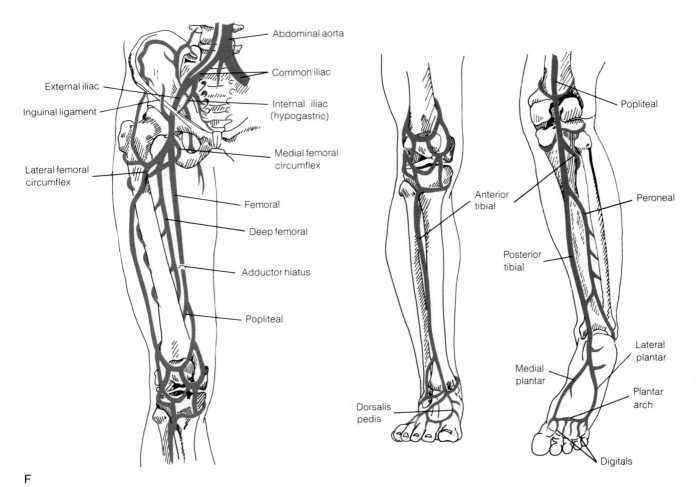

F

FIGURE 4–17. *Continued.* (*D*) Arteries of the upper extremity. (*E*) Arteries of the thorax and abdomen. (*F*) Arteries of the lower extremity. (From Gaudin AJ, Jones KC: Human Anatomy and Physiology. Orlando, Harcourt Brace Jovanovich, 1989, pp. 590, 592, 593, 595, and 597.)

TABLE 4–6. Key Arteries and Their Locations Used for Pulse Points and Pressure Points

Palpable Arteries	Location
Carotid*†	Lateral to the thyroid cartilage at the sternocleidomastoid muscle
Temporal*	Just anterior to the top portion of the ear
Facial*	At the angle of the jaw
Brachial*†	Anterior-medial surface of the elbow, just proximal to the crease
Radial†	Radial aspect of wrist, anteriorly
Ulnar†	Ulnar side of the wrist, anteriorly
Femoral*†	Inguinal ligament, midway between the iliac crest and the symphysis pubis
Popliteal†	Posterior crease of knee
Posterior tibial†	Posterior to the medial malleolus
Dorsalis pedis†	Mid-anterior surface of the tarsal bones

* *Used as a pressure point.*
Note: The carotid artery is used as a pressure point for life-threatening hemorrhage in the neck that is not controlled by direct pressure.
† *Used for pulse check.*

external jugular veins empty into the *subclavian veins* at the level of the sternoclavicular joint. These veins are often referred to as the neck veins and are used during physical assessment.

The superficial veins of the arm are illustrated in Fig. 4–18*D*. The *basilic* and *cephalic* veins and their distal branches are commonly used for placement of an intravenous line. They ultimately join together and become the subclavian veins that meet with the jugular veins to form the *superior vena cava*, the major vein that returns blood from the upper body to the heart.

LOWER EXTREMITIES, ABDOMEN, AND THORAX

As can be seen from Figure 4–18*E*, the veins returning from the lower extremities bear names similar to the arteries to which they correspond. They meet after entering the lower abdomen to form the *inferior*

Text continued on page 182

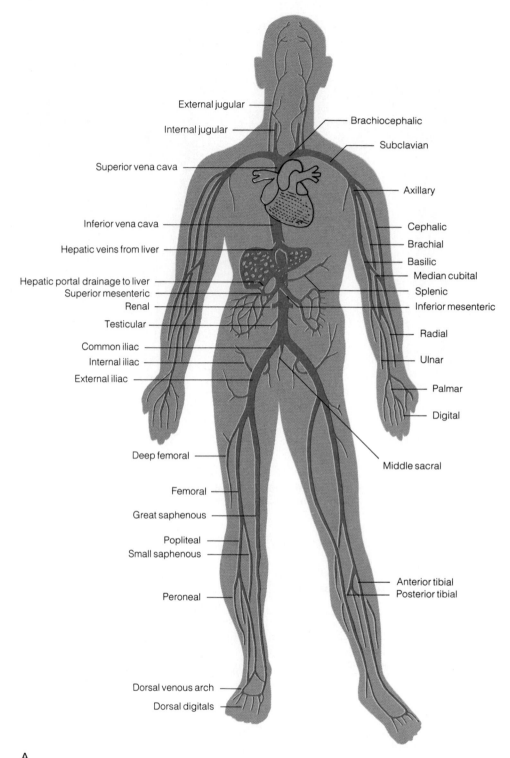

A

FIGURE 4–18. (*A*) Major veins. (*B*) Veins of the head and neck. (*C*) Venous sinuses of the brain.

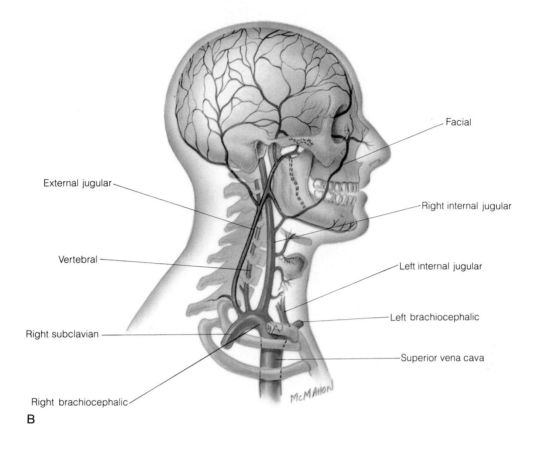

External jugular

Facial

Right internal jugular

Vertebral

Left internal jugular

Left brachiocephalic

Right subclavian

Superior vena cava

Right brachiocephalic

B

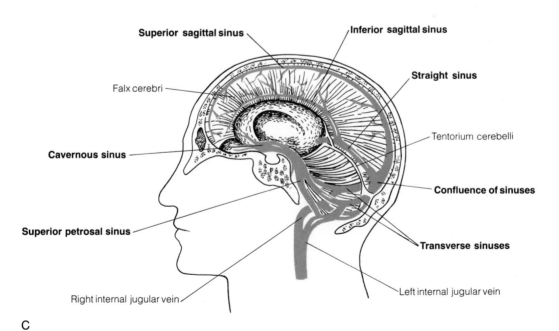

Superior sagittal sinus

Inferior sagittal sinus

Falx cerebri

Straight sinus

Cavernous sinus

Tentorium cerebelli

Confluence of sinuses

Superior petrosal sinus

Transverse sinuses

Right internal jugular vein

Left internal jugular vein

C

FIGURE 4–18. *Continued. Illustration continued on following page*

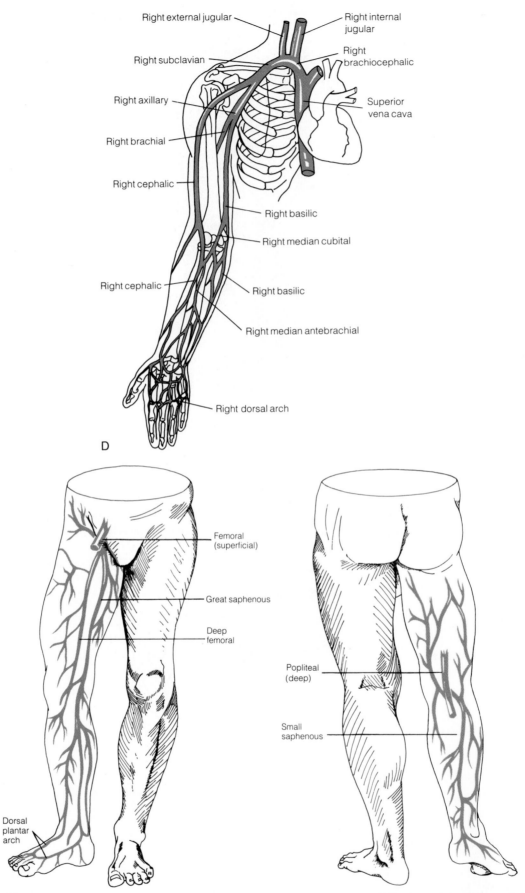

Right external jugular

Right internal jugular

Right subclavian

Right brachiocephalic

Right axillary

Superior vena cava

Right brachial

Right cephalic

Right basilic

Right median cubital

Right cephalic

Right basilic

Right median antebrachial

Right dorsal arch

D

Femoral (superficial)

Great saphenous

Deep femoral

Popliteal (deep)

Small saphenous

Dorsal plantar arch

E

FIGURE 4–18. *Continued.* *(D)* Veins of the upper extremity. *(E)* Veins of the lower extremity. *(F)* Veins of the thorax and abdomen. *(G)* Veins of the hepatic portal system. (From Gaudin AJ, Jones KC: Human Anatomy and Physiology. Orlando, Harcourt Brace Jovanovich, 1989, pp. 598–603.)

180

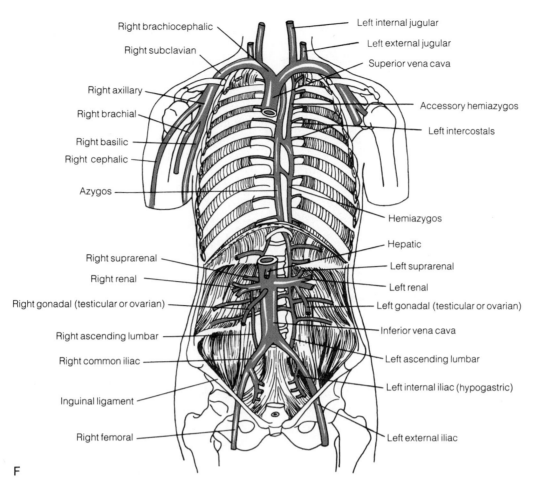

Right brachiocephalic
Right subclavian
Right axillary
Right brachial
Right basilic
Right cephalic
Azygos
Right suprarenal
Right renal
Right gonadal (testicular or ovarian)
Right ascending lumbar
Right common iliac
Inguinal ligament
Right femoral

Left internal jugular
Left external jugular
Superior vena cava
Accessory hemiazygos
Left intercostals
Hemiazygos
Hepatic
Left suprarenal
Left renal
Left gonadal (testicular or ovarian)
Inferior vena cava
Left ascending lumbar
Left internal iliac (hypogastric)
Left external iliac

F

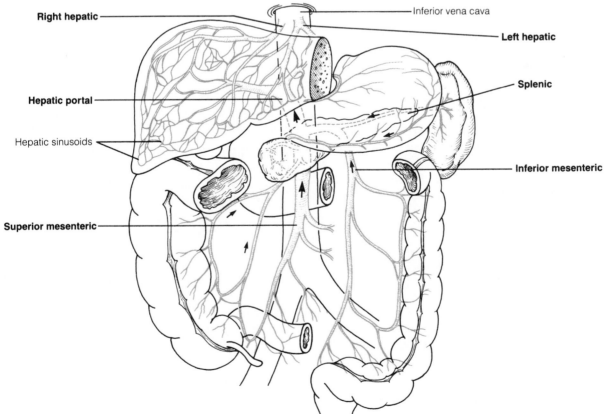

Right hepatic
Hepatic portal
Hepatic sinusoids
Superior mesenteric

Inferior vena cava
Left hepatic
Splenic
Inferior mesenteric

G

FIGURE 4–18. *Continued.*

vena cava. The inferior vena cava receives the branches from the various organs and tissues in the abdomen and trunk, and empties into the right atrium (Fig. 4–18*F*).

The veins draining the liver need special emphasis for clinical purposes. This *portal system*, as it is called, is especially important because it receives branches from the esophagus, stomach, and small intestine (Fig. 4–18*G*). It brings blood to the liver for conversion and storage of nutrients and for removal of waste products. With severe liver disease such as cirrhosis or cancer, blood flow through the liver is obstructed, and blood backs up through the connecting branches. One of these sets of branches is composed of the *esophageal veins.* When blood backs up, the veins dilate and push through the esophageal wall into the food pipe itself, a condition known as esophageal varices. These veins are then exposed to digestive juices and acid from the stomach and may rupture, resulting in massive and life-threatening bleeding.

The Microcirculation

The entire circulatory system is designed to bring blood to the tissues of the body in sufficient amounts to meet their needs for oxygen and other nutrients. The capillaries are in close proximity to the body's cells, separated by the fluid that bathes them, which is called the *interstitial fluid.* The capillaries are so narrow that the red blood cells must squeeze through one at a time. Pores in the capillaries allow solutes (small particles in solution, such as glucose, sodium, potassium, oxygen, and so on) and water to diffuse into the interstitial fluid. Likewise, waste products, other solutes, and water in the interstitial fluid may diffuse through the capillary wall into the blood. (Normally, larger molecules and red blood cells cannot pass across the capillary wall. Special mechanisms allow white blood cells to migrate through capillary walls at sites of infections.) Forces involved in the movement of blood through the capillary beds (*microcirculation*) include diffusion, osmosis, and the capillary blood pressure.

DIFFUSION

Diffusion is the flow of a solute or particle from an area of higher concentration to an area of lower concentration to reach equilibrium. If a particle or gas molecule is able to pass through the capillary membrane, that particle will flow across the capillary from the side of higher concentration to the side of lower concentration. The concentration gradient of each individual particle determines the direction of flow (see Fig. 2–4).

DIFFUSION OF OXYGEN AND CARBON DIOXIDE. For example, oxygen diffuses from the capillaries into the interstitial fluid and then into the cells because of the concentration gradient. The concentration of oxygen is higher in the capillaries than in the cells where it is used for fuel; therefore, the direction of flow is from the blood to the cells.

For the same reason, carbon dioxide flows from the cells into the capillaries since the concentration of carbon dioxide is higher in the cells. Carbon dioxide is the waste product of cellular metabolism. The blood brings carbon dioxide from the cells, where it is produced, to the lungs, where it is removed (see Fig. 3–9).

CAPILLARY BLOOD PRESSURE, OSMOSIS, AND MICROCIRCULATION

This continuous movement of fluids and solutes out of the capillaries and then back in from the interstitial fluid is called the *microcirculation.* The driving pressure on the bloodstream from the heart pushes the blood forward and against the capillary walls. This force drives water and solutes out through the capillary walls. Remember that this can only happen at the capillary level because the walls of the arteries and veins are too thick to allow the escape of components of the blood.

What brings the fluid back into the capillaries? Here, a basic understanding of osmosis is helpful. Osmosis is a process whereby water (or a solvent) moves across a membrane from an area of lower concentration of particles to an area of higher concentration of particles. Every particle in a solution holds water molecules near it. If two different concentrations of particles in water are separated by a membrane that permits the flow of water but not the particles across it, the water moves toward the side with the higher concentration of particles. It moves until it results in an equal distribution of water to particles (an equal concentration) on each side of the membrane (see Fig. 2–4).

PLASMA PROTEINS. Plasma proteins (found predominantly in blood) exert a holding or pulling force on water and counterbalance the driving force of the capillary blood pressure.

The capillary wall allows most particles to diffuse across it. The concentrations of most of the solutes in the blood and the interstitial fluid (the fluid that bathes the cells) are remarkably similar. There is one striking difference, however—the plasma proteins. These large molecules are found primarily in the blood, and not in the interstitial fluid. These proteins also exert an osmotic force or hold on water molecules. The plasma proteins use this osmotic force, called *oncotic pressure,* to "hold" onto or pull water back inside the capillary.

BALANCE OF FORCES. These are the forces that permit a microcirculation to take place. The hydrostatic pressure or blood pressure forces water and its solutes out of the capillaries. The oncotic pressure of plasma proteins brings water and solutes back into the capillaries.

The result is a balance of forces that helps maintain an equilibrium of water and blood solutes.

CAPILLARY BLOOD PRESSURE. The blood pressure at the arterial end of a capillary is greater than the oncotic pressure of plasma proteins. This difference drives water and solutes from the blood across the capillary into the interstitial space. When the blood flows through the capillary, the pressure is further reduced so that by the time the blood reaches the venous end of the capillary, the pressure is less than the oncotic pressure of the plasma proteins. This difference now pulls water back into the capillary from the interstitial space. Difference of forces in opposite directions permits the microcirculation to take place (Fig. 4–19). Just remember that when the balance is disrupted, the microcirculation is not balanced, and this becomes apparent clinically. The clinical signs of edema and dehydration can be explained by a disruption in the balance of these forces.

LIVER DISEASE. If there are fewer plasma proteins than normal in the blood, the oncotic force becomes less, and less water is pulled back within the capillary at the venous end of the *microcirculation*. Extra water accumulates in the interstitial fluid, which becomes clinically apparent as edema.

Some patients with severe liver disease have an abnormally low level of plasma proteins. These patients also have significant *edema* (Fig. 4–20). Malnutrition can also result in low plasma proteins and edema.

VENOUS OBSTRUCTION. If a vein is obstructed by a thrombus or blood clot, the blood pressure in the vein rises distal to the obstruction. This increased pressure is transmitted back through the veins to the capillary level. When hydrostatic forces exceed the oncotic pressure of the plasma proteins, fluid accumulates in the interstitial space and edema results. An EMT may see patients with clots of the deep veins of the leg who present with obvious tibial and ankle edema.

HEART FAILURE. When the heart fails, blood backs up in the venous circulation and the resulting increase

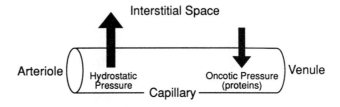

Liver Disease

FIGURE 4–20. The effect of liver disease upon microcirculation. Liver disease can cause a decrease in the number of plasma proteins. This results in a decrease in the oncotic pressure; thus less fluid is pulled back into the capillary and remains in the interstitial space. This results in a buildup of edema in the interstitial space.

in venous pressure is likewise transmitted to the capillary level. Again, if this pressure exceeds the oncotic pressure within the capillary, a net loss of water to the interstitium results, which is evident clinically as edema. Either the systemic or the pulmonary circulation can be affected, depending on whether the patient has right- or left-sided heart failure.

DEHYDRATION. The body's loss of water or blood can cause dehydration.

Water Loss. Dehydration can be caused by prolonged vomiting and diarrhea. As water is lost, the concentration of the plasma proteins is greater, since there is less water to dilute them. The "more concentrated" plasma proteins draw fluid away from the tissue to restore the plasma volume. The patient with vomiting and diarrhea develops dry skin because the capillaries pull fluid from the entire body (Fig. 4–21).

Blood Loss. A great blood loss causes the arterial pressure to fall. This results in low pressure on the arterial side of the capillary. The oncotic pressure in the capillary then pulls tissue water into the bloodstream in an attempt to restore the blood volume to normal. This replacement of blood volume is effective if blood loss is minor or occurs slowly over a period of time. However, it is not

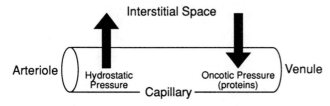

Normal

FIGURE 4–19. Normal microcirculation. At the arteriole end of the capillary, the hydrostatic pressure is greater than the oncotic pressure, and fluid is pushed into the interstitial space. At the venule end of the capillary, the oncotic pressure is greater than the hydrostatic pressure, and fluid is drawn into the capillary. The net effect results in a relatively equal movement of fluid in and out of the capillary. (After Rosen P, Barkin RM: Essentials of Emergency Medicine. St. Louis, Mosby-Year Book, Inc., 1991, p. 39.)

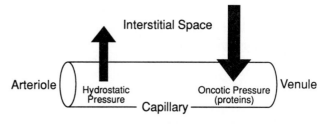

Dehydration

FIGURE 4–21. The effect of dehydration on microcirculation. With excessive water loss caused by vomiting, diarrhea, or other problems, the proportion of plasma proteins becomes greater in relation to fluid in the capillary. As a result, fluid is pulled into the capillary in an attempt to maintain the blood volume. This movement of fluid from body cells results in signs of dehydration (e.g., dry skin and mucous membranes).

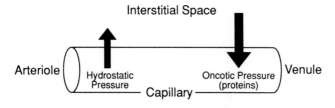

Interstitial Space

Arteriole Hydrostatic Pressure Capillary Oncotic Pressure (proteins) Venule

Blood Loss

FIGURE 4–22. The effect of blood loss on microcirculation. When a person experiences severe blood loss, the hydrostatic pressure drops below the oncotic pressure. As a result, fluid is pulled back into the capillary in an attempt to restore blood volume.

an effective method of replacing blood volume in the case of hemorrhage or rapid and continuous bleeding (Fig. 4–22).

Lymphatics

Some plasma proteins do escape from the capillaries. These proteins do not ordinarily re-enter the capillary in the microcirculation process, but are instead returned to the bloodstream by the *lymphatic circulation.*

The lymphatic system is similar to the blood vessels in that it consists of a network of lymph capillaries that drain into larger and larger vessels until they ultimately drain into the right and left subclavian veins. The lymphatic capillaries allow components of the interstitial fluid, including the proteins, to enter through their walls. The pressure exerted by the surrounding tissues on the lymphatic vessel walls is a major force in the movement of lymphatic fluid. It is a low-pressure system, and, as in the veins, the flow is helped by contraction of surrounding muscles that squeeze fluid forward, as well as by a series of one-way valves. The largest lymphatic vessel, the *thoracic duct*, also helps carry to the bloodstream some products that have been absorbed from the digestive tract.

The lymphatic system has another function besides returning fluid and protein to the bloodstream. Along its network, lymphatic vessels pass through the *lymph nodes*. Bacteria and foreign matter can enter the lymph capillaries and are filtered during passage through the lymph nodes. Here, specialized cells are present that engulf and destroy bacteria and foreign material. If they need help, more of these specialized cells are called to the affected lymph nodes.

This phenomenon becomes apparent, for example, with a sore throat, when glands or lymph nodes in the neck are swollen. These nodes are located throughout the body. In most infections, only the nodes that drain a given area become swollen. They filter the lymph fluid effectively, preventing the spread of bacteria. These nodes help contain infections.

In some infections that attack many parts of the body, swelling of the lymph nodes may occur in many areas. Mononucleosis is a common disease that presents with generalized *lymphadenopathy* (swelling of the lymph nodes in many areas).

THE SPLEEN AS A SOURCE OF LYMPHATIC TISSUE

The spleen, located under the left diaphragm, contains lymphatic tissue. It is designed to filter the blood and produce lymphatic cells. In conditions such as mononucleosis it is also swollen. Since the spleen with its blood filtering function is rich in blood vessels, physicians are always careful to palpate the left upper quadrant of the abdomen very carefully.

If an injury has occurred to the upper left quadrant of the abdomen or to the lower ribs that protect it, one must consider the possibility that the spleen has been injured. Injuries to the spleen often result in extensive blood loss. Be aware that this blood-rich organ is both delicate and vulnerable. Palpation of the left upper quadrant during your physical assessment should be done very carefully. Remember that injuries to the lower left ribs or left upper abdomen may have caused the spleen to rupture, which can result in a fatal hemorrhage.

SUMMARY

Knowledge of anatomy and physiology provides the foundation for understanding the assessment and treatment of the patients discussed in the following chapters. As you read on, compare normal anatomy and physiology with the conditions that are discussed to better appreciate the relevance and rationales of care.

REVIEW EXERCISES

1. List three components of the circulatory system and the function of each.
2. Describe the location of the heart.
3. List the major structures of the heart and the function(s) of each.
4. Describe how a valve works.
5. List the steps of electrical firing within the conduction system and the mechanical events associated with them.
6. List the components of blood and their functions.
7. Describe how oxygen is transported in blood.
8. Define the following concepts:
   Stroke volume
   Cardiac output
   Starling's law

Blood pressure
Pulse pressure
Osmosis

9. State the basic difference between sympathetic and parasympathetic stimulation of the heart.

10. Describe the structure and function of arteries, capillaries, and veins.

11. List the major arteries in the chest, abdomen, head, neck, and extremities.

REFERENCES

Guyton AC: Textbook of Medical Physiology, 8th ed. Philadelphia, WB Saunders, 1991.

Passmore R, Robson JS (eds): A Companion to Medical Studies, vol 1. Oxford, Blackwell Scientific Publications, 1969.

Raynor J: Anatomy and Physiology. Hagerstown, MD, Harper & Row, 1977.

Zuidema GD, Rutherford RB, Ballinger WF: The Management of Trauma, 4th ed. Philadelphia, WB Saunders, 1985.

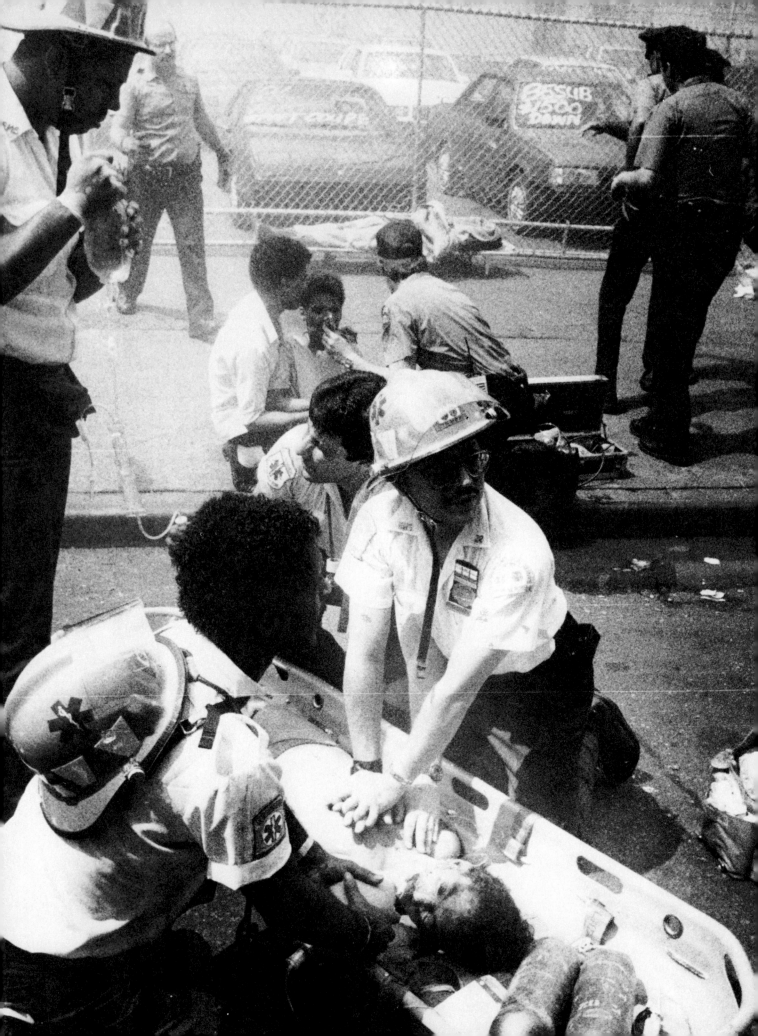

Hypovolemic Shock Secondary to Hemorrhage

The most life-threatening cause of hypovolemic shock is rapid and profuse bleeding, or *hemorrhage*.

EFFECT OF BLOOD LOSS

As stated before, the blood is important for its oxygen-carrying ability, its volume, and its various components. Acute and heavy bleeding results in a loss of all of these. It leaves a person depleted of red cells and hemoglobin (necessary to carry oxygen), blood volume (necessary to fill the vascular space), and platelets and clotting factors (necessary to stop bleeding).

If left untreated, individuals who suffer the acute loss of about half their blood volume experience circulatory arrest and die. It is the loss of volume rather than of hemoglobin that is the earliest cause of shock and death in the bleeding patient.

LOSS OF BLOOD CELLS. Normally, a person has three or four times the amount of red blood cells and hemoglobin necessary to sustain life. Many patients with chronic disease live with levels of hemoglobin that are about half what is normal. Patients with a low supply of hemoglobin are said to be *anemic*. They do not have

the energy or oxygen reserve to sustain periods of exercise, but they can tolerate the more modest activities of daily living, provided that their anemia is not too severe.

When anemia (loss of red blood cells) develops slowly, the body can make adjustments to maintain a normal blood volume. Tissue fluids move into the blood vessels through the capillaries, and a patient's blood volume is maintained. Blood pressure is maintained as long as enough oxygen is available to feed the pump.

The lower number of red blood cells in an anemic patient causes a change in the normal skin color (Fig. 5–2). With a diminished amount of hemoglobin, the pink color of oxygenated hemoglobin visible in the superficial areas of the body is less intense, leading to pallor. The skin, nail beds, creases in the palms, and conjunctivae of the eyes appear pale. Because the vessels leading to the skin are not constricted, the temperature and moisture of the skin are not affected, and they appropriately reflect environmental temperatures and other conditions. The anemic person may complain of weakness and drowsiness. The compensatory mechanisms of the circulatory system might manifest as tachycardia.

LOSS OF BLOOD VOLUME. Hemorrhage results in equal loss of both blood volume and hemoglobin. While the body can make adjustments to the loss of half of its

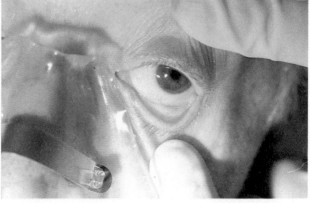
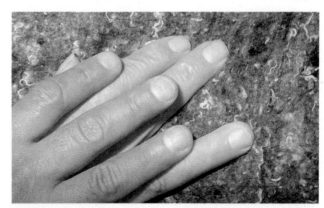

A

B

C

FIGURE 5–2. Anemia. The nail beds and conjunctivae are checked for pallor. Pale coloring of the nail beds and conjunctivae can indicate a deficiency of red blood cells and their pigment, hemoglobin. (*A*) This patient with the pale nail beds has only one-third of the normal amount of red blood cells. (*B*) The patient (bottom hand) has one-half of the normal amount of red blood cells. Note contrast of patient's nail beds with the examiner's hand (top hand). Regardless of skin pigment, the nail beds provide a quick check during the respiratory and circulatory assessment. (*C*) Note pallor of conjunctiva in patient with severe anemia (low blood hemoglobin).

hemoglobin over a period of time, which results in anemia, a sudden loss of half of its blood volume causes circulatory arrest. With the simultaneous loss of both hemoglobin and blood volume, there is enough hemoglobin to meet the tissues' oxygen needs, but not enough blood volume to perfuse the body's tissues, and therefore shock results. Even though the body is able to limit the areas that are perfused when blood loss occurs, with the loss of half its normal blood volume, there is not enough blood to fill the smallest possible system, and circulation ceases. Patients in cardiac arrest caused by hemorrhage cannot be resuscitated until their blood volume is restored.

Within EMS systems, this knowledge has led to the use of intravenous fluids to begin resuscitation of patients suffering shock secondary to hemorrhage. Common volume expanders include salt and other plasma-like solutions administered before blood is available, since patients may still have more than half of their normal amount of hemoglobin—enough to maintain life.

LOSS OF CLOTTING FACTORS. In addition to the loss of red blood cells and blood volume, the hemorrhaging patient is losing the clotting factors and platelets that are necessary for blood to clot. After extensive blood loss, transfusion of red cells, clotting factors, and platelets is required for the patient to survive.

EXTERNAL BLEEDING—RECOGNITION

By noting several important details about a patient who is losing blood, the EMT is better able to evaluate and treat the patient.

QUALITY OF BLOOD FLOW. If the blood vessel walls are severed, bleeding results. The rate of bleeding that occurs depends on the size and type of vessel injured. The arteries, being high-pressure vessels, bleed the fastest, and blood will spurt or pulsate from the wound. The veins exhibit continuous blood flow. The capillaries also show a continuous flow but because of their small size, the blood seems to ooze forth. The larger the vessel severed, the faster the rate of blood loss. In fact, when the largest vessels (such as the aorta) are severed, death results in seconds.

COLOR. Recognizing the types of external bleeding is also aided by the color of the blood flowing from a wound. Arterial blood is red since its hemoglobin is oxygen rich. Venous blood is a darker red because it contains less oxygen. Capillary blood is a color between these two.

TYPE OF VESSEL INJURY. In cases of trauma to the arterial vessels (where there is a significant muscular layer), the type of laceration encountered may influence the amount of bleeding. When smaller arteries are com-

pletely severed, the circular muscle within the arterial wall tends to constrict and thereby prevents further blood loss. Small veins also tend to collapse on themselves if they are completely severed. In the larger arteries where the middle wall of the vessel is made of tissue more elastic than muscle, such collapse does not occur. The worst type of laceration to an artery is one that severs only part of the wall. In such case, the muscle cannot fully constrict to prevent blood loss since the continuous surface of the rest of the artery holds it open.

LOCATION. External veins tend to be more superficial (closer to the body's surface) than arteries. Arteries tend to run deeper in the body and along bony surfaces, which makes them vulnerable to injury caused by fractures. The arteries are forced to come toward the surface at the joints of long bones. In an earlier discussion about the common pulse points, the locations of the superficial arteries were given. The location and depth of a wound can help predict the type of bleeding to expect. Table 5–5 summarizes the types of external bleeding.

CLOTTING. Clotting begins soon after the injury occurs, generally within 4 to 6 minutes. It is faster for smaller vessels, especially veins and capillaries, whose blood pressure is lower. Capillaries have a tendency to clot faster than other vessels. A partially severed artery is least likely to clot, because of the high pressure of the blood flowing through it. Clotting may not occur if very large vessels are lacerated, because the continuous flow of blood displaces the clotting elements.

BLEEDING CONTROL

Loss of blood volume and hemoglobin is a critical event. Thus, recognition and control of external bleeding are part of the primary survey. Obvious external hemorrhage requires immediate attention and is treated in conjunction with airway control and breathing as part of the ABCs.

Control of bleeding is a key concern for the EMT (Table 5–6). This is accomplished primarily with the application of direct pressure. In severe cases, application of pressure over a major artery may be required to assist in bleeding control; as a last resort, application of a tourniquet may be necessary. If the site of bleeding is

TABLE 5–5. Types of External Bleeding

Vessel	Flow	Color	Location
Artery	Pulsatile or spurting	Red	Deeper vessels, except at joints
Capillaries	Continuous oozing	Less red	Superficial
Veins	Continuous flow	Dark red or purple	Superficial compared with arteries

TABLE 5-6. Methods of Bleeding Control*

Direct pressure
Elevation
Pressure points
Tourniquet

* Correct order of methods to establish control of bleeding.

an extremity, control may be assisted by splinting and elevation.

DIRECT PRESSURE. The best and first measure used to control bleeding is the immediate application of direct pressure. Ideally a sterile dressing should be applied to any open wound to minimize the possibility of infection. Control of bleeding is of such high priority, however, that any clean cloth, such as a scarf, a shirt, or even the EMT's gloved hand, should be used if the sterile dressing is not immediately available (Fig. 5–3).

The object of direct pressure is to compress the bleeding vessels so that they collapse and obstruct further loss of blood. The amount of pressure required to control the hemorrhage is relative to the type of bleeding present. While minimal pressure will control capillary bleeding, more force is necessary to control bleeding from an artery.

PRESSURE BANDAGE. To allow yourself to attend to other tasks, once bleeding has been controlled with direct pressure, a bandage should be applied circumferentially to form a pressure dressing. Use sufficient sterile

gauze pads to cover the wound, then place additional dressings on top of the sterile pads. You can use additional gauze pads or other dressings such as sanitary napkins to build up the dressing. Adding bulk over the dressing focuses the bandage's pressure more directly over the wound.

A 3- to 4-inch–wide roll bandage can be rolled over the dressing three or four times and then secured by tying it or affixing tape. For wounds on an extremity, a blood pressure cuff might serve this same purpose. If the pressure dressing is not adequate to maintain bleeding control, or if the site of injury does not permit application of a circumferential dressing, continue to apply direct pressure manually. Use caution when applying direct pressure to the skull. In general the pressure should be distributed over a larger surface area to avoid the risk of depressing bone fragments.

The ideal pressure dressing should be tight enough to control all bleeding yet loose enough (if possible) to permit some blood flow to the structures beyond. When circumferential pressure dressings are applied around a limb, be careful to check for distal pulses and evidence of distal blood flow. If the distal pulse site is covered by the bandage, you can use the capillary refill test to gauge blood flow to the distal extremity. If no distal pulses are felt, the dressing is acting as a tourniquet, which is the method of last resort in bleeding control.

Do not remove the dressing once it is in place. To do so might disrupt some blood clots and cause bleeding to recur. If the dressing becomes soaked with blood, add other dressings on top of the original and reapply direct pressure (Fig. 5–3).

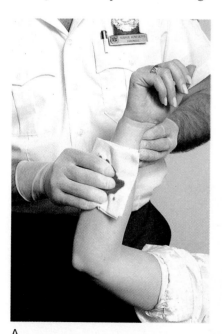 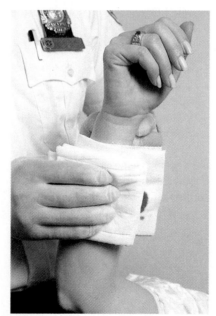 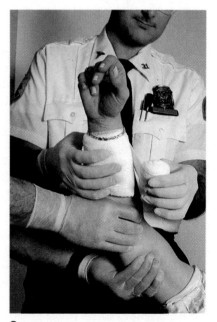

A   B   C

FIGURE 5-3. (*A*) Direct pressure is applied evenly over the wound site (with elevation) with sufficient pressure to control bleeding and not to obstruct distal arterial flow. (*B*) The dressing can be reinforced to aid in the clotting process, and (*C*) a pressure bandage can be applied to provide continued direct pressure.

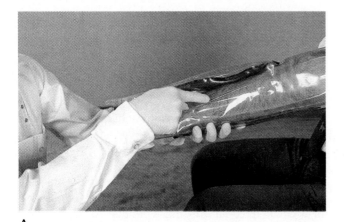
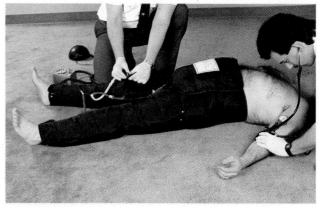

A B

FIGURE 5–4. (*A*) Air splint and (*B*) MAST can be used for continued direct pressure to control bleeding.

DIRECT PRESSURE DEVICES

Air splints and military antishock trousers (MAST) may be used to apply direct pressure over an extremity. They may be useful for situations in which there are extensive lacerations or underlying fractures. The MAST are particularly useful when controlling external bleeding in extremities whose injuries are associated with hypovolemic shock. They can cover a large surface area while at the same time immobilizing the affected limb (Fig. 5–4). The application of air splints is discussed in Chapter 8, on the musculoskeletal system.

ELEVATION. To control bleeding from the extremities, elevation is used in conjunction with direct pressure. This is recommended unless contraindicated by certain types of fractures (e.g., of the humerus). The limb can be elevated with a sling, a pillow, or a rolled blanket so that the wound is above the level of the heart.

SPLINTING. Broken bone fragments may continue to grate on blood vessels and increase bleeding if they are not immobilized. Muscular activity can also increase the rate of blood flow, and thus the bleeding, in an extremity. It is therefore useful to splint an extremity as part of the approach to bleeding control when fractures are suspected or the laceration is deep into the muscular tissues. Air splints and MAST sometimes accomplish both bleeding control and extremity immobilization simultaneously. Otherwise splints can be applied after the pressure bandage has been secured.

PRESSURE POINTS. At times, bleeding is difficult to control with direct pressure alone. Depending on the location of the wound, it may be useful to apply pressure directly over a major artery that feeds that area of the body. Pressure can be applied at the common pulse points where arteries can be palpated. For bleeding from the extremities, pressure over the brachial or the femoral artery may be useful. Compress the brachial artery (Fig. 5–5) against the humerus with your fingers. Use the

heel of your hand over the femoral artery to compress it against the pelvis (Fig. 5–6).

The pressure applied collapses the arteries and reduces or stops the blood flow. Pressure points are an adjunct to direct pressure in the control of bleeding. For example, while one EMT holds a pressure point, a second EMT should try to apply or reinforce a direct-pressure dressing.

Severe bleeding from the scalp is controlled with pressure over the temporal artery. Be careful that the temporal bone has not been injured. Facial bleeding might be reduced by compression of the facial artery, providing that the mandible has not been fractured. For life-threatening hemorrhage in the neck, pressure may have to be applied to the carotid artery. However, because the carotids are also the main suppliers of blood to the brain, the carotid artery should never be obliterated un-

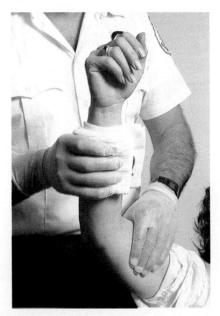

FIGURE 5–5. The pressure point for the upper extremity is located on the medial aspect of the upper arm.

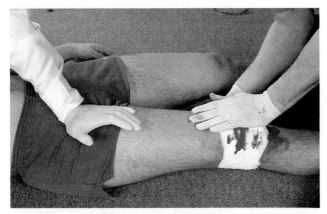

FIGURE 5–6. The pressure point for the lower extremity is located halfway between the pubic bone and the iliac crest. Place the heel of your hand in that location while maintaining direct pressure.

less life-threatening hemorrhage that cannot be controlled with any other means is present. To review other common pressure points, see Table 4–6.

TOURNIQUETS

As a last resort for uncontrolled bleeding, a tourniquet might be required. The tourniquet is a constricting band applied over an extremity with enough pressure to completely obliterate blood flow beyond the site of application. It is similar to inflating a blood pressure cuff to 140 mm Hg pressure on the arm of a person with a systolic blood pressure of 120 mm Hg. The lumen of the arteries is obliterated because the external pressure is greater than the pressure within. No blood can flow beyond.

PROCEDURE 5–1   APPLYING A TOURNIQUET

1. Place a 3- to 4-inch–wide piece of soft material, such as a folded triangular bandage or a commercial tourniquet, next to the wound.

   Note: If an improvised piece of cloth is used, it should be six to eight layers thick.

2. Wrap material around the extremity twice, then secure with a half knot (Fig. 5–7A).
3. Place a stick or pencil in the half knot and secure with a square knot (Fig. 5–7B).
4. Twist the stick until bleeding stops, then securely attach it next to the extremity (Fig. 5–7C).
5. Clearly note on the prehospital record that a tourniquet has been applied and the time of application so that it is not overlooked by hospital personnel during subsequent resuscitation efforts.
6. Mark "TK" and the time of application on the patient's forehead, use a tag on the extremity, and expose the extremity and tourniquet on arrival to the emergency department.

   Note: Once a tourniquet is applied, it is only removed by hospital personnel. Table 5–6 summarizes the sequence of methods undertaken to establish bleeding control.

7. Relay directly to hospital personnel that a tourniquet has been applied.

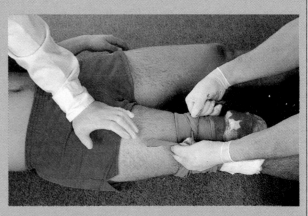

A

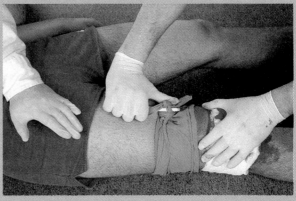

B

FIGURE 5–7. Applying a tourniquet. (*A*) Wrap a thick piece of cloth around the extremity and tie a simple knot. (*B*) Place a rigid stick over the knot, secure it in place with an additional knot, and tighten until the bleeding stops.

Continued

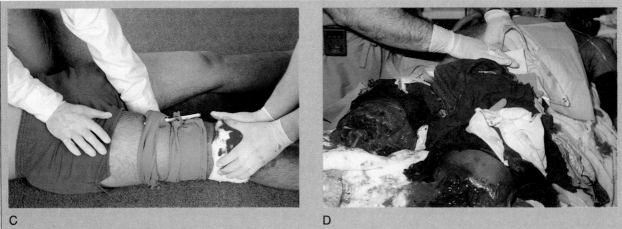

C   D

FIGURE 5–7. *Continued.* (*C*) Secure the stick proximal to the wound with a piece of cloth. (*D*) Prehospital application of tourniquets to amputated legs.

HARMFUL EFFECTS. Because a tourniquet completely stops blood flow, thereby starving the distal tissues of oxygen, a possible complication from prolonged use of a tourniquet is loss of the extremity. The pressure of the tourniquet is transmitted to the nerves as well. Nerves can tolerate pressure for only a short period of time before permanent damage ensues. Furthermore, the nerves are more susceptible to injury at some sites than they are at others, such as the elbow or knee, where they must surface to cross the joint.

THE RISK/BENEFIT CONSIDERATION. The first and major question to ask before applying a tourniquet is whether it is the only means available to accomplish bleeding control. While the possibility of permanent disability or loss of a limb may be an acceptable risk to take to sustain life, it is important to first try every other measure because the application of a tourniquet does carry with it the real risk of causing tissue and nerve damage and tissue death.

INFECTION CONTROL ISSUES

While controlling external bleeding, the EMT must be aware of universal precautions related to blood and bodily fluids. Because some diseases are transmitted through blood-to-blood contact, simple precautions are used to reduce the chances of disease transmission. These precautions include the use of gloves, goggles, and gowns to prevent the patient's blood from coming in contact with open sores or mucous membranes on the EMT's body. Chapter 12 (medical emergencies) discusses these and other universal precautions in detail.

COMPLICATIONS OF OPEN WOUNDS

Open wounds leave the body vulnerable to the possibility of being invaded by such outside substances as bacteria and foreign bodies.

INFECTION. Any open wound carries with it the possibility of introducing infection from foreign bacteria directly into the tissues below the wound. Infection spreads through the vascular system to other parts of the body. If the bones below an open wound are fractured, bacteria can enter within the bone and cause infections that are difficult to cure. The EMT tries to minimize infection by the use of sterile dressings. When a sterile dressing is not available, bleeding control must be initiated with a clean cloth or even a gloved hand if necessary. If conditions permit, however, a sterile dressing should be used.

AIR EMBOLISM. When large veins are lacerated in the upper chest or neck region, air may be sucked in because pressure is greater in the atmosphere than within the chest cavity during inspiration, a condition known as negative pressure. This air bubble can become lodged within the circulatory system and obstruct distal flow, creating an air embolism. In instances where a large vein laceration is suspected, an occlusive dressing consisting of petroleum jelly gauze, plastic wrap, or aluminum foil should be placed directly over the wound. Tape can be placed over the occlusive material and applied securely on all sides to prevent air from entering the wound. The patient should be positioned with the leg elevated and head down to prevent air from entering the wound (Fig. 5–8*A* and *B*).

INTERNAL BLEEDING

Signs of internal bleeding are obvious when a patient is vomiting blood or has heavy vaginal or rectal bleeding. After injury, bleeding in the subcutaneous tissues is indicated by the appearance of large contusions on the skin that are swollen and ecchymotic (black and blue). Suspect internal bleeding if there is swelling of a limb, such as occurs with a fracture of the femur.

The EMT must also be aware of the possibility of internal bleeding from either the mechanism of injury or

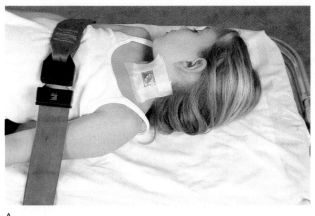
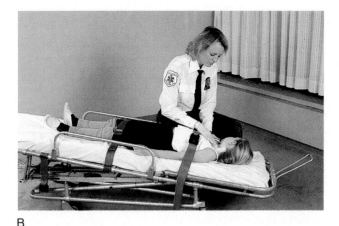

A   B

FIGURE 5–8. (A) Place adhesive plastic wrap or other airtight material over the wound and tape it on all four sides to prevent air from entering the vein. (B) Place the patient in the head down position.

the typical complaints that are associated with diseases causing rapid blood loss.

Major trauma, be it blunt or penetrating, always dictates that signs of bleeding should be searched for closely. Fractures may have large amounts of blood loss, especially fractures of the femur and pelvis. Skull fractures rarely result in significant bleeding, unless there is an open wound or the patient is an infant, in which case the sutures of the bones of the skull are still not joined.

Medical conditions such as ulcers of the stomach and duodenum or a history of an abdominal aneurysm should alert the EMT to consider internal bleeding as the reason for a patient's complaint of weakness. In women of childbearing age, a ruptured ectopic pregnancy should always be considered. Tables 5–7 and 5–8 list conditions and sites, respectively, of internal bleeding.

Regardless of whether bleeding is internal or ex-

ternal, the EMT must be familiar with the early signs of *hypovolemia*, or abnormally decreased blood volume. The body compensates for blood loss so effectively that the initial loss of blood may not be appreciated on first assessment, without a high level of suspicion and a knowledge of the compensatory mechanism. Yet continued bleeding at the same rate might lead to rapid deterioration of the patient's condition.

Compensatory Mechanisms After Blood Loss

The loss of blood results in dynamic changes in the circulatory system as the heart and the vessels attempt to compensate for the diminishing blood volume. Many compensatory mechanisms are available. They are recruited as necessary, in an additive manner, in the face of progressive blood loss. The degree of blood loss determines the type of compensatory mechanisms the body uses to maintain blood flow. In turn, these mechanisms alter the clinical presentation of the patient. The EMT estimates the severity of blood loss from his or her findings on physical assessment and acts according to local protocol.

Because the goal is to recognize and treat significant blood loss as rapidly as possible, the EMT should be familiar with the various presentations likely to be encountered. By learning the signs of early shock, the EMT often can prevent a patient from entering the hypotensive phase by providing appropriate treatment at the scene and rapid transport to the hospital.

TABLE 5–7. Conditions Causing Internal Blood Loss

Traumatic
  Blunt and penetrating injury
Medical
  Gastrointestinal bleeding
    Ulcers
    Hemorrhoids
    Aneurysms
  Ectopic pregnancy
  Vaginal bleeding

TABLE 5–8. Sites of Hidden Blood Loss*

Site	Amount	Percentage of Total Blood Volume
Hemithorax	2 liters	40
Abdomen	≥3 liters	≥50
Femur	≥1 liter	20
Pelvis	0.5 liter/fracture	10/fracture
Skull	Not significant unless infant	

* Calculated for a 70-kg man with a total blood volume of 5 liters. Large amounts of blood may fill various body cavities without external signs.

Stages of Hypovolemic Shock

The body compensates for acute hemorrhage in different ways, depending on the amount of blood loss.

BLOOD LOSS OF 10 TO 15%

The first response to blood loss is constriction of the circular muscle in the venous system. The venous system contains more than half of the total blood volume. Constricting the veins reduces the size of the total vascular space that the remaining blood volume has to fill. Venous return to the heart is unchanged. No other compensatory mechanisms are necessary.

The veins can change the space that the blood has available to occupy to compensate for the loss of 15% of the total blood volume. Thus, there may be no signs and symptoms of blood loss, provided that the total volume lost is less than 15%.

For example, a blood donor may donate 250 to 500 ml of blood over a short period of time. This can amount to 5 to 10% of the total blood volume. The donor usually is encouraged to get up slowly, is given some supplemental fluids, and is told not to exert himself or herself excessively. The donor usually returns to routine daily activities and experiences no adverse symptoms. It would be hard to detect that the donor had just lost a considerable amount of blood volume.

With few or no accompanying signs or symptoms, a blood loss of less than 15% (or the first 700 ml of blood) is the hardest amount to evaluate. Look for blood in the surrounding area from external bleeding, for signs of internal bleeding such as vomiting blood, and for the mechanism of injury, as a patient with up to a 15% loss of blood volume may show no other signs or symptoms.

BLOOD LOSS OF UP TO 30%

When bleeding surpasses 15% of blood volume, constriction of the venous space is insufficient to compensate. This will result in a decrease of venous return to the heart and a smaller stroke volume. Cardiac output begins to fall as a result. The baroreceptors sense an imminent fall in blood pressure, and the nervous system acts to maintain the blood pressure and blood flow to vital organs. This is accomplished through increased discharge of the sympathetic nervous system and release of epinephrine.

The heart rate is increased, and the pumping power of the heart is augmented to make up for the smaller stroke volume in an attempt to return the cardiac output to normal. The arterial vessels constrict to further decrease the size of the vascular space and help maintain the blood pressure. At the same time, there is a redistribution of blood flow. The arterial system severely reduces the flow to the skin, muscles, and digestive system so that the remaining blood is available to perfuse the vital organs.

SIGNS AND SYMPTOMS. The blood pressure is maintained by these compensatory mechanisms within normal ranges. However, signs of epinephrine release are evident. The patient has a rapid and thready pulse and the pulse pressure is narrowed, reflecting the smaller stroke volume. Because of the redistribution of blood away from the skin, the skin is cool, pale, and clammy. The patient is alert (and apprehensive), since blood is sent preferentially to the brain.

The breathing is rapid and shallow. Some of the body's tissues become starved for oxygen because of the redistribution of blood flow. The patient is weak, since the skeletal muscles have less perfusion and little oxygen to sustain contractions. The respiratory system senses *hypoxia*, or reduced oxygen supply to the tissues, and increases its rate to bring in more oxygen and rid the starved tissues of waste products.

If the patient is further stressed by attempting to sit or stand from the lying position, he or she feels weaker and has to lie back down. The heart is unable to maintain the blood pressure any longer against this added force of gravity or may be able to maintain the blood pressure only with a still greater increase in heart rate. Normally the heart rate is about 5 to 10 beats a minute greater when a person stands than when he or she lies down. *Orthostatic change* is the name given to alterations caused by a change from the recumbent to the sitting or standing position, be they signs of weakness, an increase in heart rate, or a fall in blood pressure. A patient is said to have orthostatic changes if, with positional changes, he or she becomes weak or dizzy, the pulse rises by more than 20 beats/min, or the systolic blood pressure falls by more than 20 mm Hg.

Do not test for the presence of orthostatic hypotension if a patient shows other signs of shock. It is an unnecessary challenge and stress to the patient. It is only useful when other signs are less clear.

Capillary refill is a useful test to help gauge blood loss. Place gentle finger pressure on a nail bed, then release it. Normally, when the nail is compressed, blood will be squeezed from the capillaries under the nail and the nail bed becomes pale. When pressure is released, the capillaries immediately refill with blood and a pink color returns. After significant blood loss, the time required for the capillaries to refill with blood increases (Table 5–9). With blood loss under 15%, the capillaries refill immediately or within 2 seconds.

However, after about 20 to 25% blood loss, the

TABLE 5–9. Capillary Refill Test*

Result	Percentage of Total Blood Loss
Normal (capillary return within 2 sec)	Minimal
Delayed (>2 sec)	Moderate
Prolonged, absent	Severe blood loss

* Correlation of capillary refill testing and percentage of blood loss.

capillaries refill more slowly. If the time for refilling is greater than 2 seconds, a person is said to have delayed capillary refill. Two seconds is about the time it takes to say "capillary return." With still greater blood loss, the time for refilling may be prolonged to the point that capillary refill seems absent. Capillary refill may be prolonged without blood loss in patients exposed to cold environments and in some older patients.

You may notice that the neck veins and the superficial veins on the arms are flat, indicating the decrease in blood volume.

The body attempts to pull additional fluid into the capillaries from the interstitial fluid to restore the blood volume. Although this is a slow process, the cells are sensitive to water loss and the patient may be thirsty. Do not allow the patient to drink fluids because of the greater danger of vomiting in the event that surgery under general anesthesia becomes necessary. Instead, to keep the patient comfortable, give him or her a moistened gauze or use glycerine lip moistener.

Do not be misled by a normal blood pressure in the supine position—all the compensatory efforts are working to maintain a sufficient perfusion pressure for the vital organs.

BLOOD LOSS OF 30 TO 45%

With still greater blood loss the compensatory mechanisms are all working to their maximum capacity, but now venous return to the heart has fallen even further. The cardiac output is but half of normal, and blood pressure falls. Hypotension is a relatively late event in blood loss, occurring only after all of the body's compensatory mechanisms are exhausted.

The mental status starts to deteriorate. There may be marked gasping for air. With further blood loss, the next most oxygen-dependent organ, the heart, will start to fail as well. The heart is beating faster and stronger in its attempt to maintain the cardiac output. This increased activity requires an increased supply of oxygen to the heart muscle. Yet now the blood pressure is falling despite the heart's efforts. Since the blood pressure is the driving force for the coronary circulation, the heart itself will begin to suffer from inadequate perfusion and lose its ability to continue both rapid and powerful contractions. In fact, the heart rate may start to fall as shock progresses.

Whereas the patient was suffering earlier from hypovolemic shock, the ability of the body to compensate has now been severely hampered by the development of cardiogenic shock as well. The bleeding has progressed to the point where hypovolemic shock has induced cardiogenic shock, and the patient is in great jeopardy.

The patient still has more than half of his or her normal hemoglobin. It is the sudden loss of volume that is critical in acute hemorrhage.

TABLE 5–10. Correlation of Signs and Symptoms with Degree of Blood Loss

Percentage of Blood Loss as Percentage of Total Blood Volume	Compensatory Effect	Signs and Symptoms
<15%	Veins contract	None or transient
<30%	Veins contract, plus epinephrine response; arteries constrict to maintain BP and reduce flow to skin, gut, and muscle	Rapid and thready pulse; cool, pale, clammy skin; nausea; thirst; weakness; anxiety; orthostatic changes; flat neck veins
	Increased heart rate	Delayed capillary refill
		BP may be "normal"
<45%	All of the above, plus decompensation, cardiac output <50% of normal	Hypotension; deteriorated mental status; rapid, shallow, "air-hungry" respirations

After Trunkey DP, Sheldon GF, Collins JA: The treatment of shock. In Zuidema GD, et al (eds): The Management of Trauma, 4th ed. Philadelphia, WB Saunders, 1985.

BLOOD LOSS OF GREATER THAN 45%

With still greater blood loss, circulatory collapse follows. The constriction of the venous and arterial vessels, which have reduced the size of the vascular space, requires muscular contraction. This contraction itself is dependent on oxygen consumption. As the patient becomes hypotensive, the constricting muscles in the vascular tree are less perfused. These muscles become exhausted and the vessels begin to dilate, causing an increase in the size of the vascular space. With loss of this valuable compensatory mechanism, a precipitous fall in blood pressure results in total circulatory collapse and then cardiac arrest. The patient must receive hospital intervention in minutes or death is certain. Table 5–10 summarizes the signs and symptoms in relation to the percentage of blood loss.

Relationship of Blood Pressure and Cardiac Output in Hemorrhage

Because of the compensatory mechanisms, the blood pressure does not fall as fast as the cardiac output.

While blood pressure measurement is a valuable tool in evaluating blood loss, remember that it may still be in a normal range even though the cardiac output is significantly diminished. Look at Table 5–10, which relates signs and symptoms and blood pressure to acute blood loss. Notice that changes in blood pressure are a late event. It is also important to note that whereas for the first 15% of blood loss there is little change in the blood pressure or cardiac output, after about 25% of blood loss, small amounts of continued bleeding will result in a rapid fall in both of these.

Treatment Modalities

After attention to airway, breathing, and bleeding control, initiate treatment for shock.

MAST

Military antishock trousers (MAST)—also called the pneumatic antishock garment (PASG)—save the lives of many patients with hypovolemic shock. The MAST found their first widespread application on battlefields, where they prolonged the lives of wounded soldiers until they could be transported to operating areas. Since then MAST have been used to treat many civilians who have suffered shock from hemorrhage and other conditions causing inadequate venous return.

MAST are basic life support devices in most areas. The National Department of Transportation Curriculum includes training in the use of MAST for all EMTs. They must be used in accordance with conditions specified by local medical control officers, and local protocols must be followed.

EFFECTS OF MAST. MAST are air-filled pants that surround the legs and the abdomen. They may come with or without gauges that show the inflation pressure (see Fig. 5–9A and B). The leg and abdominal sections (bladders) can be inflated to pressures up to 100 mm Hg. By their application and inflation, the bladders transmit their inflated pressure circumferentially to structures within the legs and abdomen. This transmitted pressure has the following effects:

- Collapses the blood vessels that have pressures lower than the MAST pressure. This reduces the effective vascular volume and increases the peripheral vascular resistance. The low-pressure veins are collapsed first. The arteries may be collapsed as well if the MAST pressure exceeds the arterial pressure.
- Shunts blood from the collapsed vessels to the heart and vital organs. The MAST increase the central

blood volume and therefore increase venous return to the heart.
- Tamponades bleeding in the legs, the pelvis, and the abdomen. MAST control bleeding both by direct pressure and by limiting blood flow under the inflated areas.
- Splints fractures in the legs and pelvis. When inflated the MAST effectively immobilize the lower extremities, and the abdominal section can be inflated to offer support to a broken pelvis.

The effects of MAST can be remarkable. A patient with a blood pressure of 50 by palpation may have a blood pressure of 100/70 once the MAST is inflated. How the MAST works has been an area of speculation and research for several years. There has been much controversy over just which effect is greater, the shunting of blood from the lower body into the central circulation or the increase in peripheral vascular resistance from the decreased effective vascular space. It appears that the amount of blood that is shunted, or autotransfused, may not be as great as was originally thought. One study showed that less than 5% of the blood volume was transferred from the legs and abdomen to the central circulation via MAST inflation (Bivins HG, et al: Blood volume displacement with inflation of antishock trousers. Ann Emerg Med 11[8]:409, August 1982).

If only small amounts of blood are actually autotransfused with the MAST, can it be expected that such profound improvements in the patient's blood pressure and clinical status can be realized from an increase in peripheral vascular resistance (PVR)? Another study has shown a 48% increase in PVR following MAST application (Gaffney FA, et al: Hemodynamic effects of medical anti-shock trousers (MAST garment). J Trauma 21[11]:931, November 1981).

The following analogy illustrates how increased PVR can affect pressure and flow. Imagine a garden hose that is laid straight across a lawn and that has been perforated with a small pin every 6 inches for sprinkling the grass. The nozzle at the end of the hose is twisted shut so that the water pressure drives water out through the pin holes only. After the water is turned on, one observes that the water rises in small streams through the pinholes to a height of 2 feet. Imagine that we take a clamp and completely close off the hose at a point halfway to the nozzle. Without changing the amount of water flowing from the faucet, we have decreased the space that it can fill. The pressure in the hose increases, and the streams emanating from the remaining holes now rise 4 feet in height.

MAST decrease the vascular space in a similar manner. The pressure in the remaining vascular space must rise, improving perfusion to vital organs.

PROCEDURE 5-2   APPLYING THE MAST

1. Examine the patient's abdomen and legs to determine the extent of injuries; once the MAST are applied these areas will not be accessible.
2. Remove the patient's trousers, socks, and other clothing if possible. If impossible, bulky objects such as a wallet, belt buckle, or keys should be removed. If folds of clothing or hard objects are left between the MAST and the skin, they may cause some local skin necrosis if the MAST are left on for a long time.
3. Lay the MAST open on the stretcher and lay the patient on the garment using a log roll procedure

(Fig. 5-9C). The top of the abdominal section of the MAST should lie below the lowest rib (Fig. 5-9D).

Note: An alternate method for applying the trousers is to slide the open garment beneath the patient (Fig. 5-9E). Another method is to place your arms through the legs of the loosely assembled garment, then grab the ankles as your partner slides them up over the patient, as you would a pair of trousers (Fig. 5-9F).

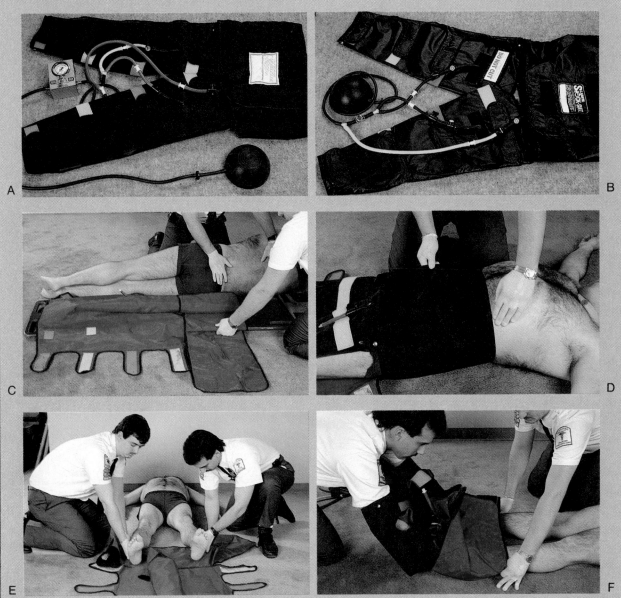

FIGURE 5-9. (*A*) MAST with a pressure gauge. (*B*) MAST without a pressure gauge. (*C*) Log roll the patient and slide the MAST beneath the patient. (*D*) Roll the patient onto the trousers and check to see that the upper margin does not cover the chest cavity. (*E*) Slide the MAST beneath the patient. (*F*) Place your arms through the legs of the trousers and have your partner slide them up the patient's extremities.

Continued

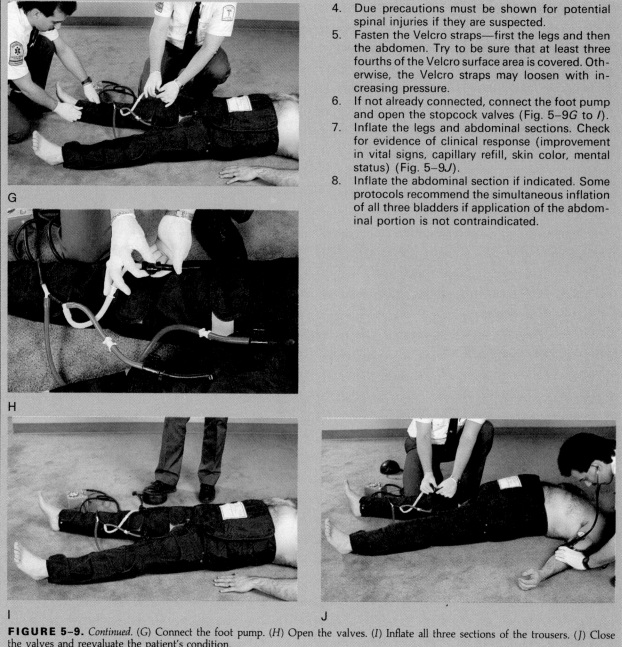

4. Due precautions must be shown for potential spinal injuries if they are suspected.
5. Fasten the Velcro straps—first the legs and then the abdomen. Try to be sure that at least three fourths of the Velcro surface area is covered. Otherwise, the Velcro straps may loosen with increasing pressure.
6. If not already connected, connect the foot pump and open the stopcock valves (Fig. 5–9G to I).
7. Inflate the legs and abdominal sections. Check for evidence of clinical response (improvement in vital signs, capillary refill, skin color, mental status) (Fig. 5–9J).
8. Inflate the abdominal section if indicated. Some protocols recommend the simultaneous inflation of all three bladders if application of the abdominal portion is not contraindicated.

FIGURE 5–9. *Continued.* (G) Connect the foot pump. (H) Open the valves. (I) Inflate all three sections of the trousers. (J) Close the valves and reevaluate the patient's condition.

REMOVAL OF THE MAST. Never deflate the MAST in the field unless instructed to do so by a physician. Sudden deflation without restoration of the circulating blood volume will result in a sudden drop in blood pressure. Usually, the MAST should be deflated only when intravenous fluids have restored an effective circulating volume. The device is deflated in stages, starting with the abdominal section first, with careful monitoring of vital signs. Some patients do not have the MAST removed until they are in the operating room.

If MAST are applied during resuscitation for cardiopulmonary arrest, they should not be removed until evidence of effective spontaneous circulation is present.

INDICATIONS. MAST are indicated for shock secondary to decreased venous return, including hypovolemic and vasodilatory shock. By decreasing the effective size of the vascular space beneath the MAST, blood pressure within the vessels above the MAST is raised. By improving blood pressure above the MAST, it is often easier to start an intravenous line to administer fluids. They are also indicated to control bleeding (internal and external) in the legs, pelvis, and abdomen. Finally, they are useful for splinting fractures in the legs and pelvis, especially if these are associated with significant bleeding.

MAST also may be useful for increasing blood flow

to the vital organs during CPR in cardiac arrest. In cardiac arrest the abdominal segment is not inflated in some emergency systems because of possible interference with ventilations (the diaphragms are pushed up), unless the patient is intubated.

Again, local protocols must be followed. Often the protocols specify both the conditions and the parameters that indicate local use of MAST.

CONTRAINDICATIONS. Because MAST increase the peripheral vascular resistance and shunt blood from the lower body into the central circulation, they can make some conditions worse. Shock from pump failure (cardiogenic shock) is considered a contraindication because the failing heart may not be able to handle additional blood volume or pump against an increased resistance. Cardiogenic shock commonly presents with pulmonary edema and hypotension. By increasing venous return, the MAST may worsen the pulmonary edema and thereby further limit the diffusion of oxygen into the blood. Thus, *the absolute contraindication to MAST is pulmonary edema.*

Other conditions might also contraindicate the use of the abdominal section of the MAST, such as late pregnancy or exposed abdominal organs. In these conditions, direct pressure from the MAST might compromise the viability of the fetus or the exposed bowel. However, local protocols might permit use of MAST in these situations if the patient's life would be lost otherwise. In such a situation the adverse effects of the MAST are a relative contraindication, because the beneficial result (saving the patient's life) outweighs them. These decisions are made by the medical control physicians and are not to be made independently by the EMT. Always be aware of the indications and contraindications for MAST according to your local protocols (Table 5–11).

CONTROVERSY. Recent studies have shown no difference in patient outcome for MAST-treated patients versus patients not treated with MAST in an urban trauma system where most victims had penetrating trauma.*

Controversy also exists regarding application of MAST in patients with severe head trauma (and increased intracranial pressure) or thoracic trauma (tension pneumothorax, cardiac tamponade, and rupture of the diaphragm). Always follow local protocols.

OXYGEN

Supplemental oxygen should be given in high concentration to patients in shock to ensure that the

---

TABLE 5–11. Contraindications to MAST Application

Pulmonary edema
Cardiogenic shock
Do not inflate the abdominal section in the event of:
    Pregnancy
    Evisceration of abdominal organs
    Impaled object in abdomen
Controversial conditions
    Severe head trauma
    Severe chest trauma with:
        Tension pneumothorax
        Cardiac tamponade
        Intrathoracic injuries

---

circulating hemoglobin is completely saturated with oxygen.

TEMPERATURE REGULATION— PREVENTION OF FURTHER HEAT LOSS

The EMT should maintain the patient's body temperature with blankets. The patient in shock will have trouble regulating his or her body temperature and cannot afford additional heat loss. When environmental temperatures exceed body temperature, the patient should be left uncovered.

POSITIONING FOR TRANSPORT

Patients with hypovolemia are suffering from decreased venous return to the heart. Therefore, transporting the patient in a supine position with the legs elevated and head down to maximize venous return is appropriate, provided that the airway and breathing are adequate or can be treated effectively in this position. Trauma patients on a long spine board may have the foot of the board elevated to accomplish this.

DECISION TO TRANSPORT

Many victims of hypovolemic shock can be resuscitated if they receive timely treatment. They are often referred to trauma centers because definitive care for many of these victims can be given only in the operating room. The ultimate therapy for a patient with hypovolemic shock is outside the bounds of the prehospital sphere.

As discussed earlier, a goal of EMS systems is to bring patients to definitive therapy as expeditiously as possible. The transport decision, or the point during the prehospital assessment when transport should begin, is one of the most important decisions that is made by the EMT.

The only acceptable delays at the scene are for therapeutic maneuvers necessary to maintain the viability of the patient en route. The EMT must consider the risks and benefits of time spent on the scene. Treatment ren-

---

* Mattox KL, Bickell W, Pepe PE, et al.: Prospective MAST Study in 911 Patients. J Trauma 29(8):1104–1112, 1989.

dered during the primary survey is mandatory. Certain aspects of the secondary survey and subsequent treatments may be best rendered while en route to the hospital, particularly if the patient is in critical condition.

Pulseless Patients

Patients in cardiopulmonary arrest from trauma are so rarely resuscitated by measures employed in the field that most EMS systems advocate a rapid transport policy for these patients. Such a policy recognizes that for pulseless patients, the only chance for survival may be rapid surgical intervention and blood and fluid therapy in an emergency department and operating room. Check with your local protocols about the procedures to be followed for traumatic cardiopulmonary arrest. These will usually include cardiopulmonary resuscitation and rapid transport.

Other Considerations

Many factors influence the field treatment of patients in shock. Some of these include the transport time to the hospital, the capabilities of the prehospital personnel, and the definitive treatment for the condition encountered.

TIME TO THE HOSPITAL

To take the extreme example, consider a patient struck by a car on a street one block from the hospital. He has suffered a possible ruptured spleen with no other apparent injuries and has signs of hypovolemic shock. His blood pressure is 80/50, and your partner asks whether you should apply the MAST. Because you are literally 20 seconds from the hospital, you decide not to apply them because from experience you know they will delay delivery of the patient by an additional few minutes. During the minutes you have saved, hospital staff not only were able to apply and inflate the MAST, but also have sent blood for cross matching, have begun transfusions of intravenous fluids, and have begun to ready the operating room for the patient's arrival.

If this same patient was encountered 30 minutes from the hospital, you would elect to apply the MAST and inflate them as soon as possible (perhaps en route), in light of the longer transport time.

CAPABILITIES OF PREHOSPITAL PERSONNEL

Besides the level of training of the EMTs on the scene, the number of trained personnel on the scene also can be a factor in deciding how much therapy can be rendered in the field without delaying transport. Consider a patient in hypovolemic shock from multiple trauma with apparent fractures of both femurs and one wrist and a blood pressure of 80/50. If two EMTs are the only available prehospital personnel, after attending to the ABCs they may elect to apply MAST (which will also help immobilize lower extremity fractures) and splint the upper extremity fracture en route to the hospital. They realize that a patient in the hypotensive phase of hypovolemic shock will soon have circulatory collapse if internal bleeding continues.

If four EMTs are on the scene, however, there may be sufficient personnel to apply MAST and splint the wrist at the scene without delay in transport.

DEFINITIVE TREATMENT

Some appreciation for the definitive treatment of life-threatening injuries can help the EMT appreciate the benefits of prehospital versus hospital care for the patients he or she is treating. For example, consider two victims of hemorrhage. One victim has suffered a laceration of the radial artery and the bleeding can be controlled with direct pressure. The other patient has been stabbed in the abdomen. Both patients have the same amount of blood loss and the same vital signs.

Control of bleeding can be accomplished for the first patient with field treatment. The patient with the abdominal wound may need surgery to control the bleeding. Both patients have a blood pressure of 100/80, with a pulse of 120, and signs of epinephrine release. Consider which patient is more likely to deteriorate further (from continued bleeding) and to become hypotensive, and for which patient the early delivery to a hospital is more important for survival.

Other conditions in which the role of early hospital treatment should be clear are tension pneumothorax and pericardial tamponade. Both of these conditions require rapid hospital treatment, which may dramatically reverse the shock state.

PROTOCOLS

The above considerations of time, capabilities of personnel, and type of treatment needed are examples of the kind of information that medical control officers use when formulating medical protocols. The ultimate goal is to render the best possible care to the patient by weighing the benefits to be gained from treatments in the field within the scope of the total needs of the patient. By appreciating the respective roles of both prehospital and hospital therapy, the EMT will be better able to recognize the point at which transport to the hospital is to begin. Because protocols are always influenced by factors that may vary from one system to another, the EMT must study the local protocols and understand the reasons for the steps in care (see Protocol: Shock).

P R O T O C O L

SHOCK

> ### NOTE!
>
> FOR THE PURPOSE OF THIS PROTOCOL, ADULT SHOCK IS DEFINED AS:
> 1. SYSTOLIC BLOOD PRESSURE OF 90 MM HG OR LESS
> 2. SYSTOLIC BLOOD PRESSURE ABOVE 90 MM HG AND SIGNS OF INADEQUATE PERFUSION, SUCH AS:
>   A. ALTERED MENTAL STATE (RESTLESSNESS, INATTENTION, CONFUSION, AGITATION)
>   B. TACHYCARDIA (PULSE GREATER THAN 100)
>   C. DELAYED CAPILLARY REFILL (GREATER THAN 2 SECONDS)
>   D. PALLOR
>   E. COLD, CLAMMY SKIN

> ### NOTE!
>
> FOR THE PURPOSE OF THIS PROTOCOL, PEDIATRIC SHOCK IS DEFINED AS SIGNS OF INADEQUATE PERFUSION SUCH AS:
> 1. ALTERED MENTAL STATE (RESTLESSNESS, INATTENTION, CONFUSION, AGITATION)
> 2. TACHYCARDIA
> 3. WEAK OR ABSENT DISTAL PULSES
> 4. CAPILLARY REFILL GREATER THAN TWO SECONDS
> 5. PALLOR
> 6. COLD, CLAMMY, OR MOTTLED SKIN
>
> THIS PROTOCOL SHOULD BE USED EVEN IF THE SYSTOLIC BLOOD PRESSURE IS NORMAL OR IS DIFFICULT TO OBTAIN.
>
> A LOW SYSTOLIC BLOOD PRESSURE MEANS THAT THE SHOCK IS SEVERE.

IF A CARDIAC CAUSE FOR SHOCK IS SUSPECTED, REFER IMMEDIATELY TO THE CARDIAC RELATED PROTOCOL!

1. Ensure that the patient's airway is open and that breathing and circulation are adequate.

> ### CAUTION!
>
> MANUALLY STABILIZE THE HEAD AND CERVICAL SPINE IF TRAUMA OF THE HEAD AND NECK IS SUSPECTED!

2. Administer high-concentration oxygen, and BE PREPARED TO VENTILATE THE PATIENT!

3. Place the patient in a face-up position.
   AND
   Elevate the patient's legs 30 degrees.

   In adults, if available, apply MAST. IF THE SYSTOLIC BLOOD PRESSURE IS BELOW 90 MM HG AND SIGNS OF INADEQUATE PERFUSION ARE PRESENT, inflate all three compartments to the maximum pressure (about 100 mm Hg) *OR* until the pop-off valves of all three compartments pop open.

   In children, if available, apply and inflate appropriate size MAST according to criteria for inflation. Inflate the leg compartments until the pop-off valves pop open.

   DO NOT DELAY PATIENT TRANSPORT TO APPLY AND INFLATE MAST!

> ### CAUTION!
>
> IF THE PATIENT HAS PULMONARY EDEMA, DO NOT INFLATE MAST!
>
> IF THE PATIENT HAS AN EVISCERATION OR AN IMPALED OBJECT IN THE ABDOMEN OR LEGS, INFLATE ONLY THE MAST COMPARTMENTS NOT OVERLYING THE EVISCERATION OR IMPALED OBJECT!
>
> IF THE PATIENT IS KNOWN TO BE PREGNANT, INFLATE ONLY THE MAST LEG COMPARTMENTS!

5. Obtain and record the vital signs, and repeat en route as often as the situation indicates.

6. Transport, keeping the patient warm.

7. Record all patient care information, including the patient's medical history and all treatment provided, on a Prehospital Care Report.

> ### NOTE!
>
> ONCE INFLATED, MAST MUST NOT BE DEFLATED IN THE FIELD WITHOUT PHYSICIAN DIRECTION!

Adapted from Manual for Emergency Medical Technicians. Emergency Medical Services Program. Albany, New York State Department of Health, 1990.

ARTERIOSCLEROTIC HEART DISEASE

Introduction

The leading cause of death in the United States is arteriosclerotic heart disease and its resulting complications. These complications include myocardial infarction, dysrhythmias, and sudden death. There are an estimated 1.5 million heart attacks, or myocardial infarctions (MIs), each year in the United States. Of this number, 500,000 victims die as a result. More than half of the deaths occur before the patient reaches a hospital. Because most of the deaths occur within the first two hours after the onset of symptoms, the public has been educated to call for help. The EMT must have a good understanding of the signs and symptoms, the treatment, and the complications arising from this disease.

ARTERIOSCLEROSIS

Like any other body tissue, the heart must have a continuous supply of oxygen. Arteriosclerosis is a progressive disease of the arteries that results in narrowing of the lumen due to deposits of fat and hardening of the arterial wall. Coronary artery disease begins when fatty deposits accumulate in the walls of the coronary arteries. As more and more of these deposits accumulate, the artery narrows, and less blood can flow through. The process is called arteriosclerosis and is known familiarly as "hardening of the arteries."

The accumulation of fatty deposits in arteriosclerosis takes many years. During the early stages of the disease, there may be no symptoms. A person is completely unaware of what is taking place in his or her body. As the arteries continue to narrow, however, less blood can pass through (Fig. 5–10).

The first indication of coronary artery disease may occur under conditions of physical or emotional stress. At such times the heart beats faster and the heart muscle needs more oxygen than the coronary arteries can deliver. Pain and discomfort in the chest develop when there is not enough oxygen delivered to the heart. This

type of coronary artery disease, which results from exertion or stress and is relieved by rest, is called *angina pectoris.*

RISK FACTORS OF HEART DISEASE.   The risk factors for coronary artery disease may be divided into two categories (Table 5–12). The first group consists of factors that are controllable or avoidable. Included in this group are unhealthy eating patterns, high blood pressure, cigarette smoking, and a physically inactive life style. As the name implies, all of these controllable risk factors have one thing in common: they can be changed to make it less likely for a heart attack to occur.

There is much evidence that smoking is a major risk factor. Cigarette smokers are much more likely to experience a heart attack than are nonsmokers, and the risk increases according to the number of cigarettes smoked. When smoking stops, that particular risk is eliminated.

People who have untreated high blood pressure also are at high risk for heart disease. With medication, however, high blood pressure can be lowered to normal levels and the risk of heart disease reduced.

Additional evidence suggests that the risk of heart attack is increased for people with high blood cholesterol levels. The presence of high blood cholesterol levels and of high blood pressure can be determined only by medical examinations. Reducing the amount of saturated fats and cholesterol in the diet may often correct the high cho-

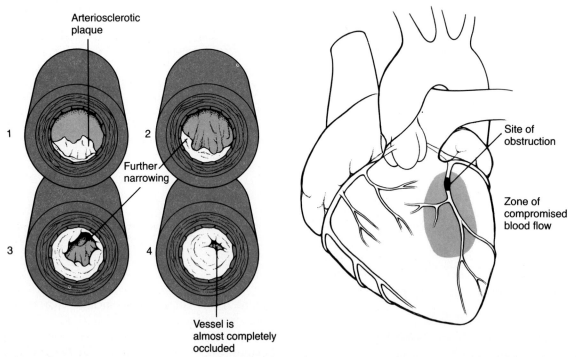

FIGURE 5–10. Progression of arteriosclerosis. An arteriosclerotic plaque forms on the intima of the vessel and projects into the lumen. As the plaque enlarges it provides a rough surface that can lead to the formation of a thrombus that further narrows the vessel lumen. Eventually the opening is too narrow to supply the heart's oxygen needs, and the surrounding tissue becomes ischemic or dies. (After American Heart Association: Health Provider's Manual for Basic Life Support. Dallas, American Heart Association, 1990, p. 17.)

T ABLE 5–12. Risk Factors for Heart Disease

Avoidable	Unavoidable
Smoking*	Age
High blood cholesterol*	Sex
High blood pressure*	Heredity
Obesity	Diabetes (can be treated)
Physically inactive life style	
Diet	

Major risk factors.

lesterol level in the blood and reduce the risk of heart attack.

Diet and eating habits in general may contribute to risk factors that can be avoided. Not only the choice of foods but also the quantity eaten is important. Overconsumption of calories without regular physical activity can lead to obesity and increased risk for cardiac disease. Regular exercise increases the ability of the heart to work efficiently.

The risk factors in the second major category are unavoidable and beyond an individual's control. These include a family history of heart disease (heredity), age, and sex.

Heart attacks become more frequent with increasing age. In fact, the death rate doubles every 10 years beyond the age of 30. Because of chemical differences that exist between men and women, men under age 60 are more likely to have a heart attack. However, women tend to catch up with men after the age of 60.

PRUDENT LIVING FOR A HEALTHY HEART. Clearly not everyone who smokes, or who has hypertension, or reaches the age of 60 will have a heart attack. Most people do not have heart attacks. The chance of having a heart attack at some time in life, however, does increase as the number of existing risk factors increases. A way to reduce the possibility of a heart attack is to reduce or eliminate as many avoidable risk factors as possible. Such prudent living, to be effective, must start at an early age.

MYOCARDIAL OXYGEN SUPPLY AND DEMAND

Ordinarily, oxygen delivered by blood flow through the coronary arteries matches the need of the heart muscle. A mismatch occurs when an increase in the heart's work is not met with a corresponding increase in blood supply. For example, if a person has narrowed coronary arteries, she may not receive adequate blood flow to the heart muscle to meet the increased oxygen needs during stress or exercise. A mismatch also can occur when the heart's ordinary needs at rest are not met because of a blockage of blood flow through the coronary arteries. A thrombus can form in a coronary artery and severely limit or obstruct blood flow to part of the heart. Then, even at rest, not enough oxygen is delivered to meet the needs of the myocardial tissue.

MYOCARDIAL ISCHEMIA AND INFARCTION

Ischemia refers to a state of decreased blood flow to an organ or tissue. *Infarction* refers to a more severe obstruction resulting in necrosis or death of heart cells. Myocardial ischemia occurs when there is not enough blood flow to satisfy the oxygen needs of the myocardium. *Angina* or *angina pectoris* is the name given to myocardial ischemia causing pain but no permanent damage. *Myocardial infarction* is the term given to severe and sustained oxygen deprivation of the myocardium that results in the death of heart cells.

ISCHEMIC CHEST PAIN

The chief complaint most common to diseases of the coronary arteries is chest pain. The term used to describe the characteristic pain resulting from inadequate blood supply to the myocardium is *ischemic chest pain*. The classic description of ischemic chest pain that follows was given in 1772 by William Heberden:

> But there is a disorder of the breast marked with strong and peculiar symptoms, considerable for the kind of danger belonging to it, and not extremely rare, which deserves to be mentioned at more length. The seat of it, and sense of strangling, and anxiety with which it is attended, may make it not improperly be called angina pectoris.
>
> They who are afflicted with it, are seized while they are walking (more especially if uphill, and soon after eating) with a painful and most disagreeable sensation in the breast, which seems as if it would extinguish life, if it were to increase or to continue; but the moment they stand still, all this uneasiness vanishes. (Heberden, William: Commentaries on the History and Cure of Diseases. London, L. Payne, News-Gate, 1802.)

Although Heberden did not connect this disease with the coronary arteries, he gave a description of the characteristics of angina pectoris that many believe is among the best descriptions ever given of this disease. The chest pain of both angina pectoris and myocardial infarction results from oxygen deprivation to heart tissue. The difference between the two types of pain is in the degree of severity and consequences. Individual patients give varying descriptions, but the sense of seriousness so well conveyed in Heberden's account is present in most cases.

Because the consequences of ischemic heart disease include severe pump failure, life-threatening heart rhythms (dysrhythmias), and sudden death, patients with complaints of ischemic chest pain are treated with the highest priority.

Myocardial Infarction

To medical personnel, myocardial infarction denotes a life-threatening condition. The patient with a myocardial infarction is at the greatest risk of fatal complications in the first hours after the onset of chest pain, and over half of those who die do so before reaching the hospital. The prevalence of this disease, its potential to cause sudden death, and the need for rapid treatment underscore the reason for an organized EMS system in the community.

PATHOPHYSIOLOGY

Usually, myocardial infarction is due to arteriosclerosis and its complications, namely, narrowing of the coronary arteries and thrombosis. It may also be caused by a vasoconstriction or spasm of the coronary vessels.

CHIEF COMPLAINT

Patients usually complain of intense, continuous chest pain described as crushing, pressing, tight, viselike, heavy, aching, or constricting. Other terms used to describe it include "burning" or "discomfort" in the chest. The pain is usually localized in the anterior chest and radiates to the neck, jaw, either arm or shoulder (more commonly the left), or rarely to the back. At times, the pain occurs primarily in areas of radiation such as the arm or jaw (Fig. 5–11). Classically, patients may describe the pain while placing a clenched fist across the chest. The pain usually lasts for several minutes, often more than 30, and is not relieved with rest or nitroglycerin (a drug used to treat patients with angina).

In a small percentage of patients, pain may not be the chief complaint. Usually, these patients are elderly, have diabetes, and complain about shortness of breath, weakness, or an altered mental state. Patients often have nausea and vomiting; they may also describe the pain as that caused by indigestion.

HISTORY OF THE PRESENT ILLNESS

A myocardial infarction can occur as a result of emotional or physical stress. It also can occur while a patient is at rest or wake a patient from sleep. Associated complaints include nausea, vomiting, weakness, shortness of breath, palpitations, lightheadedness, sweating, dizziness, and loss of consciousness.

MEDICAL HISTORY

Upon questioning, the patient may be found to have risk factors for heart disease. The patient may have a history of angina, prior myocardial infarctions, other

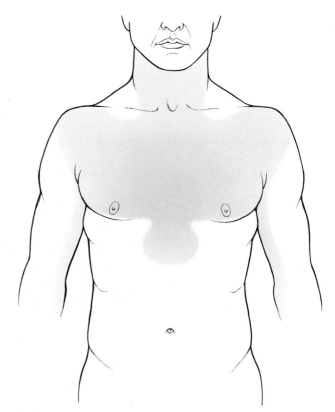

FIGURE 5–11. Possible pain patterns in myocardial infarction.

heart disease, diabetes, or hypertension. The medication history might reveal cardiac or hypertensive drug therapy. Myocardial infarctions often recur. If a patient has had a previous myocardial infarction or a history of angina, inquire if the present symptoms are similar to those experienced in the past.

PHYSICAL ASSESSMENT

The patient may be apprehensive, anxious, or fearful. Conversely, the patient may deny that the symptoms he or she is experiencing are serious. If the mental status is altered and the patient is lethargic, drowsy, or cannot be aroused, it may be an indication of low cardiac output from associated heart failure or dysrhythmias.

A range of vital signs may be encountered. The range can be attributable to associated preexisting medical conditions such as hypertension, the patient's psychologic response to the chest pain, the location of the infarction, and epinephrine release. Rapid and slow pulses are common, as are variations in the blood pressure. Some patients present with normal vital signs.

The skin may appear pale and feel cool and sweaty. The lungs should be auscultated for the presence of rales or wheezing. The patient should be closely monitored en route to the hospital for changes in mental state or vital signs.

DIAGNOSIS

The diagnosis of myocardial infarction in the prehospital setting rests primarily with the history. Although the symptoms will vary, any patient who has ischemic chest pain should be treated for myocardial infarction until proved otherwise.

In the absence of chest pain, the diagnosis may be suspected on the basis of any of the other signs or symptoms of myocardial infarction that have been discussed. Again, these include pale, cool, or sweaty skin; dizziness; altered mental status; and a *sudden* feeling of weakness, numbness, tingling, or pain in the jaw or arm.

TREATMENT

The main objective when treating a patient with myocardial infarction is based on the supply and demand concept of myocardial blood flow. Basically, seek to reduce heart work and enhance oxygen delivery. Each step in the treatment plan has its own defined objectives and indications. Through an understanding of the therapeutic objectives, you will know when to use them and be able to follow the patient's response to therapy.

As always, the first consideration is the ABCs of the primary survey. The following treatment is for uncomplicated myocardial infarction (MI):

1. Reduce anxiety and activity.
2. Provide supplemental oxygen (4 to 6 liters/min cannula [COPD 24% Venturi or 2 liters/min cannula]).
3. Carry the patient to the ambulance.
4. Prioritize transport.
5. Transport the patient in position of comfort.
6. Monitor the patient's vital signs and condition en route.
7. Use sirens only if necessary.

DECREASING BODY OXYGEN REQUIREMENTS. Reduce the oxygen need by limiting anxiety and any unnecessary activity. Psychologic stress and fear can cause release of epinephrine. Part of the effects of epinephrine are to increase the heart rate and the force of the heart's contractions. Both of these effects increase myocardial oxygen needs.

Always act in a professional manner. Be calm and reassuring; show that you care. Let the patient be aware that treatment has begun. Act efficiently and quickly to address the patient's problems without displaying your own emotions.

During care of the cardiac patient, you may have to deal with denial. To deny that one's life may be in jeopardy is a common human response. It has led many victims of heart attacks to delay seeking medical care

and helps account for the high number of deaths that occur outside the hospital. Many times you find that a patient's relative or a bystander has made the call for help. The patient may feel "better" and deny previous complaints. Dealing with denial is a real skill. You might ask the patient to describe the complaints in more detail. If you think that the patient has experienced ischemic chest pain, an honest response is to tell the patient that you cannot be sure whether he or she has a heart problem, and inform the patient that the greatest risk lies in the next 2 hours. Advise him or her to accompany you to the hospital for evaluation. Patients with compromised respiratory or circulatory systems are carried to the ambulance in a position most appropriate for their condition. Patients who are alert or experiencing shortness of breath should be placed in a position of comfort (usually the sitting position). Patients who are in shock or who are exhibiting signs of poor circulation and oxygenation to the brain, such as alterations of mental status, should be placed in the supine or coma position (left lateral recumbent).

SUPPLEMENTAL OXYGEN. In patients with suspected ischemic chest pain who have no evidence of altered mental status, hypoxia, or shock, the American Heart Association recommends 4 to 6 liters of oxygen delivered by nasal cannula or face mask. If the patient has chronic obstructive pulmonary disease (COPD), use the Venturi mask to deliver 24% oxygen or use a nasal cannula with 2-liter flow. If the patient has evidence of hypoxia (e.g., cyanosis, altered mental status) or dyspnea, give a high concentration of oxygen. The concentration for the COPD victim may be increased slowly, watching for relief of pain and signs of hypoventilation. If evidence of hypoventilation develops, it may be necessary to institute positive-pressure breathing.

MONITORING EN ROUTE. The MI patient is subject to a variety of complications. The patient should be continually reevaluated while en route to the hospital. Check vital signs and monitor the mental status and the response to therapy. Check for continuation of pain and dyspnea, and monitor the rhythm and quality of the pulse. To avoid delay in the event of a sudden cardiac arrest, the monitor–defibrillator, and mechanical aids for CPR (bag-valve mask, suction, and backboard) should be readily available. In some systems, patients with chest pain are monitored en route. This allows for the earliest detection of ventricular fibrillation and the timely application of electric shock therapy.

TRANSPORTATION. Transportation should be rapid but quiet. Avoid the use of sirens whenever possible. The hospital should be notified of the imminent arrival of all unstable patients to allow for adequate preparation.

Angina

Ischemic heart disease is a progressive disease. It ranges from the angina patient with ischemia to the myocardial infarction patient who suffers irreversible damage to part of the heart. Because many patients you encounter will have angina, you should be familiar with this condition.

Angina is a name given to ischemic chest pain, which is usually caused by exertion or stress and relieved by rest. It results from a *temporary* inadequacy of blood flow to the myocardium. The definition of angina stresses the word *temporary.* For a brief time, usually 1 to 5 minutes, and almost always less than 10 minutes, the patient experiences chest pain because the blood supply to the heart cannot meet the heart's oxygen needs. When the patient rests, the heart works less and needs less oxygen, so the pain goes away. In addition to exertion, emotional stress, exposure to cold, and heavy meals also may trigger anginal pain.

NITROGLYCERIN

Patients can live with angina for a long time. They learn to limit their activity so that they have fewer attacks. They take nitroglycerin to help relieve anginal pain when it occurs. Nitroglycerin is usually taken in the form of a pill that is placed under the tongue, where it is rapidly absorbed (Fig. 5–12). It works, along with rest, to reduce the work of the heart. It helps dilate the coronary arteries to improve blood flow to the affected area. Also, nitroglycerin dilates the larger veins, allowing more blood to pool in the dependent areas of the body.

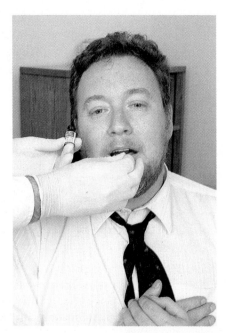

FIGURE 5–12. Nitroglycerin is administered beneath the patient's tongue.

This results in less venous blood returning to the heart, decreased cardiac output, and decreased heart work. With less work, less oxygen is required and the blood supply to the heart becomes adequate to meet the heart's oxygen demands. Because it dilates the vessels in the head as well, patients often complain of headaches (especially throbbing pain) after they take nitroglycerin. Patients learn to sit or sometimes lie down when they place a nitroglycerin tablet under the tongue because of the venous pooling effect. They may feel lightheaded if they continue to stand. Many patients have nitroglycerin patches that they apply to their skin to help prevent anginal attacks. The skin absorbs the nitroglycerin slowly over several hours, giving the benefit of sustained action.

CHIEF COMPLAINT

The typical patient with angina complains of chest pain. Again, the pain usually is pressure-like and continuous and similar to that experienced with MIs. Key to the diagnosis of angina are identifiable causes and relieving factors. It is caused by exertion or emotional stress and relieved by rest or by taking nitroglycerin.

HISTORY OF PRESENT ILLNESS

The duration of the pain, by definition, is short, usually less than 5 minutes. Pain lasting more than 5 minutes should be considered a myocardial infarction until proved otherwise.

Establish whether the pain was caused and relieved in its typical pattern. *If there has been a change in the pattern of pain or its response to rest and medication, consider it as serious as a myocardial infarction.* Ask the patient if more nitroglycerin than usual was required to relieve the pain. (*Note:* Nitroglycerin may lose its potency with time and if tablets become moist during storage.) Figure 5–13 summarizes the precipatating factors associated with angina pectoris.

MEDICAL HISTORY

The patient has a medical history of similar pains, which follows a usual pattern. The patient may take cardiac drugs and use sublingual nitroglycerin to relieve acute attacks. Such patients often have risk factors for arteriosclerotic heart disease, including high blood cholesterol, high blood pressure, a long smoking history, and a family history of cardiovascular illness.

PHYSICAL EXAMINATION

The patient is anxious and concerned. He may feel lightheaded if he has taken nitroglycerin. The patient is sitting down and looking apprehensive if still in pain.

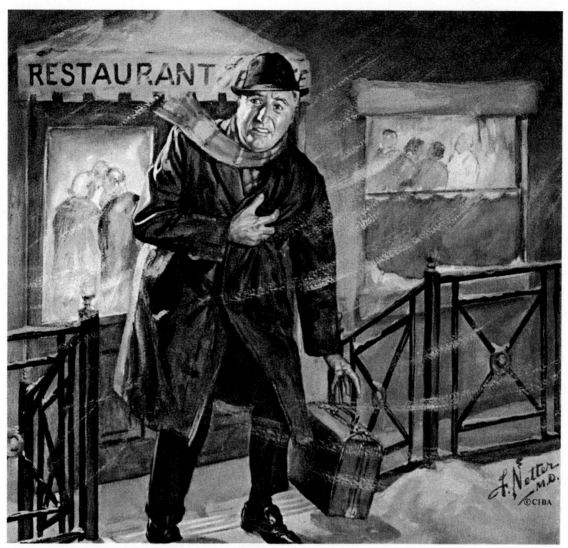

FIGURE 5-13. Factors that precipitate angina pectoris include heavy meals, physical exertion, emotional stress, and environmental stresses such as extreme cold. (From Netter F: CIBA Collection of Medical Illustrations, Vol. 5, The Heart. Summit, NJ, CIBA, 1969.)

The blood pressure, pulse, and respirations are usually within normal range. Variations are encountered. If the patient has taken nitroglycerin and is somewhat hypotensive from the venous pooling, he should be placed in a supine position.

Usually, the findings on the physical examination are normal. If the patient is exhibiting signs of hypoxia, shock, or pulmonary edema, it is cause for concern.

DIAGNOSIS

Many patients with angina may refuse transportation to the hospital. There are several factors to consider when deciding which patients to encourage to seek additional evaluation. First, you should be concerned that the patient with a history of angina has decided to call for help. You should ask how this event differs from previous anginal attacks. Patients with angina who (1)

have more frequent attacks than usual, (2) have a longer duration of pain, (3) have pain precipitated by less exertion or at rest, or (4) require more nitroglycerin than usual to relieve their pain should be encouraged to go to the hospital for further evaluation. The American Heart Association recommends that a patient with known angina who requires three or more nitroglycerin tablets over a 10-minute period to relieve pain receive hospital evaluation. A patient without a history of angina whose pain is typical of ischemic heart disease and lasts for 2 minutes or longer should also receive emergency medical evaluation.

Sometimes, bystanders might call for an ambulance because they see the anginal patient experiencing chest pain and know this is a warning sign for a heart attack. The episode may be no different from the patient's usual pattern. The patient may therefore refuse your assistance. Try to ascertain whether this event was consistent with the patient's usual pain pattern. Offer your assistance, but do not be surprised if your services are declined.

TREATMENT

You should assist the patient who still has pain as follows: calm the patient and any bystanders and be sure the patient sits or reclines. Administer supplemental oxygen at 4 to 6 liters per minute until the pain subsides. Assist the patient with medications he or she may carry for anginal attacks. If the patient becomes faint, light-headed, or hypotensive, lie him or her down and elevate the legs.

(*Note:* If the patient becomes hypotensive from the medication, it is usually transient, lasting only a few minutes. If the hypotension is sustained, cardiogenic shock should be considered.)

Sudden Cardiac Death

At times sudden death is the first indication of ischemic heart disease. Patients may have a spontaneous onset of ventricular fibrillation or asystole that causes cardiac arrest. Often these patients have risk factors for heart disease. They may have no known history of angina, myocardial infarction, or other heart problems.

Sudden death can be caused by decreased blood supply to the conduction system of the heart. This could be due to an obstruction from a thrombosis or spasm of a coronary artery. Before or shortly after pain develops, the patient suffers a dysrhythmia and loss of consciousness, breathing, and pulse. Unless treatment is rendered within minutes, death is certain.

Other causes of sudden death include electric shock, electrolyte abnormalities of the blood, drowning, and drug overdose. Effective EMS system dispatch protocols attempt to identify patients at risk for sudden death and patients who have already suffered cardiac arrest. Some systems provide "phone-directed" instructions on CPR performance to bystanders or family members who call for help. Other systems have developed broad-based community training in CPR or have trained the family members of persons at high risk for sudden death. All of these efforts recognize the importance of the two main variables associated with successful resuscitation—CPR and early defibrillation.

PUMP FAILURE, ANEURYSMS, AND TRAUMA

The heart may fail as a pump because of mechanical or electrical reasons. Either the power of the pump may be affected or the conducting system may malfunction and cause *dysrhythmias* (abnormal heart rhythms). Not only can heart failure lead to poor cardiac output but it can also cause a back-up of blood returning in the veins. First, the consequences of the heart losing its intrinsic power of contractions will be considered. The consequences of abnormal heart rhythms will be discussed later.

Introduction

Various conditions cause the heart to lose its power. Most patients with heart failure that EMTs encounter are those with either acute myocardial infarction or long-standing and progressive weakness of the heart muscle from prolonged hypertension or past MIs. In acute myocardial infarction, massive destruction of the myocardium reduces the amount of viable muscle available to perform the heart's work. Previous myocardial infarctions cause substantial scarring of the ventricular walls and a similar loss of viable heart muscle. Longstanding conditions such as hypertension and valvular disease (and COPD) may have caused the heart to overstretch to the point where Starling's law is no longer effective and failure occurs. In either case, the same kinds of problems—reduced cardiac output on the left side of the heart and back-up of blood in the venous system—may occur.

Other causes of heart failure are less common in occurrence. A patient may have taken an overdose of a cardiotoxic drug, or may have metabolic problems that result in poor heart contraction.

Pathophysiology of Heart Failure

Whatever the cause, when the ventricle cannot expel the blood in its chamber, the blood returning to the heart through the connecting atrium and venous system backs up.

RIGHT SIDE

If the right ventricle fails, the back-up occurs in the right atrium and its connecting veins; the inferior and superior venae cavae return blood from the systemic circulation. The pressure resulting from this back-up then is transmitted to the capillaries in the systemic circulation, and fluid is driven out of the vascular space, causing tissue edema.

LEFT SIDE

If the left ventricle fails, the pressure backs up through the left atrium and into the pulmonary veins. This pressure is transmitted through the pulmonary capillaries, and pulmonary edema can develop.

TABLE 5–13. Signs and Symptoms of Left-Sided
Heart Failure: Arterial Side

Sign or Symptom	Rationale
Weakness	Poor cardiac output
Altered mental status	
Fainting	
Dyspnea on exertion	Inadequate cardiac output for muscular activity
Tachycardia	Epinephrine release (compensatory) Increased cardiac output
Pale, cool, clammy skin	Increased peripheral resistance and redistribution to maintain blood pressure
Thready pulse	Low stroke volume
Narrow pulse pressure	
Hypotension	Poor cardiac output not compensated by above responses

POOR CARDIAC OUTPUT

On the forward or arterial side of the circulation, the weak heart does not eject or pump a normal stroke volume into the arteries. With a smaller stroke volume, the cardiac output will fall. To compensate, the sympathetic nervous system increases the heart's rate and force of contraction. In addition, to maintain the blood pressure in the face of low cardiac output, peripheral vasoconstriction is increased. The effects of these mechanisms lead to findings of tachycardia and pale, cool, and clammy skin on physical examination; in severe cases, hypotension may be present if the above mechanisms are not adequate to compensate (Table 5–13).

Right and Left Ventricular Failure

This section discusses the signs and symptoms of left and right ventricular failure.

LEFT VENTRICULAR FAILURE

The signs of heart failure are attributed to the resultant pressures in the arterial and venous systems. With left-sided failure, the arterial pressure is diminished. The patient has an altered mental status or complains of weakness. The body may compensate for the failing ventricle by increasing the heart rate or through vasoconstriction to maintain the blood pressure. Because the stroke volume is decreased, the patient has a rapid and thready pulse and shows pallor and cool, clammy skin.

If the patient's cardiac output is inadequate for him or her to sustain physical activity such as walking, he or she may notice becoming tired quickly and feeling short of breath on exertion. Inadequate oxygen is delivered to the muscles to sustain continuous muscular contraction. This relative lack of oxygen is sometimes

perceived by the body as though the respiratory efforts are inadequate, and it is known as dyspnea on exertion.

If blood backs up into the pulmonary veins, the increased pressure in the venous capillaries results in loss of fluid into the alveoli. This fluid loss can be heard as rales and occasionally as wheezing. When edema fluid enters the alveoli and the lungs become congested, the work of breathing is increased. The patient may appear to be in respiratory distress and complain of shortness of breath. In severe cases he sits upright and uses his accessory muscles of respiration. Because it is more difficult for oxygen to diffuse through wet lungs, the oxygen content of the blood may be decreased, leading in severe cases to cyanosis. The edema in the lungs is irritating, and coughing may be present. In severe cases, the patient may cough up foamy, pink-tinged sputum. Many authorities reserve the term pulmonary edema to describe patients with the most severe and life-threatening stage of congestive heart failure characterized by coughing of this foamy, pink-tinged sputum (Table 5–14).

RIGHT VENTRICULAR FAILURE

Because the circulatory system is a closed circuit, left ventricular failure ultimately leads to right ventricular failure. The most common cause of right-sided heart failure is pre-existing left-sided heart failure. Diseases in the lungs (such as emphysema) sometimes lead directly to right ventricular failure because of damage to the pulmonary vessels from the lung disease. Whatever the cause, when the right ventricle fails, the principle findings are explained by a back-up of blood in the great veins that raises the venous pressure. This pressure is transmitted throughout the systemic circulation. When high pressures are reached in the capillaries, plasma fluid is driven outside the capillaries, resulting in tissue edema (peripheral edema).

EFFECT OF GRAVITY. Edema first becomes obvious in the most dependent portions of the body (i.e.,

TABLE 5–14. Signs and Symptoms of Left-Sided Heart
Failure: Venous Side*

Sign or Symptom	Rationale
Sitting upright	To compensate for increased work of breathing
Using accessory muscles of respiration	
Dyspnea	Fluid in alveoli and small bronchioles
Rales	
Wheezes with normal expiratory phase	
Cyanosis	Decreased oxygen diffusion through wet alveoli
Coughing	Edema fluid irritates respiratory tract; leakage of some red cells
Pink, frothy sputum	

* Not all of these signs will necessarily be present in any one patient.

below the level of the heart). If a patient with right-sided heart failure is on his or her feet most of the day, he or she will first notice foot (pedal) edema and ankle edema. It may not be present in the morning after the patient has slept because the feet were not as dependent during the night. As the condition progresses, the patient notices edema higher up the legs (Fig. 5–14A). It may still be decreased by changing position, as when sleeping, but not as much as before. Some edema in the legs may still be present in the morning.

If a patient is bedridden, the most gravity-dependent portion of the body is the posterior surface or back. This is where edema fluid collects and the patient has sacral edema (Fig. 5–14B). In severe cases, edema fluid may be noted throughout the body. This condition is called anasarca.

PAROXYSMAL NOCTURNAL DYSPNEA. Consider what might happen to a patient with progressive pedal and ankle edema from heart failure when he or she goes to sleep and the legs are no longer the most dependent portion of the body. The extra fluid in the legs re-enters the circulation when the effect of gravity is decreased by lying down or elevating the legs. If the right-sided heart failure is associated with left-sided heart failure, a sequence of symptoms develops. The extra fluid reentering the vascular space results in an increased venous return to the heart. If the left ventricle cannot handle this extra volume, blood will back up into the pulmonary circulation. The patient will find that a few hours after having fallen asleep he or she awakes short of breath. Because this happens suddenly and usually at night it is described as paroxysmal nocturnal dyspnea (sudden nighttime shortness of breath). The patient should sit up or stand and remain so until the dyspnea is relieved through gravitational forces again. The fluid constantly shifts and redistributes itself with respect to the forces of gravity.

ORTHOPNEA. The patient soon learns that he sleeps better if he does not lie down completely and sleeps with his head elevated. The degree of elevation required for a good night's sleep may vary from two to four pillows. Some patients may have to sleep sitting upright in a chair. This condition is described as orthopnea. A patient giving a history of orthopnea may tell you how his heart failure has progressed by describing how he has gradually had to continue elevating his head at night to avoid paroxysmal nocturnal dyspnea until he finally must sleep in a chair.

NECK VEINS. Ordinarily, when a person is sitting upright the neck veins should not be distended. When examining patients with heart failure, however, neck vein distention may be seen. This neck vein distention is a sign of back pressure within the venous system (Fig. 5–14C). The neck veins should be bilaterally distended.

There may or may not be use of accessory muscles of breathing. Table 5–15 summarizes the signs and symptoms of right ventricular failure.

DIGOXIN. Often patients with chronic heart failure take the drug digoxin. Digoxin increases the power of the heart muscle contraction, especially in failing hearts. Digoxin also can affect the conduction system of the heart and is prescribed for certain conduction disturbances. Taken in overdose, digoxin usually affects the conduction system adversely.

History and Physical Findings in Patients With Heart Failure

This section discusses the history and physical findings encountered when assessing a patient with heart failure.

CHIEF COMPLAINT

The most common complaint of patients with heart failure is dyspnea, or shortness of breath. Chest pain may be the predominant complaint in some patients if the origin of the heart failure is an acute myocardial infarction. Other complaints usually are related to decreased cardiac output such as weakness, altered mental status, and fainting. Other complaints such as orthopnea and dyspnea on exertion are more apt to be elicited during the history of present illness. By themselves, they usually do not require a call for emergency ambulance assistance.

HISTORY OF PRESENT ILLNESS

Recent associated complaints and events include dyspnea on exertion (with normal activity), paroxysmal nocturnal dyspnea, orthopnea, cough (possibly productive of pink-tinged, frothy sputum), progressive fatigue, and systemic edema. The patient may also complain of ischemic chest pain or palpitations.

CHRONIC HEART FAILURE. The chronology of events varies. Typically the patient with chronic heart failure will complain of a gradual worsening of shortness of breath associated with the other symptoms of right- and left-sided heart failure. The patient may have a history consistent with paroxysmal nocturnal dyspnea, the patient awakening with acute shortness of breath 2 or 3 hours after going to sleep.

FAILURE SECONDARY TO A MYOCARDIAL INFARCTION. On the other hand, heart failure resulting from an acute MI presents differently. A patient experiencing an MI is likely to present with an episode of acute substernal chest pain followed by other symptoms of

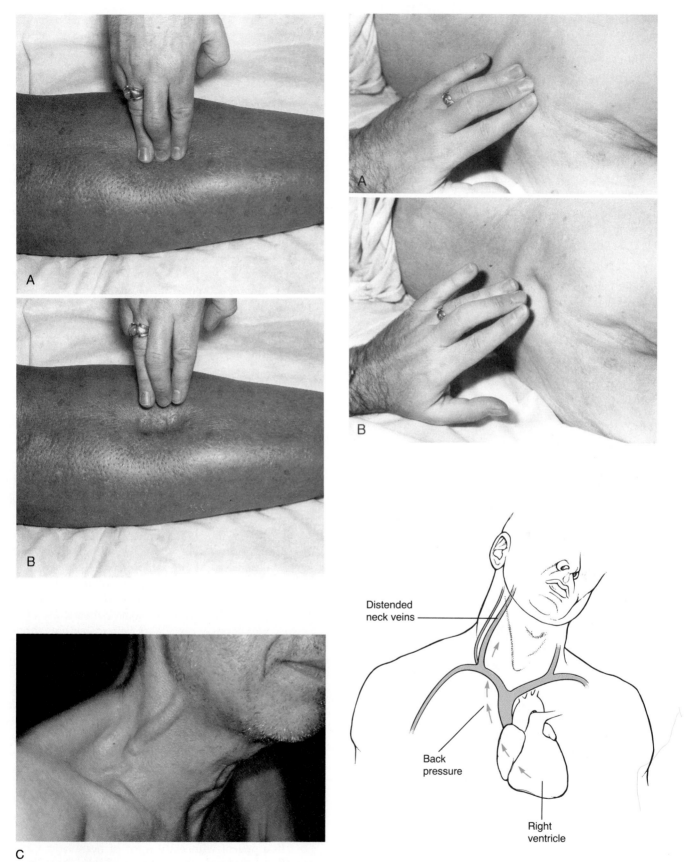

FIGURE 5–14. (*A*) Edema in the area of the tibia. (*B*) Pitting edema of sacrum. (*C*) Neck vein distention caused by a back-up of pressure from the right ventricle. (*A* and *B* and photograph in *C*, from Swartz MH: Textbook of Physical Diagnosis: History and Examination. Philadelphia, WB Saunders, 1989, p. 277 and Plate X.)

TABLE 5–15. Signs and Symptoms of Right-Sided Heart
Failure

TABLE 5–15. Signs and Symptoms of Right-Sided Heart
Failure

Sign or Symptom	Rationale
Edema of most dependent areas (e.g., pedal, ankle, sacral)	Back pressure felt greatest in gravity-dependent areas, causing fluid displacement into tissue (positional)
Anasarca (throughout body)	Severe cases
Neck vein distention in upright position	Back pressure in venous system causing distention

With associated left-sided heart failure
    Paroxysmal nocturnal dyspnea
    Orthopnea
	Reabsorption of systemic edema fluid into vascular space with changes in position; results in left heart failure and back-up in pulmonary veins and edema in lungs

failure, including shortness of breath and generalized weakness. The acute obstruction of blood flow to the myocardium causes the pain. As the destruction of the myocardium occurs, the pumping ability of the heart is compromised and failure results.

MEDICAL HISTORY

The medical history may reveal a longstanding history of cardiac problems, including angina, previous myocardial infarctions, hypertension, and congestive heart failure. The patient may be taking medications consistent with these types of problems. Digoxin may have been prescribed to improve the pumping ability of a failing heart. Furosemide (Lasix) and other diuretics may have been prescribed to reduce the blood volume. Other medications for angina and hypertension are common. Elicit a COPD history, since heart failure is a common complication of longstanding COPD.

GENERAL APPEARANCE

The EMT notices that the patient is sitting upright, struggling to breathe. The use of accessory muscles of respiration is evident. Noisy gurgling sounds accompany breathing.

MENTAL STATUS

Dyspnea causes patients to be highly agitated, anxious, and restless. This is caused by hypoxia as well as the subjective feeling of breathlessness. As hypoxia becomes more pronounced, the patient becomes lethargic and even unresponsive. These signs are ominous and require aggressive intervention with positive-pressure ventilation and supplemental oxygen.

VITAL SIGNS

Vital signs may vary. Tachycardia usually accompanies hypoxia. Likewise, the respirations tend to be rapid, deep, and labored. Take note that as a person tires, the respiratory rate may slow secondary to exhaustion.

In severe cases, when the hypoxia is more pronounced, signs of organ failure occur. Brain hypoxia manifests first with an altered mental status, but ultimately the centers of respiration are affected as well and respiratory efforts are slower and more shallow. The heart, the second most oxygen-sensitive organ after the brain, is unable to sustain a rapid rate and starts to slow as well.

Blood pressure is determined by the pumping ability of the heart and the peripheral vascular resistance. It must be interpreted in light of the present and past medical history and other physical findings. Hypertension is not uncommon. A history of this disease might be elicited or there may be evidence of severe peripheral vasoconstriction (i.e., pale, cool, clammy skin). Hypotension, on the other hand, is an ominous finding. It indicates either a myocardial infarction with severe destruction of the ventricle or such severe hypoxia that the oxygen demands of the heart muscle are no longer balanced, resulting in weak contractions.

HEAD-TO-TOE SURVEY

The head-to-toe survey will identify many of the signs of heart failure discussed previously.

SKIN. Check first for cyanosis, especially of the mucous membranes, lips, and nail beds. Then look for signs of epinephrine release such as cool, pale, clammy skin.

NECK. A quick assessment of the neck veins in the sitting position tells you if there is significant right ventricular failure. At the same time, note whether the patient is using accessory muscles of respiration (i.e., bulging of the sternocleidomastoids), signifying increased work at breathing. In some patients, use of accessory muscles may cause neck vein distention without right ventricular failure. Therefore, the significance of neck vein distention must be judged in conjunction with other signs of right ventricular failure.

BREATH SOUNDS. In patients with congestive heart failure, rales are commonly heard when fluid collects at the alveoli. Rales are the fine crackling sounds similar to what is heard when rolling pieces of your hair between your fingers next to your ear. The rales from heart failure are usually symmetrical and heard to the same level in both lung fields. If rales are heard on one side only, they are more likely due to another process (such as pneumonia).

In a patient with early signs of heart failure, rales are often heard only at the bases of the lungs. This is especially true if the patient has been sitting upright. This is because of gravity's influence on the blood's pressure throughout the vascular tree. In a patient who is sitting, the base of the lungs is the most dependent portion of the pulmonary circulation and has the highest venous pressure. (The base of the lung is *below* the heart in the sitting position.)

You will also encounter patients who are bedridden, such as patients in nursing homes, who become short of breath. Since they have been lying on their backs for some time, rales may be heard along the entire posterior surface of the lung fields. When lying down, the posterior aspect of the lungs is the most dependent portion (below the heart) and the pulmonary circulation is under higher pressure in this area.

DESCRIBING RALES. Rales are usually described by location. It is important to note if they are symmetrical (bilaterally equal) or heard in one area only. The term "bibasilar rales" describes the patient who has rales in both lungs, which are heard at the bases only. If they persist halfway up both lungs, they are described as "rales in both lungs, halfway up." The description is adapted for rales extending to the base of the scapula, the nipple line, and so on. Be descriptive. If they extend to the top of the lungs, they can be described as "rales in both lungs to the apices." The apex of the lung is its highest point.

It is best to auscultate the lungs with the patient in the sitting position. Lung sounds are distorted if the patient is supine. If the patient's condition permits, try to get help to position the patient upright so you can listen posteriorly to the lungs. An option is to lie the patient on each side and listen to the superior lung.

Note that individuals who have not been using a portion of their lungs may have atelectasis (collapsed alveoli) and rales upon initial auscultation. By having the patient take deep breaths the atelectatic portions of the lungs will open and the rales will disappear. This is not important if the patient is in obvious respiratory distress and is working hard at breathing. Patients who are bedridden or inactive, however, may have atelectatic areas, and you should have them breathe deeply a few times to see if the rales remain or disappear.

FLUID IN THE LUNGS. Some patients with long-standing heart failure may have collections of fluid within the lungs. Portions of the lungs bathed in this fluid will be quiet areas during ascultation. Because of gravity, fluid collects at the base in the sitting position and layers out posteriorly when recumbent. If the breath sounds are not heard as inferior as you might expect, it may be because of fluid.

WHEEZING. Congestive heart failure may present with wheezing rather than rales. The fluid from heart failure may irritate the airway and cause some broncho-constriction. If the clinical picture suggests heart failure, it is important to remember that the wheezing you hear may be from fluid in the lungs and not asthma. The clinical picture usually allows you to determine the cause of wheezing.

PINK, FROTHY SPUTUM. Patients with pulmonary edema may present with coughing and expectoration of pink, frothy sputum. The pinkness comes from leakage of some red blood cells through the strained pulmonary capillaries. Fluid in the airway is irritating and stimulates the coughing reflex. You will note that the frothy appearance of the expectoration in pulmonary edema makes it easily distinguishable from the thick, tenacious sputum produced by pneumonia and other respiratory infections.

EDEMA. The extremities should be checked for edema. Often it is obvious upon inspection. When edema is not obvious and you are considering heart failure as a possible diagnosis, gently press the skin of a dependent portion of the body with your finger. If you leave an impression with your finger, it is a sign of edema. The edema is described by location, such as pedal or ankle edema, edema to the knees, and so on. When evaluating bedridden patients, check the sacral area in the same manner. Figures 5—15 and 5—16 illustrate key signs and symptoms associated with left and right ventricular failure.

Treatment of Congestive Heart Failure

Prehospital treatment is directed toward patients with left ventricular failure, and specifically those patients with evidence of pulmonary congestion as evidenced by dyspnea, rales or wheezing, cyanosis and other signs of hypoxia, and signs of increased work of breathing.

The three primary goals of treatment are to *increase oxygen delivery, decrease oxygen demand,* and *decrease venous return.* Increasing oxygen delivery involves supplemental oxygen, use of gravity, and positive-pressure ventilations if necessary. Decreasing oxygen demand is done as for any patient with ischemic chest pain. Decreasing venous return reduces the amount of blood returning to the central circulation by using maneuvers and treatments that tend to localize relatively more blood in the extremities.

INCREASE OXYGEN DELIVERY

Oxygen delivery is increased by establishing airway patency, ensuring adequate ventilation, administering supplemental oxygen, and positioning the patient properly.

VENTILATION AND OXYGENATION. The mainstay of treatment is ensuring adequate oxygenation. The airway's patency should be ensured with proper positioning, airway devices, and suctioning if secretions are present in the upper airway. Give moderate to high

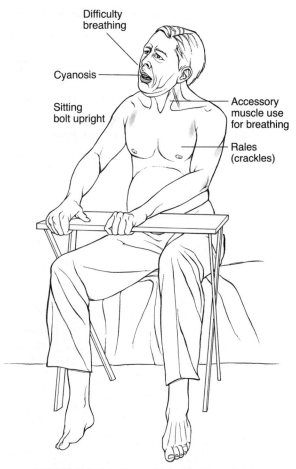

FIGURE 5–15. Signs of left-sided heart failure.

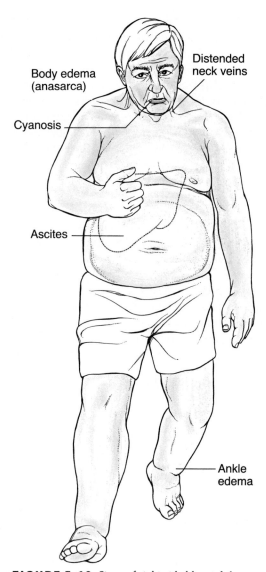

FIGURE 5–16. Signs of right-sided heart failure.

concentrations of supplemental oxygen, depending on the status of the patient. For example, if the patient has bibasilar rales and is experiencing mild dyspnea with a normal respiratory rate, you might begin with moderate oxygen concentrations (40 to 50%). If the patient's status deteriorates, increase to high-concentration oxygen with a non-rebreather mask. On the other hand, if the patient is in distress, has signs of hypoxia, is cyanotic, has rales up to the apices, or has pink, frothy sputum, a non-rebreather mask or a demand valve device should be used initially. Any patient with a depressed mental status and signs of congestive heart failure should receive high-concentration oxygen and positive-pressure assistance if indicated.

Administration of oxygen to patients with COPD and moderate distress might be started at 24 to 28% by a Venturi mask with stepwise increases if there is no improvement or a deterioration in status. Oxygenation of patients with severe distress should be started at higher concentrations.

The cardinal sign to watch for with COPD patients who receive oxygen therapy is *hypoventilation*. The EMT must carefully monitor the rate and depth of ventilations. If signs of hypoventilation are present, assist with positive-pressure ventilation. Once positive-pressure ventilation is begun, high concentrations of oxygen should be used for all patients.

Oxygen diffusion through the alveoli is compromised as fluid collects in the lungs. If this process is not corrected, the resulting hypoxia further weakens the heart and can lead to rapid deterioration and cardiac arrest. Patients in severe distress need high concentrations of supplemental oxygen so it can cross the wet alveoli and enter the blood. If there is any indication that ventilatory efforts are inadequate, immediately provide positive-pressure ventilations.

POSITION

The preferred position for patients with heart failure is the sitting position. This enables full excursion of the chest and diaphragm and localizes the edema at the bases of the lung. The seated position helps keep the alveoli in the upper lung fields dry and permits air exchange through nonedematous portions of the lungs. Patients with hypotension or depressed mental status, however, cannot tolerate this position. These patients should be treated in the supine position and receive necessary positive-pressure ventilations with 100% oxygen.

In general, patients with respiratory distress do not assume the supine position voluntarily unless their mental status is significantly depressed or they are profoundly weak from hypoxia or hypotension. Be prepared to assist or provide ventilatory support for any patient with heart failure and pulmonary edema who is supine.

DECREASE OXYGEN DEMAND

Patients with congestive heart failure and pulmonary edema are usually anxious and restless. More alarming are the patients who are lethargic or less responsive. While limiting all unnecessary physical activity, maintain verbal contact with the patient for reassurance and to elicit cooperation with therapy. Encourage him or her to continue breathing efforts. Prolonged respiratory distress is exhausting.

You will encounter patients with respiratory distress in need of oxygen who resist the application of a face mask because they perceive it as suffocating. Some of these patients will better tolerate a nasal cannula. Use whatever device they will tolerate.

DECREASE VENOUS RETURN

The failing heart cannot eject all the blood returning to it. By limiting venous return, the amount of blood returning to the heart is decreased and more closely matches the ejection potential of failing ventricles. The goal of this therapy is to minimize the back-up of blood into the lungs.

Positioning the patient in the sitting position allows more blood to pool in the veins of the lower extremities. This again is the preferred position for all patients with congestive heart failure who can tolerate it. The patient who cannot sit is in critical condition, and rapid and aggressive intervention is essential for survival. Table 5–16 lists treatments and rationales for acute pulmonary edema.

Aneurysms of the Aorta

An aneurysm, or outpouching, of the wall of the aorta can form and lead to dissection (the thoracic aorta) or rupture (the abdominal aorta). A *thoracic (dissecting) aneurysm* results when blood enters the wall of the aorta itself from a tear in the inner wall and continues to flow

TABLE 5–16. Treatments and Rationales for Pulmonary Edema

Treatment	Rationale
Supplemental oxygen	Increases alveolar oxygen levels
Positive-pressure ventilation	Ensures adequate ventilation
Sitting position	Limits venous return
	Localizes edema at lung bases
	Permits maximal ventilatory excursions

between the inner and outer walls of the vessel. This may result in occlusion of branching arteries. The blood continues to dissect the inner from the outer wall of the vessel as it travels through this newly formed passage within the wall of the aorta itself (Fig. 5–17). An *abdominal aortic aneurysm* has more of a tendency to leak

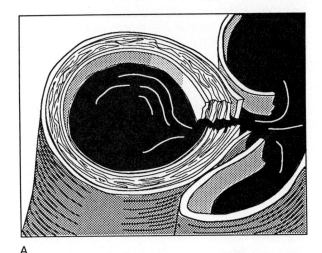

A

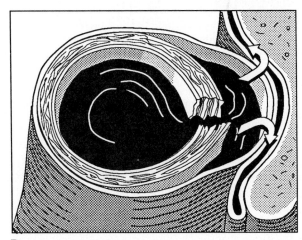

B

FIGURE 5–17. Mechanism of dissecting aortic aneurysms. (*A*) Both the inner (intima and media) and outer (adventitia) linings of the aorta as well as the covering of the mediastinum are torn. Bleeding is rapid and lethal. (*B*) The inner (intima and media) linings of the aorta are torn but the outer lining contains the bleeding. These patients require immediate surgical intervention or rupture may occur. (From Naclerio EM: Chest Injuries. Orlando, Grune & Stratton, 1971.)

or rupture, causing blood to pour into the abdomen. Both thoracic aneurysms and abdominal aortic aneurysms are caused by arteriosclerosis, which alters the integrity of the vessel. As with arteriosclerosis in general, most patients are not aware of aneurysm formation until dissection or rupture occurs. However, some patients may know they have an aneurysm from previous examinations.

RECOGNITION OF ANEURYSMS

It is important to be aware of aneurysms because they must be considered when a patient complains of chest or abdominal pain. Early recognition and proper treatment are important for survival.

Typically both thoracic and abdominal aneurysms present with pain. The pain is usually described as sudden, tearing or searing, and radiating to the back. The thoracic aneurysm presents with chest pain that radiates or is localized in the back of the thorax and radiates downward. The abdominal aneurysm often presents with pain localized in the lower abdomen, radiating to the lower back. Many patients with aneurysms also have histories of hypertension.

Because of the different manifestations and treatment considerations, thoracic and abdominal aneurysms are best discussed separately.

THORACIC (DISSECTING) ANEURYSM

As noted above, blood dissects the inner wall from the outer wall of the aorta and flows between them, forming a false passage. The formation of this false passage may lead to occlusion of the vessels branching off the aorta and may occlude the aorta itself. The dissection can continue into the abdomen or the blood flow may re-enter the true lumen of the aorta at a distal point. Or, it may rupture through the entire wall of the aorta, leading to massive internal hemorrhage. If the blood from the aneurysm enters the pericardium, *pericardial (cardiac) tamponade* may occur.

HISTORY. Thoracic aneurysm typically presents as a sudden onset of tearing, ripping, or searing chest pain radiating to the back and continuing downward into the abdomen. Many times, however, the pain is difficult to distinguish from that of an MI. There also may be complaints due to occlusion of the vessels branching off the thoracic aorta. Because these vessels include branches feeding the head and both upper extremities, the patient may faint, show signs of a cerebrovascular accident (stroke), or complain of numbness in the arms due to ischemia. Some patients experience a temporary loss of consciousness. In these situations pain may not be de-

scribed. The patient may have a history of hypertension or a known aneurysm.

PHYSICAL FINDINGS. Pertinent physical findings are related to the manifestations that occur in any given patient. They include signs and symptoms related to (1) occlusion of vessels, (2) hemorrhage, and (3) pericardial (cardiac) tamponade.

Occlusion of Vessels. Look for a disparity or asymmetry of pulses. Look for pulse deficits. Are pulses equal and symmetrical in the arms? Is there an absent or weak carotid pulse on one side? Examine the carotids gently, one at a time. You might find the blood pressure in both arms is different. Small variances are normal. A marked disparity is cause for concern. Focal neurologic findings on the motor and sensory examination may be related to occlusion of a major artery supplying the brain. (See Chapter 7 for asymmetrical findings.)

Hemorrhage. Check for tachycardia and signs of epinephrine release. Check neck veins for filling. Check capillary refill for delayed filling. If the patient is conscious and the systolic blood pressure is greater than 100, check for postural hypotension.

Pericardial (Cardiac) Tamponade. Occasionally, dissection of the aorta can continue toward the heart and blood can enter into the pericardial sac, resulting in pericardial tamponade. As the blood accumulates, it compresses the heart's chambers and prevents adequate filling. This results in obstructive shock with its accompanying signs: distended neck veins, narrowed pulse pressure, and general signs of shock. This condition requires rapid surgical intervention. Transport should be immediate.

TREATMENT CONSIDERATIONS. The diagnosis of dissecting aneurysm of the thoracic aorta has therapeutic implications that differ from other forms of noncardiogenic shock. Elevated blood pressures may worsen the dissection process. If patients are hypotensive and have evidence of poor brain perfusion, the MAST are inflated slowly until systolic pressures reach the 80 to 100 range. Most of these patients are hypertensive or normotensive. Findings consistent with dissection are signs of shock in the presence of a normal or elevated blood pressure. Hospital intervention often includes lowering the blood pressure as an initial part of therapy. High-concentration oxygen and rapid transport are the important aspects of prehospital treatment.

ABDOMINAL AORTIC ANEURYSM

A leaking abdominal aneurysm usually presents with sudden onset of lower abdominal pain that radiates or localizes to the lower back. Blood leaking into the abdomen may cause peritoneal signs such as abdominal tenderness, rigidity, and guarding (see Chapter 8). If the aorta ruptures, severe and often fatal hemorrhage results (see Fig. 5–17A). Abdominal aortic aneurysm occurs primarily in older patients. Recognition rests on the finding of tearing pain going to the back and on evidence of hypovolemia.

PERTINENT FINDINGS. The patient's mental status and cardiovascular examinations are consistent with the amount of hemorrhage. Look for signs of hypovolemic shock.

Abdominal aortic aneurysms may be discovered during the abdominal examination. A pulsatile mass found midline in the abdomen suggests an aneurysm. Pulsations may be felt normally, however, particularly in thin people. The diagnosis of abdominal aortic aneurysm does not rest with findings on the abdominal examination, because many patients may not have classical findings, as a result of obesity or other factors. Furthermore, all examiners are advised to use caution when examining the abdomen of a patient with a suspected abdominal aortic aneurysm. A working diagnosis can be made from the sudden onset of typical pain and signs of hypovolemia.

As in all hypovolemic cases, rapid transport to surgical intervention is essential. MAST may be useful in these cases, not only to elevate blood pressure, but also to tamponade bleeding.

Pulmonary Embolism

An embolism lodged in the pulmonary artery gives rise to complaints of dyspnea or chest pain. Venous thrombosis is the source of most emboli. They occur in patients with inflamed veins (thrombophlebitis), in patients requiring prolonged bedrest after surgery, or in patients taking birth control pills. Another source is fat emboli from fractures of long bones. Because of reflex changes in the lungs, patients with a pulmonary embolism may become suddenly and severely hypoxic. If large or multiple, pulmonary emboli that obstruct a major pulmonary artery can cause acute right ventricular failure.

The diagnosis is suspected from a patient's medical history, since the physical findings are so variable and nonspecific. Prehospital treatment consists of oxygen administration and transport.

CHIEF COMPLAINT AND HISTORY OF PRESENT ILLNESS

Patients commonly report dyspnea or sudden onset of chest pain that is usually sharp and pleuritic and may be unilateral. Associated complaints include cough and possibly *hemoptysis* (bloody expectorations). There may be a history of phlebitis, unilateral leg swelling or calf tenderness, prolonged bedrest or travel (car trip), recent surgery, or use of birth control pills.

PHYSICAL FINDINGS

The physical findings often are normal. Tachypnea is almost always present, however. A "rubbing" sound may be heard over the area of pain, but lung sounds usually are normal. Tachycardia and hypotension are present in severe cases. If there is significant obstruction of blood flow out of the right ventricle, the back-up may cause neck vein distention and other signs of heart failure. Signs of hypoxia, including cyanosis and altered mental status, may be present.

TREATMENT

High-concentration oxygen should be administered. If there are signs of severe hypoxia or hypotension or distention of neck veins, the condition is severe and requires rapid transport.

Dysrhythmias

Abnormal heart rhythms are the most common cause of sudden death in patients suffering from arteriosclerotic heart disease and myocardial infarction. In addition they often are the cause of heart failure that results in pulmonary edema and cardiogenic shock. Treatment of dysrhythmias usually requires the administration of drugs, electric shock, or pacemaker therapy, as well as treatment of the underlying cause.

Without an electrocardiographic (ECG) monitor, the EMT must rely on physical findings, especially pulse rate, quality, and rhythm, to suspect the presence of dysrhythmias.

The EMT is limited in the ability to recognize and deal with lethal and prelethal dysrhythmias and must rely on supportive therapy to minimize their effects. The supportive therapy may be sufficient to abolish some abnormal heart rhythms. For example, hypoxia can cause dysrhythmias.

It is important to have a basic understanding of how dysrhythmias can affect cardiovascular function. Even without knowledge of ECGs, the EMT can appreciate the potential consequences of commonly encountered abnormal rhythms. A simple classification system includes slow, fast, and irregular rhythms and the resultant effects on cardiac output.

SLOW RATES: BRADYCARDIA

By following the formula for cardiac output, it is clear that if the heart rate falls, so does the cardiac output.

Let's consider, for example, a man whose normal heart rate is 70 beats a minute and whose normal stroke volume is 70 ml of blood. This is matched to meet his needs for normal daily activities.

$$CO = HR \times SV, \text{ or } 70 \times 70 = 4900 \text{ ml/min}$$

What happens if his heart rate falls to 40 beats per minute? Applying the formula, we see:

$$CO = 40 \times 70, \text{ or } 2800 \text{ ml/min}$$

It would not be surprising if this man felt weak and complained that he had no energy.

The EMT will encounter individuals who complain of weakness or who have passed out and have slow pulse rates and perhaps an associated low blood pressure. Their symptoms may be caused by the heart rate's being too slow to maintain adequate cardiac output.

FAST RATES: TACHYCARDIA

From reviewing the cardiac output equation, it would seem that a rapid pulse could result only in a still greater cardiac output. The ability to increase heart rate is a built-in response to stressful conditions and is used as part of the compensatory response to conditions such as hypovolemia.

If the heart rate exceeds 180 beats per minute, however, the cardiac output no longer increases and may even begin to fall. Two factors make excessively fast rates counterproductive. One factor is ventricular filling time, and the other relates to the increased oxygen needs of the rapidly beating myocardium.

VENTRICULAR FILLING TIME.   Most (70%) of ventricular filling occurs during diastole. The remaining 30% of ventricular filling occurs during atrial contraction. As the heart rate increases, the time spent in diastole (at rest between beats) decreases, leaving less time for filling of the ventricle. At rates greater then 180 beats per minute, the ventricular filling is less; the stroke volume then decreases, and the cardiac output begins to fall. Extremely fast heart rates lead to markedly decreased cardiac output, and evidence of hypoperfusion may be present.

HEART RATE AND MYOCARDIAL OXYGEN NEEDS.
Like any other muscle, the heart must have periods of rest. The rest period of the heart is during diastole. At a heart rate of 75/min the heart spends about 40 seconds of each minute at rest (diastole). At a heart rate of 200/min the heart spends only 28 seconds of each minute at rest.

When the heart beats more often it must receive more oxygen from the coronary circulation to meet the increased workload. Some areas of the left ventricle are perfused with blood only during diastole. The fast heart

requires more oxygen but has less time to receive it. At very high heart rates some patients experience chest pain from insufficient oxygen delivery to the myocardium.

If the heart rate is so fast that cardiac output falls, the patient is at even greater risk. Remember that the pressure of blood in the aorta is the driving force for the coronary circulation. Table 5–17 illustrates the relationship between a very fast heart rate and myocardial ischemia.

PALPITATIONS.   It is not uncommon for patients who experience rapid heart rhythms or extra beats to describe the sensation of palpitations. Other descriptions include "skipping," "jumping in the chest," and "runaway heart." The significance of palpitations is related to their effect on cardiac output and perfusion. A patient who shows signs of hypoperfusion should be treated as a patient with cardiogenic shock. Other secondary effects include all those attributable to heart failure and myocardial infarction, such as syncope, dyspnea, dizziness, and so forth.

IRREGULAR RHYTHMS

An EMT may note an irregularity when checking the pulse. Some irregular rhythms may cause a fall in cardiac output. Others may be stable and require no intervention. Still others may be precursors of fatal events. The EMT is not able to decipher the rhythm without an ECG. He or she must be able to judge the hemodynamic significance of the dysrhythmia by the general condition of the patient and treat conditions requiring emergency care. Dysrhythmias may cause conditions such as pulmonary edema or cardiogenic shock. Treatment should be instituted as described for these conditions, with ultimate evaluation and treatment of the dysrhythmia in the hospital.

When encountering ischemic chest pain, the EMT must realize that dysrhythmias are the most common cause of death (regardless of whether an irregular pulse is encountered). The presence of an irregular pulse in the

TABLE 5–17. Very Fast Heart Rate and Myocardial Ischemia

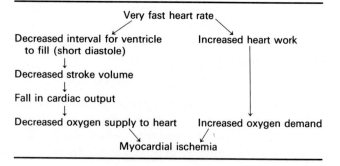

patient with an MI may be indicative of an even greater risk of sudden death.

SYNCOPE

Syncope, or a sudden loss of consciousness, should always call to mind the possibility of dysrhythmias, especially if there was no warning period and the patient cannot remember feeling ill before losing consciousness. A prolonged pause between heartbeats or a sudden occurrence of an extremely rapid rhythm in which significant fall in cardiac output occurs can cause syncope.

If an irregular pulse is encountered, the patient should be treated and transported without undue delay.

Some patients may complain of dizziness, which describes a number of different sensations. Words used to convey this awkward feeling include "confusion," "giddiness," "lightheadedness," "blacking out," "graying of vision," and "unsteadiness." This feeling may precede syncope. It can be caused by a number of conditions, and the diagnosis may be difficult to make even in the hospital. Look closely for other signs of cardiovascular or central nervous system disease.

PACEMAKERS

Mechanical pacemakers are implanted to control certain dysrhythmias, to provide a back-up if the heart's own pacemaker fails, or to serve in place of the organic pacemaker itself. Mechanical pacemakers also can fail. In such cases, the heart returns to its own rhythm. Most of the time this rhythm is too slow for adequate cardiac output. The presence of a pacemaker should in no way alter your assessment and treatment of a patient.

TRAUMATIC CARDIAC EMERGENCIES

Cardiac contusions and pericardial (cardiac) tamponade are two conditions of which the EMT should be aware when evaluating an injured patient.

Cardiac Contusion   ~bruised heart.~

Blunt trauma to the chest cavity can be transmitted to the heart. Like any other tissue, the heart bruises with injury. The contusion may range in severity from a mere bruise with no complications to disruption of the myocardium with bleeding into the pericardial sac (pericardial tamponade) or into the chest cavity itself. Most cardiac contusions do not result in severe complications. Some, however, manifest as dysrhythmias, which may or may not complicate other injuries.

✠ P R O T O C O L ✠

CARDIAC-RELATED PROBLEM

> **CAUTION!**
>
> BE PREPARED TO DEAL WITH RESPIRATORY AND CARDIAC ARREST!

1. Ensure that the patient's airway is open and that breathing and circulation are adequate.

2. Administer high-concentration oxygen.

3. Place the patient in a position of comfort, while reassuring the patient and loosening tight clothing.

4. Obtain and record the vital signs, and repeat en route as often as the situation indicates.

5. Transport, keeping the patient warm.

6. Record all patient care information, including the patient's medical history and all treatment provided, on a prehospital care report.

7. IF CHEST PAIN IS PRESENT AND IF THE PATIENT POSSESSES NITROGLYCERIN PRESCRIBED BY HIS/HER PHYSICIAN AND HAS A SYSTOLIC BLOOD PRESSURE OF 90 MM HG OR GREATER, the EMT may assist the patient in self-administration of sublingual nitroglycerin as indicated on the medicine container.

From Manual for Emergency Medical Technicians. Emergency Medical Services Program. Albany, New York State Department of Health, 1990.

CAUSE

The most common cause of cardiac contusion is impact with the steering wheel of an automobile (Fig. 5–18). Evidence of bruising or fracture of the sternum is particularly suggestive of cardiac contusion in such patients.

SIGNS AND SYMPTOMS

Cardiac contusion is suspected from the mechanism of injury and signs of trauma over the anterior chest. It cannot be diagnosed definitively in the field. An irregular pulse or a slow pulse in the context of blunt chest trauma should increase the suspicion that cardiac contusion has occurred.

TREATMENT

There is no definite treatment for cardiac contusion in the field. The EMT should be aware of the possibility of tamponade developing from blunt injury (much rarer than from penetrating wounds) and the possibility of

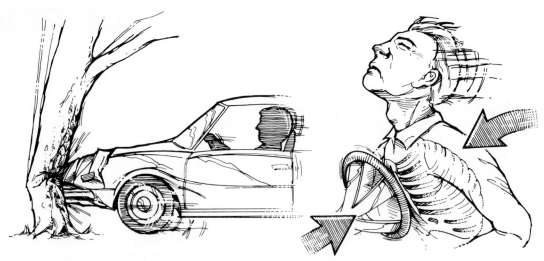

FIGURE 5–18. When the chest wall strikes the steering wheel of a car during deceleration, the heart can strike the sternum and rib cage, resulting in a cardiac contusion. (From Cardona VD, Hurn PD, Mason PJB, et al: Trauma Nursing from Resuscitation Through Rehabilitation. Philadelphia, WB Saunders, 1988, p. 116.)

cardiogenic shock in a trauma victim when the signs and symptoms of shock do not fit those of hypovolemia.

Pericardial (Cardiac) Tamponade

When the chest has sustained penetrating wounds, the heart may bleed into the pericardium (see Fig. 5–1). Signs of pericardial tamponade develop at different rates depending on the size of the wound and the chamber that is ruptured. Wounds made by ice picks or small knives produce slow bleeding, particularly if a low-pressure chamber such as an atrium or the right ventricle is the site of puncture. In fact, many of the wounds through the anterior chest hit the right rather than the left ventricle because the heart is rotated slightly in the chest so that the right ventricle is anterior to the left. Gunshot wounds, particularly large caliber, usually cause rapid and fatal hemorrhage if the ventricles are penetrated.

SIGNS AND SYMPTOMS

In addition to suspecting the injury from the site of wounds to the chest, the recognizable signs in the field that aid in making a diagnosis are signs of shock with neck vein distention. The capillary refill test may be normal because the vascular system may be full. The veins on the arms might be noticeably distended as well.

TREATMENT

The treatment of choice for pericardial tamponade is rapid transport to the hospital. In many cases, tamponade can be relieved and the shock state reversed while the wound is repaired. When the diagnosis is considered, rapid transport is indicated. Patients with

pericardial tamponade who reach the hospital alive have a good chance of survival.

One study with animals with experimentally induced cardiac tamponade found the MAST useful in the decompensated animals but noted that well-compensated animals might be made worse.* This is because increases in the venous pressure would be expected to increase the rate of bleeding from the heart. When the animals were hypotensive, the added pressure from the MAST raised cardiac output; this effect could conceivably gain some time for the moribund patient. Of course, local protocols should be consulted.

INTRAVENOUS THERAPY

Intravenous (IV) therapy has been used in prehospital care since the early development of advanced life support programs. There are essentially two reasons for starting an IV in the field: (1) to administer replacement fluid to patients who are hypovolemic or (2) to provide an IV access for the administration of medications.

Risk–Benefit Considerations

Fluid replacement is a temporary resuscitation measure used to help restore the vascular volume lost from hemorrhage or dehydration. The decision to start an IV in the field is covered by local protocol under the direction of medical control. Factors considered in local

---

* Davis JW, McKone TK: Hemodynamic effects of MAST in experimental cardiac tamponade. Ann Emerg Med 10:(4), 185, 1981.

protocols include time to a hospital, the condition of a patient, and the relative skills of the prehospital personnel. With severe and continuing internal bleeding, the time needed to start an IV at the scene may not be justifiable: more blood volume may be lost than can be restored during prehospital care. To avoid time delays in attempting to accomplish this procedure, many systems adopt guidelines calling either for one attempt at the scene or starting an IV during transport to the hospital. The latter strategy seeks to accomplish the dual goal of restoring intravascular volume and ensuring rapid transport to definitive care.

Types of Fluid

CRYSTALLOIDS. Crystalloids are solutions that contain water, electrolytes (electrically charged ions such as sodium, potassium, chloride, and so forth), and glucose. These solutions can diffuse across the capillary membrane. They are useful in replacing fluid and electrolytes lost during dehydration states or hemorrhage or to establish venous access for the administration of medications. Common solutions include 5% dextrose, normal saline, and lactated Ringer's solution. A 5% dextrose solution is used to keep veins open to maintain an access route for administration of intravenous medications. Normal saline (0.9% sodium chloride) and lactated Ringer's (containing sodium chloride, potassium chloride, calcium chloride, and sodium lactate) are used to expand plasma volume. Concentrated solutions of glucose (50% glucose) are used to treat hypoglycemia in adults; less concentrated solutions must be used in children and infants.

COLLOIDS. Colloids are solutions that contain large molecules that cannot diffuse out of the capillary and therefore hold or even "pull" fluid into the vascular space. They are used for the treatment of acute hemorrhage when whole blood is not immediately available. Examples of colloids are Plasmanate, albumin; and Dextran.

Neither crystalloids nor colloids can carry oxygen, and the severely hemorrhaging patient may require transfusion of blood cells. The role of these agents in hemorrhage or hypovolemia is to restore volume.

Intravenous Equipment

The equipment necessary for intravenous administration includes the solution, connecting tubing, a needle (and catheter) to gain access into the vein, and accessory equipment to cleanse the site and secure the needle and tubing in place.

An IV administration set connects the solution to the IV catheter. At the top of the set is a connector that inserts into the end of the IV bag and a drip chamber

to regulate and monitor flow rates. Depending on the purpose of IV therapy, a microdrip or a macrodrip may be connected. A macrodrip has a wide-diameter opening and allows for a faster flow rate and more rapid volume replacement. The rate of flow is adjusted by turning a stopcock and counting the number of drops per minute (10 drops equals 1 ml). In prehospital care of adult patients in shock, fluids are administered at a wide-open setting (flowing as fast as possible) for rapid restoration of volume. When used as access for medications, an infusion to keep the vein open would flow at the rate of 3 to 5 drops per minute.

Calculations of flow rates may be necessary during a prolonged transport, when treating children, or during a transfer of a patient with an IV in place.

Calculations to guide flow are best conducted in two steps.

1. First calculate the number of milliliters to be given per minute.

Example: The physician orders 180 ml per hour.

---

ml/hour = ml/60 minutes
180 ml/hour = 180 ml/60 minutes, or 3 ml/minute

---

2. Next convert number of milliliters per minute to drops per minute.

Example:

If 1 ml = 10 drops (for a given IV administration set) then 3 ml/minute = 30 drops/minute

---

In this example, assuming an IV administration set that delivers 10 drops per milliliter, to give 180 ml of fluid per hour one must deliver 3 ml or 30 drops per minute. The EMT would adjust the stopcock until it was set at the corresponding drip rate.

To have a better control of the rate of administration, microdrip administration sets can be used. Since the flow must pass through a narrow-diameter channel in the drip chamber, it is easier to control the infusion rate. With microdrips, 60 drops per minute equals 1 ml of fluid. The calculations would be done as above, substituting the different ratio of 60 drops = 1 ml. If one wanted to keep a vein open with a minidrip set-up, one could administer 15 drops per minute.

Another way to control the amount of fluid is to use Volutrols or Burotrols, which are small-volume chambers that contain no more than 100 ml and can be used to serve as the reservoir between an IV bag and the IV administration tubing. One can fill the Volutrol and then clamp the tube between the solution bag and the Volutrol, thereby limiting the maximal amount available for infusion. Volutrols are often used for medication administration.

Extension sets are lengths of IV tubing that can be inserted between the IV tube and the catheter. They provide a greater overall length, can be used to administer medications, and make it easier to change solutions.

CATHETERS

The most commonly used needle/catheter for prehospital care is the catheter-over-the-needle set (Fig. 5–19A). A plastic catheter rests over a needle. The needle is inserted in the vein and then withdrawn as the catheter is advanced into the lumen of the vein. The needle is removed and placed in a safe container, and the IV tubing is connected to the catheter. Sizes of IV catheters range from the largest 12-gauge catheters to small 25-gauge catheters. Since flow is directly proportional to the 4th power of the radius of the tube (or catheter) and inversely proportional to the length of the tube, larger catheters are preferred for rapid volume administration (e.g., 14 to 16 gauge). For example, compared to an 18-gauge catheter, a 14-gauge catheter will allow for twice the flow and a 12-gauge will allow for three times the flow.

A butterfly needle, a short needle with plastic wings that can be held during insertion, is more easily inserted but is usually reserved for situations where IV cannulation is very difficult but administration of intravenous medications is critical. It is not commonly used in prehospital care.

Text continued on page 236

P R O C E D U R E   5 – 3   ESTABLISHING AN INTRAVENOUS LINE

1. Check for and assemble the necessary equipment (Fig. 5–19B).

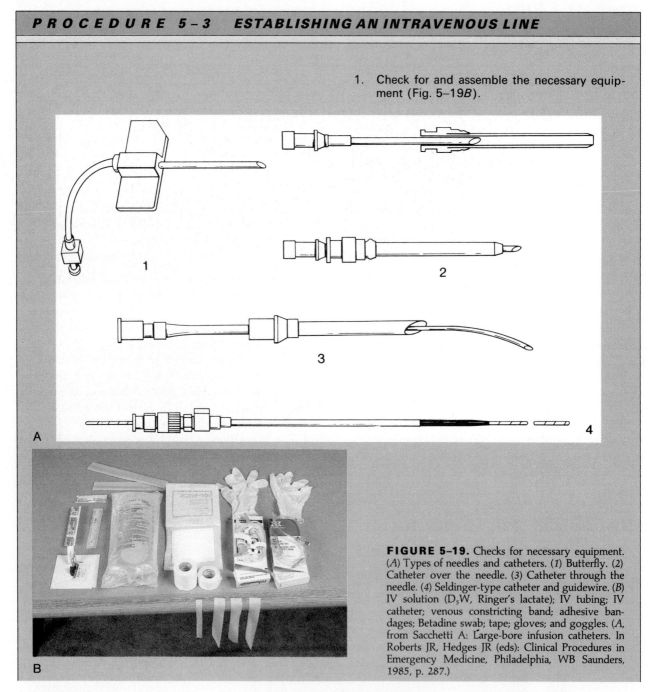

FIGURE 5–19. Checks for necessary equipment. (A) Types of needles and catheters. (1) Butterfly. (2) Catheter over the needle. (3) Catheter through the needle. (4) Seldinger-type catheter and guidewire. (B) IV solution (D$_5$W, Ringer's lactate); IV tubing; IV catheter; venous constricting band; adhesive bandages; Betadine swab; tape; gloves; and goggles. (A, from Sacchetti A: Large-bore infusion catheters. In Roberts JR, Hedges JR (eds): Clinical Procedures in Emergency Medicine, Philadelphia, WB Saunders, 1985, p. 287.)

2. Examine the IV bag for leaks, the type of solution, contamination, and expiration date (Fig. 5–20).

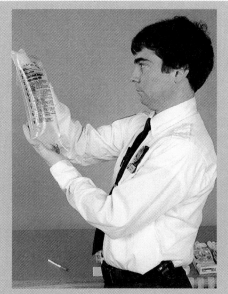

FIGURE 5–20. Properly examine IV bag for leaks, type of solution, contamination, and expiration date.

3. Connect the IV tubing to the solution aseptically (Fig. 5–21).

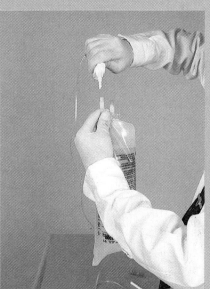

FIGURE 5–21. Connect IV tubing and solution aseptically.

4. Squeeze the drip chamber until it is half full of solution and then allow the solution to flow through the entire length of the IV tubing, making sure there is no air in the tubing (Fig. 5–22).

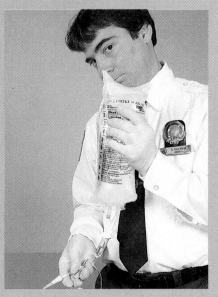

FIGURE 5–22. Correctly prepare IV solution and administration set: drip chamber half full and IV solution in tubing without air.

Continued

5. Prepare the patient psychologically, explaining that you will be inserting a needle into the vein and securing the tubing in place to administer fluids or medications. Apply a venous constricting band tight enough to obstruct venous flow but *not* arterial flow (check distal pulse) (Fig. 5–23*A* and *B*).

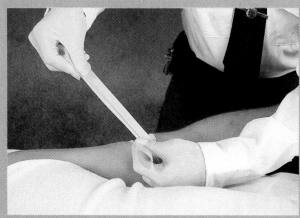 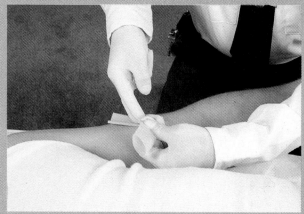

A   B

FIGURE 5–23. Apply venous constricting band.

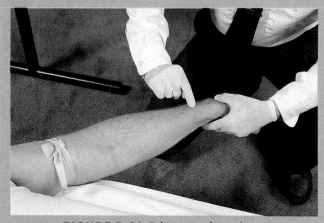

FIGURE 5–24. Palpate vein for resilience.

6. Select a site for IV insertion in the hand, forearm, or crease of the elbow. Palpate the vein for resilience and cleanse the puncture site with an antiseptic swab (e.g., Betadine) by making increasingly larger concentric circles, spiraling outward from the site of insertion (Figs. 5–24 and 5–25).

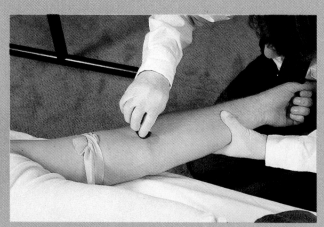

FIGURE 5–25. Cleanse puncture site area with Betadine in increasingly larger *concentric circles* that spiral outward.

7. Stabilize the vein aseptically with the thumb, stretching the skin distal to the point of insertion, and enter the skin aseptically with the needle at a 45° angle with the over-the-catheter needle bevel up (Fig. 5–26).

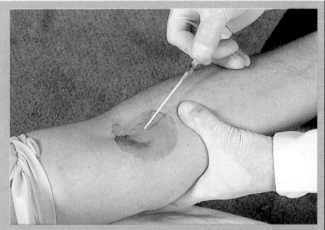

FIGURE 5–26. Stabilize vein aseptically with thumb and fingers.

8. After entering the skin, keep the needle parallel with the vein, inserting through the vein either from the side or above. Upon entering the vein you will feel "give" or a "pop" while observing for flashback of blood into the proximal chamber of the needle (Fig. 5–27).

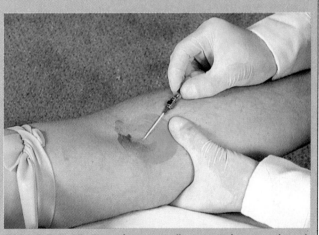

9. Hold the needle in place and advance the catheter into the vein while stabilizing the needle (Fig. 5–28).

FIGURE 5–27. Enter skin aseptically at a 45-degree angle with the over-the-catheter needle bevel-up.

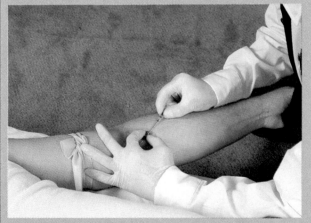

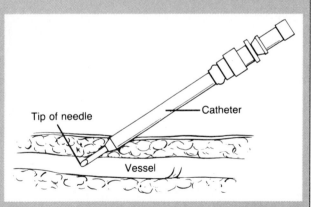

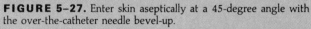

Tip of needle — Catheter
Vessel

FIGURE 5–28 Puncture the vein. Observe for flashback, and advance the over-the-needle catheter 1 mm more into vein. (*Right*, from Sacchetti A: Large-bore infusion catheters. In Roberts JR, Hedges JR (eds): Clinical Procedures in Emergency Medicine, Philadelphia, WB Saunders, 1985, p. 287.)

Continued.

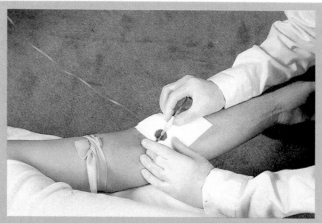

FIGURE 5–29. Withdraw the needle while applying digital pressure proximal to the venipuncture site to inhibit bleeding. Connect the IV tubing to the IV catheter.

10. Withdraw the needle while applying pressure proximal to the insertion site with your finger to inhibit bleeding. Dispose of the needle in a special container for sharp objects (Fig. 5–29).

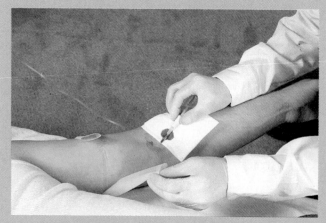

FIGURE 5–30. Remove the venous constricting band.

11. Connect the IV tubing to the IV catheter and remove the venous constricting band (Fig. 5–30).

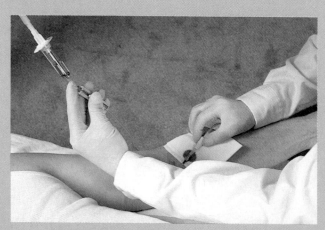

FIGURE 5–31. Open the drip chamber clamp to ensure free flow, lower the IV bag and observe for backflow of blood, and then adjust to appropriate keep-vein-open (KVO) drip rate (1 drop every 4 seconds).

12. Open the drip chamber clamp or stopcock to ensure free flow and lower the IV bag to observe for backflow of blood. Adjust the flow rate to the appropriate KVO (keep vein open [1 drop every 4 seconds]) (Fig. 5–31).

13. Apply a bandage over the puncture site and anchor the IV catheter with a chevron (criss-crossing of tape around the catheter connector) (Figs. 5–32 and 5–33).

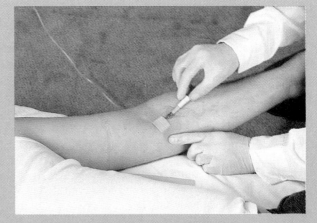

FIGURE 5–32. Apply an adhesive bandage over the puncture site.

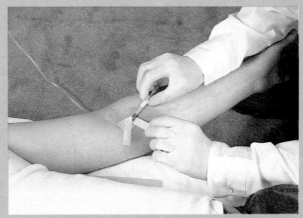

FIGURE 5–33. Anchor the IV catheter with a chevron.

14. Secure the tubing with tape, leaving the tubing/catheter junction exposed. If the IV site is at a joint, apply a rigid armboard to prevent flexion and obstruction of flow (Figs. 5–34 and 5–35).
15. Recheck the drip rate or adjust the flow according to orders. Label the IV puncture area with the catheter gauge, length, date, time, and your initials.

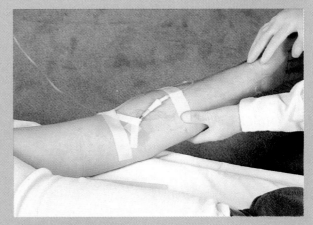

FIGURE 5–34. Secure the tubing with tape, leaving the tubing/catheter junction exposed.

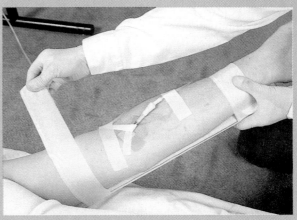

FIGURE 5–35. Apply an armboard if the venipuncture site is a flexion point on an extremity.

Complications

Complications of IV therapy should be understood. The complications and some causes are listed.

INFECTION

Breach of sterile technique can introduce foreign matter, including bacteria, from the patient's or your skin or from a contaminated needle directly into the patient's bloodstream. This is prevented by careful sterile technique. If for any reason sterile technique is breached and the catheter must remain in the patient as a critical "life line," be sure to inform hospital staff.

PYROGENIC REACTION

Patients can have an adverse reaction to an IV solution or more likely to contaminants within the solution. This can manifest as sudden fever, chills, vomiting, backache, or even cardiovascular collapse.

Stop the IV and change to a different solution if this is suspected.

INFILTRATION

Fluid can leak into subcutaneous tissue near the IV insertion site. This is most commonly caused by a misplaced IV or rupture of the vessel. It manifests as swelling around the catheter tip; the IV will stop running, and the patient may complain of swelling or pain. Bleeding from the vein may cause a hematoma at the site.

Remove the IV and hold direct pressure over the site. Then start a new IV proximally or on the other arm.

THROMBOPHLEBITIS

Inflammation of the vein can be caused by prolonged IV therapy.

CIRCULATORY OVERLOAD

A runaway IV can cause overload of circulatory volume. This is prevented by using small bags of IV solution and monitoring fluid closely. It is a special concern with heart disease patients.

AIR EMBOLISM

Air embolism is caused by air leaking into the IV line. Be sure to clear IV tubing and syringes of air prior to administration. A large bolus of air can cause embolism to the heart and lungs.

CATHETER SHEAR

Tearing of the catheter with the needle can occur, and the catheter tip can dislodge and travel distally, causing an embolism. Do not reinsert the needle into the catheter once it is withdrawn, and avoid twisting the catheter about the needle, which are the most common causes of this problem.

ARTERIAL PUNCTURE

Accidental insertion into an artery can cause arterial puncture. Should this occur, withdraw the needle and apply firm pressure over the site for at least 5 minutes. Avoid venipuncture over pulsatile areas, especially where the common pulse points in the upper arm are located.

EMT Safety

Be careful to avoid unnecessary self-contamination with blood by wearing gloves and other personal safety equipment. Make certain that you dispose of contaminated needles in an appropriate "sharps" container (see Chapter 12, Medical Emergencies). Carry the sharps container with you to the patient to facilitate proper disposal of needles.

SUMMARY

Cardiac emergencies may result in rapid and irreversible sudden death. Conditions such as shock and myocardial infarction require careful attention to airway, breathing, and circulation and rapid transport to the hospital. The protocol included in this chapter summarizes the proper approach to the cardiac patient. It is important to know and follow the protocols in your local region.

REVIEW EXERCISES

1. Define *shock* and explain its effect on the body cells.
2. List three signs of epinephrine release.
3. List four types of shock and provide one example of a cause for each.
4. Given a percentage of blood loss, indicate the likely associated signs and symptoms.
5. List four methods for controlling bleeding and describe the technique for each.
6. List uses for military antishock trousers (MAST).
7. List the contraindications to the use of MAST and three reasons for not inflating the abdominal section of the garment.
8. Describe the application process for the MAST.
9. List the signs and symptoms of pericardial tamponade and cardiac contusion and describe emergency care for each.
10. Define *arteriosclerosis* and *atherosclerosis*.

11. List the three major controllable risk factors of coronary heart disease.

12. Define the following terms:
    Angina
    Myocardial infarction
    Ischemic chest pain

13. List signs and symptoms of angina and the steps of its management.

14. Explain two ways that nitroglycerin works to relieve chest pain.

15. List signs and symptoms of myocardial infarction and the steps of its management.

16. Define *cardiogenic shock, chronic congestive heart failure,* and *pulmonary edema.*

17. List signs and symptoms of pulmonary edema and the steps of its management.

REFERENCES

American Heart Association: Advanced Cardiac Life Support Manual. Dallas, American Heart Association, 1985

Bates B: A Guide to Physical Examination, 3rd ed. Philadelphia, JB Lippincott, 1983

Guyton AC: Textbook of Medical Physiology, 8th ed. Philadelphia, WB Saunders, 1991

Morton R, Frumkin K: Pneumatic anti-shock garment. In Roberts JR, Hedges JR (eds): Clinical Procedures in Emergency Medicine, 2nd ed. Philadelphia, WB Saunders, 1991, pp 421–431

Prehospital Trauma Life Support Committee of the National Association of EMTs: Pre-hospital Trauma Life Support. Akron, Ohio, Emergency Training, 1986

Rosen P, et al (eds): Emergency Medicine: Concepts and Clinical Practice. St Louis, CV Mosby, 1983

Safer P, Bircher NG: Cardiopulmonary Cerebral Resuscitation, 3rd ed. Philadelphia, WB Saunders, 1988

Standards and guidelines for cardiopulmonary resuscitation and emergency cardiac care. JAMA 255(21):2905–2984, 1986

Zuidema GD, Rutherford RB, Ballinger WF (eds): The Management of Trauma, 4th ed. Philadelphia, WB Saunders, 1985

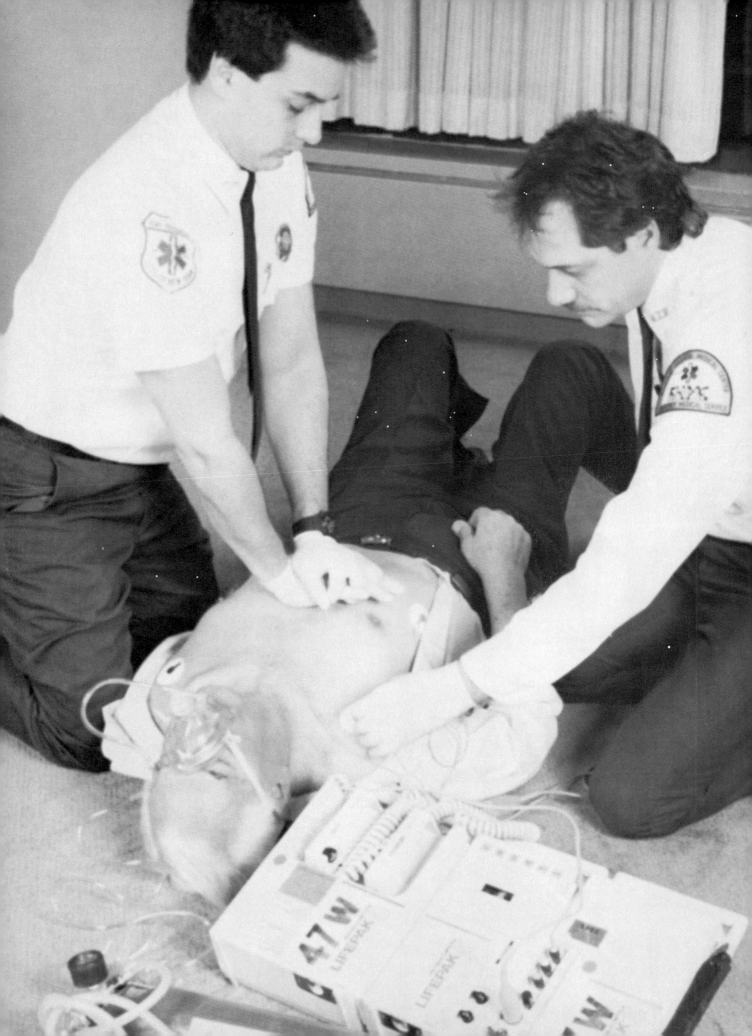

CHAPTER 6

CPR AND EMT DEFIBRILLATION

O B J E C T I V E S

At the conclusion of this chapter the reader will be able to:

1. Demonstrate on a manikin one-rescuer CPR for an adult, infant, and child.

2. Describe the switch from one-rescuer CPR to two-rescuer CPR.

3. Explain under what circumstances CPR should be started.

4. Define "ECG," "electrodes," and "leads."

5. Explain which two factors are used jointly to determine the need for defibrillation.

6. List the basic steps in the defibrillation procedure.

7. Identify the basic differences between manual, automatic, and semiautomatic defibrillators.

CARDIOPULMONARY RESUSCITATION

Introduction

Cardiopulmonary arrest is the cessation of heart function and ventilations. The patient in cardiopulmonary arrest has no ventilations and no pulse, and is clinically dead. The process of biologic death begins as the cells are deprived of oxygen. If the patient remains in cardiopulmonary arrest for longer than 4 to 6 minutes, irreversible brain damage is likely to occur. The longer the patient remains in this state, the lower the chance for survival. Because the brain is more sensitive to oxygen deprivation than any other organ, resuscitation after prolonged cardiac arrest may result in restoration of the heart beat but not of brain function.

The importance of prompt treatment, namely cardiopulmonary resuscitation and further treatments to restore heart function, cannot be overemphasized. *Cardiopulmonary resuscitation* (CPR) is a technique employing artificial ventilations and circulation designed to provide some oxygenation and perfusion of the body until measures to restore a functional heart beat can be implemented. CPR forestalls biologic death, gaining time for the brain until advanced life support (ALS) can be administered. With CPR a patient suffering cardiac arrest may recover without irreversible brain damage even after prolonged periods of cardiac arrest. ALS includes defibrillation, fluid and drug administration, and surgical techniques as necessary to resuscitate a patient. The exact type of ALS required depends on the cause of cardiac arrest. Time from the onset of cardiac arrest to the commencement of CPR and ALS is the major factor in determining the outcome for patients in cardiac arrest.

In some cases, CPR itself may resuscitate a patient in cardiac arrest. These cases usually are caused by ventilatory problems such as an obstructed airway or drowning (and some cases of primary heart disease) wherein CPR is begun shortly after the patient's heart stops beating. For example, in a case of cardiac arrest secondary to airway obstruction, by relieving the obstruction and then providing ventilation and circulation for the victim, oxygenated blood can perfuse the brain and heart, which may be adequate to restore spontaneous heart activity.

It is infrequent, however, that CPR by itself restores a functional heart rhythm. The best chance of survival from cardiac arrest is when both CPR and ALS measures are begun promptly.

The type of ALS required depends on the cause of cardiac arrest. For example, if cardiac arrest is secondary to hemorrhage, restoration of blood volume and surgical intervention are the only chance for survival. Likewise, an obstructed airway unrelieved by ALS maneuvers may require cricothyroidotomy or a tracheostomy. If the cardiac arrest is secondary to a myocardial infarction and its dysrhythmias, such as ventricular fibrillation, early defibrillation and/or drug therapy is the critical intervention.

Causes of Cardiac Arrest

The cause of cardiac arrest should be determined whenever possible. While CPR is initiated, quickly look for signs of hemorrhage or trauma, and ask any bystanders for a brief history of the events preceding cardiac arrest. An obstructed airway will be evident as you attempt to ventilate.

The local protocols of your EMS system determine your strategy regarding the site of further ALS treatment and patient transport decisions while CPR is continued. For example, you have a patient with a history of myocardial infarction before cardiac arrest. If the paramedics can arrive in 8 minutes and the hospital is 15 minutes away, your protocols may call for performing CPR at the scene to allow for earlier ALS intervention. On the other hand, if the patient showed signs of profuse internal bleeding, such as the vomiting of large amounts of blood before cardiac arrest, your actions should include rapid transport to the closest facility capable of blood volume restoration and surgical intervention. Children almost always suffer cardiac arrest secondary to respiratory problems, trauma, or hypovolemia. Because the cause is so rarely cardiac in nature, almost all systems call for rapid transport to a medical facility while performing CPR en route.

Again, local protocols dictate the procedure to follow. While CPR is continued, subsequent treatment and transport decisions are undertaken. Key to making the appropriate decision, however, is the EMT's diagnosis of the most probable condition that led to cardiac arrest.

Definitive Treatment for Ischemic Heart Disease, Dysrhythmias, and Cardiac Arrest

When cardiac arrest is the result of dysrhythmias such as ventricular fibrillation secondary to ischemic heart disease, studies have proved the benefit of early CPR in conjunction with ALS on patient survival. *Ventricular fibrillation*, a disorganized and nonproductive quivering of the heart muscle, is the most commonly encountered rhythm in victims of sudden death who are reached within minutes of cardiac arrest. Ventricular fibrillation results in no cardiac output, and patients are pulseless

TABLE 6-1. Survival Rate from Cardiac Arrest due to Ventricular Fibrillation as Related to Promptness of Initiation of CPR and ALS

Initiation of CPR (minutes)	Arrival of ALS (minutes)	Survival Rate (%)
<4	<8	43
<4	16	10
8-12	<16	6
8-12	>16	0
12	>12	0

(Data from Seattle Heart Watch and American Heart Association: Textbook of Advanced Cardiac Life Support. Dallas, American Heart Association, 1981, p. II-7.)

and require CPR. This dysrhythmia is a leading cause of sudden death, and its victims usually have no evidence of myocardial infarction. If these patients can be resuscitated, they can often lead full lives, without any disability.

Resuscitation of patients experiencing cardiac arrest and ventricular fibrillation is a goal of EMS systems. As shown in the example in Table 6-1, studies emphasize the need for prompt application of CPR (by laypersons as well as professionals) and early initiation of ALS (be it prehospital or hospital-based) if a large percentage of victims are to survive. When CPR was initiated within 4 minutes and ALS within 8 minutes, 43% of the patients with cardiac arrest and ventricular fibrillation survived. As the time lapse before CPR and ALS lengthened, the survival rate dropped drastically.

Traumatic cardiac arrest requires rapid hospital treatment. Early transport of patients with potentially fatal traumatic injuries should be a high priority before decompensation and cardiac arrest ensue. One study reported on patients with penetrating heart wounds who were judged capable of being saved with rapid operating room treatment. These patients all had potentially lethal injuries and signs of life when the ambulance arrived. The group of patients who received more extensive prehospital therapy at the expense of extra time in the field (average of 25 minutes in the field) had no survivors, whereas similar patients who received more limited prehospital therapy and spent less time in the field (average of 9 minutes) had a 67% survival rate. Although the study was small, it emphasized the importance of prompt transport of patients with penetrating heart wounds (Gervin and Fischer, 1982).

Systems Approach

Resuscitation of patients in cardiac arrest requires a systems approach to emergency care. One goal is to recognize conditions that might lead to cardiac arrest and institute appropriate treatment before it occurs. Once cardiac arrest occurs, CPR is begun along with efforts to effect prompt delivery of ALS. The selection of the type of ALS intervention depends on the EMT's assessment of the most likely cause of the arrest. Local protocols should be followed after ascertaining the cause of cardiac arrest.

One-Rescuer CPR

Obstruction of the airway, respiratory depression or arrest, and circulatory problems are always of primary concern to the EMT and are therefore addressed first in the primary survey. When encountering an unconscious patient, you must be systematic and carefully assess and treat the patient according to this prescribed sequence. The purpose of CPR is to provide oxygenation and perfusion to patients in respiratory and cardiac arrest. This is accomplished through airway maintenance, artificial ventilation, and chest compressions.

One-rescuer CPR is necessary when only two EMTs are available for the resuscitation. CPR is maintained using the one-rescuer method while equipment is readied to transport the patient to the hospital.

The first step in CPR is to establish unresponsiveness (see Fig. 6-1). Gently shake the patient and shout, "Are you okay?" To avoid aggravation of a potential neck injury in patients with suspected spinal injury, you should apply a painful stimulus such as a pinch rather than shaking the patient. Note the response of the patient to verbal and painful stimuli. If the patient is alert and responsive, no further interventions are necessary. This phase of assessment quickly rules out the need for the next phase of CPR. If the patient is unresponsive, continue with the next step of CPR—the call for help.

Call for help. The call for help recognizes that most cardiac arrest victims are discovered by laypersons. It alerts others within the sound of your voice that assistance is required. This assistance includes activation of the EMS system and participation in CPR performance by others trained in this skill. For an EMT, the call for help relates to the call for additional personnel to assist in the resuscitation and patient transport, or the dual response of EMT-paramedics.

Place the unresponsive patient in a supine position. Use the log roll or a modification of the log roll to turn the patient over, as available help permits. Be careful to support the head if you suspect injuries of the cervical spine (see Fig. 2-26).

AIRWAY AND BREATHING ASSESSMENT

When the patient is supine you must ensure a patent airway. The most common cause of airway obstruction occurs when the tongue falls against the back of the throat as the muscles of an unconscious victim relax. The tongue is attached to the lower jaw. Bringing the jaw forward lifts the tongue away from the back of the throat and opens the airway. Use either the head tilt/chin lift or jaw-thrust maneuver to open the airway.

HEAD TILT/CHIN LIFT. Place the fingers of one hand along the bony margin of the patient's lower jaw. Lift the patient's jaw anteriorly without closing the mouth while performing a head tilt with the other hand (see Fig. 6–2A).

JAW THRUST (Without Head Tilt). The jaw thrust maneuver should be used when dealing with patients who have a suspected cervical spine injury. Without tilting the patient's head, place your index and middle fingers beneath the angle of the patient's jaw (just below the ears), and your thumbs on the cheekbones (see Fig. 6–2B). The thumbs are used for the counterpressure needed to displace the jaw without tilting the head. Displace the jaw upward with your fingers.

If ventilations are ineffective in the neutral position, it might be necessary to slightly extend the neck.

BREATHING. Once the airway is open, evaluate the effectiveness of breathing. *Place your ear over the patient's mouth and nose,* and *look toward the patient's chest and abdomen.* In this position you can *look* for the chest to rise and fall, *listen* for air escaping during exhalation, and *feel* the victim's breath on your cheek (see Fig. 6–3).

If the patient is breathing spontaneously, continue to ensure airway patency by manual maneuvers or the insertion of an oropharyngeal or nasopharyngeal airway, as required.

If you cannot see, hear, or feel the patient breathing, or if the ventilations are inadequate, begin positive-pressure ventilations.

VENTILATIONS. Positive-pressure ventilations can be administered by several methods. In situations where devices capable of delivering forced air are not immediately available, begin mouth-to-mouth or mouth-to-nose resuscitation. More often you will use mechanical aids such as the pocket mask, bag-valve mask, or manually triggered demand valve resuscitator to deliver high-concentration oxygenation.

MOUTH-TO-MASK VENTILATION. Seal the mask around the patient's face, using two hands, while maintaining a head tilt/chin lift to keep the airway open. Take a deep breath, and seal your mouth around the port of the mask. Administer two smooth breaths while observing for chest rise.

Chest excursion is the best indicator of an effective ventilation. Chest rise signals the end-point of each breath to avoid overinflation and gastric distention (air in the stomach). In an average adult, visible chest excursion correlates with a tidal volume of approximately 700 to 800 ml of air.

After each breath, remove your mouth from the mask's port and inhale. Each breath should take about 1 to 1.5 seconds to deliver, and the volume of air required is about 800 to 1200 ml (see Fig. 6–4).

If you encounter resistance to ventilation, reopen the airway and attempt to ventilate again. You may wish to try a different airway maneuver.

If the head tilt/chin lift maneuver initially was ineffective, the jaw thrust might prove more effective. If this maneuver is unsuccessful, the obstructed-airway procedure should be followed (see Chapter 3).

PULSE CHECK

The absence of a pulse is the primary indicator of cardiac arrest. Absence of ventilatory efforts, unresponsiveness, dilated pupils, skin color, and even electrocardiographic (ECG) tracings are only supportive indicators of cardiac arrest. A check for pulselessness must be done for 5 to 10 seconds. This is important because a slow heart rate may otherwise be mistaken for cardiac arrest. The pulse used is the carotid pulse in the neck.

Locate the larynx in the midline of the neck, above the suprasternal notch. Slide your index and middle fingers down the groove created by the larynx and sternocleidomastoid muscle on the side of the patient at which you are kneeling. Palpate gently for 5 to 10 seconds (see Fig. 6–5).

If you feel a pulse, continue to maintain the airway and provide positive-pressure ventilations, if necessary, at a rate of 1 breath every 5 seconds. Reevaluate the pulse periodically. If no pulse is felt in the unresponsive patient with no ventilations, cardiac compressions need to be performed.

ACTIVATION OF EMS SYSTEM. The activation of the EMS system is the next step of CPR. Three diagnostic checks have been made in these first few seconds: responsiveness, breathing, and pulse. This information, along with the history of events leading to the cardiac arrest, allows the dispatcher to determine the most appropriate response within the system.

EXTERNAL CARDIAC COMPRESSIONS

External cardiac compressions provide blood flow in two ways. The first is through changes in the intrathoracic pressure during the compression and relaxation phases of the compression cycle. The second, by squeezing the heart between the sternum and the spine, contributes to blood flow. The exact forces that provide blood flow are being investigated and may vary in degree from patient to patient.

The blood flow provided during external compressions is usually not sufficient to support consciousness (although some patients may be conscious).

PATIENT POSITION. For chest compressions to be effective, the patient must be in the supine position on a hard surface. If the patient is in a bed, he should be transferred to a rolling cot stretcher with a spine board placed beneath the head and back. This minimizes the absorption of compressions by the stretcher mattress. If a stretcher or backboard is not immediately available, the patient should be moved from the bed to the floor. CPR should not be stopped while waiting for a backboard.

HAND POSITION. Position yourself to the side of the patient with your knees close to the patient and slightly separated, so that you can easily move from compressions to ventilations. The proper location of the hands while performing cardiac compressions is on the lower half of the sternum, about one fingerbreadth above the xiphoid process. To locate this position, use the index and middle fingers on the hand closest to the patient's feet, find the lower margin of the rib cage in the upper abdomen (see Fig. 6–6A), and slide your fingers upward to the inferior tip of the sternum (see Fig. 6–6B). With your two fingers on the lowest tip of the sternum, place the heel of your other hand immediately adjacent to the index finger on the sternum (see Fig. 6–6C). Only the heel of the hand should be in contact with the breast bone so that the force of compressions is directly over the sternum. Place the heel of your other hand directly on top of the hand on the sternum (see Fig. 6–6D). Keep your fingers up and off the chest wall. You may interlock your fingers to pull them away from the chest wall.

Proper hand position results in more effective compressions and minimizes injuries that may result from improper placement of the hands (and fingers) on the xiphoid or rib cage during chest compressions.

BODY POSITION. Position your shoulders directly over the lower half of the patient's sternum and lock your elbows. There should be a straight line from your shoulders to the heel of your hand, perpendicular to the patient's sternum. This position allows for more effective use of your body—bending at the hip while performing compressions (see Fig. 6–7).

Compress straight down, bending slightly at the hips during the downward thrust. Pressure should be applied only with the heel of your hand, compressing the sternum about 1.5 to 2 inches in adult patients. After compressing, release all pressure and allow the sternum to rise completely without removing your hands from the sternum. Each compression should be smooth and rhythmic, with about half of the time spent in the compression phase and half of the time in the release phase.

RATE AND RATIO. With one-rescuer CPR, continuous cycles of 15 compressions and two ventilations are performed after the initial two breaths. The compressions are performed at a rate of 80 to 100 per minute. To maintain this rate you can use a counting method. A commonly used counting method that can achieve this rate is "1 and 2 and 3 and 4 . . . and 15." The count should be rhythmic to reinforce the 50/50 distribution of the compression and relaxation phases during each compression. At the end of 15 compressions, two ventilations are administered, again observing chest rise to ensure delivery of an adequate volume of air. The 15:2 compression ratio is maintained throughout the performance of one-rescuer CPR.

PULSE CHECK. After the completion of four complete cycles (1 minute), the EMT should reevaluate the patient to determine if he is still in cardiopulmonary arrest. At this time, give two breaths and check the pulse. If the pulse is still absent, two more ventilations are administered, and compressions are continued. Thereafter, the pulse is checked every few minutes but without interrupting CPR for more than 5 seconds with each check. Table 6–2 summarizes the performance of one-rescuer CPR.

TABLE 6–2. Summary of One-Rescuer CPR

Establish unresponsiveness
Call for help
Position the victim
Open the airway
Check for breathing
Deliver two breaths and watch for chest rise
Check the carotid pulse
Activate the EMS system
Begin external chest compression on a hard surface
    Hand position/landmark check
    Depth: 1.5–2 inches
    Rate: 80–100 per minute
    Ratio: 15 compressions/2 ventilations
    Rhythm: "*One* and *two* and . . . *fifteen*"
Reevaluate pulse at 1 minute and then every few minutes

PROCEDURE 6–1   PERFORMING ONE-RESCUER CPR

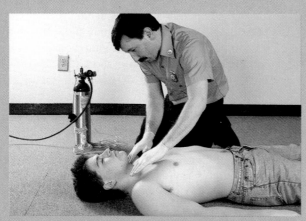

FIGURE 6–1. Checking for responsiveness.

1. Establish unresponsiveness and position the patient (Fig. 6–1).

2. Open the airway using head tilt/chin lift or jaw-thrust maneuver (Fig. 6–2A and B).

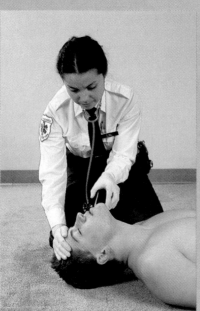

A

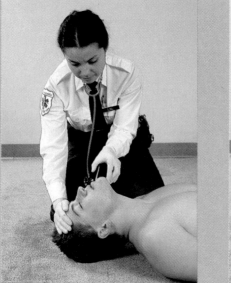

B

FIGURE 6–2. (A) Head tilt/chin lift. (B) Jaw thrust.

3. Look, listen, and feel for breathing (Fig. 6–3).

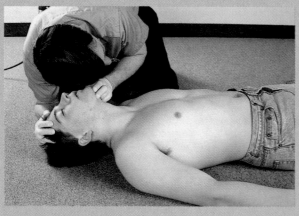

FIGURE 6–3. Establishing breathlessness.

4. Provide positive-pressure ventilation (2 breaths) and observe chest rise (Fig. 6–4).
5. Check for a carotid pulse (Fig. 6–5).

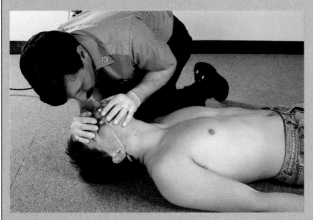

FIGURE 6–4. Mouth-to-mask ventilation.

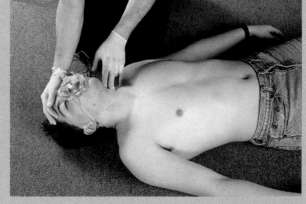

FIGURE 6–5. Check for carotid pulse.

6. Locate the correct hand position (Fig. 6–6*A* to *C*).
7. Keep fingers off chest wall (Fig. 6–6*D*).

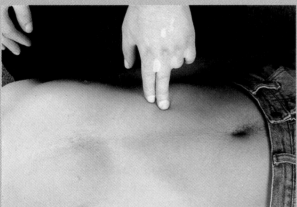

A

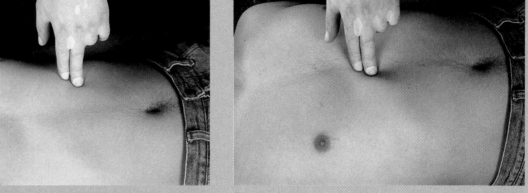

B

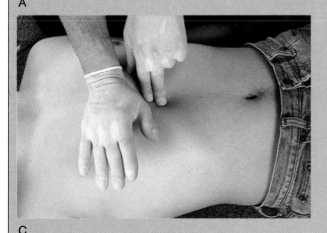

C

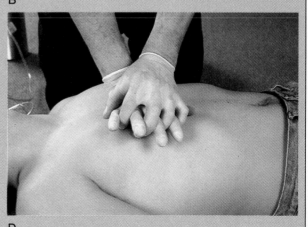

D

FIGURE 6–6. Locate the correct hand position by (*A*) placing your index and middle fingers of the hand closest to the patient's feet along the margin of the ribs and (*B*) sliding up to the bottom of the breast bone. (*C*) Place the heel of the hand closest to the patient's head next to your fingers, and (*D*) place the heel of the other hand directly over the hand on the sternum and interlock your fingers to avoid pressure in the area of the ribs.

Continued

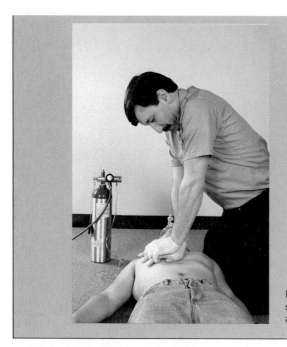

8. Maintain correct body position (Fig. 6–7).
9. Perform 4 cycles of 15 compressions/2 ventilations.
10. Recheck the pulse after 4 cycles and every few minutes thereafter.

FIGURE 6–7. While performing chest compressions, your shoulders, elbows, and the heels of your hands should be in alignment directly over the patient's sternum.

Two-Rescuer CPR

There are several advantages to having two rescuers to perform CPR. It is less fatiguing, it increases the frequency of ventilations per minute (12 instead of 8), and it permits the employment of mechanical aids and supplemental oxygen. It also permits the second rescuer to evaluate the effectiveness of cardiac compressions by checking for a transmitted pulse.

When two EMTs arrive to find a patient in cardiac arrest, one may begin one-rescuer CPR while the other readies the monitor-defibrillator and other necessary equipment for treatment and transport, radios for paramedic assistance at the scene, and so forth. When the number of available personnel permits, two-rescuer CPR should be started immediately.

TRANSITION OF ONE-RESCUER CPR TO TWO-RESCUER CPR

One-rescuer CPR may be necessary while a second rescuer readies equipment or calls for help, or it may be in progress on arrival at the scene. To minimize interruption of CPR during the integration of a second rescuer, a universal approach has been developed. As a second rescuer, advise the first rescuer that you will assist and position yourself on the opposite side of the patient from the first rescuer, and ready yourself to begin compressions.

The first rescuer then completes the compression cycle, gives two breaths and checks the pulse. If there is still no pulse, the first rescuer gives one breath and signals you to begin compressions (Fig. 6–8 and Table 6–3).

COMPRESSIONS AND VENTILATIONS

The rate and ratio of compressions to ventilations, administration of a breath, and switching from one rescuer to the other are covered in this section.

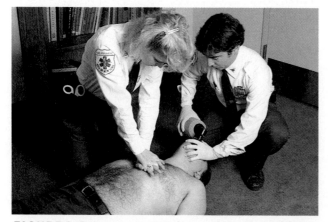

FIGURE 6–8. Two-rescuer CPR showing the positions of the two rescuers.

TABLE 6–3. Summary of Transition of One-Rescuer CPR to Two-Rescuer CPR

Rescuer 2 positions himself for compressions
Rescuer 1 administers 2 breaths and checks for a pulse
Rescuer 1 administers one breath
Tells rescuer 2 to resume compressions
Compressions and ventilations
    Ratio: 5 compressions/1 ventilation
    Rate: 80–100 per minute
    Pause after fifth compression for ventilation
Switch and pulse check

RATE AND RATIO.   In two-rescuer CPR the ratio of compressions to ventilation is 5:1. The compression rate in two-rescuer CPR is also 80 to 100 compressions per minute. At the end of 5 compressions, the compressor pauses to allow the ventilator to give one breath and then CPR is resumed. Use a rhythmic cadence to help maintain the 50/50 distribution of the compression cycle.

ADMINISTERING A BREATH.   Breaths are administered after the fifth compression. The ventilator is ready to ventilate when the compressor says "5-...."; the ventilator then administers the breath as the compressor pauses. Chest rise is again the indication that an adequate ventilatory volume has been administered. The compressor can then start the first compression of the next cycle with little interruption.

THE SWITCH AND PULSE CHECK.   CPR, especially the compression of the patient's chest, is a physically fatiguing process. For this reason, a procedure has been developed so that the rescuers can switch roles, thus sharing the role of compressor.

At the direction of the *compressor*, the switch is initiated. The ventilator administers one breath after the fifth compression and then repositions himself for compressions. At the same time, the compressor moves toward the head, checks the pulse for 5 seconds, administers one breath, and tells the new compressor to resume compressions.

The switch should be performed every few minutes or when the compressor becomes fatigued.

TWO RESCUERS STARTING TOGETHER

When two rescuers start together, one assumes the role of ventilator and the other the role of compressor.

All initial evaluation procedures (check for unresponsiveness, breathing, and pulse) are performed by the ventilator. On documenting breathlessness, the ventilator administers two breaths and checks the pulse. If there is no pulse, the ventilator signals the beginning of compressions and the two rescuers proceed as described above.

Infant CPR

For purposes of CPR performance, an *infant* is defined as someone less than 1 year of age; a *child* is defined as someone between the ages of 1 and 8 years. These are only guidelines. Most cardiac arrests in infants and children are the result of accidents or respiratory problems. Below the age of 1 year, congenital malformations, infections, and sudden infant death syndrome (SIDS) are the leading causes of cardiac arrest. In children over age 1, accidental and violent injuries are the leading cause. Rapid transport to a hospital is a high priority. Airway obstruction, severe blood loss, and head injuries are conditions that may require rapid surgical intervention. Excessive time spent on the scene is likely to decrease the chances for survival.

The following procedures are designed to provide a chronologic, prioritized, and systematic approach to an unconscious infant. There are steps of assessment you should take, followed by treatments appropriate to the problem. For example, mouth-to-mouth and mouth-to-nose breathing is administered only after cessation of breathing has been documented. Cardiac compressions are administered after the pulse check. You should adhere carefully to the prescribed sequence to ensure the early treatment of the most life-threatening problems.

P R O C E D U R E   6 – 2   *PERFORMING CPR ON AN INFANT*

1. *Establish unresponsiveness.* Gently shake the infant and briskly tap the bottom of the feet or apply a painful stimulus such as a pinch. During this phase of assessment, you should give careful consideration to the possibility of spinal injury.

   Note the response of the infant to the shaking and painful stimuli. If the infant becomes responsive, no further interventions may be necessary. This phase of assessment may quickly rule out the need for the next phase of CPR. Should the patient not respond, continue with the next step of CPR—the call for help.

2. If a patient is unresponsive, place him on the back to perform further evaluation. Turn the patient

carefully to avoid spinal injury. This is particularly important if an injury caused the unconsciousness.

3. Establish a clear airway. Airway obstruction occurs most commonly when the tongue falls to the back of the throat as the muscles of an unconscious victim relax. Because the tongue is attached to the lower jaw, bringing the jaw forward lifts the tongue away from the back of the throat and opens the airway. With the infant, hyperextension of the neck should be avoided. Rather, tilt the head into a sniffing or neutral position. The head tilt/chin lift or jaw thrust without head tilt maneuvers may be used.

Continued

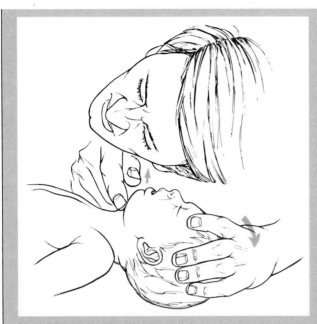

FIGURE 6–9. Chin lift in infant.

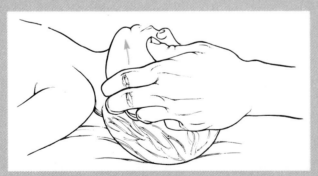

FIGURE 6–10. The jaw thrust-without head tilt.

4. Place one finger at the base of the chin while tilting the head backward, being careful not to overextend. Then lift the chin, being careful not to close the mouth (Fig. 6–9) or

5. Without tilting the head, place your thumbs on the cheek bones of the patient. Place your index and middle fingers beneath the angle of the jaw (just below the ears). Then displace the jaw upward with your fingers while maintaining counterpressure with your thumbs and opening the mouth. This technique should be used when dealing with patients with suspected spinal injury in the neck region. IMPORTANT: DO NOT TILT HEAD BACK. It might be necessary to slightly extend the neck if ventilations are ineffective with the neck in the neutral position (Fig. 6–10).

6. Once the airway is open, evaluate for breathing. Place your ear over the patient's mouth and nose, and look toward the patient's chest and abdomen. In this position you can *look* for the chest to rise and fall; listen for air escaping during exhalation; and feel the patient's breath on your cheek.

   If the patient is breathing spontaneously, continue to ensure a clear airway by manual maneuvers. If you cannot see, hear, or feel the patient breathing, or if the breathing is inadequate, begin mouth-to-mouth-and-nose breathing.

7. After establishing breathlessness, administer two slow breaths. While maintaining an open airway, seal your mouth around the infant's mouth and nose. Administer two slow breaths sufficient to cause the chest to rise, using caution not to overventilate (Fig. 6–11).

Note: Chest rise is the indication to stop an individual breath to avoid overinflation and gastric distention (air in the stomach).

8. After each breath, remove your mouth from the patient's mouth and inhale. Each breath should take about 1 to 1.5 seconds to deliver, and the volume of air required is small. If you encounter an obstruction to ventilation, reposition the airway, being careful not to overextend, and attempt to ventilate. If you still encounter resistance, follow the obstructed airway sequence and consider infectious respiratory disease as a possible cause.

Note: You might wish to try a different airway maneuver. If the head tilt/neck lift failed initially, the chin lift or jaw thrust maneuver might prove more effective. If this technique is still unsuccessful, the obstructed airway procedure should be followed.

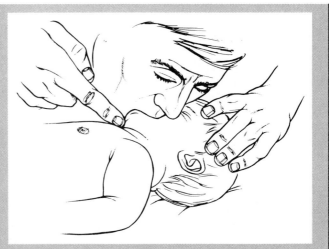

FIGURE 6–11. Infant mouth-to-mouth-and-nose ventilations.

PULSE CHECK

The absence of a pulse is the definitive proof of cardiac arrest. Absence of breathing efforts, unresponsiveness, dilated pupils, skin color, and even ECG tracings are only supportive indicators of cardiac arrest. A careful pulse check must be done for a sufficient time (5 to 10 seconds) to confirm cardiac arrest. The pulse of an infant is felt over the *brachial artery*. The brachial artery is located on the inner side of the upper arm between the elbow and the axilla. (Fig. 6–12A). Gently palpate with your index and middle fingers for 5 to 10 seconds to determine the presence of a pulse (Fig. 6–12B).

If you feel a pulse, continue to maintain the airway and provide mouth-to-mouth-and-nose breathing at a rate of 1 breath every 3 seconds if necessary and reevaluate the pulse periodically. If no pulse is felt in the unresponsive infant with no ventilations, the need for cardiac compressions has been established.

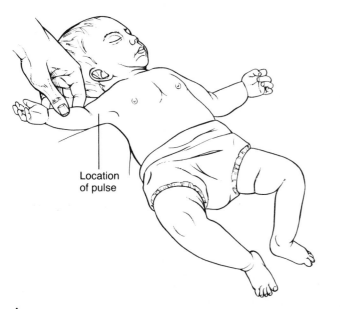

Location of pulse

A

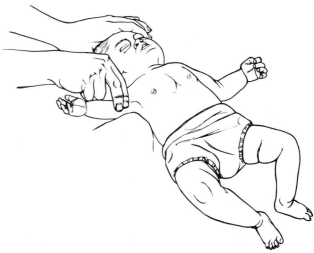

B

FIGURE 6–12. Infant pulse check. (A) The infant's pulse is located on the medial aspect of the upper arm. (B) Place two fingers over the medial aspect of the upper arm halfway between the elbow and the axillary region.

EXTERNAL CARDIAC COMPRESSIONS

External cardiac compressions provide blood flow (1) by squeezing the heart between the sternum and the spine and (2) by changing the pressure within the chest cavity during the compression and relaxation phases of the compression cycle. The exact forces that provide blood flow are being investigated and may vary in degree from patient to patient.

Blood flow during CPR is affected by variables such as rate and depth of compressions, ratio (time spent in compressions versus time spent in relaxation), and hand position. Blood flow studies have indicated that some 20 to 30% of normal output of blood is achieved during cardiac compressions. Other studies suggest that flow to the brain may be even less. The blood flow during external compressions is usually not sufficient to support consciousness (although some patients may have some response). In any case, it is important that the chest compressions be performed properly.

PATIENT POSITION

For chest compressions to be effective, the infant must be on a *hard surface*. If the patient is in a bed, he or she should be transferred to a table, floor, or other firm surface. This will minimize the absorption of compressions by the mattress.

P R O C E D U R E   6 – 3   PERFORMING CHEST COMPRESSIONS IN AN INFANT

1. After placing the infant on a hard surface, position your hand closest to the infant's head on the forehead. This will maintain an open airway while providing cardiac compressions.
2. Place three fingers over the middle of the infant's sternum with your index finger at the nipple line, then lift your index finger, leaving your middle and ring fingers on the breast bone. Use the tips of these two fingers to compress down $\frac{1}{2}$ to 1 inch at a rate of 100 compressions per minute (Fig. 6–13). The ratio of compressions to ventilations is 5:1.

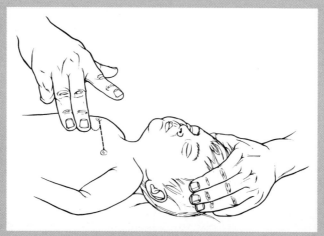

FIGURE 6–13. To locate the correct position for compressions in an infant, place your index, middle, and ring fingers of the hand closest to the infant's feet just adjacent to the nipple line. Then lift the index finger.

3. .Pause briefly after 5 compressions and breathe while observing for chest rise (Fig. 6–14).

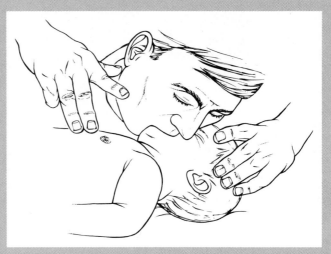

FIGURE 6–14. Provide compressions at a depth of $\frac{1}{2}$ to 1 inch and at a rate of 100 compressions/minute. Pause to administer 1 breath after every 5 compressions. Continue the 5 : 1 ratio of compressions and ventilation for approximately 10 cycles and reevaluate the pulse.

Pulse Check. After performing CPR for 1 minute, you should reevaluate the infant to determine if he or she is still pulseless. After one breath is given, the pulse is checked for 3 to 5 seconds. If the pulse is still absent, one more breath is administered and compressions are continued. Thereafter, the pulse is checked every few minutes but *without interrupting CPR for more than 5 seconds for each check.* Table 6–4 summarizes infant CPR.

MOVING THE INFANT TO AN AUTOMOBILE

Because of the infant's size, a special technique can be used by lay people and first responders to carry the infant to the automobile while continuing CPR performance. This should be used only when waiting for an ambulance would result in a significant delay or when hazards such as fire require rapid movement.

TABLE 6–4. Summary of Infant CPR

Establish unresponsiveness
Call for help
Position the victim
Open the airway—head in sniffing or neutral position
Check for breathing
Deliver two breaths (mouth-to-mouth-and-nose) and watch for chest rise
Check the brachial pulse
Activate the EMS system
Begin external chest compression on a hard surface
    Hand position/landmark check—two fingers on sternum, placed one fingerbreadth below nipple line
    Depth: 0.5–1 inch
    Rate: 100 per minute
    Ratio: 5 compressions/1 breath
Reevaluate pulse at 1 minute and then every few minutes

Place one arm midline along the infant's back and head with your elbow in the groin and your hand supporting the back portion of the infant's head. This allows you to walk with the infant to the automobile while maintaining ventilations and compressions. Someone should guide you to avoid obstacles and tripping.

CPR in Children

The major differences in CPR performance for children (aged 1 to 8 years) relate to breathing technique, checking the pulse, hand position, depth of compression, and compression rate. The initial sequence remains the same:

1. Check for unresponsiveness
2. Call for help
3. Position the victim.
4. Use head tilt/chin lift or jaw thrust without head tilt maneuvers to open the airway and establish breathlessness with the look, listen, and feel method of evaluation (Fig. 6–15A and B). Tilt the head of a small child to a neutral position or slightly farther back.

VENTILATIONS

When administering breaths to a child, mouth-to-mouth breathing is used rather than mouth-to-mouth-and-nose ventilation. While maintaining the head tilt/chin lift, pinch the nose with the fingers of the hand on the forehead. Seal your mouth around the child's mouth and administer two slow breaths. Again, observe chest rise to determine the appropriate amount of air. If re-

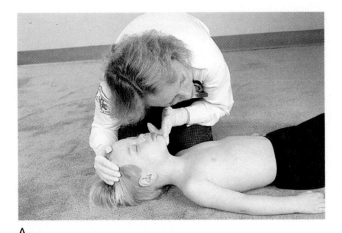

A

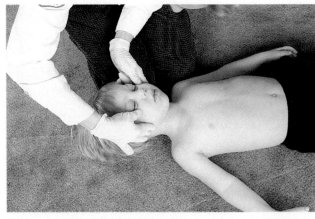

B

FIGURE 6–15. Airway opening in the child and establishing breathlessness. (*A*) The head tilt/chin lift while establishing breathlessness. (*B*) The jaw thrust-without head tilt.

sistance is encountered, reopen the airway and try again. If the patient still cannot breathe, follow the obstructed airway sequence (Fig. 6–16).

PULSE CHECK

The pulse in the child is evaluated by palpating the *carotid artery* in the neck. Using two or three fingers, locate the Adam's apple (voice box) and slide your fingers in the groove between the voice box and the muscles in the side of the neck (Fig. 6–17). Always check the pulse on the side of the child at which you are kneeling. Apply firm, gentle pressure so as not to occlude the artery and check the pulse for 5 to 10 seconds, as in an infant. If there is a pulse, provide one breath every 4 seconds. If the pulse is absent, proceed to cardiac compressions.

CARDIAC COMPRESSIONS

In the child, the heel of one hand is placed over the lower half of the sternum. Place two fingers of the hand closer to the feet on the margin of the ribs and

follow the ribs to the base of the breast bone; place the heel of that hand on the breast bone just above the location of the fingers (Fig. 6–18).

BODY POSITION.   Position yourself to the side of the patient with your knees close to the patient and slightly separated, so that you can move easily from compressions to ventilations. Position your shoulder directly over the hand on the lower half of the patient's sternum and lock your elbow. There should be a straight line from your shoulder to the heel of your hand, perpendicular to the patient's sternum. At the same time, the hand closer to the patient's head maintains a head tilt (Fig. 6–19).

DEPTH, RATE, AND RATIO.   Compress downward about 1 to $1\frac{1}{2}$ inches at a rate of 80 to 100 compressions per minute. Use a 5:1 ratio of compressions to ventilations. Compress vertically, bending slightly at the hips during the downward thrust. Pressure should be applied

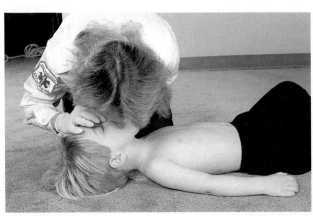

FIGURE 6–16. Mouth-to-mouth breathing in a child.

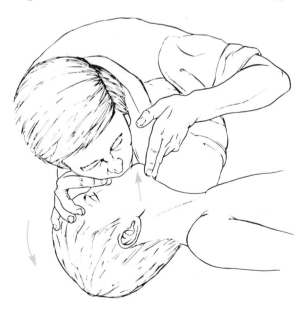

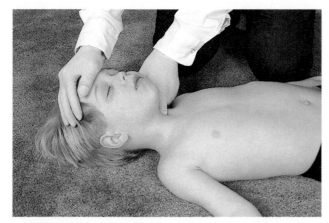

FIGURE 6–17. Checking the carotid pulse of a child.

only with the heel of your hand. After compressing, release all pressure and allow the patient's breast bone to rise completely without removing your hand. Each compression should be smooth and rhythmic, with about half of the time spent in the compression phase and half of the time in the release phase. At the end of five compressions, a chin lift is performed and one breath is administered, again observing chest rise to ensure delivery of an adequate volume of air. When proceeding with the subsequent cycles of compressions you do not have to check the landmark, but care should be taken to

ensure the correct position on the patient's breast bone. The 5:1 compression-to-ventilation ratio is maintained throughout CPR rescuer performance. Table 6–5 summarizes differences in CPR in children versus infants.

Special Considerations

This section deals with special factors to consider when initiating, stopping, and evaluating CPR, as well as complications that can result from CPR.

WHEN TO START CPR

CPR performance includes built-in assessment and treatment steps to be used for every apparently unresponsive patient. If breathing is absent or ineffective, rescue breathing should be administered. If the pulse is absent, cardiac compressions should be initiated. As a rescuer you should not concern yourself with the question of "biologic death." If an infant or child has been in cardiac arrest for a prolonged period, you should start CPR and allow hospital personnel to determine whether irreversible brain death has occurred.

In all cases of cardiac arrest, begin CPR. It is too difficult to establish with certainty the length of time that a patient has been "clinically dead", and the esti-

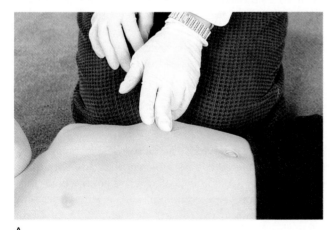

A

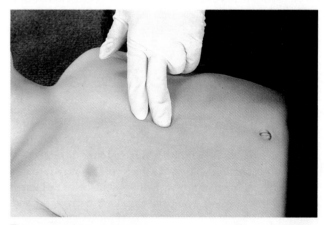

B

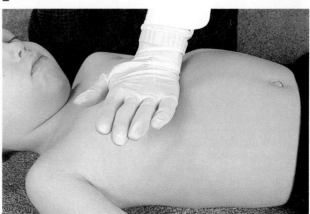

C

FIGURE 6–18. Locating the correct hand position in a child. (A) Locate the margin of the rib, (B) slide to the base of the sternum, and (C) place the same hand next to the finger location.

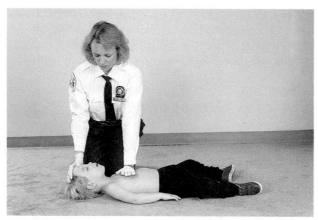

FIGURE 6–19. Body position of the rescuer during child CPR. The head tilt is maintained during the performance of compressions. During ventilations a chin lift is performed and the rescuer's hand is returned to the correct position on the sternum without rechecking the landmark.

mation of time given by the family and bystanders may be unreliable. Children, victims of drowning, and hypothermic (injuries resulting from the cold) patients have an even better chance of survival after extended periods of cardiac arrest. Children are more resilient to many disease processes than are adults, including cardiac arrest. A drowning victim may have enhanced chances because of factors such as hypothermia and because circulatory function continues for a few minutes after respiratory arrest. The hypothermic patient has less oxygen needs because low temperature slows metabolism.

EVALUATING EFFECTIVENESS OF CPR

During CPR, certain signs may be helpful in judging its effectiveness. They are essentially signs of oxygenation and circulation. Chest rise is used to monitor correct breathing technique. Signs of effective oxygenation and circulation include improvement in skin color (pinking of skin, or reversal of cyanosis), pupillary narrowing and reactivity to light, pulse return, and signs of spontaneous breathing, patient movement, and responsiveness.

When patients are successfully resuscitated, they usually experience the return of normal function gradually. For example, a patient may have return of pulse and then spontaneous respiratory efforts that may be

TABLE 6–5. (Differences from Infant) CPR in Children

Airway—slight head tilt
Breathing: Mouth-to-mouth breathing
Pulse: Carotid pulse in the neck
Compressions: Landmark—lower half of the sternum
   Check landmark only on initial cycle
   Heel of one hand
   1–1.5 inch compression
   80–100 compressions per minute
   5:1 ratio of compressions to ventilations

inadequate to support life. The airway and the breathing must be monitored and mouth-to-mouth ventilation provided as necessary.

WHEN TO STOP CPR

There are five circumstances when CPR may be stopped:

1. Primary rescuer is relieved by another rescuer.
2. Physician or physician-directed team assumes responsibility for the patient.
3. Rescuer is exhausted and unable to continue.
4. Patient is delivered to emergency department and care is transferred to emergency department personnel.
5. Patient develops spontaneous breathing and a pulse.

COMPLICATIONS OF CPR

There are many complications of CPR. Some are the result of improper performance, others may occur even with proper technique. The most frequent complication is broken ribs. Fracture of the sternum, cardiac contusions, lung lacerations, and lacerations of the liver are all possible complications of CPR. The chances for the occurrence of these complications are minimized by using the correct technique, especially by paying attention to the landmark check, hand position, and the force and depth of chest compressions. Overventilation might result in gastric distention and vomiting.

Mechanical CPR Devices

Mechanical devices that aid in CPR range from simple hand-operated units, which deal strictly with chest compressions, to sophisticated oxygen-powered machines that compress, ventilate, and, in short, perform the technique of a two-rescuer CPR team (Fig. 6–20A). When used properly, they are capable of providing excellent CPR technique under a variety of conditions. If applied improperly or left unattended, however, they have the potential of being ineffective or may cause severe complications from rib or sternum fractures.

ADVANTAGES OF MECHANICAL CPR DEVICES

The obvious advantage of mechanical CPR is avoiding rescuer fatigue. Gas-powered units have the potential to perform consistent, optimal compressions as long as there is an adequate supply of oxygen. In the case of prolonged resuscitation, such as during long transports in rural EMS systems or while rewarming hypothermic patients, mechanical CPR is invaluable. It is also very useful when CPR is performed in a moving ambulance.

DISADVANTAGES OF MECHANICAL CPR

The disadvantage of mechanical CPR is the possibility of injuring the patient as a result of operator error or inattentiveness. If the patient's position on the backboard changes, the piston may continue to compress at an improper site unless checked by the operator. Also, the compression depth may be set deeper than necessary.

These factors again reinforce the need for EMTs to remain well versed in the operation of any mechanical device they use in treatment.

TECHNIQUE OF OPERATION

The method of operation of mechanical CPR devices varies from unit to unit. For the purposes of illustration, we will use a gas-powered device to outline the sequential steps to follow. Regardless of the type of device, however, certain rules are universal:

1. Never delay a resuscitation while preparing to apply CPR devices. Manual CPR should always be started while a second rescuer readies the mechanical device.

2. When applying the device, do not interrupt CPR for extended periods. As a rule, cardiac compressions should not be stopped for more than 30 seconds. Frequent practice, however, should further reduce this period.

3. Place the patient on the CPR board and continue manual CPR (Fig. 6–20B to E). The piston arm is then attached to the CPR board.

4. Slide the device into the CPR board and lock the compressor arm in place (Fig. 6–20F and G).

5. The compression piston should be positioned cautiously in the same location as the hand position for manual cardiac compressions. (Fig. 6–20H to J).

6. The compression piston is engaged according to the manufacturer's criteria, to avoid overcompression. The unit should be constantly monitored to avoid accidental displacement of the compression piston that might occur from patient movement or a rough ride (Fig. 6–20K and L).

7. The ventilation device can be attached to the mask or endotracheal tube for the administration of positive pressure from the device, or positive pressure can be applied from a system outside the device.

8. Because the device is powered by gas, the oxygen source must be monitored closely.

Special Resuscitation Situations

From time to time, the EMT will encounter resuscitation situations that require modification of the approach to the patient. In all instances, however, the goal of CPR remains the same: to ensure adequate oxygenation of tissues.

MOUTH-TO-STOMA VENTILATION

When the EMT encounters individuals who breathe through a stoma (surgical opening) in the neck, he or she must provide mouth-to-stoma breathing directly through the opening. The stoma may or may not communicate with the mouth and nose. In cases where the opening can communicate with the upper airway, air might leak out of the upper airway during mouth-to-stoma ventilation. If leakage occurs, the mouth and nose should be sealed during ventilation. Again, chest excursion should be used to check effectiveness.

DROWNING

When attempting to rescue a drowning person, the EMT's first concern is his or her own safety. When possible, a floatable rescue device should be tossed to the drowning person. In instances where the distance to the person or the patient's status prevents such actions, a boat or raft should be used to effect a rescue. Finally, if the EMT must swim to the victim, he or she should be aware of his or her own abilities and limitations and act accordingly.

If the drowning victim is unresponsive, evaluation of ventilations and breathing should begin as soon as possible. Obviously, external chest compressions should not be attempted while the victim is in the water. Positive-pressure breathing, however, should be started as soon as possible. It can be started when the EMT can stand in shallow water. It also can be started if the victim can be placed on a floating object in deep water.

If the victim has suffered a possible neck injury, the neck should be supported in a neutral position, and the victim should be floated onto a backboard (when available) before being removed from the water. Keep the head, neck, and chest aligned to prevent further serious injury. Positive-pressure ventilation can be performed with the head in a neutral position. To do so, use the modified jaw thrust maneuver without head tilt.

Cardiac compressions should begin as soon as the victim is on a hard surface. The length of time that the victim has been submerged should not affect the decision to resuscitate. Many drowning victims have successfully recovered after long periods of submersion. Hypothermia (low body temperature) and the mammalian diving reflex are two factors that may be present in victims of near drowning and that retard brain death.

During drowning, large quantities of water may be swallowed or enter the lungs. Water in the mouth can be removed by turning the patient. Water in the stomach need not be attended to unless excessive gastric distention interferes with ventilation efforts. Should this occur,

Text continued on page 258

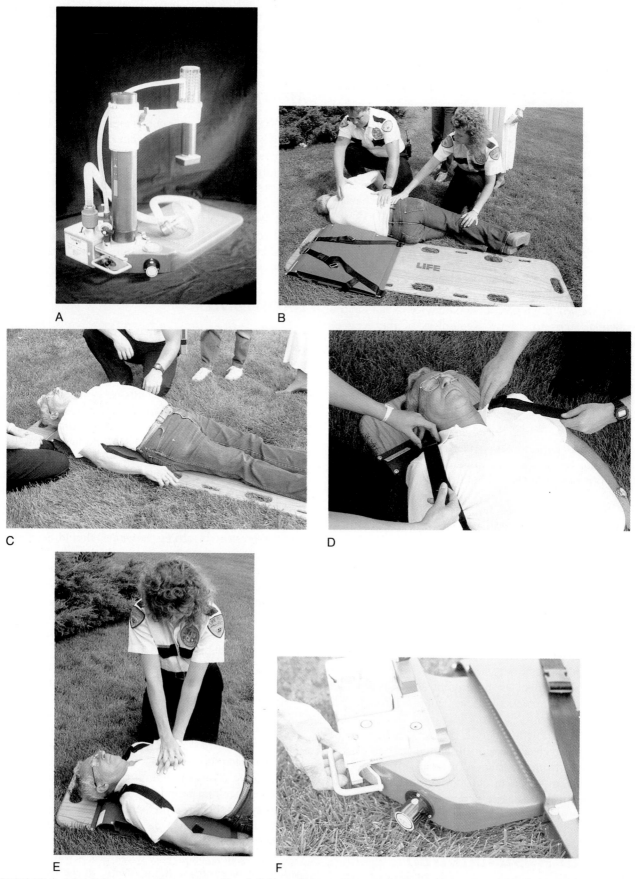

FIGURE 6–20. (*A*) Gas-powered compressor. (*B* and *C*) Log roll the patient onto the CPR and spine board. (*D*) Secure the patient to the board and (*E*) resume CPR. (*F*) Slide the compression unit into the board and (*G*) attach the compression arm. (*H*) Position the piston on the the sternum in the same location as a cardiac compression. (*I, J,* and *K*) Adjust the height and tighten the arm in place. (*L*) Monitor the unit closely. (Courtesy of Michigan Instruments, Grand Rapids, MI.) *Illustration continued on opposite page*

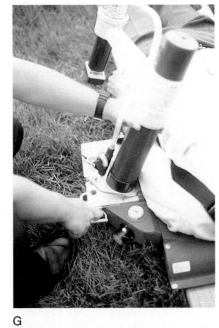

G

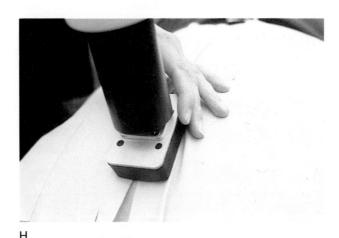

H

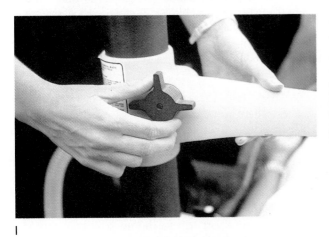

I

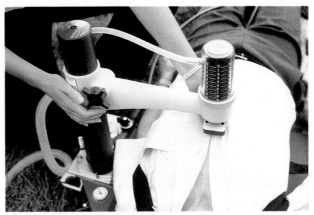

J

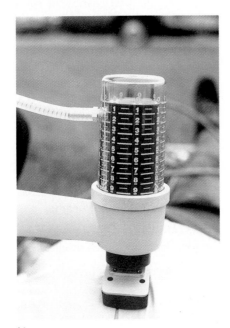

K

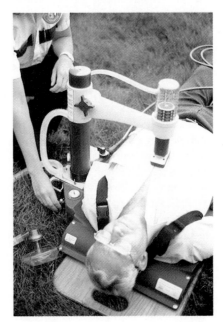

L

FIGURE 6–20. *Continued*

the patient should be rotated onto the side and gentle pressure should be applied to the upper abdomen. During this procedure, suction apparatus, if available, should be readied to minimize the chance of aspiration.

ELECTRIC SHOCK

Electric shock may cause either respiratory or cardiac arrest. In either instance, there may be further injuries including internal and external burns and trauma resulting from falls. In the latter situation, approach the patient with appropriate concern for possible injuries to the cervical spine.

If the victim is still in contact with or near the source of electricity, the wire should be cleared away from the patient with a nonconductive object such as a dry stick. In instances in which the electric current is fixed or cannot be moved, the patient must be separated from the electrical source with a nonconductive object.

CPR During Movement

Performing effective CPR under even optimal conditions requires a focused and diligent approach. Maintaining effective CPR technique while moving the patient down stairs, through doorways, along walkways, and in a moving ambulance is one of the most difficult tasks facing the EMT. Most patients go through several phases of movement during transport to the hospital. The goal is to provide the best CPR possible while still effecting rapid transport. For each phase of movement, specific methods should be used. In all circumstances, however, the most important factor is maintaining an awareness of the effectiveness of CPR and the time frames in which no CPR is possible.

DECISION TO TRANSPORT

In systems in which advanced life support (ALS) units with additional ALS modalities (e.g., intubation, pharmacology) are available, it frequently is better to wait for their arrival before moving the patient who has experienced a myocardial infarction or "sudden death." The goals are (1) to provide good CPR and defibrillation and (2) to deliver the most rapid additional ALS available. If transport to the hospital takes less time, then it is the appropriate decision if effective CPR can be continued. The rationale for selecting either strategy is based on the time that will transpire from the onset of cardiac arrest to defibrillation and ALS versus the logistical considerations associated with moving the patient.

Consider the following situations (assume both patients complained of severe chest pain and then suffered cardiac arrest).

•   **C A S E   H I S T O R Y   1**   •

You respond to a call and find a 55-year-old man in cardiopulmonary arrest on the fifth floor of a building without an elevator. You are told that the patient clutched his chest, fell to the floor, and lost consciousness about 2 minutes before your arrival. You provide complete CPR and contact the dispatcher about the availability of a paramedic unit while your partner performs CPR. The dispatcher advises you that the paramedics are responding and will be at the scene within 4 minutes. You decide to wait.

•   **C A S E   H I S T O R Y   2**   •

On arrival at a call two blocks away from the hospital, you find a 60-year-old victim of cardiopulmonary arrest. You start CPR but the patient remains in cardiac arrest. With the help of the police, you place the victim in the ambulance and deliver him to the emergency department within 3 minutes.

These two cases illustrate two distinct circumstances where good judgment was exercised. In Case History 1, the trip down five flights of stairs would have resulted in a significant transport delay and interruptions in effective CPR. The decision to wait for an ALS unit while performing effective CPR made a great deal of sense.

In Case History 2, the easy access to the ambulance and the timely short trip to the hospital probably give the patient the best chance for survival. If a paramedic unit were a minute away, however, this strategy might be altered.

It is obvious that these cases represent relatively well-defined situations. Most cardiac arrest calls probably fall between these two extremes, making the judgment to transport or to wait on the scene a little more difficult. These decisions are based on the availability of resources within your own system.

MOVEMENT STRATEGIES

Once having made the decision to transport, the following strategies are helpful.

STAIRWAY.   When moving a patient down stairs, the following principles should be adhered to:

1. Secure the patient to the device selected for transport.

2. If possible, transport of the patient should be done with no less than four people, including EMTs and helpers.

3. CPR should be done on each landing. As quickly as possible, the patient should be moved to the next landing. If possible, this should be achieved in less than 30 seconds, but each instance will vary. Ordinarily, manual CPR is not possible when moving patients down stairs. The main concern is safe patient movement.

4. When the patient has been delivered to street level, he or she can be placed on a cot stretcher that ideally is raised about halfway to the full upright position. This facilitates CPR along the pathway to the ambulance.

GROUND LEVEL AND INTO THE AMBULANCE. The following techniques should be used during ground movement and lifting into the ambulance:

1. With the rolling cot stretcher at the halfway upright position, CPR should continue. Two helpers who are not participating in CPR should position themselves at the top and bottom ends of the cot stretcher.

2. On command, so that the CPR participants can prepare to move, the stretcher should be advanced with the patient's feet first toward the ambulance so that the EMT who ventilates the patient is walking forward. Preparation for movement off stairs or curbs should occur as each obstacle is encountered, minimizing any slight interruptions in technique. The ventilator should direct the movement (Fig. 6–21).

3. At the ambulance, the helpers positioned at the head and foot of the stretcher should lower the stretcher to its lowest position while CPR continues.

4. To lift the patient into the ambulance, CPR should be stopped briefly while the compressor and one helper lift the stretcher from the side position. The ventilator can wait inside the ambulance and resume CPR as soon as the stretcher is locked in place. Again, the patient should be hyperventilated after any period when CPR was interrupted.

CPR DURING TRANSPORT. While the ambulance is in motion, the following protocol should be followed.

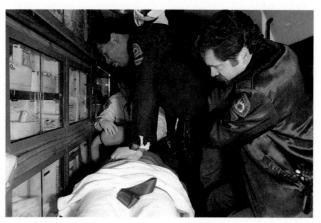

FIGURE 6–22. CPR during transport.

Ideally, four people should be involved to provide both effective CPR and safety for the EMTs:

1. One person should be positioned at the head of the patient, producing mechanical ventilation. A second EMT should be administering cardiac compressions, while a third helper supports the compressor from behind to provide enough stability to minimize loss of balance (Fig. 6–22).

2. To avoid abrupt movements, the driver should exercise great care during departures and when stopping. The compressor is in great jeopardy of injury should a short stop or collision occur; thus, every precaution should be taken.

3. On arrival at the hospital, the driver and helper can receive the stretcher while the compressor and ventilator briefly interrupt CPR. Movement into the emergency department should proceed as described previously.

Transfer care to the hospital's emergency staff as you describe the circumstances surrounding the cardiac arrest.

Summary

Emergencies in general are anxiety provoking and sometimes cause rescuers to panic and act inappropriately. This is even more likely when infants or children are involved. The best method for preventing panic is preparation. This includes intensive practice during your initial training as well as continuing your emergency medical education. You should practice as often as possible on a training manikin. Refresher training biannually or annually is the best method for ensuring retention of critical information.

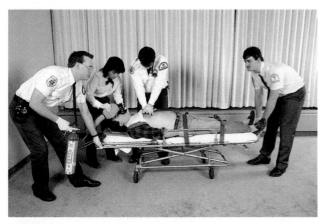

FIGURE 6–21. CPR during movement.

EMT DEFIBRILLATION

Introduction

The most common and treatable cause of sudden death is *ventricular fibrillation* from ischemic heart disease. Up to 70% of victims of sudden death experience this rhythm. In diseases such as myocardial infarction, the conduction system may lose control of the myocardial cells. Because the cells in the heart have automaticity, the ability to depolarize and discharge on their own, the uncontrolled cells may act independently of the conduction system and of each other. This may result in the chaotic rhythm known as ventricular fibrillation. No effective synchronized contraction of the heart is possible; no blood is pumped. The pacemaker has lost control.

The useless quivering of the heart in ventricular fibrillation can be stopped by depolarizing the myocardial cells simultaneously and making them all repolarize (recharge) simultaneously. The fastest cells to recharge are those that compose the pacemaker. Being the first part of the heart ready to discharge, the pacemaker can resume control.

The forced discharge, or firing, of the heart's cells can be accomplished by *defibrillation*, the external application of an electric shock that travels across the heart. Sufficient energy must be delivered to most of the heart to ensure successful defibrillation.

Many patients who receive early defibrillation can be saved. Without defibrillation, ventricular fibrillation deteriorates to cardiac standstill or *asystole* (no contraction). Resuscitation of patients with *asystole* (no contraction) is far less likely than if the patient has ventricular fibrillation.

Evolution of Concept

Before the 1960s, patients who suffered sudden death outside the hospital rarely survived. When they arrived at the hospital by ambulance, most were pronounced dead. In the early 1960s, the technique of cardiopulmonary resuscitation (CPR) was developed to provide artificial ventilation and circulation for victims of cardiac arrest until they could receive advanced care in a hospital setting. Hospital care consisted of both CPR and advanced life support (ALS). ALS consists of defibrillation of the heart, administration of drugs, placement of pacemakers, and application of specialized airway management techniques like intubation of the trachea. It was clear from hospital experience that the early application of both CPR and ALS (especially defibrillation) resulted in a higher patient survival rate. With the development of portable defibrillators, also in the 1960s, application

of defibrillation in the field became technologically feasible. Efforts began to bring hospital care to victims of sudden death in the field, saving critical minutes from the time of cardiac arrest to the application of defibrillation and other advanced skills.

PREHOSPITAL EMERGENCY CARDIAC CARE AND DEFIBRILLATION

Pioneers such as Pantridge in Belfast, Northern Ireland, and Grace in New York City introduced the concept of mobile intensive care units that brought the "hospital" to the patient's side. Early paramedic programs in Miami, Pittsburgh, Seattle, and other cities extended hospital care through nonphysician medical personnel. Through the use of portable defibrillators, airway adjuncts, and emergency cardiac drugs in conjunction with CPR, it was demonstrated that more victims of cardiac arrest could be saved. Because of the impact of this approach on sudden death from heart disease, ALS units became part of EMS system development. As mentioned earlier, in 1973, the federal Emergency Medical Services Systems legislation stimulated growth of EMS and ALS across the country.

Studies of care rendered by paramedics and advanced EMTs documented the effectiveness of prehospital ALS systems. Survival rates of 43% were reported when victims of cardiac arrest secondary to ventricular fibrillation received prompt CPR (less than 4 minutes) and prompt ALS (less than 8 minutes). Yet, these skills were in the hands of a small number of prehospital providers and therefore available to only a minority of patients. Training time for advanced EMT programs was lengthy. Learning rhythm recognition and pharmacology required additional training time for prehospital personnel. This precluded wide application of the ALS programs, particularly in areas where volunteers provided the bulk of the personnel.

Looking closely at the most important elements necessary to resuscitate the clinically dead patient, the time that elapsed between onset of cardiac arrest and initiation of CPR and defibrillation stood out. In the 1970s, Eisenberg, Copass, and others from Seattle studied the use of defibrillation by basic EMTs. Again, an increase in the survival rate was noted. Many other programs in urban, rural, and suburban settings have demonstrated the effectiveness of EMTs performing defibrillation.

WHY EMTS? EMTs represent the largest group of providers of prehospital emergency care in the United States. To resuscitate victims of sudden cardiac death, most EMTs must rely on CPR and transport to a medical facility or the arrival of paramedics at the scene. Any increase in time from cardiac arrest to the application of

ALS (especially defibrillation) increases the likelihood of death. The outcome for cardiac arrest victims who receive CPR alone is well known to practicing EMTs. Despite vigorous and physically challenging efforts to continue CPR, death is often almost certain without advanced therapy.

Many communities have developed EMT-defibrillation (EMT-D) programs in recognition of the value of early defibrillation. These programs teach the necessary essentials of ECG recognition and defibrillation to permit the safe application of lifesaving therapy. The programs are relatively short and can be given as a supplementary course to EMTs. This focused approach permits the training of personnel who, because of time restraints, may not be able to attend an advanced EMT course. The selection of defibrillation as the focus for additional training recognizes the following facts:

- The most common and most treatable rhythm encountered early in cardiac arrest is ventricular fibrillation.
- Defibrillation is the definitive treatment for ventricular fibrillation and can be taught as a distinct module in a relatively short time.
- Time from cardiac arrest to defibrillation is the most important variable in the successful treatment of ventricular fibrillation.
- EMTs are the most likely medical personnel to initially encounter the sudden death victim.

CONCEPTUAL FRAMEWORK. The knowledge necessary to administer lifesaving defibrillation includes recognition of signs of cardiac arrest, ability to perform CPR, basic ECG recognition, and monitoring and defibrillation techniques. EMTs administer defibrillation under the authorization and orders of a physician who assumes responsibility for medical control. It is administered as part of an EMS system response.

The following section is organized to provide the necessary knowledge needed to understand the role of defibrillation in the treatment of cardiac arrest. The content is intentionally limited to the essential information needed for the EMT-D provider.

Most cases of ventricular fibrillation occur in connection with ischemic heart disease. By understanding the normal mechanisms of electrical conduction within the heart, one can better appreciate electrocardiograms and the rationale for defibrillation.

The principles of ECG monitoring and interpretation are presented to provide a foundation for understanding the ECG and defibrillation. Only essential rhythms necessary to understand the decision to defibrillate are emphasized.

In the defibrillation section, techniques are presented using the conventional manual monitor–defibrillator for illustration purposes. Understanding operation of the manual monitor–defibrillator will lead to better appreciation of the automatic and semiautomatic defibrillators popular today. Anatomy and physiology of the heart's conduction system are discussed in Chapter 4.

Electrocardiogram

The electrical activity generated by the depolarization and repolarization of the heart is detected, amplified, and displayed as an *electrocardiogram* or *ECG*. An ECG machine is connected to the body's surface by electrodes and cables. The electrodes pick up the heart's signal, and the cables transmit the signal to the ECG machine. The signal is then amplified and displayed on a monitor or paper readout.

ELECTRODES AND ECG LEADS

Electrodes can be placed at various locations on the body depending on the purpose of the ECG reading. The placement of electrodes creates a *lead*, which receives the electrical events of the heart. Standard monitoring leads contain a positive electrode, a negative electrode, and an electrode that serves as a reference or ground. As the wave of depolarization across the heart occurs, the electrical event is received by the electrodes. If the wave of depolarization is toward the positive end of a lead, the deflection or wave form is directed upward on the ECG monitor or readout. If the wave of depolarization moves toward the negative end, the deflection is directed downward. If the wave travels at a right angle to the two electrodes, the deflection is directed both upward and downward (Fig. 6–23).

Electrodes for monitoring leads are placed so as to form a triangle around the heart. Depending on what you are monitoring, they can be attached to the extremities or to the torso near the extremities. When monitoring cardiac patients, electrodes are placed on the left and right upper chest and the lower left chest wall. For rhythm interpretation, the most commonly used leads are called *leads I, II,* and *III.* The standard placement of electrodes for these leads is displayed in Fig. 6–24. Generally, lead II is selected because it gives positive deflections in the normally depolarizing heart. The selection of leads is done by turning a switch on the ECG machine: the electrical orientation of the electrodes (positive, negative, or reference) is changed within the ECG machine, resulting in a new lead.

ECG MONITOR

The device used to display an ECG is called a *monitor,* or *oscilloscope.* Some ECG machines also

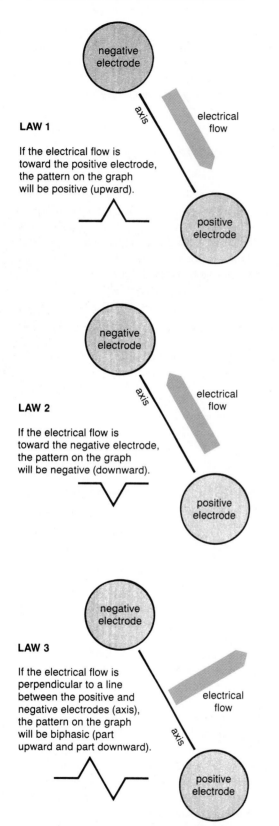

LAW 1

If the electrical flow is toward the positive electrode, the pattern on the graph will be positive (upward).

LAW 2

If the electrical flow is toward the negative electrode, the pattern on the graph will be negative (downward).

LAW 3

If the electrical flow is perpendicular to a line between the positive and negative electrodes (axis), the pattern on the graph will be biphasic (part upward and part downward).

FIGURE 6–23. Electrical flow, electrode placement, and ECG readings. (From Weiderhold R: Electrocardiography: The Monitoring Lead. Philadelphia, WB Saunders, 1988, p. 36.)

transcribe the wave onto paper for analysis and record keeping.

SCREEN (CATHODE RAY TUBE). The screen portion of an ECG is a cathode ray tube (CRT). This device is similar to a television or computer screen. It presents a blue or green background with the waveforms superimposed as bright lines. The screen is used to determine the basic ECG rhythm and to observe for significant changes while monitoring a patient. Some monitors allow the operator to "freeze" or stop the wave on the screen for closer observation.

PAPER READOUT. To record the ECG rhythm, most monitors have a paper readout. A hot stylus serves as a pen to record ECG waves on heat-sensitive paper. The stylus heat can be adjusted if the readout is too light or too dark. The paper is pulled under the stylus at a predetermined speed. Lines on the paper permit calculation of rate, size, and duration of the waveforms. The readout provides a permanent record for future reference and documentation (Fig. 6–25).

AMPLIFICATION AND STANDARDIZATION. The ECG amplifies electrical signals from the heart so they can be seen. The size of the wave forms can be adjusted to amplify weak signals. A standard marker allows one to measure the heights of the ECG waves against a standard reference voltage.

The standard marker makes a mark on the recording to allow you to check the machine and record the standard voltage. Standardization is usually calibrated so that a 10-mm deflection (10 small boxes on the ECG paper) corresponds to 1 millivolt (Fig. 6–26). It is important to push the standard button to check your reference deflection each time you use the monitor. If the amplification is inadvertently turned all the way down, all recordings may appear as flat lines and the rhythm would be misinterpreted.

ATTACHING THE ELECTRODES. Monitoring electrodes come prepackaged for easy application. They consist of thin foam pads with a central pregelled electrode. The gel substance improves the conduction at the skin-electrode interface. The electrode is surrounded by an adhesive border for attachment to the patient's skin (Fig. 6–27). A protective covering seal, which prevents drying of the gel and adhesive, is pulled away just before attachment to the patient. The outer surface of the electrode has a metal protruding stub that is connected to the cable.

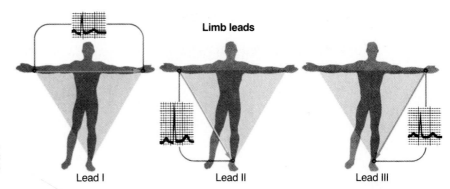

Limb leads

Lead I   Lead II   Lead III

FIGURE 6–24. ECG leads I, II, and III. (From Wiederhold R: Electrocardiography: The Monitoring Lead. Philadelphia, WB Saunders, 1988, p. 34.)

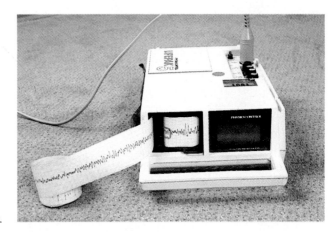

FIGURE 6–25. Paper read-out and monitor.

Calibration Marks

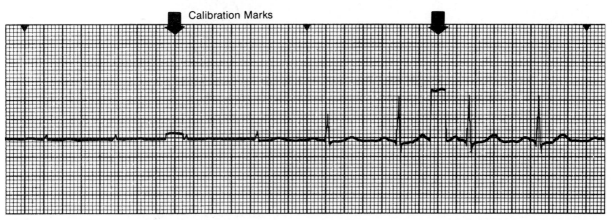

FIGURE 6–26. Note calibration marks (*arrows*) and corresponding size of ECG waves. Usually the calibration marks are adjusted to 10 small boxes. (From Wiederhold R: Electrocardiography: The Monitoring Lead. Philadelphia, WB Saunders, 1988, p. 29.)

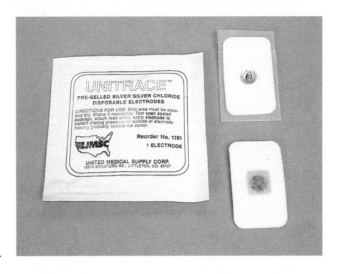

FIGURE 6–27. Electrodes.

P R O C E D U R E   6 – 4   ATTACHING THE ELECTRODES

1. To ensure good contact and adhesion, remove any perspiration from the patient's skin surface with a gauze pad before attaching the electrode. Check to be sure the gel on the electrode has not dried.
2. Attach the electrodes to the patient to form a triangle around the heart (as described earlier) (Fig. 6–28A).
3. Attach the cables to the electrodes. Cables are color-coded and have abbreviations such as RA (right arm), LA (left arm), and LL (left leg) to prompt correct placement (Fig. 6–28B).
4. If the patient is conscious, instruct the patient to lie still and not touch metal during monitoring, so as to avoid interference in the tracing.

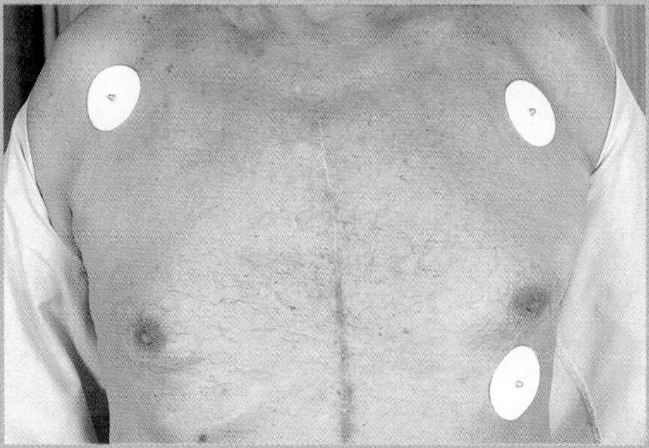

A 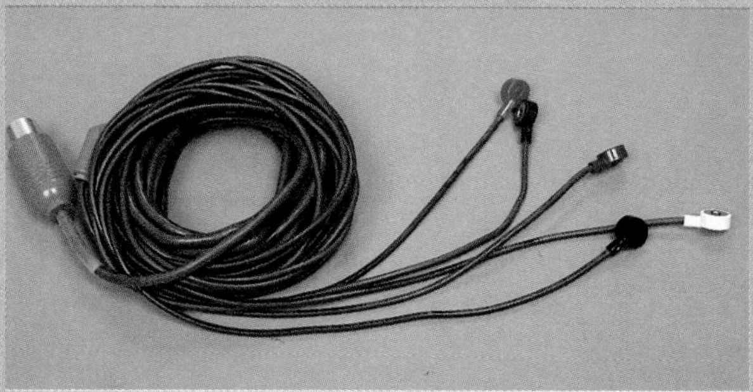   B

FIGURE 6–28. (A) Electrode placement in triangle around heart. (B) Patient cable.

PADDLE MONITORING.   Some monitor–defibrillators permit monitoring through the defibrillator paddles to permit rapid rhythm assessment and defibrillation. The paddles act as the monitoring electrodes. The lead select switch must be turned to *paddle mode* to use paddles as the monitoring electrodes. Some medical directors discourage use of paddle monitoring because of the potentially poorer quality of the ECG tracing. If paddles are used, one must be particularly alert to ensure that the lead select is on paddle rather than lead I, II, or III. If inadvertently, the lead select is not on paddle, the monitor will register a flat line, leading the EMT to an incorrect rhythm assessment.

P R O C E D U R E   6 – 5   OPERATING THE MONITOR

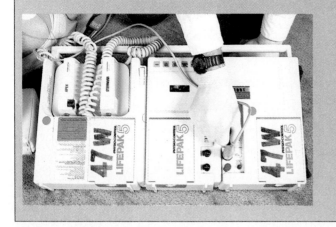

1. Turn on the machine and select lead II for routine monitoring (Fig. 6–29).
2. When the rhythm appears on the screen, turn on the recorder and press standard button. For normal standardization, adjust the amplitude so that the deflection is about 10 mm in height (10 small boxes). Observe the rhythm on the screen and paper readout. If necessary, adjust the amplitude and the stylus heat with the respective controls.

FIGURE 6–29. Select lead II for routine monitoring.

Many monitors have an audible beep that alerts the EMT to the rate of the rhythm. The sound is initiated by the ECG complex. The sound intensity can be adjusted with the systolic volume control switch.

ECG RECOGNITION

An ECG is the recording of the electrical events of the heart on a paper tracing or monitor. There are standard deflections and intervals that represent different electrical events of the heart's rhythm. The letters assigned to the waves or deflections seen on a normal heart beat are arbitrarily chosen as P, Q, R, S, T, and U. The *P wave* represents depolarization of the atria. It is usually a positive wave in lead II. The *QRS complex* represents depolarization of the ventricles. The *Q wave* is the first downward deflection that occurs before the *R wave*, or first positive deflection. The negative deflection following the R wave is called the *S wave*. This complex takes various forms but is always referred to as the QRS complex even though some parts of the wave may not be seen (Fig. 6–30). The *T wave* represents ventricular repolarization. In some patients, a *U wave* may follow the T wave. Its significance is unclear in normal hearts, but it is known to appear in patients taking certain drugs or with electrolyte disturbances.

The *PR interval* is the time from the beginning of the P wave to the first deflection of the QRS complex. It represents the time from sinoatrial (SA) node discharge to ventricular depolarization. The normal PR interval is between 0.12 and 0.20 second. Longer intervals reflect delay or blocked conduction through the atrioventricular (AV) node. The QRS wave is normally less than 0.12 second in duration. A prolonged QRS wave represents abnormal conduction. Figure 6–31 summarizes the relationship of the complexes and intervals to the mechanical events of the cardiac cycle. Note that the complexes will appear differently in different leads. The QRS complex may show the greatest variation.

ANALYZING RATE. The ECG is recorded on paper over time. By knowing the speed of the recording, one can use markings on the paper to determine the rate of a rhythm. Some ECG machines permit you to vary the speed, which changes the time value of the markings. For EMT-D and most medical purposes, the paper runs at the standard speed setting at 25 mm/second. At this speed the following methods are useful to estimate rate.

SIX-SECOND STRIP. There are marks on the top of the paper for every 3 seconds of the ECG tracing. By counting the number of ventricular (QRS) complexes within two of these markings, one can estimate the rate of heart beats per minute by multiplying by 10. This is no different than taking a pulse rate. The marks on the paper are used to time the components of the heart rhythm (Fig. 6–32).

Number of complexes within 2 top marks	=	number in 6 seconds
Multiply this number × 10	=	number of complexes in 60 seconds

LARGE-BOX METHOD. ECG paper is scored with vertical and horizontal lines that form boxes to permit measurement of rate and amplitude of the ECG tracing. The dark vertical markings correspond to 0.2 second. Five dark lines represent 1 second (5 × 0.2 second = 1 second); 300 dark lines represent 1 minute (300 × 0.2 second = 60 seconds). Find a QRS complex that lines up with a dark vertical line and count the number of dark lines to the next QRS complex. (The tip of the R wave usually is used so that the same point within a complex is used as the reference point.) Divide 300 by the number of dark lines between complexes to find the rate per minute. The values for successive large boxes are 300, 150, 100, 75, 60, and 50, which are the results of dividing 300 by 1, 2, 3, 4, 5, and 6 (Fig. 6–33). One can easily memorize and recall the successive value that each dark line represents. When using this system the complexes must occur at regular intervals.

SMALL-BOX METHOD. Each large box contains five smaller boxes. Because the large box represents 0.2 second, each small box represents 0.04 second. There are 1500 small boxes in 1 minute (1500 × 0.04 second = 60 seconds). Rates can be determined as with the large box method by finding a complex that lines up on a vertical line, counting the number of small boxes to the same point of the next complex, and dividing it into

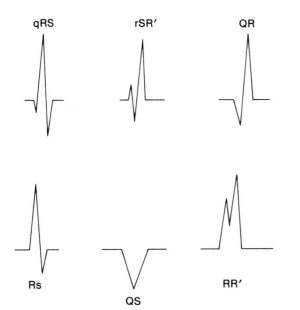

FIGURE 6–30. Different variations of the QRS complex. (From Johnson R, Swartz MH: A Simplified Approach to Electrocardiography. Philadelphia, WB Saunders, 1986, p. 20.)

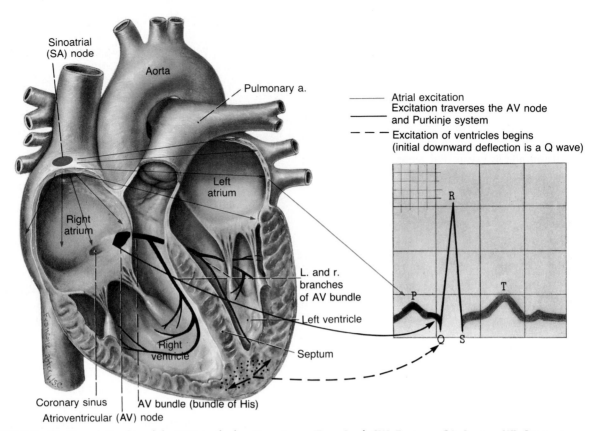

FIGURE 6–31. The relationship of the ECG to the heart's anatomy. (From Jacob SW, Francone CA, Lossow WJ: Structure and Function in Man, 5th ed. Philadelphia, WB Saunders, 1982.)

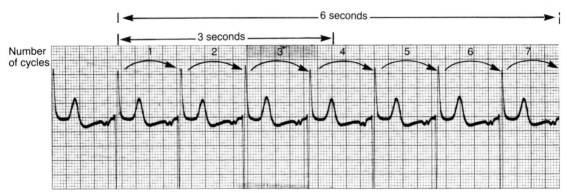

FIGURE 6–32. Six-second strip calculation. (From Johnson R, Swartz MH: A Simplified Approach to Electrocardiography. Philadelphia, WB Saunders, 1986, p. 19.)

1500. Always measure between similar points of a complex (Fig. 6–34).

INTERVALS. Small boxes also are used to measure intervals between complexes. For example, the QRS interval is ordinarily less than 0.12 second, or three small boxes. By counting the number of small boxes within a QRS interval, one can rapidly estimate the duration by multiplying by 0.04 second (the time represented by one small box). If the QRS complex is 0.12 second or longer (more than three small boxes), it is abnormal. Knowing the intervals (and even the rate) is not necessary for EMTs to perform defibrillation, but their determination is included here as part of a basic conceptual framework.

RHYTHM

Terms used to describe rhythms are *regular*, *irregularly irregular*, and *regularly irregular*. Look for patterns over several seconds of the ECG tracing.

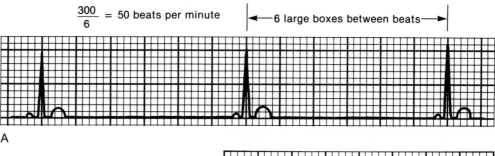

$$\frac{300}{6} = 50 \text{ beats per minute}$$ |← 6 large boxes between beats →|

A

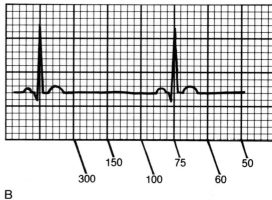

150   75   50
300   100   60

B

FIGURE 6–33. Large-box method for calculation. (*A*) Divide number of large boxes between beats into 300 to determine rate. (*B*) Memorize the value of each large box to estimate rate. (From Johnson R, Swartz MH: A Simplified Approach to Electrocardiography. Philadelphia, WB Saunders, 1986, p. 19.)

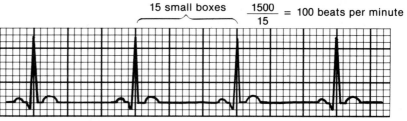

15 small boxes $\frac{1500}{15} = 100$ beats per minute

FIGURE 6–34. Small-box method for calculation. (From Johnson R, Swartz MH: A Simplified Approach to Electrocardiography. Philadelphia, WB Saunders, 1986, p. 19.)

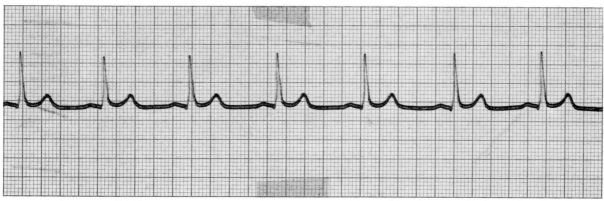

FIGURE 6–35. A regular rhythm (normal sinus rhythm). (From Council on Nursing, Carlson V, Ungvarski P (eds): ECG Workbook for Arrhythmia Recognition, 2nd ed. New York, American Heart Association, New York City Affiliate and Heart Fund, 1982.)

REGULAR. Most people have regular rhythms, with P waves and QRS complexes occurring at regular intervals. Normal sinus rhythm is an example of a regular rhythm (Fig. 6–35).

IRREGULARLY IRREGULAR. Other rhythms have no predictable pattern. It is not possible to predict accurately where the next complex will appear. Atrial

fibrillation is an example of this type of rhythm (Fig. 6–36). The QRS complexes occur randomly without order and with no fixed relationship to the rapidly depolarizing atrium.

REGULARLY IRREGULAR. Some rhythms have an irregular but distinct pattern that recurs at periodic intervals. This may be caused by extra beats that are

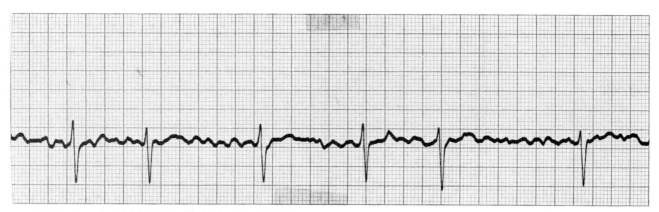

FIGURE 6–36. An irregularly irregular rhythm. Atrial fibrillation. (From Council on Nursing, Carlson V, Ungvarski P (eds): EKG Workbook for Arrhythmia Recognition, 2nd ed. New York, American Heart Association, New York City Affiliate and Heart Fund, 1982.)

coupled with every first or second normal beat (Fig. 6–37).

RELATIONSHIP BETWEEN THE P AND QRS WAVES

Normally a P wave and QRS wave are coupled together. The PR interval is relatively constant, representing the time from SA node firing to ventricular depolarization. The rate for P waves and the rate for QRS complexes are the same.

Extra beats can occur for many reasons. Patients with ischemic heart disease commonly have beats that originate in the ventricle rather than the SA node. In this case, the resulting P and QRS complexes may not be related or no P waves may be seen (Fig. 6–38).

Rhythm Recognition and the Decision to Defibrillate

To defibrillate, an EMT needs to know basic *patterns* of a few rhythms. Knowing the rate of a rhythm or the names of individual complexes is not necessary to identify ventricular fibrillation. In fact, ventricular fibrillation has no rate at all. There are no QRS complexes and no discernible rhythm.

The decision to defibrillate is based on pulselessness and the recognition of ventricular fibrillation on an ECG tracing. Distinguishing ventricular fibrillation from most organized rhythms is usually not difficult. On an ECG tracing, ventricular fibrillation has a disorganized appearance, whereas most organized rhythms have well-defined ventricular complexes (Fig. 6–39).

Before defibrillation is performed, both pulselessness and ventricular fibrillation must be present. Ventricular fibrillation is not capable of producing a pulse. ECG and physical findings are used *jointly* to determine the need for defibrillation.

Both criteria must be met because the following circumstances can occur. First, some ECG rhythms resemble ventricular fibrillation, but a pulse is present. Second, some ECG rhythms are encountered in cardiac arrest that have organized ventricular complexes, but no pulse is present. In these two cases, defibrillation is not indicated. These situations reinforce the need to base the judgement to defibrillate on both ECG and physical findings.

Important Rhythms for EMT-D

The important rhythm patterns to recognize (not specifically name) include the following:

- Rhythms with organized ventricular complexes such as normal sinus rhythm

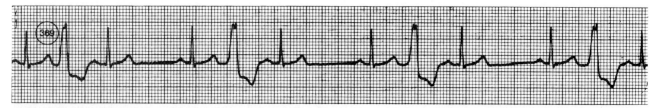

FIGURE 6–37. Regularly irregular rhythm. (From Phillips RE, Feeney MK: The Cardiac Rhythms: A Systematic Approach to Interpretation, 3rd ed. Philadelphia, WB Saunders, 1990, p. 426.)

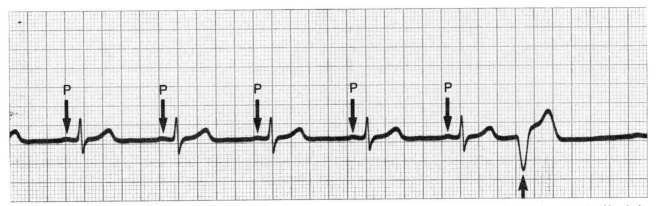

FIGURE 6–38. A ventricular beat without a P wave. (From Council on Nursing, Carlson V, Ungvarski P (eds): EKG Workbook for Arrhythmia Recognition, 2nd ed. New York, American Heart Association, New York City Affiliate and Heart Fund, 1982.)

- Rhythms associated with cardiac arrest (there are four basic types)
- Potentially confusing rhythms that might resemble ventricular fibrillation at first glance

RHYTHMS WITH ORGANIZED VENTRICULAR COMPLEXES.

When an ECG tracing has all of the previously described parts of a normal ECG that repeat at a rate of 60 to 100 times a minute, it is called normal sinus rhythm (Fig. 6–40). This is the most common example of an organized rhythm. Sinus tachycardia has an ECG appearance that is similar to sinus rhythm except the rate is greater than 100 beats per minute. Sinus bradycardia also has a similar appearance except the rate is less than 60 beats per minute.

RHYTHMS ASSOCIATED WITH CARDIAC ARREST.

Four basic rhythms are associated with cardiac arrest. One type is *ventricular fibrillation*. A second is *pulseless ventricular tachycardia*, which often degenerates to ventricular fibrillation. A third is *asystole*, which, as described earlier, appears as a flat line or isoelectric line. A fourth type is called *electrical mechanical dissociation* (EMD), which is characterized by the appearance of organized complexes on the ECG without associated heart contraction and pulse. Treatment for ventricular fibrillation and ventricular tachycardia (in some EMT-D systems) employs defibrillation. Treatment for asystole and EMD requires drug therapy, and defibrillation is of no value.

VENTRICULAR FIBRILLATION. Ventricular fibrillation is characterized by wide, multiformed complexes that vary in size and regularity, giving a jagged, dis-

organized, chaotic appearance on the ECG. This chaotic activity reflects the disorganized firing of various parts of the ventricles. There is no organization, no synchronized electrical or mechanical event, and no cardiac output. Depending on the amplitude of the electrical activity, ventricular fibrillation is commonly called *coarse* or *fine*. There is no absolute criterion for these two terms, but coarse ventricular fibrillation generally is seen in the first minutes after cardiac arrest and is more easily defibrillated. Look carefully at the tracings in Figure 6–41.

VENTRICULAR TACHYCARDIA. Ventricular tachycardia is a rapid dysrhythmia (rate 100 to 220) that originates within the ventricles. It *may or may not* be capable of producing a pulse. Ventricular tachycardia is characterized by wide ventricular complexes often without discernible P or T waves (Figure 6–42). P waves may be noted but they are not initiating the QRS complexes. Most tracings of ventricular tachycardia show a regular appearance, but occasionally they may be irregular. Ventricular tachycardia may be prolonged or interspersed between more regular-appearing complexes of normal sinus rhythm. Defibrillation is performed when ventricular tachycardia is pulseless and continuous. When a rhythm appears that has the appearance of ventricular tachycardia but has a pulse, defibrillation is not indicated. Ventricular tachycardia often is a precursor to ventricular fibrillation. Some EMT-D programs do not advocate defibrillation for this rhythm because it can be confused with other abnormal rhythms for which defibrillation is not indicated.

ASYSTOLE AND AGONAL RHYTHM. The term *asystole* simply means *without contraction*. There is no electrical or mechanical heart activity. Other descriptive terms are *cardiac standstill* and *flat line*.

Asystole may be the initial cardiac arrest rhythm

Text continued on page 272

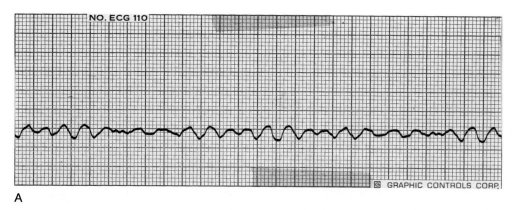

A

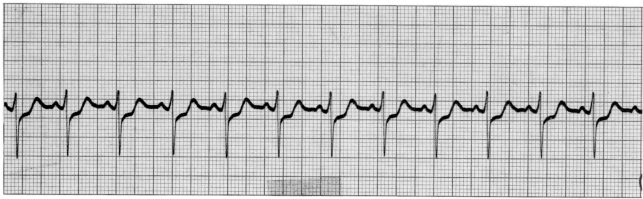

B

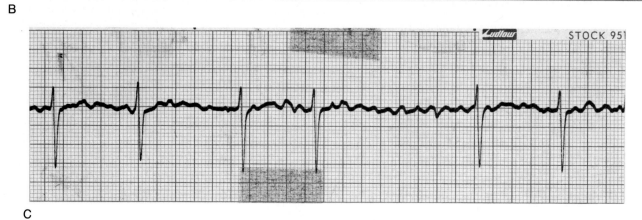

C

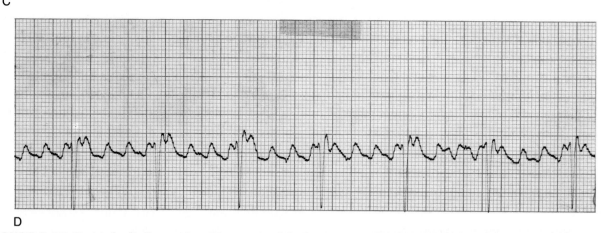

D

FIGURE 6–39. Ventricular fibrillation (A) and four organized rhythms (B to D). (E) Baseline drifting from patient movement. (A to D, from Council on Nursing, Carlson V, Ungvarski P (eds): EKG Workbook for Arrhythmia Recognition, 2nd ed. New York, American Heart Association, New York City Affiliate and Heart Fund, 1982; E, from Phillips RE, Feeney MK: The Cardiac Rhythms: A Systematic Approach to Interpretation, 3rd ed. Philadelphia, WB Saunders, 1990, p. 71.) *Illustration continued on following page*

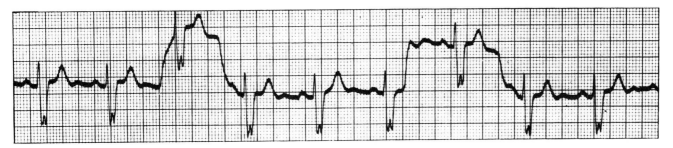

E

FIGURE 6–39. *Continued*

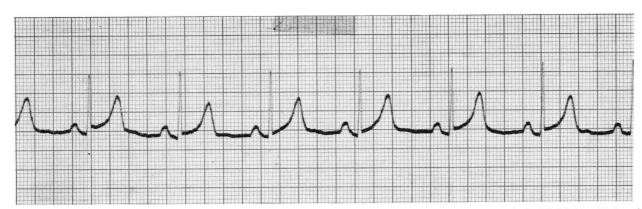

FIGURE 6–40. Normal sinus rhythm. (From Safer P, Bircher N: Cardiopulmonary Cerebral Resuscitation, 3rd ed. Philadelphia, WB Saunders, Bailliere Tindall Book, 1988, p. 184.)

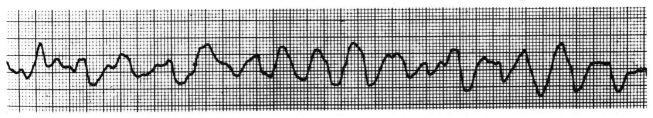

A

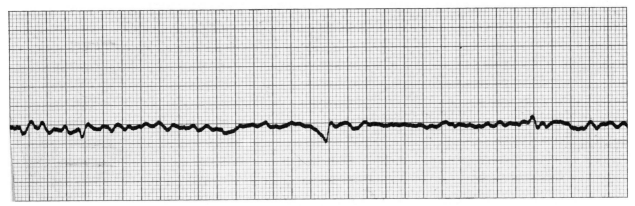

B

FIGURE 6–41. Ventricular fibrillation. (*A*) Coarse and (*B*) fine ventricular fibrillation. (*A*, from Phillips RE, Feeney MK: The Cardiac Rhythms: A Systematic Approach to Interpretation, 3rd ed. Philadelphia, WB Saunders, 1990, p. 401; *B*, from Council on Nursing, Carlson V, Ungvarski P (eds): EKG Workbook for Arrhythmia Recognition, 2nd ed. New York, American Heart Association, New York City Affiliate and Heart Fund, 1982.)

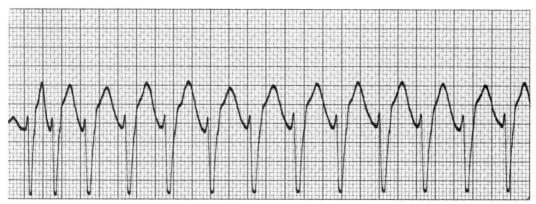

FIGURE 6–42. Ventricular tachycardia. (From Council on Nursing, Carlson V, Ungvarski P (eds): EKG Workbook for Arrhythmia Recognition, 2nd ed. New York, American Heart Association, New York City Affiliate and Heart Fund, 1982.)

or it may appear after several minutes in cardiac arrest. Sometimes the dying heart produces wide beats at a very slow rate with long pauses in between. This is referred to as *agonal* (pertaining to dying) *rhythm* (Figs. 6–43 and 6–44).

Ultimately, all cardiac arrest rhythms progress to asystole if left untreated. A patient is never pronounced dead because the rhythm is asystole, since treatment with CPR and ALS may resuscitate some patients. When asystole is the first rhythm encountered, recheck the monitoring equipment to make sure all leads are attached and the amplitude setting is proper.

Because it is possible (although not common) for ventricular fibrillation to appear as a flat line in one lead, turn the lead select to another setting and take a second look at the rhythm from a different vantage point. There are times when fine ventricular fibrillation may be apparent in another lead. If there is any confusion between very fine ventricular fibrillation and asystole, medical directors often advocate treating the patient for ventricular fibrillation.

ELECTRICAL MECHANICAL DISSOCIATION. EMD is characterized by organized electrical activity without a pulse. In some instances, the tracing will have the P, QRS, and T components seen in normal sinus rhythms;

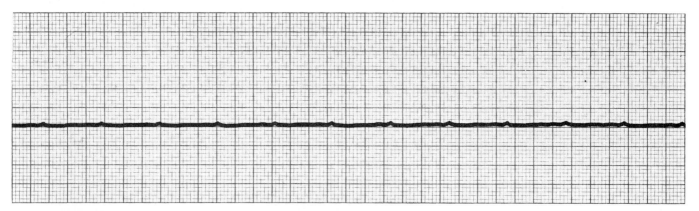

FIGURE 6–43. Asystole. (From Council on Nursing, Carlson V, Ungvarski P (eds): EKG Workbook for Arrhythmia Recognition, 2nd ed. New York, American Heart Association, New York City Affiliate and Heart Fund, 1982.)

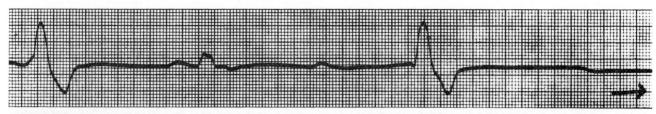

FIGURE 6–44. Agonal rhythm. (From Phillips RE, Feeney MK: The Cardiac Rhythms: A Systematic Approach to Interpretation, 3rd ed. Philadelphia, WB Saunders, 1990, p. 410.)

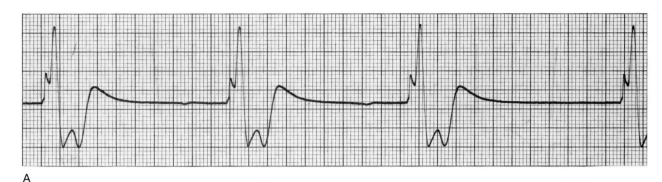

A

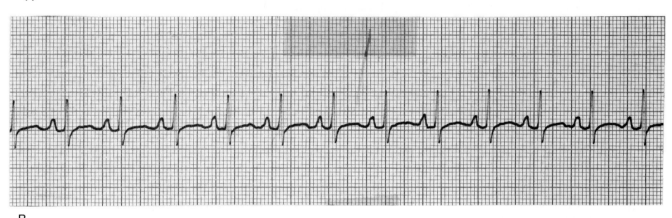

B

FIGURE 6–45. Electrical mechanical dissociation (EMD). Complexes are seen on ECG, but there is no pulse. (From Council on Nursing, Carlson V, Ungvarski P (eds): EKG Workbook for Arrhythmic Recognition, 2nd ed. New York, American Heart Association, New York City Affiliate and Heart Fund, 1982.)

at other times, only ventricular complexes may exist (Fig. 6–45).

The appearance of EMD should cause a careful search for conditions such as hypovolemia, tension pneumothorax, and cardiac tamponade, which require early hospital intervention.

POTENTIALLY CONFUSING RHYTHMS

Although ventricular fibrillation is usually easy to recognize, three rhythms may appear similar at first glance: *artifact, atrial fibrillation,* and *atrial flutter.* The key to differentiating these rhythms from ventricular fibrillation is, again, a careful search for QRS complexes, an equipment check, and the presence or absence of a pulse.

ARTIFACT. Artifact is *disturbance* in the ECG tracing caused by many conditions such as electrical interference, patient or cable movement, dislodging of the cables, muscle tremors, and seizures.

During electrical interference, the cable acts like an antenna and can pick up an electrical current from an AC outlet. The cable may be in contact with an electric bed or metal.

Other causes of artifact include poor attachment of the electrodes to sweaty patients, placement of electrodes over bony prominences, defective pads, patient contact

by the EMT or another person, and performance of CPR. Occasionally, the wiring of the cable itself may be defective. For this reason, it is useful to carry extra cables and electrodes. Figure 6–46 illustrates different types of artifact.

ATRIAL FLUTTER. Atrial flutter is a rhythm where the atria discharge at a rate between 220 and 350 times a minute. Here an abnormal electrical mechanism or pacemaker has taken charge, suppressing the normal pacemaker (SA node). The ventricular complexes are usually rapid (150 per minute) but can vary in rate, and they sometimes are difficult to see because of the predominant overriding pattern of the flutter waves. Flutter waves have a saw-tooth pattern that can mimic ventricular fibrillation. Atrial flutter can be distinguished by the presence of a pulse and the presence of a QRS complex on closer inspection (Fig. 6–47).

ATRIAL FIBRILLATION. Atrial fibrillation occurs when the abnormal discharge of the atria exceeds 350 per minute. No organized contraction of the atria is possible. As in flutter, the fibrillatory waves may be mistaken for ventricular fibrillation. The amplitude of the waves will vary from coarse to fine patterns. Some patterns are so fine that they may appear as a straight line. The ventricles still contract, however, and ventricular complexes are present.

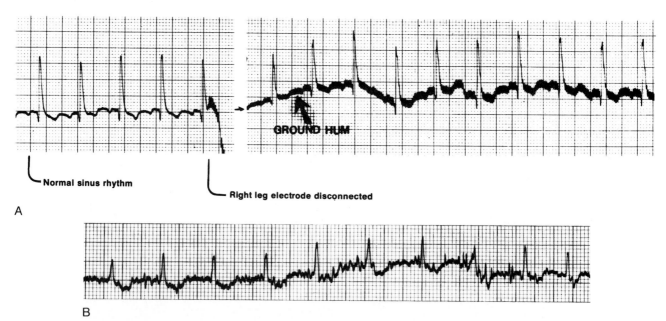

A

B

FIGURE 6–46. Different types of artifact: (*A*) 60-cycle interference; (*B*) muscle tremor. (From Phillips RE, Feeney MK: The Cardiac Rhythms: A Systematic Approach to Interpretation, 3rd ed. Philadelphia, WB Saunders, 1990, pp. 70, 71.)

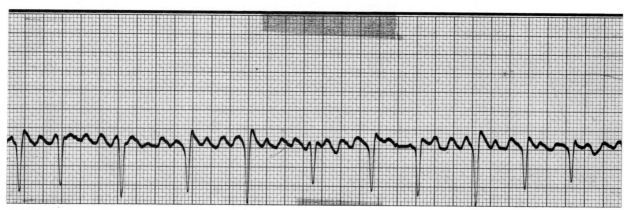

FIGURE 6–47. Atrial flutter. (From Council on Nursing, Carlson V, Ungvarski P (eds): EKG Workbook for Arrhythmia Recognition, 2nd ed. New York, American Heart Association, New York City Affiliate and Heart Fund, 1982.)

Because the AV node is being bombarded by impulses from the atria in excess of 350 times a minute, the AV node is incapable of transmitting each impulse through to the ventricles. Instead, the ventricles respond in an irregularly irregular pattern, and the ultimate rate of ventricular discharge will vary (Fig. 6–48).

PACEMAKER SPIKES IN PRESENCE OF VENTRICULAR FIBRILLATION

Patients with permanent pacemakers may produce ECG spikes that are seen even in the presence of ventricular fibrillation (Fig. 6–49). This can confuse some automatic defibrillators and some EMTs. If there is no pulse and CPR is indicated, these patients should be defibrillated with paddles placed at least 5 inches from the pacemaker box if it is imbedded in the left side of the chest.

Many other rhythms may appear. It is not necessary to know every rhythm to make the correct decision to defibrillate. The diagnostic process remains the same. The patient who has no pulse and ventricular fibrillation or ventricular tachycardia on the ECG is defibrillated. Again, clinical findings and ECG findings together make the diagnosis.

Figure 6–50 summarizes the decision to defibrillate.

Defibrillation Devices

Essentially three types of monitor-defibrillators are available for EMT-D. All allow for rhythm evaluation, defibrillation, and the recording of rhythm and voice on a dual channel tape cassette. Common features of the portable defibrillators used in prehospital care include a battery power source, capacitors to store direct current,

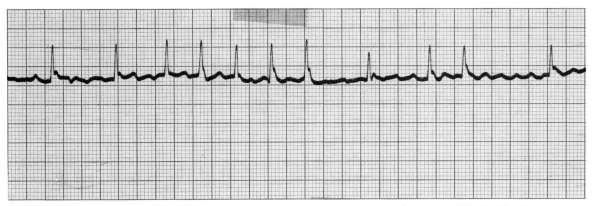

FIGURE 6–48. Atrial fibrillation. (From Council on Nursing, Carlson V, Ungvarski P (eds): EKG Workbook for Arrhythmia Recognition, 2nd ed. New York, American Heart Association, New York City Affiliate and Heart Fund, 1982.)

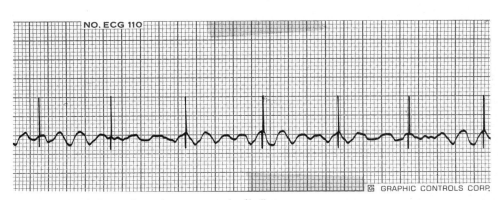

FIGURE 6–49. Pacemaker spikes in ventricular fibrillation.

energy-select switches, charge switches, and discharge switches to allow the current to flow from the capacitor to the electrodes. Many types of monitor–defibrillators have been introduced over the past few years. Recognizing that successful resuscitation of victims of ventricular fibrillation is time dependent, may new devices use new technology to analyze rhythms, determine the need for defibrillation, charge the capacitors, and even discharge the current through the chest electrodes. Terms applied to the three types of monitor–defibrillators include *manual, automatic,* and *semiautomatic.* The manual type requires the EMT to analyze the rhythm, determine the need for defibrillation, select proper energy and charge the paddles, and then defibrillate the patient by activating the discharge switch or button (Fig. 6–51). The semiautomatic type analyzes the rhythm, identifies ventricular fibrillation and some ventricular tachycardias as needing defibrillation, advises the EMT on the need to defibrillate, and simultaneously selects charge energy and charges the capacitors, but it requires user interaction to deliver the shock to the patient. The automatic type identifies ventricular fibrillation and some ventricular tachycardias, charges the paddles at preselected energy levels, and defibrillates the patient after advising the user to stand clear.

No one type of monitor defibrillator is the "best." Many circumstances influence the decision about what device to use in any particular EMS system, including the amount of time available for training and retraining, the number of arrests that an EMT is likely to encounter, and the preferences of providers and medical directors. Regardless of what device is selected, it is imperative that the EMT be thoroughly familiar with its operation, care, and maintenance. In this chapter the manual monitor–defibrillator is used for illustration of the multiple steps involved. The automatic and semiautomatic machinery incorporate all the steps of the manual defibrillator, except that some of the steps are done automatically.

Technique Using Conventional Defibrillators

All of the following procedures assume that the operator is using a manual monitor–defibrillator. The technique employed in defibrilliaton requires practice. The basic components necessary for successful defibrillation include rhythm recognition, correlation of clinical

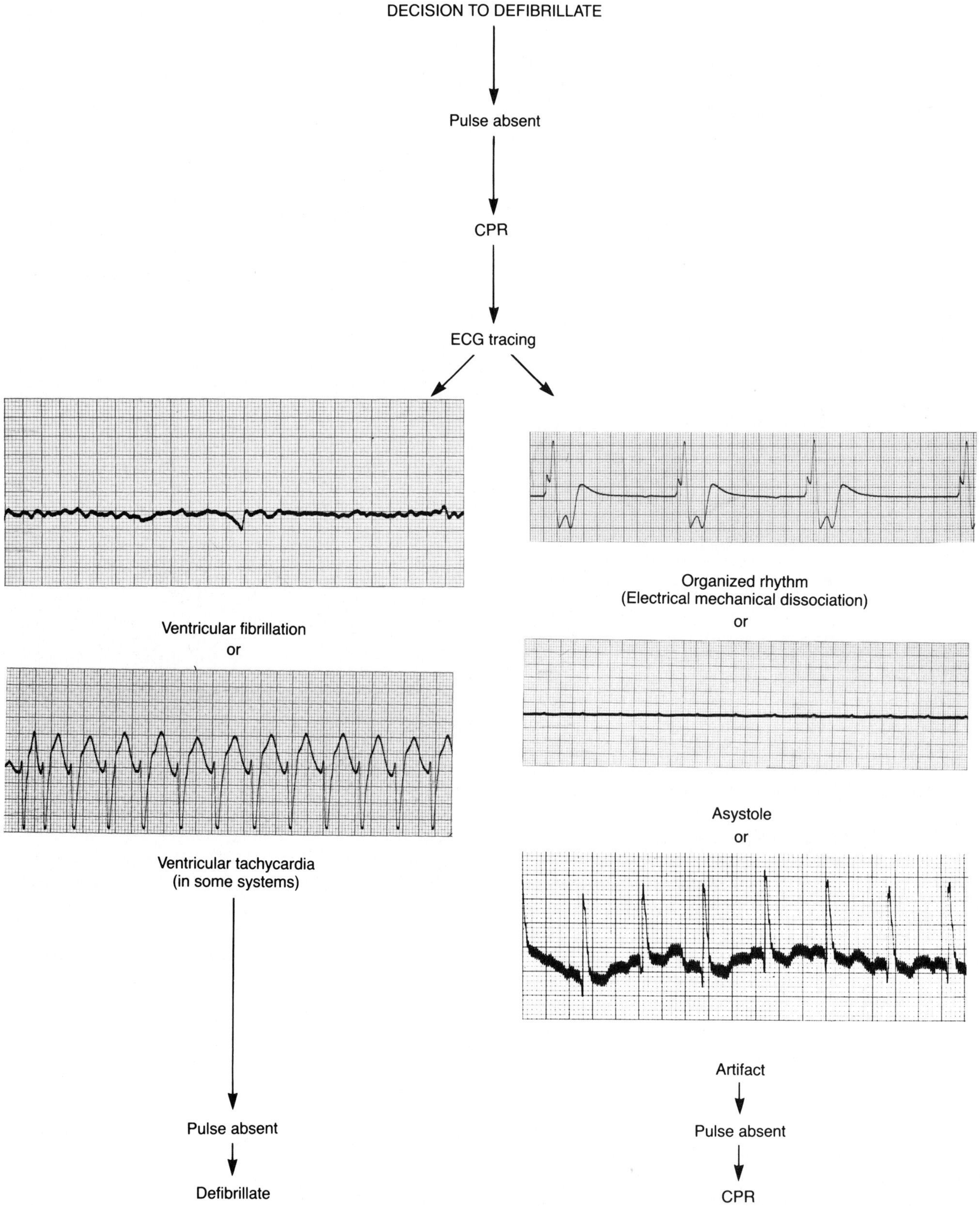

FIGURE 6–50. Decision to defibrillate. (*Top* and strips at *left* and *top right*, from Safer P, Bircher N: Cardiopulmonary Cerebral Resuscitation, 3rd ed. Bailliere Tindall Book, 1988, p. 194; *middle right*, from Council on Nursing, Carlson V, Ungvarski P (eds): EKG Workbook for Arrhythmia Recognition, 2nd ed. New York, American Heart Association, New York City Affiliate and Heart Fund, 1982; *bottom right*, from Phillips RE, Feeney MK: The Cardiac Rhythms: A Systematic Approach to Interpretation, 3rd ed. Philadelphia, WB Saunders, 1990.)

signs, application of a conductive gel, paddle placement and pressure, energy selection, energy delivery, and post-defibrillation evaluation. During defibrillation of the patient, the EMT is responsible for ensuring that rescuers and bystanders are not in contact with the patient.

RHYTHM RECOGNITION. Use of the monitor has been discussed. In the case of cardiac arrest, one should confirm pulselessness for at least 5 seconds. Again, it is this diagnostic check, together with recognition of ventricular fibrillation (or pulseless ventricular tachycardia), that leads to the decision to defibrillate.

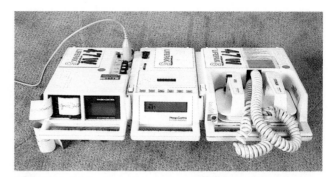

FIGURE 6–51. Manual monitor–defibrillator for EMT-D. (*Left*) Monitor; (*center*) medical control recording device; (*right*) defibrillator.

PROCEDURE 6–6 OPERATING THE MONITOR

1. Attach the patient cables to the electrodes, which are placed in standard positions on the patient (Figs. 6–28*A* and 6–52).
2. Turn on the main power switch. A line or ECG tracing appears on the screen. Turn the paper recording switch to on and press the standardization button. Adjust the standardization to about 10 mm, if it is not already preset. Turn on the medical control recording device if it is not turned on automatically.
3. Make sure the lead selection button is in the cable mode, usually lead II (see Fig. 6–29).
4. Observe the ECG on the monitor and the paper. If the monitor tracing is not bright enough or the paper readout is not dark enough, adjust these elements by turning the appropriate dials. Evaluate the ECG pattern and recheck the pulse. If a flat line appears, recheck the equipment and amplitude setting or select another lead.
5. Verbally describe important events as you proceed, such as ascertaining pulselessness, rhythm interpretation, energy selection, energy delivery, and postdefibrillation rhythm and pulse.

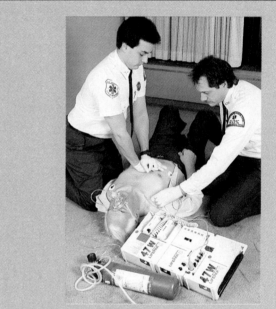

FIGURE 6–52. Attach electrodes.

MONITOR–DEFIBRILLATOR ELECTRODES. Some machines use one set of electrodes for both monitoring and defibrillation. These electrodes are placed below the right clavicle on the right sternal border and to the left of the nipple at the mid-axillary line.

As with standard monitoring electrodes, combination electrodes are attached using adhesive pads with gel covering the electrode. If there is excessive sweating, wipe the area before application to ensure good contact Avoid attachment over bony prominences.

PRECORDIAL THUMP. In instances of ventricular fibrillation or ventricular tachycardia it may be necessary to administer a *precordial thump*. A precordial thump is used when the defibrillator is not immediately available in a witnessed cardiac arrest. It is administered in the mid-sternum with the side of a closed fist. From a height of 8 to 12 inches, deliver a single blow, and evaluate the pulse and ECG (Figs. 6–53 and 6–54).

DEFIBRILLATOR OPERATION. Defibrillation is performed by the placement of paddles on the anterior chest wall in such a way as to maximize electrical energy delivery through the heart. The energy is a short burst of direct current generated by batteries that charge energy-storage capacitors within the machine. The capacitors are connected to the paddles, which are placed on the chest wall in a configuration that delivers the current through the heart when the current is released.

ENERGY SELECTION

Energy selected for defibrillation is expressed in *joules*, or watt-seconds (Fig. 6–55). Energy settings cur-

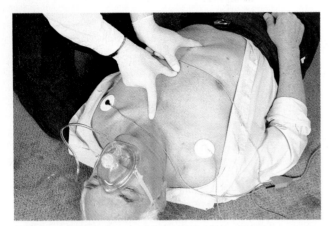

FIGURE 6–53. Measure halfway between the top and bottom of the sternum.

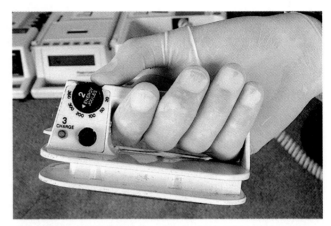

FIGURE 6–55. Select the appropriate energy.

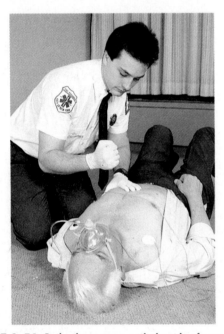

FIGURE 6–54. Strike the sternum with the side of your clenched fist from an 8- to 12-inch distance.

rently recommended by the American Heart Association are 200 joules for the first defibrillation, and, if ventricular fibrillation persists, 200 to 300 joules for the second defibrillation and 360 joules for the third defibrillation. When the selection has been made, the internal capacitors are charged by pushing a charge button. The charge button and energy selection switch are located on the machine and also on the paddles (Fig. 6–56). An audible noise or flashing light may indicate the machine is charging. The machine takes several seconds to become fully charged. When the device indicates that the capacitors are fully charged, the energy can be released from the paddles by simultaneously depressing two buttons on the paddles or a button on the machine.

Some machines cannot hold a full charge for long periods. If energy leaks from the capacitors, the machine may disable the discharge switch to prevent the operator from delivering less than the selected energy. When energy leaks, some machines automatically recharge, whereas others may require user interaction. Be aware of the specific characteristics of your machine.

DISARMING THE DEFIBRILLATOR

Should the patient's rhythm change so that defibrillation is no longer indicated, the EMT must safely discharge the paddles according to manufacturer's instructions. For some manual defibrillators, this can be easily done by turning the energy select button, turning the power off, or dumping the charge into the test device or paddle cradle on the machine. Know the specific characteristics of the monitor used in your program.

ENERGY DELIVERY

Generally, 200 joules of energy are used initially for adult defibrillation. Maximum output for the portable machines is generally 360 to 400 joules. Use doses recommended in your local protocols.

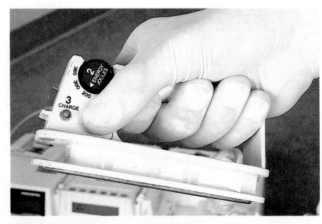

FIGURE 6–56. Charging the defibrillator paddles.

To maximize energy delivered through the heart, the operator must use proper technique and procedure to minimize the resistance of the chest wall. Proper paddle placement, use of a conductive gel interface between the paddles and the skin, and sufficient paddle pressure are important for the delivery of the energy selected.

PADDLE PLACEMENT

Defibrillator paddles are placed in two locations on the anterior chest wall. One paddle is positioned just below the right clavicle on the right sternal border. The other paddle is placed just to the left of the left nipple on the mid-axillary line (Fig. 6–57).

Paddle placement is important because the position of the paddles directs energy flow. If the paddles are placed too close to each other, only a small portion of the myocardium may be defibrillated. In hospital settings, and less commonly in prehospital settings, anterior-posterior placement of paddle electrodes is sometimes used. Again the heart is between the two contacts for electrical flow. The anterior paddle should be placed on the precordium just to the left of the sternal border, whereas the other paddle is placed posteriorly, behind the heart beneath the scapula and lateral to the spine. Figure 6–58 illustrates the pathway of energy with correct paddle placement.

CONDUCTIVE MEDIUMS

To improve conduction across the skin, a conductive gel or medium is used (Fig. 6–59A and B). You can use saline-soaked gauze pads, special conductive gels or creams, or pregelled monitor defibrillator pads that are attached to the skin. Regardless of the conductive medium selected, care must be taken so that bridging does not occur. *Bridging* is the transfer of electricity from one paddle to another by the conductive medium, sweat, or other forms of moisture on the chest wall. This can result from excessive conductive gel being spread across the chest's surface or from too much saline pooling above the sternum and running toward the other paddle. The electric energy (taking the path of least resistance) bridges across the skin surface rather than through the chest wall. Defibrillation is then ineffective. Bridging can be recognized by the appearance of sparks on the chest wall or a muffled explosive sound after energy discharge. If this occurs, wipe the skin surface dry and repeat the correct procedure.

PADDLE PRESSURE

The pressure should be sufficient to ensure firm contact between the paddle and the surface of the skin. About 25 pounds of muscular pressure is recommended. Use arm pressure instead of body weight to avoid slip-

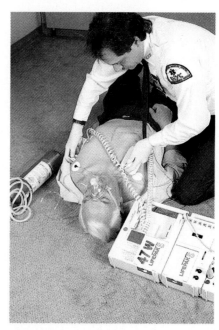

FIGURE 6–57. Paddle placement.

ping and coming in contact with the patient or stretcher during energy discharge.

PADDLE SIZE

Paddle size can influence energy delivery. Most equipment used by EMTs is designed for adult patients. Smaller paddles are indicated for children (8 cm diameter) and infants (4.5 cm diameter) (Fig. 6–60). However, ventricular fibrillation is rare in children and infants, in whom most deaths are caused by respiratory problems or trauma. In the rare situation in which defibrillation may be warranted (if authorized in your system) the energy setting for children should be 2 joules per kilogram of body weight (about 1 joule per pound).

ENERGY DELIVERY

After determining the need for ventricular defibrillation and charging the paddles, make sure that all personnel stand clear of the patient, the bed or stretcher, or any equipment touching the patient. Say out loud, "Stand clear," then observe to make sure no one (including you) is in direct or indirect contact (Fig. 6–61). When you are sure that all are clear, depress both paddle discharge buttons simultaneously. The electrical energy is transmitted across the chest wall and through the heart. Energy delivery usually causes the patient to have a transient muscle spasm and movement. After every defibrillation, check for pulse and reassess the rhythm. Immediately following defibrillation, recheck the pulse and ECG (Fig. 6–62).

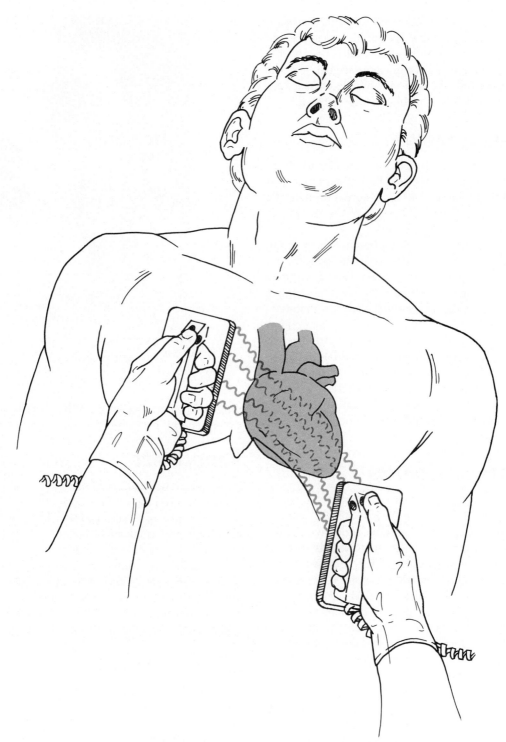

FIGURE 6–58. Pathway of energy during defibrillation.

DEFIBRILLATION

Timely defibrillation is the most important treatment in successful resuscitation of cardiac arrest victims who have suffered ventricular fibrillation or pulseless ventricular tachycardia. Practice with your partner and use mock scenarios to reduce the time from arrival at the scene to application of the first defibrillation. Ideally this should take place as soon as possible. Local protocols should be followed, but basic steps are outlined in Procedure 6–7.

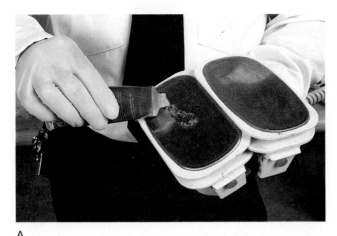

A

FIGURE 6–59. Applying gel to paddles.

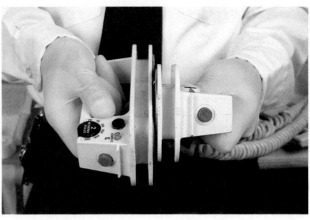

B

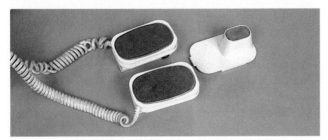

FIGURE 6–60. Adult and pediatric paddles.

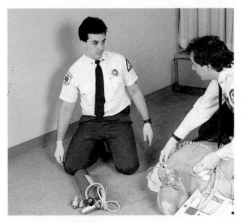

FIGURE 6–61. Clear personnel prior to defibrillation.

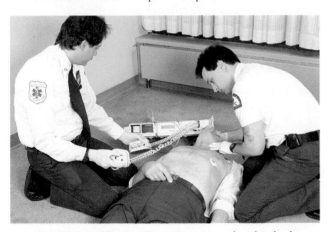

FIGURE 6–62. Reevaluate the patient after the shock.

PROCEDURE 6–7
DEFIBRILLATION

1. If pulselessness is detected, initiate CPR.
2. As soon as a monitor-defibrillator is available, attach leads and turn on the recorder and the medical control recording device.
3. Assess rhythm. If ventricular fibrillation or pulseless ventricular tachycardia is present, check for pulse (for at least 5 seconds) and charge paddles to 200 joules.
4. Apply paddles to correct location, using conductive gel and firm (25-pound) pressure.
5. Operator announces, "Stand clear" and makes sure no one is in contact with patient, stretcher, or patient equipment.
6. Press the discharge buttons on the paddles to defibrillate.
7. Reevaluate pulse and rhythm.
8. If the patient is still in ventricular fibrillation, repeat steps 3 through 7 with 200 to 300 joules.
9. If the patient is still in ventricular fibrillation, repeat steps 3 through 7 with 360 joules.
10. If the rhythm changes, always evaluate the need for CPR.

Defibrillation and the ECG

Immediately after defibrillation, an isoelectric (flat) line may be observed for a short interval on the ECG. This corresponds with the forced rest period after the simultaneous discharge of the myocardial cells caused by defibrillation. The isoelectric line represents the whole purpose of defibrillation. Defibrillation stops the chaotic and disorganized firing of fibrillation and forces all the cells to take a rest at the same time. This rest gives the pacemaker a chance to assume control of the heart's rhythm again.

Postdefibrillation Care

The results of defibrillation vary from case to case, but three general possibilities can be anticipated:

- The patient remains in cardiac arrest with ventricular fibrillation or ventricular tachycardia.
- The patient remains in cardiac arrest but shows a rhythm of asystole or EMD.
- The patient has a pulse and a rhythm with organized ventricular complexes.

PATIENTS REMAINING IN VENTRICULAR FIBRILLATION OR TACHYCARDIA

Many patients remain in ventricular fibrillation or tachycardia after defibrillation. The recommended response is to deliver a second defibrillation immediately after verifying that the dysrhythmia persists and that a pulse is not present. The second defibrillation is sometimes more effective. This is because the first defibrillation reduces chest wall resistance (permits energy to flow more freely), allowing more energy to be delivered across the heart. If the patient remains in ventricular fibrillation or tachycardia after the second defibrillation, the energy delivered during the third defibrillation can be increased to 360 joules.

If after three defibrillations, the patient still remains in ventricular defibrillation or tachycardia, he or she will probably require ALS, including drug therapy, before he or she can be resuscitated. The appropriate response at this point is to continue CPR and render further ALS to the patient as soon as possible.

Some protocols may call for a second series of three defibrillations after a short period of CPR. The EMTs should deliver CPR for 1 to 2 minutes and administer 100% or high-concentration oxygen during ventilations. The patient may be too hypoxic or acidotic (from waste products building up during cardiac arrest) for defibrillation to be effective. By delivering CPR with ventilations supplemented with 100% oxygen, the patient may be more responsive to the next defibrillation series.

PATIENTS CONVERTING TO ASYSTOLE OR EMD

Frequently, after defibrillation, patients remain in cardiac arrest but show a rhythm of asystole or EMD. Defibrillation is not indicated for either of these rhythms. (Always reassess your equipment and try a second lead when asystole first appears.) Drug therapy is needed to treat these rhythms. Continue CPR and get the patient to the closest hospital. Always try to assess the cause of the cardiac arrest. Not every case is caused by myocardial infarction. Consider as possible causes hypovo- lemia, tension pneumothorax, and other conditions requiring rapid definitive hospital treatment. Follow local protocols. Monitor the rhythm en route to the hospital while continuing CPR. If ventricular fibrillation reappears, local protocols may direct you to render another defibrillation attempt.

PATIENTS WHOSE PULSE RETURNS

Patients whose pulse returns show varying clinical and ECG responses. Of greater importance is the fact that a pulse is now present. Continue to monitor ventilations closely and administer positive-pressure ventilations as indicated.

IMPROVEMENT IN CLINICAL STATUS. A lapse usually occurs between the reappearance of a pulse and the return of spontaneous respirations and consciousness. Your handling of the airway and ventilatory status is critical at this point. Ensure adequate oxygenation and ventilations. Usually a patient's speed of recovery is related to the length of time he or she was in cardiac arrest. Patients who are defibrillated immediately after a witnessed cardiac arrest are the most likely to have rapid return of spontaneous ventilations and consciousness. Patients who have spent a longer time in cardiac arrest may require continued respiratory support and have no return of consciousness in the prehospital setting. Care of their airway and ensuring ventilations are the important factors leading to their survival after a pulse has returned.

TYPES OF RHYTHMS. Patients whose pulse returns may show various rhythms on the ECG. Patients may respond to defibrillation with the return of rapid rhythms with organized complexes. Atrial fibrillation or atrial flutter is not uncommon. The appearance of these latter rhythms after successful defibrillation reinforces the importance of the pulse check and careful ECG evaluation after each defibrillation attempt. Some patients may respond with very slow rhythms. With good oxygenation, their pulses often get stronger and faster.

Refibrillation

If a patient converts from ventricular fibrillation to an organized rhythm and then returns to ventricular fibrillation, a repeat attempt at defibrillation is warranted. Energy selection for treatment of recurrent fibrillation should be similar to the amounts last used to convert the rhythm. Recurrent ventricular fibrillation usually indicates a need for antiarrhythmic drug therapy. The strategy should be to seek such therapy in the shortest possible time.

Recorder

Documentation of the rhythm before and after defibrillation is an important part of the medical record. As noted, the devices used with conventional defibrillators have a built-in recorder that documents ECG, defibrillation, and voice (Fig. 6–63). EMTs should record their actions verbally during all phases of assessment and treatment. This recording serves as part of the medical record and is essential for quality assurance. This enables the defibrillation program to proceed with *standing orders* under proper medical control. The recording is part of the record review and allows for accurate recording of the events leading up to and following defibrillation. Accurate prehospital records (as achieved through recording devices) allow for reviews and studies that lead to improvements in both EMS systems and in the performance of individual EMS providers.

Medical Control

Medical control is an essential part of any EMT-D program. Physicians must assume responsibility for the program. The essential components requiring physician direction include education, protocol development, continuing education programs to ensure skill retention, case review, and evaluation of outcome.

Usually, standing orders are used in EMT defibrillation programs. Standing orders are written protocols directing the actions of EMTs to save valuable time in administering advanced therapy when they encounter critically ill patients. Standing orders are especially important in conditions such as ventricular fibrillation, in

which prompt application of defibrillation makes a difference in outcome. The following is a sample protocol for patients in cardiac arrest with ventricular fibrillation or ventricular tachycardia.

✚ P R O T O C O L ✚

DEFIBRILLATION OF PATIENTS WITH CARDIAC ARREST AND VENTRICULAR FIBRILLATION OR VENTRICULAR TACHYCARDIA

1. Begin CPR (if you witness cardiac arrest, give a precordial thump if a defibrillator is not immediately available).

2. As soon as a monitor–defibrillator is available, evaluate rhythm.

3. If ventricular fibrillation or ventricular tachycardia is observed, and no pulse, defibrillate at 200 joules.

4. Reassess pulse and rhythm; if no pulse and if ventricular fibrillation or ventricular tachycardia is still present, defibrillate at 200 to 300 joules.

5. Reassess pulse and rhythm; if no pulse and if ventricular fibrillation or ventricular tachycardia is still present, defibrillate at 360 or 400 joules.

6. Reassess pulse and rhythm continue CPR if necessary.

7. If cardiac arrest persists, perform CPR for 1 minute and perform up to three more defibrillations at 360 joules.

8. Follow local strategy to obtain earliest ALS.

Automatic and Semiautomatic Defibrillators

This section gives a general explanation of how automatic and semiautomatic defibrillators operate.

AUTOMATIC

As mentioned earlier, some defibrillators are fully automatic. They can interpret ventricular fibrillation and, in some cases, ventricular tachycardia and spontaneously initiate defibrillation. Automatic defibrillators remove the necessity of ECG rhythm recognition and minimize concerns about EMT error (Fig. 6–64).

Automatic defibrillators are attached to the patient and turned on; the EMTs then stand clear of the patient. An audible signal notifies the rescuers of the impending defibrillation. Extreme caution should be exercised to avoid inadvertently shocking rescuers or bystanders (see Fig. 6–64).

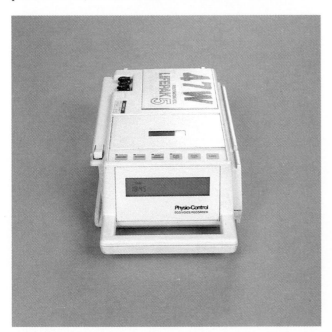

FIGURE 6–63. Medical control recorder.

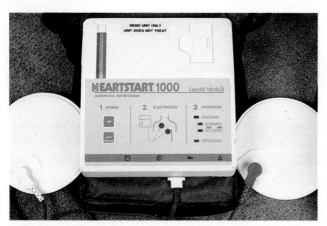

FIGURE 6–64. Automatic defibrillator.

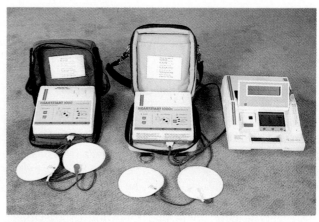

FIGURE 6–65. (*Left* and *middle*) Automatic defibrillator. (*Right*) Semiautomatic defibrillator.

SEMIAUTOMATIC

Semiautomatic defibrillators are similar to automatic defibrillators in that they are capable of recognizing ventricular fibrillation and some cases of ventricular tachycardia (Fig. 6–65). However, they differ in that the rescuer must initiate the defibrillation. Some program medical directors prefer this type of device since it theoretically reduces the chances of injury to rescuers and bystanders.

Semiautomatic defibrillators vary slightly in their operation. A typical protocol for the operation of a semiautomatic defibrillator follows.

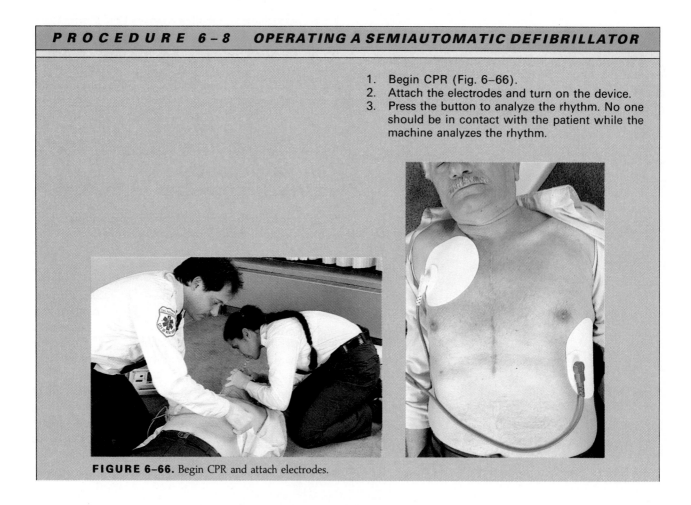

P R O C E D U R E 6 – 8   OPERATING A SEMIAUTOMATIC DEFIBRILLATOR

1. Begin CPR (Fig. 6–66).
2. Attach the electrodes and turn on the device.
3. Press the button to analyze the rhythm. No one should be in contact with the patient while the machine analyzes the rhythm.

FIGURE 6–66. Begin CPR and attach electrodes.

4. If ventricular fibrillation is present, the machine automatically charges to 200 joules while sounding an audible alarm and/or a voice recording directing bystanders to stand back (Fig. 6–67).
5. The machine then advises you to press the defibrillation button.
6. Make sure that everyone is clear of the patient and deliver the shock. Say "I'm clear, you're clear, everybody's clear" while carefully observing the area around the patient.
7. Following the shock, push the analyze button.
8. If the machine advises to shock, repeat procedures 5 through 7.
9. If ventricular fibrillation persists after the second shock, the energy level can be increased to 200 to 300 joules before initiating the next defibrillation and to 360 joules for the third shock, if necessary.

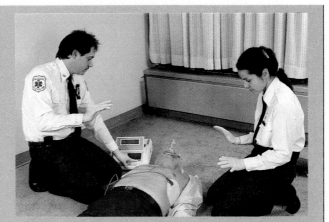

FIGURE 6–67. Machine charges, advises shock, all clear.

The American Heart Association recommends three "stacked" defibrillations followed by 1 minute of CPR. If the defibrillator continues to advise defibrillation, another set of three "stacked" defibrillations is provided, followed by 1 minute of CPR. This process is continued until the machine no longer advises to defibrillate or until ALS measures are available (i.e., drug therapy, intubation, and so forth). If the patient is within a few minutes' transport time to ALS, then it may be appropriate to transport after two sets of stacked shocks. However, if transport would be prolonged, defibrillations would be continued until the machine no longer advises defibrillation.

If the patient regains a pulse, evaluate ventilation and provide positive-pressure ventilation and/or supplemental oxygen as needed.

Defibrillator Maintenance

The defibrillator must be carefully maintained to ensure readiness and prevent operational failure. Following the manufacturer's instructions, set up and adhere to a regular schedule of maintenance, visual checks, and testing of delivered energy. Keep a log to record these maintenance functions.

MEDICAL CONTROL MODULE

At the completion of the call, the EMT must document the events by completing a patient record and providing the medical control physician with the medical control module. This module records the events of the call and allows the physician to produce a record that includes the serial ECG tracings, the times of defibril-

lation, and the time of transport. This type of record provides the primary basis for quality assurance.

VOICE RECORDER

The voice recorder of an automatic defibrillator is maintained as is any tape cassette system. A fresh tape should be placed in the machine at the beginning of every tour. If tapes are to be saved for call review sessions, they should be labeled and modified to prevent overtaping.

BATTERIES

Battery maintenance varies from machine to machine; regardless of the individual machine, however, all batteries should be tested on a regular basis to ensure an adequate charge. Back-up batteries and battery chargers should be available in sufficient numbers to ensure that fresh batteries are at hand if needed.

TROUBLE SHOOTING

Table 6–6 lists the key trouble-shooting steps for one type of defibrillator. Know appropriate steps to take for the equipment you use.

Summary

Defibrillation is a dramatic intervention that has been proven to save lives of victims of cardiac arrest. Because EMTs are overwhelmingly the largest group of medically trained personnel to reach emergency patients, EMT-D offers a great advance in prehospital care. With

TABLE 6-6. Trouble and Corrective Action

Trouble	Steps to Correct	Trouble	Steps to Correct
Unit fails to turn on	1. Verify battery is fully installed 2. Install a fully charged battery and recheck operation	Service mandatory	1. Turn device off, then on 2. Replace battery with fully charged battery 3. If message remains, discontinue use and follow medical protocols to continue patient care 4. Remove device from use and request repair
Check electrode message	1. Attach electrodes to patient 2. Press electrodes down on patient's chest 3. Verify cables are connected to electrodes 4. Verify electrodes have not reached their expiration date 5. Apply a new set of electrodes 6. If message continues, impedance may not permit defibrillation and patient should be treated according to medical protocols	Self-check does not indicate OK	1. Turn device off, then on. If message "Self-test OK" still does not appear, follow medical protocols to continue patient care 2. Remove device from use and request repair
Memory module?	1. Verify medical control module is installed and fully seated in receptacle 2. Replace medical control module with new or empty module	Needs service message	1. Replace medical control module
		Controls do not operate	1. Install a fully charged battery 2. Control is defective, request service
Needs service, battery low messages	1. Battery is nearly depleted, replace with fully charged battery if available 2. Continue to operate if replacement battery is not available	Clock time is wrong	1. Reset clock, check date 2. Reset date
		Clock cannot be set	1. Check that medical control module has been removed from device 2. If unable to set, remove device from service and request repair
Service mandatory, battery low messages	1. Battery is depleted, unit will no longer operate, replace with fully charged battery 2. Follow medical protocols to continue patient care if replacement battery is not available	Check recorder	1. Ensure tape cassette is installed 2. Ensure cassette is not at end of tape 3. Ensure tape door is closed fully

(From Laerdel Heartstart 2000 Operating Manual, Laerdel Corporation, Armonk, NY.)

some basic understanding of the ECG and the principles of defibrillation, the EMT is asked to distinguish ventricular fibrillation and pulseless ventricular tachycardia from asystole and electrical mechanical dissociation in pulseless, clinically dead patients. EMTs who master the necessary knowledge can offer defibrillation in addition to CPR to cardiac arrest patients and greatly enhance the chances of successful resuscitation.

To stay current in this skill, attend case review and skill retention sessions. Review the text, your protocols, and specific operating procedures for your monitor-defibrillator. Be thoroughly familiar with the use and maintenance of your equipment and know its abilities and its limitations.

REVIEW EXERCISES

1. Describe the correct steps of performance for:
   One-rescuer CPR
   Two-rescuer CPR

2. Describe the appropriate actions for performing CPR under the following conditions:
   Moving a cardiac arrest patient down a stairway
   At ground level
   In a moving ambulance

3. Describe the history of prehospital defibrillation.

4. Explain why EMTs are an ideal population to provide prehospital defibrillation.

5. Explain the following concepts related to the function of the heart (Chapter 4):
   Automaticity   Repolarization
   Depolarization   The rest period
   Conductivity

6. Define the following terms:
   Electrodes
   Leads
   Standardization

7. Describe the operation of the monitor.

8. Explain how to calculate rate using the following methods:
   Six-second strip
   Large-box method
   Small-box method

9. Correctly label an ECG complex and explain its relationship to mechanical events within the heart.

10. List your actions when presented with the following ECG rhythms with conventional and semiautomatic defibrillators:
    Asystole
    An organized rhythm without a pulse (EMD)
    Ventricular tachycardia without a pulse
    Ventricular fibrillation

11. Describe the operation of a conventional defibrillator.

12. State the American Heart Association recommended energy levels for defibrillation.

13. Describe the care of the patient following successful defibrillation.

REFERENCES

American Heart Association: Advanced cardiac life support manual. Dallas, American Heart Association, 1985.

Cummins RO, Eisenberg MS: Pre-hospital cardiopulmonary resuscitation. Is it effective? JAMA 253:2408–2412, 1985.

Eisenberg MS, et al: Treatment of out-of-hospital cardiac arrest with rapid defibrillation by emergency medical technicians. N Engl J Med 302(25):1379, 1980.

Gervin AS, Fischer RP: The importance of prompt transport in salvage of patients with penetrating heart wounds. J Trauma 22:443–448, 1982.

Prehospital Trauma Life Support Committee of the National Association of EMTs: Pre-hospital trauma life support. Akron, Ohio, Emergency Training, 1986.

Safer P, Bircher N: Cardiopulmonary cerebral resuscitation, 3rd ed. Philadelphia, WB Saunders, 1983.

Standards and guidelines for cardiopulmonary resuscitation and emergency cardiac care. JAMA 255:2905–2985, 1986.

Zuidema GD, Rutherford RB, Ballinger WF: The Management of Trauma, 4th ed. Philadelphia, WB Saunders, 1985.

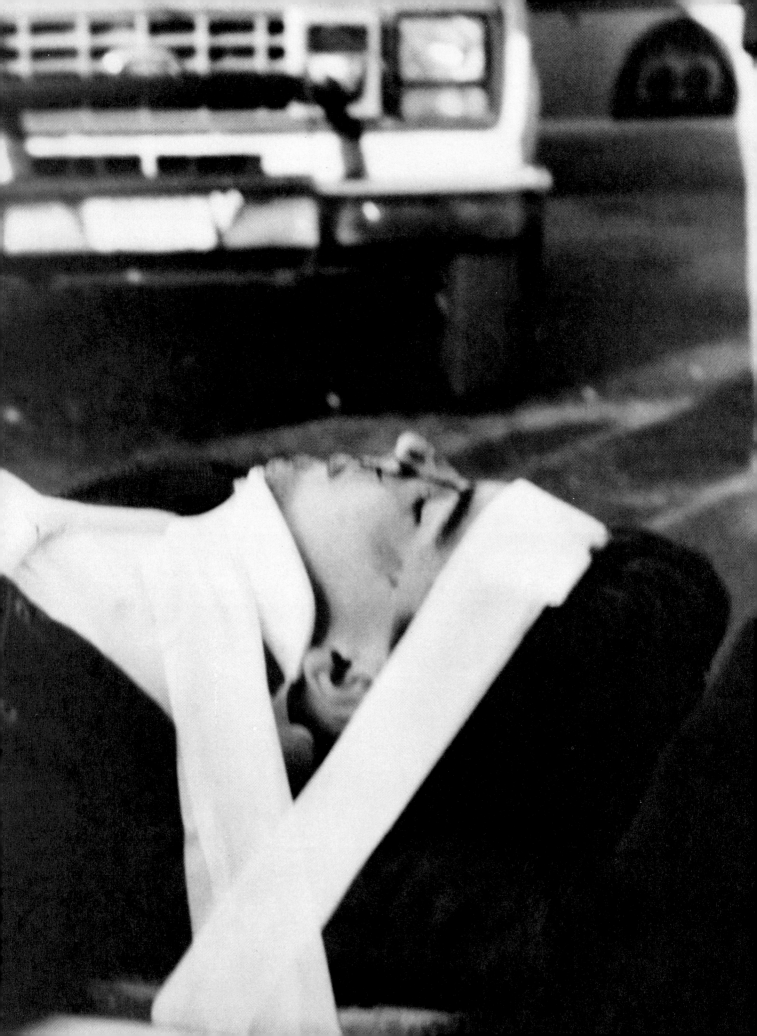

CHAPTER 7

CENTRAL NERVOUS SYSTEM EMERGENCIES

OBJECTIVES

At the conclusion of this chapter the reader will be able to:

1. Describe how the brain is protected from injury.

2. List three functions of the central nervous system.

3. List two signs and symptoms of possible basilar skull fracture.

4. Demonstrate how to open an airway in a patient with a suspected neck injury.

5. Demonstrate how to evaluate an unconscious patient with a suspected spinal injury

6. Demonstrate how to properly immobilize the cervical spine.

7. Demonstrate a four-person log roll for the patient with a suspected spinal injury.

8. Demonstrate how to "package" a patient with a suspected spinal injury to ensure no movement when the board is turned or tipped.

9. Demonstrate the proper helmet removal technique.

10. List the steps to be taken in the emergency care of a patient during and after a seizure or a convulsion.

INTRODUCTION

One of the major goals of emergency care is to ensure brain viability. This underscores the need for the EMT to be familiar with the functions of the nervous system. A large majority of deaths due to trauma result from direct injury to the nervous system. In addition, because the brain is the controlling center for other vital organ systems, such as respiration and circulation, brain dysfunction may result in cardiopulmonary failure and death. Because of the interdependence of the heart, lungs, and brain, signs of brain function are used to assess the status of other vital organs.

The *nervous system* is the controlling organ of the body. It is the center of consciousness and the intellectual, emotional, and behavioral functions that make up much of the characteristics of personality and human behavior. It receives and interprets stimuli from the internal and external environment, and it directs and regulates other organs and tissues. Some of its activity is conscious or willful, while much of the brain activity is unconscious or involuntary in response to the environment.

DIVISIONS OF THE NERVOUS SYSTEM

Central and Peripheral Nervous System

The nervous system is composed of two main divisions: the *central nervous system* and the *peripheral nervous system*. The central nervous system is the computer, and the peripheral nervous system is the communicator. The central nervous system is made up of the brain, the brainstem, and the spinal cord (see Fig. 2–17).

The central nervous system (CNS) receives information about the outside environment and about functions within the body itself. In turn, it organizes and analyzes this information and formulates a response that directs the activities of the organs, muscles, and other tissues.

The CNS receives and transmits information via nerves or special tracts of nerve tissue that extend through the CNS and extend out into the peripheral nervous system. The peripheral nervous system is composed of the nerves outside the central nervous system, which extend from both the brainstem and spinal cord. Peripheral nerves leaving from the brainstem are called *cranial nerves*, and those leaving from the spinal cord are called the *spinal nerves*. The peripheral nervous system carries messages to the spinal cord and brain via *sensory nerves*, and it carries messages back to the muscles and various organs via the *motor nerves*.

Voluntary and Autonomic Divisions

The nervous system can also be divided by function. Divisions include voluntary or willful activities, such as running to catch a train, and involuntary activities. The *autonomic nervous system* (ANS) is concerned with control of involuntary body functions. This includes control of the heart, smooth muscles within organs such as the digestive tract, and the glands.

VOLUNTARY DIVISION

The voluntary nervous system connects the central nervous system with sensory nerves that receive information from the skin and special sense organs (i.e., senses of sight, hearing, smell, taste, pain, and so forth). We are aware of these sensations. The motor nerves of the voluntary nervous system then carry information back to the body, directing conscious actions such as the control of our skeletal muscles. As the name implies, the voluntary nervous system controls activities that require willful or conscious action. For example, when lifting the lid off a hot pot of soup on the stove, the voluntary nervous system gauges how long your hand can tolerate the heat from the handle while you stir the soup before you must put the lid back down.

AUTONOMIC NERVOUS SYSTEM

The involuntary or autonomic nervous system is composed of the special tracts of nerves and nerve centers that control vital body functions such as heart rate, constriction and dilation of blood vessels, digestion, heat regulation, and other vegetative processes. Sensory nerves carry information such as the oxygen content in the blood, the blood pressure, and body temperature to special centers in the brain, where this information is analyzed. In response, the brain sends messages via the motor nerves back to the various organs and tissues directing or modifying their activity. Such activities may result in a change in heart rate, respiratory rate, or the amount of sweating from the skin; release of hormones; and constriction or dilation of the muscle in the walls of the blood vessels. The autonomic nervous system functions "automatically," without our conscious control.

PARASYMPATHETIC AND SYMPATHETIC DIVISIONS. There are two main divisions of the autonomic nervous system, the *parasympathetic* and *sympathetic*. In general, these two divisions within the autonomic nervous system usually have opposite effects upon a given organ or tissue. For example, as discussed earlier, the parasympathetic division *will slow* the heart's rate, whereas the sympathetic will speed it up. These two divisions, with their opposite effects, tend to counterbalance each other.

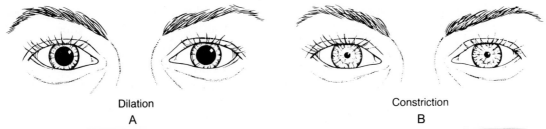

Dilation
A

Constriction
B

FIGURE 7-1. Effects of the sympathetic and parasympathetic nervous systems on pupil diameter: (*A*) Increased sympathetic stimulation results in dilation of the pupil. (*B*) Increased parasympathetic stimulation results in constriction of the pupil.

They allow the brain to *modulate* an organ's activity to meet the body's needs at any given time.

Control of the size of the pupil is a result of this balance between sympathetic and parasympathetic nerves. The parasympathetic nerve to the eye constricts the iris muscle, while the sympathetic nerve causes it to dilate, as shown in Figure 7-1.

Parts of the Nervous System That Can Regenerate After Injury

Practically speaking, one has a chance of regenerating new nerve tissue if a peripheral nerve is damaged. However, once nerves within the central nervous system die, they are lost forever. This explains why a patient with an amputated limb may eventually regain nervous control of the reattached parts after successful reimplantation. However, if a patient suffers a gunshot wound to part of the brain, the cells that are destroyed in the path of the bullet will not regenerate. Other parts of the brain may take over some of the lost cells' functions, but the patient is likely to have some permanent disability.

The Nervous System's Dependence on Oxygen and Glucose

The nerve cell is very dependent on an adequate supply of oxygen and glucose, but it is most dependent on an adequate supply of oxygen. If complete cessation of oxygen delivery occurs, as in cardiac arrest, central nervous system activity ceases in about 5 seconds and the patient will become unconscious. If some oxygen is not delivered to the brain within about 4 to 6 minutes, irreversible brain damage occurs. Herein lies the importance of the early application of cardiopulmonary resuscitation. Other conditions such as hypoxia or hypotension, which result in inadequate delivery of oxygen to the brain, can cause cell damage.

Patients who are hypoxic have altered brain function. The most sensitive areas are those concerned with intellect, behavior, and consciousness. Changes in one's behavior, ability to reason, judgment, and level of consciousness are often referred to as alterations in mental status. In fact, *altered mental status is the most sensitive indication of inadequate oxygen* and explains why the check for responsiveness is the first element in the primary survey. One form of altered mental status is agitated or even combative behavior. This can be confused with intoxication or psychiatric disorders. The finding of unresponsiveness or altered mental status must raise the question of whether adequate oxygen is being delivered to the brain. The EMT then assesses the respiratory and circulatory systems, the next steps in the primary survey.

Patients with a low blood glucose can present with a variety of symptoms and signs—from abnormal behavior to coma or complete unresponsiveness. Patients who present with abnormal mental status but who are able to swallow are often given sugar in recognition of the brain's dependency on this nutritional substance (see Hypoglycemia in Medical Emergencies, Chapter 12).

Hypoxia and *hypoglycemia* (low blood glucose) must be considered in all patients with an altered mental status. The reason is straightforward. If brain cells are not functioning because of an inadequate supply of oxygen or glucose, continued deprivation can lead to irreversible brain damage. Since in most cases administration of oxygen or glucose will do no harm, many systems have protocols that call for the administration of oxygen and glucose to all patients with an altered mental status. At the very least, assessment of the adequacy of these nutrients must be considered.

Nerve Cells and Pressure

Nerve cells are very sensitive to pressure. If an outside force is applied to the nerves, nerve function becomes compromised. Both the amount of pressure transmitted to the nerve cells and the period of time over which it is applied will affect the amount of nerve damage that occurs. A sudden force, applied over a few milliseconds, may disrupt nerve or brain function temporarily or permanently, depending on the *amount of force* applied. Lesser forces sustained over long periods of time result in damage in proportion to the *length of time over which the force is applied.*

Patients who have bleeding within the skull suffer from increased pressure on the brain. They may have little or no permanent damage if the accumulated blood and blood clots can be evacuated early by surgery. The same problem, if left untreated for a longer period of time, may result in permanent brain damage and death.

Another example of the effect of pressure on the nerves is a condition called Saturday night palsy. The drunken party-goer may fall asleep on his arm which is draped over the back of a chair. If he is not too inebriated, he may awake in an hour with pain and a burning sensation in his arm. He may feel at first that he is unable to move his arm effectively. This will resolve in a short time. If he is so intoxicated that he does not awake until the morning, he may note that he cannot move his arm at all. The nerve has been subjected to the same amount of pressure for a longer period of time, and it may take days for the full return of normal function.

Protection of the Brain and Spinal Cord

Because the brain and spinal cord are of such central importance and so sensitive to pressure, they are protected and encased within strong bones that make up the skull and vertebral column. Under the bones are three layers of membranes that separate bone from the brain and spinal cord, and that offer further protection. In addition, between the two innermost membranes lies the cerebrospinal fluid, which can absorb shocks from sudden blows and adds still another layer of protection. The clear, colorless spinal fluid serves to provide some nutrition to the nerve cells as well.

THE SKULL

The *skull* is made up of several bones that compose cranium, the face, and the lower jaw or mandible (Fig. 7–2). It is important to know the names of several of the bones to enable accurate recording and communication of the location of injuries.

The bones making up the cranium are flat, irregularly shaped bones that are separate at birth to allow for passage of the skull through the birth canal. Over time, they fuse together at suture lines. The bones making up the outer surface of the cranium include the *frontal* bone anteriorly (the forehead), the *occipital* bone posteriorly, and the *parietal* and *temporal* bones, which form the lateral surfaces of the cranium. The parietal bone sits superior to the temporal bone, which is above and behind the ear—remember the temporal artery.

After birth and during infancy, there are two sites where the bones do not meet and soft spots are present.

These are the anterior and posterior *fontanelles* and are located in the midline of the top of the skull at either end of the parietal bones (Fig. 7–3).

THE BASE OF THE SKULL.   The largest part of the brain, the cerebrum, sits within the cranium and rests on numerous bones that are fused together, forming the *base of the skull*. In the midline of the base of the skull is an opening called the *foramen magnum*. The lower part of the brain, *the brainstem*, travels through the foramen magnum as it leaves the cranium to connect with the spinal cord (Fig. 7–4).

The space *within* the cranium holds about 1 liter. After infancy, when the cranial bones are fused together, the cranial space is nonexpandable. This space is filled almost entirely with brain tissue, the rest being spinal fluid and circulating blood. If bleeding should occur within this nonexpandable space, pressure will be transmitted to the brain tissue itself. Since brain tissue is very susceptible to pressure, this will cause loss of brain function. If the pressure is severe, the brain may herniate (be forced down) through the only opening in the cranium, the foramen magnum. This is a dire emergency calling for prompt neurosurgical evaluation. The diagnosis of this *herniation* of the brain is discussed later in this chapter.

THE FACIAL BONES.   The orbits that surround the eyes and the nasal bones and the maxilla make up the front of the skull. The zygomas connect the temporal bone with the maxilla and are easily palpated where the cheek meets the temple just anterior to the ear. The *mandible* or lower jaw is connected to the rest of the skull at the temporomandibular joints (Fig. 7–5).

THE SPINAL COLUMN

The spinal column consists of 33 vertebrae extending from the base of the skull to the *coccyx* (tail bone). Most vertebrae are held together by ligaments and separated by cartilaginous discs that serve as cushions. The ligaments allow for movement such as bending and rotation while maintaining proper alignment of the vertebral column. Proper alignment is essential, since the spinal cord passes through the vertebral column.

The vertebrae are named by their location and structure. Starting from the head, the first seven vertebrae are named the *cervical* vertebrae. The next 12 vertebrae are the *thoracic* vertebrae and are the main support for the rib cage, with each pair of ribs joining the corresponding vertebrae. The next five vertebrae are the *lumbar*. They extend to the *sacrum*, which consists of five vertebrae fused together. Extending from the sacrum are four fused vertebrae, which make up the coccyx or tailbone (Fig. 7–6).

The vertebrae have an anterior body and a posterior spinous process that allow for attachment of ligaments. Arcs of bone connect the body and spinous process of

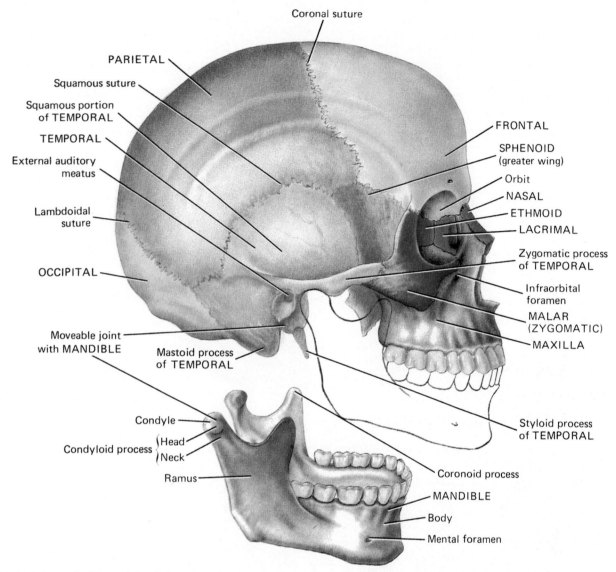

FIGURE 7–2. The bones of the skull. (From Solomon EP, Phillips GA: Understanding Human Anatomy and Physiology. Philadelphia, WB Saunders, 1987, p. 81.)

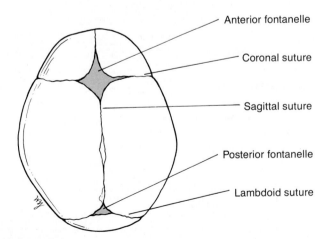

FIGURE 7–3. Soft spots or fontanelles on the infant skull. (From Swartz MH: Textbook of Physical Diagnosis: History and Examination. Philadelphia, WB Saunders, 1989, p. 553.)

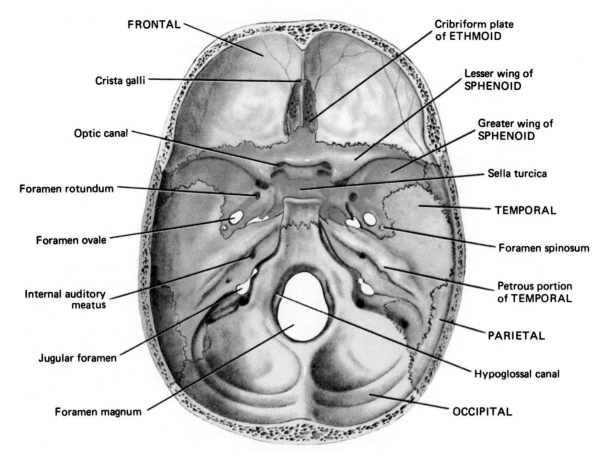

FRONTAL

Crista galli

Optic canal

Foramen rotundum

Foramen ovale

Internal auditory
meatus

Jugular foramen

Foramen magnum

Cribriform plate
of ETHMOID

Lesser wing of
SPHENOID

Greater wing of
SPHENOID

Sella turcica

TEMPORAL

Foramen spinosum

Petrous portion
of TEMPORAL

PARIETAL

Hypoglossal canal

OCCIPITAL

A

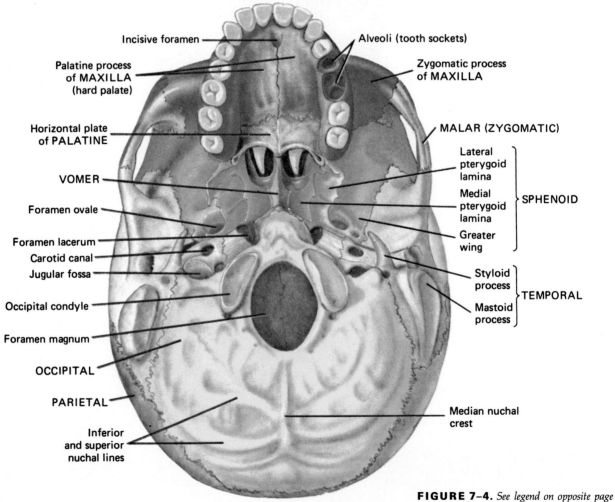

Incisive foramen

Palatine process
of MAXILLA
(hard palate)

Horizontal plate
of PALATINE

VOMER

Foramen ovale

Foramen lacerum

Carotid canal

Jugular fossa

Occipital condyle

Foramen magnum

OCCIPITAL

PARIETAL

Inferior
and superior
nuchal lines

Alveoli (tooth sockets)

Zygomatic process
of MAXILLA

MALAR (ZYGOMATIC)

Lateral
pterygoid
lamina

Medial
pterygoid
lamina

Greater
wing

SPHENOID

Styloid
process

Mastoid
process

TEMPORAL

Median nuchal
crest

B

FIGURE 7-4. *See legend on opposite page*

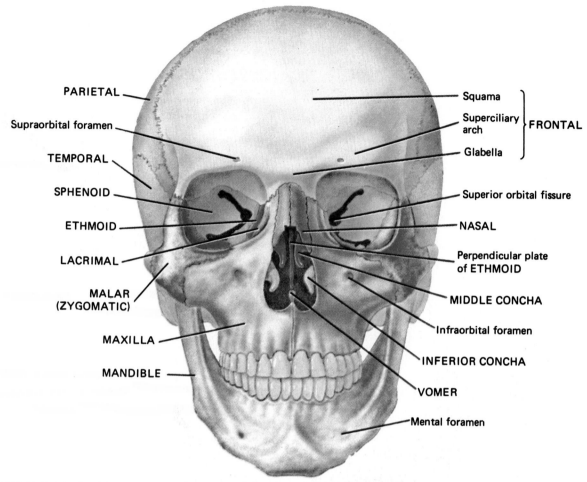

PARIETAL

Supraorbital foramen

TEMPORAL

SPHENOID

ETHMOID

LACRIMAL

MALAR
(ZYGOMATIC)

MAXILLA

MANDIBLE

Squama

Superciliary
arch

Glabella

} FRONTAL

Superior orbital fissure

NASAL

Perpendicular plate
of ETHMOID

MIDDLE CONCHA

Infraorbital foramen

INFERIOR CONCHA

VOMER

Mental foramen

FIGURE 7–5. The facial bones. (From Solomon EP, Phillips GA: Understanding Human Anatomy and Physiology. Philadelphia, WB Saunders, 1987, p. 80.)

each vertebra, leaving a central opening through which the spinal cord travels. At the level of each vertebra are openings through which the peripheral nerves leave the spinal column and travel to the various parts of the body (Fig. 7–7).

At birth, the spinal cord fills most of the spinal column. However, as one ages, the cord grows more slowly than the bony spinal column until, at adult age, the cord itself ends at the level of the first lumbar vertebrae. The nerves to the lower parts of the body extend down from this level until they exit at the appropriate lumbar or sacral vertebrae.

THE MEMBRANOUS COVERINGS

The *meninges* or membranous coverings of the brain and cord have three layers. The outer layer closest to the skull and vertebral column is a tough, leathery layer called the *dura*. Arteries travel along the skull between the bone itself and the dura. If they are severed, bleeding can result between the dura and the bone. This bleeding is named for the space it occupies—outside the dura, hence *epidural* (above dura). The middle layer is called the *arachnoid* layer. Between the dura and the arachnoid

FIGURE 7–4. Base of skull: (*A*) superior view; (*B*) inferior view. The base of the skull is made up of several fused bones. The brain exits through the foramen magnum, which is located in the center. This is the site of herniation when swelling or bleeding occurs within the skull. (From Solomon EP, Phillips GA: Understanding Human Anatomy and Physiology. Philadelphia, WB Saunders, 1987, pp. 82, 83.)

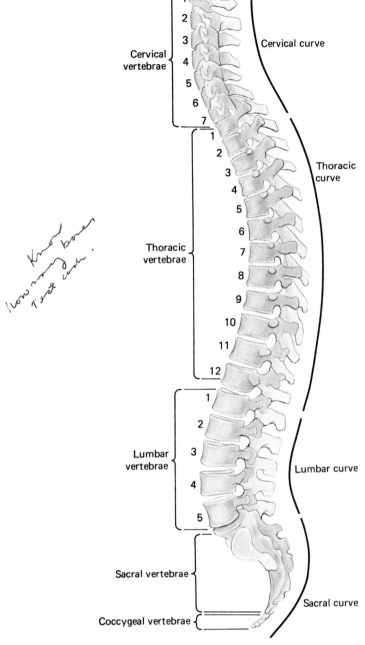

FIGURE 7–6. The vertebral column and structure of the vertebrae. (From Solomon EP, Phillips GA: Understanding Human Anatomy and Physiology. Philadelphia, WB Saunders, 1987, p. 85.)

layer are many veins and venous sinuses. Venous bleeding following injury may occur in this space between the dura and the arachnoid membranes. This bleeding is also named for its location with respect to the dura—under the dura, hence *subdural.* The innermost layer is called the *pia mater,* which is adherent to the brain tissue

itself. It is between the arachnoid and the pia mater that cerebrospinal fluid circulates (Fig. 7–8).

CEREBROSPINAL FLUID

The *cerebrospinal fluid* helps protect and cushion the brain and acts like a liquid shock absorber. It is continually being formed and absorbed from blood-rich plexuses. It serves a nutritional role as well, as it circulates around the brain and spinal cord, within *ventricles* (hollow cavities) within the brain, and within the innermost center of the spinal cord itself.

The Central Nervous System and Its Parts

The central nervous system (CNS) is composed of the brain, brainstem, and spinal cord (Fig. 7–9).

The brain is the central computer. It processes sensory input from sensory nerves and organizes responses that are then transmitted back to the body by outgoing motor nerves. Sensory input includes sight, hearing, smell, taste, and (touch). Temperature, pain, touch, pressure, and tickle are all variations of feeling. Special receptors in the ear and special nerve pathways relay input concerning balance and equilibrium. In addition, the brain receives input about the oxygen and carbon dioxide content of the blood, as well as about the body's circulatory and nutritional status. All this information is processed at incredible speeds, as evidenced by one's reaction to a startling noise or noxious taste or odor. So much information is received by the brain at any one time that ordinarily we are conscious of only about 1% of the sensory input.

THE CEREBRUM

The largest and most superior portion of the brain is called the *cerebrum.* The cerebrum is divided down the middle into right and left halves called *hemispheres.* Generally, the right hemisphere controls the left side of the body and vice versa. The two hemispheres communicate with each other through a special pathway called the *corpus callosum.* The convoluted hemispheres are further subdivided into different *lobes* or sections that have specific and distinct functions. They are named by their location with respect to the overlying skull bones, i.e., the frontal lobe is the area responsible for intellectual functions and motor control of skeletal muscles, whereas the parietal area is the center for sensory perception. The occipital area is the center for receiving and processing visual stimuli and the temporal area receives smell and hearing signals. The different lobes communicate with each other (Fig. 7–10). Loss of brain tissue in a specific

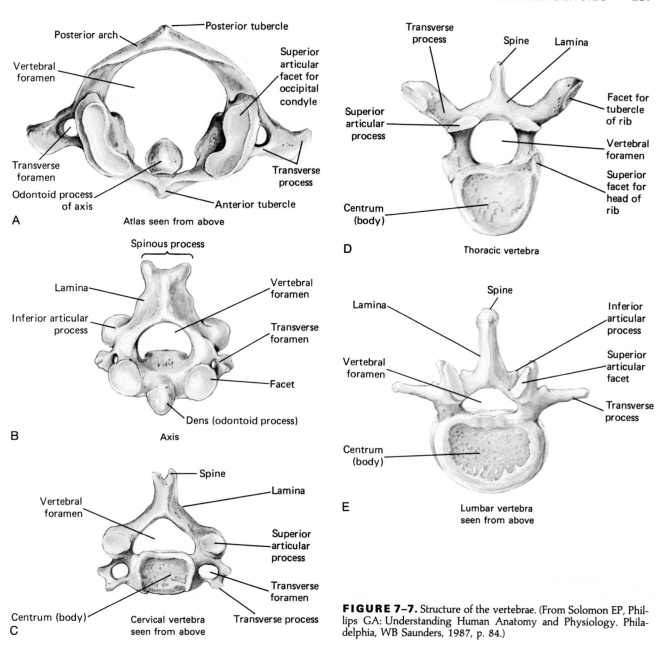

FIGURE 7–7. Structure of the vertebrae. (From Solomon EP, Phillips GA: Understanding Human Anatomy and Physiology. Philadelphia, WB Saunders, 1987, p. 84.)

area can result in distinct and limited losses of function, which again points to the subdivision of labor within the brain itself.

THE HOMUNCULUS. Within the various lobes, one can see further subdivisions of function. Specific portions of brain tissue carry out distinct and different tasks. This can be appreciated when one maps out the division of labor at the junction of the frontal and parietal lobes. This is where sensory and motor signals governing skin sensation and movement are received and processed. The schematic drawing equating each body part to the corresponding brain cells in this area is known as the homunculus. Consider the drawing in Figure 7–11 and compare the amount of brain dedicated to the hand and face and throat with that dedicated to the hips and abdomen. The use of the hand is a complex task and more cells are necessary in its control than one would require for a simpler function such as bending at the waist. Likewise, speech and eating involve integrated functioning of multiple muscles in a complex sequence, and therefore more brain cells are delegated to these tasks.

INNER STRUCTURE OF THE BRAIN. The outermost layer of the cerebrum contains the cell bodies, which act

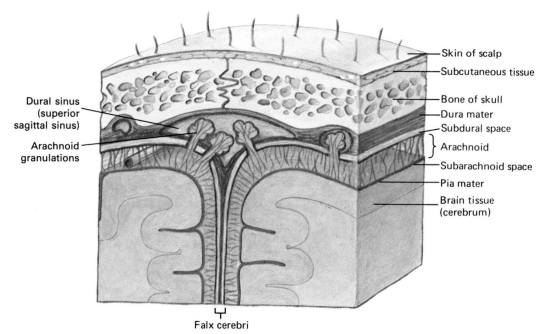

FIGURE 7–8. The meninges provide a layer of protection for the brain and spinal cord. They may also become locations for the collection of blood following trauma or spontaneous rupture of cerebral vessels. (From Solomon EP, Phillips GA: Understanding Human Anatomy and Physiology. Philadelphia, WB Saunders, 1987, p. 141.)

as the computers or decision makers. The communicating portions of the nerve bodies travel together in nerve tracks as they journey down through the brainstem and into the spinal cord to their point of communication with the corresponding peripheral nerve. The nerve tracts begin to cross over to the opposite side at the level of the brainstem, explaining why the right brain controls the left side of the body and vice versa.

The cell bodies are different in appearance from the nerve tracts. The former is sometimes referred to as *gray matter* and the latter as *white matter.*

You may begin to view the inner structure of the brain as a complex control box with a specific wiring diagram. Use is made of this anatomical knowledge in tracing signs and symptoms of neurologic disease to the most likely site of disruption, much as an electrician would investigate a problem by referring to the wiring diagram.

For example, nerve tracts from the area displayed in the homunculus drawing travel tightly together as they leave the cerebrum. They must travel closely together since all the nerves leaving the brain must travel down through the hole in the base of the skull—the foramen magnum. Damage to a relatively small area, where nerves from the hemisphere are tightly packed, can therefore result in catastrophic consequences—such as loss of sensation and motor function in an entire half of the body. You will see this condition many times

when you care for patients who are victims of strokes (see the medical CNS section at the end of this chapter).

THE BRAINSTEM

The brainstem is the lower part of the brain. It is made up of bundles and tracts of nerves traveling down to the spinal cord from the cerebrum. It has distinct nerve cell centers of its own as well. Some nerve centers located in the brainstem control muscles of the eyes and iris. They communicate by peripheral nerves called cranial nerves, which originate in the brainstem and travel through the skull. Other nerve centers in the brainstem monitor and direct respiratory and circulatory function. Because these areas are so close together, *loss of function of structures innervated by the cranial nerves (such as control of pupillary size or eye movement) raises great concern that the neighboring centers that control respiration and much of circulation will be damaged as well,* leading to loss of vital function. Checking the pupils is part of the patient survey for patients with a head injury and also in patients with an altered mental status or loss of nerve function.

Damage to certain parts of the brainstem can result in characteristic breathing patterns. The respiratory patterns that may present include Cheyne-Stokes; central neurogenic hyperventilation; and irregular patterns such as apneustic, ataxic, and Biot's. By putting together signs such as breathing patterns and the function of specific

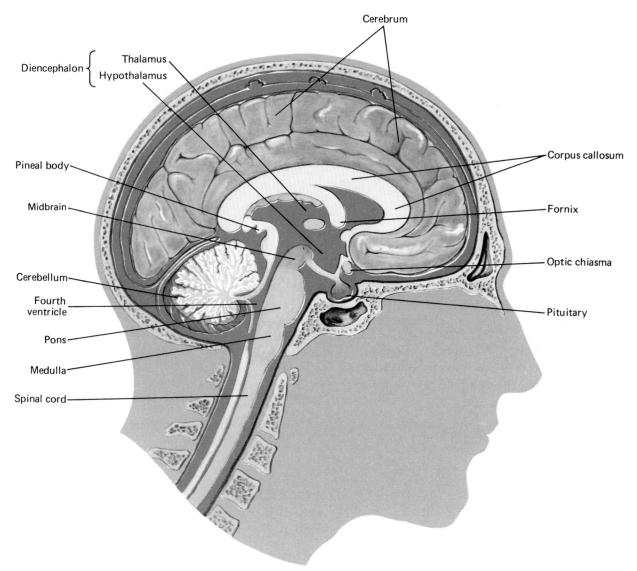

FIGURE 7-9. Parts of the central nervous system. (From Villee CA, Solomon EP, Martin C, Martin D: Biology, 2nd ed. Philadelphia, Saunders College Publishing, 1989.)

cranial nerves (such as those to the eyes), physicians are able to judge whether the brainstem is working properly. Some of this information, particularly relating to the pupils and breathing patterns, can be elicited by the EMT. It provides important baseline information that will later help a physician determine whether a patient's condition is improving or deteriorating.

THE CEREBELLUM

The cerebellum is an outpocketing of the brain located behind or posterior to the brainstem. It is primarily concerned with coordination of movement and balance.

THE SPINAL CORD

The spinal cord emerges from the brainstem and is a continuation of nerve tracts from all parts of the brain. It has its own processing centers as well. One example is its reflex action. For example, touching a red hot iron will cause an *immediate* reaction to remove one's hand *before* the brain receives the message that damage has occurred (Fig. 7-12). This type of action can occur through the reflex arcs along each segment of the spinal cord. Because of the importance of spinal injuries, this area is discussed in greater detail in the next section of this chapter along with the peripheral nervous system.

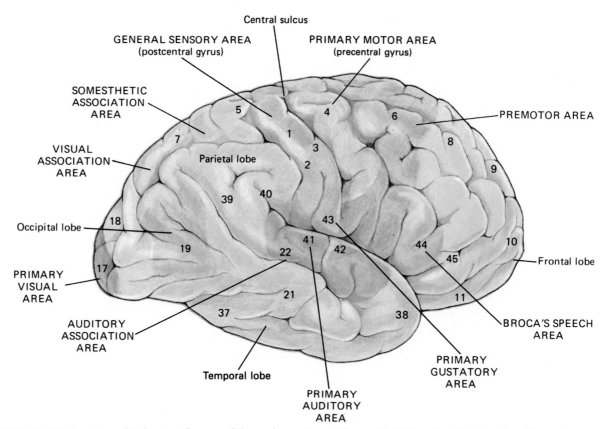

FIGURE 7–10. Functions related to specific areas of the cerebrum. (From Solomon EP, Phillips GA: Understanding Human Anatomy and Physiology. Philadelphia, WB Saunders, 1987, p. 135.)

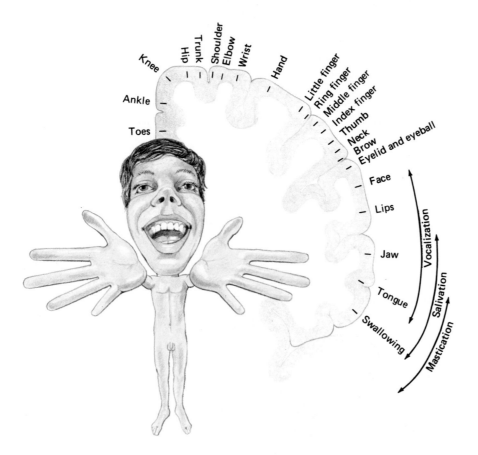

FIGURE 7–11. The distorted appearance of *homunculus* is in proportion to the amount of brain surface area devoted to a particular body function. (From Solomon EP, Phillips GA: Understanding Human Anatomy and Physiology. Philadelphia, WB Saunders, 1987, p. 127.)

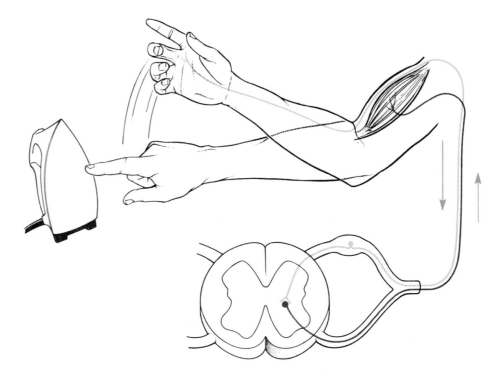

FIGURE 7–12. The rapid removal of one's hand from a hot iron, before the pain is actually felt, is an example of a reflex action. The motor response is mediated through the spinal cord.

Types of Action Mediated by the CNS

We can summarize some of the complex activities of the central nervous system by looking at the types of activities that it controls. Types of action mediated by the nervous system include automatic, reflex, and conscious actions and the voluntary and involuntary control of muscles.

AUTOMATIC ACTION

Breathing, control of heart rate and blood pressure, and temperature regulation are all examples of automatic activities handled by the autonomic nervous system.

REFLEX ACTION

The withdrawal of the body from pain, as in the example of the hot iron given earlier, is an example of a reflex action. The stretching of a tendon, as occurs when a physician strikes the patellar tendon below the knee with a reflex hammer, results in an immediate extension movement of the leg. This extension of the leg in turn shortens the tendon (which was stretched by the hammer) back to its normal length. The testing of reflexes assesses reflex activity at the level of the spinal cord via its reflex arc.

CONSCIOUS ACTION

Playing a game of basketball requires the processing of sensory input from our eyes, ears, and other general senses (finger position, touch, balance). One remembers how much effort and control is needed to shoot a jump shot from 15 feet. Memory and sensory perception are integrated as the brain directs the body while a player dribbles into position, avoids defensive players, and shoots the ball.

VOLUNTARY CONTROL OF MUSCLES

The skeletal muscles that cause the body's movement are under conscious control and respond to the will to contract or relax.

INVOLUNTARY CONTROL OF MUSCLES

Contraction or relaxation of the smooth muscle that is present in our blood vessels or digestive tract cannot be controlled by will. Such smooth muscles relax or contract in response to the body's needs, which are determined by processing information about blood pressure, oxygen needs, and nutritional status.

Blood Supply to the Head

Most of the blood supply to the brain *(80%) is provided by the carotid arteries* (Fig. 7–13). That is why one never palpates both carotid pulses at one time. Carotid pulse checks should be done gently, especially in elderly patients, since one might dislodge arteriosclerotic plaques. These could produce emboli that can obstruct

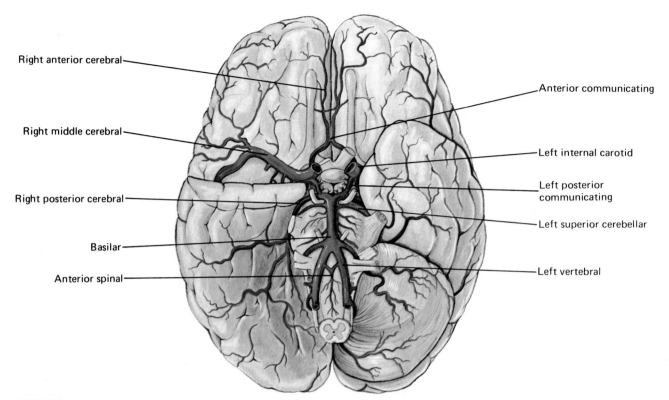

FIGURE 7–13. As you view this illustration, try to imagine the effects of an obstruction or rupture of a given artery. (From Solomon EP, Phillips GA: Understanding Human Anatomy and Physiology. Philadelphia, WB Saunders, 1987, p. 232.)

smaller arteries to the brain above. The rest of the brain's blood flow comes from two vertebral arteries that merge to form the *basilar* artery and feed the brainstem. The basilar artery then joins the two carotid arteries to form a network that feeds the rest of the brain.

After the carotids and basilar arteries meet, specific arteries branch off to feed specific portions of the brain. This specificity of blood supply explains why the obstruction of a single artery results in a specific loss of function, such as weakness and sensory loss on one side of the body. The consequences of sudden obstruction to blood flow to the brain is commonly referred to as a stroke.

Pathophysiology

STRUCTURAL AND METABOLIC INJURIES

Injuries to the nervous system can occur in two general ways. A disease or injury may affect only a portion of the nervous system (damage to the structure, e.g., a gunshot wound) or the entire nervous system can be affected by a generalized problem (damage to the cells' metabolism, e.g., hypoxia).

STRUCTURAL INJURIES. Injuries to the brain that cause disruption of *specific* sections of brain tissue or nerves result in loss of specific functions. Damage can

occur to one area while other parts of the nervous system may still function. Injuries that involve specific areas are said to be *structural injuries*. These injuries may be traumatic or nontraumatic.

For example, a penetrating wound to the head may disrupt the tracts of nerves on the left side of the brain only and leave the right side of the brain functionally intact. Because the nerves cross to the other side of the body, the patient with a wound to the left brain may not have use of the right side of the body, but the left side of the body may still function.

Some medical conditions can be classified as structural as well. This situation is commonly encountered in patients who have suffered a disruption of the blood supply in one artery supplying a particular area of the brain (stroke). Such a patient can experience weakness and loss of sensation on one side of the body. He or she has suffered an insult (interruption of blood flow) to part of the structure of the brain.

METABOLIC INJURIES. When the energy processes necessary for the patient's life are compromised, the patient has experienced a *metabolic injury*. The best example of this is the lack of oxygen following a cardiac arrest. All the brain's cells are affected. The patient loses consciousness, does not respond to stimuli such as pain, has no ability to move, and loses control of vital functions such as breathing. The cells on both sides of the body are affected equally.

How can the EMT tell if a patient has a structural

or a metabolic problem? One clue to structural injury is an asymmetry of findings. The EMT notes *a difference when comparing one side of the body to the other*, almost as if *certain* wires had been cut on an electrical diagram. Contrast this with metabolic injuries, which *affect all central nervous system tissues equally*. Both sides of the brain are equally affected. Such an injury affects the metabolism of all cells. Examples include hypoxia from any cause, low blood sugar, shock, and poisoning. For example, you would not expect the victim of cyanide poisoning to be able to move one side of the body better than the other. Both sides of the brain have been poisoned. Figure 7–14 illustrates the motor and sensory findings for metabolic versus structural problems.

SECONDARY COMPLICATIONS FOLLOWING BRAIN INJURY

After direct injury to the brain, later complications can occur that lead to further damage to brain tissue. These secondary complications include hypoxia, hypotension, hypoglycemia, infections, and increased intracranial pressure. They can follow the primary event and

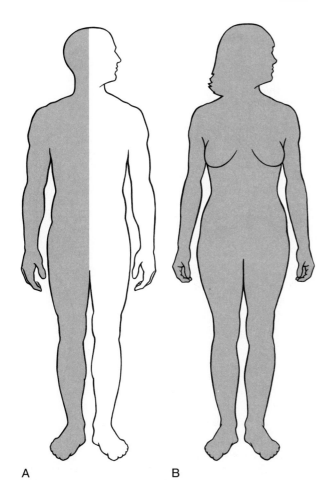

FIGURE 7–14. (*A*) Structural injuries result in one-sided or lateralizing signs. (*B*) Metabolic problems affect all portions of the brain equally and result in global physical findings.

further compromise the ability of the injured nerve tissue to heal or regain function. These secondary processes may even exacerbate the original injury, resulting in more extensive damage or death.

These complications can result from a loss of the brain's ability to control vital organ systems following injury, such as loss of breathing control following a blow to the head. They may also arise from other injuries such as bleeding or chest trauma that can lead to hypoxia or hypotension. Swelling or bleeding within the skull is another example of secondary brain injury. Since the brain is contained in a nonexpandable space, swelling or bleeding within the skull results in increased pressure on the brain (increased intracranial pressure). As you will remember, the brain is very sensitive to pressure. While the bleeding or swelling is a result of the initial injury, the damage from increased pressure occurs later. Some examples that illustrate these processes follow.

HYPOXIA. A patient suffering multiple trauma may suffer both a head injury and a flail chest. The resulting hypoxia from the flail chest is a further insult to the damaged brain tissue.

HYPOTENSION. A patient suffering head trauma and severe hemorrhage from a ruptured spleen may have both hypotension and direct brain damage. The hypotension aggravates the brain injury by decreasing perfusion of the brain with oxygen.

HYPOGLYCEMIA. As an example, consider a diabetic patient who was working on his roof through the afternoon. He missed a meal, became faint, and fell from the roof, sustaining a head injury. If damage to brain tissue occurs from the fall, the chance of healing is further compromised by the lack of a vital brain nutrient—glucose.

INCREASED INTRACRANIAL PRESSURE. A patient may have suffered a head injury with a loss of consciousness, recovered, and then experienced a sudden deterioration in his or her mental status. Such a patient may have suffered a laceration to an artery, which resulted in bleeding within the cranium. This increase in intracranial pressure was the cause of additional brain injury and occurred after the patient had apparently recovered from the initial event. (See epidural hematoma later in this chapter.)

INFECTION. A patient with an open skull fracture recovers from the brain injury only to suffer from an infection of the brain.

The importance of recognition and management of secondary brain injury cannot be overemphasized. Little can be done for recovery of brain tissue that was destroyed as a result of direct trauma (such as a gunshot wound). However, there may be other areas of brain tissue that, while damaged, may heal if no further insult is suffered. Neurosurgical centers have found that

TABLE 7–1. Secondary Brain Injury

Hypoxia*
Hypotension*
Low blood sugar*
Increased intracranial pressure†
Infection‡

* Primary treatment is begun in the field.
† Treatment may be started in the field in some instances.
‡ Treatment is primarily preventative.

the increased ability to save patients with severe head injuries results from careful attention to and treatment of these secondary processes.

How the EMT addresses these problems in the field will be considered under treatment, later in this chapter. Table 7–1 summarizes the secondary complications of brain injury and prehospital treatment.

HEAD INJURIES

Mechanism of Injury

More than half of all head injuries in the United States are the result of motor vehicle accidents. Other common sources of injuries include falls, home and sports accidents, and penetrating wounds from knives and guns.

BLUNT TRAUMA — STATIC AND DYNAMIC FORCES

It is important to recognize that a head injury may be caused by either static or dynamic forces. Most blunt head injuries are a combination of both.

An example of a *static* injury would be a car falling off a jack onto the head of a mechanic lying on the ground. The force of the injury is applied in only one direction. The head and brain do not move about following the impact but rather are crushed between the car and ground.

Dynamic forces causing head injury are those that follow the initial blow. They are caused by movement of the brain within the skull, which has been set in motion by the impact. Dynamic forces can be applied even without a direct blow to the skull. The most common example may be in car accidents where the driver is wearing a seat belt and the driver's head does not strike any part of the car. However, the deceleration forces following the collision cause the head and its contents to be subjected to rotational or shearing forces.

Usually, the effects of the two types of forces, static and dynamic, are additive. In fact, it has been determined that if rotation of the skull can be prevented, it takes a much greater blow to result in the same amount of brain damage.

The important thing to remember is that a direct blow to the head is not necessary for brain damage to occur. As in situations such as car accidents, a patient securely restrained by a seat belt might not suffer a direct blow to the head. However, the head is subject to acceleration and deceleration forces. It might rotate with considerable speed about the neck when the car suddenly stops. Areas of diffuse damage can occur throughout extensive areas within the brain.

Often, with these types of injuries, the head is spun about its axis, resulting in injuries to the inferior portion of the cerebrum. The inferior portion of the cerebrum can strike against the edges of the many little bones that make up the base of the skull.

CONTRECOUP. Because of the dynamic components of head injury, injuries may occur on the side of the brain opposite the site of the blow. The brain continues to move within the skull after the initial impact and can strike the opposite side of the skull. This *coup* or blow is *contra* or opposite to the site of the external trauma and hence is called a *contrecoup* injury (Fig. 7–15). An example might be a patient who sustains a blow to the frontal bone and complains of visual disturbances because the brain continued to move until the occipital lobe struck the inside of the occipital bone.

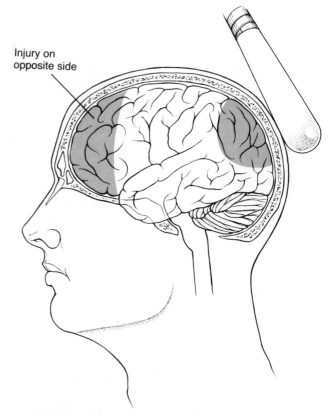

Injury on opposite side

FIGURE 7–15. As the brain moves within the skull following a blunt trauma (e.g., head struck with baseball bat) the opposite side of the brain can strike the inner lining of the skull, causing a contrecoup injury.

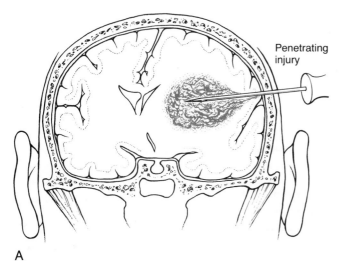

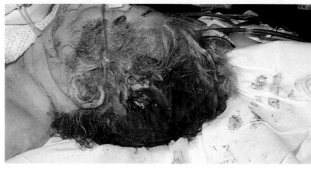

A   B

FIGURE 7–16. (*A*) Example of penetrating wound to the brain. (*B*) Deep laceration of scalp caused by fall on street after being struck by car. This patient suffered a subdural hematoma underneath the area of the external laceration.

PENETRATING INJURY

Most penetrating injuries are the result of gunshot and knife wounds. Besides destroying brain tissue in the path of the missile or penetrating object, associated bleeding and later swelling can extend the injury zone to brain tissue surrounding the path of penetration. Bullets cause shock waves that widen the area of damage in proportion to the speed and weight of the bullet (Fig. 7–16*A*).

Head Injury and Associated Cervical Spine Injury

The possibility of a cervical spine fracture is associated with a traumatic head injury. Although only a small percentage of patients with a head injury have fractures of the cervical spine, those who do run the risk of paralysis and death if the cervical spine fracture is not handled properly. Because of their awareness of the fact that head and neck injuries are often *associated injuries*, EMTs should be highly suspicious that patients with a head injury may also have an injury to the cervical spine.

Scalp Wounds

Many head injuries result in scalp lacerations. There may or may not be associated skull fractures and injury to brain tissue (Fig. 7–16*B*). The scalp has numerous small blood vessels, and significant bleeding can occur from scalp lacerations. As with other wounds, control of bleeding from the scalp is best controlled with direct pressure. The pressure should be applied gently and be just sufficient to control the bleeding; it should be dis-

tributed over a wide area with a wide dressing and bandage. Because of the rich vessels in the scalp, hematomas commonly occur, which on palpation are difficult to distinguish from depressed skull fractures. (See depressed skull fractures later in this chapter). By applying the direct pressure over a broad area, one is less likely to displace loose bone fragments downward into the brain. If a depressed skull fracture is suspected, apply pressure to the edges of the intact portion of the skull.

One can bleed to death from scalp lacerations. Often, when patients are found hypotensive, active bleeding from scalp wounds may have ceased. Look at the amount of obvious bleeding on the ground or floor. The patient may not bleed again from the wound until the blood volume is replaced and the hypotension corrected.

Apply direct pressure to the wound with a sterile bandage. Do not attempt to clean the wound or irrigate it with sterile saline in the field. Since it is difficult to know whether a skull fracture is also present, one runs the risk of the irrigation fluid carrying debris and foreign bacteria into the brain itself.

Do not attempt to explore inside the margins of the wound to determine whether a skull fracture is present. This knowledge serves no useful purpose in the field and runs the risk of disrupting blood clots and introducing bacteria. Table 7–2 summarizes the correct treatment of scalp lacerations.

Skull Fractures

Although it takes a significant force to cause a fracture of the skull, a skull fracture in itself does not mean that significant or any brain damage has occurred. A patient with a skull fracture may have remarkably little

TABLE 7–2. The Treatment of Scalp Lacerations

Do	Don't
Use gentle direct pressure to control bleeding	Explore the wound
Apply the pressure over the edges of the intact bone if a depressed fracture is suspected	Irrigate the wound
Distribute the pressure over a wide area if possible	
Estimate and record the degree of blood loss as evident from external bleeding	

or no other signs of injury except for abnormal x-ray findings. On the other hand, patients without skull fractures may suffer lethal head injuries.

There are certain areas where skull fractures do more damage than others. One region is the temporal area, where a major artery—the middle meningeal artery—travels along a groove on the inside surface of the temporal bone. If the sharp bony fragments of the fracture lacerate this artery, significant bleeding can occur inside the skull.

Monitor the patient closely when the injury is sustained over the temporal bones (Fig. 7–17A).

OPEN VERSUS CLOSED FRACTURES

Like other fractures, skull fractures may be open or closed. An open fracture is one where the skin over the fracture site is not intact, allowing communication between the outside environment and the brain or its meninges. This results in an increased risk of infection. A closed fracture is one where the skin above the fracture site is still intact.

TYPES OF SKULL FRACTURES

LINEAR. A *linear* fracture is a simple line or crack along a bone of the cranium. Most skull fractures are of this type. Sometimes the line can be seen if there is an extensive scalp laceration over it (Fig. 7–17B).

COMMINUTED. A *comminuted* fracture has multiple cracks radiating outward from the point of impact. Usually, more force is necessary to cause this type of injury.

DEPRESSED. When greater forces strike the skull, especially if they are applied over a small surface area (as with a hammer blow), the bone fragments may be depressed downward toward the brain. The *depressed* skull fracture may be confused with a hematoma, since both will have a soft center that is easily depressed on palpation.

With open wounds, the depressed fracture may be obvious. A *penetrating wound* through the scalp may cause

a depressed skull fracture. Bullets in particular can drive skull fragments forward and into the brain. Do not attempt to remove penetrating objects that are lodged within the skull (Fig. 7–17B).

BASILAR SKULL FRACTURE. The *basilar* skull fracture is a crack in the *base* or floor of the skull. Basilar skull fractures are usually diagnosed by characteristic signs. These include leaking of clear cerebrospinal fluid from the nose or ear, since these structures are contingent with bones of the base of the skull. Sometimes the cerebrospinal fluid that leaks from the nose or ear is mixed with blood.

Place a loose sterile dressing over any leaking cerebrospinal fluid or blood from the nose or ear. Do not attempt to obstruct or block the flow, since it might cause foreign bacteria to back up through the fracture site and lead to infection within the brain. The main purpose of the dressing is to minimize further contamination by outside debris or bacteria. Do not obstruct the nasal passage (Fig. 7–17B).

Other signs of basilar skull fracture include black and blue areas or *ecchymosis* below the eyes (raccoon's sign) (Fig. 7–18) or behind the ear (Battle's sign). The usefulness of these signs (raccoon's and Battle's) has been apparent to many EMTs who have been called to the scene where they have found a seemingly drunk man lying on the sidewalk, only to discover on closer inspection that he was unconscious from a basilar skull fracture and not just sleeping it off. Alcoholics are at high risk for sustaining skull fractures and their complications (e.g., subdural hematoma).

Brain Injuries

CONCUSSION

A *concussion* is defined as a transient loss of consciousness or neurologic function due to a blow to the brain. The blow to the brain sends shock waves that temporarily disrupt brain function. The diagnosis of concussion can be made only after the patient is again fully conscious and has recovered all neurologic function. It is a reversible injury that by itself causes no permanent damage to the brain.

There are many degrees of concussion. The least severe and most common is a momentary loss of function immediately following impact, in which case the patient may not even be sure that consciousness had been lost. The patient might suffer a short period of confusion but will have full recall of events up to or after the point of impact.

Also common are brief periods of *amnesia* (memory loss). The patient cannot recall events just prior to impact or in the period immediately following the blow. The patient may experience retrograde (before the impact)

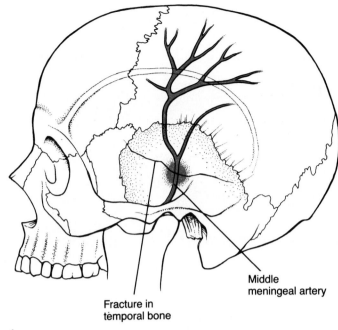

Middle
meningeal artery

Fracture in
temporal bone

A

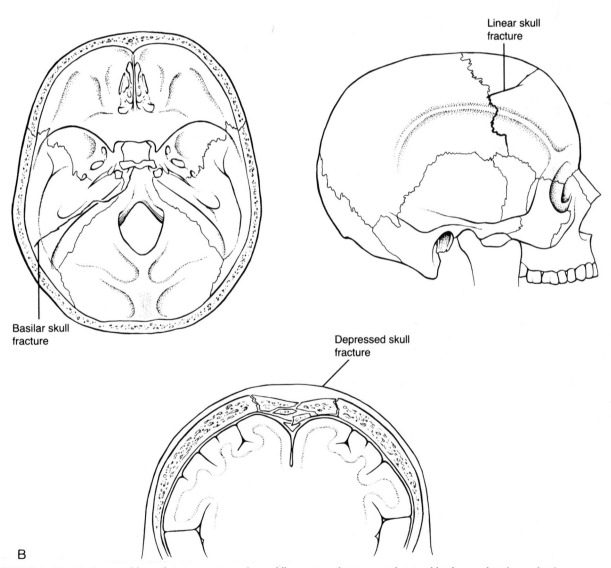

Linear skull
fracture

Basilar skull
fracture

Depressed skull
fracture

B

FIGURE 7-17. (*A*) Temporal bone fractures can tear the middle meningeal artery, resulting in bleeding within the epidural space. (*B*) Types of skull fractures.

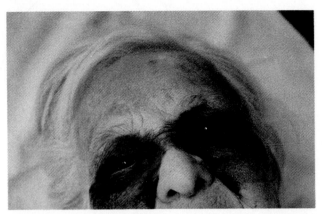

FIGURE 7–18. Raccoon's sign, indicating possible basilar skull fracture. (Courtesy of P. Viccellio, M.D.)

or antegrade (after the impact) amnesia. The brain is not able to store these events in its memory.

More severe concussions can result in unresponsiveness or coma for longer periods of time, some even lasting longer than 24 hours. These patients are at risk of additional brain damage from secondary complications.

CEREBRAL CONTUSIONS

More severe injuries cause direct damage, with bruising or contusion of the brain. Bruised brain tissue does not function properly. There may be specific localized findings that correlate with the site of injury. Depending on the location of the bruise or contusion, this might manifest as loss of motor ability on one side or perhaps an isolated visual disturbance.

CEREBRAL HEMATOMAS

Bleeding can take place following head injury either within the brain tissue itself or in the spaces between the meningeal layers that cover the brain. A major complication of bleeding within the skull is the resultant increase in intracranial pressure.

INTRACEREBRAL HEMATOMAS. Intracerebral hematomas can follow penetrating wounds that tear or sever vessels within the brain. In the case of a lacerated artery, this can result in decreased flow to brain tissue distal to the injury. Bleeding will first affect brain tissue in the immediate proximity of the hematoma. If the bleeding is severe it can raise the pressure within the entire cranium and affect the rest of the brain as well.

SIGNS OF INCREASED INTRACRANIAL PRESSURE

As pressure within the cranium rises, certain signs and symptoms appear. The conscious patient may complain of *headaches, nausea, and vomiting.* Sometimes the vomiting is *projectile,* meaning that the vomitus is ejected from the mouth with considerable force.

The *level of consciousness may begin to deteriorate.* The patient who was previously alert now gets sleepy or more confused and is more difficult to arouse. Instead of responding to verbal commands, the patient may eventually respond to painful stimuli only.

Children are more likely to experience drowsiness and nausea and vomiting after even minor head injuries. The seriousness of these signs can be determined only after a careful neurologic examination. In the field the EMT must regard these signs as possible indications of increasing intracranial pressure.

The most sensitive indicator of increasing intracranial pressure is a changing (deteriorating) level of consciousness. After suffering a head injury, the damage due to the direct blow—concussion or contusion or disruption of the blood supply—has been completed. Signs present immediately following the injury can be attributed to the blow itself.

Any worsening of the condition can no longer be explained as due to the initial impact but must be considered the result of secondary forces—such as increased intracranial pressure from bleeding or swelling within the skull. This is especially the case if there are no other complications such as hypoxia or hypotension to explain the deterioration in status.

EYE AND MOTOR FINDINGS. Other signs of increased intracranial pressure may be due to herniation of brain tissue through the only opening available, the foramen magnum. Since the nerves to the eyes leave the brainstem in this area, they are often compressed between the herniating brain and bony structures. One might note eye findings such as a dilated pupil on one side. The dilated pupil may not constrict when a light is shined in it. The eyelid over the dilated eye may begin to droop as well. Since nerve tracts bearing sensory and motor nerves to the entire body can be compressed as well, the EMT might note that the patient has weakness, paralysis, and sensory loss on one side. Often the dilated pupil is on the same side as the brain lesion, and the motor loss is on the opposite side. However, other presentations do occur.

As the pressure increases, the motor and sensory findings may extend to both sides. With further deterioration, the patient may assume abnormal body positions or postures. The classical postures are *decorticate,* in which the *arms are flexed* but the legs are extended, and later *decerebrate,* in which the *arms are extended* and internally rotated at the shoulders with the wrists flexed and the legs extended (Fig. 7–19A and B). These postures may be assumed spontaneously by the patient or in response to pain. If herniation of the brain continues, there may be no body movement whatsoever, with the limbs *flaccid,* the muscles being limp and without tone.

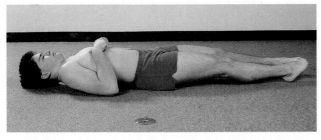 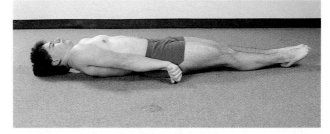

FIGURE 7–19. (*A*) *Decorticate posturing*—arms and wrists flexed, legs and feet extended. (*B*) *Decerebrate posturing*—arms extended and internally rotated at the shoulders with wrists flexed. The legs are extended.

There are cases of herniation of the brain where there is simultaneous compression of both right and left brain through the foramen magnum. This will result in loss of function of both pupils and sides of the body simultaneously. However, the patient will deteriorate in a manner similar to that described above.

VITAL FUNCTIONS. With transmission of increased pressure to the brainstem, the centers controlling vital functions are affected as well.

RESPIRATIONS. Abnormal respiratory patterns might occur, indicating damage to different levels of the brain. These patterns—Cheyne-Stokes respirations, central neurogenic hyperventilation, and apneustic, ataxic, and Biot's patterns of breathing—are presented in Figure 7–20. You may more often see Cheyne-Stokes and central neurogenic hyperventilation patterns, since these patterns are encountered in other diseases as well. Mimic the patterns in Figure 7–20 and practice drawing them in a similar form. You can then record the pattern in this same manner when you encounter it in the field, and the observation can be transmitted to hospital personnel.

PULSE AND PRESSURE. A late sign of increased intracranial pressure is a rising blood pressure with a slow pulse. The rising pressure within the cranium tends to collapse the blood vessels, and it is more difficult for blood to overcome this added resistance to flow. The brain makes a last-ditch effort to receive blood by a drastic rise in the blood pressure (especially the systolic) to overcome this increased intracranial pressure collapsing the blood vessels. Blood pressure receptors outside the head note this increase in blood pressure and tell the heart to slow down—hence the sign is *increasing blood pressure and slowing pulse*. This sign, called Cushing's reflex, is a late sign.

There are many different presentations of increased intracranial pressure. Some types do not present with a unilateral dilated pupil at any time. The possible signs that might be encountered are summarized in Table 7–3.

In addition to intracerebral hematomas, there are two other classic types of intracranial hematomas: epidural and subdural.

EPIDURAL HEMATOMA. Laceration of the arteries traveling along the inner surface of the cranium can lead to hematomas in the space *outside* the dura—hence, *epidural hematomas* (Fig. 7–21). Since the bleeding is arterial, the blood accumulates rapidly and can lead to rapid deterioration of the patient's neurologic status. This

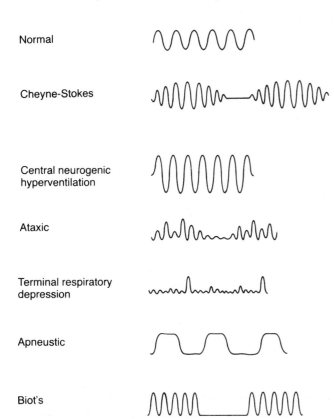

FIGURE 7–20. Diagrams illustrating the patterns of abnormal respiration that may be present following brain injury.

Normal

Cheyne-Stokes

Central neurogenic hyperventilation

Ataxic

Terminal respiratory depression

Apneustic

Biot's

TABLE 7–3. Signs of Increased Intracranial Pressure

Deteriorating level of consciousness on sequential examinations
Complaints of headache and nausea in the conscious patient
Vomiting (may be projectile)
Deteriorating GCS score
Dilation of one pupil (may be unresponsive to light and associated with eyelid droop)
Rising blood pressure with falling pulse rate

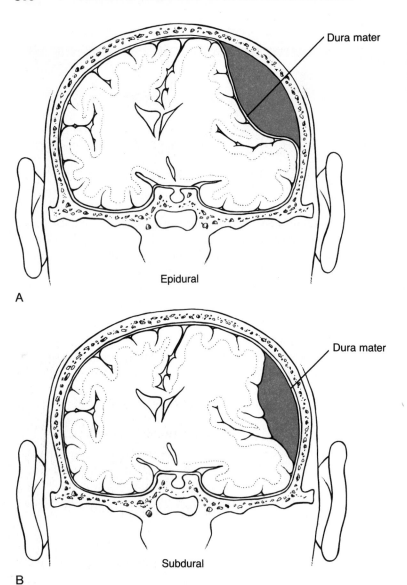

A

B

FIGURE 7–21. (*A*) Epidural hematomas occur in the space between the dura and the skull and result from arterial bleeding. (*B*) Subdural hematomas occur in the space between the dura and the arachnoid and result from venous bleeding. Bleeding within the meninges requires rapid identification so that the bleeding can be stopped and the clot can be removed.

makes early recognition of signs of intracranial pressure important, since the bleeding must be stopped and the clot promptly evacuated surgically to prevent further morbidity and death.

Classically, epidural hematomas are taught as presenting with a short period of unconsciousness after blunt trauma to the head, followed by a lucid interval where the patient regains consciousness. Shortly thereafter, the patient shows a deterioration in the level of consciousness and has a dilated pupil on the side of the blow and weakness and sensory impairment on the opposite side of the body. Within a short time, the patient manifests abnormal respiratory patterns, abnormal posturing, perhaps the Cushing's reflex (high blood pressure and a slow pulse), and then death if left untreated.

•   C A S E   H I S T O R Y   •

A 15-year-old catcher in a softball game is struck on the left side of the head (over the temporal bone) with the bat. She falls unconscious across home plate. After

30 seconds, she regains consciousness and is brought to the bench where she says she feels "all right." A short time later, she states she has a headache and vomits. She acts sleepy and soon it is difficult to arouse her. An ambulance is called for. The EMT finds the youngster comatose and unresponsive to verbal stimuli. She is breathing adequately and has a normal pulse and blood pressure. She has no related past medical history.

On neurologic examination, she is noted to have a dilated pupil on the left side that reacts sluggishly to light. She shows no spontaneous movement, but after a painful stimulus, shows withdrawal of the right arm.

During transport to the hospital, a subsequent examination reveals the patient to have rapid and deep ventilations, fixed and dilated pupils on both sides, spontaneous bilateral decerebrate posturing, and a rising blood pressure and slow pulse.

The youngster is taken to a neurosurgical center nearby. An epidural hematoma is diagnosed and the patient is taken to the operating room to have the bleeding stopped and the hematoma evacuated.

This presentation reveals many aspects of head injury. A blow was suffered sufficient to result in loss of consciousness for a short time. However, the patient soon regains consciousness and it appears as if she has suffered no more than a concussion. The initial injury is over. When the patient deteriorates, the change in condition must be explained by a secondary process. Since she has not been hypoxic or hypotensive and has no history suggesting a low blood sugar, the change in condition is most likely due to increased intracranial pressure. The blow sufficient to cause loss of consciousness was also sufficient to fracture the skull.

The temporal bone, in addition to being more easily fractured than other cranial bones, covers a major artery—the middle meningeal. The resultant arterial bleeding from the laceration of the underlying artery caused the patient's epidural hematoma.

However, patients with epidural hematomas may show symptoms in three different ways. Some patients with epidural hematomas have a loss of consciousness, a lucid interval, and then subsequent deterioration. Some patients are unconscious and remain so from the time of impact. Others never lose consciousness from the initial blow but later lose consciousness when the epidural hematoma expands and causes an increase in pressure within the skull.

Not only do emergency care workers have to look for signs of both primary and secondary types of head injuries, they must also be highly suspicious when a patient has sustained a significant traumatic injury and yet appears "all right."

• CASE HISTORY •

A 40-year-old man was struck by a van on a city street. He reportedly was thrown 30 feet by the impact. According to bystanders, the man had never lost consciousness. When the ambulance arrived, the patient refused medical evaluation and treatment. He was sitting on the curb, alert and a bit agitated. The EMTs took a look at the van, noting a dent in the front caused by the blow. They took another look at the victim and noted blood coming from his nose and ear. They insisted that the man accompany them to the hospital for further evaluation. The patient went along reluctantly but refused any medical attention whatsoever en route. One of the physicians at the hospital questioned the EMTs as to why they had brought the man to the emergency department. They reported the mechanism of injury and the signs of skull fracture that they had observed. About one hour later, the patient suffered a deterioration of consciousness and a dilated pupil with weakness on the opposite side. The patient had an epidural hematoma that was evacuated in the operating room, and he left the hospital after making a full recovery.

SUBDURAL HEMATOMAS. Underneath the dura lies a rich venous network. When veins in this area are ruptured following trauma, bleeding is confined to the space between the dura and the arachnoid membrane, resulting in subdural hematomas. Although bleeding from veins is under lower pressure than is arterial bleeding, if either large veins or many smaller veins are ruptured, blood can accumulate rapidly. If smaller veins bleed, it will take a longer time for the same amount of blood to accumulate in the subdural space.

With rapid bleeding, subdural hematomas show signs of increased intracranial pressure in a very short time. Acute subdural hematomas carry the highest mortality of all expanding lesions following head trauma.

Slower bleeding can result in subdural hematomas that are not apparent for a longer period of time. The period from the time of injury until signs of increased pressure appear can range from days to months. In these latter cases, there is usually more time to seek medical attention and therefore the mortality from these "chronic" subdurals is much less (see Fig. 7–21).

It is not possible for the EMT to distinguish the type of underlying lesion that is causing signs of increased intracranial pressure. However, awareness of the rapidity with which epidural hematomas and acute subdural hematomas cause death should result in early transport of victims with these signs to hospitals with facilities to treat neurologic injuries. Not all conditions with increased intracranial pressure can be helped by operations. In fact, a great number of cases of increased intracranial pressure following trauma are from generalized swelling of the brain. Many patients with nonoperable lesions, however, are saved by treatment of the increased intracranial pressure itself.

Nevertheless, the decision as to whether a patient with signs of intracranial pressure is a candidate for surgery must be made quickly in most cases. This decision is aided tremendously by an accurate and knowledgeable record of the mechanism of injury, the initial symptoms, and subsequent evaluations of the patient's status en route to the hospital. All these are the role of the EMT.

Assessment of Patients with Head Injuries

THE HISTORY

The mechanism of injury should be discovered as completely as possible. In motor vehicle accidents, an estimation of the speed of impact, the point of impact, the position of the victim in the car, and whether the patient was wearing a seat belt are all significant factors.

The following are pertinent questions to ask.

WHEN DID THE INJURY OCCUR? Was there immediate loss of consciousness? Was there a lucid interval if loss of consciousness did occur? As we have seen, a lucid interval following loss of consciousness followed by a deterioration in mental status points to a secondary process.

WAS THE INJURY A DIRECT BLOW? If so, this would lead you to suspect a possible complication of a skull fracture, e.g., an epidural hematoma. Was the patient wearing a seat belt so that the head did not strike directly? If so, subsequent deterioration may more likely be due to diffuse brain swelling from rotational forces.

WAS THERE A DOCUMENTED PERIOD OF APNEA OR CYANOSIS AT THE SCENE? The patient may have suffered sufficient hypoxia before help arrived to cause loss of all neurologic function. This knowledge will aid interpretation of subsequent neurologic examination. For example, the patient may have an expanding bleed within the skull, but the typical findings one might expect are masked by the deprivation of oxygen to ALL brain cells due to inadequate ventilations.

DID BLOOD EVIDENT AT THE SCENE SUGGEST SEVERE BLOOD LOSS? Is the patient at risk for hypovolemic shock from a scalp laceration?

ARE THERE ANY KNOWN DISEASES THAT MAY HAVE CONTRIBUTED TO THE ACCIDENT? Is the patient a known diabetic? Was the fall secondary to low blood sugar? If so, the patient is at risk for secondary brain damage due to this condition. Did the patient complain of chest pain and pass out before the accident?

PHYSICAL EXAMINATION

The physical examination should be brief so as not to delay transport, yet complete enough to determine the necessary prehospital treatments and record the patient's baseline status. This is accomplished by practicing the components of the examination as described below.

PRIMARY SURVEY. As with all cases, assessment begins with the primary survey. The establishment of the airway, breathing, and circulation are the first concerns. Approach all injured patients with the assumption that a cervical spine injury exists. Ideally, the cervical spine is immobilized manually as the primary survey proceeds.

CERVICAL SPINE CONSIDERATIONS. Because the cervical spine may have been injured by the same mechanisms that led to the head injury, due concern must be shown to prevent further injury to the spinal cord. All patients who are unconscious or who have altered mental status from either the head injury or alcohol or drugs must be assumed to have suffered a possible cervical spine injury.

The airway maneuver of choice is the modified jaw thrust. Unconscious patients may require the insertion of an oropharyngeal or nasopharyngeal airway. If a patient cannot be ventilated, then you may have to slightly extend the neck. The inability to ventilate takes precedence over a "possible" injury to the spine.

Suction must be available to aid in keeping the airway clear. The patient with a head injury is likely to vomit. Associated injuries to the face may cause bleeding or swelling, which can also compromise the airway.

SECONDARY SURVEY. Because terms such as lethargic, stuporous, and semicomatose can have different meanings to various observers, it is better to avoid their use. (See medical CNS emergencies later in this chapter, under altered mental status). More objective methods of assessing a patient's mental status have been developed and are currently employed. One method currently used by most emergency personnel and neurosurgeons is the Glasgow Coma Scale.

THE GLASGOW COMA SCALE

The *Glasgow Coma Scale* (GCS) is an assessment method utilizing three parameters—eye opening, verbal response, and motor ability. By carefully defining the parameters of measurement, use of the GCS promotes intraobserver reliability in assessing and describing patients with altered mental status. While the GCS was introduced earlier in the patient assessment chapter, it is repeated here because of its particular usefulness in assessing head injury patients.

While designed initially with the head trauma patient in mind, the GCS is a useful tool in evaluating and describing the neurologic status of all unresponsive patients because of its intraobserver reliability. *It enables health personnel at all levels to speak the same language.*

GENERAL TECHNIQUE. Remember that this score is intended for patients with an altered mental status. These patients range from individuals who are well-oriented and able to obey commands to patients who are deeply comatose and unable to respond to any stimuli. Accordingly, stimuli are applied sequentially, starting with *verbal questions and commands* and followed by administration of a *painful stimulus* if there is still no response.

The patient is then scored according to set criteria within the three general parameters. There are four possible eye responses, five possible verbal responses, and six motor response criteria. The best score is *15*, while the most unresponsive patient receives *3*.

To apply a pain stimulus, the developers of the scale recommend applying pressure to the nailbed. Another technique used by many emergency department and prehospital personnel is to pinch the skin over the forearms or trapezius to administer a painful stimulus. The pain stimulus should be applied bilaterally, since there may be a sensory deficit on one side.

EYES. If the eyes are open upon your arrival or OPEN WITHOUT STIMULI, the patient receives a score of 4. If they OPEN UPON VERBAL COMMAND, "Open your eyes!" the score is 3, and if they OPEN FOLLOWING PAINFUL STIMULI, the score is 2. If they DO NOT OPEN in response to pain, the score is 1. A score of 1 is the lowest score for each subcomponent.

VERBAL. The *alert* and oriented patient receives the highest score of 5. A patient who is *confused* but is able to respond in a conversational manner receives a 4. A patient who cannot maintain a conversation and gives *inappropriate* responses to questions posed by the examiner receives a score of 3. This patient may respond in a disorganized fashion with exclamatory or profane language. However, the key in distinguishing the confused from the inappropriate response is whether the attention of the patient can be maintained. The *confused patient will converse with the examiner and the patient's attention can be maintained. The inappropriate patient will drift off* and will not answer the examiner's questions without repeated verbal stimulation. This patient has a more depressed mental status than the patient who is confused.

The patient who responds with *incomprehensible* sounds and moaning and no recognizable words receives a 2. The patient who does NOT RESPOND verbally at all receives a 1.

MOTOR. The score of 6 is given to a patient who *obeys verbal commands*, such as "Move your arms," by making the appropriate movement. It is assumed, of course, that there are no fractures or other wounds of the extremities that will affect motor function. The GCS is concerned with brain function, not the status of any other components necessary for movement.

For example, a patient with a spinal injury that leaves the legs paralyzed would receive a GCS score of 6 if he or she is able to move an arm in response to a verbal command. This is evidence that the brain is intact. The fact that the patient's legs cannot move is a result of damage to a lower structure, in this case the spinal cord.

The other possible scores are elicited after application of painful stimuli. If a patient can *localize to pain* a score of 5 is given. Localizing pain is evidenced by an attempt on the part of the patient to reach for or remove the source of painful stimulus. For example, if the left trapezius is pinched as a painful stimulus, a patient might reach a hand up toward the examiner's fingers.

If the patient does not reach up for the examiner's hand but rather pulls away from the pain stimulus, the patient is said to *withdraw*. A withdrawal response is given the score of 4.

Some patients respond with flexion of one or both arms in response to pain. This is called a decorticate response and indicates that the higher brain centers are damaged. This flexion of the arms will be accompanied by extension of the legs in most cases. The *flexion* response receives a score of 3 (see Fig. 7–19).

With deeper coma or more extensive brain damage, a patient may respond to pain with the extension of both the arms and the legs. The extension of the arms is quite characteristic. The shoulders rotate internally, and the wrists flex. This response is also known as a decerebrate response. It indicates that the entire upper brain is functionally separate from the brainstem and the rest of the nervous system. The *extension* response receives a score of 2.

The lowest score of 1 is given if NO RESPONSE is observed from verbal or painful stimuli.

A patient is graded according to the response that would give the highest score. It does not have to be bilateral. That is, if the patient could not move one side, but responded on the other side with a flexion response, the motor score would receive a grade of 3 for the flexion that was observed. Remember to apply a pain stimulus on each side.

COMMUNICATING THE FINDINGS OF THE GLASGOW COMA SCALE

The EMT should be very familiar with the GCS. It enables accurate assessment of brain function with a very brief examination. While the EMT should know the numerical values of the signs, it is more important to communicate this assessment by describing the findings that were observed. This enables other health personnel to picture the patient more vividly and quickly than if they had to translate numerical scores back to responses. By describing the findings, one is less apt to misrepresent or misinterpret a patient's condition.

Always describe the patient and record your findings according to the subcomponents of the score. Your records may have space for the score such as:

GCS ____V,	____M,	____E =	____ (total)
(1–5)	(1–6)	(1–4)	(3–15)

When presenting the patient, do so in the following manner:

• C A S E   H I S T O R Y •

We have a 30-year-old man who was shot in the head. No other injuries are evident. There is a wound over the right temporal bone and no exit wound is visible. The patient was injured 10 minutes prior to our arrival. He was found to be breathing spontaneously, with deep ventilations at a rate of 26 per minute with no cyanosis. BP is 120/80 and the pulse is 60/min, regular and of normal quality. The patient is not responsive without application of pain. *The Glasgow Coma Scale shows eyes opening to pain, incomprehensible sounds, and extension as the best motor response.*

From this description, other health personnel can picture the patient's mental status more vividly than if the patient is described as comatose or as having a GCS of *6.* Furthermore, this manner of presentation indicates that the EMT has a good working knowledge of the GCS. If the patient's initial condition can be accurately described, the EMT's baseline examination takes on more meaning to other health personnel. This is especially important if signs change on subsequent examinations during transport or in the hospital.

Some EMS systems use the total score to help guide therapy. For instance, they may recommend hyperventilation for scores lower than *8.* Other systems might use the total score to decide whether a patient should be transported to a receiving hospital that has neurosurgical capabilities. These decisions are made by local medical control.

The GCS has been used to predict the outcome from head injuries once all treatable secondary conditions have been corrected. The EMT should never draw conclusions about a patient's chance of survival from the score in the field. There are two good reasons for this. First certain secondary conditions (e.g., increased intracranial pressure) that will lower the GCS can only be treated in a hospital setting. Second, it is quite common to find patients who have *both* head injury and a metabolic problem, such as the drunk driver or the patient with low blood sugar who falls down a flight of stairs. Metabolic causes of coma will result in a low GCS. A patient who is "dead drunk" may have no response to verbal or painful stimuli and receive a total GCS of *3.*

SPECIAL SITUATIONS

Some patients cannot be assessed for all three components. For example, if a patient has extensive wounds and swelling about the eyes, it may be difficult to assess his or her eye opening ability. Or if a patient is intubated with an endotracheal tube, it is not possible to assess his or her verbal performance. Such patients are best described by the subcomponents of the score that can be assessed. For the intubated patient, this would be:

    GCS: motor—flexion
         eye—no response
         verbal—not applicable, patient intubated

For the patient with massive injuries about the eyes:

    GCS: verbal—incomprehensible sounds
         motor—withdraws
         eyes—not tested because of swelling

VITAL SIGNS

As previously discussed, there are many variations in the vital signs resulting from head trauma and damage to the central nervous system. These variations may be present initially or they may be elicited on subsequent examinations. Sometimes they correspond with a level of brain function, as is the case with some abnormal respiratory patterns. At other times, they reflect a specific complication such as increased intracranial pressure (Cushing's reflex). Obviously, they must be interpreted in light of associated injuries outside the CNS as well. Because injuries may evolve both within and outside the nervous system, *vital signs should be checked at frequent intervals.*

RESPIRATIONS. While assessing the respiratory rate and depth, observe carefully for any abnormal respiratory patterns.

TEMPERATURE. The brain controls regulation of temperature. In some cases of brain injury, the patient is unable to control body temperature and feels cold or hot to the touch. The general aim is to help the patient maintain body temperature.

PULSE AND BLOOD PRESSURE. In cases of trauma, look for signs of *hypovolemia* from other associated injuries. A rapid and weak pulse and a narrowed pulse pressure (with or without hypotension) point to hypovolemia. If these are present, the EMT should look outside the head for other injuries causing blood loss. A good rule of thumb is that shock is never caused by bleeding *within the head.* There are only two exceptions: (1) An infant may have bleeding within the head sufficient to cause hypovolemic shock because the infant's skull is much larger in relation to the body. Also, the infant's skull may expand, allowing more blood to accumulate, since the suture lines between the bones have yet to fuse. (2) Severe damage to the brainstem itself may cause shock because of damage to centers controlling heart function and constriction of the blood vessels.

Treatment of hypovolemia takes priority over the treatment of associated head injuries. It is the more immediate threat to life.

A rising blood pressure with a slowing pulse should raise suspicion of increased intracranial pressure. This is usually a late sign and found in patients with low GCS scores.

HEAD AND SCALP

Examine the scalp for signs of fractures such as wounds, swelling, crepitus, or other deformities. Gently palpate any swellings since depressed skull fractures may be present. Use direct pressure to control bleeding. Look carefully for signs of basilar skull fractures such as raccoon's eyes and Battle's sign and for CSF leaking from the ears and nose.

PUPILS

The pupils should be evaluated for their size, their responsiveness to light, and their equality or symmetry. The pupils should always be checked because they give an indication of brainstem function. They are easily and readily evaluated and have good intraobserver reliability.

SIZE. The size of the pupils is described as midposition, constricted, or dilated. They can be expressed more specifically in terms of their diameter in millimeters (see Fig. 2–41).

Normally, the pupil varies in diameter in response to changing light conditions. It dilates when it is dark and constricts in response to bright sunlight.

A common cause of dilation of the pupils is hypoxia. A common cause of constriction of the pupils is narcotics. Another common cause of pupillary constriction is eyedrops used to treat glaucoma. Various drugs also affect the size of the pupils. Their effects will be considered in Chapter 12 on poisoning.

Older patients may have had surgery for cataracts, during which the iris muscle, which controls the diameter of the pupil, is dissected. They are often left with an irregularly shaped pupil that is more dilated than the normal eye.

EQUALITY. The pupils are generally equal to one another in size. If the pupils are not the same size, they are said to be unequal. The finding of unequal pupils usually means that *part of the brain* has been injured. It is important to be aware that *about 5%* of the population has slightly unequal pupils. This condition, called *anisocoria*, is just a normal variance of which most people are unaware. That is because in most cases of anisocoria, the difference between the pupils' diameters is only 1 to 2 mm.

When the unilateral dilated pupil is a sign of increased intracranial pressure, there usually are other abnormal neurologic findings as well. Furthermore, the difference in pupil size is usually greater than 2 mm.

REACTIVITY TO LIGHT. Much information can be gained by shining a penlight or flashlight into the pupils. Normally, pupils constrict when light is shined into the eye, and this response is described as *reactive to light*. The normal response is for both pupils to react equally when light is shone into one eye. This is because of connecting pathways between the left and right portions of the brain. Because the connecting pathways may be damaged, always shine your light into both eyes. If both pupils do not react equally, describe your findings.

When this simple test is done for patients in a coma, the results often can help determine if the coma is due to structural or metabolic problems. Most of the time,

if coma is due to a metabolic problem such as low blood sugar or an overdose, *the pupils react to light.* (One important exception is severe deprivation of oxygen, when the pupils are usually dilated and nonreactive to light.) There are a few other exceptions that are due to drugs, which will be discussed in Chapter 12. When the pupils do not react to light, physicians look for an underlying structural problem, i.e., damage to a part of the brain.

Bilaterally nonreactive pupils may be dilated and nonreactive, midposition and nonreactive, or constricted and nonreactive, depending on what part of the brain or brainstem is injured.

TRAUMATIC IRITIS. One common situation that affects both the size of a pupil and its ability to react to to light is *trauma to the eye itself*. Often, after blunt trauma to the eye, the iris muscle is in spasm. This results in a midposition or slightly dilated pupil that responds *sluggishly to light, if at all*. Usually, the white part of the eye is noted as having dilated blood vessels. There may be swelling or other signs of injury as well.

RECORDING AND DESCRIBING PUPILLARY FINDINGS. The eye findings should always be recorded and described according to these three parameters. The following examples serve to illustrate possible eye findings in three patients:

- As may be found in a normal person when practicing the eye examination: Pupils midposition, equal, and equally reactive to light
- As may be found in a patient in cardiopulmonary arrest: Pupils 7 mm in diameter, equal, and nonreactive to light
- As may be found in a patient with severe head trauma whose brain is herniating: Pupils, left, 8 mm and nonreactive to light; right, 4 mm and reactive to light

NECK AND SPINE ✓

If a patient is alert and awake, ask if there is any pain in the neck or along the cervical, thoracic, or lumbar spine. Gently palpate the entire spine. Is there any tenderness? Is there a deformity present or other signs of fractures such as *crepitus* or swelling and wounds over the spine? All patients with any alteration in mental status, intoxication, or with a significant mechanism of injury should have their spines immobilized. The neck should be kept in the neutral position and immobilized at the scene. A cervical collar can be applied at this time. Immobilization should be maintained until further evaluation can take place in the emergency department.

Immobilization is best accomplished with the help of a short or long spine board. The short board may be used to extricate the patient from an automobile. Other patients should be splinted to a long board. The head should be attached in a neutral position with the aid of the straps and supported with a rolled blanket or other suitable device. The torso should be attached first and then the head.

Once a patient is attached to a spine board, EMTs may have to turn the patient as a unit onto one side if vomiting should occur, to prevent aspiration of the vomitus into the lungs. Figure 7–22 illustrates the technique for suctioning the airway of a properly immobilized patient.

Blankets are used to help prevent head movement to the side. Further support can be provided by using long strips of tape or straps across the patient's forehead, which are attached on either side to the back board or stretcher. Cervical collars by themselves offer incomplete immobilization.

There may be uncooperative or combative patients who are difficult to immobilize. One EMT should attempt to keep the head in the neutral position by staying behind the patient and applying gentle inline immobilization (in the same direction as the spine).

The spine and spine injuries are covered in detail later in this chapter.

MOTOR AND SENSORY EXAMINATION

The neurologic examination for motor and sensory function should be brief in the field. Basically, the examination is to grossly determine (1) whether motor ability and sensation are intact and then (2) whether they are equal on both sides of the body.

The conscious patient should be touched on each side, first on the hands and then on the feet, and asked if the examiner's touch can be felt. By touching the hand and the foot, the examiner is testing the *most distal* portions of the extremities and is reasonably sure that sensation above is also intact. (See spinal injuries section at the end of this chapter.)

The patient is then asked to move both hands and then the feet. The motor examination should also begin with the hands and feet because:

- As with the sensation test, the most distal nerves will be tested.
- The patient may have other injuries that would make movement of the rest of the extremities painful or inadvisable.

Providing the patient has no other injuries in the extremities or spine, or conditions that would otherwise preclude further examination, ask the patient to flex an elbow or knee. This can be followed by asking the patient to raise an arm at the shoulder or a leg at the hip. Generally, this is sufficient.

Remember that if a patient cannot move because of pain, refrain that patient from further attempts at movement. As a general rule, pain on movement should cause the EMT to search for injuries outside the central nervous system.

The sensation of unconscious patients is assessed by applying a painful stimulus to the hands and feet. Depending on the degree of coma, any of the motor responses seen on the GCS may occur.

The patient is carefully observed to see if the motor and sensory responses are symmetrical, i.e., equal on both sides. As mentioned previously, asymmetrical responses imply that part of the structure of the nervous system has been damaged.

SEIZURES

It is not uncommon for patients with head injuries to suffer generalized convulsions or seizures. The rec-

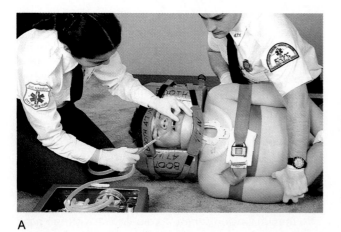
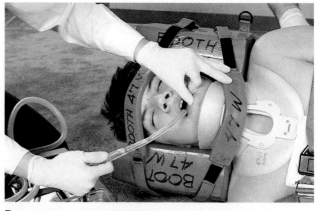

A   B

FIGURE 7–22. (*A* and *B*) Once the patient is firmly secured to a long spine board, the board is rotated to the lateral position and suction is applied. The lateral position allows for the free flow of vomitus and secretions to prevent aspiration.

TABLE 7-4. Prehospital Documentation of Central Nervous System Function

Time (minutes)	0		5		10		15	
Respiration								
Pulse								
Blood pressure								
GCS								
Eyes								
Verbal								
Motor								
Eyes	R	L	R	L	R	L	R	L
Size (in mm)								
React to light								
Motor								
Arms								
Legs								
Sensory								
Arms								
Legs								
Abnormal respiratory pattern								

(Adapted from Committee on Trauma, American College of Surgeons: Early Care of the Injured Patient, 2nd ed. Philadelphia, WB Saunders, 1976.)

ognition and management of seizures are covered in the last section of this chapter.

SERIAL EXAMINATIONS

Vital information is gained from repeating the neurologic examination and the vital signs. Whether a patient's status improves, deteriorates or stays the same in the prehospital phase of treatment is important information for both emergency department personnel and the neurosurgeon. Repeat examinations should be performed every 5 to 10 minutes and recorded. These examinations should include the GCS, vital signs, eye findings, and sensory and motor examinations. Neurologic flow sheets are recommended; there are several models that have been used. One example is that suggested by the American College of Surgeons (Table 7-4).

Become familiar with the record keeping used in your system. With practice, you will be able to perform this brief neurologic examination in about 30 seconds.

Treatment

As in all patients, priority treatment of patients with head injuries is directed toward ensuring patency of the airway, adequate ventilations, and effective circulation.

AIRWAY

Again, the airway maneuver of choice for the patient with a head injury is the modified jaw thrust. Any blood or secretions in the oropharynx should be suctioned and the presence or absence of a gag reflex evaluated. Patients without a gag reflex should have an oropharyngeal or nasopharyngeal airway inserted. The spine should be immobilized and the suction equipment should be readily available. If the patient has a return of the gag reflex, the oropharyngeal airway should be removed, as it may cause the patient to vomit. In EMS systems where an esophageal airway or an endotracheal tube is used, care should be taken to maintain the neck in a neutral position while the tube is inserted. Endotracheal intubation is discussed in Chapter 3. You should check local protocols.

VENTILATIONS

If ventilations are inadequate, assist with positive-pressure ventilation. Avoid extension of the head and neck. Good ventilations for patients with a head injury are important, not only to ensure an adequate supply of oxygen, but to prevent a buildup of carbon dioxide as well.

Both the oxygen content and the carbon dioxide content of the blood have an effect on the cerebral blood vessels. When the blood's oxygen content is decreased, the cerebral vessels dilate to permit more blood flow to the brain. Likewise, when the carbon dioxide level in the blood increases (as occurs with hypoventilation), the cerebral vessels also dilate. The brain senses that something may be wrong with its oxygen delivery system. By dilating the vessels, more blood will flow through the brain. Remember that oxygen delivery is dependent on both the oxygen content of the blood and the amount of blood flowing through an area. However, in patients with head injuries, bleeding within the skull translates into greater intracranial pressure. This follows from the fact that the pressure in the nonexpandable skull is proportional to the sum of its contents, namely brain, spinal fluid, and blood.

On the other hand, when the carbon dioxide level in the blood is low, the cerebral blood vessels constrict, allowing less blood to flow to the brain. The carbon dioxide content of the blood is low during hyperventilation.

We can use this principle in treating patients with increased intracranial pressure. By hyperventilating a patient, you can reduce the carbon dioxide content of the blood while maintaining the oxygen content and thereby reduce blood flow to the head. Since the pressure within the skull is the sum of its contents—i.e., brain, spinal, fluid, and blood, by reducing the amount of blood entering the head, the pressure within the skull is reduced.

In some EMS systems, hyperventilation is incorporated in prehospital treatment protocols. For example, in head-injured patients with a GCS score of less than 8, the patient is ventilated at a rate of 25 times a minute. This should be checked with local protocols.

The importance of maintaining adequate oxygenation and ventilation cannot be overemphasized for the reasons mentioned earlier. When in doubt about the depth or relative adequacy of a patient's ventilations, it is usually more prudent to assist with positive-pressure ventilations.

OXYGENATION

All patients with severe head injuries, and especially those requiring positive-pressure ventilations, should receive high-concentration supplemental oxygen. In patients with COPD, local protocols should be consulted to determine the appropriate oxygen delivery system.

CIRCULATION

Treatment of shock is a high priority. Bleeding must be controlled, and for head injury wounds, care should be taken when applying direct pressure to avoid compounding depressed skull fractures. MAST, leg elevation, and other shock treatments should be used. Hypotension can result in inadequate oxygen delivery to an already damaged brain.

TREATMENT OF SECONDARY HEAD INJURIES

Ensuring oxygenation, providing adequate ventilations, and treating hypotension will address three of the major causes of secondary head injuries. While these treatments are important in and of themselves, they help maintain the viability of the damaged brain as well. Two additional treatments involve glucose administration to patients with suspected hypoglycemia and the prevention of infection. Some EMS systems permit the use of oral glucose to conscious patients suspected of having a low blood sugar. Others permit administration of glucose intravenously or glucagon intramuscularly in known diabetics (see Medical Emergencies, Chapter 12). Early prevention of infection is a general goal of wound care. Table 7–5 summarizes the causes of secondary head injuries and related evaluation and treatment considerations.

IMMOBILIZATION AND POSITION OF TRANSPORT

All patients with head injuries must be evaluated for spinal injuries and treated accordingly.

The conscious patient with an isolated head injury

TABLE 7–5. Evaluation and Treatment of Secondary Head Injuries

Causes	Evaluation	Treatment Prehospital
Hypoxia	Look for cyanosis, bleeding in upper airway, chest injuries	Oxygen Assist ventilations Suction
High CO_2	Inadequate ventilatory efforts result in high blood CO_2 and dilation of cerebral vessels, raising intracranial pressure	Positive-pressure ventilations
Hypotension	Obvious external or suspected internal bleeding, pulse, blood pressure, spinal shock	Control bleeding Elevate feet MAST and IV fluids as per protocol
Increased intracranial pressure	Deterioration in mental status, nausea, vomiting, unequal pupils, increased blood pressure, slow pulse, deteriorating GCS	Local protocols may recommend hyperventilation
Low blood sugar	Hard to evaluate, gather history of diabetes	Follow local protocol Oral or IV glucose, IM glucagon
Infection	Prevention	Use sterile techniques

may be transported in the semisitting position. This decreases the gravitational effect on cerebral blood flow and allows the patient to more easily clear the airway if vomiting should occur.

In instances where definitive spinal immobilization is necessary, such as when the use of a short spine board is required, the supine position is the position of choice. It is essential that the patient be secured adequately to the device to allow for rotation in the event of vomiting. Again, suction should be readily available.

Some texts recommend that the lateral recumbent coma position be used during transport. This allows for easier drainage of blood or secretions from the mouth and nose. However, if this position is utilized, great care should be taken to maintain good cervical alignment.

The priorities to consider when deciding which position to use in transport remain airway and ventilation, circulation, and the possibility of spinal injury.

NOTIFICATION AND TRANSPORT

Patients with severe head injuries, like trauma patients, require definitive care in the hospital setting. With head injuries, the timely evaluation and treatment by a neurosurgeon are essential to save certain patients. Early notification of the hospital permits the mobilization of the necessary team members. An accurate and precise description of the neurologic findings and the mechanism of injury are invaluable. Some systems may direct the ambulance to transport the patient to the most appropriate and not necessarily the closest hospital facility. Since this is based on the EMT's findings and the description of the patient, assessment and presentation of the patient with a head injury are important aspects of the care rendered by the EMT.

SPINAL INJURIES

At present, the incidence of spinal cord injuries is between 3 to 5 per 100,000 population. While the number of spinal injuries may be small, the impact on the lives of patients and their families can be devastating. Careful management in the prehospital phase of treatment frequently makes the difference between a good recovery or a lifetime of paralysis or even death. The possibility of spinal injury should always be foremost in the minds of EMTs to ensure proper management of the trauma victim.

Anatomy and Physiology

THE SPINAL COLUMN

Since the spinal cord is well protected by the spinal column, injuries to the cord are usually associated with injuries to the bony vertebrae as well. The basic structure of the vertebral column is reviewed here. The spinal column consists of 33 vertebrae extending from the base of the skull to the tip of the coccyx. The individual vertebrae are held together by ligaments and separated by discs of cartilage. This allows for movement and bending while at the same time maintaining the alignment of the vertebral column. Most of these vertebrae are separate bones; however, some are fused together. There are 7 cervical vertebrae extending from the base of the skull. There are 12 thoracic vertebrae (one for each pair of ribs), which give posterior support to the rib cage or thoracic cavity. There are 5 lumbar vertebrae, which form the mid to lower back. These are connected to 5 sacral vertebrae, which are fused together (and called the sacrum) and form the posterior portion of the pelvic girdle. Extending from the sacrum are 4 coccygeal vertebrae, which are also fused and constitute the rudimentary tailbone. They are collectively called the coccyx.

Basic Components of the Vertebrae

Most of the individual nonfused vertebrae have a common structure. They are made up of an anterior body that gives support to the column. Posteriorly, they have a spinous process that can be felt particularly well in the lower cervical, thoracic, and lumbar regions. Connecting the anterior and posterior portions are the transverse processes. The anterior, posterior, and transverse bones form a circular canal called the *vertebral foramen* or spinal canal. The vertebral foramen is where the spinal cord lies.

There are processes on each vertebral body that serve as the points of contact or joints between adjacent vertebrae. The vertebrae are attached by ligaments on the anterior, lateral, and posterior surfaces. These ligaments hold the vertebrae in position while allowing a limited degree of movement. The vertebrae are separated from each other by intervertebral discs made of fibrocartilage. These smooth discs allow the vertebrae to move slightly upon one another. Because they can withstand compression, the discs also act as shock absorbers, cushioning the spine from injury.

Between the adjacent vertebrae on each side are openings through which spinal nerves and vessels exit. These nerves exit at each vertebral level. There are 31 pairs of spinal nerves grouped as follows: 8 cervical (C), 12 thoracic (T), 5 lumbar (L), 5 sacral (S), 1 coccygeal (Co). The abbreviations C, T, L, S, and Co followed by the appropriate numeral are used to identify the individual nerves. There are 8 cervical nerves because the first exits above the first cervical vertebra. The spinal cord actually ends at the level of the first lumbar vertebra, after which the spinal nerves travel distally together until each pair exits at the appropriate level in the lumbar, sacral, and coccygeal area.

There are some variations from this common structure. For example, the first and second cervical vertebrae are altered to some degree to provide for a wide range of movement of the head. The thoracic vertebrae have an additional surface where the ribs are attached. The sacrum and coccyx are fused for added support in the pelvic girdle. However, collectively they provide central support for the entire body and protection for the spinal cord and nerves (Figs. 7–23 and 7–24).

SPINAL NERVES

Each spinal nerve has both sensory and motor components. One spinal nerve leaves from each side of the vertebral column. There are therefore 31 pairs of spinal nerves in all. Together with the 12 cranial nerves (leaving the brainstem), they constitute the peripheral nervous system. The function of the peripheral nervous system is to provide a means of communication between all structures of the body and the central nervous system. These peripheral nerves continue to subdivide until they form an extensive network that *innervates* or connects with the various tissues, organs, and muscles.

The sensory branches bring information to the spinal cord and brain. The motor nerves transmit information from the brain and spinal cord to organs, muscles, and tissues, regulating their activity. Since the spinal nerves are the communicating wiring to and from the

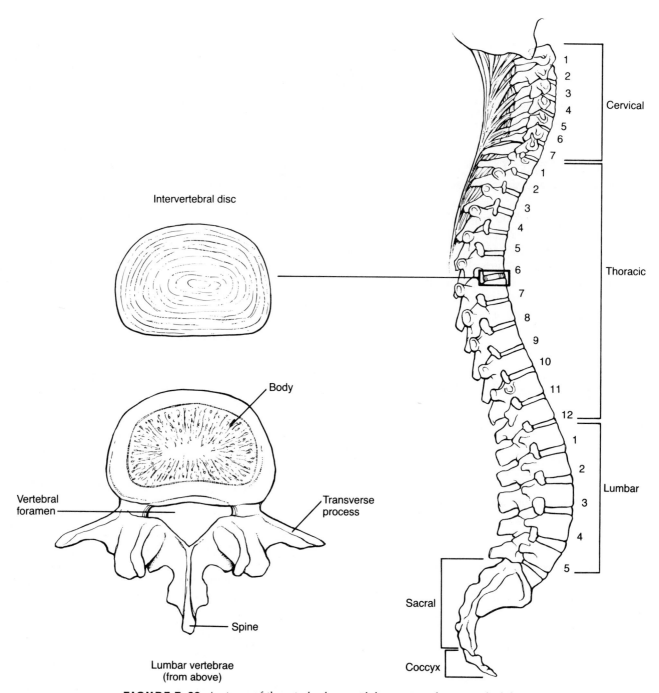

Intervertebral disc

Body

Vertebral
foramen

Transverse
process

Spine

Lumbar vertebrae
(from above)

Cervical

Thoracic

Lumbar

Sacral

Coccyx

FIGURE 7–23. Anatomy of the spinal column with ligaments and intervertebral discs.

brain, any disruption along the nerve pathways can result in loss of sensory and motor function. This loss always occurs distal to the site of injury.

Dermatomes—The Sensory Component

Knowledge of the anatomy of the spinal cord and peripheral nerves helps determine the level of injury. Following the wiring diagram of the nervous system, we find that particular segments of skin or *dermatomes* are innervated by nerves exiting from nearby segments

of the vertebral column. The same is true for skeletal muscles. The sensory components of the nerves follow dermatome patterns as is seen in Figure 7–25.

As you can see from the diagram, sensation from the skin over the collar bone anteriorly is transmitted through the nerve entering the vertebral column at the fourth cervical vertebra. Sensation from skin around the nipple is transmitted through the spinal nerve entering the vertebral column at the fourth thoracic vertebra. If the vertebral column were damaged and it crushed the

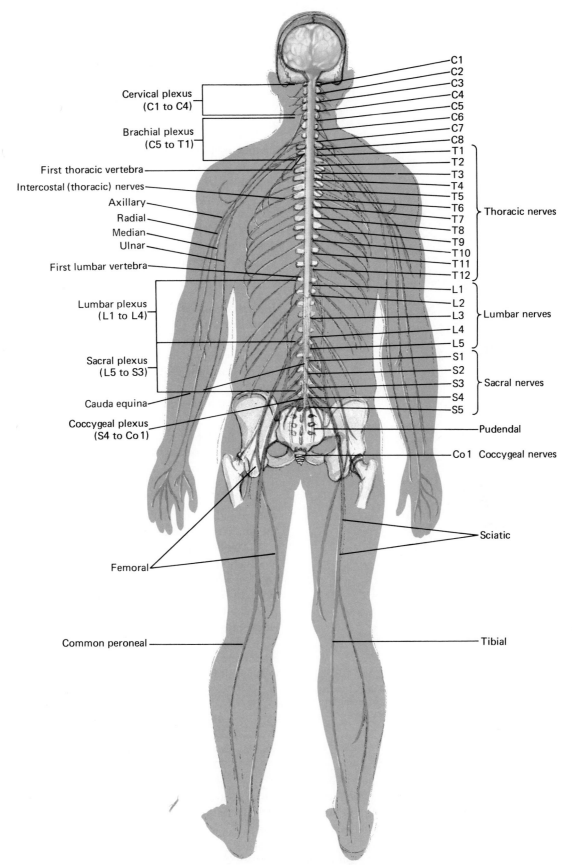

FIGURE 7–24. Spinal nerves. (From Solomon EP, Phillips GA: Understanding Human Anatomy and Physiology. Philadelphia, WB Saunders, 1987, p. 153.)

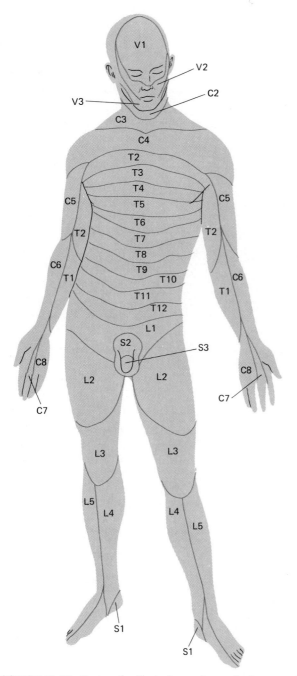

FIGURE 7–25. Review the illustration and note the location of the following dermatomes: C4, clavicle; T4, nipple line; T10, navel; and L1, groin. (From Solomon EP, Phillips GA: Understanding Human Anatomy and Physiology. Philadelphia, WB Saunders, 1987, p. 155.)

spinal cord at the first thoracic vertebra, function below or distal to the injury would be lost. Such a patient could still feel sensation over the collar bone (C4), but would not be able to appreciate sensation in the nipple dermatome (T4).

The EMT is not expected to memorize the entire dermatome chart. However, the EMT should commit to memory certain key dermatomes. They are easily re-

TABLE 7–6. Key Dermatomes

C4	Sensation anteriorly over the clavicle, including the shoulder
T4	The nipples
T10	The umbilicus
L1	The groin or inguinal region

membered because they relate to anatomical landmarks, such as the collar bone C4, nipple T4, umbilicus T10, and groin L1 (Table 7–6).

Knowledge of these key dermatomes helps clue the EMT to recognize possible respiratory complications resulting from spinal cord injury. This is because the motor components of the nerves innervating these key areas (except the groin) innervate various muscles of respiration.

Innervation of Muscles—The Motor Component

Skeletal muscles are also innervated by nerves from nearby segments of the vertebral column. Because there are so many muscles involved in movement of an extremity, many nerves are required for coordinated movement of the arm or leg. As can be seen from Table 7–7, the muscles of the arm and shoulder are innervated by the nerves from segments C4-T1. An intact nerve from C5 is necessary to flex the arm at the elbow. An intact nerve from C7 is necessary to extend the elbow. Therefore, patients with a cervical spine injury damaging all nerves below C6 will be able to flex their arms but not extend them. The muscles for the legs come from the lumbar and sacral segments.

The EMT is not expected to remember the precise innervation of each muscle group. However, the rescuer will be asked to test for motor function and muscle strength of both the lower and upper extremities. Table 7–7 is intended to give you a general idea of the relationship between spinal nerves and motor function. This table also includes the muscles of respiration: the diaphragm, the intercostals, and the abdominal muscles, which will be discussed below.

TABLE 7–7. Spinal Nerves and Motor Functions

Muscle or Motor Function	Spinal Cord Segment
Diaphragm*	C3–5
Flex elbow	C5
Extend elbow	C7
Finger motion	C8+
Intercostals*	T2–8
Abdominal	T8–12
Flex knee	L5
Extend knee	L3
Move toes	L5–S1

* *Muscles of respiration.*

Peripheral Nerves and the Muscles of Respiration

A major concern with spinal cord injury is respiratory function. All of the nerves that innervate the respiratory muscles pass through the cervical and thoracic portions of the spinal column. Therefore, injuries to the cervical and thoracic spine may affect, in some ways, a patient's ability to breathe. The main muscle of respiration, the diaphragm, is innervated by the phrenic nerve, which arises from branches off the third, fourth, and fifth cervical vertebrae (C3-C5). The intercostal muscles are innervated by nerves from T2-T8, and the abdominal muscles from T8-T12.

Here we review how injuries to various levels of the spinal cord affect the ability to breathe. If the spinal cord is damaged at the level of the third cervical vertebra, all the muscles of respiration are paralyzed. There are no spontaneous respirations. The EMT must provide total respiratory support in this situation.

Injuries below C5 result in loss of both the intercostal and abdominal muscles of breathing, resulting in diaphragmatic breathing only. The diaphragm will continue to function because the nerves have already exited from the spinal cord above the level of injury. The loss of the intercostal and abdominal muscles may result in smaller tidal volumes. The patient must compensate for the decreased tidal volume by increasing his or her respiratory *rate*. The EMT notes abdominal movement only. Supplemental oxygen is required and possible assistance of ventilations with positive pressure may be necessary. When the intercostals and the abdominal muscles are paralyzed, the patient is unable to cough as effectively and experiences more difficulty in clearing secretions, blood, or vomitus. Suction must be available and used to keep the oropharynx clear. Table 7–8 summarizes the level of spinal cord injury in relation to the respiratory status of the patient and treatment.

Autonomic Nervous System

One of the critical concerns with spinal injuries is the autonomic problems that can result. A knowledge of the autonomic pathways aids the EMT in anticipating and appreciating the potential complications and associated signs.

There are two main divisions of the autonomic nervous system, the parasympathetic and the sympathetic. In many instances, their actions tend to counterbalance each other. One illustration is their opposite effect on the heart's rate; the sympathetic tends to increase the rate, whereas the parasympathetic system slows it down. Another illustration is the effect on the pupils. The parasympathetic system constricts the pupils, whereas the sympathetic system dilates the pupils.

The parasympathetic effects tend to be relatively localized; that is, their effects take place at the specific organs that they innervate. The sympathetic system tends to be more concerned with a *"mass response."* It affects many parts of the body at the same time. The best example is its ability to prepare the body to respond to crisis. Simultaneously, the sympathetic nervous system can increase the heart rate, increase the blood flow to skeletal muscles, regulate the blood pressure, and decrease circulation to the skin and digestive system. It preferentially directs blood flow to the muscles, heart, and brain where it will be needed to flee from danger or to do battle—the so-called *flight or fight* response.

Anatomically, the sympathetic nervous system coordinates this activity by communication along a chain of nerves (ganglia) just outside the thoracic and upper lumbar spinal cord—the *sympathetic chain*. Here, branches of spinal nerves concerned with sympathetic actions group together with sympathetic branches from neighboring vertebrae. *Thus, when the spinal cord is severed at or above the upper thoracic level, sympathetic influence may be lost.* Parasympathetic nerves, on the other hand, arise directly from the brainstem and the sacral nerves. Adjacent branches do not intermingle to form a coordinated response.

NEUROGENIC SHOCK. If a patient suffers an injury to the cord at C7 and loses function of the sympathetic chain, there may be no sympathetic activity remaining. There are two significant ramifications from such an injury.

1. The patient may become hypotensive from vasodilation. The sympathetic nerves control the tone of the blood vessels. With loss of sympathetic tone, the blood vessels dilate. This results in more space for the blood to occupy than normal and results in vasodilatory shock. This condition is known as neurogenic shock and, if severe, can result in underperfusion of vital organs. Many patients with this type of shock have systolic blood pressures in the range of 70 to 80 mm Hg. Their pulse rate appears normal in the range of 60 to 80. They cannot compensate by increasing their heart rate since that, too, is a function of the sympathetic nervous system. Also, because the vessels are dilated, the skin may be

TABLE 7–8. Level of Spinal Cord Injury in Relation to Respiratory Status and Treatment

Level of Injury	Respiratory Status	Treatment
Above C3	Complete paralysis of all muscles of respiration	Positive-pressure ventilations, O$_2$
Below C5	Paralysis of intercostals and abdominal muscles, causing:	Supplemental O$_2$
	Decreased tidal volume	May require positive-pressure ventilations
	Ineffective cough	Suction of airway

warm and perhaps flushed, in marked contrast to the cool, pale, and clammy skin of the patient with hypovolemic shock who has a normal sympathetic nervous system.

Key signs are hypotension, slow or normal heart rate, and warm, well-perfused extremities (variable).

2. The patient may have associated injuries causing internal bleeding and hypovolemic shock. Because the blood vessels cannot constrict or the heart rate increase, the patient is unable to compensate for the hypovolemia. Worse yet, because key signs of internal bleeding (tachycardia, pallor, cool skin, and sweating) are absent, the hypovolemia may not be appreciated in the field.

Diagnosis of internal injuries in such a patient is further complicated by the fact that other signs such as pain or tenderness may be absent because of the loss of sensation.

Therefore, the EMT must have a high index of suspicion of internal bleeding whenever a patient with spinal cord damage from multiple trauma is evaluated.

PRIAPISM.   Another sign of spinal cord injury is *priapism* (sustained penile erection). This is also explained by loss of sympathetic influence. The parasympathetic nerves causing dilation of the penile vasculature are unopposed by the sympathetic nerves that constrict these vessels.

BLADDER DYSFUNCTION.   Patients with spinal cord damage may be unable to urinate. Since they will also have lost sensation, they will not be aware that the bladder is full and that they are retaining urine. This urinary retention is usually not a problem in the prehospital sphere. However, if you are called to transfer a patient hours after injury to another facility, you will note that a *urinary catheter may be placed* to prevent distention of the urinary bladder.

BOWEL DYSFUNCTION.   Some patients no longer have normal peristaltic function of the gastrointestinal tract. They may require a nasogastric tube to help decompress the stomach to prevent vomiting. Again, this situation is encountered during transfers rather than in the acute phase in the field.

Mechanism of Injury

As mentioned, most injuries to the spinal cord occur because of damage to the spinal column that protects the cord. The cord is a soft tube that can be torn, crushed, or contused when the bony vertebrae are broken or displaced from their normal alignment. There are two types of injuries—open and closed. Open injuries are produced by penetrating wounds—primarily from gunshot wounds or knives. The EMT is more apt to encounter patients who suffer from closed injuries

secondary to fractures or dislocations of the spinal column. These injuries are most often the result of motor vehicle accidents or falls.

The most common cause (greater than 50%) of spinal cord injury is motor vehicle accidents, followed by falls and sports-related accidents. Diving accidents are a common cause of sports related injuries.

VULNERABLE VERTEBRAE

The spinal column can be crushed, displaced in any direction, or broken. While injuries can occur at any site along the spinal column, there are certain sections of the column that are more vulnerable than others. *The most common sites of vertebral injury are where vertebrae that allow motion meet vertebrae that are fixed.* The thoracic vertebrae are fixed by the ribs and allow little motion. The cervical vertebrae are highly mobile, allowing a greater range of motion of the head and neck. Therefore, one can visualize the results of a sudden deceleration injury, as in a car accident. A driver wearing a seat and shoulder belt experiences little movement of the thorax. However, the head continues to move forward with the velocity prior to impact. The junction of lower cervical vertebrae and upper thoracic vertebrae becomes the fulcrum at which maximum stress is applied. This junction is the site of both bony fracture and tearing of the supporting ligaments.

With this concept in mind, we see that the same potential exists at the other end of the thoracic vertebrae. Here, the fixed thoracic vertebrae T1-T10 meet the more mobile lower two thoracic vertebrae T11 and T12 (remember the 11th and 12th ribs are "floating" ribs that are not attached to the sternum anteriorly). Again, mobile and fused vertebrae meet. A common site of injury is from T10 to L1.

Since the sacrum is composed of vertebrae that are fused together, another site of potential injury exists where the lower lumbar vertebrae meet the sacrum.

Sites where mobile vertebrae meet fixed vertebrae include either end of the fixed thoracic vertebrae, where the lower cervical vertebrae meet T1, and where the upper lumbar and "free" thoracic vertebrae meet T10. The lower lumbar vertebrae are also prone to injury where they meet the sacrum. Table 7–9 summarizes the common sites of fracture where fixed and mobile vertebrae meet.

SPECIFIC MECHANISMS

There are many types of mechanisms of injury. In addition to direct blows, the EMT must appreciate the dynamic forces that are set in motion after impact. As with head injuries, these dynamic forces often do more damage than the blow itself. By appreciating these potential mechanisms, the EMT maintains the appropriate

TABLE 7-9. Common Sites of Spinal Injury

Mobile	Fixed
Lower cervical, C5–7	Thoracic, T1–10
Lower thoracic, T10–L1	Thoracic, T1–10
Lower lumbar, L4–5	Sacrum

level of suspicion when approaching accident victims. Since most spinal cord injuries are closed injuries, there may be little gross evidence of damage to the spinal column. The mechanism of injury should be documented and relayed to hospital personnel so they can continue to check for related complications while further evaluation (e.g., x-ray studies) proceeds. Different mechanisms of injury are associated with particular types of fractures. Knowing the mechanism of injury helps hospital personnel piece together the clinical presentation and x-ray findings with the history of injury.

COMPRESSION FORCES. Compression forces occur when one spinal vertebra is driven onto another. The force may be transmitted from above (the head) or below. Examples include accidents when diving into shallow water when the head and neck are in normal alignment (not flexed) or falls from a height with the victim landing on his or her feet or buttocks. These forces often compress vertebrae to the point where the bones burst. Damage to the spinal cord follows when the resulting bone fragments impinge on the soft vulnerable cord (Fig. 7–26).

FLEXION INJURIES. Flexion forces usually involve fixed and mobile vertebrae. Here the head is driven forward by sudden deceleration (as described above) or when force is applied to the back of the skull. The bodies of the adjacent vertebrae are wedged together anteriorly with resulting fracture to the body of the vertebrae. In some instances, this type of injury can tear the posterior ligament that supports the spine, allowing one vertebra to slide forward onto another, compressing the cord in between.

As mentioned, flexion forces occur when the head is jolted forward in a head-on collision from deceleration forces or when the top of the head strikes the windshield with the neck in a flexed position. Flexion injuries also can result from falls when the spine is sharply flexed, and jackknifes at the waist. A final example includes lap belt injuries, where the pelvis is held stationary and the deceleration forces place maximal stress on the thoracic and the lumbar vertebrae (Fig. 7–27).

EXTENSION INJURIES. Hyperextension injuries can occur when the head is suddenly jolted backward. An example would be striking the windshield of a car with the face. The anterior ligaments supporting the spine can tear with consequent swelling and possible instability resulting in dislocation.

In other cases, the cord can be contused against structures within the spinal column. The elderly are particularly prone to this type of injury. The blood supply to the cord may be compromised in hyperextension injuries as well. These latter two examples show how cord injury can occur without a broken neck.

Whiplash injury is a common term used to describe hyperextension of the neck resulting from motor vehicle accidents. This injury occurs when the head is jolted backward suddenly when a car is struck from behind. The muscles in the anterior of the neck try to overcome this violent change in head position and can tear if sufficient force is exerted. Usually, these whiplash injuries cause more muscle soreness and stiffness than column or cord injury. However, it is impossible to reliably establish the severity at the scene, and cervical immobilization should be instituted (Fig. 7–28).

OPEN WOUNDS—MISSILE INJURIES. Gunshot wounds may damage the spinal cord directly or drive bone fragments into the spinal canal. The course of a bullet within the body is unpredictable. It may ricochet off other bones and change course. Knife wounds may enter the spinal canal between vertebrae and damage the cord. Fortunately, these injuries are less common than those previously described.

It is important to reconstruct the mechanism of injury during the 10-second survey and conceptualize the forces that may have caused spinal injury. In some cases, where there is no external evidence of injury, the mechanism of injury provides the rationale for immobilization and treatment.

Types of Injuries

Types of injuries that can occur to the spinal cord are similar in many respects to injuries that occur to the brain. They can range from concussion, or a temporary loss of function, to complete laceration and disruption of the cord, resulting in permanent damage.

As with concussion to the brain, where there may be a temporary period of total unresponsiveness, concussion to the upper cord may disrupt nerve tracts that control movement of the entire body, resulting in temporary but complete paralysis. It is impossible at the scene to determine whether a patient has suffered a temporary concussion or total disruption of the spinal cord.

Other patients may have contusions of the cord following trauma in which the spinal cord is bruised against the bony spinal column. Specific areas of the cord may be damaged, resulting in various degrees of motor and sensory loss.

Bleeding may also occur within the spinal column, in the epidural and subdural spaces, or within the cord itself. Unlike the brain, however, epidural and subdural

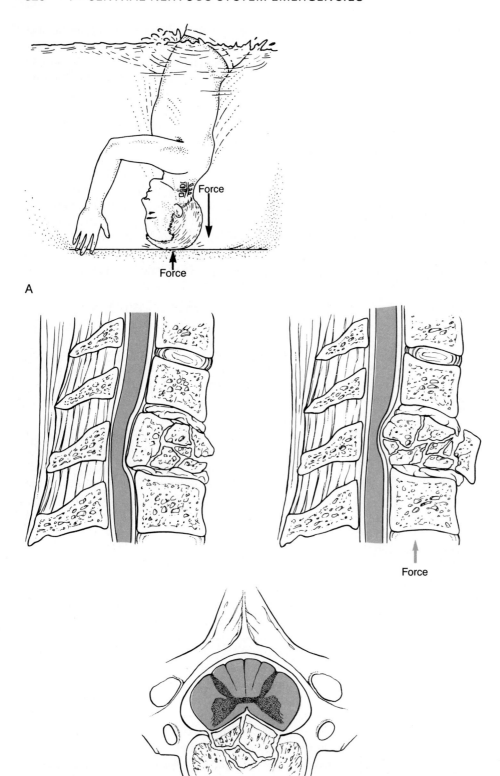

A

B

FIGURE 7–26. (*A* and *B*) When a force is applied directly along the path of the vertebral column, the vertebrae are compressed onto one another, causing fractures of the vertebral body. (*A*, from Kitt S, Kaiser J: Emergency Nursing: A Physiologic and Clinical Perspective. Philadelphia, WB Saunders, 1990, p. 458.)

bleeding does not usually result in compression of the cord because the blood may disperse along the entire length of the spinal canal. Bleeding within the cord itself results in damage because of localized compression and disruption of the vascular supply.

Compression of the cord results mostly from trauma to the bony vertebral column and the discs and ligaments that support it, with the extruding of bone or supporting tissue into the space normally occupied by the cord. If this occurs with tremendous force, the entire cord can be disrupted.

Bony fragments or penetrating injuries can lacerate

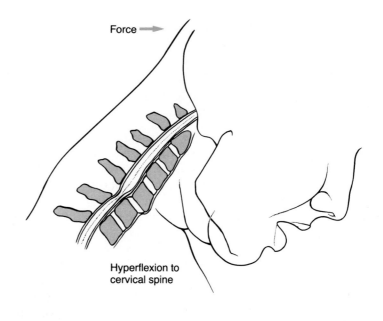

Force →

Hyperflexion to
cervical spine

FIGURE 7–27. As the spine is
exposed to extreme flexion forces,
the supporting posterior ligaments
can tear, allowing the vertebrae to
be pushed anteriorly.

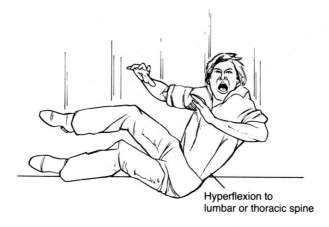

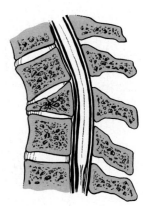

Hyperflexion to
lumbar or thoracic spine

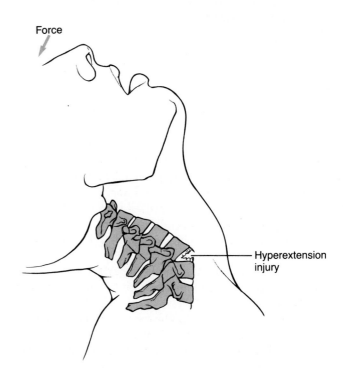

Force

Hyperextension
injury

FIGURE 7–28. When forces are applied to the forehead or face,
hyperextension injuries can occur. This figure illustrates an example
of a hyperextension force and the related displacement of vertebrae.

the cord. Again, the degree of laceration varies from minor wounds to complete transection of the cord. Open wounds run the additional risk of secondary infection.

COMPLETE AND INCOMPLETE INJURIES TO THE SPINE

Injury to the spinal cord may be complete or incomplete. With complete injury, no nerve function below the level of the spinal cord is evident. Only those structures innervated by spinal nerves leaving the spinal column above the level of injury will function. There is no motor or sensory function below the level of the injury. With incomplete injury, some nerve tracts at the site of injury are damaged while others are spared. This results in normal findings above the level of injury with *variable* sensory or motor losses below. Any loss of sensory or motor function indicates the need for spinal cord immobilization. This underscores the importance of a thorough secondary survey.

A knowledge of the types of injuries aids the EMT in appreciating the need for proper assessment and the importance of maintaining a high index of suspicion. Positive neurologic findings do not indicate permanent damage. On the other hand, the absence of neurologic findings does not mean that an injury to the spinal column has not occurred.

Patient Assessment

The goals of patient assessment are to determine if the possibility of spinal injury exists and, if it does, to determine and document the level of injury. Appreciation of the possibility of spinal injury leads to proper care and handling at the scene and immobilization prior to and during transport to prevent further injury. Knowledge of the presence and level of spinal injury helps to identify and anticipate the complications requiring respiratory and circulatory support.

SCENE SURVEY

During the scene survey, attempt to determine the mechanism of injury. Try to conceptualize what types of forces occurred during the accident. Could the patient have suffered a compression, extension, or flexion type injury to the spine? *Assume that all unconscious accident victims have suffered a possible spinal injury.* If the patient was a victim of motor vehicle accident, a significant fall, or a sports-related injury, approach the patient with a high level of suspicion. This is important to prevent aggravating a possible injury during the assessment phase.

Look at the patient. Bruising or lacerations about the head, face, and forehead should raise your suspicion. So should signs of trauma to the shoulders or pelvis,

since forces causing these injuries may be transmitted to the spine.

The burden of proof rests with the EMT, not with the patient, in eliminating the possibility of injury to the spine. Frequently, accident victims deny or minimize their injuries. A primary goal is to *prevent further injury from occurring.*

THE PRIMARY SURVEY

- When spinal injury is suspected, the primary survey is modified to provide immediate support to the cervical spine. Do not move the patient to establish unresponsiveness. If the patient is unresponsive, log roll the patient as a unit, then proceed with the survey.
- Open the airway with the modified jaw thrust in order to PREVENT HYPEREXTENSION OF THE NECK. If a patient is found with his or her head flexed, return it to the neutral position and support the head. If resistance is encountered in returning the neck to the neutral position, evaluate the adequacy of ventilations in the position found. In certain types of dislocation injuries, the vertebrae can become locked in a dislocated position.
- If the patient is hypoventilating or apneic, provide positive-pressure ventilations, again avoiding extension of the neck if possible.
- Look for and control external bleeding and seal open chest wounds. Life-threatening injuries take priority and call for early transportation.
- With possible spinal injuries, it is generally accepted that extra time should be spent in immobilizing the patient securely prior to transport unless signs of inadequate ventilation and circulation exist that are outside the bounds of prehospital care.

For example, consider a patient with inadequate ventilations from a drug overdose who fell down a flight of stairs and has injuries to the face and neck. The mechanism of injury and the physical signs raise the suspicion of spinal injury. If adequate ventilations can be administered with positive-pressure ventilations at the scene and no evidence of circulatory problems exist, it would be advisable to take a few extra minutes to secure the patient to a spine board prior to transportation to the hospital.

Contrast this with a patient who has a possible spine injury and an identified tension pneumothorax, who must be transported immediately since the identified threat to life cannot be treated in the field. *Definitive treatment of a life-threatening condition always takes precedence over a possible spinal injury.* While attempts should be made to maintain the spine in a neutral position on a firm board, basic life support and transportation to definitive care are the higher priority.

HISTORY

Reconstruct the mechanism of injury and the events leading up to the accident. You may need the help of bystanders or witnesses to reconstruct the events surrounding the accident. In cases where the victim is unconscious, this may be the only means available. The condition of the patient may dictate that the history is obtained at the same time that treatment is rendered. However, do not overlook these important data.

Important questions to consider and observations to note are:

- When did the injury occur?
- What was the position of the patient at the time of injury? Was he thrown by the impact (e.g., pedestrian struck)?
- In motor vehicle accidents, what does the car look like? Estimate the speed of impact and determine the position of the victim in the car. Was he or she wearing a seat belt? Has he or she been moved? Did he or she move initially?
- Did the patient pass out prior to the accident?
- Was there a period of cyanosis or apnea?
- In falls, estimate the height of the fall, and note the surface the patient struck upon landing.
- Do you suspect alcohol or drug use?
- What is the previous medical history? Is it in any way related to the cause of the accident (e.g., a diabetic with hypoglycemia, fainting, etc.)?

THE SECONDARY SURVEY— VITAL SIGNS

RESPIRATIONS. Look closely at the rate and depth of respirations. Shallow breathing may indicate that the muscles of respirations are impaired. Look at the type of breathing. Is it abdominal breathing only? Ask the patient to take a deep breath to check for the effectiveness of the intercostals. Does the chest rise and expand? You can also ask the patient to exhale vigorously or cough to check abdominal muscle function.

PULSE AND BLOOD PRESSURE. Is there evidence of neurogenic shock (hypotension with a normal or slow pulse)? Trauma sufficient to cause cord damage may well have caused other injuries. *Since signs of hypovolemic shock may be masked by the simultaneous presence of neurogenic shock, look carefully for signs of injuries known to be associated with significant blood loss.* This includes bruising and fractures of the ribs, especially over the liver and spleen, and fractures of the pelvis and femur. Remember that these patients also have sensory loss and may not complain of pain or tenderness.

TEMPERATURE. There is loss of thermoregulatory mechanisms with some severe spinal injuries. The patient who is vasodilated exchanges heat more easily with the environment. If the environmental temperature is lower than normal body temperature, the patient loses heat and needs to be covered with blankets. The patient who loses the ability to sweat may also be unable to regulate the body's temperature. Proper care is guided by an understanding of the body's thermoregulatory mechanisms. See heat emergencies in Chapter 11, Environmental Emergencies, for further discussion.

HEAD-TO-TOE SURVEY. Pay special attention to the spine. Slide your hand under the patient, assessing the cervical, thoracic, and lumbar spine for tenderness or deformities. Look for bruises on the shoulders or pelvis.

Take a close look at the neck before a cervical collar is applied. Look closely for any obvious injuries. Are the larynx and trachea intact? Are they deviated to one side? Check the neck veins closely. Are they flat or distended? Remember that patients with multiple trauma may have significant bleeding or obstructive shock (from pericardial tamponade or tension pneumothorax). The neck veins provide valuable clues. If the condition changes and signs of shock are present, you may wish to remove the collar to reevaluate the position of the trachea and the fullness of the neck veins while maintaining cervical immobilization.

MOTOR AND SENSORY EXAMINATION. A brief examination of the sensory and motor functions should be performed prior to transportation. Both feet and hands should be checked for the ability to feel touch and pain and for motor function.

It is important to be systematic in order to identify the level of injury. Compare one side with the other. Begin distally and work up toward the head. Check for sensation in the feet, then move up the legs, abdomen, and torso, and then proceed to the hands and up the arms. Document the findings. Note and describe any level where sensory findings change. Be descriptive, e.g., 2 inches below the nipple, and so forth. Draw a mark with a pen at the site.

If a line of demarcation appears where the skin is moist or clammy above and dry below, note this in the same manner. It may be the only clue in an unconscious patient. (Loss of sympathetic nerve activity affects the sweat glands below the level of injury.)

For motor function, ask the patient to move the toes up and down and lift both feet 3 to 4 inches off the ground. Then place your hands against the soles of both feet. Have the patient try to push your hands away, using only the toes, in order to gauge the patient's strength. You may then ask the patient to flex and extend the knees. Tell the patient to stop the movement if any pain is encountered. If there are fractures in the lower extremities or pelvis, do not ask the patient to move the legs.

The muscle strength should be noted as absent, weak, or present. For example, a patient who has weak function may be able to flex an arm against gravity but not if the examiner applies a slight counterforce opposing the movement.

Note that a patient with a complete lesion at C6 may be able to flex an arm (C5) but may not be able to extend it (C7) if the examiner places it in the flexed position.

Proceed in the same way with the arms, starting at the hands. First check for sensation and then for movement. Have the patient grasp your fingers in the palm of one hand and squeeze to check for strength. Ask the patient to flex and extend an arm at the elbow. Again, compare the two sides and document your findings (Figs. 7–29 and 7–30).

UNCONSCIOUS PATIENT.   If the patient is unconscious, use a pin or sharp object to stimulate the feet and then the hands. Check the face for any grimacing while observing the limbs for signs of movement. The type of movement in unconscious patients should be described. Use of the classifications of motor testing for the Glasgow Coma Scale, i.e., localization, withdrawal, and flexion and extension responses, is recommended for consistency. Be sure to check both sides.

Even if it is obvious on initial inspection and assessment that the patient cannot move or feel the upper limbs, be sure to check the lower extremities. *Do not assume* that because upper body function is compromised that the entire cord is damaged. If the patient has an incomplete lesion the nerve tracts to more distal areas may have been spared. Sparing of distal portions has great relevance in determining subsequent treatment in the hospital.

One must also check all areas distal to a loss of sensation most carefully for the presence of fractures and other injuries, since the patient will be unaware that this part of the body is injured.

RESPIRATORY IMPLICATIONS OF THE MOTOR AND SENSORY EXAMINATION.   If a sensory level is found, think about the level of spinal cord function in terms of implications on the muscles of respiration. Use your knowledge of key dermatomes to help determine whether the muscles of respiration may be affected (Table 7–10).

PERFORM SEQUENTIAL EXAMINATIONS.   The neurologic examination and checking of vital signs should

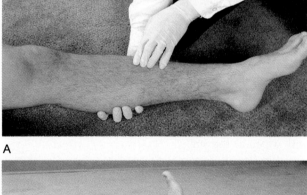

A

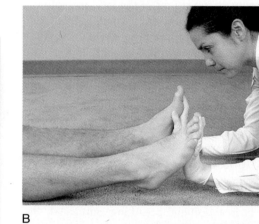

B

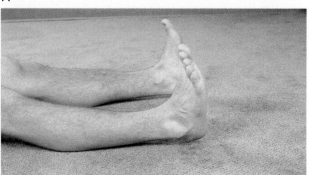

C

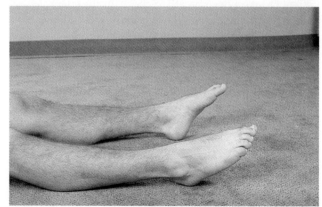

D

FIGURE 7–29. *Sensory examination:* (A) Have the patient close his eyes and provide stimuli to the lower extremities using a pinch or touch with a blunt object. Have the patient indicate when he feels the stimuli. If the patient is unable to speak, observe for responsiveness while applying stimuli. When conducting a sensory examination, note sensory loss on one side of the body as compared to the other and, when appropriate, check for levels of sensory functions at the clavicle, nipple line, navel, and groin (key dermatomes). *Motor examination:* (B) Holding the balls of the feet, ask the patient to apply downward pressure with his feet. (C) Have the patient flex his ankle. (D) Have the patient extend his feet. When checking for motor function, note the differences in motor strength, as well as the ability to move one extremity or the other (lateralizing signs).

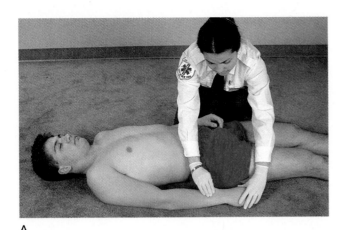

A

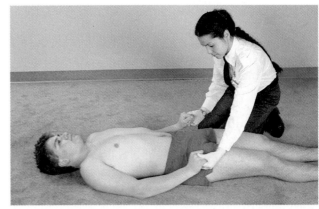

B

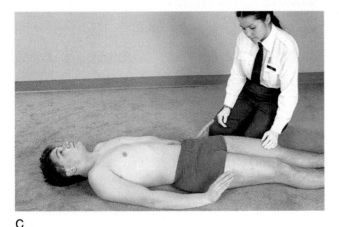

C

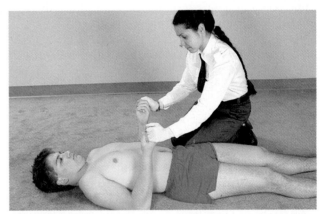

D

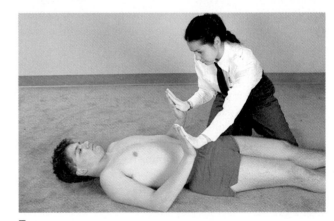

E

FIGURE 7–30. *Sensory examination:* (*A*) Have the patient close his eyes and provide stimuli on both surfaces of the upper extremities using a pinch or touch with a blunt object. Have the patient indicate when he feels the stimuli. If the patient is unable to speak, observe for responsiveness while applying stimuli. *Motor examination:* (*B*) Have the patient hold both of your hands at the same time and squeeze with equal pressure. (*C*) Have the patient extend his hands. (*D*) Have the patient flex his elbows against resistance. (*E*) Have the patient extend his elbows against resistance.

TABLE 7–10. Association Between Sensory/Motor Examination Findings and Function of Respiratory Muscles

Sensory Dermatome	Motor	Muscles of Respiration
C4	Quadriplegia*	All muscles of respiration may be affected
T4	Paraplegia†	Diaphragm is intact Loss of intercostals (partial) and abdominals
T10	Paraplegia	All intact

* *Quadriplegia = paralysis of all four extremities.*
† *paraplegia = paralysis of the lower extremities.*

be repeated periodically. Record your findings on a form similar to that used for patients with head injuries. Pay particular attention to changes in the level of motor or sensory function.

Treatment

GETTING TO THE PATIENT

Most victims who sustain spinal injury do so in motor vehicle accidents. Many may still be trapped in the vehicle when help arrives. *Therefore, gaining access and initiating lifesaving measures are often the first steps in the rescue.*

Patients who are still in an automobile should be evaluated, with due attention given the cervical spine. One EMT must return the head and neck to the neutral position and hold them there while supporting the weight of the head. This is true for both conscious and unconscious patients. If the primary survey shows there is no immediate danger to life, the ideal means of extrication is to apply a rigid cervical collar and immobilize the spine via a short spine board prior to removal of the patient. Rigid collars should be used rather than soft collars, as the former offers better immobilization. Once removed, the patient should then be affixed to a long spine board in anticipation that injuries to the thoracic or lumbar spine may also have occurred.

When the primary survey shows that CPR or other lifesaving measures are needed, or another hazard such as a fire exists, there will be no time to employ the use of the short spine board. (See the emergency patient lifts and carries in Chapter 16.) Whenever there are enough personnel, one rescuer should maintain traction on the patient's head and neck while the other rescuers remove the patient from the accident area.

In all instances, the cardinal principle is to maintain and support the cervical spine in a neutral position at all times. This requires that the EMT supporting the patient's head must serve as the team leader when the patient is to be moved. This enable's the EMT to be in a position to continue to support the head. The handling should be gentle, with support of the weight of the head so that alignment of the head and neck is maintained in the neutral position. Be careful not to allow the patient's head to repeat the mechanism of injury.

Combative patients who are thrashing about may require that one person be assigned to support the head throughout the prehospital phase. Always consider the possibility of hypoxia as the explanation for agitated or combative behavior, and administer supplemental oxygen.

OXYGEN

Patients with altered mental status or with any evidence of neurologic dysfunction should be given high-concentration oxygen. The provision of an adequate airway and attention to secretions that may obstruct the airway are major concerns. If there is any doubt about the adequacy of ventilations, assist with positive-pressure devices. It is *essential* to ensure adequate oxygen delivery to damaged nerve tissues.

Have suction ready, since the airway may have to be cleared while the head is still immobilized. If the patient vomits while immobilized on a spine board, be ready to move the patient as a unit onto one side to prevent aspiration. Patients with adequate ventilations who have a clear potential for airway compromise due to bleeding or vomiting should be placed on the side to prevent aspiration while supporting the cervical spine (see Fig. 7–22). The alternative is to securely package the patient on a long spine board that is then tilted on its side to allow secretions to clear. Again, considerations about the airway and breathing are the higher priority.

IMMOBILIZATION

As with all suspected fractures, the patient with possible spinal injuries should be immobilized prior to movement.

PATIENT FOUND LYING ON THE GROUND. An essential part of assessment is to check for deformities of the spine. If minor deformities are found, immobilize the patient without attempting to correct the deformity. However, if there is especially abnormal angulation, this will sometimes prevent proper immobilization. An attempt should be made to gently return the patient to the neutral position. *However, forceful manipulation must be avoided.* If resistance is encountered, then immobilize the patient to the board in the position in which he or she is found.

Patient should be log rolled to a supine position onto a long spine board or lifted with a scoop stretcher. The patient must be secured by the use of straps that prevent movement during carry or if the patient must be turned as a unit should vomiting occur. (See lifts and carries in Chapter 16 for specific techniques.)

THE LOG ROLL

The log roll is a suitable movement technique for potential spinal injury victims. It is used to place a patient on a spinal immobilization device without disturbing the alignment of the spinal column.

It is essential that the log roll be performed slowly and carefully. The team leader must observe the team closely to ensure that good alignment is maintained during movement.

The principles and techniques used in preparing patients for spinal immobilization follow. More information about lifts and carries can be found above and in Chapter 16.

PROCEDURE 7-1 LOG ROLL

1. The team leader maintains gentle in-line immobilization to the cervical spine, taking care to support the weight of the patient's head and the normal alignment.
2. Apply cervical collar (Fig. 7-31A).
3. Three other rescuers are positioned along one side of the patient while the spine board is placed on the opposite side (Fig. 7-31B and C).
4. On command from the team leader, the patient is rolled toward the three rescuers who support the spinal column (Fig. 7-31D).
5. The rescuers then position the board behind the patient, checking for proper position (Fig. 7-31E).
6. Roll the patient onto the spine board upon the command of the team leader (Fig. 7-31F).
7. Securely attach the patient to the spine board across the upper chest, pelvis, legs, and at the head. This will provide maximum immobilization during transport (Fig. 7-31G to J).

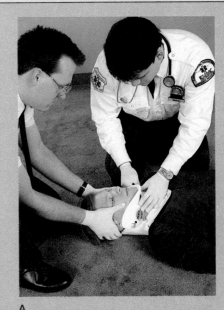

A

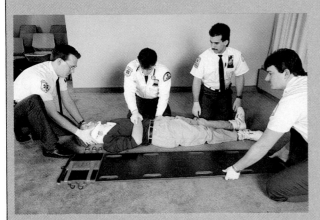

B

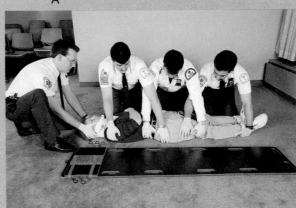

C

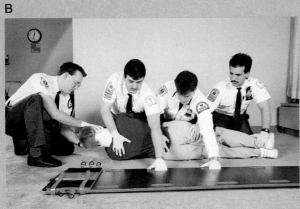

D

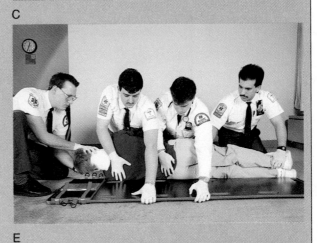

E

FIGURE 7-31. (A) The lead EMT is positioned at the patient's head, maintaining in-line immobilization, and a cervical collar is applied to the patient. (B) The spine board is placed along the patient's side. (C) Three assisting personnel line up alongside the patient (with the strongest rescuers at the patient's shoulder and hip) with the spine board on the opposite side. The rescuers on the side reach across the patient and place their hands evenly spaced along the side of the patient. (D) Upon command from the EMT at the patient's head, they smoothly rotate the patient to a 90-degree angle. (E) While maintaining support with one hand, the spine board is wedged beneath the patient's arm and leg.

FIGURE 7-31. Continued

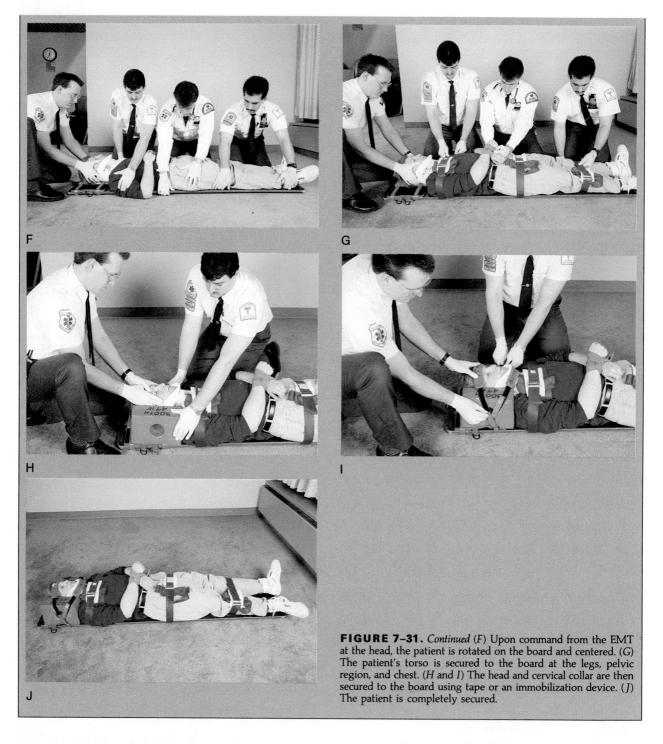

FIGURE 7–31. *Continued* (F) Upon command from the EMT at the head, the patient is rotated on the board and centered. (G) The patient's torso is secured to the board at the legs, pelvic region, and chest. (H and I) The head and cervical collar are then secured to the board using tape or an immobilization device. (J) The patient is completely secured.

Spinal Immobilization

GENERAL PRINCIPLES

- Assume spinal injury in the presence of an appropriate mechanism of injury.
- Manual immobilization of the cervical spine should be done as the first step of assessment for all suspected trauma victims.
- Immobilize the patient before moving him or her, except in the setting of a hazardous condition, e.g., fire, toxic fumes, and so forth. Otherwise, use manual immobilization techniques.
- Do not delay transport of patients in shock or extremis for the sake of comprehensive immobilization, e.g., a short spine board.
- Neurologic deficits need not exist to suspect spinal injury.

- A cervical collar alone does not constitute spinal immobilization. Attachment to a board should be done as well.
- Be prepared should the patient start vomiting. Be ready to log roll the patient and have suction ready.

OVERALL APPROACH TO SPINAL INJURY

- Cervical in-line immobilization
- Jaw thrust for airway maintenance or oropharyngeal or pharyngeal airway
- Cervical collar
- Attach to immobilization device and anticipate vomiting.
- Suction—rotate patient and immobilization device if needed.
- Transport slowly if possible.

WATER ACCIDENTS

Victims who are still in the water following diving accidents should be floated on their back into the shallow water. Be careful to support the head and not allow hyperextension if mouth-to-mouth resuscitation is necessary. Place a long spine board or other board (e.g., surfboard) under the patient and allow it to float up.

Treatment for Shock

The treatment for shock is of high priority and should be instituted when shock is recognized. Patients with evidence of hypovolemic shock must have the appropriate treatments initiated as early as possible. If signs of rapid uncontrollable bleeding are encountered, or if the patient has suffered from extensive blood loss, transport to the hospital should take precedence over elaborate immobilization. However, when signs of spinal cord injury are present, it may be difficult to recognize the cause of shock. Recognition of the cause of hypotension, if it exists, is important because it will influence decisions regarding both treatment and transport.

NEUROGENIC SHOCK

When findings of neurogenic shock are encountered, the EMT must use all available information to determine what type of treatment is necessary (i.e., none, leg elevation, MAST) and whether significant hemorrhage has also taken place.

Neurogenic shock occurs with injuries to the upper spinal cord (cervical through upper thoracic), which disrupts the sympathetic influence on the heart and blood vessels. This results in extensive vasodilation. There is not enough blood volume to fill the increased vascular space, and the blood pressure falls. In addition, because the sympathetic nerves have been damaged, the heart cannot increase its rate to compensate by increasing cardiac output.

RECOGNITION. In a patient with findings of spinal cord injury, the presence of hypotension without other cardinal signs of shock (tachycardia and pale and clammy skin) suggests neurogenic shock. These patients have normal or slightly slow heart rates. Many of these patients do not exhibit signs of poor organ perfusion. Their mental status may be normal and the skin may be warm, dry, and pink below the level of injury. A few neurogenic shock victims have poor perfusion. They may have altered mental status and cool cyanotic extremities.

Treatment is directed toward ensuring adequate perfusion to support the brain circulation. Patients with neurogenic shock who have adequate perfusion of the brain may require no additional circulatory support in the field. On the other hand, patients with signs of poor perfusion (altered mental status, cool cyanotic extremities) should be treated by measures that increase venous return (elevated leg portion of long spine board, IV fluids, MAST) or decrease the vascular space (MAST).

Local protocols may call for implementation of the MAST. It must be remembered, however, that the lesion causing neurogenic shock is a cervical or high thoracic lesion, and the muscles of respiration may be affected to varying degrees. The patient may be relying totally upon the diaphragm to breathe. Only the leg portions of the MAST should be inflated, at least initially, since inflation of the abdominal section may infringe upon the diaphragm by displacing abdominal contents upward. If the abdominal section must be inflated, it may be necessary to assist with positive-pressure ventilations to compensate for its effect upon the diaphragm.

Check your local protocols regarding use of MAST for neurogenic shock from spinal injury. Do a careful assessment of the mental status, respiratory efforts, and level of function and relay this information to the medical control officer.

Note: Studies with MAST have shown that little respiratory compromise takes place in normal individuals even with inflation of the abdominal portions. As discussed earlier, during inhalation the diaphragm contracts and *pushes* the abdominal contents down into the abdomen. During exhalation, the diaphragm relaxes and the abdominal contents then help return the diaphragm to the relaxed position higher in the thoracic cavity. If the diaphragm is weak or paralyzed, the rescuer must provide positive-pressure ventilations to displace it downward into the abdomen to allow the lungs to expand. If the abdominal segment of the MAST is inflated, the rescuer must displace the diaphragm against this additional external pressure of the abdominal MAST suit as well.

HYPOVOLEMIC SHOCK IN THE SETTING OF NEUROGENIC SHOCK. Any patient with neurogenic shock has to be assessed for the possibility of internal bleeding. Trauma sufficient to cause a cord injury is capable of causing other associated fractures and damage to internal organs. Signs ordinarily associated with hypovolemic shock (tachycardia; cool, pale, and clammy skin) are masked. Furthermore, the patient is not able to perceive pain in areas of injury that might be sites of internal bleeding. Therefore, signs such as pain and tenderness over the abdomen and fracture sites may not be present. One must look closely for other possible evidence of internal bleeding. This includes swelling and lacerations; bruising or evidence of rib fractures, especially over the spleen and liver; and evidence of pelvic and long bone fractures.

When neurogenic shock is present, it is very difficult to evaluate by physical examination whether there is significant internal hemorrhage. This is true not only in the field but in the hospital as well. In one group of patients with cervical spine damage and neurogenic shock, it was impossible to distinguish those with ruptured spleens and livers from those with no other injuries from vital signs and the abdominal examination. Therefore, when patients with neurogenic shock are encountered, and the mechanism of injury suggests the possibility of internal bleeding, early transportation to a hospital is a high priority.

Psychological Support

Often, patients with fractures of the spine and paralysis are still conscious. Understandably, they are very distressed. When you evaluate patients and ask them to perform tasks they are unable to do—"Do you feel me touching you? Can you move your hand?"—you are further confirming their fears about their injury. Be thorough and attentive and finish your assessment. Your evaluation is an essential part of the medical evaluation and treatment. Since whether a patient will recover can never be determined in the field, it is most important to maintain a positive attitude. Do not draw conclusions and then transmit them to the patient. This interferes with your own performance and generates fear and negative feelings in a patient who is already experiencing considerable anguish.

Helmet Removal

Following motorcycle accidents it may be necessary to remove helmets so that proper assessment and treatment may be instituted. The process of helmet removal must be done with extreme caution to avoid movement of the cervical spine.

P R O C E D U R E   7 - 2   REMOVING A HELMET

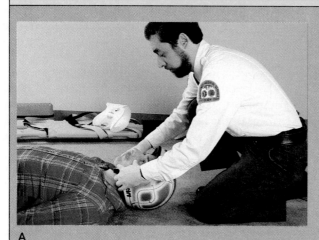

A

FIGURE 7–32. (*A*) One EMT is positioned at the patient's head, maintaining in-line immobilization with the hands along the edge of the helmet and fingers supporting the jaw line. (*B*) A second EMT removes the helmet strap by releasing the connections or cutting the strap. (*C*) The second EMT then reaches beneath the patient's neck with the hand closest to the head and stabilizes the head with the index finger and thumb supporting the mastoid processes on each side. The elbow of this hand should rest on the floor to provide the necessary support to the patient's head when the helmet is removed. (*D*) The hand closest to the feet should cup the chin of the patient to maintain alignment and stabilization during helmet removal. (*E*) Upon command, the EMT holding the helmet should spread the helmet, using lateral pulling forces. Legend continued on opposite page.

1. One EMT should be placed above or behind the patient and place one hand on each side of the helmet. Grasping the patient at the angles of the mandible, the EMT maintains in-line immobilization (Fig. 7–32*A*). Remove chin strap (Fig. 7–32*B*).
2. The rescuer holds the patient's head, with one hand under the neck at the occiput. The other hand is over the anterior face with the thumb supporting one angle of the mandible, and the index and middle fingers supporting the other angle of the mandible (Fig. 7–32*C* and *D*).
3. The first EMT then carefully manipulates the helmet off by lifting each side over the ear and gliding it off the head. Full face helmets have to be tilted back to clear the nose. Move the helmet, NOT THE HEAD, during the procedure (Fig. 7–32*E* and *F*).
4. After the helmet is removed, the first rescuer assumes control of in-line immobilization while the second EMT applies a cervical collar and the other measures to immobilize the neck (Fig. 7–32*G* to *I*). Again, extreme caution should be exercised not to move the cervical spine.

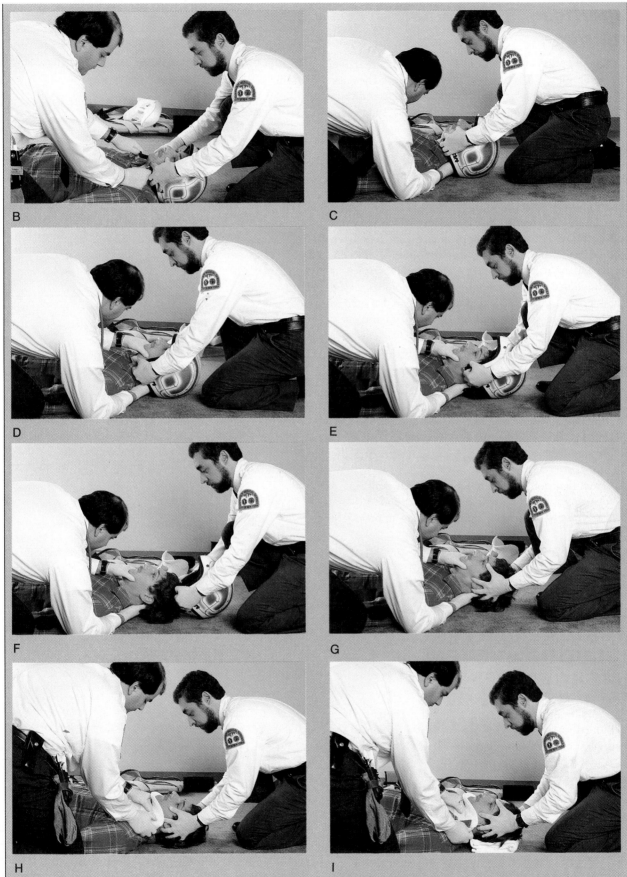

FIGURE 7–32. *Continued* (*F*) Slide the helmet carefully off the head. Helmets that have face pieces may require slight backward rotation of the helmet during removal to clear the patient's nose. (*G*) Once the helmet has cleared the top of the head the second EMT can resume in-line immobilization. (*H*) The head is carefully lowered to the floor or (*I*) supporting pad. The use of a pad is dictated by the posture of the patient. If the neck will be placed in the hyperextended position when released, a pad should be utilized.

Significance of Spinal Injuries

Many spinal injuries result in death prior to arrival at the emergency department. This is because they are associated with other severe injuries or because injuries to the upper cervical spine cause disruption of the nerves necessary for ventilations. Other injuries result in permanent impairment when improper handling at the scene or late recognition in the hospital setting delays diagnosis and treatment. The spinal cord, like the brain itself, is susceptible to a secondary injury from hypoxia, hypotension, and increased pressure. These secondary injuries can result in permanent loss of function, which may not have occurred if early and appropriate care had been rendered. Still other injuries may not be apparent initially and depend on the EMT being appropriately suspicious of a significant injury and properly immobilizing the patient. Specialty referral hospitals have been designated in many regions, in recognition of the need for early application of definitive care to maximize a victim's chance for recovery. The scope of care in the field includes:

- Maintenance of a high level of suspicion after assessing the mechanism of injury, so that due caution can be taken in handling, evaluating, and immobilizing the patient's spine
- Prevention of further injury by immobilizing the spine
- Treatment of associated injuries that will cause death or further disability if left unattended
- Early delivery of the patient to the appropriate facility
- Gathering of key data such as the findings from the initial and subsequent neurologic examinations

MEDICAL CENTRAL NERVOUS SYSTEM EMERGENCIES

An alteration in a patient's central nervous system (CNS) function is a common reason why people call for emergency medical care. Because the CNS controls the rest of the body, dysfunction can result in loss of consciousness, sensation, motor ability, and vital functions. There are two general mechanisms by which normal function of the nervous system can be altered. There are disease processes originating in the central nervous system itself, such as cerebrovascular accidents within the brain (strokes). There are also many conditions that initially affect organ systems other than the CNS but that result in CNS disturbances, such as hypoxia, hypoglycemia, and certain poisonings.

⚕ P R O T O C O L ⚕

SUSPECTED HEAD OR SPINAL INJURIES (NOT MEETING MAJOR TRAUMA CRITERIA)

1. Establish and maintain airway control while manually stabilizing the cervical spine.

2. Assess the patient's ventilatory status.

    a. Suction as necessary.

    b. Assist the patient's ventilations as necessary.

    > IF HEAD INJURY IS SUSPECTED, THE PATIENT IS NOT ALERT, THE ARMS AND LEGS ARE ABNORMALLY FLEXED AND/OR EXTENDED (NEUROLOGIC POSTURING), OR THE PATIENT IS SEIZING OR HAS A GLASGOW COMA SCALE OF LESS THAN 8, HYPERVENTILATE THE PATIENT.

    c. Administer high-concentration oxygen.

3. Assess the patient's circulatory status.

4. Obtain and record the initial vital signs, including the Glasgow Coma Scale and a neurologic assessment, i.e., level of consciousness (AVPU), pupils, and sensory and motor function in the extremities, before and after spinal immobilization.

5. Immobilize the patient's head and spine with a rigid cervical collar and an appropriate immobilization device, i.e., a KED, Kansas Board, XP1, or short board if the patient is sitting or a long board if the patient is in a face-up position.

    > *NOTE!*
    >
    > THE TECHNIQUE OF *RAPID EXTRICATION* IS NOT INTENDED FOR STABLE PATIENTS WITH ISOLATED HEAD OR SPINAL INJURIES! *RAPID EXTRICATION* IS INTENDED FOR MAJOR TRAUMA PATIENTS.

6. Repeat and record the vital signs, including the Glasgow Coma Scale and level of consciousness, en route as often as the situation indicates.

7. Transport, keeping the patient warm.

8. Record all patient care information, including the patient's medical history and all treatment provided, on a prehospital care report.

(Adapted from Manual for Emergency Medical Technicians. Emergency Medical Services Program. Albany, New York State Department of Health, 1990.)

The general goals of prehospital care for patients with altered CNS function are to ensure adequate ventilations and circulation, rule out the possibility of trauma (or if trauma exists, support the cervical spine), give supplemental oxygen and perhaps glucose, and assess and treat the underlying cause.

Altered Mental Status

Often the first indication of central nervous system problems is an alteration or change in the patient's mental status. This can range from mild confusion and abnormal behavior to deep coma, where the patient is totally unresponsive to verbal or painful stimuli. Upon finding an alteration in mental status, the EMT must immediately assess the adequacy of ventilations, since control of vital functions such as breathing and circulation may be compromised. For example, with an overdose from a CNS depressant (such as a narcotic or barbiturate), a patient may at first appear sleepy or lethargic and then gradually enter into a more depressed and unresponsive state (coma). Continued depression of the nervous system can affect the ability to breathe, and the patient may suffer hypoventilation and respiratory arrest. In fact, the most common cause of death from overdose is failure of the respiratory system.

Respiratory problems are also the first concern for patients with conditions such as strokes or seizures. Loss of control of the musculature may allow the tongue to fall back into the pharynx, blocking the airway. Loss of reflex actions such as the ability to gag or clear the airway places the patient at risk for aspiration of any secretions or vomitus. In fact all patients who are unresponsive are subject to complications from airway obstruction, aspirations, and respiratory failure.

Terminology and Degrees of Altered Mental Status

There are many terms used to describe an alteration in mental status. Commonly used terms to describe altered levels of consciousness include lethargy, stupor, semicoma, and coma.

LETHARGY. Sluggishness or sleepiness. The patient is easily aroused but drifts into a sleepy state without continued stimulation.

STUPOR. A state of lessened responsiveness. The patient can be aroused but more stimuli are required than for the lethargic patient. In addition, with arousal, the stuporous patient does not reach a normal level of consciousness and function. For example, speech may be slurred or garbled and motor ability may be sluggish and uncoordinated.

SEMICOMA. A condition of unconsciousness or lack of awareness of one's environment from which the patient may be aroused.

COMA. A lack of responsiveness to the environment. The patient is unconscious and cannot be aroused by external stimuli.

Although these terms are commonly used to describe patients' conditions, their use has certain disadvantages. For example, the same patient may be described as semicomatose or stuporous by different observers. Furthermore, an EMT will have difficulty in assessing *changes* in a patient's condition using these terms alone. For this reason most authorities recommend using more concrete descriptions of a patient's ability to respond to stimuli. This is the reason that such methods as the Glasgow Coma Scale are used.

Some patients evolve by degrees from an alert state to a coma, as happens with the gradual but continued absorption of a toxic drug or chemical. Other patients may suddenly become comatose secondary to conditions such as a generalized seizure or a bursting blood vessel within the brain. This is why the history of the event is so important.

In conscious or uncooperative patients there are also degrees of intellectual and memory function. One can quickly determine whether a patient is oriented to the environment. The patient is assessed as to orientation to *person, time,* and *place*. A confused patient may not be aware of the time of day, date, or even year. Likewise, a patient may not be aware of the immediate surroundings. Less common are patients who are not aware of their own name. Patients are described as "oriented times three" if they are aware of all three variables. If they are not aware of one of the variables, they are said to be "oriented to person and place but not to time," and so forth. As often happens with patients who have suffered a concussion, loss of memory can also occur. Patients may not be able to remember the immediate events preceding or following their illness.

Causes of Altered Mental Status

There are numerous causes of altered mental status. As described previously, CNS problems have either a structural or a metabolic origin. This basic understanding helps the EMT appreciate physical findings that may provide a rationale for treatment in either the prehospital or hospital phase of care.

STRUCTURAL CAUSES. The most common structural problem encountered by the EMT is a stroke or *cerebrovascular accident*. When the blood supply to part of the brain is disrupted, that portion of the brain fails to function from lack of oxygen. Since only part of the brain has been damaged, the patient may have findings on the physical examination that are one-sided or asymmetric. This is because only one portion of the brain has been affected. Many victims of stroke have an altered mental status. The presence of asymmetric motor and sensory findings in the medical patient with an altered mental status should suggest a structural condition such as a cerebrovascular accident. Another possibility to explore is whether the patient has a history of recent head

TABLE 7–11. Causes of Altered Mental Status

Structural	
Cerebrovascular accident (CVA)	
Recent Head Trauma	

Metabolic	
External	*Internal*
Poisonings	Hypoxia
Overdoses	Hypotension
Hypothermia or hyperthermia	Diabetic states
Infections	Organ failure

trauma. Consider whether the patient could be suffering from an expanding subdural hematoma originating from a head injury that occurred a week or a month before.

METABOLIC CAUSES. The majority of patients with altered mental status suffer from metabolic problems. These problems usually originate outside the CNS. While they can affect brain function by many different mechanisms, they affect both sides of the brain equally. Therefore, the physical findings are generally bilateral and diffuse rather than one-sided.

The sources of metabolic problems may be external or internal. Examples of external problems include poisonings, overdoses, or environmental conditions such as hypothermia or hyperthermia (abnormally low [hypo] or high [hyper] body temperature). Infectious organisms that invade the CNS are another example. All these conditions are caused by agents or factors outside the body. Examples of internal problems include all respiratory or circulatory conditions that result in hypoxia or hypoperfusion of the brain. Other internal problems are diabetic states and failure of the liver or the kidneys, which causes a buildup of toxic substances. Table 7–11 provides examples of structural versus metabolic problems.

Specific Medical Emergencies Involving the Central Nervous System

Since there are many causes of altered mental status, the following discussion focuses on the presentation of CNS emergencies where the disease process often originates within the CNS itself. We also include infection of the brain and its meninges. Other conditions that affect the CNS indirectly or that are a result of diseases of other organs are discussed more thoroughly in the appropriate chapters throughout this text.

CEREBROVASCULAR ACCIDENTS

A *cerebrovascular accident* (CVA) or stroke is defined as a blockage or disruption of blood flow in an artery feeding the brain. This can occur by obstruction of the vessel (by a thrombus or embolus) or by rupture of the vessel itself (Fig. 7–33). In the case of an obstruction, the brain tissue distal to the obstruction is deprived of oxygen and nutrients. This results in damage to the section of the brain supplied by that artery. Therefore, one would expect that the functions controlled by that part of the brain would be affected. When a vessel in the brain ruptures, not only is the distal brain affected, but bleeding within the brain can result in increased pressure and damage to surrounding structures. If bleeding is extensive, herniation and massive destruction of brain tissue can occur.

The patients most likely to suffer CVAs are those with the risk factors for arteriosclerosis and heart disease (see arteriosclerosis in Chapter 5). Therefore, patients with high blood pressure, increased blood cholesterol, and a smoking history are at increased risk for stroke.

Causes

THROMBUS. The most common cause of a CVA is thrombus or blood clot formation within a cerebral artery. The signs and symptoms correlate with the part of the brain being deprived of blood flow. For example, if a vessel supplying the occipital lobe were involved, the patient may complain of visual disturbances. If the frontal lobe were involved, the patient may experience intellectual or motor disturbances. If the CVA involves flow to the parietal area, sensory loss may occur. In some instances when a major artery is blocked, the loss of function is widespread.

TRANSIENT ISCHEMIC ATTACKS. Frequently, a stroke (particularly a thrombotic stroke) is preceded by a *transient ischemic attack* (TIA). A TIA is a temporary loss of brain function secondary to diminished blood supply to part of the brain. The diagnosis is made when a patient presents with a neurologic deficit that completely resolves within 12 hours. Again, the type of deficit reflects the region of the brain supplied by the diseased artery. The patient who presents with a stroke may give a history of prior neurologic signs and symptoms that resolved on their own.

EMBOLUS. A less common cause of CVAs is *embolus*. An embolus is a substance that travels through the circulation until it lodges in an artery that has a smaller diameter than the embolus. Blood flow distal to the obstruction is then compromised. Signs and symptoms occur suddenly.

HEMORRHAGE. When a cerebral artery bursts, the onset of signs and symptoms is rapid. With continued

FIGURE 7–33. Types of stroke (*A*) *Thrombus*—due to the loss of a smooth inner surface, clots (thrombi) form at the site of arteriosclerosis. Eventually, the narrowed vessel can become totally occluded, resulting in a stroke. *Embolus*—a stroke due to an embolus occurs when a small clot from the heart or central vessel comes loose and travels to a vessel within the brain (that is smaller than the clot), becomes lodged, and obstructs distal flow through the vessel. Strokes caused by thrombus or embolus may be preceded by a transient ischemic attack (TIA). (*B*) *Hemorrhage*—a hemorrhagic stroke results from a rupture of a vessel within the brain. The symptoms of a hemorrhagic stroke tend to be more abrupt and more severe than the other types of stroke.

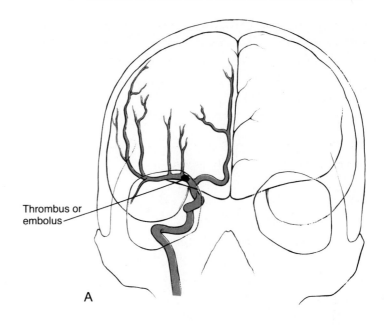

Thrombus or embolus

A

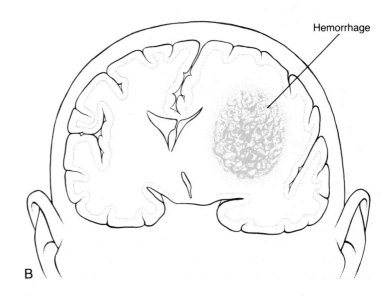

Hemorrhage

B

bleeding, the signs may progress and the neurologic examination can change. These patients often complain of headache. Bleeding may be confined within the brain tissue or it may spread along the subarachnoid space. In this latter instance, called *subarachnoid hemorrhage*, patients may exhibit signs of neck stiffness. They may resist flexion of the neck because the blood in the subarachnoid space irritates the meninges. This resistance to neck flexion is called *nuchal rigidity*. It may be noted even in unconscious patients if an attempt is made to flex the neck to elicit this sign.

Hemorrhagic strokes and subarachnoid hemorrhage have the highest mortality rates of all types of CVAs. Complaints of headache and neck stiffness and signs of nuchal rigidity should alert the EMT to impending com-

plications from continued bleeding. These patients may require lifesaving surgery and therefore warrant early transport.

Signs and Symptoms of Cerebrovascular Accidents

The signs and symptoms of strokes are quite varied, as they reflect the portion of the brain that is deprived of blood. Motor and sensory findings are usually asymmetric. CVAs in many patients are recognized immediately by the presence of one-sided sensory and motor loss. The body on the opposite side of the lesion can be weak or completely paralyzed. This can include facial paralysis, which is evident by the drooping of the eyelids and mouth. The eyes themselves may drift to one side.

✚ P R O T O C O L ✚

CEREBROVASCULAR ACCIDENT

SPECIAL ASSESSMENT CONSIDERATIONS

1. Perform Glasgow Coma Scale and record all findings.

2. Document any neurologic deficits.

3. Note medical history—especially diabetes, hypertension.

Treatment

1. Maintain ABCs and intervene as required.

2. Administer high-concentration oxygen.

3. Place patient in a semisitting position, if the patient is conscious.

4. DO NOT PERMIT PHYSICAL ACTIVITY!

5. Monitor the patient's condition and document vital signs as indicated.

6. Transport the patient to the appropriate hospital.

7. If the patient is unconscious, transport him or her in a coma position.

8. Record all patient care information, including the patient's medical history and all treatment provided on the patient care record.

(Adapted from Basic Life Support Protocols. New York City Emergency Medical Services, 1990.)

Some patients with CVAs have intellectual impairment and difficulty in communicating, with or without associated motor and sensory findings. They may have trouble with verbal expression or comprehension. They may not be able to recognize or name common objects. The entire range of alterations in mental status may be encountered, from alert and oriented to deep coma.

Other signs and symptoms of CVA include urinary and fecal incontinence (loss of sphincter control) and nausea and vomiting. Some patients may have seizures or convulsions.

Management Considerations

The patient with sensory or motor loss must have the affected portions of the body protected during movement and transport. The patient who is having difficulty with communication requires patience and understanding.

SEIZURES

A *seizure* is defined as a temporary alteration in behavior due to abnormal electrical activity in the brain. Other names for seizures are *convulsions* and *epilepsy.*

Seizures have many causes. Several of the causes of altered mental status mentioned previously can result in seizures. A scar on the brain or on its meningeal covering from previous head trauma is one identifiable cause. Other causes include drug or alcohol withdrawal, eclampsia (toxemia of pregnancy), and trauma. Many other patients have a history of seizures for which no cause can be found. They are often given anticonvulsive drugs such as phenobarbital or phenytoin to prevent seizures from recurring. If they stop taking these medications, they are prone to suffer a convulsion.

What is the result of this abnormal electrical activity? Again this depends on what portions of the brain are stimulated. The most dramatic seizures are those that involve the motor cortex, resulting in spasmodic contractions of the skeletal muscles. However, there are types of epilepsy that affect only the cognitive portion of the brain.

Types of Seizures

GRAND MAL. A *grand mal* seizure is the type most people think of when they use terms such as convulsions or epilepsy. A grand mal seizure usually has three phases, the *tonic* phase, the *clonic* phase, and a *postictal* period. During the tonic phase there is a sustained contraction of all voluntary muscles. This usually results in extension of the body and the extremities. This phase lasts for up to 30 seconds. Ventilations are compromised because of the sustained contraction of the respiratory muscles. This is followed by the *clonic* phase, characterized by intermittent contractions and relaxations of the skeletal muscles, which results in rapid jerking movements. During this period the patient may become injured from striking surrounding objects. The clonic phase lasts from seconds to a few minutes. Again, the spasms of contractions and relaxations interfere with ventilations, and the patient can become cyanotic. These spasms may be followed by a short period (up to 30 seconds) of flaccid paralysis while breathing is slowly reestablished. The patient may suffer loss of urine while in the tonic phase and may bite his or her tongue during the clonic phase. The final phase of a seizure is the *postictal* phase, in which the patient shows a depressed level of consciousness and confusion. The patient slowly awakes but may feel confused and drowsy and fall asleep for a short period. Afterward, the patient may complain of headache, some muscle aching, and perhaps a sore tongue.

AURA. Some seizures *originate* in one part of the brain, producing early warning signs peculiar to the site of origin. Some patients may become aware of strange smells, visual or auditory sensations, or motor events in only one part of the body. These sensations or activities may herald the onset of a generalized convulsion. These preliminary events are referred to as *aura.*

FOCAL SEIZURES. Some patients have *focal seizures* that do not generalize and involve the entire brain. These may affect only a portion of the body or may manifest as an alteration in consciousness with bizarre behavior.

STATUS EPILEPTICUS. A rapid succession of epileptic attacks without an intervening period of consciousness is called *status epilepticus.* This is a definite threat to life because of the sustained respiratory compromise.

FEBRILE CONVULSION. The term *febrile convulsion* is used to describe a seizure in a child between 6 months and 6 years of age, which is precipitated by a high temperature in the setting of an infection. Febrile convulsions occur in up to 5% of children.

PETITE MAL. *Petite mal* seizures are brief lapses of attention and awareness lasting from 10 to 20 seconds. They are more common in childhood but sometimes persist into adulthood. Petite mal seizures can occur many times a day. The child may suddenly stare, with the eyes turned upward or to the side, accompanied by fluttering eyelids. The episode is always brief (seconds) and the child can continue or return to previous activities as if nothing happened.

Management Considerations

The general goals of management are the same as those for any patient with altered mental status. However, patients with seizures also require some special interventions.

AIRWAY. Following a grand mal seizure, the patient may need assistance in establishment of an airway during the postictal phase. The patient may have a short period of flaccid paralysis or significant depression of the nervous system. If there is no gag reflex, an oropharyngeal airway may have to be inserted to keep the tongue from obstructing the airway. As the patient's reflexes return, this airway must be removed to prevent the person from gagging, which may induce vomiting.

If the seizure does not remit within 5 minutes or if recurrent seizures occur (status epilepticus), respiratory compromise becomes the major concern. High oxygen concentrations should be given and, if possible, assistance with positive-pressure ventilation. However, because of the intensity of the muscle contractions, only small and inadequate tidal volumes may be delivered by positive-pressure breathing. The patient is at risk of death or brain damage from ventilatory failure. Appropriate treatment calls for administration of drug therapy that can stop seizure activity within a minute of the drug injection. Therefore, *rapid transport is of high priority* to minimize the time from the start of the seizure to administration of drugs to stop seizure activity, enabling the return of adequate ventilations.

In EMS systems where prehospital advanced life support exists, paramedics may be called upon to administer such drugs on the scene. This is recommended only when the estimated time of arrival of the paramedics is less than the transport time to the hospital, and when it is consistent with local protocols.

⚜ P R O T O C O L ⚜

SEIZURES

MANAGEMENT OF THE PATIENT WHO IS SEIZING

1. Protect the patient from harm, AND remove hazards from the patient's immediate area, AND avoid unnecessary physical restraint.

2. Ensure that the patient's airway is open.

> DO NOT FORCE THE PATIENT'S MOUTH OPEN OR FORCE AN ORAL AIRWAY OR ANY OTHER DEVICE INTO THE PATIENT'S MOUTH IF IT IS CLENCHED TIGHTLY DURING THE SEIZURE! A NASAL AIRWAY MAY BE USED.

3. Suction the airway as needed. Avoid stimulation of the posterior pharynx during suctioning because this may cause vomiting.

4. Administer high-concentration oxygen and ventilate if necessary.

5. Transport immediately, keeping the patient warm.

6. Obtain and record the vital signs, and report en route as often as the situation indicates.

7. Record all patient care information, including the patient's medical history and all treatment provided, on a prehospital care report.

MANAGEMENT OF THE POST-SEIZURE PATIENT

1. Ensure that the patient's airway is open and that breathing and circulation are adequate.

2. Suction the airway as needed. Avoid stimulation of the posterior pharynx during suctioning because this may cause vomiting.

3. Administer high-concentration oxygen.

4. Treat injuries sustained during the seizure.

5. Be prepared for additional seizures.

6. Obtain and record the vital signs, and repeat en route as often as the situation indicates.

7. Transport, keeping the patient warm.

8. Record all patient care information, including the patient's medical history and all treatment provided, on a prehospital care report.

(Adapted from Manual for Emergency Medical Technicians. Emergency Medical Services Program. Albany, New York State Department of Health, 1990.)

Psychological Aspects

Patients who have recurrent seizures may be very sensitive to the perceptions of those around them after they have recovered from an attack. The reliability of information solicited during the history may be affected by the refusal of the epileptic patient to acknowledge the disease in the presence of coworkers or friends. Concern for this sensitivity can be shown by clearing crowds away from the patient and creating a relatively private environment before any interviewing takes place.

MENINGITIS

Infections of the central nervous system can be life threatening and require prompt evaluation and therapy. They can be caused by bacteria or viruses. The most common infection is called *meningitis*, since it involves the meningeal coverings of the brain and can present with signs of meningeal irritation. Meningitis usually follows an infection in another area of the body, which spreads via the bloodstream. Many cases of meningitis follow infection of nearby structures such as the upper respiratory tract and the inner ear. Some cases follow head trauma, where fractures of the skull allow bacteria access to the CNS.

Signs and Symptoms

The onset of meningitis can be abrupt or gradual. The symptoms include a change in mental status, severe headache, stiff neck, photophobia (bright light irritates the eyes), nausea, loss of appetite, and fever. Initially, the patient may be irritable but depression of the mental status can be rapidly evolving. Signs include nuchal rigidity (resistance to flexion of the neck), seizures, and loss of peripheral nerve functions—particularly the cranial nerves controlling eye movement and hearing. Some patients may have a rash characterized by small red spots or small sites of hemorrhage visible under the skin. The patient may give a history of having a previous infection with a sudden worsening of the condition, with the signs noted above. Once the CNS is involved, some patients will deteriorate rapidly.

Signs leading to early recognition can be lost in coma. Infants often will have few signs other than high fever, vomiting, and irritability or convulsions. Later they may have a depressed mental status. In addition, they may have bulging of the fontanelles.

NUCHAL RIGIDITY. The finding of nuchal rigidity is elicited by flexing the neck forward 45 degrees with the patient in the supine position (Fig. 7–34). If nuchal rigidity is present, the patient responds by flexing the legs at the hip and the knee. This finding is caused by irritation of the pain-sensitive spinal nerves. Patients complaining of stiff neck may assume a fetal position posture when left alone. Nuchal rigidity is also encountered in cases of subarachnoid hemorrhage. Table 7–12 summarizes the signs and symptoms of meningitis in adults and infants.

Special Consideration

Some patients have a viral meningitis for which there is no specific treatment. They usually do well with supportive therapy while the disease runs its course. Other patients with bacterial meningitis may have a rapid and fulminant progression of the disease. They will die without early administration of antibiotic therapy. Diagnosis is made by examination of the cerebrospinal fluid. Since the presentations of meningitis are variable, all patients with evidence of this disease deserve early transport to the hospital for timely evaluation and therapy.

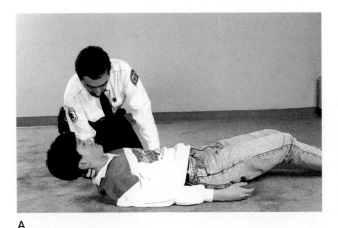
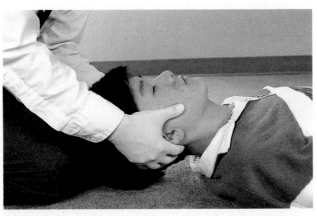

A   B

FIGURE 7–34. (*A*) When the neck is flexed in a patient with meningeal irritation, the lower extremities may be drawn up, or (*B*) the patient may resist flexion (nuchal rigidity). NECK FLEXION SHOULD NEVER BE PERFORMED ON ANY PATIENT SUSPECTED OF TRAUMA.

TABLE 7–12. Signs and Symptoms of Meningitis

Adults	Infants
Alteration in mental status	Alteration in mental status
Stiff neck	Fever
Fever and chills	Vomiting
Seizure	Seizures
Headache	Bulging fontanelles
Vomiting	
Focal neurologic signs	

Prophylaxis

The EMT in rare situations may be advised to take drug therapy to minimize the chance of contracting one particular type of bacterial infection that can lead to meningitis. There are many different bacteria and viruses that cause meningitis. One type of bacteria, the meningococcus, has been known to cause infections that lead to meningitis in EMTs who have been in close contact with infected patients. The bacteria is spread by respiratory droplets and requires close contact such as kissing or confinement in a closed space (family members) to spread. The health care provider who delivers mouth-to-mouth or mouth-to-mask ventilations is therefore at increased risk of contracting the bacteria.

Being in close contact with respiratory droplets from a patient with meningococcal meningitis does not mean that a health worker will contract meningitis. Actually the risk is quite small. First the bacteria must infect the upper respiratory tract, and then only a few spread to the central nervous system. Some individuals carry this bacteria in the nasopharynx. They do not contract a disease but may spread it to others. Therefore, it is prudent for an EMT who has been in contact with a patient who has meningitis to ask his or her physician if prophylaxis with an antibiotic is advisable. Decontamination of the ambulance and your equipment should follow standard procedures, as covered in Chapter 12 on infectious diseases.

Approach to the Patient with a Central Nervous System Medical Emergency

Because so many problems can result in altered mental status, identification of the underlying cause is an extremely difficult task. However, delay in identification of certain causes results in unnecessary morbidity if treatable conditions are overlooked. Some of these conditions can be treated in the field, others in the hospital. Regardless of the site of treatment, the evaluation

in the field is often the only chance to gather data and clues leading to early diagnosis. The EMT must develop a systematic approach that identifies the most life-threatening conditions early, followed by a search for clues to other common and treatable conditions. Assessment and treatment must be integrated in a way that avoids unnecessary delays in transport. At times the history and secondary survey are best completed while en route to the hospital.

PRIMARY SURVEY

The primary survey recognizes the role of the CNS in directing vital functions by the check for responsiveness. As always, the identification and treatment of life-threatening conditions takes precedence. Obviously, all unconscious patients are at risk of airway obstruction, and manual techniques as well as mechanical airway devices should be utilized to ensure the patency of the airway. The need for ventilatory support should be quickly established, as these two conditions, airway and ventilatory compromise, represent the greatest threat to life in the prehospital phase. The possibility of head trauma should be assessed during this phase to allow for alteration of airway techniques and early immobilization of the spine if that is indicated.

SECONDARY SURVEY

The secondary survey, incorporating the history and physical examination, provides the rationale for prehospital treatment and early transport decisions. Furthermore, early hospital therapy is often determined on the basis of prehospital findings and clues. A systematic approach that always includes key questions maximizes information gathering in a timely manner. For example, always collecting a medication history and bringing the patient's medications to the hospital will provide important information to the hospital staff.

HISTORY. With medical patients, the history is often the primary rationale for treatment. A patient may have no positive physical findings other than an altered mental status. In such a case, a history of diabetes provides the rationale to administer glucose. Likewise, a history of febrile illness followed by headaches and change in mental status might lead to an early diagnosis of meningitis. There are certain key areas for questioning that provide much valuable information.

HISTORY OF PRESENT ILLNESS

Was the change in mental status rapid or slow? Was there an abrupt onset? A rapid deterioration in mental status would point to a sudden progressive process such as *hemorrhage* within the brain, whereas a gradual deterioration might suggest continued absorption of a poison or drug. The time from the patient's last normal level of function to the present condition should be ascertained. Furthermore, any changes in the patient's condition that occurred prior to your arrival and during your care should be noted. Is the mental status improving, deteriorating, or does it remain the same? Did the therapy you instituted (e.g., oxygen, glucose) make the difference?

The presence of *associated complaints*, the *chronology of events*, and a history of *similar past experiences* are invaluable in identifying the underlying cause. For example, the patient with rapid onset of altered mental status and *associated complaints* of headache and neck stiffness might suggest the presence of a subarachnoid bleed. Another patient may present with a deterioration of consciousness and have a history of recent head injury. This *chronology* might point to the possibility of a subdural hematoma. *Similar past experiences* are especially helpful in identifying chronic or recurrent conditions such as hypoglycemia and seizures.

PAST MEDICAL HISTORY

Always ask about heart disease, hypertension, diabetes, and chronic obstructive pulmonary disease. The first three conditions are all risk factors for strokes. The history of diabetes, as mentioned before, is essential to elicit in the patient with an altered mental status. If a history of psychiatric disease is elicited, never *assume* that an alteration in mental status is secondary to the psychiatric disorder. Many organic problems might result in depressed, agitated, and combative states with bizarre behavior. However, in the presence of a psychiatric history, the possibility of an overdose should not be overlooked. Epilepsy is another condition to ask about. A seizure may not have been witnessed. Patients in the postictal phase have depressed CNS function, and a wide range of findings may be encountered.

Look for medic alert tags. Ask about previous hospitalizations or whether the patient is under a physician's care. This will uncover significant past illness or conditions that still require treatment. Bring the patient's current medications to the hospital.

Obtain an allergy history. If the patient's condition changes, this may not be possible later on.

It is especially important to question witnesses about the pattern, activity, and duration of any seizures that are described. Did the patient have a focal seizure initially (limited activity in one area of the body) that evolved into a grand mal seizure? This kind of information might aid the physicians in determining the cause.

VITAL SIGNS

Are there abnormal respiratory patterns? Cheyne-Stokes breathing is encountered in many patients with CVAs. Other abnormal patterns point to possible brainstem dysfunction or metabolic disturbances (Kussmaul's respiration; see diabetes in Chapter 12).

Note the character of the pulse and the blood pressure. Is there evidence of adequate perfusion? Are there signs of hypovolemia present? Is the blood pressure high and the pulse normal or slow, as in Cushing's reflex (a sign of increased intracranial pressure)?

The temperature should be checked to assess the possibility of infectious causes, hyperthermia, or hypothermia. At times an alteration in temperature may be the result of CNS disease, whereas at other times it may point to the diagnosis.

MENTAL STATUS

Assess the mental status by categorizing the patient as alert and oriented to person, place, and time. If abnormal mental status is present, assess verbal response according to the Glasgow Coma Scale for verbal ability.

HEAD-TO-TOE SURVEY

Skin color and moisture should be checked to help identify hypoxia (cyanosis) and hypoperfusion (pale and clammy). Warm, hot, dry skin would suggest heat stroke.

Note abnormal smells on the breath. An odor of alcohol might be noted. A fruity odor would suggest diabetic acidosis.

Pupils should be checked as you would in the patient with a head injury. Note their size, equality, and reactivity to light.

Check the neck for nuchal rigidity by attempting to flex the neck by bringing the chin toward the chest. If the patient resists flexion or flexes the legs at the hips, this is a positive finding suggesting meningeal irritation (meningitis versus subarachnoid bleeding). If there is any question of cervical spine injury, this maneuver is contraindicated.

The patient is checked for motor and sensory function in the same manner as is the patient with a head injury. Check both sides of the body, looking for equal strength and sensation on each side. Classify abnormal responses according to the Glasgow Coma Scale.

As with the patient with head injuries, periodically reevaluate the vital signs and the neurologic condition and record your findings.

Treatment

Specific management considerations for patients with seizures, CVAs, and meningitis were discussed previously. However, they bear further emphasis and discussion. These are generally applicable to all patients with altered mental status or obvious CNS dysfunction.

AIRWAY

The most treatable and one of the most common hazards faced by patients with altered mental function is airway compromise. Either obstruction secondary to the tongue or inability to clear secretions can place the patient in jeopardy. Airway patency is achieved through a combination of appropriate manual airway techniques and mechanical airway devices. The presence or absence of a gag reflex should be checked in all unconscious patients. If it is absent, an oropharyngeal or nasopharyngeal airway should be used. Secretions and vomitus are cleared from the airway via a combination of suctioning and proper positioning. All nontraumatic unconscious patients who are adequately ventilating are routinely placed in the coma position in recognition of these concerns (Fig. 7–35).

VENTILATION AND SUPPLEMENTAL OXYGEN

All patients with altered brain function should be assumed to have inadequate oxygen delivery to the brain until proved otherwise. Supplemental oxygen is indicated and the respiratory rate and depth must be carefully assessed to identify the need for positive-pressure breathing. If there is any doubt about the adequacy of ventilations, assist the patient. Patients with cyanosis or evidence of respiratory disturbance should receive high concentrations of oxygen. Other patients who are unresponsive may benefit from oxygen delivery via the nasal cannula, allowing easier access to the airway in case of vomiting and easier management of the patient in the coma position. Patients who are agitated or combative may be oxygen deprived and likewise should receive supplemental oxygen if it is tolerated.

GLUCOSE ADMINISTRATION

Because diabetes is so prevalent, hypoglycemia as a cause of altered mental status must always be considered. Since lack of glucose causes brain cell death, and supplemental glucose causes no harm, most hospitals and many EMS systems routinely administer glucose to all patients with an altered mental state when the diagnosis is not clear. Following such a regimen allows for treatment of patients with hypoglycemia in cases in which the history is unavailable and at the same time does no harm to those who have normal or elevated blood glucose levels. In EMS systems that do not utilize IV glucose or IM glucagon, oral high-concentration glucose solutions may be administered to patients who are capable of swallowing and have a gag reflex (see Chapter 12 on Medical Emergencies).

Never administer an oral agent to an unconscious patient or a patient with no gag reflex.

TRANSPORT DECISION   5 - 3 - 94

In the nontraumatic patient, certain findings dictate an early transport decision. The decision to transport has to be considered as part of the patient's treatment. As with uncontrollable internal hemorrhage, there are certain CNS disorders that require early hospital treatment. These include subarachnoid hemorrhage, meningitis, and suspected subdural hematomas secondary to an old head injury. Positive meningeal signs (neck stiffness, nuchal rigidity) and signs of increased intracranial pressure are both indications for an early transport decision.

The following are general goals of management for patients with altered mental status:

- Ensure adequate airway and ventilation.
- Rule out head trauma—otherwise support cervical spine.
- Ensure adequate circulation.
- Treat with supplemental oxygen.
- Treat for hypoglycemia—if according to local protocol.
- Assess for possible cause of coma.
- Perform baseline and serial neurologic examinations.

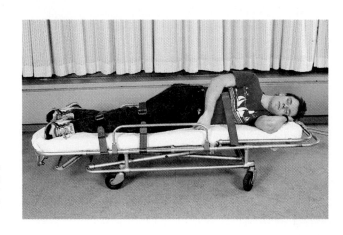

FIGURE 7–35. During transport, the patient can be placed in the left lateral recumbent position (coma position): lying on the left side with the left hand beneath the head (this stabilizes the patient's upper body by using the arm as a support frame). Suction should be ready to clear secretions or vomitus.

- Transport early in the position best suited to maintain a patent airway and ventilations.
- Maintain an airway and ventilations en route.

Summary

Central nervous system problems are among the most common type of emergencies encountered by EMTs. Both traumatic and medical problems arising from the CNS can result in paralysis or death. Therefore, you must be prepared to quickly recognize the problem and provide immediate and lifesaving prehospital care and rapid transport to an appropriate medical facility. Take time to review the protocols relating to CNS emergencies, which summarize the key steps of assessment and management.

❊ P R O T O C O L ❊

ALTERED MENTAL STATUS (NONTRAUMATIC AND WITHOUT RESPIRATORY OR CARDIO-VASCULAR COMPLICATIONS)

> *NOTE!*
>
> THIS PROTOCOL IS FOR PATIENTS WHO ARE VERBALLY RESPONSIVE, RESPOND TO PAINFUL STIMULI, OR ARE UNRESPONSIVE.

1. Ensure that the patient's airway is open and that breathing and circulation are adequate, and suction as necessary.

2. Administer high-concentration oxygen. In children, humidified oxygen is preferred.

3. Obtain and record the vital signs, including determining the patient's level of consciousness.

4. IF THE PATIENT IS UNRESPONSIVE OR RESPONDS ONLY TO PAINFUL STIMULI, transport immediately, keeping the patient warm.

   IF THE PATIENT IS CONSCIOUS, HAS A GAG REFLEX, AND IS ABLE TO DRINK WITHOUT ASSISTANCE, provide glucose or a sugar solution (if available) by mouth, then transport, keeping the patient warm.*

5. Repeat and record the vital signs, including the level of consciousness and Glasgow Coma Scale en route as often as the situation indicates.

6. Record all patient care information, including the patient's medical history and all treatment provided, on a prehospital care report.

(From Manual for Emergency Medical Technicians. Emergency Medical Services Program. Albany, New York State Department of Health, 1990.)

Review Exercises

1. List the bones of the skull and spinal column.
2. Describe how the brain is protected from injury.
3. List the parts and functions of the central and peripheral nervous system.
4. List the divisions and functions of the autonomic nervous system.
5. List the signs and symptoms and the treatment of a skull fracture.
6. List four types of brain injury and how they occur.
7. List the signs and symptoms and the treatment for subdural and epidural hematoma.
8. List five types of "secondary" brain injury.
9. State the body locations for the following dermatomes:

Cervical—4	Thoracic—4
Thoracic—10	Lumbar—1
Lumbar—5	

10. List the steps of assessment for a patient with head and spinal injury.
11. Describe proper spinal immobilization for the following patients:
    Stable automobile accident victim
    Unstable automobile accident victim
12. Describe the proper steps for removing a helmet from a suspected spinal injury victim.
13. Define stroke.
14. List three causes of stroke.
15. Describe the steps of assessment and the treatment of a stroke patient.
16. List two types of seizure disorders and describe their effects.
17. List steps in the emergency care of a patient during and after a convulsion.
18. Describe the treatment for status epilepticus.
19. Describe the approach to the patient with an altered mental state.

References

American College of Surgeons, Walt J (ed): Early Care of the Injured Patient, 3rd ed. Philadelphia, WB Saunders, 1982.

Bates B: A Guide to Physical Examination, 3rd ed. Philadelphia, JB Lippincott, 1983.

Guyton AC: Textbook of Medical Physiology, 8th ed. Philadelphia, WB Saunders, 1990.

Hughes S: The Basis and Practice of Traumatology. Rockvilla, MD, Aspen, 1984.

Nakum A, Melvin J: The Biomechanics of Trauma. Norwalk, CT, Appleton-Century-Crofts, 1985.

Neuman T: Unusual Forms of Trauma. In Baxt WG (ed): Trauma: The First Hour. Norwalk, CT, Appleton-Century-Crofts, 1985.

Passmore R, Robson JS (eds): A Companion of Medical Studies, vol 1. Oxford, Blackwell Scientific Publications, 1969.

Prehospital Trauma Life Support Committee of the National Association of EMTs: Pre-hospital Trauma Life Support. Akron, OH, Emergency Training, 1986.

Rayner K (ed): Atlas of the Body, Chapters 14 and 15. New York, Rand-McNally, 1980.

Raynor J: Anatomy and Physiology. New York, Harper & Row, 1977.

Rosen P et al (eds): Emergency Medicine: Concepts and Clinical Practice. St. Louis, CV Mosby, 1983.

Zuidema GD, Rutherford RB, Ballinger WF: The Management of Trauma, 4th ed. Philadelphia, WB Saunders, 1985.

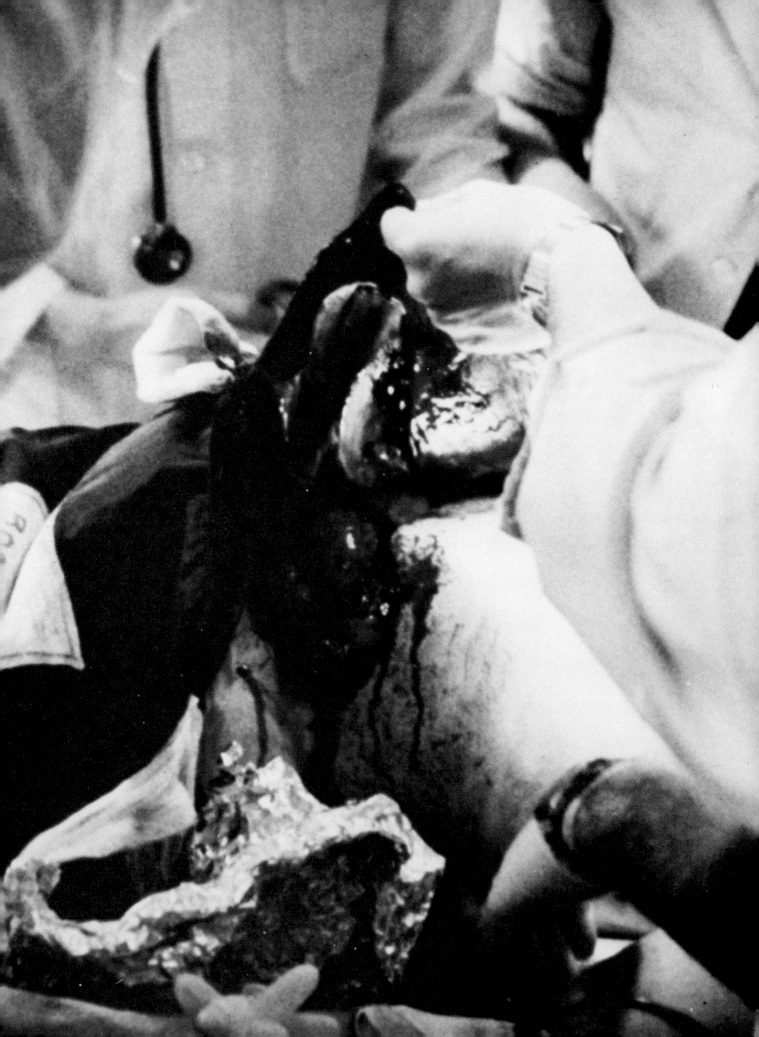

CHAPTER 8

ABDOMINAL EMERGENCIES

OBJECTIVES

At the conclusion of this chapter the reader will be able to:

---

1. Define acute abdominal distress (acute abdomen).

---

2. List the steps that should be followed in the treatment of a patient with acute abdominal distress.

---

3. List the boundaries and contents of the abdominal cavity.

---

4. Demonstrate the assessment of a patient with an abdominal injury.

---

5. Demonstrate the care of a patient with abdominal evisceration.

---

6. Demonstrate the care of a patient with an impaled object in the abdomen.

---

7. Demonstrate the care of a patient with a blunt abdominal injury.

---

8. List the external male genitalia.

---

9. List the external female genitalia.

---

10. Describe the emergency care of injuries to the male genitalia.

---

11. Describe the emergency care of a rape victim.

INTRODUCTION

Patients with complaints relating to the abdomen are frequently encountered in the prehospital setting. Problems with the abdomen may involve common medical disorders that arise from the abdominal organs such as bleeding ulcers or appendicitis or from complications from blunt or penetrating injuries. Occasionally, diseases outside the abdomen may have abdominal pain as their chief complaint.

A primary concern when faced with a complaint of abdominal pain or injury to the abdominal wall is the potential for *internal hemorrhage*. The abdomen contains large vessels, including the aorta and vena cava, as well as highly vascular organs such as the spleen and liver. You must be alert for signs of internal bleeding and hypovolemic shock. A second major concern is *peritonitis* or inflammation of the peritoneum, the internal lining of the abdominal cavity, which can be a sign of many different life-threatening conditions. You will be expected to recognize signs of this "acute abdomen." Both internal hemorrhage and peritonitis require early hospital intervention.

An understanding of the anatomy and basic physiology of the abdomen and genitalia is helpful in interpreting signs and symptoms found in patients with abdominal complaints.

Common complaints offered by patients with abdominal problems include pain, bleeding, nausea and vomiting, a change in eating and bowel habits, and *jaundice* (a yellowing of the skin or sclera of the eyes). Because the abdomen is such a large cavity, internal bleeding can cause shock with little external evidence. Other signs of hypovolemic shock must be searched for.

A word of caution: it is very difficult, even for experienced physicians, to diagnose all abdominal emergencies. It is not expected that EMTs will make a definitive diagnosis. In fact, a detailed and extensive history taking and physical examination in the field may be counterproductive if it delays transportation to the hospital. Rather, EMTs should appreciate the severity of some abdominal conditions, elicit preliminary findings in the field, institute shock treatment when appropriate, and concentrate on rapid movement of the patient to the hospital. Further questioning, a physical examination, and repeat evaluations can be done while en route to the hospital.

MEDICAL EMERGENCIES OF THE ABDOMEN

Overview

There are some general categories of medical problems that can aid the EMT in understanding abdominal conditions. These include hemorrhage, infection, organ failure, peritonitis, obstruction, perforation, and ischemia.

HEMORRHAGE

The most common cause of hemorrhage within the abdomen is bleeding from the wall of the digestive tract, as from stomach ulcers in the upper gastrointestinal (GI) tract, or diverticulitis in the lower digestive tract. Aneurysms arising from the abdominal aorta may leak or rupture as discussed previously in Chapter 5.

INFECTIONS

There are various causes of infection in the abdominal cavity. Infections can involve the digestive, urinary, or reproductive organs. One possible cause is when a tubular structure such as the appendix becomes obstructed and cannot drain, allowing bacteria to invade the compromised wall of the appendix. Another mechanism is when the wall of the large bowel perforates, allowing normally present bacteria to pass through the open wound. The bacteria cause an infection once outside the bowel that can spread through the abdominal cavity and cause peritonitis.

ORGAN FAILURE

Any of the abdominal organs may fail to function because of a variety of reasons. For example, the liver may fail due to the excessive ingestion of alcohol. If this occurs, dangerous toxins can build up in the blood, producing harmful effects to body cells.

OBSTRUCTION

Many of the abdominal organs are tubular structures that are designed to allow substances within to pass through. When these tubes are obstructed, problems necessarily result.

For example, a blockage can occur anywhere along the gastrointestinal tract, causing a backup of food or fluid. The intestine above the obstruction becomes distended, which results in hypovolemia and at times ischemia of the bowel wall. Causes of obstruction include a twisting of the intestine around a surgical scar, the trapping of the intestine within a hernia, a tumor encroaching upon the lumen of the intestine, or massive swelling secondary to inflammation.

Blockage of a *ureter* (draining tube from the kidney to the bladder) by a kidney stone will cause a back-up of urine.

PERFORATION

An ulcer in the stomach or duodenum can perforate or pierce through the gastrointestinal tract and lead to leakage of bowel contents into the peritoneum. This produces an inflammation of the peritoneum (peritonitis) that can be life threatening. Perforation may also lead to hemorrhage if vessels are in the path of the perforation.

PERITONITIS

As explained earlier, the peritoneum is the internal lining of the abdominal cavity. Peritonitis is an inflammation of this lining. This occurs when foreign material such as stomach acids, intestinal contents, bacteria, bile, or urine comes in contact with the peritoneum. Peritonitis is an acute emergency. Because of the patient's profound distress, findings of abdominal tenderness and guarding, and the possible need for immediate surgical attention, patients with peritonitis are often said to have an "acute abdomen."

ISCHEMIA

Like any other organ, abdominal organs are dependent on an adequate blood supply. Emboli can block and thrombi can form in the arteries feeding the abdominal organs; herniation of intestinal tissue can strangulate the blood supply to part of an organ; or a loop of bowel (or the testicle) may twist, compromising the blood supply and causing gangrene. These are examples of mechanisms that cause ischemia to abdominal organs. Consider ischemia an emergency problem, which usually requires prompt surgical attention.

Anatomy, Physiology, and Pathophysiology

Knowledge of the anatomy and physiology of the abdominal cavity is useful when trying to discover the type of medical problem or injury the patient may have suffered. The following section integrates a review of the major organs and structures within the abdominal cavity and some common disorders associated with them. Since so many different medical problems may arise from the abdomen, you are not expected to be able to diagnose a specific problem. The aim is to recognize signs of some potentially life-threatening conditions, such as intra-abdominal hemorrhage, peritonitis, and gastrointestinal bleeding. The following discussion provides some insight into the different causes of abdominal problems and should help you in the expedient evaluation and treatment of patients (Fig. 8–1).

THE ABDOMINAL CAVITY, PELVIC CAVITY, AND PERITONEUM

The abdominal cavity is defined as the space bordered by the diaphragm above and the pelvic inlet below. The anterior wall of the abdomen is formed by the

abdominal wall muscles, the sides by muscles and iliac bones, and the posterior by the lumbar vertebrae and posterior portions of the iliac bones, muscles, and diaphragm. The pelvic cavity is formed by the pelvic bones and is separated from the abdominal cavity by an imaginary plane from the sacrum to the symphysis pubis (See Fig. 2–11). Within the abdomen lie the greater part of the gastrointestinal tube, the liver, pancreas, spleen, kidneys, gallbladder, ureters, adrenal glands, and major blood vessels and nerves. Within the pelvis lie the distal parts of the ureters, the bladder, the sigmoid colon and rectum, and internal genitalia (Fig. 8–2A to D).

The lining of the inner abdominal cavity is called the *peritoneum.* The peritoneum is a smooth membrane that lines the abdominal wall and the contents of the abdomen. It has two parts, the *parietal* peritoneum which lines the abdominal and pelvic walls, and the *visceral* peritoneum, which covers most of the intra-abdominal organs. The space between the visceral and parietal peritoneum is called the peritoneal cavity (Fig. 8–3).

The peritoneum suspends abdominal organs from the walls of the abdominal cavity via ligaments and folds of tissue called *mesentery* and *omentum.* The peritoneum and its folds carry nerves and vessels to the organs they cover and support. Some organs are fixed in position, while others, such as the small intestine, are mobile to allow for freedom of motion. The relative differences in mobility of the abdominal organs lead to points of stress and shearing during abrupt deceleration of the body, as in a collision.

The visceral and parietal peritoneum are innervated with different types of sensory nerves. These nerves are the source of the pain associated with abdominal conditions and peritoneal inflammation. Because of the extensive scope of the peritoneum, "peritonitis" can result in diffuse pain, sometimes encompassing the entire abdomen.

It is important to remember that the superior abdominal border is the diaphragm and that some of the upper abdominal organs are under the lower ribs. Since the diaphragm is mobile, penetrating wounds to the lower chest may enter the abdominal cavity. With forced expiration, for example, the upper portion of the right diaphragm can extend as high as the 4th costal cartilage anteriorly to the 8th rib posteriorly, the left diaphragm being slightly lower than the right (Fig. 8–4).

The pelvic bone can bleed heavily and cause injury to pelvic organs when fractured (Fig. 8–5).

The space behind the peritoneum is called the *retroperitoneal* space. Bounded anteriorly by the peritoneum and posteriorly by the spine and muscles, it contains the kidneys, ureters, adrenal glands, pancreas, portions of the duodenum (intestinal tract), the major vessels, particularly the abdominal aorta and the inferior vena cava. Bleeding occuring within the retroperitoneal space may not be apparent from examination of the anterior abdomen (see Fig. 8–2A).

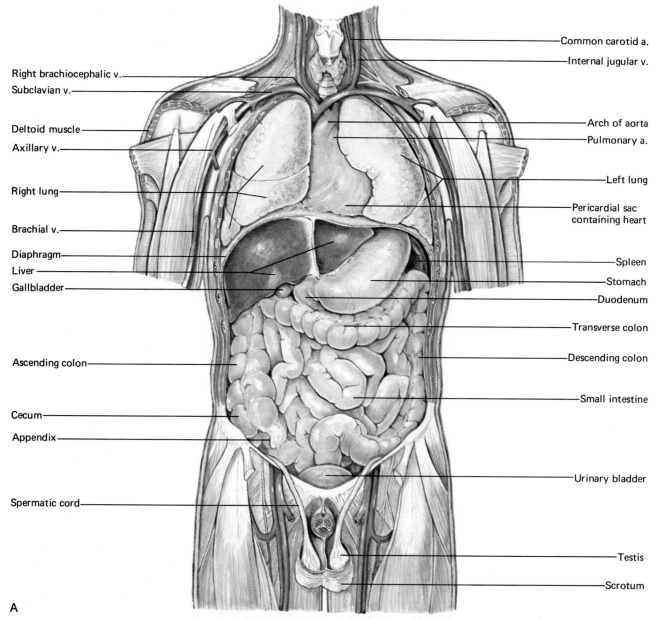

Common carotid a.
Internal jugular v.
Right brachiocephalic v.
Subclavian v.
Deltoid muscle
Axillary v.
Arch of aorta
Pulmonary a.
Right lung
Left lung
Pericardial sac containing heart
Brachial v.
Diaphragm
Liver
Gallbladder
Spleen
Stomach
Duodenum
Transverse colon
Descending colon
Ascending colon
Small intestine
Cecum
Appendix
Urinary bladder
Spermatic cord
Testis
Scrotum

A

FIGURE 8–1. (*A*) Anterior view of the body with rib cage and greater omentum removed. (*B*) Deeper anterior view of the body with small intestine removed. (From Solomon EP, Phillips GA: Understanding Human Anatomy and Physiology. Philadelphia, WB Saunders, 1987, pp. 17–18.)

Illustration continued on opposite page

ABDOMINAL REGIONS

Anteriorly, we can divide the abdomen into four quadrants by two imaginary lines through the umbilicus: the left upper quadrant (LUQ), the right upper quadrant (RUQ), the left lower quadrant (LLQ), and the right lower quadrant (RLQ). This allows us to describe areas of pain or injury and relate those findings to the anatomic structures beneath. For example, right lower quadrant pain

may be caused by inflammation of the appendix, which is located in that quadrant (Fig. 8–6).

Other terms are also used to refer to areas of the abdomen. The area just below the xiphoid process is commonly called the *epigastrium*. A patient complaining of pain in this region is said to have "epigastric pain." The area surrounding the umbilicus is called the *periumbilical region*, and the region just above the groin is commonly called the *suprapubic region* (Fig. 8–7).

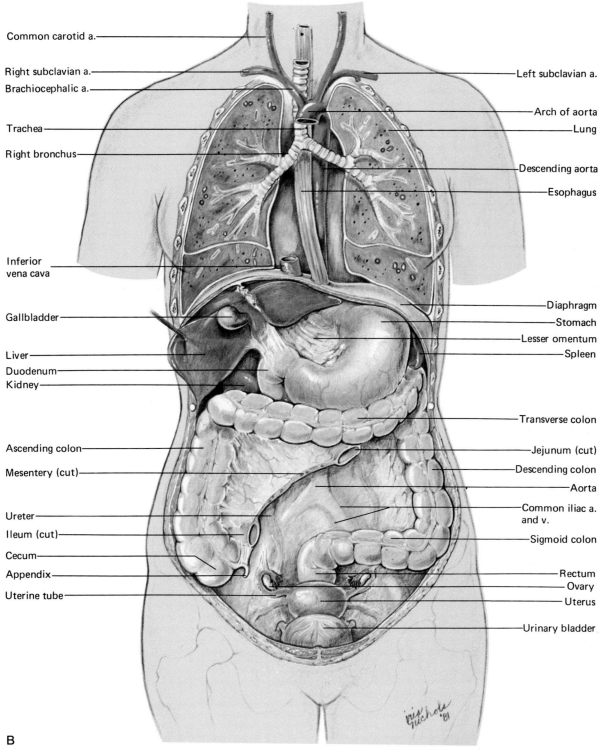

Common carotid a.

Right subclavian a.
Brachiocephalic a.

Trachea

Right bronchus

Inferior
vena cava

Gallbladder

Liver
Duodenum
Kidney

Ascending colon

Mesentery (cut)

Ureter

Ileum (cut)

Cecum

Appendix

Uterine tube

Left subclavian a.

Arch of aorta
Lung

Descending aorta

Esophagus

Diaphragm
Stomach
Lesser omentum
Spleen

Transverse colon

Jejunum (cut)
Descending colon
Aorta
Common iliac a.
and v.
Sigmoid colon

Rectum
Ovary
Uterus
Urinary bladder

B

FIGURE 8–1. *Continued*

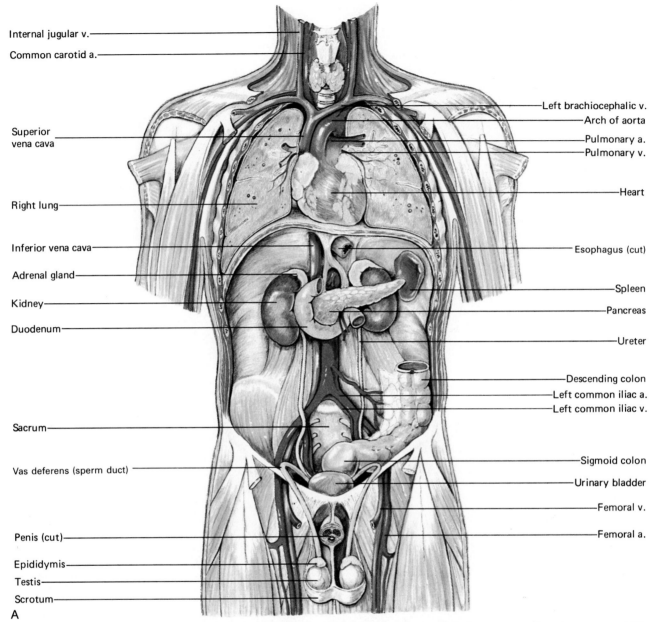

Internal jugular v.

Common carotid a.

Superior vena cava

Right lung

Inferior vena cava

Adrenal gland

Kidney

Duodenum

Sacrum

Vas deferens (sperm duct)

Penis (cut)

Epididymis

Testis

Scrotum

Left brachiocephalic v.

Arch of aorta

Pulmonary a.

Pulmonary v.

Heart

Esophagus (cut)

Spleen

Pancreas

Ureter

Descending colon

Left common iliac a.

Left common iliac v.

Sigmoid colon

Urinary bladder

Femoral v.

Femoral a.

A

FIGURE 8–2. (*A*) Deep anterior view of the body. The stomach, small intestine, and most of the large intestine have been removed. The kidneys, pancreas, and other deep structures are visible. (*B*) Posterior view of the body. Muscles have been removed to show the skeletal structures and position of the kidneys. (From Solomon EP, Phillips GA: Understanding Human Anatomy and Physiology. Philadelphia, WB Saunders, 1987, pp. 19–20.)

Illustration continued on opposite page

Surface landmarks that can be felt include the xiphoid and the costal margins. The costal margin is formed by the costal cartilages, beginning with the 7th, to the tips of the 12th rib. A distinct step is felt when the 10th rib is encountered. Sometimes it is difficult to find the tip of the 12th rib, which terminates in abdominal wall muscles. Other important bony landmarks are the iliac crest; the anterior superior iliac spine; and the inguinal

ligament, which passes from the anterior superior iliac spine to the pubic tubercle.

BLOOD SUPPLY

The primary artery within the abdomen is the abdominal aorta. It is located behind the peritoneum, in the midline. Several major arteries arise from the aorta

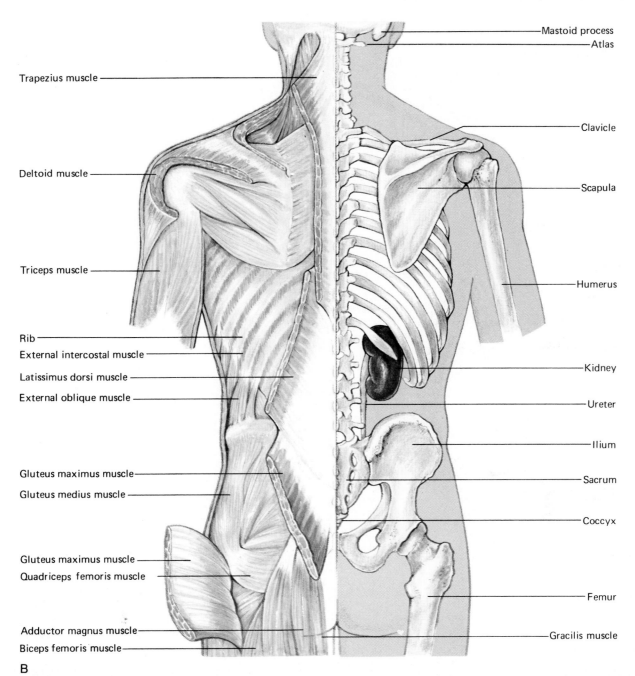

Trapezius muscle

Deltoid muscle

Triceps muscle

Rib

External intercostal muscle

Latissimus dorsi muscle

External oblique muscle

Gluteus maximus muscle

Gluteus medius muscle

Gluteus maximus muscle

Quadriceps femoris muscle

Adductor magnus muscle

Biceps femoris muscle

Mastoid process

Atlas

Clavicle

Scapula

Humerus

Kidney

Ureter

Ilium

Sacrum

Coccyx

Femur

Gracilis muscle

B

FIGURE 8–2. *Continued*

to feed the organs within the abdomen (see Fig. 4–17*E* and *F*). The abdominal aorta branches to become the common iliac arteries within the pelvic cavity. The common iliacs continue on to feed the lower extremities. The abdominal aorta is a common source of aneurysms, which may leak or rupture.

There are two major venous drainage systems within the abdomen. The digestive organs drain their blood into the portal venous system, which brings it to the liver so that nutrients absorbed through the GI tract can be processed and blood can be detoxified. This blood is then emptied into the vena cava. The retroperitoneal and pelvic organs feed their returning blood directly into the vena cava. The vena cava is the major vein in the abdomen and is located in the retroperitoneal space next

Text continued on page 360

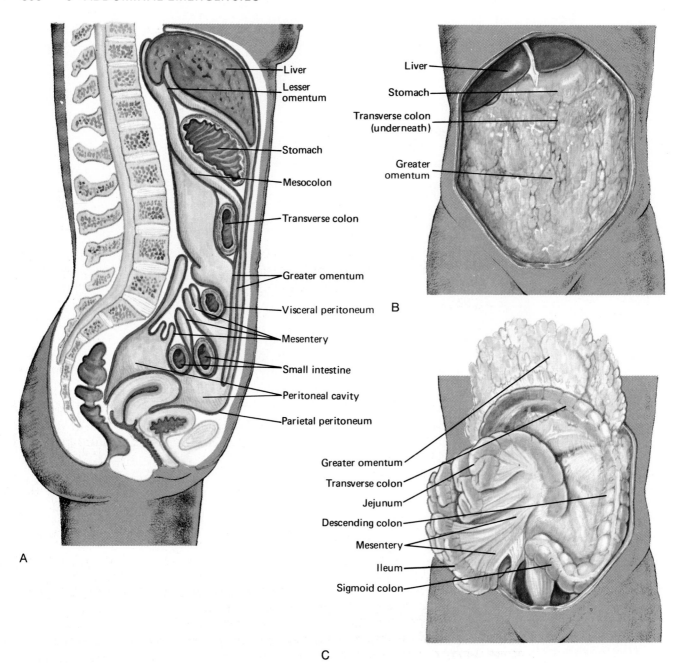

Liver
Lesser omentum
Stomach
Mesocolon
Transverse colon
Greater omentum
Visceral peritoneum
Mesentery
Small intestine
Peritoneal cavity
Parietal peritoneum

A

Liver
Stomach
Transverse colon (underneath)
Greater omentum

B

Greater omentum
Transverse colon
Jejunum
Descending colon
Mesentery
Ileum
Sigmoid colon

C

FIGURE 8–3. The peritoneum lines the abdominal cavity. The visceral peritoneum covers the organs and suspends many by ligaments and folds of tissue called mesentery and omentum. Nerve fibers in the visceral and parietal peritoneum register different types of pain, an important fact to remember in the evaluation of abdominal pain. The peritoneal cavity contains most of the abdominal organs. Behind the peritoneum is the retroperitoneal space. (*A*) Sagittal section through abdomen and pelvis. (*B*) Frontal view of abdomen. (*C*) Frontal view of abdomen with transverse colon and greater omentum lifted to show mesentery. (From Solomon EP, Schmidt RR, Adragna PJ: Human Anatomy and Physiology, 2nd ed. Philadelphia, Saunders College Publishing, 1990, p. 577.)

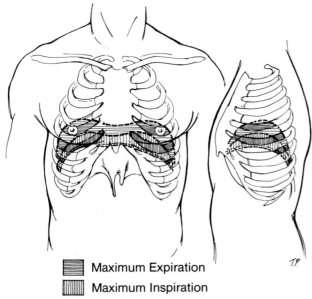

■ Maximum Expiration

▥ Maximum Inspiration

FIGURE 8-4. The level of the diaphragm varies with respiration and may be as high as the 4th costal cartilage. Penetrating wounds in the lower thorax may enter the abdominal cavity and injure the liver or other organs in the upper abdomen. (From Cardona VD, Hurn PD, Mason PJB, et al: Trauma Nursing from Resuscitation Through Rehabilitation. Philadelphia, WB Saunders, 1988, p. 120.)

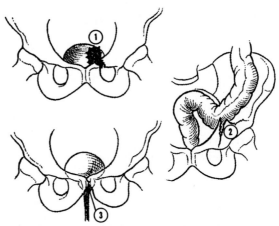

FIGURE 8-5. Examples of injuries secondary to a fractured pelvis (*1*) ruptured bladder; (*2*) tears of the bowel; and (*3*) tears of the urethra. (From Connolly JF: DePalma's The Management of Fractures and Dislocations: An Atlas. Philadelphia, WB Saunders, 1989 p. 76.)

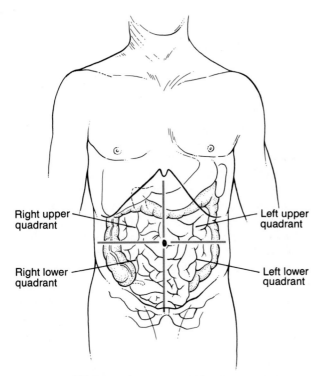

FIGURE 8-6. The abdominal quadrants and related organs. (From Swartz MH: Textbook of Physical Diagnosis: History and Examination. Philadelphia, WB Saunders, 1989, p. 320.)

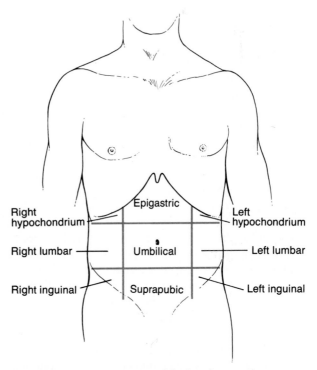

FIGURE 8-7. Epigastric, periumbilical, and suprapubic are terms commonly used to describe locations of pain and tenderness and also the location of bruises and other wounds. (From Swartz MH: Textbook of Physical Diagnosis: History and Examination. Philadelphia, WB Saunders, 1989, p. 320.)

to the aorta (see Fig. 4—18C). Find the femoral pulse that lies halfway between the anterior superior iliac spine and the symphis pubis.

PAIN AND NERVE INNERVATION

One reason that the diagnosis of abdominal conditions is difficult is that abdominal pain is transmitted by two distinct pain pathways. One pathway, the *visceral pathway*, gives perceptions that are imprecise as to both the quality of the pain and its actual location. The second pathway, the *somatic pathway*, is perceived more clearly, the pain having a sharp, even knifelike quality—and is localized anatomically near or over the organ from which it emanates. Unfortunately, the pain perceived in the early stages of abdominal diseases is usually via visceral pathways, making early diagnosis more difficult.

VISCERAL PAIN. Visceral pain fibers innervate the visceral peritoneum and travel via the autonomic nervous system to the spinal cord and brain. Visceral or organ pain is initiated by stretching or distention of an organ as occurs, for example, with an intestinal obstruction. Other conditions that give rise to visceral pain include chemical damage to the organ or ischemia. Visceral pain is perceived as diffuse, cramping, and aching. Patients may have difficulty in finding adjectives to describe this pain.

Rather than being attributed to the organ itself, a patient may feel the pain in an area quite removed from the anatomical source. The location of the referred pain is often the dermatome corresponding to the segment of the body from which an *organ originally developed in embryo*. While the organ moved to a different location as the embryo and fetus developed, it continued to share nervous innervations with structures from its point of origin. The brain confuses the pain as arising from the original spinal dermatome. For example, the diaphragm originated from the cervical plexus, and is innervated by nerves from the 3rd, 4th, and 5th cervical segments, the phrenic nerve. Pain can be referred from the diaphragm to the shoulder. Likewise, pain from the heart can be referred to the neck, jaw, and arm, shared points from its developmental origin. Figures 8—8 and 8—9 illustrate some common areas of referred pain from visceral organs. An example of nerve pathways associated with the pain of appendicitis is seen in Fig. 8—10.

Because visceral pain arises from the autonomic nervous system, it may be accompanied by symptoms such as nausea, vomiting, sweating, changes in heart rate (fast and slow), lowered blood pressure, and contractions of the abdominal wall muscles.

Early in the presentation of appendicitis, only the visceral pain fibers may be stimulated. Instead of pain in the right lower quadrant, where the appendix is usually

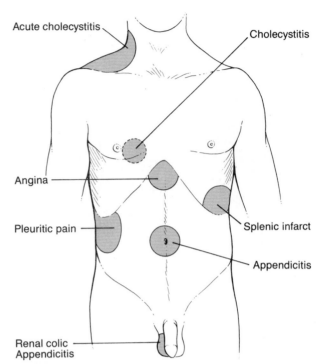

FIGURE 8–8. Anterior surface areas of referred pain. (From Swartz MH: Textbook of Physical Diagnosis: History and Examination. Philadelphia, WB Saunders, 1989, p. 324)

located anatomically, the patient may first complain of periumbilical pain and nausea and vomiting.

SOMATIC PAIN. Somatic pain fibers innervate the parietal peritoneum and abdominal wall and travel through spinal nerves. Somatic pain occurs when nerve fibers in the parietal peritoneum are stimulated by inflammation from an adjacent abdominal organ. The brain perceives a *sharp* pain localized to the abdominal wall overlying the involved organ, and may initiate a reflex contraction (guarding) of the overlying musculature. For example, when appendicitis begins to cause inflammation of the overlying parietal peritoneum, the patient complains of sharp pain in that area. Palpation of this area reveals tenderness and may stimulate guarding. In an attempt to avoid pain, the patient will often become "immobilized", resisting and wary of any movement, sometimes with the thighs flexed to "relax" the abdominal peritoneum. If the palpating fingers are suddenly removed from the abdomen, the patient may feel excruciating pain (rebound tenderness), a sign of peritoneal inflammation.

The Digestive System

The function of the digestive system is to break down foods, absorb them into the blood stream, and process them into useful forms for energy, growth, and

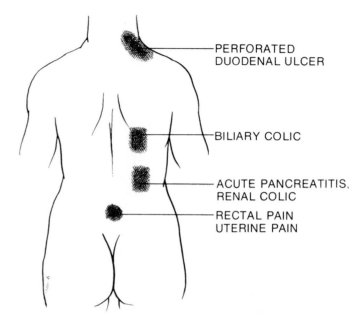

FIGURE 8-9. Posterior surface areas of referred pain. (From Schwartz GR, Safar P, Stone JH, et al: Principles and Practice of Emergency Medicine, 2nd ed. Philadelphia, WB Saunders, 1986, p. 726.)

other body functions. Food is broken down both mechanically and chemically. It is mechanically made smaller by chewing in the mouth and churning in the stomach and intestines. Food is chemically broken down by acids and enzymes that are secreted into the mouth, stomach, and intestines. As food travels through the digestive tract, it becomes smaller and smaller until it is either absorbed or excreted as feces.

MOUTH

The digestive tract begins with the mouth and teeth. Here, mechanical breakdown of food begins during chewing. Salivary glands secrete enzymes rich in saliva, which moistens food and begins the chemical breakdown. In the posterior portion of the mouth, the food is directed into the esophagus by the epiglottis. The importance of the epiglottis in preventing aspiration as discussed in Chapter 3. Normally, as food or liquid enters the posterior pharynx, the epiglottis closes over the trachea, and muscles direct the substance into the esophageal opening (Fig. 8-11).

ESOPHAGUS

The esophagus travels through the chest cavity just posterior to the trachea. It enters the abdominal cavity through the diaphragm. It is a muscular tube that propels food from the mouth to the stomach through the process of peristalsis. Peristalsis is a muscular action that moves food in a coordinated manner through the entire diges-

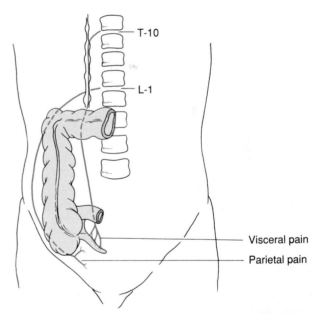

FIGURE 8-10. The pain pathways that may be stimulated in a "typical" case of appendicitis. Visceral and parietal transmission of pain from the appendix. Visceral pain is perceived as coming from the T10 or umbilical area. Somatic pain is perceived as coming from the right lower quadrant in the L1 dermatone. Both types of pain are caused by appendicitis. Initially, only a dull continuous periumbilical pain may be perceived, accompanied by nausea and perhaps vomiting and anorexia. Later, as the appendix becomes inflamed, the covering of the parietal peritoneum is stimulated and pain is perceived as sharp and localized to the right lower quadrant. It may be accompanied by guarding. Most people would be able to guess that appendicitis was a probable cause if they saw a patient with somatic pain. However, when only visceral pain is present, it would be a more difficult diagnosis. (From Guyton AC: *Textbook of Medical Physiology.* 6th ed. Philadelphia, WB Saunders, 1981, p. 619.)

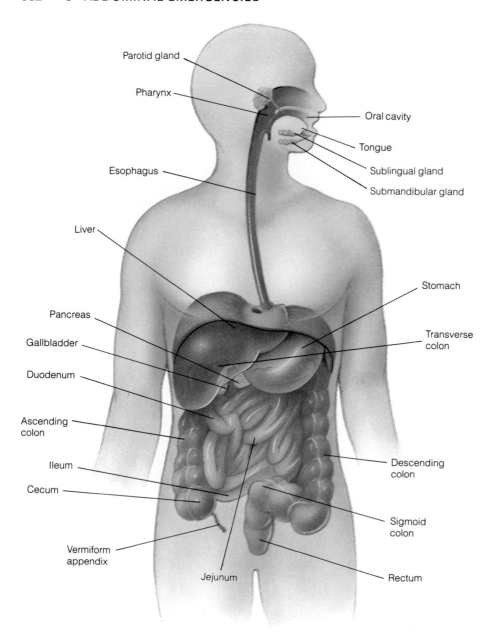

FIGURE 8–11. Organs of the digestive system. (From Gaudin AJ, Jones KC: Human Anatomy and Physiology. Orlando, Harcourt Brace Jovanovich, 1989, p. 441.)

Parotid gland

Pharynx

Oral cavity

Tongue

Esophagus

Sublingual gland

Submandibular gland

Liver

Stomach

Pancreas

Transverse colon

Gallbladder

Duodenum

Ascending colon

Descending colon

Ileum

Cecum

Sigmoid colon

Vermiform appendix

Jejunum

Rectum

tive system. Sequential muscular contractions along the esophagus and intestines squeeze food along (Fig. 8–12). The lower end of the esophagus acts as a one-way valve to prevent a reflux of stomach contents into the esophagus.

Esophageal disorders may cause complaints such as indigestion or heartburn. Gastric acid may reflux into the esophagus, causing irritation of the esophageal wall, resulting in a burning sensation or chest pain. Esophageal disorders can be confused with myocardial infarction. It is important to carefully collect the history relating to the character of the chest pain and the past medical history. Some patients may have taken antacids. Inquire whether or not this relieved the pain. Pain related to this disorder may also be reduced or relieved while sitting. When in doubt, treat for myocardial infarction. Remem-

ber that it is not uncommon for patients with ischemic chest pain to attribute their discomfort to "indigestion."

The esophagus may also be the site of hemorrhage. Patients with severe liver disease, often related to heavy alcohol use, may have *esophageal varices*. Esophageal varices are balloon-like blood vessels that can protrude through the lower esophageal wall, where they can be subject to erosion from gastric acids. A varice may rupture and result in massive bleeding. Signs of esophageal bleeding include *hematemesis* (vomiting blood) and possibly melena (blood in the stool that appears black with a tarry consistency and a distinct foul odor).

The esophagus can also perforate from a variety of mechanisms. Forceful vomiting or retching may cause tears in the esophagus, causing profuse bleeding. Ingestion of caustic or corrosive substances can cause per-

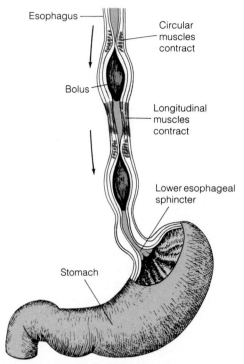

FIGURE 8–12. Peristalsis occurs by the sequential contraction and relaxation of smooth muscle along the digestive tract. (From Gaudin AJ, Jones KC: Human Anatomy and Physiology. Orlando, Harcourt Brace Jovanovich, 1989, p. 450.)

foration. Esophageal perforation is life threatening and requires immediate surgical intervention.

STOMACH

The stomach is a J-shaped organ, located in the left upper quadrant (LUQ). Most of the stomach is protected by the ribs. When distended, the stomach can be easily palpated in the LUQ. It has two openings, one connecting with the esophagus and the other leading to the *duodenum*, the first phase of the small intestine. The volume of the stomach varies tremendously. It has the ability to expand to 10 times its empty size. The stomach stores food and breaks it down mechanically via contraction and relaxation of muscles, and chemically via strong acids and enzymes.

It is the action of the stomach acids on blood that causes it to have a black and tarry appearance in stool. Since stomach acid is neutralized as food enters the small intestine, melena is a sign of upper GI bleeding—above the duodenum.

Peptic ulcer disease and gastritis are common disorders in which the digestive action of the gastric juices begins to work on the organ's own lining. Under a variety of conditions, the acidic gastric juice bores a hole in the wall of the stomach or duodenum. This hole causes pain in the epigastric region or in the back, depending on the

location of the crater. The pain may be relieved by the administration of antacids or milk. Aspirin ingestion or coffee may aggravate or precipitate the pain. The pain may be described as burning or indigestion. The patient often has a past medical history of ulcers or gastritis. Common medications that the patient may be taking include Tagamet (cimetidine), Zantac (ranitidine), Pepcid (famotidine), and antacids. Ulcer disease can cause several complications. Of greatest concern is bleeding. The ulcer may bore through a blood vessel and cause massive bleeding. Abdominal pain associated with hematemesis, melena, or signs of hypovolemic shock should make you suspicious of bleeding ulcers. Gastritis means inflammation of the gastric mucosa and can result in multiple small erosions of the stomach lining, causing a diffuse, burning epigastric pain that can be accompanied by severe bleeding.

SMALL INTESTINE

Food travels from the stomach into the small intestine. The small intestine is located in the central part of the abdominal cavity throughout all four quadrants. The small intestine ranges from 10 to 20 feet in length and provides the large surface area through which nutrients are absorbed. The small intestine is divided into three segments. The first area is the *duodenum*, which extends from the stomach. It is U-shaped, leaving the stomach to the right and hooking back to the left, where it connects to the second phase of the small intestine, the *jejunum*. Attached to the duodenum is the drainage tube from the liver, pancreas, and gallbladder. The jejunum connects with the *ileum*, the third part of the small intestine. The ileum ends at the ileocecal junction, where the large and small intestines meet. The small intestine is relatively mobile and suspended from one point like a fan by folds of the peritoneum. The only exception to this is the duodenum, which is fixed in position as it meets the stomach, making it subject to tears during deceleration accidents.

The most common emergency arising from the small intestine is duodenal ulcers. The second most common is obstruction. Obstruction can occur because of external compression or internal blockage, or from twisting or kinking of the intestine around scar tissue from previous abdominal surgery. External compression includes the condition of incarcerated hernia.

Hernias are outpocketings of the peritoneum into abnormal openings in the abdominal wall. The most common is an inguinal hernia, and patients may complain of pain or a swelling in the groin (Fig. 8–13). With inguinal hernia, the bowel enters the inguinal canal and can present as swelling anywhere along the entire path of the canal and even into the scrotum in males. This is a common condition and does not by itself constitute

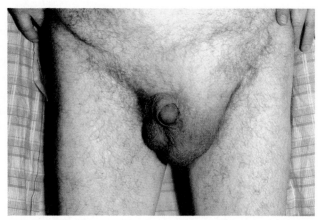

FIGURE 8–13. Inguinal hernia. (From Swartz MH: Textbook of Physical Diagnosis: History and Examination. Philadelphia, WB Saunders, 1989.)

an emergency as long as the bowel can easily slide back into the peritoneal cavity. However, if the small intestine becomes trapped or incarcerated, a blockage of flow through the small intestine occurs, and the blood flow to the trapped segment of bowel can be compromised. Other sites where a hernia can become incarcerated include the femoral canal (swelling just above the femoral artery) or umbilicus. These are more likely to occur in women.

Intestines can also twist around scars from previous abdominal surgery, and this is a common cause of intestinal obstruction. Internal obstruction can occur anywhere in the small intestine when a foreign body becomes lodged in the lumen. The smallest portion of the intestine is the ileocecal junction, and it is often the point of blockage.

The initial symptom of obstruction is crampy abdominal pain that comes and goes. The pain is diffuse and cannot be described as arising from a particular area but may be centered in the area of obstruction. As the buildup continues, the pain becomes more steady and severe, with marked abdominal distention and vomiting as intestinal contents back up. The vomitus varies. Initially, stomach or gastric contents may be seen. Depending on the site of obstruction, the vomitus may be bilious (containing bile), greenish yellow, or even feculent (brownish and smelling of feces) if the obstruction is very low.

If you suspect intestinal obstruction, you should inquire about the last bowel movement or the passage of gas. Patients with obstruction have a history of no recent bowel movements or gas.

Peritonitis can cause a paralysis of peristaltic movement. This becomes a type of obstruction, since there is no movement of intestinal contents, and is typified by marked dilation with no signs of intestinal activity.

Ischemia to the intestine can occur if the blood supply is compromised by formation of clots or occlusion from emboli. The degree of ischemia can be partial or complete, leading to intestinal infarction. The patient will experience pain, which may be of sudden onset, particularly if there is complete occlusion from an embolus. Emboli usually come from the heart and are not uncommon in patients with atrial fibrillation who have an irregularly irregular rhythm to the pulse.

PANCREAS

The *pancreas* has two general functions. First, it secretes digestive enzymes into the digestive tract to aid in the breakdown of food, and second, it secretes the hormone insulin into the blood to regulate the use of glucose by the body's cells. The pancreas extends across the upper abdomen behind the stomach and in front of the spine, in the retroperitoneal space. Ulcers on the posterior surface of the stomach can sometimes bore back through to the pancreas. The main pancreatic duct travels through the pancreas and delivers digestive secretions from the pancreas to the duodenum as it joins the common bile duct at the ampulla of Vater (see the discussion on the gallbladder later in this chapter).

A normal pancreas produces an odorless, colorless fluid that is rich in enzymes and bicarbonate. Bicarbonate neutralizes the gastric acid that would otherwise be injurious to the small intestine. Bicarbonate also aids the action of the pancreatic enzymes on food in the small intestine. Severe pancreatic insufficiency can lead to malabsorption.

In its role as an endocrine organ, the pancreas secretes the hormone insulin, which regulates glucose metabolism. The most common medical problems related to the pancreas are *diabetic states* and *pancreatitis*. Diabetes is the disease that results from failure of the pancreas to produce a sufficient amount of insulin. This is covered in Chapter 12, Medical Emergencies.

Pancreatitis exists in two forms: *acute* and *chronic*. Pancreatitis can be life threatening. The basic abnormality is the inflammation of pancreatic tissues. It has many causes but the most common are heavy alcohol consumption and gallstones that block pancreatic duct outflow.

The attack of pancreatitis can begin with sudden severe epigastric pain, which may radiate to the back. In some patients it is perceived as either right or left upper quadrant pain. The character of the pain is variable, but is often described as knifelike. The pain may be aggravated by lying down and be somewhat relieved by sitting up. Eating or drinking may worsen the symptoms. Vomiting, fever, and tachycardia are other common signs of the disease. Ecchymosis may be seen in severe cases in the periumbilical region or over the flank. Ultimately, the patient may develop hypovolemic shock.

LIVER

The *liver* is a large, solid, soft organ located in the right upper quadrant of the abdomen, just below the diaphragm and partially protected by the lower ribs. The liver has several functions. It produces bile, which it secretes into the intestine to aid in the digestion of fatty foods. It plays a major role in the metabolism of carbohydrates, proteins, and fats.

One of the main functions of the liver is to filter out toxins from the blood. It detoxifies drugs, alcohol, and other potentially poisonous substances. When the liver is overwhelmed by toxins, liver failure may occur. This may occur with chronic alcohol ingestion or by an overdose of certain drugs such as acetaminophen. Patients who have reduced liver function may need adjustments during drug therapy due to their decreased ability to detoxify the substance. The liver also produces proteins that play an important role in fluid balance and blood clotting. Patients with severe liver disease are at increased risk for bleeding.

As with pancreatitis, alcohol consumption is a major cause of liver disease, leading to *hepatitis* (inflammation) or *cirrhosis* (scarring). Other causes of liver disease are infections and drug reactions. Infectious hepatitis is of concern to EMTs and all health workers (see Communicable Diseases in Chapter 12).

Liver disease may be accompanied by jaundiced (yellow) skin or mucous membranes. The earliest jaundice tends to appear at the sclera (the white portion of the eyes) or mucous membranes. Jaundice is caused by a buildup of bilirubin in the blood. Bilirubin is a breakdown product of red blood cells that is processed and excreted by the liver into the small intestines. Extensive liver damage or blockage of the normal excretion (along the pathway of bile ducts) can contribute to jaundice (Fig. 8-14). (Excessive breakdown of red blood cells can also cause jaundice.) Other signs and symptoms of liver failure may include vomiting, lethargy, and anorexia. End stages of liver failure can result in hepatic coma due to a buildup of toxins in the blood, which alters brain function.

GALLBLADDER

The *gallbladder* is an organ that stores and concentrates bile produced by the liver. It is located under the liver in the right upper quadrant of the abdomen. Bile leaves the liver via the hepatic ducts. The hepatic ducts and the cystic duct from the gallbladder form the common bile duct. The common bile duct joins with the pancreatic duct and empties into the duodenum at the ampulla of Vater (Fig. 8-15).

Bile is ordinarily stored in the gallbladder. The presence of fatty food in the duodenum stimulates the gallbladder to secrete bile into the small intestine. Depending on the site of obstruction in the duct system, the patient may develop problems related to the gallbladder, the liver, or the pancreas.

The major medical emergency related to the gallbladder is cholecystitis (inflammation or low-grade, chronic infection of the gallbladder). This usually occurs when gallstones, or rocklike concretions of cholesterol, bile pigment, and calcium, block the bile exit from the

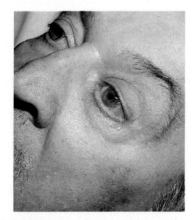

FIGURE 8-14. Note jaundice in the eyes of a patient with severe liver disease.

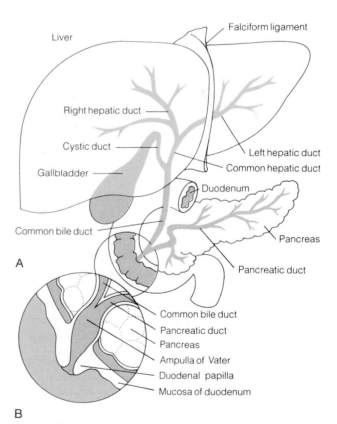

FIGURE 8-15. (A) The ducts of the liver, gallbladder, and pancreas. (B) Note how a blockage at the ampulla of Vater may affect all three organs. (From Gaudin AJ, Jones KC: Human Anatomy and Physiology. Orlando, Harcourt Brace Jovanovich, 1989, p. 458.)

gallbladder. The gallbladder can become distended and inflamed.

Initially, the patient with gallbladder disease may complain of right upper quadrant pain, which is aggravated by the ingestion of fatty foods. The pain may be located in the right upper quadrant or referred to the right subscapular region posteriorly, and may be confused with pancreatitis or ulcer disease. The patient with acute cholecystitis may also exhibit vomiting, fever, and jaundice from blockage of the bile duct by gallstones. On palpation, the right upper quadrant may be tender; the pain may be aggravated with inspiration. Some patients may describe pain similar to that of myocardial infarction. Finding tenderness on palpation of the abdomen in the right upper quadrant would be more suggestive of gallbladder disease.

LARGE INTESTINE

The *large intestine* begins in the right lower quadrant, continuing the flow of digestive contents from the ileum. It begins with the *cecum* and the *appendix*, then the *ascending colon*, the *transverse colon*, the *descending colon*, and the *sigmoid colon*. The cecum is the junction between the ileum and the ascending colon. The appendix is a worm-like outpocketing of the cecum with an extremely narrow lumen and no known function. The colon wraps around the boundary of the peritoneal cavity, first up the right side (ascending) and then across (transverse) the upper portion of the abdomen anterior to the duodenum, pancreas, ileum, and jejunum. It then travels down the left side (descending) of the abdomen to meet the sigmoid colon. The sigmoid colon travels into the pelvis, is relatively mobile, and leads into the rectum. The sigmoid colon varies in length. Some patients suffer twisting of the sigmoid colon, which results in obstruction.

The function of the large intestine is the absorption of water and electrolytes from contents delivered by the small intestine and the formation of feces. With constipation, the colon contains feces for a longer time and absorbs an excess amount of water, resulting in hard stools. With diarrhea, the colon absorbs little water and sometimes has increased secretions (at times with blood). The colon that is not functioning at all does not absorb water and does not move feces along, becoming massively dilated, a condition called *megacolon*. The colon normally contains bacteria that make up a considerable portion of the feces. Many diseases that you may encounter arise from the large intestine.

DIVERTICULA.   Diverticula of the bowel are quite common and are usually asymptomatic. A diverticulum is an outpouching of the inner wall of bowel tissue into the muscle layer of the bowel (Fig. 8–16). Diverticula most often occur on the left side of the large intestine. Diverticula that occur near arteries may cause painless bleeding. This bleeding may become severe and is responsible for the majority of cases of massive lower GI bleeds. Bleeding can have a sudden onset. The diverticula may become clogged with feces and pus and lead to an infection of the large intestine. This is called *diverticulitis*. It causes mild to moderate pain, usually located in the left lower quadrant. The character of the pain is dull or aching and may be associated with anorexia and nausea. Fever is also common. The patient may have left lower quadrant tenderness and other signs of peritoneal inflammation. Complications of diverticulitis include obstruction secondary to massive swelling, perforation of the bowel, peritonitis, and bleeding. The victim may have developed hypovolemic or septic shock, depending on the duration and extent of the problem.

DIARRHEA.   Diarrhea, sometimes bloody, may be associated with many different diseases. The most common cause is a viral or bacterial infection. There are more serious and less common causes including parasitic infections, ulcerative colitis, and infarction of the large intestine. Patients with severe diarrhea develop dehydration and hypovolemia.

Infectious conditions that cause both vomiting and diarrhea are called *gastroenteritis*. Here fluid losses are exacerbated by the inability to retain fluids by mouth.

OBSTRUCTION.   Obstruction of the large intestine occurs for a variety of reasons. The bowel may twist on itself in areas where it is mobile, such as the sigmoid colon. A cancerous tumor can encroach on the lumen and the patient may note narrow stools for a period of time prior to complete obstruction. Fecal impactions are another cause of obstruction. Victims of large bowel obstruction have pain, a failure to pass gas and stool, and abdominal distention. In contrast to small bowel obstruction, vomiting does not usually occur, due to the distance from the upper GI tract and the fact that the ileocecal junction acts as a valve, which prevents a backflow of material.

INTUSSUSCEPTION.   Intussusception is a surgical emergency that occurs most often in very young children, usually under the age of 2 years. It occurs suddenly, often at night, and usually in a well-nourished child. The mechanism of the problem relates to the peristaltic action of the bowel, which literally telescopes one portion of the intestine into the other through the peristaltic movement. The site of intussusception is usually the ileocecal junction, with the small intestine telescoping into the large bowel. The small intestine drags its mesentery and blood vessels along as it continues to enter the colon by peristaltic action. Compression of the bowel and its mesenteric veins leads to edema and obstruction, and there is increased mucus production and capillary bleeding, which manifest as the patient passes a bloody mucoid stool that appears like "currant jelly" (Fig. 8–17).

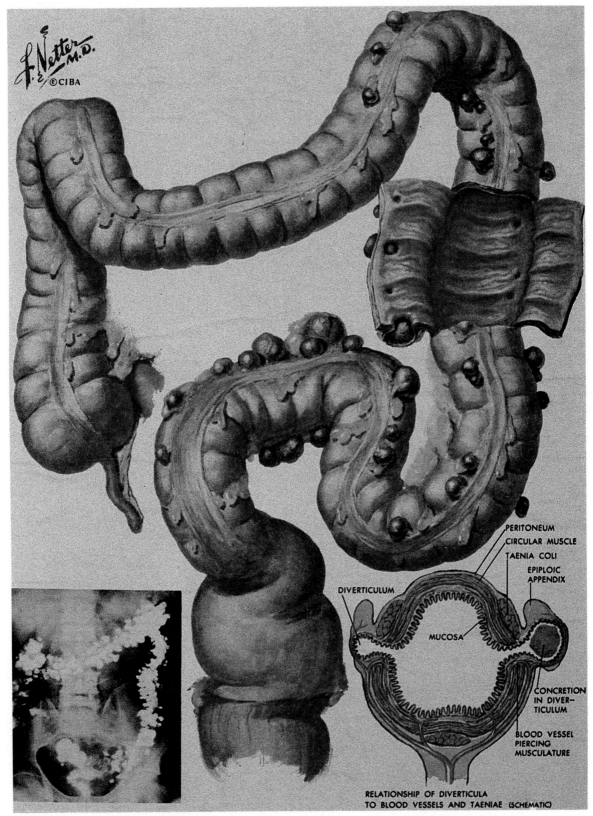

FIGURE 8-16. Diverticula are herniations of mucosa through the muscular wall of the large intestine. (From Netter FH: CIBA Collection of Medical Illustrations, Vol 3, Digestive System, Part II. Summit, NJ, CIBA Pharmaceutical Co, 1962, Sec XII, Plate 19, p. 130.)

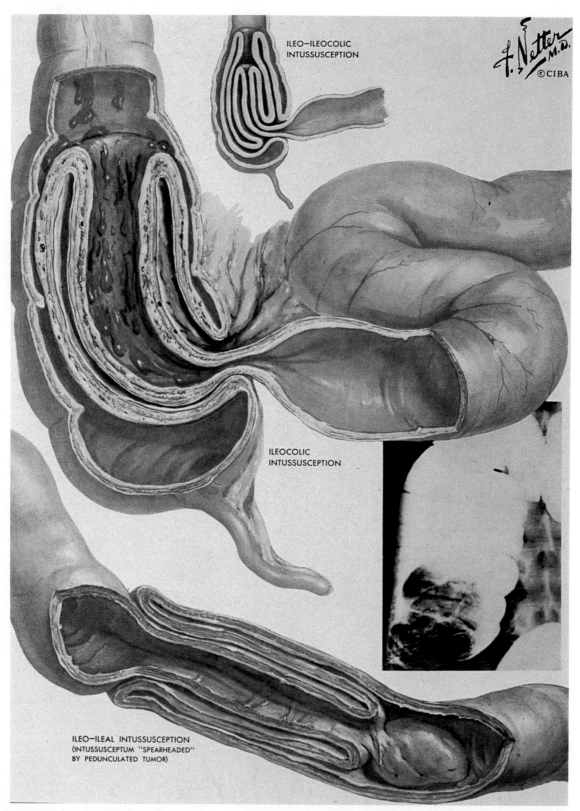

FIGURE 8–17. The typical site of intussusception is at the ileocecal junction. The peristaltic wave telescopes the bowel and its mesentery into more distal bowel. Note the swelling of the bowel and the bleeding that will lead to mucoid "currant jelly" stool. (From Netter FH: CIBA Collection of Medical Illustrations, Vol 3, Digestive System, Part II. Summit, NJ, CIBA Pharmaceutical Co, 1962, Sec XII, Plate 23, p. 1.)

The pain of intussusception may be intermittent, the child awakening with severe pain and the knees drawn up, only to return to normal activity between pains. On physical examination, a "sausage-like" mass may be palpated in the right upper quadrant.

APPENDICITIS. Appendicitis is the most common surgical emergency. It is thought that appendicitis occurs when bowel contents become clogged in the lumen of the appendix. As the normal mucosal secretions continue to collect within the blocked appendix, it distends. Nerve fibers produce a mild vague pain that is usually interpreted as being in the umbilical region by the patient. As times passes, and further distention develops, there is more severe pain and an associated loss of appetite, with nausea and vomiting. As the intestinal wall is compromised from the swelling and bacteria begin to invade the tissue, signs of infection such as fever develop. Now that the parietal peritoneum is stimulated, pain localizes in the right lower quadrant. The combination of right lower quadrant pain, fever, nausea, and vomiting is highly suggestive of appendicitis. If the appendix goes untreated, it can become gangrenous and rupture, spilling its contents into the peritoneum.

Upon physical examination the patient may complain of right lower quadrant tenderness, and there is voluntary guarding of the abdomen. As the disease progresses, peritonitis may develop and the patient may present with acute pain and flexion of the lower extremities. The definitive therapy for appendicitis is surgery. The main complication is perforation, which spills pus into the peritoneal cavity. At first the pus irritates the right lower quadrant and the pain is local, but ultimately it spreads to a larger area of the abdomen. As the infection progresses, septic shock may develop. Once the infection spreads, the pain markedly increases and the fever rises. The physical examination shows peritoneal signs, including diffuse tenderness localized to the right side, involuntary guarding, rebound tenderness, and distention. At this point, the disease becomes life threatening.

RECTUM AND ANUS

The *rectum* connects the sigmoid colon to the *anus*. The rectum is the storage container for feces, terminating in the anus, a 2-inch canal. They are lined with a series of sphincter muscles that control the evacuation of fecal contents. Hemorrhoids are a common medical problem that relates to these structures. *Hemorrhoids* are ballooning of the veins that drain the rectal area. They can occur in any adult and rarely cause problems that come to the attention of the EMT. When they do, it is usually because of massive rectal bleeding as the hemorrhoids burst. Hemorrhoids occur more frequently with alcoholics and other victims of liver disease, as well as in pregnant

women in whom the venous return is obstructed by the bulk of the fetus.

Occasionally, you may encounter patients who have foreign bodies entrapped in the rectum. Such objects have included bottles, light bulbs, and vibrators. You should not attempt to remove the foreign body in the field, since objects may inadvertently be displaced further up the GI tract or break, causing more serious complications. The patient should be placed in the position of comfort and transported to the hospital.

The Urinary System

The urinary system is composed of two kidneys, two ureters, the urinary bladder, urethra, and external genitalia. The role of the urinary system is to regulate fluid volume and blood salt concentration, and to filter the blood of toxins.

KIDNEYS AND URETERS

The *kidneys* are located in the retroperitoneum, high up on the posterior abdominal wall just under the diaphragm. A large portion of the kidneys is protected by the posterior rib cage. They are connected to the urinary bladder by tubes called *ureters* (Fig. 8–18). The kidneys are slightly mobile and can move with respiration. They are highly vascular organs. The kidneys play a very important role in regulating fluid levels in the body. When the body is overhydrated, as occurs during excessive fluid intake, the kidneys excrete larger volumes of water, a process known as diuresis. When the body is dehydrated, the kidneys conserve water and urine output is restricted. In severe hypovolemic states caused by bleeding, diarrhea, or other problems, the kidneys may shut down completely, resulting in no urine output.

The control of *electrolytes* (salts) in the bloodstream is another important function of the kidneys. Common salts include sodium and potassium. When blood flow to the kidneys is reduced, as in hypovolemia, heart failure, or any form of shock, the kidneys automatically retain sodium salt. The retention of sodium by the kidneys allows them to retain water, thereby increasing blood volume.

The kidneys also act as filters of toxins in the blood. They filter poisons, medications, and also a byproduct of metabolism called urea.

Kidney, or renal, failure can be acute or chronic. The causes of each are numerous. Acute renal failure can be caused by decreased blood flow in a shock-like state, intrinsic renal disease caused by infection, drug reactions (adverse reactions to antibiotics), or uncommon systemic diseases. It can also be caused by obstructions to the outflow of urine, either at the ureter, as caused by a stone or tumor, or at the urethra, as caused by enlarge-

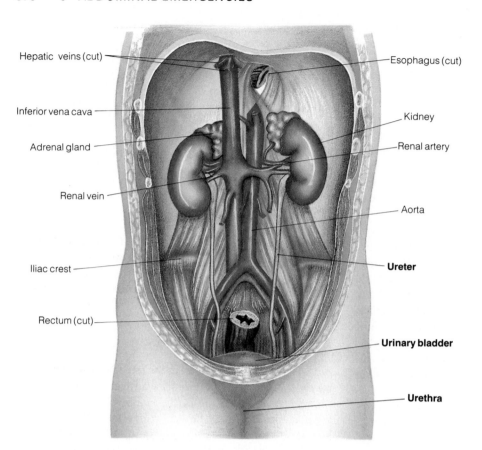

Hepatic veins (cut)

Inferior vena cava

Adrenal gland

Renal vein

Iliac crest

Rectum (cut)

Esophagus (cut)

Kidney

Renal artery

Aorta

Ureter

Urinary bladder

Urethra

FIGURE 8–18. Organs of the urinary system. (From Gaudin AJ, Jones KC: Human Anatomy and Physiology. Orlando, Harcourt Brace Jovanovich, 1989, p. 647.)

ment of the prostate gland. Chronic renal failure can be caused by diabetes, hypertension, intrinsic renal disease, and uncommon systemic diseases. Patients in renal failure require dialysis. Dialysis is a method that is used to artificially filter the blood. Patients in acute renal failure generally receive their treatment in a hospital setting. Dialysis is also offered in specialized clinics built specifically for this purpose. Patients in chronic renal failure may require this procedure several times a week.

Patients with a new onset of renal failure or those who fail to receive their dialysis therapy exhibit signs of *uremia*. Uremia is caused by a buildup of urea in the bloodstream. Also building up at this time are dangerous combinations of electrolytes, acids, and drugs. The uremic patient has a decreased or total absence of urine output, an altered mental state, seizures, tachycardia, deep and rapid respirations, pallor, congestive heart failure, and pulmonary edema. As urea builds up within the system, the body attempts to sweat this substance out of the body pores, so that a white powder forms on the skin, known as uremic frost. This is irritating and causes itching if the patient is conscious at this stage. The breath also becomes foul and smells strongly of urine. Dialysis can prevent these problems but patients require regular treatment. Dialysis patients are most apt to have problems if they miss a dialysis session. Then they may suffer

from overhydration, congestive heart failure, and electrolyte abnormalities that can cause weakness and even cardiac arrhythmias.

The most common emergency related to the kidney is *pyelonephritis*. This is an infection of the kidney that is more common in females but that may occur in either sex. Pregnancy, neurologic conditions that affect the bladder (as in quadriplegics), and diabetes are factors that increase the risk. This is a severe infection, which may present with very high fevers, shaking chills, abdominal and back pain, nausea, vomiting, diarrhea, and dysuria. Affected patients often have pain posteriorly in the flanks (below the ribs and above the ilium). The urine usually contains pus or blood, and septic shock may occur.

Kidney stones are hard, stone-like substances that are formed when there are excessive amounts of certain products in the urine. Renal colic is caused by passage of a stone from the kidney into the ureters, causing partial or total obstruction to urine flow. With peristaltic waves of the ureter come spasms of intermittent pain, causing the patient to roll and move around in an attempt to find a position of comfort. The pain is felt in the back or along the path of the urinary system, sometimes radiating into the groin or testicle. The condition may be accompanied by blood in the urine.

This condition occurs more often in men than in

women, in a 3:1 ratio, with most cases occurring between the ages of 20 and 50. The back-up of urine can cause kidney damage.

URINARY BLADDER AND URETHRA

The *bladder* is located anteriorly, low in the pelvis. When distended with urine, the bladder can be felt in the lower abdomen. Ureters bring urine to it from the kidneys. The purpose of the bladder is to store urine. It releases urine under voluntary control by relaxation of sphincter muscles at its junction with the *urethra*. The urethra is a tube through which urine is expelled. It is short in women, exiting above the vagina in the external genitalia. It is longer in men, passing through the prostate gland at the neck of the bladder and then through the penis. Bladder emergencies may result from infections. They occur more often in females and rarely are serious enough to require the assistance of an EMT, but left untreated they can ascend and involve the kidneys. Patients who complain of pelvic pain, with difficulty urinating, and who describe blood in the urine, along with fever, suprapubic tenderness, and voluntary guarding, should be suspected of having a bladder infection.

Acute urinary retention, usually caused by obstruction of the urethra, is a painful condition with suprapubic pain and a feeling of distress. Enlargement or hypertrophy of the prostate, common in nearly all elderly men, may cause obstruction of the urethra, which passes through the prostate as it leaves the bladder. The distended bladder may be felt suprapubicly. Relief is gained by insertion of a urinary catheter through the penile urethra into the bladder. There are many other causes of urinary retention, including infections, neurologic disorders, and adverse drug reactions.

You will encounter patients who have indwelling urinary catheters inserted through the penile urethra. These may be placed for temporary relief of urinary retention pending surgery on the prostate gland. Other patients may have permanent indwelling catheters. Sometimes the catheter is placed suprapubicly, through the abdominal wall. Such patients are prone to develop urinary infections. If left untreated, the infection can ascend up the urinary tract and cause infection of the kidney.

The Reproductive System

MALE REPRODUCTIVE SYSTEM

The *male reproductive system* includes the *testicles* and *epididymis*, the *seminal vesicle*, the *prostate gland*, the *penis*, the *urethra*, the *vas deferens*, and the *scrotum*. The scrotum is a pouch in which lie the testes and the epididymis. The testicles are suspended in the scrotum by the spermatic cord, which passes down from the abdomen through the inguinal canal. The left testicle usually lies slightly lower in the scrotum than the right testicle. The testicles produce the male hormone *testosterone*, as well as *sperm* and *semen* (seminal fluid). The sperm are transported via the vas deferens up through the spermatic cord to the base of the bladder. Here the vas deferens joins the seminal vesicle (which stores semen) to form the ejaculatory duct, which travels through the prostate where it opens into the prostatic portion of the urethra. The prostate gland secretes fluid that mixes with the semen. The penis is a highly vascular organ that becomes erect during sexual arousal for insertion into the vagina during sexual intercourse. Through the penis passes the urethra, a tube through which both urine and semen pass (Fig. 8–19). During ejaculation, only semen passes through the urethra.

Medical complaints involving the male urinary/reproductive system encountered by EMTs may include acute urinary retention, testicular torsion, and infections.

Torsion of the testicles is most common in younger men and adolescents. The testicle can twist within the scrotum about the spermatic cord, which not only supports but carries the vas deferens, arteries, and veins to the testicle. The blood supply to the testicle can be shut off with torsion. This is a surgical emergency. If the torsion is not relieved within hours, gangrene of the testicle can result. There may be swelling in the scrotal area and marked pain, which is referred to the testicle, but sometimes only abdominal pain accompanied by nausea or vomiting may be present.

Infections can cause pain and burning on urination and pain and swelling of the testes and epididymis. Infections can involve the prostate, the urethra, the bladder, and the testicles and epididymis. Complaints offered by patients with urinary tract infections include *dysuria* (painful urination), *hematuria* (blood in the urine), frequency of urination, and discharge of pus from the urethral opening.

FEMALE REPRODUCTIVE SYSTEM

The *female reproductive system* consists of the *uterus, ovaries, fallopian tubes, vagina,* and *external genitalia.* (See also Chapter 13.) The female external genitalia, or *vulva*, include folds of skin called the *labia majora* and *labia minora*, the *clitoris, vaginal orifice*, and *urethral orifice*. The labia minora enclose the clitoris. The urethral orifice lies behind the clitoris. Bartholin's glands are mucous-secreting glands lying deep to the posterior part of the labia majora.

The vagina travels upward to surround the cervix

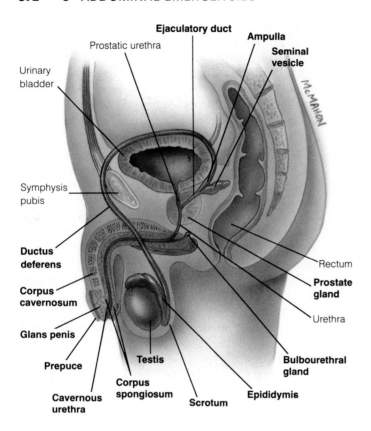

FIGURE 8–19. Organs of the male reproductive system. (From Gaudin AJ, Jones KC: Human Anatomy and Physiology. Orlando, Harcourt Brace Jovanovich, 1989, p. 699.)

of the uterus. The uterus is a pear-shaped muscular organ that lies between the bladder and the rectum. The cervix of the uterus extends into the vagina (Fig. 8–20). The cervix has a central opening, or os, which is normally plugged with mucous. It opens to permit menstrual blood flow and dilates during delivery of a baby. The fallopian tubes (oviducts) extend from both sides of the uterus to receive an *ovum* (a specialized cell) from the ovaries, which have both reproductive and endocrine functions. During ovulation, a mature egg is released from one ovary and travels through the fallopian tube, which guides its passage to the uterus (see Chapter 13). The female hormones, estrogen and progesterone, are produced by the ovary and control menstruation and influence the sexual characteristics of women.

Major medical emergencies that may present as abdominal or pelvic pain include *ectopic pregnancy, vaginal bleeding,* and *infections.*

Ectopic pregnancy is defined as an implantation of the fertilized ovum in an area outside the uterus, usually in the fallopian tubes. As the implanted ovum outgrows the tube and ruptures, abdominal pain and internal bleeding occur.

Common complaints of patients with ectopic pregnancy include abdominal pain, a missed menstrual period, and, depending on the severity of bleeding, signs of shock. Often, it is accompanied by vaginal bleeding, but this is not universal. In some studies, almost one-third of the patients with ectopic pregnancy did not have vaginal bleeding with other symptoms. Ectopic preg-

nancy is a life-threatening condition. Death results from internal bleeding. Always consider the possibility of ectopic pregnancy in a woman of childbearing age who presents with sudden abdominal pain and signs of shock.

Vaginal bleeding can occur for multiple reasons. The causes of vaginal bleeding in pregnancy are presented in Chapter 13. Other causes include severe menstrual bleeding, endometriosis, and threatened abortion or miscarriage. Treat for shock if signs are present. Do not attempt to control vaginal bleeding by stuffing pads into the vagina.

Pelvic inflammatory disease (PID) can cause severe abdominal pain and peritonitis. It is caused by bacterial infection of the female reproductive organs. It may be accompanied by fever and abdominal or pelvic pain. Since the fallopian tubes enter the peritoneal cavity, infection from the reproductive organs can result in peritonitis.

Other conditions, such as a twisted ovarian cyst, can cause severe abdominal and pelvic pain. It is not productive to attempt to diagnose these conditions in the field. They are part of a differential diagnosis in women who present with lower abdominal pain. You may hear about these and other conditions as patients describe their past medical histories.

The Endocrine System

The endocrine system consists of many hormone-secreting organs throughout the body. Those located in the abdomen include the adrenals, pancreas, and the

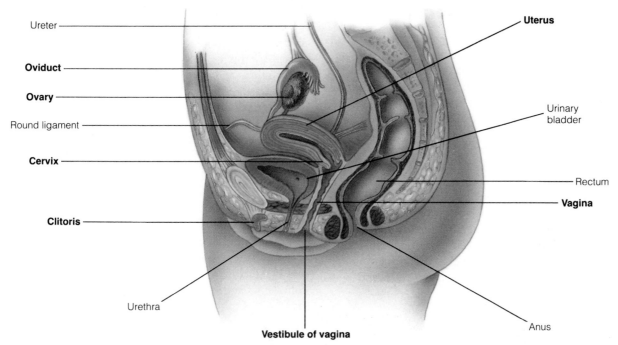

FIGURE 8-20. Organs of the female reproductive system. (From Gaudin AJ, Jones KC: Human Anatomy and Physiology. Orlando, Harcourt Brace Jovanovich, 1989, p. 709.)

ovaries. The testicles are located outside the abdomen in the scrotum.

There is one adrenal gland located above and attached to each kidney. The adrenal glands are responsible for the secretion of several hormones. Epinephrine (adrenaline) is one of the major hormones and is discussed throughout the text.

Spleen

The spleen is a highly vascular organ located in the left upper quadrant and protected by the ribs. The main concern for the EMT is injury, since the injured spleen can cause fatal hemorrhage. Designed to filter broken red blood cells, its tasks can be assumed by other organs if it is removed. The spleen can be swollen in conditions such as mononucleosis or severe liver disease.

Abdominal Aortic Aneurysm

Abdominal aortic aneurysms, almost always caused by atherosclerosis, can leak and rupture and cause life-threatening hemorrhage. At the time of rupture, patients may experience sudden pain and syncope. They present with abdominal pain and/or back pain, often described as tearing and usually continuous in nature. Patients may offer a history of this condition. The leaking aortic aneurysm can be felt as a wide, palpable, pulsating mass in the midline in the upper abdomen above the iliac crests.

Avoid deep palpation if this is encountered. Remember, however, that it is not uncommon to feel a pulsation from the abdominal aorta in normal patients, particularly if they are thin. See Chapter 5 for more discussion of aneurysms.

Other Causes of Abdominal Pain

There are other diseases that may cause a patient to present with abdominal pain. These causes include pneumonia; myocardial infarction; muscular strains; severe diabetic ketoacidosis; sickle cell crisis; toxins such as lead, arsenic, thallium, or organophosphates; drug withdrawal; and spider bites.

Fluid Shifts and Hypovolemia in Abdominal Pain

Obstruction and peritonitis may result in a shift of fluid to the abdomen. Fluid shifts to the abdomen result in a loss of circulating blood volume and hypovolemia. This can occur for various reasons. The findings are signs of hypovolemia manifested by rapid pulse and lowered blood pressure. These patients need volume replacement in the hospital setting.

Loss of fluids from vomiting and diarrhea also produce hypovolemia.

The Acute Abdomen

The patient with unremitting abdominal pain of recent onset is often said to have an "acute abdomen." Others reserve this term for patients with peritonitis. This is a general term that is commonly used to signify the importance of early diagnosis of these patients. Not all patients with acute abdominal pain have catastrophic conditions. However, as a general rule, it is a useful reminder that for many patients with acute abdominal pain, their outcome is dependent on early diagnosis and surgical intervention.

Signs of an acute abdomen include a patient lying still, with knees drawn up, avoiding any movement, and breathing shallow breaths—all attempts to avoid movement of the abdomen; complaints of abdominal pain; findings of local or diffuse abdominal tenderness or guarding; and with hypovolemia, rapid pulse and perhaps lowered blood pressure.

APPROACH TO THE PATIENT WITH ABDOMINAL PAIN

Because it is extremely difficult to diagnose the cause of abdominal pain in the field, and because many patients may need timely hospital interventions, the EMT should focus on identifying life-threatening conditions and act to bring these patients to the hospital as quickly as possible. Life-threatening conditions include bleeding and the acute abdomen. The bleeding patient may present with signs of shock with or without obvious evidence of blood loss.

An acute abdomen is one that may require rapid surgical intervention, administration of antibiotics, and restoration of fluid balance and blood. It is noted in the prehospital arena by findings such as the following:

- Patient positioned to avoid any movement of the abdomen (supine or on the side with knees raised, and shallow breathing)
- A distended and tense abdomen
- Abdominal tenderness
- Abdominal guarding (voluntary or involuntary)

While additional historical and physical information may be helpful to the physician in making a diagnosis, accumulation of such data should not delay hospital transport. Rather, data can be gathered en route to the hospital or at the hospital.

Primary Survey

As with all patients, the primary survey is the first approach to the patient. If signs of shock are present, rapid transport is indicated. Establishing an airway and administration of supplemental oxygen should be early steps. The position of choice during transport is determined by the mental status of the patient, the position of comfort, and the need to maintain the airway to prevent aspiration, particularly if the patient is vomiting. Transporting with the legs elevated may be indicated if the patient is hypotensive, with due precautions to care for the airway in the presence of nausea or vomiting. Application of MAST should be considered according to local protocols.

History

Pain or bleeding are common chief complaints. Others may be weakness, vomiting, change in bowel habits, and inability to urinate. Information pertinent to these complaints and others follow.

ABDOMINAL PAIN

Abdominal pain has different manifestations.

LOCATION.   The pain may be diffuse and poorly localized or the patient may be able to point to an area of the abdomen. Does the pain radiate? Remember that a patient's pain may be referred to another area even outside the abdomen. Figure 8–21 summarizes some locations of abdominal pain by illness. Figure 8–22 adds examples of different characteristics of abdominal pain that may be encountered.

QUALITY.   Use the patient's own words to describe the quality of the pain. Is the pain severe or relatively mild? What adjectives does the patient use to describe it: knifelike, tearing, dull, or crampy?

DURATION.   When did the pain begin? Was it gradual in onset or sudden and acute? Were there other symptoms associated with the onset of pain such as syncope or faintness, nausea and vomiting, or an urge to move the bowels? Is the pattern of pain continuous and steady or intermittent and crampy? Did it change in quality or location? If so, when?

AGGRAVATING AND RELIEVING FACTORS.   Are there relieving or aggravating factors? Has the patient taken medications such as antacids? Does eating aggravate or relieve the pain? Look at the position of the patient. Is the patient lying immobile in one position, trying to avoid any movement? Or is the patient writhing about, trying without success to find a position of comfort?

BLEEDING.   Bleeding from the mouth, rectum, urinary tract, or vagina may be present. What are the characteristics of the bleeding? Vomiting resulting from upper GI bleeding may be manifested by bright or dark

FIGURE 8-21. Abdominal pain by location. (From Schwartz GR, Safar P, Stone JH, et al: Principles and Practice of Emergency Medicine, 2nd ed. Philadelphia, WB Saunders, 1986, p. 725.)

(A) Right upper quadrant (RUQ):
Hepatitis
Cholecystitis, biliary colic
Duodenal ulcer
Pyelonephritis
Pancreatitis (bilateral)
Myocardial infarction, ischemia
Pneumonia with pleural reaction

(B) Left upper quadrant (LUQ):
Ruptured spleen
Gastric ulcer
Duodenal ulcer
Pancreatitis
Pyelonephritis
Gastritis
Splenic enlargement
Myocardial infarction, ischemia
Pneumonia with pleural reaction
Ruptured aortic aneurysm
Perforated colon (tumor, foreign body)
Renal pain

(C) Right lower quadrant (RLQ):
Appendicitis
Ectopic pregnancy
Diverticulitis
Kidney stone
Intestinal obstruction
Leaking aneurysm
Twisted ovarian cyst
Pelvic inflammatory disease
Incarcerated hernia
Renal pain

(D) Left lower quadrant (LLQ):
Ectopic pregnancy
Diverticulitis
Kidney stone
Appendicitis
Leaking aneurysm
Renal pain
Incarcerated hernia
Perforated colon
Pelvic inflammatory disease
Intestinal obstruction

(E) Epigastric:
Duodenal and gastric ulcer
Esophagitis
Myocardial infarction
Gallbladder

(F) Periumbilical:
Intestinal obstruction
Appendicitis
Pancreatitis
Abdominal aortic aneurysm
Diverticulitis

(G) Suprapubic:
Urinary tract infection
Pelvic inflammatory disease
Acute urinary retention

(H) Diffuse pain:
Peritonitis
Acute pancreatitis
Early appendicitis
Sickle cell crisis
Mesenteric thrombosis
Gastroenteritis
Dissecting or rupturing aneurysm
Colitis
Intestinal obstruction
Uremia, diabetes mellitus
Diverticulitis
Strangulated groin hernia

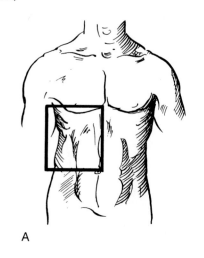

A

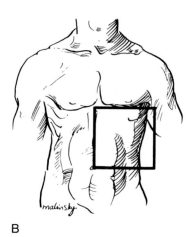

B

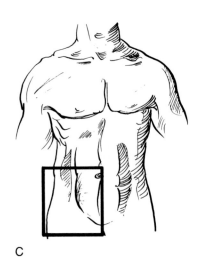

C

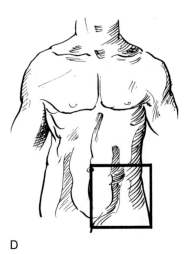

D

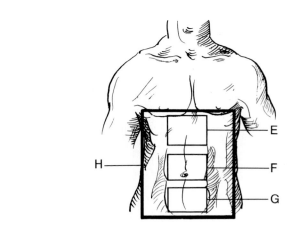

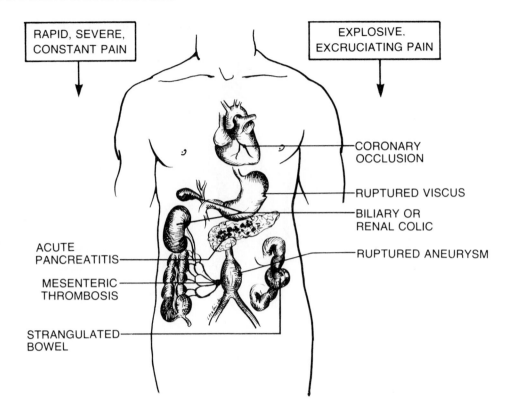

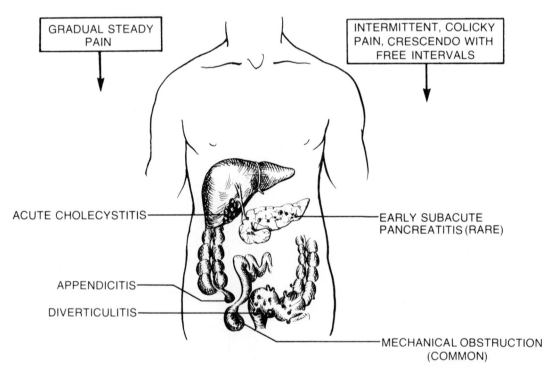

FIGURE 8–22. Quality and character of arising abdominal pain caused by various disease entities. (From Schwartz GR, Safar P, Stone JH, et al: Principles and Practice of Emergency Medicine, 2nd ed. Philadelphia, WB Saunders, 1986 p. 728.)

red blood, alone or mixed with vomitus, or as material that looks like coffee grounds. A sample may be brought to the hospital to be tested for the presence of blood.

Blood from the rectum may appear as melena, a black or tarry stool with a distinct foul odor; bright red blood; or blood mixed with stool.

Are there complaints of vaginal bleeding? Are they associated with abnormal pain? Is vaginal bleeding occurring during the menstrual period or outside the normal cycle? Does the patient think she may be pregnant?

JAUNDICE. A yellowish tinge to the sclera of the eyes or skin is known as jaundice. The color can range from a faint yellowish tinge to marked orange texture to the skin. Jaundice often indicates liver disease or gallbladder disease. Did the patient notice jaundice? If so, when?

NAUSEA AND VOMITING. Ask the patient if there was any nausea or vomiting. When did vomiting begin? Is it associated with pain? What was present in the vomitus? Undigested food, mucous, bile, coffee-ground material, blood? Was there a feculent smell to the vomitus, signifying a lower GI obstruction?

ANOREXIA. Has the patient been eating and drinking? When was the last meal or fluids taken?

DIARRHEA AND CONSTIPATION. Diarrhea is the presence of frequent watery stools. It may be tinged with blood. Constipation is a difficulty in passing stools, accompanied by a feeling of urgency or rectal fullness. Inquire whether recent bowel habits were normal?

CHILLS AND FEVER. Ask the patient about fever or chills consistent with an infectious process.

URINARY SYMPTOMS. Are there problems related to the urinary tract, such as *dysuria* (burning on urination), *hematuria* (blood mixed with the urine), *frequency* (an urge to urinate more often than usual), *polyuria* (frequent urination with large amounts of urine)? (Note that diabetic ketoacidosis can present as abdominal pain.) Does the patient note the presence of a discharge from the penis or vagina?

CARDIOPULMONARY SYMPTOMS. Does the patient have complaints that may be associated with the cardiopulmonary systems, especially in the face of upper abdominal pain? Remember that pneumonia can cause abdominal pain, particularly in children. Also remember that myocardial infarction can present with abdominal pain and vomiting.

Past Medical History

The past medical history may be informative. In addition to the usual questions about heart disease, COPD, hypertension, and diabetes, does the patient have a history of abdominal disease such as liver disease, ulcers, or urinary tract infections? Has the patient ever had abdominal surgery? Does the patient have a history of abdominal aneurysm?

Has the patient experienced similar episodes in the past? If so, what was the diagnosis?

Medications and Allergies

Is the patient taking medications for abdominal problems? What other medications is the patient taking?

Physical Examination

After the primary survey and vital signs are taken, look for findings associated with abdominal complaints during the secondary survey. Is there jaundice in the sclera or skin? Are there signs of dehydration? Any unusual odors?

From your first approach to the patient, note whether the patient is lying still, with signs of peritonitis, or is writhing about trying, without success, to find a position of comfort.

Inspect the abdomen, looking for obvious distention and scars from previous surgery. Lightly touch the abdomen and feel whether it is tense or soft. If the muscles are rigid, ask the patient to try and relax them.

Ask the patient to point to any area of pain and begin palpation away from that quadrant, examining this area last. Gently palpate the abdomen using the pads of your fingertips (Fig. 8–23) (Some examiners choose to use two hands to palpate the abdomen. One hand is placed on top of the other. The examiner concentrates on feeling with fingerpads of the lower hand while gentle pressure is applied with the superior hand.) Move your fingers gently and smoothly from one area to another,

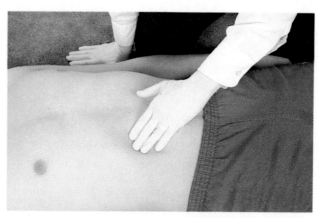

FIGURE 8–23. Palpation of the abdomen should begin away from the area of pain with gentle palpation. Note rigidity and tenderness.

avoiding abrupt movement. Watch the patient's face for reaction as you gently palpate all four quadrants. Note areas of tenderness. Is there any rigidity of the abdominal wall muscles? In what quadrants? Ask the patient to try and relax the muscles to see if the guarding is voluntary or involuntary. Note the presence of any midline pulsatile mass that might indicate an abdominal aneurysm. Note whether there is abrupt pain when your fingers are withdrawn (rebound tenderness), but do not purposely try to elicit this finding.

Key findings you are looking for are the patient's position and reaction to movement, distention of the abdomen (Fig. 8–24), the presence and location of tenderness and abdominal muscle wall rigidity (voluntary versus involuntary), the presence of blood, signs of shock or dehydration, jaundice, and the presence of a pulsating mass.

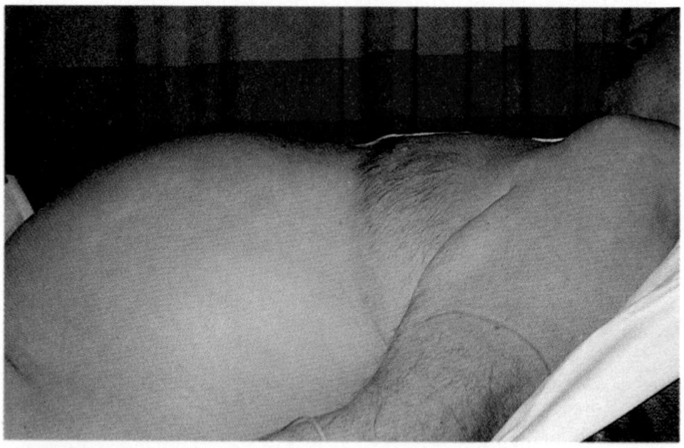

FIGURE 8–24. (*B*) Abdominal distention. In this case, the distention is due to accumulation of fluid in abdomen from liver failure (ascites).

Treatment of Medical Abdominal Emergencies

Treatment for major abdominal emergencies takes place in the hospital. Rapid transport and shock treatment may be required by some patients.

✠ P R O T O C O L ✠

TREATING ABDOMINAL EMERGENCIES

1. *Maintain an airway*, especially in the presence of vomiting. Patients with altered mental status and vomiting should be placed in the left lateral recumbent position, with suction on standby to aid in keeping the airway clear en route.

2. *Administer high-concentration oxygen* if there are signs of shock or peritonitis (to compensate for the associated shallow breathing).

3. *Treat shock if it is present*. Maintain body temperature, elevate legs, and consider using the MAST.

4. *Place the patient in a position of comfort* if this is not contraindicated by the need to control the airway or treat the patient for shock. Patients with peritoneal signs may find the most comfort by being transported supine, or on their side, with hips and knees flexed. A pillow may be placed under the knees to support the weight of the legs.

5. *Give nothing by mouth*. The patient with an abdominal emergency may require surgery, and a full stomach adds to the risk of aspiration when anesthesia is administered.

6. *Complete your examination while en route to the hospital*. Repeat vital signs as indicated. Record your findings. Notify the hospital of your impending arrival with a critical patient.

TRAUMA TO THE ABDOMEN

Extent of the Problem

Because of the large vessels and highly vascular organs within the abdomen, injuries can result in rapid blood loss and death. Since the abdomen is such a large cavity, distention of the abdomen may not be apparent, even after significant abdominal bleeding. Because of this, the EMT must maintain a high level of suspicion when encountering patients with abdominal trauma.

Abdominal trauma may result from blunt or penetrating forces. People involved in automobile accidents and pedestrians who have been struck by a vehicle account for most cases of blunt trauma to the abdomen, which has a significant mortality rate. Other common causes of abdominal trauma are blows to the abdomen and falls. Many deaths from abdominal trauma occur before the patient receives surgical intervention.

Penetrating injuries may result from stab wounds or missile injuries. Stab wounds are caused by assault with knives or other sharp objects, self-inflicted wounds, or impalement on objects following a collision or fall. Missile injuries may result from gunshot wounds, shotgun wounds, or explosive fragmentation devices.

The primary goal of prehospital care for abdominal injuries is to quickly recognize life-threatening injuries and provide rapid transport while administering essential life-support treatments en route. Most serious abdominal injuries require surgical intervention and cannot be stabilized in the field. In most regional EMS systems, a patient with a penetrating injury to the abdomen is a trauma center candidate.

Mechanism of Injury

The mechanism of injury is an important means of suspecting the presence of intra-abdominal injuries. Internal bleeding may not be obvious, and one must remain alert for signs of compensated shock. Tears or perforations of hollow organs can cause spillage of contents into the peritoneum, and signs of peritonitis may be present.

BLUNT ABDOMINAL TRAUMA

Blunt trauma may result in injuries from compression or deceleration type forces.

COMPRESSION INJURIES. Compression injuries occur when two opposing forces compress intra-abdominal organs, resulting in contusions, tears, or rupture. For example, in automobile accidents the unbelted driver may be thrown against the steering wheel, fixing the anterior wall of the chest and abdomen. As the rest of the body moves forward, the posterior abdominal wall and spine compress the intra-abdominal organs within. Solid organs such as the spleen, liver, and kidneys are fragile and highly vascular. When torn or ruptured, they can bleed profusely, causing hypovolemic shock. The pancreas, extending across both upper quadrants, can be compressed by the vertebral bodies. When hollow organs such as the stomach or intestines burst or are torn or ruptured, their contents may be spilled into the peritoneal cavity, resulting in severe inflammation and infection.

Compression of the abdominal contents can exert such pressure that the abdominal cavity itself is violated. One such example is rupture of the diaphragm, with the abdominal contents squeezed upward into the thorax.

DECELERATION INJURIES. Deceleration injuries result when organs or vessels tear at a point of attachment during a sudden cessation of motion.

After a car hits a wall and the occupant strikes the steering wheel or dashboard, the mobile organs within the body will continue to move. Initially, they all move at the same velocity. Their rate of deceleration and the distance they move depend on their relative mobility within the body, and these differences create shearing forces that can tear and rupture organs. For example, the liver, a relatively mobile organ, is attached to the abdominal wall by a fixed ligament (ligamentum teres). During deceleration, the liver continues to move beyond its supporting ligament and literally splits or tears over it (Fig. 8–25).

The kidneys are attached by the ureter and the vascular pedicle (carrying major vessels to the kidney) off the aorta and vena cava. With deceleration, shearing forces can cause tears in the renal artery (Fig. 8–26). The intestines and spleen are other organs within the abdomen affected by this type of injury.

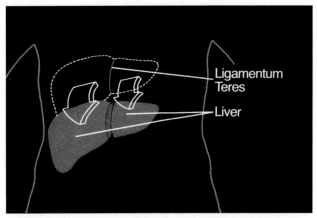

FIGURE 8–25. During deceleration the liver can tear over the ligamentum teres, which is attached to the abdominal wall. (From Prehospital Trauma Life Support, 2nd Ed. PHTLS Committee in cooperation with Committee on Trauma of the American College of Surgeons. McSwain NE Jr, Butman Am, McCornell WK, Vomacka, RW (eds). Copyright © Emergency Training, Akron, Ohio, 1990.)

Deceleration injuries can be deceiving, since there may be no external evidence of trauma to the abdominal wall.

SEAT BELT INJURIES. A properly applied seat belt is applied across the pelvis between the anterior-superior iliac spine and the femur at a 45-degree angle with the floor. If tight enough to remain in that position, the bony pelvis will protect soft organs within. If the seat belt is improperly positioned, forces can be transmitted to the abdominal wall, compressing the organs within (Fig. 8–27). Abrasions, contusions, and ecchymosis in a band across the abdominal wall are indications of the point of compression of a seat belt. If a lap belt is worn without a shoulder belt, it serves as a fulcrum for extreme flexion of the spine, and compression fractures of the T12 to L2 vertebrae can result. Even if the

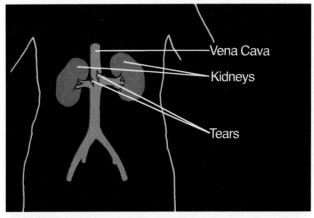

FIGURE 8–26. The vessels attached to the kidneys can tear at the point of attachment as the kidneys move forward during deceleration. (From Prehospital Trauma Life Support, 2nd Ed. PHTLS Committee in cooperation with Committee on Trauma of the American College of Surgeons. McSwain NE Jr, Butman Am, McCornell WK, Vomacka RW (eds). Copyright © Emergency Training, Akron, Ohio, 1990.)

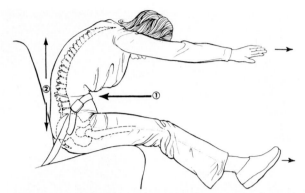

FIGURE 8–27. Lap belts can cause compression and injury of the bowel and other structures within the abdomen during deceleration. (From Connolly JF: DePalma's The Management of Fractures and Dislocations: An Atlas. Philadelphia, WB Saunders, 1989, p. 76.)

seat belt is properly worn, one must be concerned about deceleration forces on internal organs.

PENETRATING INJURIES

Stab wounds can range in severity from simple superficial punctures and lacerations of the skin to penetration of major organs and vessels.

The structures that are punctured or lacerated are determined by the location of the wound, the size of the object, and the direction at which it entered the abdominal cavity. Obviously, objects that puncture major vessels such as the aorta or vena cava are more likely to result in massive blood loss and death. It is important to know what instrument caused the stabbing. When possible, you should bring the object to the emergency department to assist the physician in determining the extent of injury.

You should always be highly suspicious that there is internal bleeding. A small puncture may appear benign and lull the EMT into underestimating the extent of injury.

MISSILE INJURIES. Missile injuries are generally more severe than stab wounds. In gunshot wounds, the muzzle velocity or speed at which the bullet travels is the major factor in determining the severity of injury and an important part of the history of the event as obtained by the EMT. Handguns have muzzle velocities of from 500 to 1,500 feet per second, as compared to military or large game hunting rifles, which have muzzle velocities of from 2,000 to 3,000 feet per second. As the bullet travels through the body, kinetic energy is displaced to the surrounding tissues, creating a zone of injury that radiates out from the penetrating cavity. The greater the velocity, the greater the kinetic energy and the larger the zone of injury. Figure 8–28 illustrates the difference in the zone of injury when comparing medium-velocity to high-velocity weapons.

The distance of the weapon to the victim also

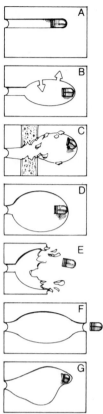

FIGURE 8–28. The zone of injury resulting from a medium-velocity versus a high-velocity weapon. (A) Low velocity, no cavitation, entrance and exit small. (B) Higher velocity, formation of cavity, arrows show direction and magnitude of acceleration of tissue. (C) Velocity as in B, but deformation of bullet and creation of secondary missiles upon penetrating bone. (D) Very high velocity, large cavity, and small entrance. Exit may be small. (E) Very high velocity, thin target, large and ragged exit. (F) Velocity, caliber, and thickness of tissue such that cavitation occurs deep inside, and entrance and exit are small. (G) Asymmetric cavitation as bullet begins to deform and tumble. (From Cardona VD, Hurn PD, Mason PJB, et al: Trauma Nursing from Resuscitation Through Rehabilitation. Philadelphia, WB Saunders, 1988, p. 118.)

determines the extent of injury. This in large part is due to the loss of velocity during the flight of the missile.

Finally, the location of the wound and trajectory of the bullet also affect the severity of the injury. However, it is extremely difficult to determine the path of a bullet or other missile since it may ricochet off bone and travel from the abdomen to the chest. You should carefully check for entrance and exit wounds when evaluating gunshot or other missile wounds.

Questions to ascertain are what type of weapon was used? What was the distance from the victim? How many shots were fired?

Patient Assessment

Since the primary injury is often hidden within the abdominal cavity, the evaluator must rely on two major factors to identify life-threatening problems: the mechanism of injury and early signs of hypovolemic shock.

MECHANISM OF INJURY

Because of the mechanism of injury, some patients will be identified as trauma center candidates, with rapid evaluation and transport the high priorities. Obtaining the mechanism of injury must be included as part of your scene assessment and patient evaluation. Someone who has fallen from a height of 20 feet or who has been shot in the abdomen need not exhibit signs of shock to be treated as having a severe injury. Often, you should rapidly transport such a patient to the local trauma center purely on the basis of the mechanism of injury. This allows for early application of definitive care in the emergency department or the operating room.

Record the mechanism of injury with sufficient details to allow hospital personnel to reconstruct your observations from the scene. Include time of injury and particular circumstances, as warranted. For example, in car accidents it is important to estimate speed, type of car, type of collision (head-on, lateral, roll-over) and deformities to the car, position of the victim in the car, whether the victim was belted, and particular damage noted to the victim's compartment (e.g., steering wheel broken, sign of collision on windshield, and so forth).

SIGNS OF HYPOVOLEMIA

The early recognition of internal bleeding relies on careful assessment during the primary survey. Delayed capillary refill, pale and sweaty skin, and rapid breathing and tachycardia are the early signs of shock, as discussed in Chapter 5. Hypotension and altered mental status are late signs of shock. Both require immediate hospital intervention.

What are the patient's complaints? Early bleeding may not cause peritoneal signs. Is the patient experiencing nausea or vomiting? What is the position of the patient? With penetrating trauma, expose the patient and look for entrance and exit wounds. If possible, reconstruct the scenario with a mind toward the type of weapon, distance, and trajectory of gunshot wounds and, for stab wounds, the type and size of instrument, angle of penetration, and position of the victim and assailant during the stabbing.

With blunt trauma, look for bruises, tire marks, and seat belt marks on the abdominal wall. Broken bones raise the suspicion of significant internal injury. Evaluate the ribs, especially noting fractures over the liver or spleen. Apply firm gentle pressure inward and then backward on the iliac crests and press on the symphysis pubis. If you feel movement of the pelvic bones, stop; movement is evidence of a pelvic fracture. Pelvic fractures

can cause significant blood loss as well as injury to pelvic organs. Is there a scrotal hematoma or blood on the penile meatus indicating a possible tear of the urethra?

Palpate the abdomen, noting tenderness and guarding in the four quadrants.

Be aware that signs of severe injury can be masked for multiple reasons. Often patients in accidents are intoxicated. There may be associated head injuries or spinal injuries with loss of pain perception and the normal sympathetic nervous system response to hypovolemia. Some studies suggest some patients with abdominal injuries may exhibit a vagal nerve response that blunts a tachycardia in response to blood loss. Is the patient elderly or on beta blockers? Age and certain drugs can limit heart rate. All these facts are important to ascertain when evaluating the patient.

Is there pain outside the abdomen, as may occur with splenic rupture and shoulder pain?

Take an ample history, noting allergies, medications, past medical history, last meal, and the events leading up to the trauma.

SPECIAL CONSIDERATIONS

EVISCERATION. Evisceration is the presence of abdominal contents, usually intestines, protruding through a laceration of the abdominal wall (Fig. 8–29). It occurs after slash injuries, where a large opening is created in the abdomen. Do not attempt to introduce the organs back into the abdominal cavity. Cover exposed organs with a moist sterile dressing or an airtight dressing to prevent the exposed bowel from drying out.

To make a moist dressing, use a large sterile multitrauma dressing moistened with sterile saline, and apply around the exposed organs (Fig. 8–30). Cover the moist dressing with a dry multitrauma dressing and tape it in place. To secure an airtight dressing, wrap the exposed bowel loosely with aluminum foil or plastic wrap and secure all edges with tape to prevent air from entering the dressing (Fig. 8–31). Transport the patient in the supine position with hips and legs flexed, placing a pillow under the knees to help maintain this position.

URINARY TRACT INJURIES. Urinary tract injuries can manifest with various presentations. Kidney injuries are suspect with bruises over the flank. There may be blood in the urine. If microscopic blood is present, it will not be apparent to the naked eye, but the urine can be tested at the hospital. Injuries to the pelvis can cause bladder or urethral tears. There may be blood at the penile meatus or a scrotal hematoma (Fig. 8–32), evident by black or bluish discoloration of the scrotum caused by blood extending downward through anatomic planes. If these signs are evident, the patient should avoid urinating until he receives hospital evaluation.

Direct injuries to the male genitalia can result in

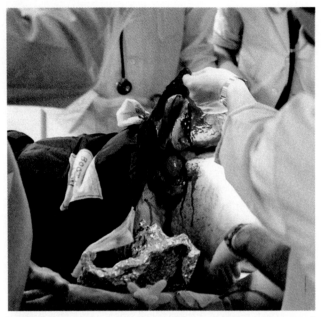
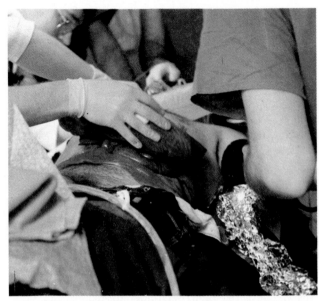

FIGURE 8–29. Evisceration caused by a self-inflicted slash wound across the abdomen. The patient also inflicted other stab wounds, causing internal hemorrhage. Prehospital treatment included covering exposed bowel with an airtight dressing (using aluminum foil) and applying MAST trousers (legs only inflated) to treat hypovolemia. (Courtesy of P. Viccellio, MD)

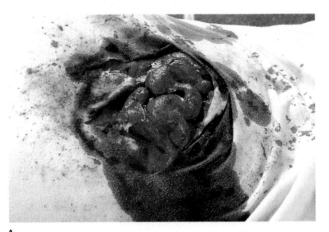

A

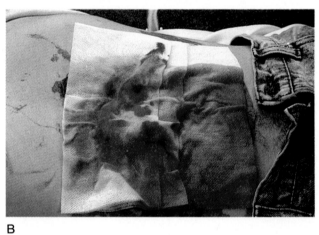

B

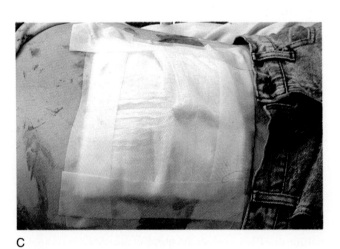

C

FIGURE 8–30. (*A*) Evisceration. (*B*) Place a moistened multitrauma around the exposed viscera, (*C*) cover with a dry, sterile dressing, and tape in place.

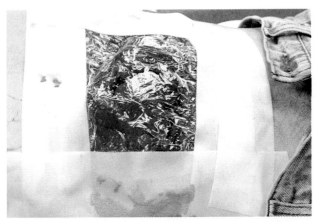

FIGURE 8–31. Wrap the exposed viscera in plastic wrap and tape completely around the border of the dressing to attain an airtight seal.

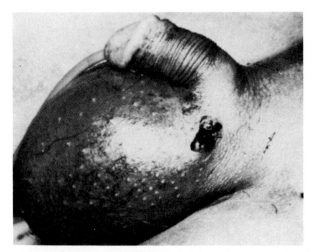

FIGURE 8–32. Scrotal hematoma. (From Wiener SL, Barrett J: Trauma Management for Civilian and Military Physicians. Philadelphia, WB Saunders, 1986, p. 262.)

lacerations, bruising, avulsion, or even amputation. Use direct pressure (moisten dressings applied to denuded or "skinned" areas) to control bleeding. Bring avulsed or amputated parts to the hospital after wrapping them in a moist sterile dressing and putting them into a plastic bag placed over ice. If genital skin is caught in a zipper, you may need to cut away part of the zipper around the entrapped skin.

Injuries to the female genitalia may manifest from direct trauma or straddle injuries—falling onto an object with the main force applied to the perineum. External bleeding may be present and should be controlled with direct pressure. Do not place dressings within the vagina. If necessary, dressings can be held in place with a triangular bandage. For blunt trauma in pregnancy, see Chapter 13.

Foreign bodies in the genitalia or urethra should be left in place for removal at the hospital.

In general, penetrating objects in the abdomen should be left in place and removed in the hospital. Stabilize the penetrating object with a stack dressing (see Chapter 9) on all sides of the object, secured by tape. If the victim is impaled on a fence post or other large object, it may be necessary to cut the object so that the patient can be moved with the impaled object stabilized in place.

Treatment of Traumatic Abdominal Emergencies

Treatment of major traumatic abdominal emergencies should be done within the hospital. Rapid transport and shock treatment may be required by some patients. Other factors to consider are listed in the following protocol.

✚ P R O T O C O L ✚

TREATING TRAUMATIC ABDOMINAL EMERGENCIES

1. *Treat the whole patient.* In the setting of multiple blunt trauma, immobilize the spine as indicated and treat life-threatening injuries.

2. *Maintain the airway,* especially in the presence of vomiting. Patients with altered mental status and vomiting should be positioned in the left lateral recumbent position, with suction on standby to aid in keeping the airway clear en route. For patients who are immobilized on a spine board, be aware that the patient may have to be turned as a unit if vomiting occurs. Suction must be available.

3. *Give high-concentration oxygen* if shock or peritoneal findings are present.

4. *Control external bleeding,* secure penetrating objects in place, and dress open wounds.

5. *Treat for shock if present.* Maintain body temperature, elevate legs, and consider the MAST.

6. *Position the patient* according to the need for spinal immobilization, airway maintenance, positive-pressure breathing, shock treatment, and comfort. Patients with abdominal injuries may find the most comfort from being transported supine, with hips and knees flexed. A pillow may be placed under the knees.

7. *Give nothing by mouth.* The patient with an abdominal emergency may require surgery.

8. *Complete the examination en route* to the hospital. Repeat vital signs as indicated. Record your findings.

9. *Select the hospital* by local protocols for trauma center candidates. Notify the hospital of the impending arrival.

Sexual Assault and Rape

Victims of sexual assault and rape need special consideration. Rape is usually defined as sexual intercourse against the will of the victim, often with force or threat of violence. Considerations beyond the medical needs of the patient include the need for psychological support and the preservation and collection of medicolegal evidence.

Rape and sexual assault may be accompanied by other injuries. Prioritize the medical response accordingly. However, from the beginning, remember that the job of EMTs is medical. Your role is never to act as a law enforcement officer. Your attitude must be exclusively that of a medical professional who shows empathy toward the plight of the victim.

PSYCHOLOGICAL CONSIDERATIONS

A rape or sexual assault victim has been subjected to a situation where control of his or her body has been taken away. It is important from the beginning to establish a relationship where the victim can regain control. Always explain your actions and only act with the victim's consent.

Unless there is an overwhelming need to examine the victim (e.g., to control profuse bleeding), the privacy of the victim should be maintained. Avoid exposing the victim's genital area. There is little to be gained from an examination in the field.

MEDICOLEGAL CONSIDERATIONS

Rape and sexual assault are crimes, yet in many states a victim (unless a minor) may refuse to press charges for many reasons. However, some evidence that may be present at the scene, such as semen on clothing or on the victim's skin, deteriorates with time. It is important to collect evidence that can then be saved, allowing the victim to decide at a later date whether to pursue the matter through the legal system. Thus, some aspect of control is returned to the victim and, by collecting the biological evidence, future options are preserved.

Rape and sexual assault victims require special care on the part of EMT. To restore the victims' sense of control, respect their wishes, explain your actions, and examine and treat with their consent. Urge them to accompany you to the hospital where full examination and treatment can be instituted. Psychological support begins with you and continues through the emergency department, with referral to community counseling services and specially trained personnel. Preserve evidence so that criminal prosecution is not hampered should the victim press charges. First and foremost, act as a medical professional.

EMT GUIDELINES IN CASES OF SEXUAL ASSAULT

- Preserve the patient's privacy as much as possible. Clear away crowds or bystanders.
- Questions should be medical and directed to obtain information to treat the patient. Do not ask questions about the assault itself beyond what is needed to institute care for the patient. A detailed history can be taken at the hospital by hospital staff and law enforcement personnel. If the patient recounts events of assault, record the patient's statements just as they are given as in "patient states 'I was raped. . . .'" Be precise. Your record will probably be scrutinized should the patient press charges, and you may be called on to testify in court. Remember, your job is that of a medical professional; you are not a legal or police authority.
- Ask the victim to come to the hospital for proper examination, treatment, and preservation of evidence. Advise the patient not to urinate, defecate, wash, shower, brush teeth, or douche prior to examination, as evidence may be lost.
- Clothing discarded at the scene should be collected and placed in a bag with as little handling as possible. Clothing may contain semen, blood, hairs, or other evidence that may help identify the rapist.
- Maintain a chain of custody of any gathered evidence. Evidence that is collected should be under the direct observation or control of the EMT or otherwise placed in a secure locked compartment. When turned over to the hospital or legal authorities, it should be signed for on the patient care record to document the chain of custody. Later, if the materials are introduced as evidence in a court of law, this documentation will aid in identifying who had control of the material.

  If for some reason, evidencial material is handed from one prehospital provider to another, written notation should be made of the transfer so that the chain of custody is documented.
- If the patient evaluation and treatment take place at the crime scene, interfere as little as possible with the scene, being careful not to litter unnecessarily with wrappings of dressings and other materials used in the care of the patient.
- *Impaled* objects in the urethra, vagina, or rectum should be treated as you would other impaled injuries, with the object left in place to tamponade possible internal bleeding and to be removed in the hospital.
- If the patient refuses care, respect his or her wishes. In rape or sexual assault cases, it is important to leave the patient with a friend or other person who can offer comfort and support. It is also important to give the victim the contact number for the local rape counseling center.

Summary

The assessment and management of abdominal emergencies represent a unique challenge to the EMT. Since the abdominal cavity has the ability to store great quantities of blood, you must maintain a high index of suspicion about internal bleeding. Vital signs should be monitored frequently; and rapid transport should be initiated when early signs of hypovolemic shock appear.

REVIEW EXERCISES

1. Define acute abdomen.
2. List five types of abdominal emergencies.
3. List the borders of the abdominal and pelvic cavities.
4. State the differences between visceral and somatic pain.
5. List the structures of the digestive system and describe their functions.
6. List the structures of the urinary system and describe their functions.
7. List the structures of the male and female reproductive systems and describe their functions.
8. List five signs and symptoms of an acute abdomen.
9. List the general steps of treatment for a patient with an acute abdomen.
10. Demonstrate care of a patient with the following trauma to the abdomen:
    Evisceration
    Impaled object
    Blunt abdominal trauma
11. Describe emergency care of injuries to male and female genitalia.
12. List the basic steps in the management of a victim of sexual assault.

REFERENCE

Bates B: *A guide to physical examination*, Philadelphia, 4th ed. JB Lippincott, 1987.

Eisenberg MS, Copass MK: *Emergency medical therapy*, 3rd ed. Philadelphia, WB Saunders, 1988.

Ellis H: *Clinical Anatomy: A revision and applied anatomy for clinical students*, 4th ed. Philadelphia, FA Davis, 1969.

Guyton AC: *Textbook of medical physiology*, 8th ed. Philadelphia, WB Saunders, 1990.

McSwain NE, Kerstein MD: *Evaluation and management of trauma*. Norwalk, Appleton-Century-Crofts, 1987.

PHTLS Committee in cooperation with Committee on Trauma of the American College of Surgeons, McSwain WE Jr, Butman Am, McConnell WK, Vomacka RW (eds): *Prehospital Trauma Life Support*, 2nd ed. Akron, OH, Emergency Training, 1990.

Rosen P, et al (eds): *Emergency medicine: concepts and clinical practice*, 2nd ed. St. Louis, CV Mosby, 1988.

Schwartz GR, et al: *Principles and practice of emergency medicine*, 2nd ed. Philadelphia, WB Saunders, 1986.

Schwartz SI, et al: *Principles of surgery*. New York, McGraw-Hill, 1969.

Soper RG, et al: *EMT manual*. Philadelphia, WB Saunders, 1984.

Swartz MH: *Textbook of Physical Diagnosis: History and Examination*. Philadelphia, WB Saunders, 1989.

Williams PL, Warwick R (eds): *Gray's anatomy*, 36th ed. Philadelphia, WB Saunders, 1980.

Zuidema GD, et al (eds): *The management of trauma*, 4th ed. WB Saunders, 1985.

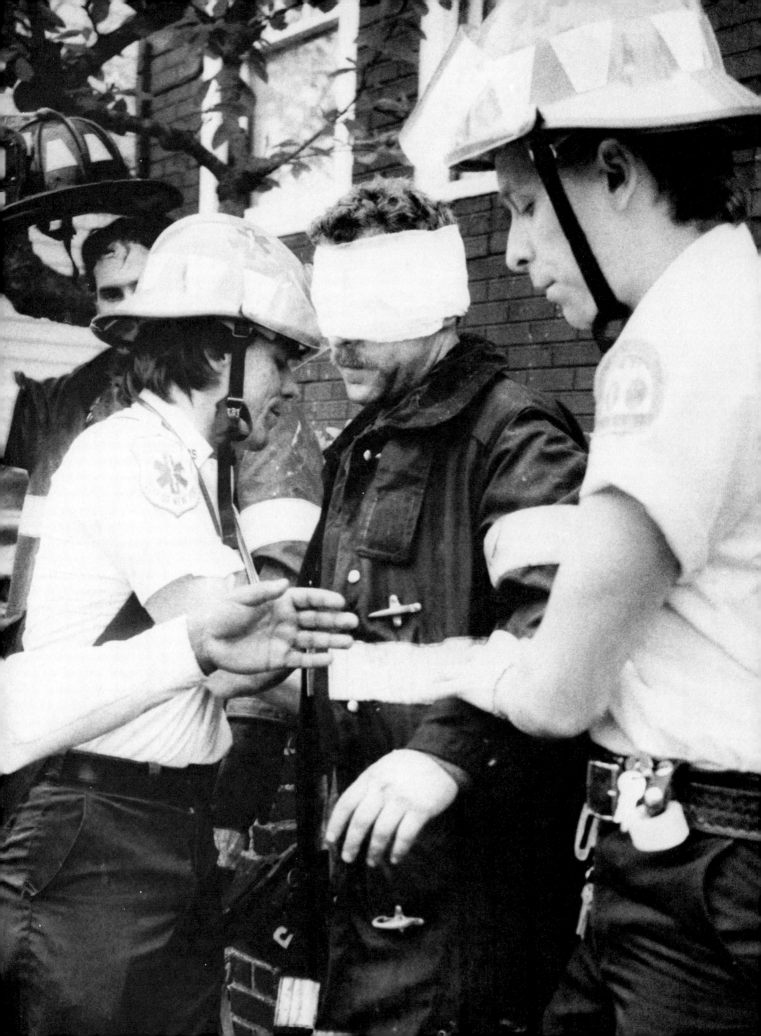

CHAPTER 9

SOFT TISSUE INJURIES

OBJECTIVES

At the conclusion of this chapter the reader will be able to:

1. Define dermis, epidermis, and mucous membranes.

2. Describe the proper handling of amputated or avulsed parts and impaled objects.

3. Demonstrate how to apply the following:
   Roller bandage
   Head bandage
   Bandage for the chest and back
   Bandage for the knee and elbow
   A dressing to an impaled object

4. Describe three common sites of facial fractures and how to recognize each.

5. Give two causes of traumatic nosebleeds and two causes of nontraumatic nosebleeds.

6. Describe how to remove foreign bodies from the eye.

7. List the three sections of the ear and give a brief description of each.

8. Describe how to manage bleeding injuries to the neck.

INTRODUCTION

Almost all trauma patients suffer injury to the skin and soft tissues at the point of impact. The soft tissues include the skin, the subcutaneous layer of fat and connective tissue beneath the skin, and the skeletal muscles, tendons, and ligaments. Injuries to the soft tissue are classified as open or closed. With open injuries the skin is broken. Closed injuries imply that the skin remains intact.

This chapter focuses on the *general* care of closed and open wounds to the skin and soft tissues and on techniques of wound dressing and bandaging. The management of soft tissue injuries to specific body areas is included in the respective chapters of this text.

To appreciate the consequences of damage to the skin and the layers of tissue beneath, one requires some understanding of its anatomy. Soft tissue injuries themselves are usually not life threatening. However, they may suggest the existence of more serious injuries to underlying organs or major blood vessels. Therefore, one should look to the skin in conjunction with the mechanism of injury for clues to the type of trauma sustained and possible underlying injuries.

ANATOMY AND PHYSIOLOGY OF THE SKIN AND SOFT TISSUES

The skin is the largest organ of the body, providing a protective covering and insulation. It separates the internal from the external environment. It is a *barrier to infection and loss of body fluids and is important for regulation of body temperature.*

Layers of the Skin

THE EPIDERMIS

The skin has two major layers, the epidermis and the dermis, which rest on the subcutaneous tissue (Fig. 9–1). The surface or outermost layer is called the *epidermis*. It is nonvascular and made up of four separate sublayers. The epidermis is impermeable which means it cannot be penetrated by microorganisms, and it is also responsible for preventing water loss from the cells underneath. The most superficial layer of the epidermis is dead tissue that is constantly rubbed or flaked away and replaced by the living cells underneath, which migrate upward. The layers of the epidermis become filled with a protein called keratin as they move upward toward

the skin surface. This protein is partly responsible for the skin's impermeable barrier.

The epidermis is also responsible for the color of the skin. It contains a special pigment called melanin, which helps protect the body from the sun's radiation. This pigment contributes to the color of the skin and is produced deep within the layers of the epidermis.

Skin color is also influenced by the blood flow in the skin capillaries contained within the dermis. Increased flow, as occurs in a hot environment, causes the skin to have a pink appearance. When blood flow to the skin is reduced (as a result of vasoconstriction in hypovolemic shock or in cold temperatures), the skin may appear pale.

THE DERMIS

The *dermis* is composed of dense connective tissue that contains the nerves, blood vessels, sweat and sebaceous glands, and hair follicles. The connective tissue gives strength to the skin and serves to anchor and support the other structures. The nerves in the dermis have various specialized endings that can perceive different sensations such as pressure, vibration, pain, warmth and cold, and so forth. If this layer of skin is completely damaged, as occurs in third-degree burns, there will be no sensory perception. The blood vessels within the dermis play an important role in temperature regulation. They can constrict to prevent heat loss to the environment and dilate when the body needs to give off heat.

The sweat glands play an important role in the regulation of body temperature as well. Evaporation is an important means of cooling, particularly in extremely hot environments or when there is a rapid buildup in internal heat production (as in exercise). The sebaceous glands secrete an oily substance called sebum, which helps moisturize the skin. The sebaceous glands are located near the hair follicles, which guide the sebum out to the surface of the skin where the oily substance spreads out. Hairs grow from these hair follicles, which are located within the dermis. Injuries that spare part of the dermis may allow for regrowth of new skin from cells that make up the hair follicles and sweat glands. Burns that destroy all structures within the dermis require skin grafting.

MUCOUS MEMBRANES

As skin continues into a body orifice, it changes its character. The keratinized layer of the epidermis is absent and is replaced by mucous membranes. Mucous membranes line the internal surface of the body such as the oropharynx, nasopharynx, ureters, bladder, lungs, intestines, and vagina. This membrane is rich in mucous glands, which secrete a lubricating fluid (mucus) to protect the body from invading organisms.

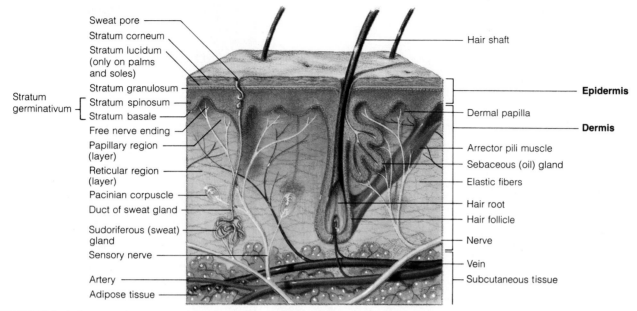

FIGURE 9–1. Layers and structures of the skin. (From Gaudin AJ, Jones KC: Human Anatomy and Physiology. Orlando, Harcourt Brace Jovanovich, 1989, p. 101.)

SUBCUTANEOUS TISSUE

Beneath the skin is a layer of fat and connective tissue called the subcutaneous tissue. It serves as a body insulator, and the fat can be utilized for energy as needed. Beneath the subcutaneous tissue is the fascia, a fibrous membrane covering that separates the subcutaneous tissue from the skeletal muscles. When we discuss burns, knowledge of the skin and subcutaneous layers will be central in the determination of their severity and complications. Table 9–1 lists the layers and functions of the skin.

WOUNDS

Wounds are considered to be either open or closed. Closed wounds are the result of blunt forces that do not break the integrity of the skin. Open wounds, by definition, are those in which the skin surface is broken.

Closed Wounds

When blunt or compression forces are applied to the skin, the capillaries or larger vessels may leak or rupture. This may be accompanied by slight swelling from leakage of plasma (edema) into the injured area. There may be tenderness or pain at the site of injury. This type of injury is commonly referred to as a bruise or *contusion*.

Contusions can be accompanied by leakage of blood from injured vessels. This bleeding may be visible just under the skin as a black and blue area and is called *ecchymosis*. The color changes to greenish brown and then to yellow over time, as the blood products break down and are absorbed. When blood *collects* beneath the skin it is known as a *hematoma* (literally a tumor or swelling containing blood) (Fig. 9–2).

Open Wounds   *Test wounds*

Any wound that results in a break in the skin is referred to as an open wound. There are several types of open wounds that range from a slight scraping of the

TABLE 9–1. Layers and Functions of the Skin   *test*

Layer	Function
Epidermis	
Outer layer (keratin)	Protective barrier to infection; prevents water loss
Melanin	Protects from sun's radiation
Dermis	
Blood vessels	Body temperature regulation; constricts to conserve heat; dilates to remove heat
Nerve endings	Sensation
Sebaceous glands (sebum)	Moisturize
Sweat glands	Temperature regulation; cools via evaporation
Hair follicles	Guides sweat and sebum to the skin surface
Subcutaneous layer	
Connective tissue and fat	Insulation; stores energy (fat)

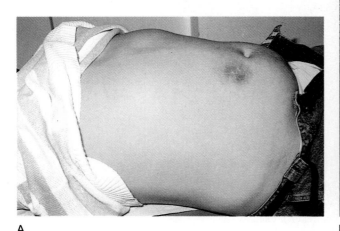

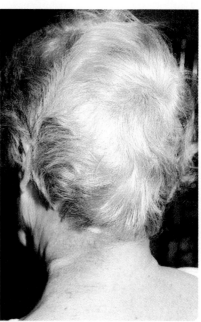

A   B

FIGURE 9-2. (*A*) Ecchymosis on abdomen caused by a kick to the abdomen one day prior. (*B*) Severe hematoma on occipital area of scalp is visible. This was caused by a fall 3 days before due to fainting. Note that blood under the scalp has gravitated down to the neck, causing ecchymosis along its path.

outermost layers of the skin to complete amputation of an extremity.

ABRASIONS

An abrasion is a scraping of the surface of the skin or mucous membrane. It may result in the breaking of superficial capillaries, causing an oozing of blood at the skin's surface. While often very painful, abrasions themselves do not usually result in significant blood loss but are subject, like other open wounds, to infection (Fig. 9–3*A*).

LACERATIONS

A laceration is a tearing of the skin or other soft tissues. It may occur as a result of a blunt tearing force or from a sharp object. The extent of surrounding tissue damage is a function of the mechanism of injury. Blunt forces that tear the skin may cause significant damage to the surrounding tissues. On the other hand, a very sharp object is more apt to cause an incision type wound and cause little damage to the tissue surrounding the wound (Fig. 9–3*B*).

AVULSION

An avulsion is a *tearing away of the skin's surface.* A complete avulsion injury may tear away a complete segment of skin. An incomplete avulsion occurs when the skin is torn back and a characteristic flap forms. This flap may be attached by a pedicle or small piece of skin.

This pedicle represents the remaining source of blood and nerve supply to the avulsed flap and should be handled carefully (Fig. 9–3*C*).

PUNCTURE

A puncture occurs when a sharp instrument is driven through the skin's outer layer. Punctures can be very deceiving. A small puncture wound may be caused by an object, such as an ice pick, that has penetrated to a significant depth, causing damage to underlying structures (Fig. 9–3*D*).

AMPUTATION

An amputation involves the *cutting away from the body of a limb or protruding structure.* Sharp or crushing forces may result in amputation (see Fig. 5–7*D*). Since the amputated part has no blood supply, the time to surgical intervention plus the care of the amputated part are important factors in successful replantation.

CRUSHING

Crushing injuries may result in both open and closed wounds. A crush injury is the result of the severe compressing force that damages and sometimes tears the soft tissues and underlying structures. An example would be a tire going over a leg, a finger caught in an old wringer-type washing machine, or an extremity caught in a meat grinder (Fig. 9–3*E* and *F*). Crushing injuries can cause significant damage to underlying structures.

Severity and Complications

The severity of a wound is dependent on the mechanism of injury, the site of injury, the extent of the injury, and the introduction of foreign bodies or contamination into the wound. It is important to consider damage to underlying structures, including blood vessels, nerves, ligaments, bones, joints, and organs within the body cavities. Common complications of wounds include bleeding, infection, and damage to underlying structures. Nerve damage, fractures, and injury to muscles, tendons, and ligaments may result in loss of function. Wounds over the major body cavities, the head, chest, and abdomen, carry the risk of damage to internal organs (Fig. 9–4).

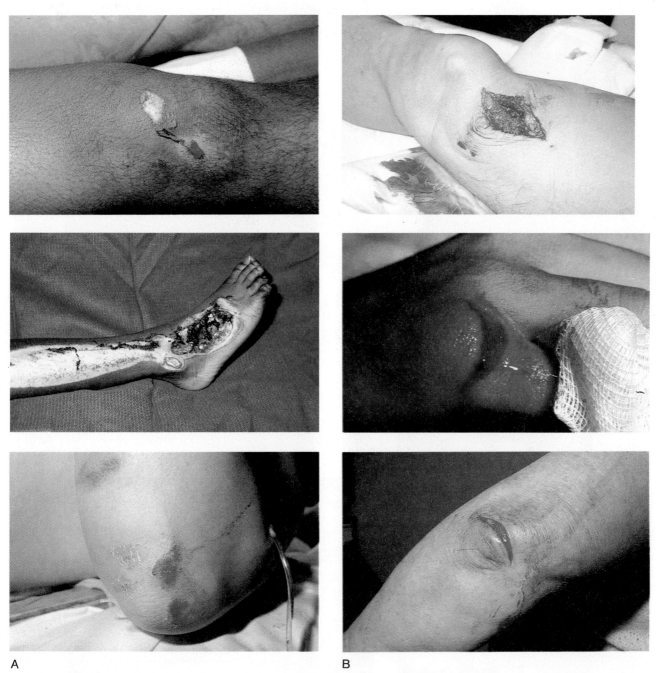

A   B

FIGURE 9–3. (*A, top*) Abrasion wounds of the kneecap caused by a fall to the ground after being struck by an automobile. (*A, center*) Deep abrasion through all levels of skin caused by being dragged by an automobile on the road. (*A, bottom*) Note severe abrasions, contusions of the elbow and arm of a patient struck by an automobile. (*B, top*) Deep laceration to the thigh caused by a circular saw. (*B, center*) Laceration over knuckle on the lateral aspect of the hand was caused when this person struck another in the teeth. Lacerations in this area suggest contamination from human bite wounds. (*B, bottom*) Laceration of the elbow caused by a fall on the street. *Illustration continued on following page*

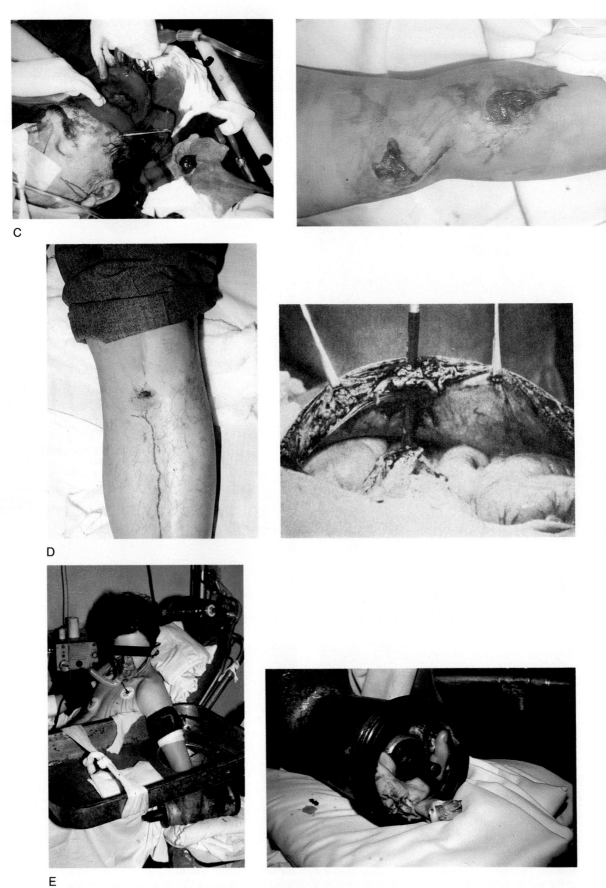

C

D

E

FIGURE 9–3. *Continued.* (*C, left*) A severe avulsion of the scalp caused by blunt trauma. (*C, right*) Avulsions over knee and lower leg. (*D, left*) Puncture wound of anterior lower leg. (*Right*) Puncture in the abdomen can result in significant damage to underlying structures. (*E*) Crush injury. A man with his arm caught in a meat grinder is brought to the hospital along with part of the grinder. (*D, right*, from Wiener SL, Barrett J: Trauma Management for Civilian and Military Physicians. Philadelphia, WB Saunders, 1986, p. 213.)

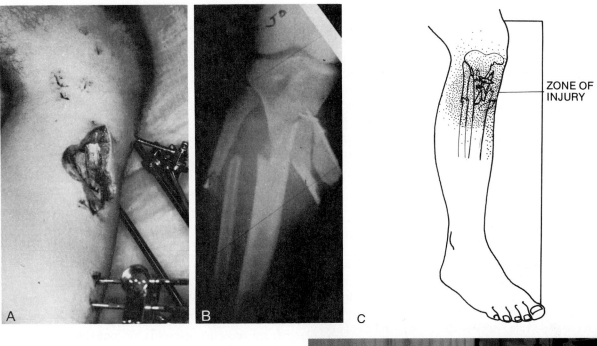

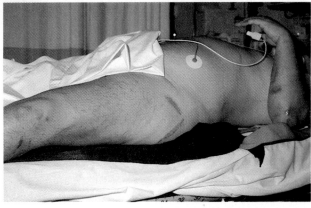

FIGURE 9–4. The extent of soft tissue damage will be determined by the mechanism of injury, location of the injury, and foreign bodies introduced into the wound. The illustration above depicts the (A) apparent soft tissue injury, (B) the x-ray film, and (C) the zone of injury resulting from a pedestrian being struck in the lower leg by a car bumper. (D) Constellation of external wounds seen on a patient struck by an automobile. External wounds raise suspicion of injuries to underlying organs and tissues. (A to C, from Zuidema GD, Rutherford RB, Ballinger WF: The Management of Trauma, 4th ed. Philadelphia, WB Saunders, 1985, p. 548.)

Assessment

A history of the mechanism of injury should be obtained. Life-threatening conditions take priority. Wounds that involve the airway or result in external hemorrhage should be recognized and treated during the primary survey. Consideration of the location of the wound may suggest underlying organ damage or internal bleeding. In the case of missile wounds, look for exit wounds. If there is loss of function, consider damage to bones and muscles as well as to nerves and vessels. Check for neurovascular function distal to the injury, and record your findings.

Management

Procedures employed in wound management include control of bleeding, prevention of further contam-
ination, immobilization of the affected part, preservation of avulsed or amputated parts, and stabilization, in place, of all impaled objects except those lodged in the cheek.

BLEEDING CONTROL

Control of bleeding should be accomplished by direct pressure, elevation, use of pressure points, and, if all else fails, the application of a tourniquet. The extent of blood loss (both internal and external) should be assessed along with a search for signs of hypovolemic shock.

Do not underestimate the significance of external blood loss in infants and small children. What would be a minor blood loss for an adult could be lethal for a small child. Control bleeding and estimate the significance of any external blood loss with consideration for the size of the child. Be sure to make an effort to reassure the child and explain your actions as much as possible.

Remember that infants have a blood volume of 80 to 100 ml per kilogram of body weight. Therefore an 11-lb, or 5-kg, baby has a total blood volume of 500 ml.

With closed wounds, little care may be necessary for minor bruises. However, with larger contusions accompanied by swelling or hematomas, counterpressure via pressure dressings may be used to prevent further bleeding beneath the skin. Application of ice or cold packs may reduce further swelling by vasoconstriction of the underlying vessels. Elevation of the extremity may cause some pain relief and minimize further swelling by its gravitational effect on blood flow. If a patient complains of pain on movement, splinting of the extremity may be appropriate, especially if a fracture is suspected. Patients should minimize their activity and movement.

Open wounds must be covered to control bleeding and minimize infection. When needed, a bulky dressing may be applied to help focus the direct pressure over the wound and to absorb heavy bleeding. Always think about the underlying organs and the mechanism of injury. As mentioned earlier, a patient is usually at greatest risk from the associated injuries, not those to the soft tissues themselves.

INFECTION

All open wounds are subject to infection. Sterile dressings should be applied when possible. In general, deeper wounds should not be washed or irrigated in the field. However, superficial abrasions that are particularly dirty may be washed gently with sterile saline or sterile water prior to dressing if there are no associated injuries of a critical nature and circumstances permit. Likewise, gross contamination and debris on avulsed flaps may be rinsed before dressing.

IMMOBILIZATION

Immobilization of the affected part serves to minimize blood flow to the immobilized area and thereby helps to reduce swelling. When feasible, elevation is used for a similar purpose. In addition, immobilization and elevation reduce pain. Check for fractures and splint any that are discovered.

PRESERVATION OF AVULSED OR AMPUTATED PARTS

In certain instances, a patient may have an avulsed portion of skin reattached to cover an open wound or even have reattachment of an amputated part. Retrieval and proper handling in the field of any separated body part increases chances of successful reattachment.

Avulsed flaps of skin must be handled gently to preserve the remaining blood supply to the flap. They may be returned to their normal anatomic position after irrigation of gross debris.

HANDLING OF AMPUTATED OR COMPLETELY AVULSED PARTS. Parts detached from the body remain viable for a few hours when left at room temperature. By cooling the part, it can remain viable for up to 18 hours. However, as with any body tissue, amputated or avulsed parts can suffer frostbite. To accomplish cooling without causing cold injury to the part itself, the severed tissue should never be placed directly on ice. Gross contamination of the detached part should be rinsed off with sterile saline or sterile water. The part should then be covered with a sterile dressing and placed in a watertight plastic bag. This bag should then be placed in another container with ice or ice and water, labeled, and transported with the patient to the hospital (Fig. 9–5).

IMPALED OBJECTS

When the EMT encounters an impaled object, he or she must act to avoid any complication to underlying structures. A knife or other type of impaled object may be implanted in such a way as to be actually occluding flow from a severed blood vessel and thereby acting to control bleeding (Fig. 9–6). Removal of such an object may precipitate active hemorrhage, which results in hypovolemic shock. Impaled objects should be stabilized in place to avoid such consequences unless the object is in the cheek. If the object is too large to be stabilized, it may be shortened.

SPECIAL CONSIDERATIONS

Wounds to the veins of the neck may lead to an air embolism. As changes in intrathoracic air pressure occur during breathing, air may be sucked into the veins during inspiration and travel through the bloodstream until the air bubble lodges in a smaller vessel. The trapped air embolism then obstructs distal blood flow. Patients are more prone to develop an air embolism if they are sitting and the wound is above the level of the heart. Such a wound should be covered with an occlusive dressing, and the patient should be transported in a supine position to reduce the chances of an air embolus (see Fig. 5–8A and B).

Chest wounds should also be covered with an occlusive dressing to prevent air from entering the pleural space.

DRESSINGS AND BANDAGES

A dressing is any material that covers a wound. It prevents introduction of further contamination into the

FIGURE 9–5. Amputated parts
should be carefully rinsed with sterile
saline or water, wrapped in sterile gauze
moistened with sterile saline and placed
in a plastic bag and transported on ice.

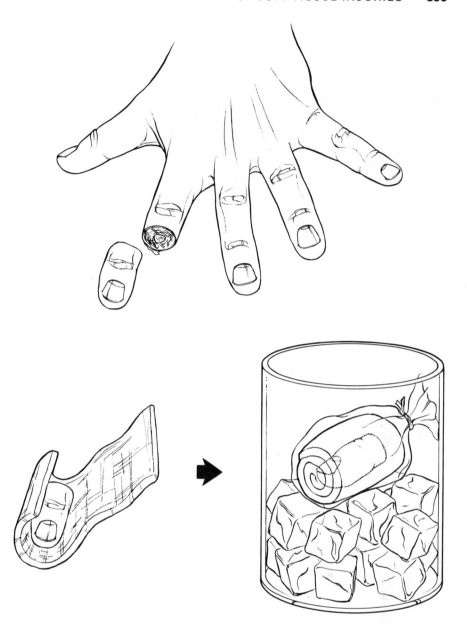

wound and aids in bleeding control. Ideally, a sterile
dressing should be used, but if one is not immediately
available, any clean material or even your gloved hand
should be used for initial control of blood loss. A bandage
is material used to secure a dressing in place and to
provide pressure over the dressing to aid in the control
of bleeding.

Dressings

Suitable dressings include any sterile material used
to cover a wound. There are many types available. The
basic dressing employs a sterile gauze or other absorbent
material that is applied directly to the wound. The dressing selected may vary in size and thickness according
to the wound. Wounds that cover a large surface area
such as extensive abrasions may require a *multitrauma
or universal dressing*. A universal or multitrauma dressing
is made of thick absorbent material, measuring 9 × 36
inches in size. It is folded upon itself and packed within
a sterile cover. This dressing is useful to cover large
areas such as abrasions or burns or for use as a pressure
dressing over long, open wounds. It is also useful as a
padding for splints.

Most punctures or lacerations can be effectively
covered with a *4 × 4 gauze dressing*. In instances where
occlusive or airtight dressings are needed, sterile plastic
wrap, sterile aluminum foil, or sterile petroleum-impreg-
nated gauze may be used. Some dressings, similar to

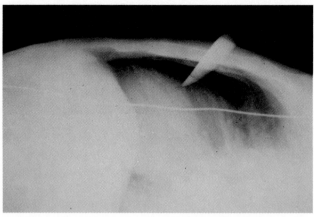

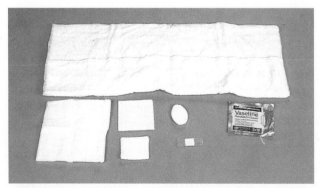

A   B

FIGURE 9–6. (*A*) Impaled knife in the anterior chest. Impaled objects are stabilized in place in the field with a bulky dressing. (*B*) Note on the x-ray film that the tip of the knife lies just short of the cardiac shadow. (Courtesy of Paul Krochmal, M.D.)

Band-Aids, come prepacked with *adhesive* around them and are ideal for small and minor wounds (Fig. 9–7).

Bandages

A bandage holds a dressing in place. It allows the EMT to attend to other tasks. It must be tight enough to control bleeding yet not so tight as to cut off circulation to the limb. There are various types of bandages.

SELF-ADHERENT BANDAGES

Self-adherent bandages come as rolls of slightly elastic, gauzelike material that can be wrapped around the dressing on the affected part or extremity. The self-adherent quality makes it easy to work with and allows for its rapid application. The elastic quality of this bandage helps in applying pressure to control arterial hemorrhage.

Ace bandages, which are used to support joints, should not be confused with self-adherent bandages. Ace bandages are much more elastic and, if not properly applied, result in uneven pressure to the limb and possible

complications from obstruction of distal blood flow and pressure on local nerves.

GAUZE ROLLER BANDAGES

The gauze roller bandage is a cotton and relatively nonelastic roller bandage that comes in various widths. It is most commonly used for extremity and head dressing applications.

TRIANGULAR BANDAGES

Triangular bandages are probably the most versatile of all bandages. Formed from cutting a 36- to 42-inch square of cloth (usually muslin) diagonally, the resulting triangle can be folded as necessary for multiple uses. This versatility allows for rapid application of direct pressure or support to almost any portion of the body. They may be used as a sling in the triangular form or may be folded and used as a cravat-type bandage. A cravat bandage, by definition, is simply a triangular bandage folded to form a band around an injured part. Triangular bandages are also used in the application of tourniquets.

ADHESIVE TAPE

Adhesive tape is utilized to secure self-adherent or roller bandages, occlusive dressings, or 4 × 4 (4-inch by 4-inch) squares of gauze. For small abrasions or less serious wounds, adhesive tape may be used to attach a dressing in place (Fig. 9–8).

AIR SPLINTS

For wounds on the extremities with associated fractures, or where immobilization is indicated, an air splint may be applied over a dressing and bandage. The air splint is an inflatable cylindrical tube. Air splints are available in various sizes to adapt to upper and lower

FIGURE 9–7. Common dressings used in prehospital care: Across the top, a multitrauma dressing. Below from left to right: a 4 × 8 inch surgical pad, 4 × 4 gauze and 2 × 2 sponges, eye patch and adhesive bandage, and petrolatum jelly gauze.

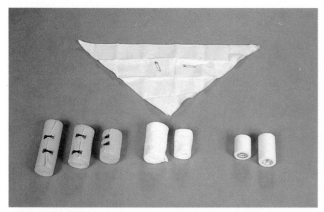

FIGURE 9–8. Common bandages used in prehospital care: Across the top, triangular bandages for slings and for holding splints in place. Across the bottom, elastic bandages, self-adherent bandages, and adhesive tape.

extremities. The pneumatic antishock garment (PASG) may be used in a similar fashion over the lower extremities and pelvis.

BLOOD PRESSURE CUFFS

In instances where added pressure is needed to control hemorrhage, a blood pressure cuff may be used as a bandage. The pressure of the cuff can be inflated until arterial bleeding is controlled. When using a blood pressure cuff or other tightly applied bandage, careful attention should be paid to <u>distal blood flow</u>. Again, *distal blood flow is evaluated by checking for the presence of a distal pulse and capillary refill.*

When applying a pressure dressing, follow the steps outlined in Procedure 9–1.

PROCEDURE 9–1 APPLYING A PRESSURE DRESSING

1. Cover the wound with the appropriate sterile dressing while applying firm pressure with your hand until the bleeding stops (Fig. 9–9A). If the bleeding continues, the dressing can be reinforced with more absorbent material and more direct pressure may be applied. In some cases it is advantageous to build up a bulky dressing over the wound to focus the pressure over the bleeding vessels (Fig. 9–9B).
2. Once bleeding is controlled, continue to apply pressure and attach a self-adherent or roller bandage around the affected part. Just enough pressure should be applied to control bleeding.
3. If bleeding recurs following application, additional dressings and bandages may be applied.
4. Following the application of the dressing and bandage, circulation <u>should be evaluated</u> by <u>checking for a distal pulse and capillary refill.</u>
5. Immobilize and elevate the affected part by using the appropriate splints and slings. If possible, care should be taken to <u>maintain sterility</u> during application of dressings and bandages.

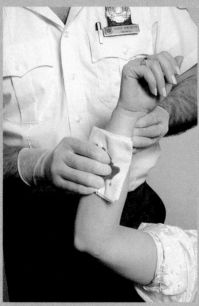

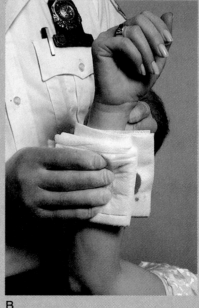

A   B

FIGURE 9–9. Applying a pressure bandage: (A) Apply direct pressure with a gloved hand and a sterile dressing, and elevate limb. (B) If bleeding continues, reinforce dressing with gauze or surgical pads, and apply direct pressure. Attach dressing with a bandage to hold in place. Applying pressure over a proximal artery (pressure point) may assist with bleeding control.

Methods of Bandage Application

There are many ways to attach dressings to various parts of the body—extremities, head, and trunk.

ROLLER BANDAGE

The roller bandage is the most common type of bandage used in prehospital emergency care. It comes in either self-adherent or gauze material and in various widths that are selected on the basis of the area to be bandaged.

P R O C E D U R E   9 – 2   **BASIC PRINCIPLES OF APPLYING A ROLLER BANDAGE**

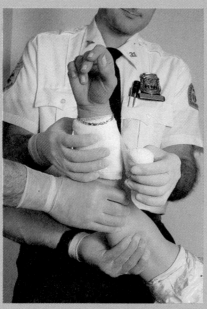

1. Working at a steady pace, roll the bandage evenly over the body surface. Maintain a uniform pressure during the application and avoid clumping of the bandage material.
2. After encircling the body part once, the bandage should be anchored in place by folding a corner end over the second layer of the bandage.
3. Cover the fold to prevent slippage with the next layer (Fig. 9–10).
4. Overlap the subsequent layers approximately halfway over the previous layer. The bandage should be tight enough to control bleeding but loose enough to allow distal blood flow.

Note: The EMT should be especially cautious when using self-adherent bandages which, because of their elastic quality, can become extremely tight.

5. Once the bandage is in place, attach the end with adhesive tape.

FIGURE 9–10. Basic principles of applying a bandage: Roll the bandage with the bulk of the roll facing away from the affected surface. Encircle the body part once and fold the corner of the bandage across the second layer. The next layer should cover the fold to anchor the bandage in place. Each subsequent layer should traverse the previous one approximately halfway across the width of the bandage. Attach the bandage in place with a piece of tape, and check for distal blood flow.

BANDAGE FOR THE EXTREMITIES

The bandages for the extremities are probably the simplest to apply. The cylindrical shape of the arm or leg lends itself to easy bandage attachment.

P R O C E D U R E   9 – 3
BANDAGING AN EXTREMITY

1. Using a simple roller bandage, anchor the bandage distally or proximally to the wound.
2. Rotate the bandage toward the wound while overlapping each previous layer halfway across the width of the bandage.
3. Once the bandage has covered the surface on both sides of the wound, reverse the direction and cover the wound again.
4. Attach the bandage in place.

PROCEDURE 9–4   APPLYING A HEAD BANDAGE

1. Apply gentle pressure to the wound with a flat hand (Fig. 9–11A).
2. Begin the head bandage by anchoring the bandage below the occipital protuberance (Fig. 9–11A to D).
3. (Circle the head completely once or twice.) Begin to traverse the bandage back and forth across the top of the head until the area with the dressing is completely covered (Fig. 9–11E and F).
4. Secure the bandage in place by circling the head once or twice and taping the bandage in place (Fig. 9–11G to H).

   Note: Application of this type of bandage takes two persons; the bandage is useful for isolated scalp lacerations where spinal injury is not suspected. In cases where rapid transport is indicated, delay at the scene to apply this type of bandage is not warranted.

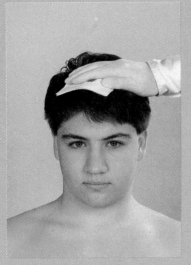

A

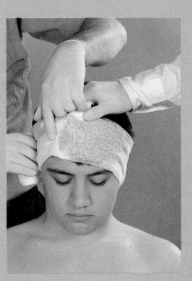

B

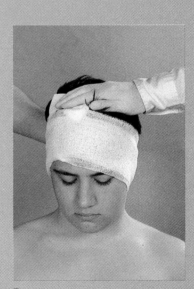

FIGURE 9–11. Applying a head bandage: (*A*) Apply direct pressure with a flat hand. (*B*) Circle the head once beneath the occipital prominence and across the forehead. (*C* and *D*) Anchor the bandage in place by folding a corner end of the first layer over the second layer and then circling once again, securing the anchor in place.

C

D

Continued

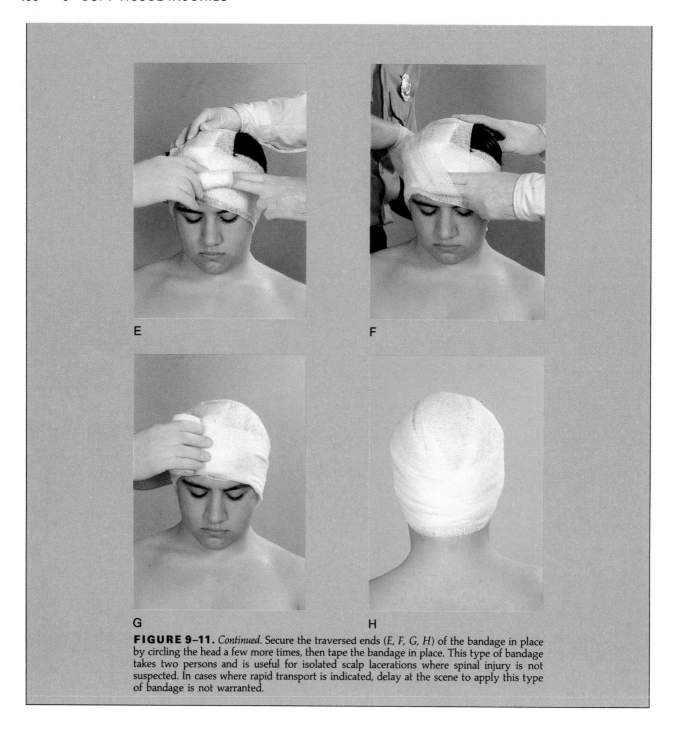

FIGURE 9–11. *Continued.* Secure the traversed ends (*E, F, G, H*) of the bandage in place by circling the head a few more times, then tape the bandage in place. This type of bandage takes two persons and is useful for isolated scalp lacerations where spinal injury is not suspected. In cases where rapid transport is indicated, delay at the scene to apply this type of bandage is not warranted.

BANDAGE FOR THE CHEST AND BACK

Most dressing applications to the chest and back can be done with tape across the skin's surface. However, at times the skin surface is sweaty or wet and it is difficult to attach tape. In these instances, a triangular bandage can be used. This bandage is used to hold dressings in place over abrasions or superficial wounds. When securing the bandage around the circumference of the chest, be careful not to exert excessive pressure that may restrict chest movement. Penetrating wounds require an occlusive dressing, and wounds with active bleeding require hand pressure.

PROCEDURE 9-5   APPLYING A BANDAGE TO THE KNEE OR ELBOW

The figure-eight bandage secures a dressing over a joint while at the same time allowing for mobility.

1. Start the roller bandage below the joint and anchor it in place (Fig. 9–12A).
2. Traverse the bandage diagonally across the joint over the dressing (Fig. 9–12B).
3. Circle the bandage above the joint. After circling the proximal portion, traverse downward to form an "X" over the dressing on the joint and continue this pattern until the bandage is complete (Fig. 9–12C to E).

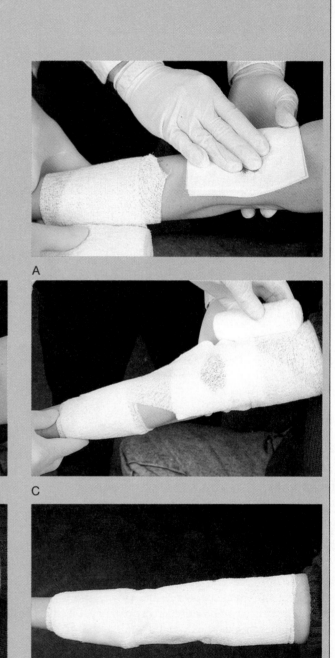

A

B

C

D

E

FIGURE 9–12. Applying a bandage over a knee or elbow: (A) Circle the extremity below the joint and anchor the bandage in place. (B and C) Traverse the joint diagonally over the dressing, and circle the extremity above the joint. (D) Traverse the extremity diagonally again, making an "X" with the bandage over the center of the joint. (E) Continue this pattern until the dressing is secure; then tape the bandage in place.

PROCEDURE 9-6 **APPLYING A DRESSING AND BANDAGES TO AN IMPALED OBJECT**

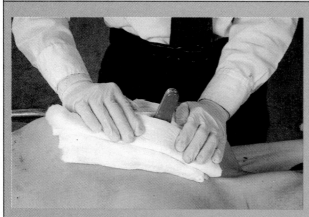

FIGURE 9-13. Stabilizing an impaled object: Place surgical pads or a multitrauma dressing on both sides of the impaled object to stabilize it in place.

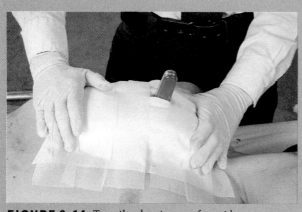

FIGURE 9-14. Tape the dressings on four sides.

1. Place a dressing around the impaled object (Fig. 9–13).

2. Place bulky pads such as multitrauma or universal dressings around the object and bandage them securely in place. The bulk should be sufficient to limit any movement of the impaled object (Fig. 9–14).

   Note: If the object is impaled in the *thoracic cavity*, an occlusive dressing should be utilized.

   Note: Never remove an impaled object unless it is penetrating the cheek. Objects impaled in the cheek should be gently removed since they may interfere with *airway/respiration*. If significant bleeding occurs in the cheek after removal, a dressing may be applied from within the mouth, with finger pressure applied to control bleeding (see Fig. 9–21).

INJURIES TO THE FACE AND SOFT TISSUES OF THE HEAD AND NECK

Your first concern when encountering a patient with injuries to the face and neck is the airway. The facial bones give structural support to the airway and loss of their integrity can compromise airway patency. Bleeding, foreign bodies, broken teeth and dentures, and vomitus can obstruct the air passage. Trying to maintain a clear airway in the presence of bleeding and foreign bodies is often difficult and may require use of many techniques. Manual extraction of foreign bodies, control of bleeding, suctioning, use of appropriate airway techniques, and positioning of the patient to permit drainage may all need to be employed in severe cases.

The face has a rich blood vessel supply, and injuries can cause extensive bleeding. Because the facial bones are part of the skull and offer protection to the brain, trauma to the face should cause the EMT to search for signs of injury to the brain and cervical spine. The facial bones also offer protection to the eye and the middle and inner ear, and the EMT must be able to institute special handling techniques for these sensitive organs.

Many vital structures are closely packed in the neck. The larynx and trachea, major arteries and veins, esophagus, and cervical spine are all prone to injury. Besides direct damage to these structures, an air embolism can result from a laceration of a major vein.

FACIAL INJURIES

Bones of the Face

The skull is composed of bones that form the cranium (encasing the brain) and the face itself. The major facial bone structures that the EMT should be familiar with include the *maxilla* (forming the upper jaw), the *mandible* (the lower jaw), and the *zygoma* (connecting the maxilla and the frontal and the temporal bones). The outer ridges of the eye socket, known as the orbit, are formed from edges of the maxilla, zygoma, and frontal bones. The nasal bones are the base from which the cartilage and soft tissues that make up the nose extend (see Figs. 7–2 and 7–5).

Soft Tissues

The skin covering the face is rich in blood vessels and nerves. While bleeding is often brisk from facial injuries, it is usually easily controlled with direct pressure. Nerves exit through foramen or small openings in the skull to innervate the muscles and skin on the face. Salivary glands that secrete saliva to aid in digestion are located on each side of the face below the ear and within the oral cavity. The facial muscles are complex and allow for facial expression and *mastication* (chewing). Because of the complexity of structures beneath the skin, careful handling is required (Fig. 9–15).

Fractures of the Facial Bones and Airway Compromise

The patency of the airway is maintained by the support of the facial bones. When the facial bones collapse following trauma, the traditional airway maneuvers may need to be modified. Standard techniques to open the airway rely on the structural integrity of the facial bones to lift the tongue forward. In the presence of facial fractures, the chin-pull maneuver and use of oropharyngeal or nasopharyngeal airways may be necessary. The head tilt is contraindicated if cervical spine fracture is suspected. In some cases, advanced airway maneuvers such as endotracheal intubation or cricothyroidotomy may be necessary to effectively secure or provide an airway.

Common causes of fractures of the facial bones include motor vehicle accidents; industrial accidents; falls; and domestic violence, including both missile wounds and blunt trauma.

Recognition of Facial Fractures. There are common sites where facial fractures tend to occur. Knowledge

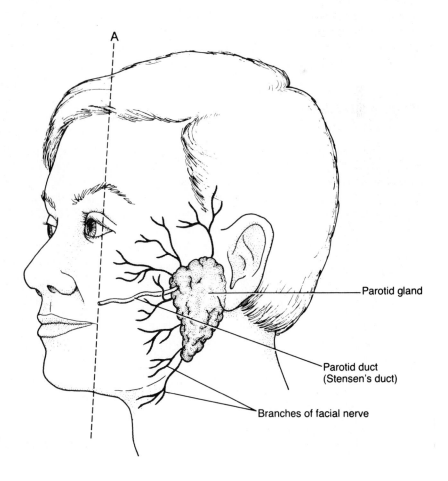

FIGURE 9–15. Laceration to the face may involve the parotid gland and duct and facial nerves and vessels. (From Kitt S, Kaiser J: Emergency Nursing: A Physiologic and Clinical Perspective. Philadelphia, WB Saunders, 1990, p. 123.)

Parotid gland

Parotid duct (Stensen's duct)

Branches of facial nerve

of these sites leads to appropriate assessment techniques to allow for early recognition of problems that may influence airway treatment.

Less force is needed to fracture facial bones than to fracture the frontal bone of the cranium. The most easily fractured are the nasal bones, which, because of their prominence and relative fragility, are the most common site of fracture in the body, after the wrist. The zygomas, the mandible, and the maxilla require a force of greater energy before fracture occurs. The frontal bones of the cranium require a significantly greater blow (Table 9–2).

Because force is absorbed by the collapse of facial bones following impact, less force is left to be transmitted to the brain. As stated by the American College of Surgeons:

> The facial skeleton is constructed so that, through sequential small bone failures, it can absorb a tremendous amount of impact energy while affording maximal protection against concussion of the cranial vault. (American College of Surgeons, Walt J (ed): Early Care of the Injured Patient, 3rd ed. Philadelphia, WB Saunders, 1980.)

For example, when the face is struck against the windshield in a high-speed automobile accident, sequential fractures of the nose, maxilla, or mandible dissipate the force imparted to the skull and the brain within. However, the airway may be compromised as a result of loss of structural support of the face and bleeding. The role of the EMT is to address the airway problems to avoid unnecessary deaths due to airway compromise.

COMMON SITES OF FRACTURES

MAXILLA. The maxilla is broken in high-speed impact accidents, where the face is thrown forward onto dashboards, windshields, or part of the steering wheel. There are points of weakness within the maxilla where fractures are most likely to occur. These were first described in 1901 by Le Fort and still carry his name. One or more Le Fort-type fractures may occur in a single patient.

Major sites of fractures include *Le Fort I*, a transverse fracture above the roots of the teeth, with instability of the upper teeth and the upper palate; *Le Fort II*, a fractured triangular segment containing the nasal bones and the frontal process of the maxilla, with instability of the nose as well as the upper teeth; and *Le Fort III*, with the fracture line extending through the maxilla, nasal bones, and zygomas, causing instability of the entire midface relative to the base of the skull (Fig. 9–16).

Sometimes with severe trauma, fractured segments of the mid-face are driven downward and impacted, causing depression of the face. Fractures may occur unilaterally and vary with the force and point of impact.

On inspection, a patient with mid-face fractures may

TABLE 9–2. Force Required to Cause Facial Fractures

	Measured in G
Nasal bones	35– 80
Zygoma	50– 80
Mandible	70–110
Central maxilla	129–180
Frontal bone	150–200

Study by Federal Aviation Agency to determine the impact forces following deceleration that produce fractures of the human face. From Edgerton and Kenney: Emergency care of maxillofacial and otological injuries. In Zuidema, GD, Rutherford RB, Ballinger WF: The Management of Trauma, 4th ed. Philadelphia, WB Saunders, 1985, p. 276.

appear to have an elongation of the mid-face with swelling and periorbital ecchymosis and edema (Fig. 9–17). Palpation may reveal tenderness and crepitus, as well as deformity. Asymmetry of the face should be noted. Instability of a segment can be assessed by gentle palpation; a Le Fort-type fracture should be suspected. Unstable mid-face fractures often are associated with damage to bones making up the base of the skull. Since both the nose and the base of the skull may be damaged when mid-face fractures are encountered, use of the nasopharyngeal airway in such cases is contraindicated.

MANDIBLE. Fractures of the mandible can cause severe airway problems. The mandible often breaks at more than one site following injury. The most common sites of fracture are shown in Fig. 9–18.

The patient with a mandible fracture may complain of pain in the jaw or problems with the teeth and be unable to bite properly. (Problems with alignment of the teeth can follow both maxilla or mandible injury.) Sometimes the patient's jaw may not close. Of greatest concern are fractures of the mandible that cause collapse of the airway. In these cases, the chin-pull (tongue-jaw lift) or insertion of an oropharyngeal airway may be required to keep the tongue away from the posterior wall of the pharynx. One may have to pull the tongue forward during the chin pull. If these maneuvers are not successful, then advanced airway maneuvers are of the highest priority (Fig. 9–19A to C and Fig. 2–27).

ORBITS. Fractures of the orbits of the eye may occur as isolated fractures or as part of a mid-face fracture. Fractures of the lower rim of the orbits can cause entrapment of the muscles that move the eye (see Eye Injuries later in this chapter). Figure 9–20 shows assessment for facial fractures. This examination should be performed in a gentle manner.

Bleeding and the Airway

Bleeding following injuries to the face is of great concern when the blood enters the airway and interferes

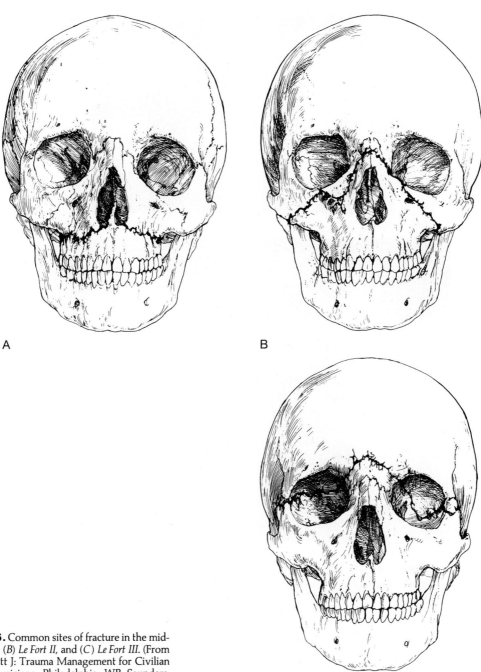

FIGURE 9–16. Common sites of fracture in the midface: (*A*) *Le Fort I*, (*B*) *Le Fort II*, and (*C*) *Le Fort III*. (From Wiener SL, Barrett J: Trauma Management for Civilian and Military Physicians. Philadelphia, WB Saunders, 1986, pp. 148–150.)

with ventilations. Blood, blood clots, loose teeth, or other foreign bodies should be removed from the airway with a finger sweep or suction. If no injury to the cervical spine is suspected, a conscious patient may be allowed to sit and should be encouraged to clear the airway by coughing. Unconscious patients may be placed in the lateral recumbent position with the head down to facilitate drainage. With possible cervical spine injury, attempts should be made to maintain cervical alignment while providing for airway clearance and drainage—as the situation dictates. Swelling and hematomas can form within the oral cavity and under the tongue, which may

compromise the airway and require advanced airway maneuvers. Partial compromise may evolve to severe compromise as swelling progresses.

BLEEDING FROM THE FACE. Bleeding from the face itself should be controlled with direct pressure. Bleeding within the oral cavity may also be controlled with direct pressure if it is within reach of your fingers. A rolled 4 × 4 gauze bandage can be pressed with the finger against oral lacerations, with counterpressure supplied by other fingers on the outside of the cheek. A rolled 4 × 4 gauze bandage, similar to that used in a

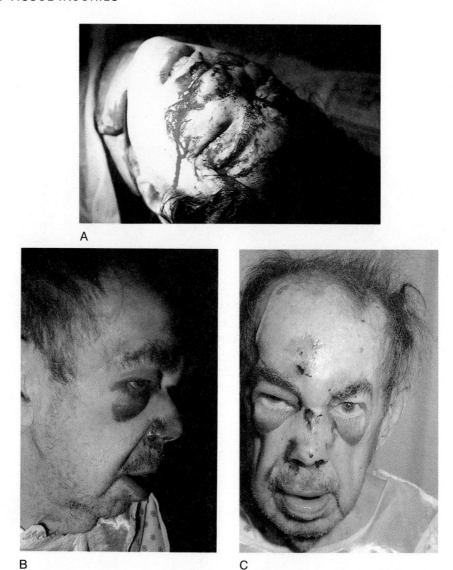

FIGURE 9–17. (*A*) A patient with severe mid-face trauma and avulsion of upper face. One must suspect mid-face fractures in such patients. (*B* and *C*) A man who suffered severe facial trauma after a fall. This man suffered orbital and nasal fractures. This pattern of ecchymosis (raccoon's eyes) may suggest basilar skull fracture.

dentist's office, can be placed between the cheek and gums of a conscious patient to control bleeding in that area.

Avulsions

Complete and deep avulsions of the facial skin with exposed underlying nerves, muscles, and tendons should be treated by placing a dressing moistened with sterile saline directly over the wound to prevent drying. Then a dry dressing and bandage should be applied over the moistened dressing to maintain bleeding control and prevent infection.

Avulsed parts (including teeth) should be rinsed of gross debris, placed in a moistened dressing, inserted in a watertight plastic bag, and, if possible, transported on ice or ice and water. Broken denture fragments should be brought to the hospital as well, since hospital staff

must assume aspiration of missing fragments unless all parts are accounted for.

Although facial lacerations can bleed briskly, they rarely are life threatening. If signs of hypovolemic shock are present, look carefully for other sites of blood loss.

Impaled objects in the cheek should be removed if

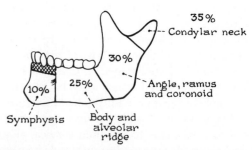

FIGURE 9–18. Common sites of fracture in the mandible. (From Zuidema GD, Rutherford RB, Ballinger WF: The Management of Trauma, 4th ed. Philadelphia, WB Saunders, 1985, p. 302.)

FIGURE 9–19. (*A* and *B*) Fractures of the mandible with posterior displacement may result in obstruction of the airway. (*C*) A tongue-jaw lift can be used to pull the tongue away from the pharynx. (From Zuidema GD, Rutherford RB, Ballinger WF: The Management of Trauma, 4th ed. Philadelphia, WB Saunders, 1985, p. 278.)

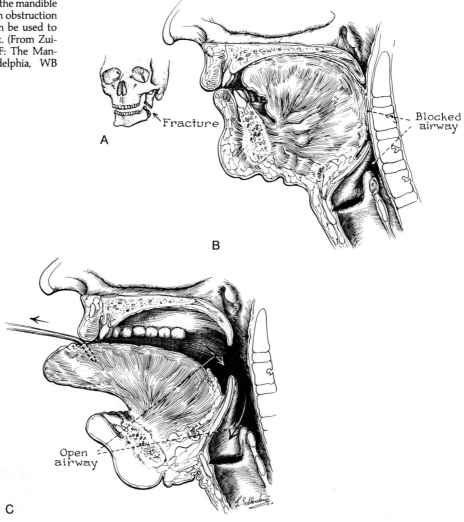

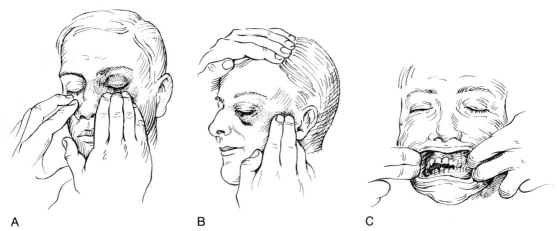

FIGURE 9–20. While examining the face you may note (*A*) irregularities or tenderness over the bones of the orbit, (*B*) deformity of the zygoma, and (*C*) a problem with alignment of the teeth, secondary to fractures of facial bones. (From Schultz RC: Facial Injuries, 2nd ed. Chicago, Year Book Medical Publishers, 1977.)

possible, since they may interfere with respiration. Gently try to pull the object back through the wound. Control bleeding as one would for other intraoral lesions (Fig. 9–21A to C). Do not use excessive force if resistance is encountered. Rather, control bleeding with the object in place, stabilize the object in place, and position the patient to allow for drainage if necessary.

Summary of Management

The primary concern for patients with facial injuries is patency of the airway. Conscious patients complaining of difficulty breathing, with noisy respirations, accessory muscle effort, or ineffective or absent air movement, require immediate attention to ensure an open airway. Assessment of the bony support of the face helps determine the need for special airway maneuvers. Patients with evidence of fracture of the mid-face should not have a nasopharyngeal airway inserted. Patients with fractures of the mandible may require use of the chin pull or insertion of an oropharyngeal airway to achieve forward displacement of the tongue. Blood and foreign debris in the airway must be cleared with a finger sweep and suction. The lateral recumbent position with the head

down may be necessary to allow for drainage. Supplemental oxygen should be given to any patient with signs of airway compromise. If the above measures are inadequate, then advanced surgical maneuvers to gain access to the airway take the highest priority.

Bleeding control is accomplished with direct pressure. Impaled objects that penetrate the cheek should be removed if possible. Since considerable impact forces are encountered in patients sustaining severe facial injuries, appropriate concern should be shown for the possibility of cervical spine fractures. Table 9–3 summarizes the problems and treatment of facial trauma.

INJURIES TO THE NOSE

The EMT is often called upon to manage patients with bleeding from the nose. Bleeding from the nose is one of the most common findings following nasal fractures. It also occurs from digital trauma in children and spontaneously in all age groups, but particularly among the elderly. Individuals with a history of bleeding disorders, liver disease, or medications that interfere with blood clotting may suffer serious nosebleeds and call for medical assistance. Although most nosebleeds are easily

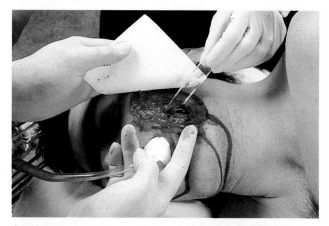

A

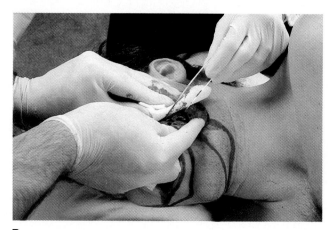

B

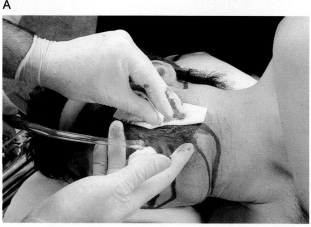

C

FIGURE 9–21. Management of an impaled object in the cheek. As the object is withdrawn, be prepared to control bleeding from the inside (*A*) and the outside (*B*) of the cheek. Manual control of bleeding may be required. (*C*) Keep suction ready.

TABLE 9–3. Treatment of Airway Problems in Patients with Facial Injuries

Problem	Treatment
Fracture	
Maxilla	Avoid use of nasopharyngeal airway
Mandible	Chin pull
	Oropharyngeal airway (if indicated)
Other	
Foreign bodies	Finger sweep and suction to clear blood, clots, loose teeth, etc.
Bleeding	Direct pressure with finger in mouth and counterpressure on outside of cheek
	Pressure points—facial and temporal arteries
Uncontrolled bleeding	Lateral recumbent position
Inadequate ventilations with above measures	Rapid access to advanced airway techniques

controlled, there are a small number that can result in serious hemorrhage and even death if left unattended.

Application of Anatomy to Bleeding Control

A working knowledge of the anatomy of the nose and its blood supply is helpful in understanding the treatment options available in the field. The nose itself consists mostly of cartilage, which extends from the nasal bones. A septum divides the nose into halves, which terminate externally as the nostrils or nares. The inner surface is lined by a thin mucosal membrane that helps moisten, warm, and filter air.

The main blood vessels are contained within the mucous membrane alongside bone and cartilage. Conditions that affect the mucous membrane such as cool, dry air and upper respiratory tract infections predispose patients to nosebleeds.

ANTERIOR NOSEBLEEDS

Nosebleeds are categorized as either anterior or posterior. Ninety percent of all nosebleeds occur in a region known as *Kiesselbach's area*, along the nasal septum, within 2 cm of the nasal tip. As can be seen from Fig. 9–22, this area receives its blood supply from all the vessels that supply the nose. Direct pressure can be applied to this general area by pinching the nostrils between the fingers over the length of the cartilaginous septum (Fig. 9–23). The patient or the EMT can apply this pressure. Generally, once applied, the pressure should not be released for 5 minutes. If bleeding persists, reapply the pressure.

As can be seen from Figure 9–22, one vessel that supplies this area where bleeding commonly occurs is the septal branch of the superior labial artery. Pressure can be applied to this artery by placing a rolled gauze between the upper lip and the gums and applying pressure on the upper lip from the outside. This method should be considered as a possible adjunct to nose pinching, since it addresses only one of the arteries feeding Kiesselbach's area.

POSTERIOR NOSEBLEEDS

Ten percent of nosebleeds are considered posterior. Posterior nosebleeds can bleed extensively and are not controlled with maneuvers in the field. They cannot be

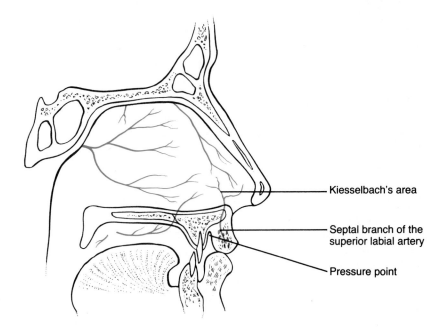

FIGURE 9–22. Blood supply to the nose. Key areas where bleeding control can be applied include Kiesselbach's area and the vessels in the upper lip (anterior nosebleeds). Deeper vessels that can cause posterior bleeding in the nose may require hospital intervention for control of bleeding. (After Kulig K: Epistaxis. In Rosen P, et al (eds): Emergency Medicine: Concepts and Clinical Practice. St. Louis, CV Mosby, 1983.)

Kiesselbach's area

Septal branch of the superior labial artery

Pressure point

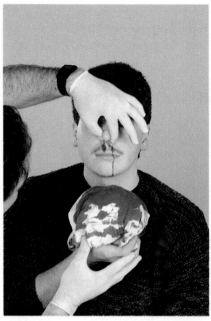 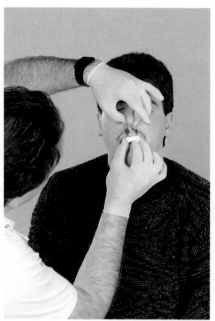 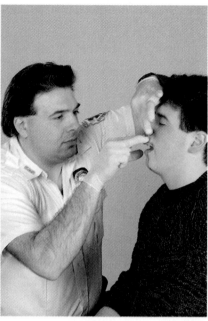

A   B   C

FIGURE 9–23. Methods of controlling anterior nosebleeds: (*A*) Apply pressure by pinching the nose closed on either side. (*B*) If bleeding is not controlled by pressure, place a small gauze square between the inside of the upper lip and the front teeth and (*C*) apply pressure to the outside of the upper lip.

distinguished from anterior nosebleeds in the field, so the nose pinch maneuver should be used in all cases.

Causes of Nosebleeds

TRAUMA

FRACTURES OF THE NOSE. Again, trauma to the nose commonly results in bleeding. Isolated nose fractures are suspected by a history of trauma, tenderness over the nose, and bleeding. Additional findings include crepitus, obvious bony deformity, swelling, and instability of the bony portion of the nose. These additional symptoms are not always found. Usually, bleeding from isolated nasal fractures is easily controlled.

NOSEBLEEDS AND LEAKAGE OF CEREBROSPINAL FLUID. It is important to remember that severe trauma to the face can cause fractures to the base of the skull, and the EMT should be alert for leakage of cerebrospinal fluid (CSF) or blood mixed with CSF. Damming up of CSF (clear fluid) or blood leakage from the brain may predispose the patient to infection and lead to increased intracranial pressure. Persistent bleeding from the nose, which is not easily controlled, may be an indication of a fracture to the base of the skull. Other signs of basilar skull fracture, if present, should likewise raise suspicion. These may include raccoon's eyes, Battle's sign, CSF or blood from the ear, or signs of increased intracranial pressure. Fractures of the nose and maxilla that result in instability to the mid-face (see Le Fort II and Le Fort III,

Fig. 9–16) also are commonly associated with leakage of CSF from the nose.

DIGITAL TRAUMA. The most common cause of nosebleeds is from self-induced exploration of the nostrils. The bleeding that results is usually minor and controlled with the nasal pinch.

NONTRAUMATIC CAUSES

There are many nontraumatic causes and associated conditions that predispose patients to nosebleeds. Some of the conditions that predispose patients to anterior and posterior nosebleeds are listed in Table 9–4. Drying (i.e., low humidity) and congestion (allergies, upper respiratory tract infections, pregnancy) of the mucous membranes are often associated with anterior nosebleeds. Foreign bodies should be suspected in children.

Posterior nosebleeds are most often seen in the elderly, who tend to have *arteriosclerosis*. Patients with inherited bleeding disorders, patients who are taking anticoagulants or "blood thinners" such as coumadin, or those who have liver disease are prone to nosebleeds

TABLE 9–4. Nontraumatic Causes of Nosebleeds

Anterior	Posterior
Upper respiratory tract infection	Arteriosclerosis
Low humidity, winter	Hypertension
Allergies	Medications and diseases
Foreign bodies	that affect blood
Spontaneous and unexplained	clotting

because of interference with blood clotting. These conditions make any nosebleed worse, and if their presence is elicited during the history, this should raise suspicion of the potential seriousness of the episode. Ask about these conditions when taking the past medical history.

Hypertension is felt by some individuals to be a predisposing factor. Others feel it is a cause of nosebleeds. The history of hypertension should be elicited as part of the past medical history.

Management of Nosebleeds

To manage patients with nosebleeds, use direct pressure to control bleeding, as discussed above. The nose pinch is the preferred maneuver. It can be performed by the patient if appropriate. Continue the pressure for 5 minutes to allow clotting to take place. Repeat if bleeding continues.

Another procedure that may be useful in some cases (in addition to the nasal pinch) is the use of the pressure point over the labial artery. Again, one uses a rolled gauze inserted upward between the upper lip and gum, with pressure exerted against the upper lip. Some protocols recommend the application of ice packs over the nose to induce vasoconstriction. Keep the patient calm and upright. The patient should remain sitting with head forward to allow clearance of blood from the mouth. This helps avoid the swallowing of blood or aspiration into the airway.

HYPOVOLEMIC SHOCK

Excessive bleeding can occur from nosebleeds, particularly posterior bleeds. It is difficult to estimate the amount of blood loss, since a patient may have swallowed considerable amounts of blood over a period of time. Pale clammy skin, tachycardia, orthostatic hypotension, hypotension, and altered mental status are indications of significant blood loss. Since posterior nosebleeds need hospital intervention, any patient with signs of hypovolemia or severe uncontrollable nasal bleeding should receive the same urgency in care and transport as would any patient with severe internal bleeding. If the patient becomes lethargic or unresponsive and unable to remain in the sitting position, place the patient in the lateral recumbent position with the head down to allow for drainage away from the airway.

EYE INJURIES

Anatomy and Physiology

The eye is a delicate organ whose unique structure demands special handling. An appreciation of the structure and function of the eye and the structures that protect and surround it help the EMT appreciate the proper steps in care. Proper treatment in the field can preserve eye function following potentially blinding injuries. Conversely, improper handling of an injured eye may result in further damage and loss of vision.

The eye is a globular structure filled with a gel-like fluid called the *vitreous humor*. It rotates within the bony orbit through the action of the orbital muscles (Fig. 9–24).

The outer layer of the eye, called the *sclera*, is composed of a tough, fibrous, and *opaque* (not transparent to light) protective membrane, except for the portion over the iris and pupils. Here the outer layer is called the *cornea*. The cornea is transparent to light so that light rays can enter the opening of the eye, the pupil. Surrounding the pupil is the pigmented or colored portion of the eye, called the *iris*. The iris is a circular muscular structure that controls the amount of light that enters the eye through the *pupil*. The iris is made of constricting and dilating muscles. Depending on the tone of these two types of muscles, the pupil changes in size. The pupil constricts in response to bright light and dilates in dim light, permitting more light to enter. It also changes in size (to a lesser degree) when one focuses on near or far objects, dilating to improve far vision and constricting when focusing on close objects. Because the muscles of the iris are directed by cranial nerves, pupillary size is often used in evaluating brain function and the effects of drugs and other factors on the central nervous system.

As light passes through the pupil it is focused by the lens onto the posterior wall of the eye or the *retina*. *Ciliary muscles* are attached to the *lens* to change its shape so light can be focused. The retina is composed of millions of sensory receptors that convert light into nervous impulses, which are then transmitted via the *optic nerve* to the brain for interpretation as a visual image.

CHAMBERS OF THE EYE

Anatomically, the eye can be divided into an anterior and posterior chamber by the lens. The anterior chamber is filled with a circulating watery fluid called the *aqueous humor*. The posterior chamber is filled with a firmer gel-like fluid called the *vitreous humor*. The aqueous and vitreous humors are under slight pressure and give shape and firmness to the eye.

THE IMPORTANCE OF THE HUMORS.   The aqueous humor is continuously formed by specialized capillaries. It circulates within the anterior chamber and then is drained and reabsorbed back into other capillaries. When drainage of the aqueous humor is obstructed, pressure builds up and causes a condition known as glaucoma. If the blockage is not corrected, the nerves can be damaged by the increased pressure, with resultant loss of vision.

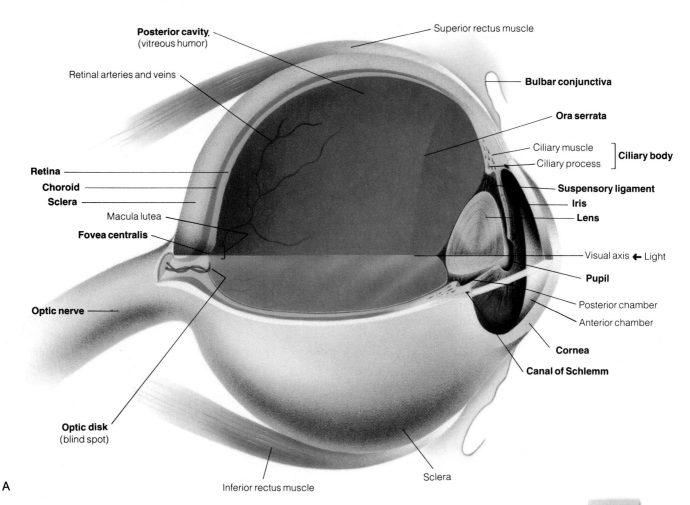

Posterior cavity, (vitreous humor)

Retinal arteries and veins

Retina

Choroid

Sclera

Macula lutea

Fovea centralis

Optic nerve

Optic disk (blind spot)

Superior rectus muscle

Bulbar conjunctiva

Ora serrata

Ciliary muscle
Ciliary process] **Ciliary body**

Suspensory ligament

Iris

Lens

Visual axis ← Light

Pupil

Posterior chamber

Anterior chamber

Cornea

Canal of Schlemm

Inferior rectus muscle

Sclera

A

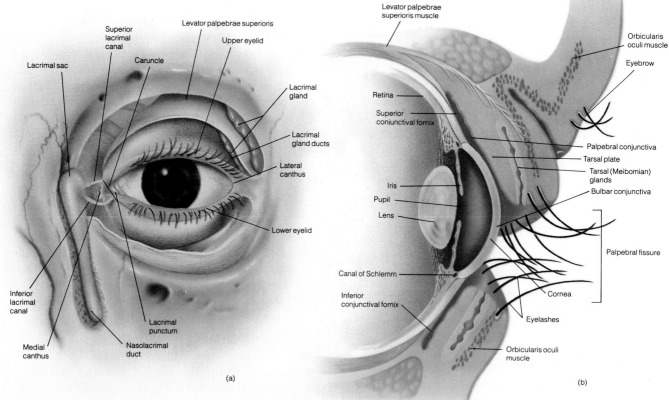

Lacrimal sac

Superior lacrimal canal

Caruncle

Levator palpebrae superioris

Upper eyelid

Lacrimal gland

Lacrimal gland ducts

Lateral canthus

Lower eyelid

Inferior lacrimal canal

Medial canthus

Nasolacrimal duct

Lacrimal punctum

(a)

Levator palpebrae superioris muscle

Retina

Superior conjunctival fornix

Iris

Pupil

Lens

Canal of Schlemm

Inferior conjunctival fornix

Orbicularis oculi muscle

Eyebrow

Palpebral conjunctiva

Tarsal plate

Tarsal (Meibomian) glands

Bulbar conjunctiva

Palpebral fissure

Cornea

Eyelashes

Orbicularis oculi muscle

(b)

B

FIGURE 9–24. (*A* and *B*) Anatomy of the eye. (From Gaudin AJ, Jones KC: Human Anatomy and Physiology. Orlando, Harcourt Brace Jovanovich, 1989, pp. 382 and 386.)

FIGURE 9–25. Major bones that make up the orbits or sockets of the eye.

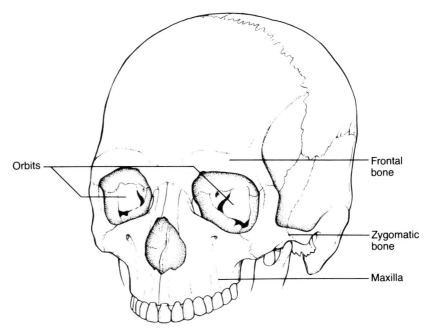

Orbits

Frontal bone

Zygomatic bone

Maxilla

The vitreous humor is not formed or drained continually. This gel-like substance cannot be lost without permanent damage. Loss of the vitreous humor from a penetrating wound to the eye can result in permanent loss of eye shape and function. Because of this fact, *direct pressure must never be applied to an injured eyeball.*

PROTECTION

The eye is set deep within orbits or sockets formed by many bones (Fig. 9–25). The outer palpable ridges are composed of parts of the frontal and zygomatic bones and the maxilla. The eye is protected in front by the eyelids. The eyelids can blink quickly to protect the eye from oncoming objects. The eyelashes aid as filters to help prevent small particles from entering the eye. The conjunctiva, a mucous membrane, lines the interior surface of the eyelids and covers the anterior surface of the eye. It changes its composition as it extends over the sclera and again over the cornea. When the conjunctiva is irritated by a foreign body or inflamed (from an infection or allergy), the capillary vessels become prominent and pink eye or conjunctivitis results (Fig. 9–26).

Tears are secreted by *lacrimal glands* located at the superior lateral surface of each eyeball. Tears are secreted continuously and serve to moisten and clean the eyeball and provide lubrication for smooth passage of the eyelids over the eyeball. Tears are drained through the lacrimal canals located at the medial portion of each eyeball.

A layer of fat behind the eye serves as an additional cushion between the eyeball itself and the bony orbit. Loss of this fat during starvation explains why eyes may appear sunken.

Injuries to the Eye

There are three important principles to remember when caring for eye injuries:

- *Avoid pressure*—No pressure should be transmitted onto an eye that may have suffered a penetrating injury.
- *Cover both eyes to limit movement*—To limit movement of one eye, both eyes must be covered.
- *The patient's cooperation is needed*—Patient cooperation is important, especially when irrigating the eye or during treatment for foreign bodies. The eye is extremely sensitive, especially following ir-

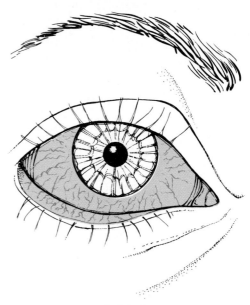

FIGURE 9–26. Conjunctivitis.

ritating injuries. Explain your actions to gain the patient's cooperation. Have the patient lie supine.

FOREIGN BODIES

Foreign bodies are very irritating and cause considerable pain. They may be noticed on the eyeball itself, on the lower eyelid, or under the upper eyelid. Foreign bodies under the upper lid may be felt by the patient upon blinking. Some foreign bodies may be very superficial and easily removed. For example, if dust or dirt falls or is blown by wind into the eye, the tearing mechanism may be adequate to remove it. Other foreign bodies may be deeply embedded and require eye surgery. For example, if a person is hammering and a piece of metal ricochets back into the eye, it may enter with considerable force and have to be removed by a physician.

Upon inspection, the lower lid and most of the eyeball are easily visualized. Have the patient look to either side and up and down so you can inspect most

of the anterior surface. At times objects become trapped under the upper lid. To fully inspect this area, the patient must cooperate by looking downward while you evert the upper lid using a cotton-tipped applicator as a fulcrum.

Have the patient look downward as you grasp the eyelashes with your thumb and finger. Make sure your hands are clean. Using a cotton-tipped applicator, place the end of the applicator in the middle of the upper lid (see Fig. 9–27). Using the applicator as a fulcrum, pull the lid forward and upward, causing it to fold back over the applicator, thus exposing the inside surface of the lid.

While maintaining the lid everted, have your partner rinse any foreign body away with irrigating solution or gently remove it with a moistened cotton-tipped swab (see Fig. 9–29).

Occasionally, you may have to remove contact lenses to properly care for the eye. Figure 9–28 demonstrates the proper technique for removing hard and soft contact lenses.

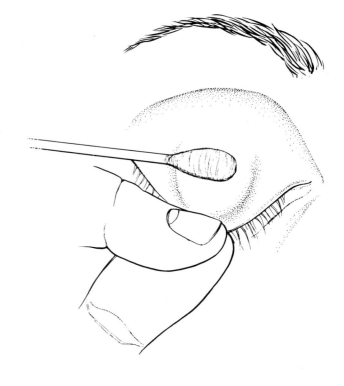

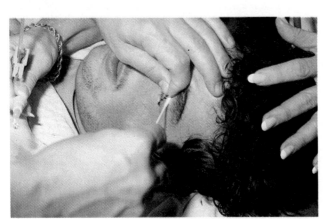

A

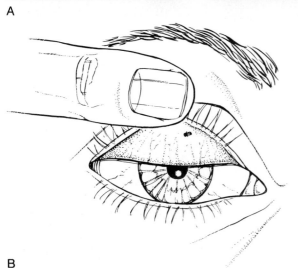

B

FIGURE 9–27. (*A* and *B*) Everting the upper lid to examine for foreign body.

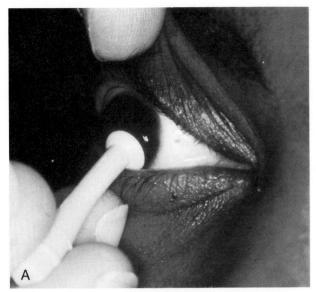
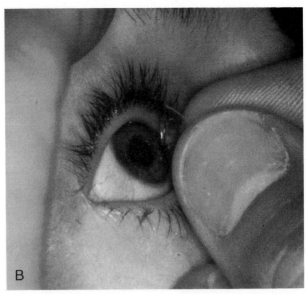

FIGURE 9-28. If it should be necessary to remove a contact lens, (A) hard lens can be removed with a special bulb contact remover, and (B) soft lens can be removed by gentle finger manipulation or irrigation. (From Cardona VD, Hurn PD, Mason PJB, et al: Trauma Nursing From Resuscitation Through Rehabilitation. Philadelphia, WB Saunders, 1988, p. 609.)

PROCEDURE 9-7 REMOVING FOREIGN BODIES FROM THE EYE

Irrigation is the preferred method for removal of foreign bodies.
1. Use sterile water or saline with an IV administration set or a specially packaged eye-irrigating solution (Fig. 9-29A).
2. Allow a gentle stream of water to pass from the medial portion of the sclera over the rest of the eyeball as you attempt to flush away the foreign body (Fig. 9-29B). Respect the delicacy of the eyeball and do not use a high-pressure stream. Rinse the affected portion of the eyelid if necessary.

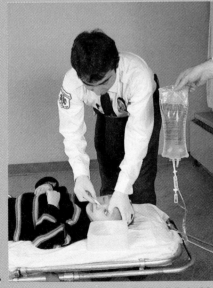
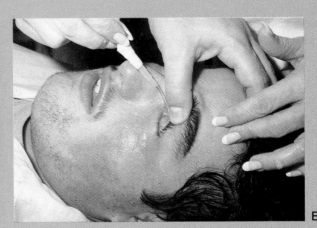

FIGURE 9-29. Removing foreign bodies from the eye.

Continued

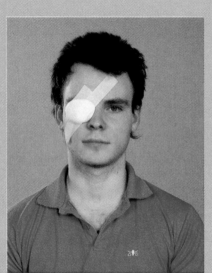

3. If removal by irrigation is not successful, an alternate method of removal is to gently wisk the foreign body off the eye with a clean, moistened cotton-tipped applicator.

Note: Do not try to use an applicator to remove foreign bodies from the cornea. Scratches to the cornea may result, causing scar formation and impairment of vision. The only method advised for removal of foreign bodies on the cornea is irrigation.

4. Once foreign bodies are removed, the eye may be patched if the patient complains of pain or foreign body sensation. Use a specially prepared eye patch, and tape it with plain cellophane tape or adhesive tape. A 4 × 4 gauze can be folded to serve the same purpose (Fig. 9–30).

5. At times foreign bodies cannot be removed in the field by the above measures. If this is the case, cover both eyes with eye patches. It is necessary to cover both eyes to limit eye movement, since the two eyes move symmetrically. It is desirable to limit eye movement, since a foreign body embedded under the upper lid may continue to scratch the eyeball that is moving underneath. Have the patient lie supine on the stretcher and remain calm.

Note: Explain to the patient why you are taking the above actions in order to gain the patient's confidence and cooperation. This is especially important with children who may be frightened by having both eyes covered.

FIGURE 9–30. Eye patch. Use two standard eye patches. Fold one in half and place it over the closed lids, then cover with a second patch and tape in place. Two patches are more effective in keeping the eyelid closed.

CORNEAL ABRASIONS

The cornea is particularly sensitive. Scratches on the cornea from brushing against a tree branch or from foreign bodies are painful. The feeling may persist even after a foreign body is removed from the cornea by irrigation. You might notice a small defect on the normally smooth corneal surface. This may be more apparent if you shine a light on the eye from the side. There may be accompanying inflammation of the conjunctiva over the nearby sclera, noticeable as pinkening from the dilating capillaries. Patching an eye with corneal abrasions is recommended and may give some pain relief.

IMPALED OBJECTS

If an impaled object is protruding from the eyeball, never remove it. To do so runs the risk of loss of the vitreous humor and permanent damage to the eye. Rather, stabilize the object with a dressing composed of several 4 × 4 gauze squares built up around the impaled object. Cover the dressing with a paper cup or piece of cardboard folded into a cone shape. Have the patient close the other eye and tell him or her not to move the eyes. Secure the cone in place with a self-adherent bandage. Cover the other eye, keeping the patient calm, and transport him or her in the supine position. The purpose of the cone-shaped dressing is twofold. One is to prevent the object from becoming more deeply embedded in the eye; the other is to prevent any pressure from being transmitted to the eyeball itself.

BURNS TO THE EYES

CHEMICAL BURNS. Chemical damage depends on the nature of the chemical and the length of time it is in contact with the eye. Alkaline and acid materials are particularly harmful. Other toxic chemicals can have variable effects. For example, the methylisocyanate gas leak in Bhopal, India, which killed thousands of people, also caused blindness in many of the survivors. Since it is often difficult to predict what effects a particular chemical may have, the rule is to immediately flush the eye with clean water or other irrigating solution such as sterile saline. The EMT can use a raised 1-liter bag of saline with an attached intravenous tubing to direct the flow over the eyeball. Irrigate in the same manner you would to remove a foreign body, that is, from the middle of the eye out toward the side. Hold the eyelids open with your fingers. Continue irrigation for at least 20 minutes and longer if the chemical agent is alkaline.

If irrigating solution is not readily available, use tap water and irrigate using any of several methods. These include having the patient's eyes held open under a gently flowing faucet, pouring water from a glass or other container onto the eyes, or placing the patient's face in a large pan of water and having the patient blink. The patient's face can be placed in a pan of sterile or clean water for short periods of time, followed by time to take a breath, and then resubmerged. The water should be changed every few minutes. Remember that the longer the chemical is in contact with the eye, the greater the chance of it causing damage.

Some patients have difficulty holding their eyes open during the irrigation process. Some EMS systems permit use of a topical anesthetic solution such as tetracaine for patients, particularly children, who cannot cooperate because of the pain. A drop or two of this solution anesthetizes the eye, allowing for adequate irrigation. Prompt irrigation is of highest priority. When conditions permit, irrigation should be done in the ambulance while the patient is en route to the hospital and then continued by the EMT until care is transferred to the emergency department staff. If possible, obtain the name of the chemical and bring the container, if available, along.

If irrigation is completed before arrival at the hospital, you should patch the eye if you have instilled anesthetic drops. The normal protective reflexes of the eye are lost due to the anesthesia, and the unprotected eye is more prone to injury from foreign bodies.

LIGHT INJURIES. Exposure to too much infrared light from the sun or to ultraviolet light from arc welding without protective goggles can result in painful burns to the cornea. The pain usually occurs a few hours after exposure. Cover the eyes with moist patches and transport the patient to the hospital.

BURNED EYELIDS. Burns to the eyelids may occur following exposure to fire and intense heat. Cover the eyelids with a moist, sterile dressing and transport the patient to the hospital.

LACERATIONS

Lacerations to the eyelids can cause brisk bleeding because of the rich blood supply (Fig. 9–31). Check to see whether there is accompanying damage to the eye itself. Use gentle and direct pressure to control bleeding from the eyelid, but avoid transmitting pressure to the eye itself. There may be associated injury to the eyeball that may not be obvious on initial inspection in the field. Loss of the internal contents of the eye by direct pressure on the eyeball can result in loss of sight. For lacerations to the eye itself, cover both eyes with loose dressings and transport the patient to the hospital in the supine position.

CONTUSIONS

Contusions of the eye can result in bleeding within the eye or on its surface. Leakage of small capillaries on the sclera can result in red blotches that look alarming but are usually quite benign (Fig. 9–32A). This condition, called *subconjunctival hematoma*, also occurs spontaneously. Bleeding within the eye is sometimes visible between the iris and the cornea (Fig. 9–32B). This collection of blood shifts with gravity and layers along the most dependent portion of the iris. If this is seen, cover the eye and transport the patient to the hospital in the supine position.

Direct trauma to the eye can cause spasm of the iris muscle and surrounding inflammation of the conjunctiva. This may be associated with other injuries of

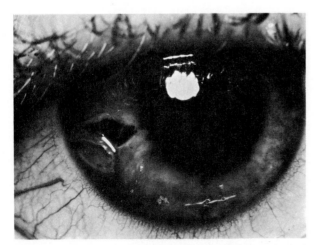
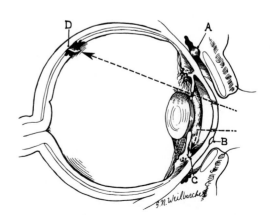

FIGURE 9–31. Laceration to the cornea can occur from small missiles and can penetrate deep into the eyeball. Sites of foreign bodies include (*A*) under upper lid, (*B*) on cornea, (*C*) within anterior chamber, and (*D*) posterior wall of eye. (From Zuidema GD, Rutherford RB, Ballinger WF: The Management of Trauma, 4th ed. Philadelphia, WB Saunders, 1985, pp. 261–262.)

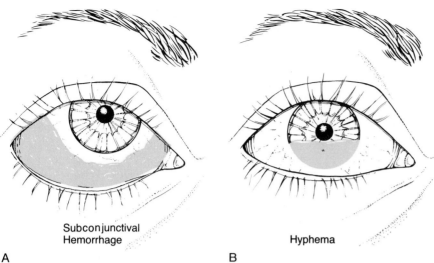

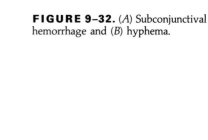

FIGURE 9–32. (*A*) Subconjunctival hemorrhage and (*B*) hyphema.

A   B

Subconjunctival
Hemorrhage   Hyphema

multiple trauma or from an isolated injury such as a tennis ball. The pupil may appear fixed in midposition or slightly dilated, and may be unresponsive to light. The term given to this traumatically induced spasm of the iris muscle is *traumatic iritis*. Such isolated injuries should not be mistaken for the unilateral fixed and dilated pupil seen with herniation of the brain. The patient with brain herniation will likely have other abnormal neurologic findings as well.

EXTRUDED EYEBALL

If the eyeball is extruding from the socket, do not attempt to replace it. Rather, place several layers of 4 × 4 gauze squares with a hole cut out of the center and moistened with sterile saline around the extruding eyeball. Attach a cup or a cone shaped from cardboard over the dressing with bandages. Then cover the opposite eye and transport (Fig. 9–33).

FRACTURE OF THE ORBIT

Significant blows to the orbit of the eye can result in fractures. The patient may have tenderness and signs of soft tissue trauma along the orbital ridge. At times, orbital fractures are complicated by impairment of eye movement and visual disturbance. Occasionally, the muscles that move the eye become entrapped in the fracture. The patient may not be able to move both eyes symmetrically in all directions. Because the eyes are not

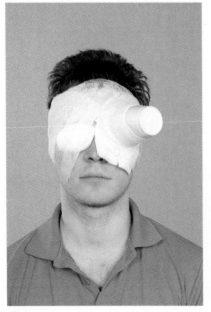

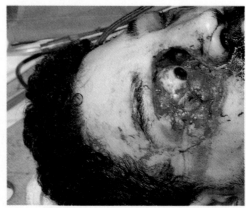

A   B

FIGURE 9–33. (*A*) Use of a cup to protect an extruded eyeball such as a patient (*B*) with severe trauma to the orbit and eye.

FIGURE 9–34. Asymmetrical eye movement secondary to fracture of the orbit and entrapment of an eye muscle. The patient may complain of double vision.

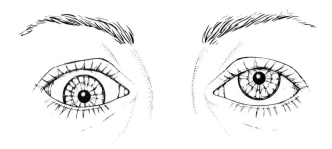

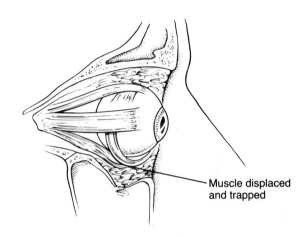

— Muscle displaced and trapped

symmetrical, the patient can experience doubled or impaired vision (Fig. 9–34).

Nontraumatic Eye Pain

Occasionally, a patient may call for an ambulance because of severe eye pain not associated with injury. Blockage of the outflow of the aqueous humor can cause a buildup of pressure in the anterior chamber of the eye, a condition known as *glaucoma*. In addition to the pain, the patient may complain of visual disturbance such as halos around lights. Often the pain is associated with headache, nausea, and vomiting. The cornea may appear hazy and steamed, and the pupil is often stuck in midposition and not responsive to light. The sclera surrounding the iris may appear pink and inflamed. This condition is a medical emergency. Transport to a hospital is required for medical and surgical treatment to reduce the pressure within the eye.

EAR INJURIES

Anatomy and Physiology

The functions of the ear include hearing, establishing position sense, and balancing. Sound waves are transmitted into fluid waves and finally into nerve impulses,

which enable the brain to "hear." Movement of the head and changes in body position cause changes in fluid-filled structures of the ear, which are relayed as nerve impulses to different parts of the brain.

Because much of the ear is enclosed within the skull, blood extruding from the ear after trauma is a sign of possible skull fracture. Also, because of the location of the middle and inner ear, infections of the ear are a potential cause of meningitis.

STRUCTURE

Each ear is composed of three sections called the *external*, the *middle*, and the *inner* ear (Fig. 9–35).

EXTERNAL EAR. The external ear is composed of the *auricle* or *pinna*, which is the outer visible ear flap, and the *external auditory canal*, a curving tube leading inward through the temporal bone to the tympanic membrane. The auricle, made up of skin and cartilage, provides protection to the opening and directs sound waves into the auditory canal. The auditory canal is lined with modified sweat glands, which secrete earwax, or *cerumen*, to trap particles and bacteria that may enter the ear.

MIDDLE EAR. The middle ear is an air-filled cavity that transmits sound waves from the external to the inner ear. It begins at the *tympanic membrane* or *eardrum* and ends at the *oval window* of the inner ear. Communicating across from the eardrum are three tiny bones

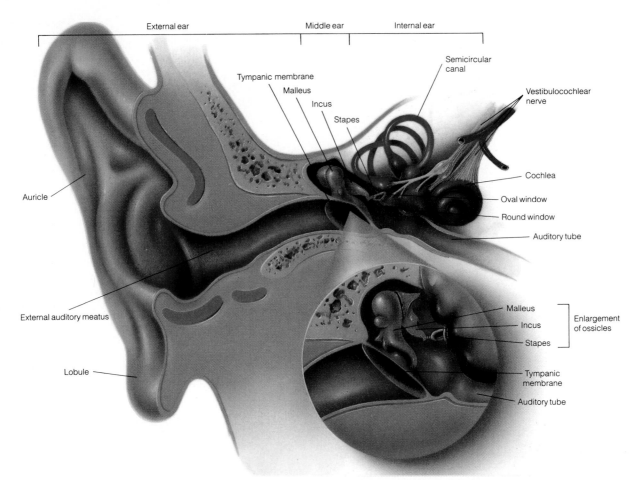

FIGURE 9–35. Anatomy of the ear. (From Gaudin AJ, Jones KC: Human Anatomy and Physiology. Orlando, Harcourt Brace Jovanovich, 1989, p. 395.)

called, in order, the *malleus* (hammer), the *incus* (anvil), and the *stapes* (or stirrup). These three small bones, known as the auditory ossicles, are attached to each other and act as a series of levers, which transmit sound waves collected at the eardrum to the inner ear.

The middle ear communicates with the nasopharynx via the eustachian tube. This tube allows the equalization of air pressure between the middle ear and the outside or atmospheric pressure. Because of this communication, infections of the pharynx can travel up the eustachian tube and cause infections of the middle ear.

INNER EAR. The inner ear is encased within the skull. It contains coiled and looped tubes that are filled with fluid and lined with special sensory cells. There are three main portions: The *central enlarged vestibule; three semicircular canals* extending at right angles to each other; and the *cochlea,* a spirally wound tube resembling a snail shell. All these structures are lined with receptor cells. The vestibule and semicircular canals are concerned with position sense. The cochlea is concerned with hearing. Nerve fibers from the receptor cells collect in bundles and travel from the ear as the *vestibular* (position and

balance) and *cochlear* (auditory or hearing) divisions of the eighth cranial nerve to respective parts of the brain.

HEARING

Sound waves are physical vibrations of air. They have amplitude and frequency characteristics. The amplitude, or size and energy of the waves, is related to loudness. The frequency, or number of vibrations (or cycles) per second, is related to the pitch of the sound. The greater the frequency, the higher the pitch. As sound waves hit the tympanic membrane, they set the interconnected ossicles in motion. The ossicles are connected to the oval window of the inner ear and thus transmit sound waves from the tympanic membrane to the inner ear. When the waves reach the inner ear, they produce an inward and outward motion of the oval window, causing a movement of fluid within the cochlea that is sensed by the receptor cells within. The receptor cells initiate nerve impulses that are sent to the brain for interpretation.

There are muscles connected to the ossicles that can dampen sound waves if they are excessively loud.

However, sudden explosions may damage the hearing mechanisms, as may continued and unprotected exposure to loud noises such as jet engines.

BALANCE AND POSITION

Fluid within the semicircular canals and the vestibule is set in motion by the turning of the head and changes in the head's position with respect to gravity. Sensitive hair cells line these tubes and detect the effect of movement and gravitation on the fluid. The hair cells send impulses through the vestibular portions of the eighth cranial nerve to the cerebrum and the cerebellum for aid in determination of position and balance.

Injuries to the External Ear

TRAUMA

Blunt trauma can cause contusions and hematoma formation in the auricle. Severe blows can also damage the eardrum, with resulting pain or bleeding from the middle ear, which may be visible in the auditory canal. Following significant trauma, blood or clear fluid from the ear should always be considered as a possible sign of skull fracture. In such cases, a loose sterile dressing should be applied.

LACERATIONS AND AVULSIONS OF THE AURICLE. Because the auricle projects outward, it is susceptible to laceration, avulsion, and complete amputation (Fig. 9–36). If possible, remove gross contamination and

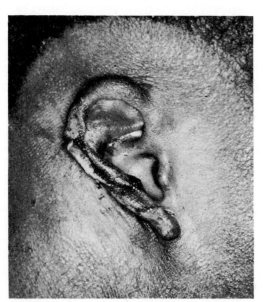

FIGURE 9–36. Avulsion of the ear. (From Zuidema GD, Rutherford RB, Ballinger WF: The Management of Trauma, 4th ed. Philadelphia, WB Saunders, 1985, p. 336.)

apply a sterile dressing. A bulky dressing should then be applied around the pinna (the external flap of the ear) before bandaging. Treat incomplete avulsed parts of the auricle by approximating their anatomical position and then holding them in place with a bulky dressing until a bandage can be applied. Treat completely avulsed or amputated parts as you would any other by removing gross contamination, wrapping the amputated part in a gauze moistened with sterile saline solution, and then placing the part in a plastic bag. Keep the part cool by placing it over ice or in water with ice added.

FOREIGN BODIES

Foreign bodies that are lodged in the auditory canal should be left for removal in the emergency department unless otherwise directed by local protocol. The eardrum is extremely sensitive, and objects that have penetrated the eardrum may cause pain and bleeding. Be careful not to obstruct blood flow from the auditory canal.

BAROTRAUMA

During exposure to changing environmental pressures (as in flying or underwater diving) the middle ear maintains equal pressure on each side of the tympanic membrane via air movement through the eustachian tubes (Fig. 9–37).

If changes in pressures occur before equalization can occur, unequal pressures on the tympanic membrane may cause distortion and rupture. This condition is called *barotrauma*. Barotrauma can occur when divers or airplane passengers change depth or altitude too quickly, without time for equalization to occur.

UNDERSTANDING THE MECHANISM OF BAROTRAUMA. A balloon descending in water serves as a good model for what happens in the ear of a diver submerging. As a balloon descends, the effective atmospheric pressure increases relative to the depth of the water. Air that fills a balloon at the surface is compressed as it descends, due to the increased pressure from the water on all sides. The tympanic membrane is also subject to these pressures. Normally, pressure on the inside of the tympanic membrane increases to match the atmospheric pressure. If a diver cannot equalize pressure on both sides of the tympanic membrane because of blockage of the eustachian tube, rupture of the eardrum can result (Fig. 9–38).

Patients with barotrauma of the ear are likely to present with pain or hearing loss. Upper respiratory tract infections may predispose patients to barotrauma during airplane trips due to clogging of the eustachian tubes, which prevents equalization. For the same reason, experienced divers do not dive when they have a cold.

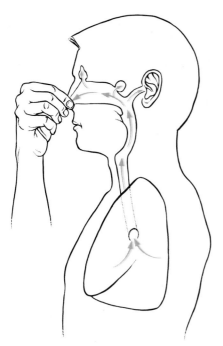
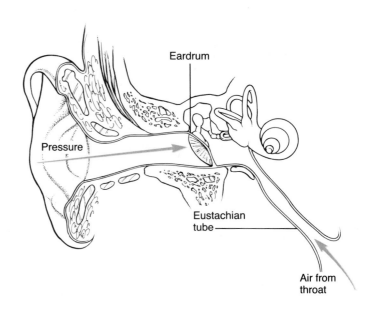

FIGURE 9–37. Unequal pressures on both sides of the eardrum may cause distortion or injury. Many people have felt this when descending from an air trip, especially when they have a cold. In this circumstance, one may attempt to exhale while closing one's nose and mouth, increasing the pressure in the internal air spaces such as the eustachian tube. (Redrawn after Neuman TS: Unusual forms of trauma. In Baxt WG: Trauma: The First Hour. Norwalk, CT, Appleton-Century-Crofts, 1985, pp. 269–270.)

There is no prehospital treatment for barotrauma of the ear.

Infections

MIDDLE EAR INFECTIONS

Because the ear communicates with the pharynx via the eustachian tube, infections of the upper respiratory tract can invade the middle ear and cause infection. These infections tend to be painful and can be associated with high fever. Children are more prone to middle ear infection because they have a short and relatively straight eustachian tube. When fluid builds up against the tympanic membrane, pressure on the membrane causes intense pain. On occasion, the tympanic membrane bursts, allowing the infection to drain through the auditory canal. This rupture usually results in relief of pain, as the pressure against the eardrum is relieved by drainage. The drainage is usually bloody *purulent* (pus-like) fluid.

Middle ear infections can lead to infection of the meninges of the brain, or meningitis. A patient who has altered mental status, neck stiffness, or other neurologic problems in the setting of a middle ear infection should be evaluated for meningitis.

NECK INJURIES

Because so many vital structures are packed together tightly in the neck, injuries to this area call for rapid assessment and intervention. The three vital systems, respiratory, circulatory, and neurologic, have critical structures passing through the neck. The major causes of death from neck injuries are airway obstruction and hemorrhage. During the primary survey, signs of airway distress and hemorrhage dictate rapid intervention. At the same time, precautions are taken for potential cervical spine injuries.

Anatomy

Respiratory components found in the neck include the pharynx, the larynx, and the trachea (Fig. 9–39). The larynx and the trachea are anterior in the neck; the larynx is palpable (and especially prominent in males) and known as the Adam's apple. The larynx and the trachea are formed of cartilage and subject to fracture and collapse. The larynx contains the vocal cords. The epiglottis is located at the superior portion of the larynx and prevents aspiration of food particles during swallowing.

The major circulatory vessels are the common ca-

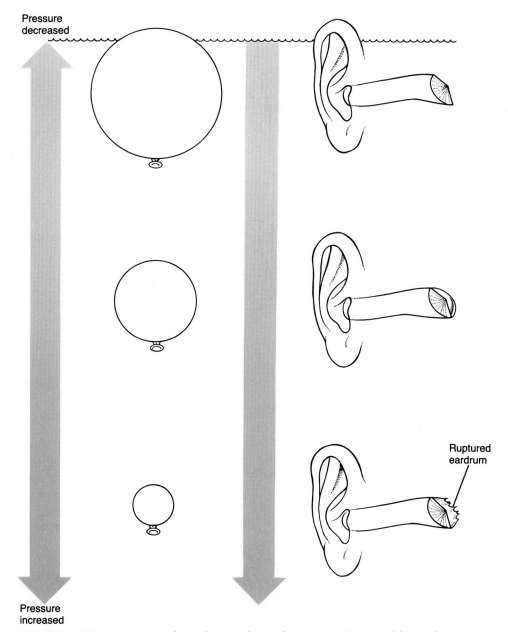

Pressure
decreased

Pressure
increased

Ruptured
eardrum

FIGURE 9–38. Barotrauma to the eardrum. (Redrawn after Neuman TS: Unusual forms of trauma. In Baxt WG: Trauma: The First Hour. Norwalk, CT, Appleton-Century-Crofts, 1985, pp. 269–270.)

rotid arteries and the internal and external jugular veins. The common carotids are located lateral to the larynx and trachea and medial (in the upper neck) and posterior (lower neck) to the sternocleidomastoid muscles. The external jugulars are located on the anterolateral aspect of the neck and are quite superficial, extending from the angle of the jaw down to the clavicle. The internal jugular veins are the major veins in the neck and are located lateral and posterior to the carotid arteries. Immediately posterior to the larynx and trachea is the esophagus. The posterior portion of the neck is made up of the cervical vertebrae and the thick paracervical muscles. These structures offer protection to the neck from behind. The cervical portion of the spinal cord passes through the cervical vertebrae. Many major peripheral nerves also pass through the neck. These nerves innervate important structures such as the vocal cords, the diaphragm, and the tongue, as well as parts of the autonomic nervous system.

Anteriorly, the neck is more vulnerable to injury. The shoulders and the jaw offer protection when the head is in the flexed position.

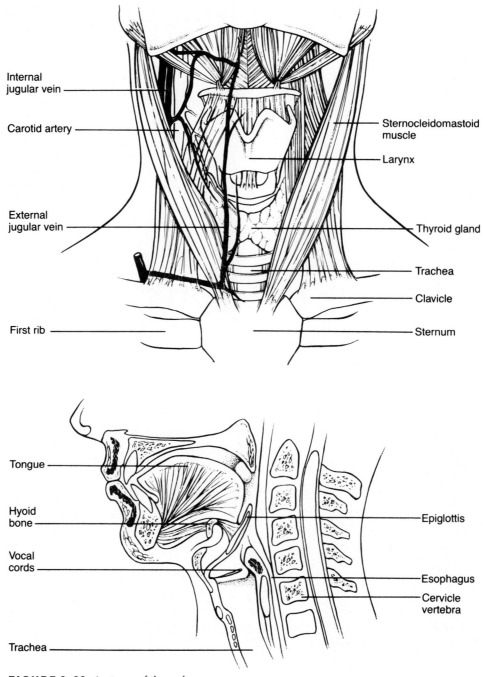

Internal
jugular vein

Carotid artery

Sternocleidomastoid
muscle

Larynx

External
jugular vein

Thyroid gland

Trachea

Clavicle

First rib

Sternum

Tongue

Hyoid
bone

Vocal
cords

Epiglottis

Esophagus

Cervicle
vertebra

Trachea

FIGURE 9–39. Anatomy of the neck.

Mechanisms of Injury

BLUNT

The most common mechanism of injury is from motor vehicle accidents, where the anterior neck is impacted on the steering wheel or dashboard. Hyperflexion and hyperextension injuries may also injure soft tissues and the cervical spine. Other causes of blunt injuries include strangling, hangings, "clothesline" injuries during sports (football), snowmobile accidents in which, for ex-

ample, the driver fails to see a chain across the road, and assaults. Blunt injuries often result in airway obstruction secondary to fracture and collapse of the larynx and trachea.

PENETRATING

Penetrating wounds can result from missile or stab wounds. Depending on the location, any of the neck structures can be affected. The most common cause of death following penetrating wounds is hemorrhage.

However, the airway may be penetrated directly or compromised due to pressure from an expanding hematoma. Additionally, interruption of carotid flow may result in signs of stroke. Laceration to the jugular veins may lead to an air embolism.

It is important to remember that missile and knife wounds, if directed downward, can enter the thoracic cavity and cause pneumothorax and hemothorax or injury to great vessels in the chest. Both blunt and penetrating injuries can lead to cervical spine fracture.

Specific Injuries

RESPIRATORY INJURIES

Following blunt or penetrating trauma, the cartilage that maintains patency of the larynx and trachea can fracture, tear, or collapse (Fig. 9–40). When lacerations of the airway occur, air can escape from the airway into the soft tissues, resulting in subcutaneous emphysema (Fig. 9–41). Swelling and expanding hematomas can cause further compromise to airway patency, with partial compromise evolving to severe compromise over time.

COMPLETE OBSTRUCTION. During the primary survey, signs of obstruction may be noted. A patient may show signs of respiratory efforts (use of accessory muscles of breathing, intercostal and supraclavicular retractions) with little or no air movement. When patients are found in respiratory arrest, an obstruction may be identified by the inability to ventilate, as evidenced by the lack of chest excursion and airway resistance during attempts to institute positive-pressure ventilations. Both of these problems suggest the presence of a complete

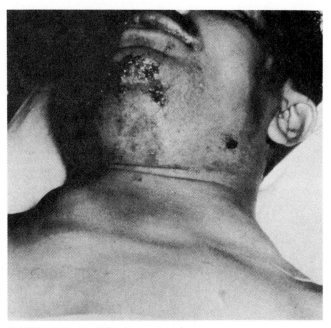

FIGURE 9–41. Subcutaneous emphysema.

airway obstruction and may require advanced airway procedures to secure a patent airway.

PARTIAL OBSTRUCTION. Partial airway obstruction may be manifested by several signs. Stridor may be heard. Dyspnea and increased work of breathing may be noted. The respiratory rate may be increased and the use of accessory muscles may be obvious on inspection. Hemoptysis (coughing up blood), subcutaneous emphysema, and evidence of a deformity of the larynx on gentle palpation may be noted. The patient may sound hoarse and experience difficulty or pain in swallowing, coughing, talking, and moving the neck.

PENETRATING INJURIES. In addition to the signs and symptoms noted above, a penetrating injury may cause bubbling of blood over the skin wound or even create a false airway.

Extreme care must be taken when handling these patients. *Palpation should always be gentle in the presence of laryngeal or tracheal trauma to avoid further disruption of the existing air passage.* Otherwise, a partially torn airway may become displaced and discontinuous, resulting in complete obstruction.

Bubbling wounds should be dressed with sterile 4 × 4 gauze squares, and careful attention must be directed at preventing blood from entering the air passage.

At times, the patient may be able to ventilate effectively through a traumatic airway. For example, a knife slash across the anterior neck may create a new and effective air passage (much like a tracheostomy). Since this new opening may be functioning as the primary point of air exchange, a dressing should not be applied that might occlude air flow.

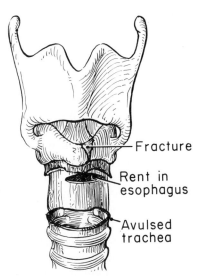

FIGURE 9–40. Injuries to the neck can fracture the cartilage of the larynx or tear the trachea or esophagus. (From Zuidema GD, Rutherford RB, Ballinger WF: The Management of Trauma, 4th ed. Philadelphia, WB Saunders, 1985, p. 366.)

Labels on figure 9-40: Fracture / Rent in esophagus / Avulsed trachea

MANAGEMENT. Open the airway with the appropriate manual maneuver and assess ventilations. In the presence of inadequate or absent ventilations, attempt to ventilate. Administer positive-pressure ventilations. If resistance is noted and there is no chest excursion, readjust the airway and attempt ventilations again. If efforts are still unsuccessful, consider the possibility of foreign body airway obstruction and initiate the appropriate procedures. However, if clear evidence of laryngeal or tracheal injuries exist, such as flattening of the larynx, subcutaneous emphysema, or open wounds, rapid transport to the hospital and access to advanced airway procedures (e.g., cricothyroidotomy) are of the highest priority.

Patients with signs of partial obstruction should receive positive-pressure ventilations (if indicated) and supplemental oxygen. In the presence of good air exchange, supplemental oxygen may be administered via a nonrebreather mask. Since bleeding often occurs with neck injuries, suctioning equipment must be kept ready. Be aware that partial obstruction can progress to complete obstruction due to swelling and associated injuries to the vocal cords and surrounding soft tissues.

In the presence of bubbling wounds, control bleeding to prevent aspiration into the airway. Since bubbling is an indication that the airway has been punctured, one may have to place the patient in a coma position with the head down to allow blood from the airway to clear through the mouth.

BLEEDING INJURIES

VASCULAR INJURIES. The major problems with vascular injuries are hemorrhage (leading to hypovolemic shock), airway compromise secondary to an expanding hematoma, air embolism, and ischemia of the brain secondary to loss of carotid blood flow.

ARTERIAL BLEEDING. The carotid arteries are the major vessels to the head and brain. Bright red blood spurting from the neck must be controlled with direct pressure. With massive hemorrhage, use of a pressure point (the carotid artery) between the wound and the heart may be necessary to control bleeding. This is the only time one uses the carotid artery as a pressure point. Pressure must be maintained manually while en route to the hospital.

VENOUS BLEEDING. Dark red blood coming from the neck indicates venous bleeding. Lacerations should be covered with an occlusive dressing to prevent air from entering the vein and traveling to the heart where it can obstruct blood flow in the heart or in a pulmonary artery (air embolism). Laying the patient in the head-down position increases venous pressure within the neck veins (relative to the heart) and reduces the chance of an air embolism.

NEUROLOGIC SYMPTOMS. The presence of neurologic symptoms (hemiparesis, facial droops, sensory loss, and so forth) following wounds to the neck may occur following interruption of carotid blood flow.

EXPANDING HEMATOMA. Severe arterial or venous bleeding can cause accumulation of blood beneath the soft tissues that can expand if not controlled. The expanding hematoma can put pressure on the airway.

MANAGEMENT. Hemorrhage is the most common cause of death from penetrating neck wounds. Direct pressure should be applied. If arterial bleeding persists, apply pressure over the carotid artery. In either case, pressure may have to be maintained by hand, since application of a pressure bandage is not feasible around the neck. Obvious venous bleeding should be covered with an occlusive dressing, and the patient should be transported with the feet elevated. Treatment for hypovolemic shock may be necessary. If bleeding cannot be controlled, rapid transport is indicated.

CERVICAL SPINE INJURIES

Cervical spine injuries must be assumed to be present when patients suffer severe blunt trauma to the neck. Certain penetrating injuries, especially from gunshot wounds, can also injure the cervical spine. When such injuries are suspected, the head should be maintained in the neutral in-line position. Sandbags and appropriate immobilization techniques should be employed to maintain the in-line position during transport. It would be impractical and inappropriate to utilize a cervical collar when bleeding or other wounds of the neck require continuous inspection and attention. The recognition of cervical spine injuries and neurologic findings resulting from damage to the spinal cord are covered in Chapter 7, on injuries to the central nervous system.

ESOPHAGEAL INJURIES

The esophagus is located just behind the trachea. It can be injured by penetrating trauma. Perforation of the esophagus can result in bleeding and the vomiting of blood. Air can escape from the pharynx through the esophagus and manifest as subcutaneous emphysema. Patients with esophageal injuries may complain of dysphagia (pain on swallowing). These findings may be seen with injuries to the airway as well. Since it is impossible to distinguish the cause of such symptoms in the field, one must assume that these findings are indicative of possible airway damage. There is no prehospital treatment for esophageal perforations. Blood from the esophagus that enters the mouth can be aspirated. Have suction ready and position the patient with the head down in a lateral recumbent position to direct drainage of continuous bleeding out of the mouth and away from the larynx.

INJURIES TO THE CHEST

Knife wounds that enter the neck are often directed from above in a downward direction. One must be alert to the possibility that such wounds can enter the thoracic cavity, particularly if the entry wound is to the lower neck. Missile wounds are notorious for altering their path after entry. Maintain a high suspicion in these cases, and look for signs of pneumothorax, hemothorax, injury to the great vessels, and tamponade.

Summary

Soft tissue injuries can result in hemorrhage, damage to vital organs, and severe infections. You must carefully assess for evidence of life-threatening conditions and be prepared to provide resuscitation and rapid transport to surgical intervention.

REVIEW EXERCISES

1. List the location and function of the layers and major structures of the skin.
2. Describe the difference between open and closed wounds.
3. Describe the appearance of the following types of wounds:

Contusion	Abrasion
Laceration	Avulsion
Puncture	Amputation
Crush injury	

4. Describe the management of the following types of soft tissue injuries:

Amputation	Avulsion
Impaled objects	

5. Describe the steps for applying a pressure bandage.
6. List the major structures of the eye and their functions.
7. Describe the management of the following eye injuries:

Foreign bodies	Corneal abrasions
Chemical injuries	Light injuries
Lacerations	Contusions
Extruded eyeball	Facture of the orbit

8. List the major structures of the ear and their functions.
9. Describe the management of the following ear emergencies:

Avulsions	Foreign bodies
Barotrauma	Infections

10. List the major bones of the face.
11. Describe the assessment and management of facial fractures.
12. Describe the management of airway compromise secondary to fractures of the mandible.
13. Describe the management of the following types of face and neck emergencies:

Esophageal injuries	Avulsions
Impaled objects	Nosebleeds
Tracheal injuries	Vascular injuries

REFERENCES

American College of Surgeons, Walt J (ed): Early care of the injured patient, 3rd ed. Philadelphia, WB Saunders, 1982.

Balkany T, Jafek B: Otological trauma. In Zuidema GD, Rutherford RB, Ballinger WF (eds): The Management of Trauma, 4th ed. Philadelphia, WB Saunders, 1985.

Balkany T, et al: Management of neck injuries. In Zuidema GD, Rutherford RB, Ballinger WF (eds): The Management of Trauma, 4th ed. Philadelphia, WB Saunders, 1985.

Cantrill S: Facial trauma. In Rosen P, et al (eds): Emergency Medicine: Concepts and Clinical Practice. St Louis, CV Mosby, 1983.

Deutsch T, Feller D: Injuries to the eyes, lids and orbits. In Zuidema GD, Rutherford RB, Ballinger WF (eds): The Management of Trauma, 4th ed. Philadelphia, WB Saunders, 1985.

Edgerton M, Kenny J: Emergency care of maxillofacial and otological injuries. In Zuidema GD, Rutherford RB, Ballinger WF (eds): The Management of Trauma, 4th ed. Philadelphia, WB Saunders, 1985.

Greene T, Yanofsky N: Common ophthalmologic problems. In Rosen P, et al (eds): Emergency Medicine: Concepts and Clinical Practice. St Louis, CV Mosby, 1983.

Hughes S: The Basis and Practice of Traumatology. Rockville, MD, Aspen, 1984.

Kaban L, Goldwyn R: Facial Injuries. In May HL: Emergency Medicine, New York, John Wiley & Sons, 1984.

Kulig K: Epistaxis. In Rosen P, et al (eds): Emergency Medicine: Concepts and Clinical Practice. St Louis, CV Mosby, 1983.

Nakum A, Melvin J: The Biomechanics of Trauma. Norwalk, CT, Appleton-Century-Crofts, 1985.

Neuman T: Unusual forms of trauma. In Baxt WG: Trauma: The First Hour. Norwalk, CT, Appleton-Century-Crofts, 1985

Ohanesian R: Injuries to the eye and adnexa. In May HL: Emergency Medicine. New York, John Wiley & Sons, 1984.

Raynor J: Anatomy and physiology. New York, Harper & Row, 1977.

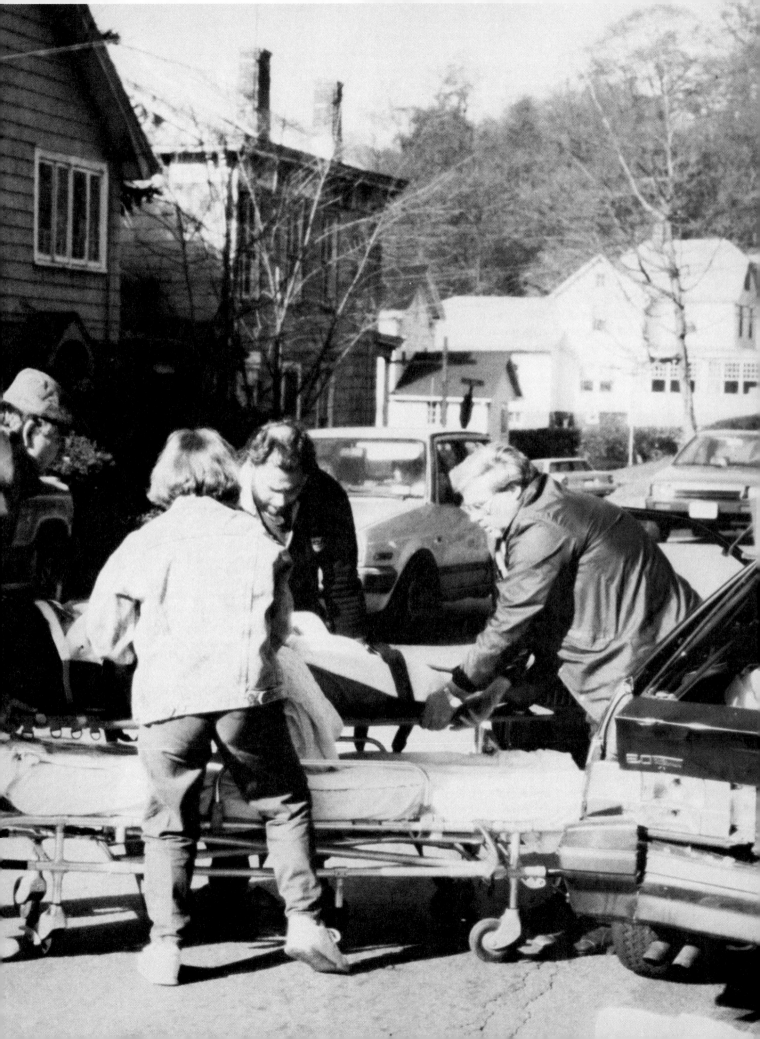

MUSCULOSKELETAL SYSTEM

O B J E C T I V E S

At the conclusion of this chapter the reader will be able to:

---

1. Explain how bones grow.

---

2. List the main bones and muscles of the upper extremities.

---

3. List the main bones and muscles of the lower extremities.

---

4. Define the following:
   Transverse fractures
   Spiral fractures
   Oblique fractures
   Greenstick fractures
   Comminuted fractures
   Impacted fractures
   Compression fractures
   Avulsion fractures

---

5. Describe how to perform a neurovascular assessment of the distal extremities.

---

6. Demonstrate how to apply the following:
   Rigid splint to the humerus and leg
   Air splint to the arm
   Hare traction splint to the leg
   Sager traction splint to the leg
   Pillow splint to the foot

---

7. Describe six signs and symptoms of fractures.

---

8. List three injuries associated with pelvic fractures.

INTRODUCTION

Fractures of bones and injuries to ligaments, tendons, and muscles account for a significant number of all injuries. Motor vehicle accidents, falls, and sports injuries are common causes. The elderly are particularly prone to fractures from weakening of the bones with age. Fractures are usually very painful and can result in deformities, temporary or permanent loss of function, and even death from the complications associated with fractures.

Bones are strong structures that give support and protection to the body. Usually, the forces required to break or fracture a bone are more than sufficient to result in damage to nearby or underlying soft tissues and organs. Complications of fractures include hemorrhage and damage to nearby vessels and nerves or underlying organs.

A working knowledge of anatomy aids recognition of fractures and their complications. Establishing the mechanism of injury and relating it to anatomical structures is the first clue to evaluation and treatment. Fractures often occur in patterns, and recognition of one fracture often raises suspicion that an associated fracture in another part of the body has also occurred. For example, a fracture of the heel following a fall alerts the EMT to the possibility of an associated fracture to the vertebral column.

Obvious fractures may distract the EMT causing more serious or associated injuries to be overlooked. The search for fractures occurs as part of the secondary survey and is aided by knowledge of the mechanism of injury, general signs and symptoms of fractures, and classic presentation of certain injuries. Treatment of fractures is directed toward immobilizing the injured part to prevent pain and further injury.

ANATOMY AND PHYSIOLOGY

Skeletal System

The skeletal system provides a framework for support and protection of the body. Muscles are attached to the skeletal system to allow movement of one part relative to another, The size and functions of bones vary widely, ranging from the tiny bones of the middle ear, which transmit sound waves for hearing, to large bones such as the femur, which must support the body's weight during walking and running. There are 206 bones that make up the skeleton (Figs. 10–1 and 10–2). Many of these bones have been discussed under previous sections of this text. Refer to Chapters 3 and 7 for review of the skull, the face, the spinal column, and the thoracic cage.

The skull and face, the spinal column, and the thoracic cavity are collectively referred to as the axial skeleton. The axial skeleton is designed primarily for support and protection of the internal organs. Some movement occurs within the vertebral column. The upper and lower extremities, the shoulder, and the pelvis make up the appendicular skeleton. The appendicular skeleton is primarily concerned with movement and support of the body in the erect position. The appendicular skeleton also offers protection to the internal organs contained within the pelvis.

The skeletal system is composed of connective tissue. The major connective tissues include bone, cartilage, ligaments, tendons, and blood marrow. Bone is a calcified connective tissue that gives strength to the skeleton. *Cartilage* is the softer precursor to the bony skeleton in the fetal stage, when formation and calcification of bone begin. Cartilage persists at the sites of bone growth (growth plates, or epiphysis) and within the bones during childhood. At the end of adolescence, after growth of the bones is essentially complete, the cartilage within the growth centers becomes calcified as well. Cartilage persists in adult life as the costal cartilage along the anterior ends of the ribs until a person reaches old age. Cartilage is present throughout life at the joints of two or more bones, where it serves as a cushion and provides a friction-free surface. The special cartilage found at joints or articulations of bones is called articular cartilage. Cartilage is also found within the respiratory tract and in the ears, where it gives support to structures such as the larynx, trachea, bronchi, nose, and pinna or outer ear.

Ligaments are tough, connective tissue bands that bind one bone to another at joints. Many extremity injuries involve the tearing or stretching of ligaments resulting in instability of the joints. Injuries to ligaments are called *sprains*. *Tendons* are tough, connective tissue bands that connect muscle to bone and serve to pull or move bones as muscles contract. Tendons can be over-stretched or torn following trauma or violent contractions of muscles. Injuries to the muscles or tendons are called *strains*.

THE ANATOMY OF BONES

A bone provides strength to withstand the forces of gravity, weightbearing, and muscular movement and, at the same time, is relatively light in weight. There are two basic types of bone tissue, called compact bone and spongy bone. *Compact bone* is more dense (heavier) and provides the greatest strength. Compact bone makes up the outer layer of all bones and the central portions (shafts) of long bones that are subjected to considerable twisting or torsional forces. *Spongy bone* (also called cancellous bone) is lighter in weight. It is lattice-like in structure (like a sponge) and provides good support against compression forces.

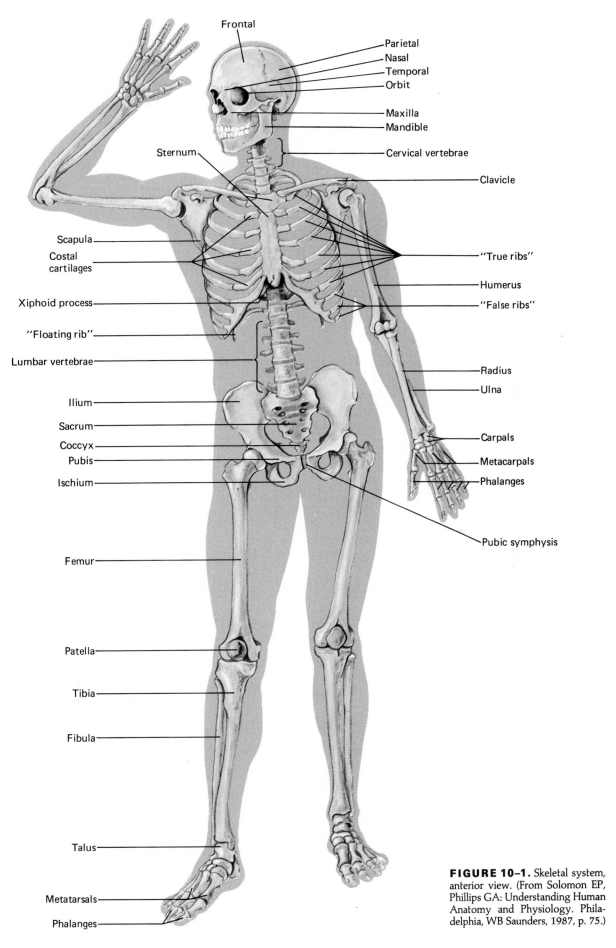

Frontal

Parietal
Nasal
Temporal
Orbit

Maxilla
Mandible

Sternum

Cervical vertebrae

Clavicle

Scapula

Costal
cartilages

"True ribs"

Humerus

"False ribs"

Xiphoid process

"Floating rib"

Lumbar vertebrae

Radius

Ulna

Ilium

Sacrum

Coccyx

Pubis

Ischium

Carpals

Metacarpals

Phalanges

Pubic symphysis

Femur

Patella

Tibia

Fibula

Talus

Metatarsals

Phalanges

FIGURE 10–1. Skeletal system, anterior view. (From Solomon EP, Phillips GA: Understanding Human Anatomy and Physiology. Philadelphia, WB Saunders, 1987, p. 75.)

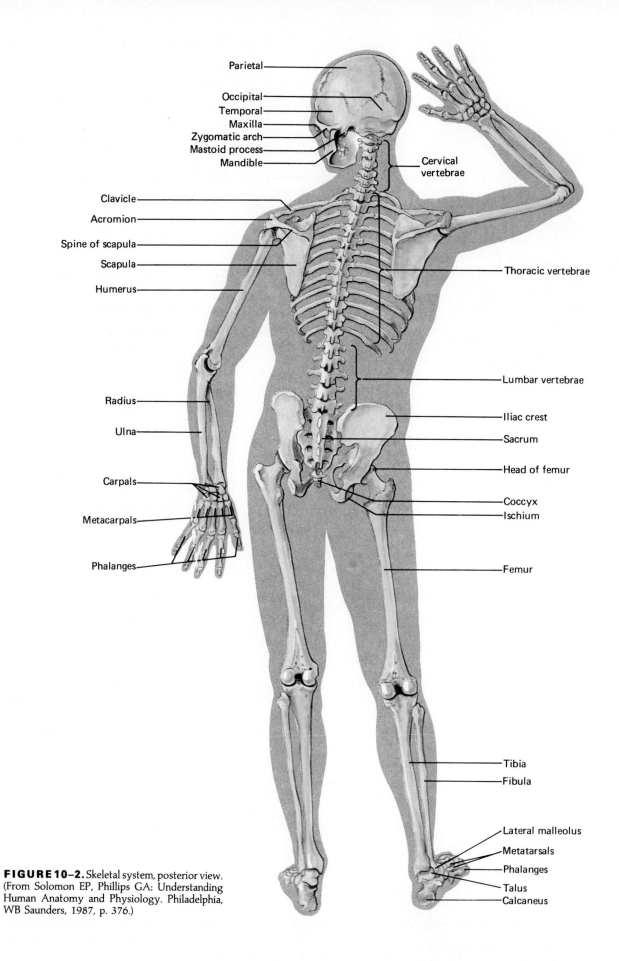

FIGURE 10-2. Skeletal system, posterior view. (From Solomon EP, Phillips GA: Understanding Human Anatomy and Physiology. Philadelphia, WB Saunders, 1987, p. 376.)

Parietal

Occipital

Temporal

Maxilla

Zygomatic arch

Mastoid process

Mandible

Cervical vertebrae

Clavicle

Acromion

Spine of scapula

Scapula

Humerus

Thoracic vertebrae

Radius

Ulna

Lumbar vertebrae

Iliac crest

Sacrum

Head of femur

Carpals

Metacarpals

Coccyx

Ischium

Phalanges

Femur

Tibia

Fibula

Lateral malleolus

Metatarsals

Phalanges

Talus

Calcaneus

BONES IN VARIED SHAPES. There are long bones, as discussed above, with a shaft made of compact bone and spongy bone at the ends. Examples of long bones include the humerus, clavicles, metacarpals, femur, and tibia. There are short bones that are predominantly spongy bone with an outer layer of compact bone. These include the carpal bones of the wrist and the tarsal bones of the ankle. There are flat bones that consist of spongy bone between two layers of compact bone. Examples of flat bones include the bones that make up the cranium and the sternum. Other bones are irregular in shape, such as the scapula and the vertebrae.

Marrow, which is the source of blood cells, is contained within the center of the shafts of long bone and within the meshwork of spongy bone. *Periosteum* is a two-layered fibrous membrane that covers bone except at the articular surface of joints. It provides the attachment point for muscles and tendons and contains the blood vessels that provide nutrition for bones. Some bones, such as long bones, have a nutrient artery that provides the major blood supply.

BONE GROWTH

The skeleton in the fetus is initially made of cartilage. After approximately seven weeks, centers of ossification (sites where cartilage is changed to bone) start transforming cartilage to calcified bone. In the long bones of the body, plates of cartilage continue to serve as the major sites of bone growth until growing is complete. These cartilage plates are also called *epiphyseal plates or growth plates.*

These epiphyseal plates represent a relatively weak point in the young. Should displacement of this plate occur following fracture, there is danger of interruption of growth or of growth in an angular direction.

The shaft of the bone has a central area known as the *diaphysis*. The ends of the diaphysis are known as the *metaphyses* (plural), which represent the more recently developed ends of the shaft. The ends of the bone are known as the *epiphyses* (plural). The epiphysis is usually an expanded area to allow a surface for articulation (joining) with other bone(s) at a joint (Fig. 10–3). Separating the epiphysis from the metaphysis is the growth plate of cartilage, also known as the epiphyseal plate. This is the site of active bone growth for the long bones. The growth plates calcify when growth is complete. The shaft is constructed predominantly of compact bone. The ends of the bone are predominantly spongy bone covered by a thin layer of compact bone. The bone is covered by the periosteum, except at the joint surface, where articular cartilage provides a friction-free cushion and interface. Blood vessels enter the bone from the periosteum and through nutrient vessels. Marrow, which produces red blood cells, fills the medullary canal of the shaft and the mesh of spongy bone (see Fig. 10–3).

BONE REMODELING. There are two different types of bone cells. One type *forms* or lays down new bone, while the other *breaks down* existing bone for purposes of repair and remodeling during growth. Obviously, during growth there is more bone formation than breakdown. During most of adult life, the processes are evenly matched. During old age, there may be more bone breakdown or resorption than formation, resulting in weaker bones—a process known as osteoporosis. Older individuals with osteoporosis are more susceptible to fractures.

Bones serve as a store of calcium for the body. The process of formation and resorption of bone is one way that calcium is stored and made available to other tissues.

BONE HEALING. Following a fracture or a break in a bone, bleeding occurs and the bone cells near the site of the fracture die. Cells capable of laying down new bone accumulate at the site of the fracture and a callus (or bony material) is formed. Cells that can break down or reabsorb bone help remodel and organize the callus into healed bone. Healing is influenced by age, the general condition of the patient, alignment of the broken bone ends, and complications such as infections and impaired blood supply.

Early and proper handling of a fractured bone is important to bone healing. Minimizing further damage to soft tissue by immobilizing the broken bone ends in the field is one of the most important steps in the care of fractures.

Muscular System

The muscles are tissues capable of contraction or shortening. They are attached and designed in such a way that the power of their contraction results in movement. There are three types of muscle: *Voluntary*, or *skeletal muscle; involuntary*, or *smooth muscle*; and *cardiac muscle*. Contraction of the voluntary muscle results in movement of the skeleton. Voluntary muscles are under the individual's conscious control. They are attached to bone directly or by tendons in such a way as to allow movement of one bone relative to another. Contraction of the smooth muscle results in automatic functions such as peristalsis, which causes movement of food through the digestive tract. Involuntary or smooth muscles are characterized by the fact that they are not under conscious control. They are found within the internal organs such as blood vessels, the digestive and urinary systems, and the respiratory system. Cardiac muscle is similar in structure to skeletal or voluntary muscle. However, it functions automatically to pump blood with each heartbeat. It is not under conscious control. Instead, it functions under control of its own pacemaker and is directed by the involuntary nervous system.

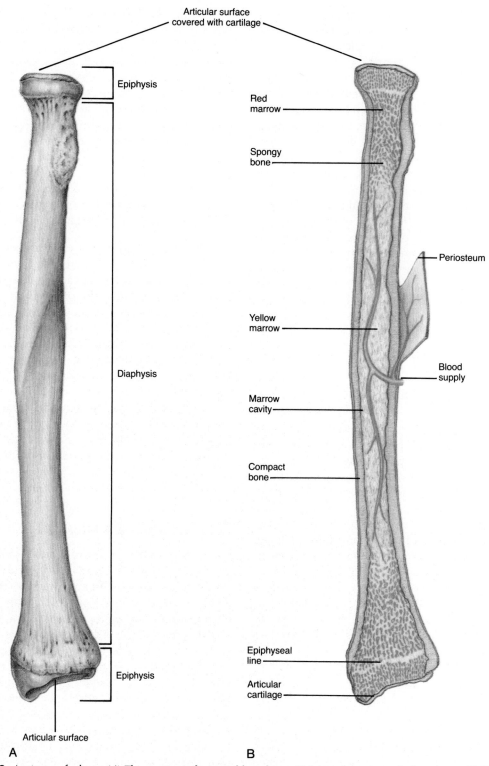

Articular surface
covered with cartilage

Epiphysis

Diaphysis

Epiphysis

Articular surface

A

Red
marrow

Spongy
bone

Yellow
marrow

Marrow
cavity

Compact
bone

Periosteum

Blood
supply

Epiphyseal
line

Articular
cartilage

B

FIGURE 10–3. Anatomy of a bone. (*A*) The structure of a typical long bone. (*B*) Internal structure of a long bone. (*C*) Three-dimensional diagram showing the microscopic appearance of a cross-section and a longitudinal section of the various components of compact bone. (From Solomon EP, Phillips GA: Understanding Human Anatomy and Physiology. Philadelphia, WB Saunders, 1987, pp. 73 and 74.) *Illustration continued on opposite page.*

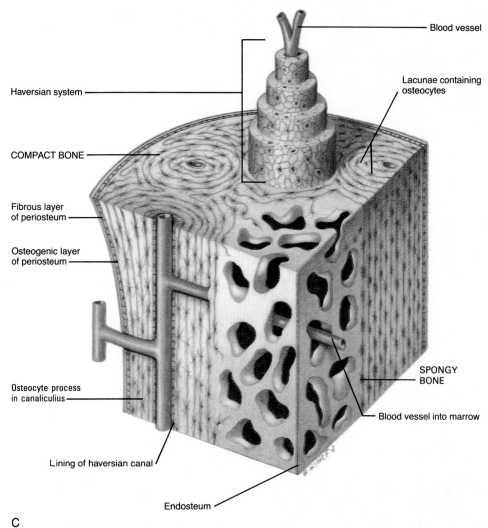

Blood vessel

Lacunae containing osteocytes

Haversian system

COMPACT BONE

Fibrous layer of periosteum

Osteogenic layer of periosteum

SPONGY BONE

Osteocyte process in canaliculius

Blood vessel into marrow

Lining of haversian canal

Endosteum

C

FIGURE 10–3. *Continued*

Specific Bones, Muscles, and Joints of the Extremities

UPPER EXTREMITIES

The upper extremities consist of the shoulder, the arm, the elbow, the forearm, the wrist, and the hand. The shoulder is formed by the articulation (joining) of the humerus with the scapula and receives support from attachments between the scapula and the clavicle (Figs. 10–4 and 10–5).

SHOULDER AND HUMERUS. The shoulder is formed by three bones and the muscles that are attached. The *scapula*, commonly known as the shoulder blade, is an irregularly shaped bone that lies on the upper part of the back. Its *acromial process* can be felt at the lateral edge of the shoulder. Just below the acromion is the *glenoid fossa* (cavity), which serves as a shallow socket for articulation with the head of the humerus. The triangular lower portion of the scapula lies over the posterior ribs, where it is covered by thick muscles, but the medial border is readily seen and felt.

The clavicle or collarbone can be palpated throughout from its attachment to the sternum to its attachment with the acromion. The clavicle serves as the attachment of the upper extremity to the axial skeleton. It is often fractured when forces that exceed the strength of the bone are transmitted from falls on the arm or shoulder.

The *humerus* is the bone of the upper arm. It is a long bone extending from the glenoid process of the scapula, where the rounded head of the humerus forms a *ball-and-socket joint*. Ball-and-socket joints permit a wide range of motion in all planes. The main portion of the humerus is referred to as the shaft. The shaft widens as it nears the elbow to form the surface for articulation with the bones of the forearm. The outer palpable projections of the lower humerus are called the medial and lateral epicondyles, which serve as the points of attachments of the muscles of the forearm. By definition, a

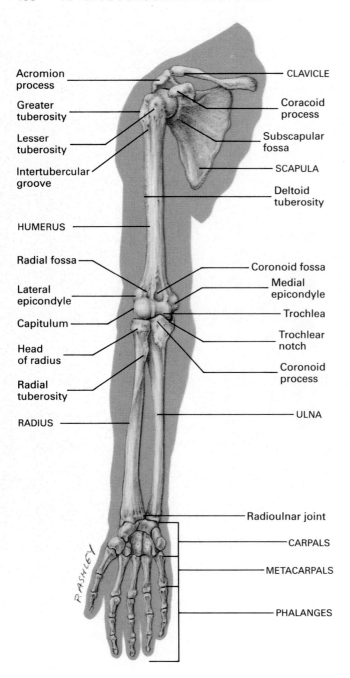

FIGURE 10–4. The upper extremity. (From Solomon EP, Phillips GA: Understanding Human Anatomy and Physiology. Philadelphia, WB Saunders, 1987, p. 88.)

condyle is a rounded projection of bone, usually for articulation with another bone, and an *epicondyle* is an eminence above a condyle for the attachment of muscle (see Fig. 10–5).

Major muscles of the shoulder include the deltoid, the pectoralis major, the trapezius, and the latissimus dorsi. The deltoid covers the shoulder, originates in the clavicle and scapula, and has its insertion point at the lateral aspect of the humerus. It serves to abduct (draw away from the median plane) the shoulder and aids flexion and extension of the arm. The *pectoralis major* is the major muscle covering the upper anterior chest wall, which inserts at the humerus, serving to adduct (draw

toward the median plane) and rotate the arm medially. The *trapezius* is a large muscle that originates from the occipital bone and the cervical and thoracic vertebrae and inserts at the lateral aspect of the clavicle and scapula, where it raises the clavicle, among other actions. The *latissimus dorsi* is a broad triangular muscle that originates from the lower half of the vertebral column and crest of the pelvis and inserts at the humerus. It adducts, extends, and rotates the arm medially (see Figs. 10–13 and 10–14).

ELBOW AND FOREARM.   The elbow is made up of the articulation of the lower humerus and the proximal

FIGURE 10–5. The humerus. (From Solomon EP, Phillips GA: Understanding Human Anatomy and Physiology. Philadelphia, WB Saunders, 1987, p. 89.)

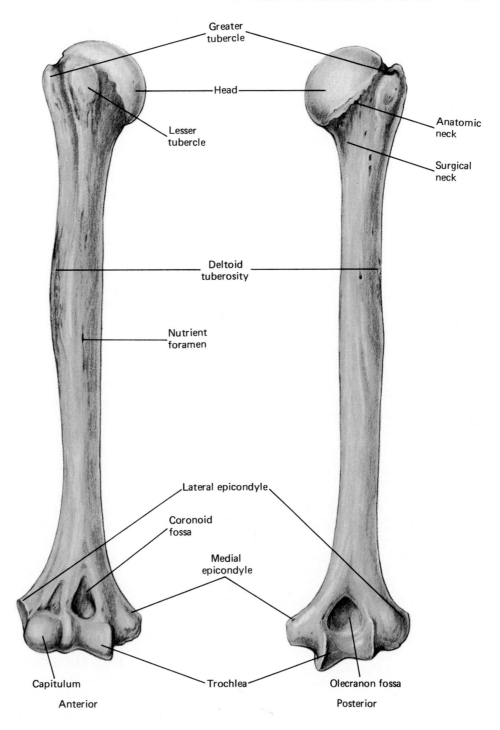

Greater tubercle

Head

Lesser tubercle

Anatomic neck

Surgical neck

Deltoid tuberosity

Nutrient foramen

Lateral epicondyle

Coronoid fossa

Medial epicondyle

Capitulum

Trochlea

Olecranon fossa

Anterior

Posterior

ends of the radius and ulna (see Figs. 10–4 and 10–6). The ulnar bone is located medially along the length of the forearm. It is a superficial bone and can be palpated along its entire length from the olecranon, or posterior point of the elbow, to the wrist. The radius lies parallel to the ulna on the lateral aspect of the arm. The radius and ulna are joined to each other by ligaments that allow rotation of the radius about the ulnar bone. Just distal to the lateral epicondyle of the humerus, the radial head

can be palpated and felt to rotate during rotation of the arm. The elbow is a complex joint, since the three bones articulate with each other in different fashions. The hinge properties of the joint (from the ulna–humerus articulation) allow for flexion and extension, while the other articulations allow for rotation of the forearm.

The muscles moving the forearm cause flexion, extension, and rotation, The principal muscle that flexes the arm is the biceps, which originates from the scapula

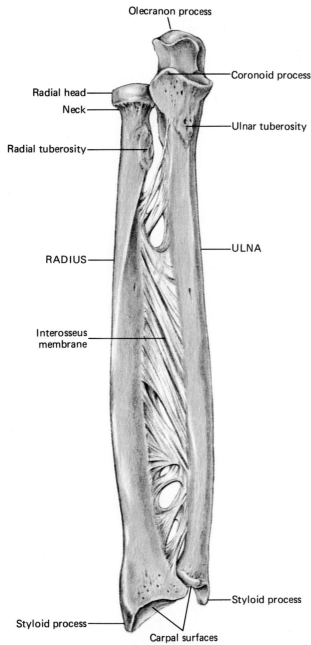

Olecranon process

Coronoid process

Radial head

Neck

Ulnar tuberosity

Radial tuberosity

ULNA

RADIUS

Interosseus
membrane

Styloid process

Styloid process

Carpal surfaces

FIGURE 10–6. The forearm. (From Solomon EP, Phillips GA: Understanding Human Anatomy and Physiology. Philadelphia, WB Saunders, 1987, p. 90.)

and inserts at the proximal end of the radius. The major muscle extending the arm is the triceps, originating from the scapula and posterior portion of the humerus and inserting on the olecranon of the ulna. Medial rotation of the arm is referred to as *pronation*, and lateral rotation is called *supination*.

WRIST AND HAND. The wrist is composed of eight small bones, called *carpal* bones, in two rows of four (see Figs. 10–4 and 10–7). These bones articulate with the radius and the ulna proximally and with the metacarpals

distally. The *metacarpals* consist of five bones that extend from the wrist to the knuckles, where they articulate with the first row of finger bones (called phalanges). The wrist is a complex joint that allows for flexion; extension; abduction; adduction; and circumduction, which is a circular motion.

LOWER EXTREMITIES

PELVIS AND FEMUR. The *pelvis* is a ringlike structure consisting of the sacrum and the coccyx posteriorly, with the two innominate (hip) bones, which join to either side of the sacrum and meet anteriorly at the pubic symphysis, completing the ring (Fig. 10–8). Each innominate bone consists of three fused bones, called the ilium, the ischium, and the pubis. The *ilium* is a winglike bone forming the superior lateral aspect of the pelvis; its uppermost portion is known as the iliac crest. The *ischium* forms the posterior portion, and the ischial tuberosity (protuberance) bears the weight of the body in the sitting position. It is palpable with the thigh flexed and the buttock relaxed. The *pubis* is composed of a body and superior and inferior pubis rami. These three bones, separate during childhood, fuse at the acetabulum, which is the socket for the hip joint. The pelvis protects the internal organs in the pelvic cavity and supports the weight of the body. The body's weight is transmitted to each femur when standing or to the ischial tuberosities when sitting.

The *femur* is the longest and strongest bone in the body (Figs. 10–9 and 10–10). It has a rounded head, which articulates with the acetabulum forming the hip joint, a true ball-and-socket joint. The femoral neck extends for about 2 inches and attaches the head of the shaft of the femur at the greater and lesser trochanters, which are projections of bone serving as attachments for muscles. The shaft of the femur widens distally before articulation at the knee joint, and the medial and lateral condyles are easily palpated.

KNEE AND LOWER LEG. The *tibia* is the major weight-bearing bone of the lower leg (Fig. 10–11A). It is widened both proximally and distally for articulation at the knee and ankle joints. The tibia runs anteriorly and superficially along the entire lower leg. Proximally, the medial and lateral tibial condyles form a surface for articulation with the femoral condyles (Fig. 10–11B). Strong ligaments hold the joint together. At the knee, the *patella*, a small flat bone, is easily palpable anteriorly. It is contained within the tendon on the quadriceps muscle. Its posterior portion is covered with cartilage and it articulates with the two femoral condyles. The knee joint is a hinge joint permitting flexion and extension and some rotation when the knee is in the flexed position.

The *fibula* is a smaller long bone running parallel,

Text continued on page 442

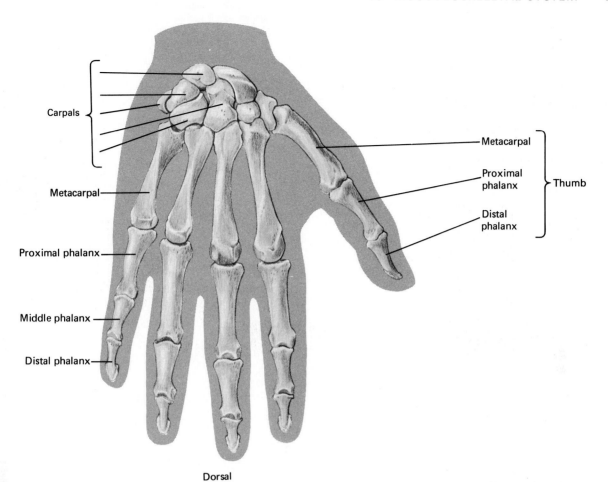

Dorsal

FIGURE 10–7. The hand. (From Solomon EP, Phillips GA: Understanding Human Anatomy and Physiology. Philadelphia, WB Saunders, 1987, p. 91.)

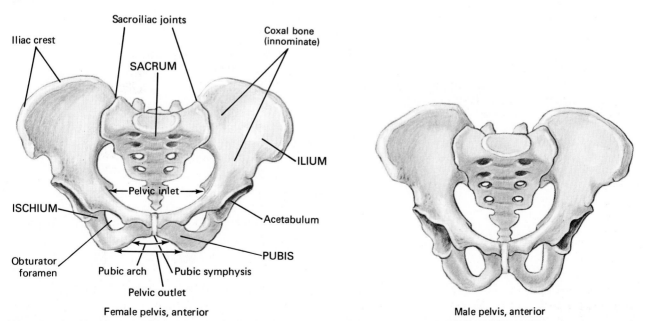

Female pelvis, anterior   Male pelvis, anterior

FIGURE 10–8. The pelvis. (From Solomon EP, Phillips GA: Understanding Human Anatomy and Physiology. Philadelphia, WB Saunders, 1987, p. 91.)

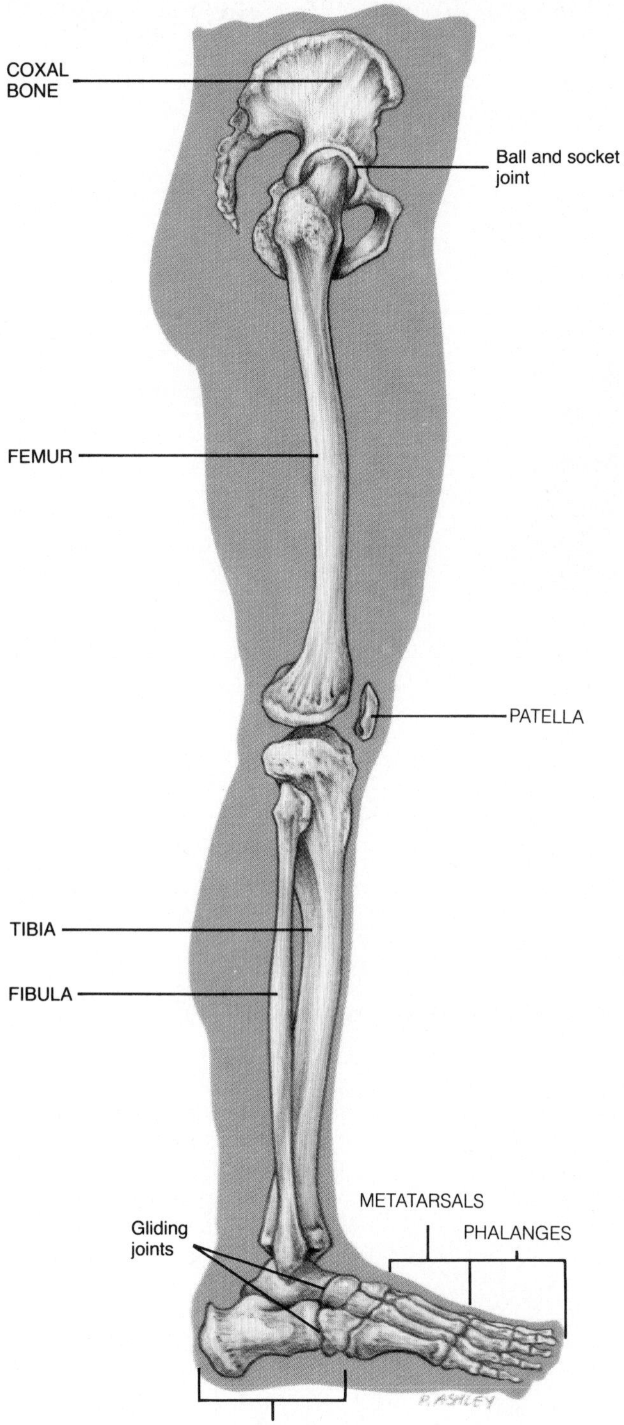

COXAL
BONE

Ball and socket
joint

FEMUR

PATELLA

TIBIA

FIBULA

METATARSALS

PHALANGES

Gliding
joints

TARSALS

R. ASHLEY

FIGURE 10–9. The lower extremity. (From Solomon EP, Phillips GA: Understanding Human Anatomy and Physiology. Philadelphia, WB Saunders, 1987, p. 92.)

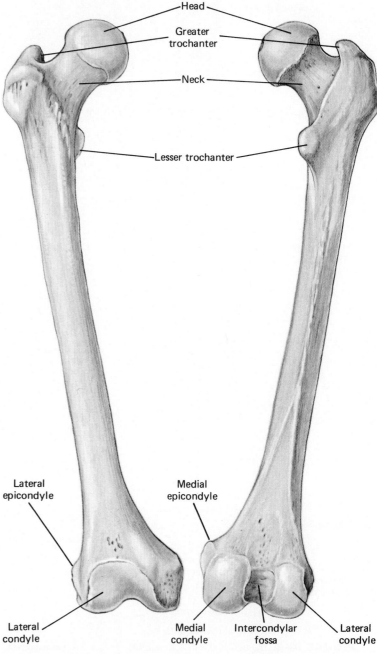

Head

Greater
trochanter

Neck

Lesser trochanter

Lateral
epicondyle

Medial
epicondyle

Lateral
condyle

Medial
condyle

Intercondylar
fossa

Lateral
condyle

Anterior

Posterior

FIGURE 10–10. The femur. (From Solomon EP, Phillips GA: Understanding Human Anatomy and Physiology. Philadelphia, WB Saunders, 1987, p. 92.)

440

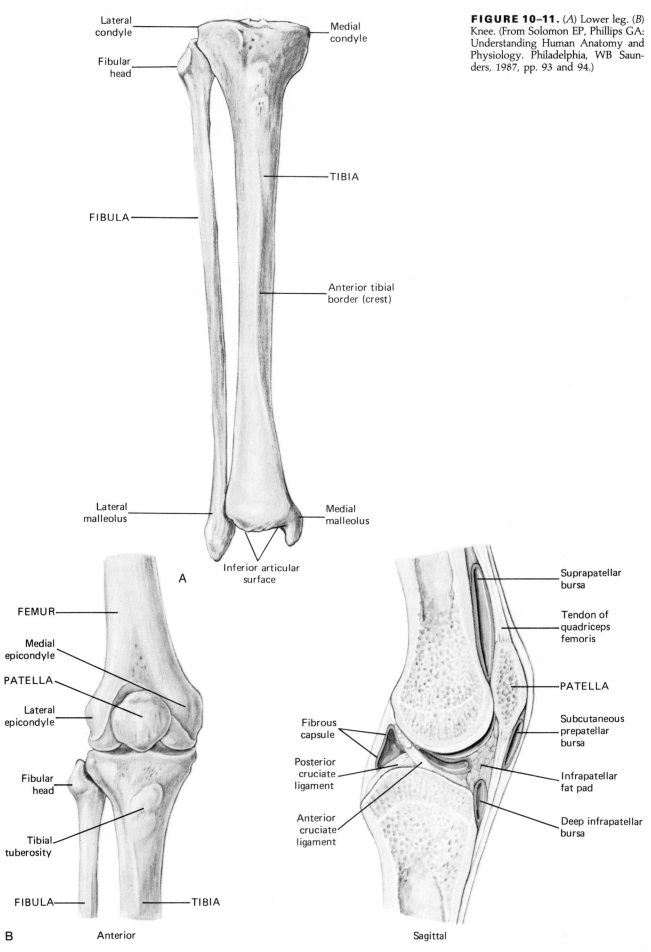

Lateral condyle

Medial condyle

Fibular head

TIBIA

FIBULA

Anterior tibial border (crest)

Lateral malleolus

Medial malleolus

Inferior articular surface

A

FIGURE 10–11. (A) Lower leg. (B) Knee. (From Solomon EP, Phillips GA: Understanding Human Anatomy and Physiology. Philadelphia, WB Saunders, 1987, pp. 93 and 94.)

FEMUR

Medial epicondyle

PATELLA

Lateral epicondyle

Fibular head

Tibial tuberosity

FIBULA

TIBIA

B

Anterior

Suprapatellar bursa

Tendon of quadriceps femoris

PATELLA

Subcutaneous prepatellar bursa

Infrapatellar fat pad

Deep infrapatellar bursa

Fibrous capsule

Posterior cruciate ligament

Anterior cruciate ligament

Sagittal

lateral, and posterior to the tibia. The proximal head of the fibula articulates with the tibia and can be palpated on the lateral and posterior aspect of the lower leg just below the knee. It is not a weight-bearing bone; rather it serves as a point of attachment for muscle and forms part of the ankle joint.

ANKLE AND FOOT. The bones of the foot include seven tarsal bones, five *metatarsal* bones, and 14 *phalanges* (Fig. 10–12). The ankle joint is formed by articulation of the tibia and fibula and the talus bone (one of the tarsals). The talus rests on the calcaneus, or heel bone, and is attached to the rest of the foot through the other five tarsal bones, transmitting the weight of the body to the foot. Ligaments attach the palpable lateral and medial malleoli to the talus and calcaneus.

The primary movement at the ankle is flexion and extension. The articulation with the talus bone permits other complex motions of the ankle and foot.

Extending from the tarsal bones are the metatarsal bones and phalanges. The foot functions as a support for the body's weight when standing and acts as a springboard when walking and running.

Major muscles of the lower limb include the gluteus maximus, quadriceps, hamstrings, gastrocnemius, and tibialis anterior (Figs. 10–13 and 10–14). The *gluteus maximus* extends from the pelvis to the femur. It extends and abducts the thigh and rotates it laterally. Flexion and adduction of the thigh is a function of adductor muscles extending from the pubis, ilium, and lower vertebrae to the femur. Extension of the leg is accomplished by the quadriceps, which extends from the ilium to the tibia. The quadriceps, with its muscular thickness, also helps protects the thigh. Flexion of the lower leg is accomplished by the hamstrings, extending from the ischium and femur to the tibia. *Dorsiflexion* (upward flexion) of the foot is accomplished by the tibialis anterior extending from the tibia to the foot. *Plantarflexion* (downward movement) of the foot is accomplished by the gastrocnemius and the soleus extending from the condyles of the femur and proximal tibia and fibula to the calcaneus.

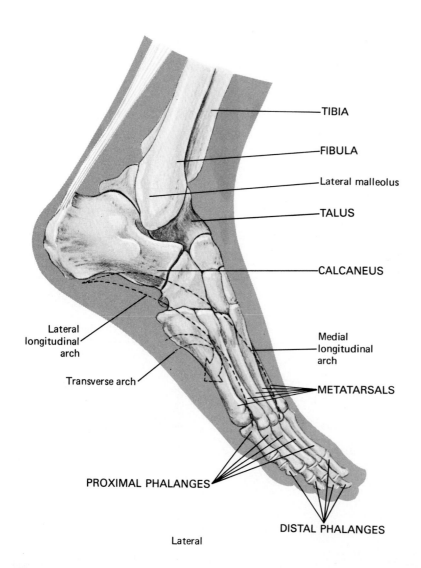

TIBIA

FIBULA

Lateral malleolus

TALUS

CALCANEUS

Lateral longitudinal arch

Medial longitudinal arch

Transverse arch

METATARSALS

PROXIMAL PHALANGES

DISTAL PHALANGES

Lateral

FIGURE 10–12. Foot and ankle. (From Solomon EP, Phillips GA: Understanding Human Anatomy and Physiology. Philadelphia, WB Saunders, 1987, p. 93.)

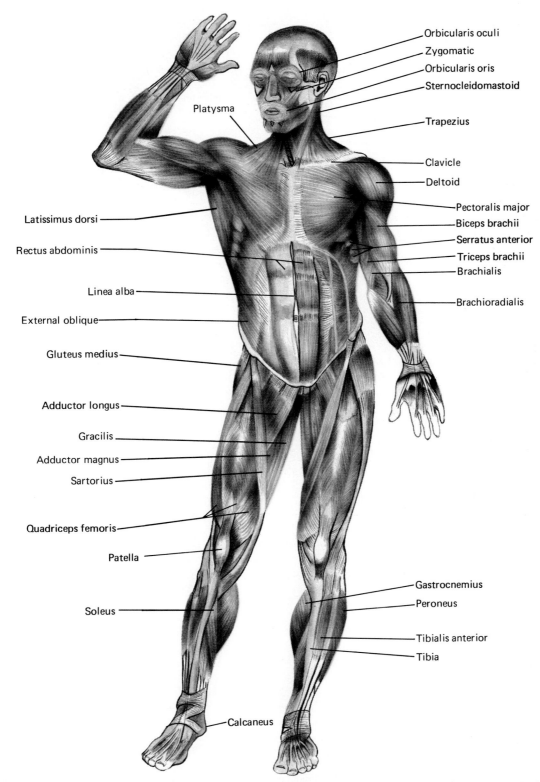

FIGURE 10–13. Muscles: Anterior view. (From Villee CA, Solomon EP, Martin C, Martin D: Biology, 2nd ed. Philadelphia, Saunders College Publishing, 1989.)

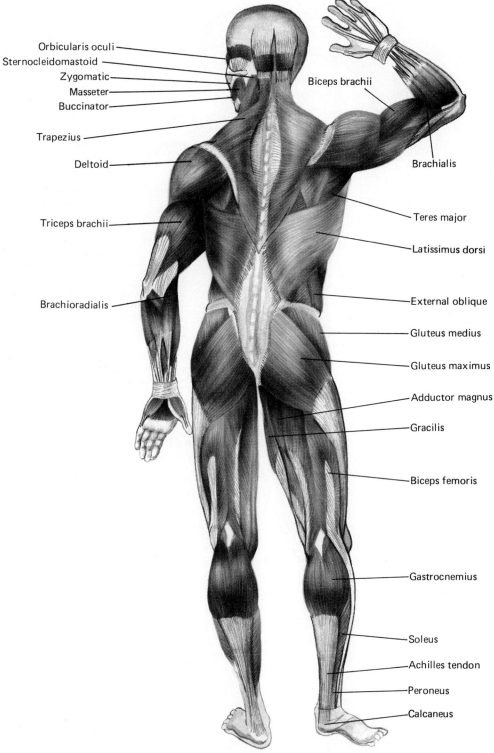

FIGURE 10-14. Muscles: Posterior view. (From Villee CA, Solomon EP, Martin C, Martin D: Biology, 2nd ed. Philadelphia, Saunders College Publishing, 1989.)

MUSCULOSKELETAL SYSTEM INJURIES

Injuries to the musculoskeletal system include fractures, dislocations, sprains, and strains. A fracture is simply defined as a break in the continuity of bone. This break may be complete, with the two ends widely separated, or incomplete, with a hairline crack along a portion of the bone. Sprains are injuries to ligaments, usually resulting from stretching forces. Strains are injuries to muscles or their tendons, again usually from overstretching or violent contractions. Sprains and strains may be minor, with only overstretching of some of the fibers, or major, resulting in complete disruption of the ligament or tendon. A dislocation is a displacement of the bones in a joint from their normal anatomical position. For a dislocation to occur, stretching or tearing of the joint ligaments must take place as well. Dislocations can be associated with fractures, sprains, and strains. The forces causing the above injuries are similar in many cases, as are many of the signs and symptoms.

Mechanisms of Injury

The mechanism of injury often helps the EMT predict the location and type of fracture. Reconstructing the mechanism of injury is the first step in assessment of the trauma victim. Such knowledge may generate a high level of suspicion of certain types and patterns of injuries. For example, you would suspect that the passenger in a front-end collision would have injuries to the head, neck, and chest, as the head and thorax are thrown against the windshield and dashboard. Furthermore, as a knee hits the dashboard, force is transmitted from the knee along the femur to the hip and pelvis, indicating the need for a search for fractures along the entire path of the transmitted force. The mechanism of injury should always be included in the patient care record and transmitted to the hospital staff. It helps them too in their search and treatment of both direct and associated injuries.

Forces that cause fractures may be direct or indirect. Examples of *direct forces* applied to a bone would include a car bumper striking the tibia of a pedestrian, a gunshot wound shattering a bone, and a falling person landing on both feet and breaking the heel bones.

Indirect forces are usually forces that are transmitted along the axis of bones, resulting in an injury at a location other than the point of impact (Fig. 10–15). For example, a person falling on an outstretched hand may have a fracture of any of the bones of the upper extremity, because different transmitted forces are generated according to the exact position of the hand and arm at the time of impact. Wherever the transmitted force exceeds the strength of the bone, a fracture may occur. Another example of indirect force is a *twisting force*. Such

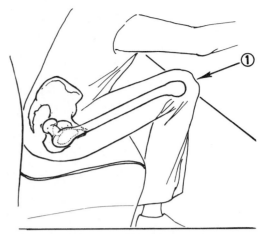

FIGURE 10–15. The force from the dashboard (*1*) is transmitted along the axis of the bone. The bone can fracture or, in this case, dislocate at the hip. (From Connolly JF: DePalma's The Management of Fractures and Dislocations: An Atlas. Philadelphia, WB Saunders, 1981, p. 5.)

an injury can occur, for example, when a skater catches one of the blades in the ice while doing a spin. The planted blade acts as a fixation point while the leg continues to rotate, transmitting a twisting force along the axis of the bones. Another indirect force that can cause fractures is the violent contraction of muscles, which tears off the bony attachment.

Pathologic fractures result when bone diseases have destroyed and weakened bone to the point where minimal stress leads to a fracture. Bone cancer, congenital diseases, and osteoporosis are examples of diseases that may lead to pathologic fractures. For patients with such diseases, the forces resulting from ordinary activities such as stepping off a curb may cause a fracture (Fig. 10–16).

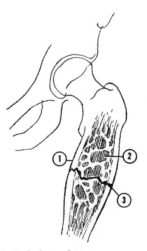

FIGURE 10–16. Pathologic fractures can occur when diseased bone weakens (*1* and *2*). The amount of force needed to cause a fracture is significantly reduced. Pain is usually not a feature of this slow-growing process until pathologic fracture occurs (*3*). (From Connolly JF: DePalma's The Management of Fractures and Dislocations: An Atlas. Philadelphia, WB Saunders, 1981, p. 2104.)

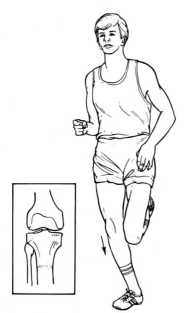

FIGURE 10–17. Stress fractures can be caused by continued repetitive loading of bone (fatigue fracture). (From Connolly JF: DePalma's The Management of Fractures and Dislocations: An Atlas. Philadelphia, WB Saunders, 1981, p. 1725.)

Stress fractures are fractures that result from overuse or continuous activity. The cumulative effect of repetitive stress resulting from activities such as jogging may lead to a stress fracture. These are likely to occur in athletes, joggers, or military recruits, and usually affect the lower extremities (Fig. 10–17).

Types of Fractures

OPEN AND CLOSED FRACTURES

Fractures can be classified as *closed or open* (Fig. 10–18A and B). A *closed* or simple fracture has no break in the skin over the fracture site, and the fracture does not communicate with the external environment. An *open* or compound fracture communicates with the external environment because the skin above the site has been broken. Open fractures run the risk of infection and should be covered with a sterile dressing. Open fractures can result from penetrating wounds, lacerations from crush injuries to a limb, or from sharp bone fragments tearing through the surrounding soft tissue and skin.

OTHER CLASSIFICATIONS OF FRACTURES

Fractures can also be classified according to the pattern and extent of fracture lines and fragments. Some of these patterns are typically caused by direct forces, while others are typical of indirect forces. The EMT should appreciate that many different conditions and forces can cause fractures.

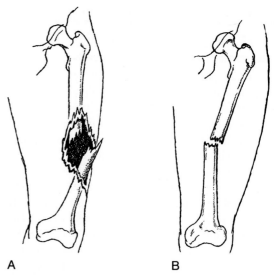

A   B

FIGURE 10–18. (*A*) Open fracture. (*B*) Closed fracture. (From Connolly JF: DePalma's The Management of Fractures and Dislocations: An Atlas. Philadelphia, WB Saunders, 1981, pp. 8 and 9.)

TRANSVERSE FRACTURES. Transverse fractures are fractures that are usually produced by a direct force applied perpendicularly to a bone (Fig. 10–19).

SPIRAL FRACTURES. Spiral fractures have long, sharp, and pointed bone ends. They are produced by twisting or by rotatory forces (Fig. 10–20).

OBLIQUE FRACTURES. Oblique fractures are produced by a twisting force with an upward thrust. The fractured ends are short and run at an oblique angle across the bone. A direct force at an angle to the bone may also cause an oblique fracture (Fig. 10–21).

GREENSTICK FRACTURES. Greenstick fractures result from compression or angulation forces in long bones of children under the age of 10, when the bones are still soft and resilient. The bone remains intact on one side and cracks on the other (Fig. 10–22).

COMMINUTED FRACTURES. Comminuted fractures have multiple (always more than two) fragments and are caused by severe direct violence (Fig. 10–23).

IMPACTED FRACTURES. Impacted fractures are caused by strong forces that drive bone fragments firmly together. The fragments move in unison and the patient may retain function of the extremity (Fig. 10–24).

COMPRESSION FRACTURES. Compression fractures result when spongy bones collapse from transmitted forces that drive bones together. For example, a common site of a compression fracture is the vertebrae that collapse when a person falls from a height and lands on the heels or buttocks.

AVULSION FRACTURES. Avulsion fractures result from forceful contraction of a muscle against resistance, with the tearing of a fragment of bone at the site of insertion (Fig. 10–25).

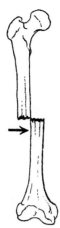

FIGURE 10–19. Transverse fracture. (From Connolly JF: DePalma's The Management of Fractures and Dislocations: An Atlas. Philadelphia, WB Saunders, 1981, p. 9.)

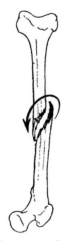

FIGURE 10–20. Spiral fractures result from torsional forces. (From Connolly JF: DePalma's The Management of Fractures and Dislocations: An Atlas. Philadelphia, WB Saunders, 1981, p. 10.)

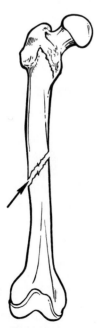

FIGURE 10–21. Oblique fracture. (From Connolly JF: DePalma's The Management of Fractures and Dislocations: An Atlas. Philadelphia, WB Saunders, 1981, p. 9.)

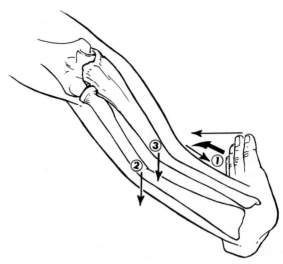

FIGURE 10–22. Greenstick fractures are incomplete fractures that occur in children due to the soft, immature bone tissue. Force vectors from supination injury (*1*) produce volar angulation of the radius (*2*) to a greater degree than angulation of the ulna (*3*). (From Connolly JF: DePalma's The Management of Fractures and Dislocations: An Atlas. Philadelphia, WB Saunders, 1981, p. 898.)

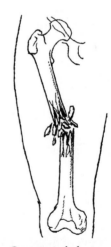

FIGURE 10–23. Comminuted fracture. (From Connolly JF: DePalma's The Management of Fractures and Dislocations: An Atlas. Philadelphia, WB Saunders, 1981, p. 10.)

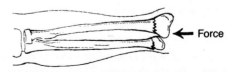

FIGURE 10–24. Impacted fracture occurs when a force is applied on the long axis of a bone causing compression of the bone into itself. (From Connolly JF: DePalma's The Management of Fractures and Dislocations: An Atlas. Philadelphia, WB Saunders, 1981, p. 10.)

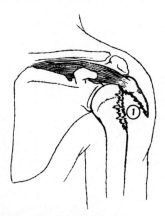

FIGURE 10-25. An avulsion fracture can occur when muscles pull on the bone segment. (From Connolly JF: DePalma's The Management of Fractures and Dislocations: An Atlas. Philadelphia, WB Saunders, 1981, p. 12.)

Signs and Symptoms of Fractures

PAIN AND TENDERNESS

Pain is probably the most common symptom of a fracture. Point tenderness at the fracture site is almost always elicited on palpation. Pain is, at times, referred distal or proximal to the site of fracture, so examination of the entire extremity is essential. (For example, a fracture of the hip may present with referred pain to the knee.)

DEFORMITY

Angulation of long bones, protuberance of the bone end against the soft tissues, and overriding or separation of bone fragments by opposing muscles can result in visible and palpable deformities (Fig. 10–26).

SWELLING AND DISCOLORATION

Fluid or blood loss at the site of injury can result in swelling or discoloration of the affected part. This can be an early sign, or it may not be apparent for some time after injury. By comparing extremities, one can gauge the extent of swelling (Fig. 10–26).

LOSS OF USE

Loss of function of a skeletal part occurs with fractures. This can result from pain on attempted movement or gross disruption of bones, ligaments, or tendons. Therefore, one should never attempt to force movement when a patient does not voluntarily move a limb. Other reasons for loss of function include neurovascular compromise, making assessment of neurovascular function distal to an injury mandatory.

CREPITUS

During palpation, the EMT may note a grating sensation or sound indicating bone fragments rubbing against one another. One should not deliberately attempt to elicit this sound but rather recognize its significance if it is encountered during the initial palpation.

EXPOSED BONE

Bone ends protruding through the skin are an obvious sign of an open fracture. However, often pain and tenderness are the only signs of fracture. Sometimes a patient is still able to use the fractured limb, particularly if it is an impacted fracture (Fig. 10–26).

Signs and Symptoms of Dislocation

A dislocation is a complete or partial separation of the bones in a joint, resulting in loss of their normal anatomic alignment (Fig. 10–27). It can result from both direct and indirect violence. Some patients have recurrent dislocations of the shoulder due to previous injuries that overstretch the joint structures, and suffer dislocation from voluntary muscle contraction without any trauma.

A dislocation may be associated with a fracture, and signs and symptoms of a fracture may be present. Signs that are more specific for dislocation include *loss of movement* and *deformity at a joint*, with the joint possibly *locked in a deformed position*. *Pain and swelling* over the joint are other findings.

Dislocations can occur at any joint, and common sites include the shoulder, the elbow, the fingers, the hip, the knee, and the ankle. Classic signs of many of these dislocations and their treatments are discussed under specific injuries.

Signs and Symptoms of Sprains

A sprain is an injury to a ligament. Minor sprains result from overstretching of ligament fibers and may be accompanied by *pain, swelling, and disability*. Major sprains can involve total disruption of the ligament with instability of the joint and possible dislocation. The most common site of sprain is the ankle joint.

Differentiating Musculoskeletal Injuries

It is often difficult to differentiate a fracture from a sprain. Pain, swelling, and disability are common to both and may be the only signs present. It is best to assume a fracture has occurred in these situations and

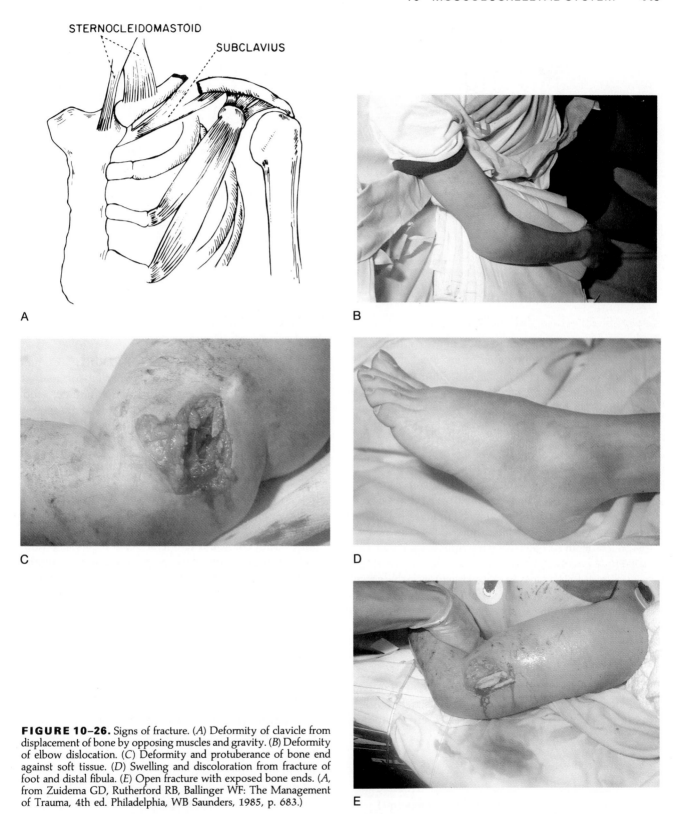

FIGURE 10–26. Signs of fracture. (*A*) Deformity of clavicle from displacement of bone by opposing muscles and gravity. (*B*) Deformity of elbow dislocation. (*C*) Deformity and protuberance of bone end against soft tissue. (*D*) Swelling and discoloration from fracture of foot and distal fibula. (*E*) Open fracture with exposed bone ends. (*A*, from Zuidema GD, Rutherford RB, Ballinger WF: The Management of Trauma, 4th ed. Philadelphia, WB Saunders, 1985, p. 683.)

treat accordingly. Certain signs are specific for fractures, such as crepitus, angulation of a long bone, and, of course, protrusion of bone ends.

Deformity of joints or locking of a joint in a deformed position are specific signs for dislocations. There may be fractures of the bones of the joint as well.

Complications

The acute complications resulting from fractures and dislocations include *blood loss, injury to nerves and vessels, injuries to underlying organs, fat embolism, and infection.* As noted above, the force necessary to cause a

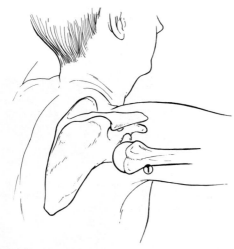

FIGURE 10-27. Shoulder dislocation. (From Connolly JF: De-Palma's The Management of Fractures and Dislocations: An Atlas. Philadelphia, WB Saunders, 1981, p. 6.)

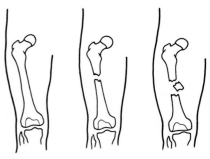

AVERAGE	40 cm. length	40 cm. length	40 cm. length
DIMENSIONS	8 cm. radius	9 cm. radius	10 cm. radius
VOLUME CHANGE	Normal	+ 2.1 liters	+ 4.5 liters

FIGURE 10-28. Blood loss in the thigh results in minimal changes in the radius. Review the values as shown. (From Zuidema GD, Rutherford RB, Ballinger WF: The Management of Trauma, 4th ed. Philadelphia, WB Saunders, 1985, p. 106.)

fracture is usually sufficient to cause injury to the adjacent soft tissues. Nerves and vessels often travel along bones and are vulnerable to damage from direct violence or broken bone ends. At joints, they are particularly vulnerable to injury. Infection is a possible complication of all open wounds.

BLEEDING

Bleeding can be a life-threatening complication of fractures, especially if there are multiple fractures or open fractures. Fractures of the pelvis and femur are particularly serious in terms of associated blood loss. The range of blood loss from certain closed fractures is shown in Table 10-1.

Signs of blood loss in closed fractures include swelling and discoloration of the limb and the signs of shock. If significant swelling is noted in the thigh, for example, it might indicate severe blood loss (Fig. 10-28).

VASCULAR INJURIES

MECHANISMS OF VASCULAR INJURY. Vessels can be pinched or torn by bone fragments, damaged directly by the violence causing the fracture (especially with

TABLE 10-1. Average Blood Loss With a Closed Fracture

Fracture Site	Amount Blood Loss (ml)
Radius and ulna	150-250
Humerus	250
Pelvis	1500-3000
Femur	1000
Tibia and fibula	500

(From Simon R, Koenigsknecht S: Orthopedics in Emergency Medicine: The Extremities. Norwalk, CT, Appleton-Century-Crofts, 1982.)

penetrating injuries such as gunshot wounds), go into spasm, be compressed by soft tissue swelling, or be occluded by thrombosis. For examples of some of these mechanisms, see Figure 10-29.

COMMON SITES OF VASCULAR INJURY. Common sites where fractures or dislocations are associated with vascular injury include dislocation of the shoulder, elbow, knee, and bones of the foot; fractures near these joints; and the temporoparietal region of the skull (middle meningeal artery) (Figs. 10-29A and B).

SIGNS AND SYMPTOMS. Vascular injuries can result in loss of blood flow to distal tissues as well as blood loss if the vessel is torn. Without early restoration of the blood supply, the limb may be lost. The presence of vascular compromise is determined by assessing distal pulses, skin color and temperature, and capillary return, and by noting signs such as pain, numbness, tingling, prickling, sensory loss, or paralysis distal to the injury. One way to remember the signs of ischemia of a limb is to keep in mind the five P's: pain, pulselessness, pallor, paresthesia (numbness or tingling, prickling), and paralysis. Always check for vascular compromise before and after applying splints.

PERIPHERAL NERVE INJURY

MECHANISMS OF NERVE INJURY. In cases of trauma to an extremity, nerves are injured more often than arteries. Injuries from mechanisms similar to those that injure arteries can range from nerve contusion to complete disruption of a nerve's function. For example, torn bone ends can tear or pinch the nerve, displaced joints can stretch or compress a nerve, and violent forces such as gunshot wounds can cause direct damage (Fig. 10-30).

COMMON SITES OF NERVE INJURY. Common sites where fractures or dislocations cause disruption of nerves include the clavicle, shoulder, humerus, elbow, wrist, hip and femur, knee, and spinal cord (Fig. 10-31).

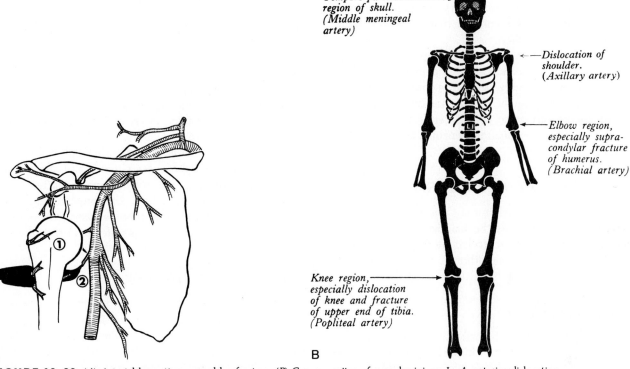

Temporo-parietal region of skull. (Middle meningeal artery)

Dislocation of shoulder. (Axillary artery)

Elbow region, especially supra-condylar fracture of humerus. (Brachial artery)

Knee region, especially dislocation of knee and fracture of upper end of tibia. (Popliteal artery)

A

B

FIGURE 10–29. (*A*) Arterial laceration caused by fracture. (*B*) Common sites of vascular injury. In *A*, anterior dislocation of the shoulder (*1*) causes the anterior humeral circumflex branch to be avulsed off the axillary artery (*2*). (*A*, from Connolly JF: DePalma's The Management of Fractures and Dislocations: An Atlas. Philadelphia, WB Saunders, 1981, p. 59; *B*, from Adams JC: Outline of Fractures, 8th ed. New York, Churchill Livingstone, 1983, p. 66.)

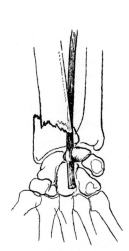

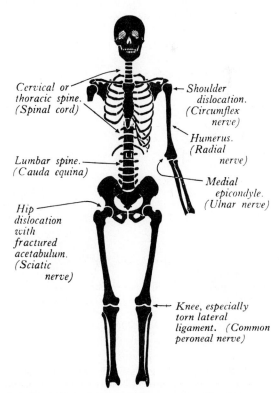

Cervical or thoracic spine. (Spinal cord)

Shoulder dislocation. (Circumflex nerve)

Humerus. (Radial nerve)

Lumbar spine. (Cauda equina)

Medial epicondyle. (Ulnar nerve)

Hip dislocation with fractured acetabulum. (Sciatic nerve)

Knee, especially torn lateral ligament. (Common peroneal nerve)

FIGURE 10–30. Injury of the median nerve due to fracture-dislocation of a bone. (From Connolly JF: DePalma's The Management of Fractures and Dislocations: An Atlas. Philadelphia, WB Saunders, 1981, p. 72.)

FIGURE 10–31. Common sites of nerve injuries. (From Adams JC: Outline of Fractures, 8th ed. New York, Churchill Livingstone, 1983).

SIGNS AND SYMPTOMS OF NERVE INJURY. The signs and symptoms of nerve injury are numbness, pain, abnormal sensation (different from that in the other limb), and loss of motor ability.

While most fractures are not complicated by nerve or vessel injury, it is mandatory that neurovascular function be evaluated in every case. Since continued swelling from the injury or from the constriction caused by tightly applied splints can cause later deterioration in neurovascular function, reevaluation of neurovascular status is required.

INJURIES TO THE VISCERA

Fractures of the pelvis may injure viscera within the pelvic cavity such as the bladder, urethra, rectum and lower intestine, and reproductive organs. Injuries to the thorax may cause hemothorax, pneumothorax, or rupture of the spleen and liver (Fig. 10–32).

FAT EMBOLISM

Small particles of fat from fractured bones can enter the bloodstream and become lodged in the lungs, causing shortness of breath. Fractures of the long bones and pelvis have been noted to cause fat embolisms, particularly after crushing injuries. Fat embolisms can cause shortness of breath even when there is no apparent injury to the lungs or any cardiovascular or cerebrovascular compromise. While the syndrome usually becomes apparent 1 to 3 days after injury, it can occur earlier in some cases, and field treatment requires supplemental oxygen.

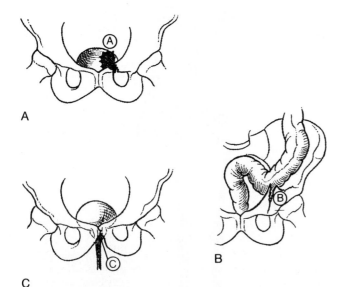

A

C

B

FIGURE 10–32. Fracture of the pelvis with rupture of the bladder (*A*), laceration of the colon or rectum (*B*), and rupture of the urethra (*C*). (From Connolly JF: DePalma's The Management of Fractures and Dislocations: An Atlas. Philadelphia, WB Saunders, 1981, p. 76.)

Physical Assessment

PRIMARY SURVEY

During the scene survey, determine the potential mechanism of injury by observing the immediate environment and briefly questioning the patient and bystanders. As always, the primary survey is undertaken while considering the possible presence of spine injuries. Assessment of the airway, breathing, circulation, control of hemorrhage, and identification of other life-threatening conditions such as open chest wounds and shock take priority over fractures. Do not become distracted by a grotesquely angulated fracture. Life-threatening conditions always come first and in some cases may require rapid transport along with primary life-support measures.

SECONDARY SURVEY

Begin the secondary survey by obtaining more information about the mechanism of injury and the conditions immediately surrounding the injury. It is very helpful to determine what was the position of an injured automobile passenger, whether a seat belt was worn, the speed at impact, the height from which a patient fell, as well as the position of the body upon impact. A history of events immediately preceding an accident might point to medical conditions that might have caused the accident. For example, did a patient trip and fall, or become dizzy, lose consciousness, and then fall?

Following a head-to-toe survey approach ensures that adequate attention is paid to the thorax, abdomen, and spine. Clothing should be opened or cut away if necessary to visualize the soft tissues and inspect the patient for abrasions, bruises, or deformities. Patterns of skin wounds and the nature of the injury may help you visualize the forces experienced by the patient during the trauma.

Some types of injuries can be anticipated by the mechanism of injury. For example, you can suspect that the motorcycle driver who is thrown over the handlebars and lands first on the shoulders or pelvis, with secondary jackknifing of the spinal column, may have suffered fracture to the thoracic and lumbar spine; or that patients with lap belt injuries may suffer a compression injury to the abdominal viscera, bruising of the abdominal wall, and a vertebral fracture from hyperflexion in the area around the lap belt (Fig. 10–33).

Other classic patterns of mechanisms of injury and their associated injuries are noted in Table 10–2 and Figure 10–34.

EXAMINATION OF THE BONY PELVIS. To quickly assess the pelvis for fractures, gently compress the two iliac crests medially and posteriorly. Stop if there is any complaint of pain or if you note instability of the pelvic

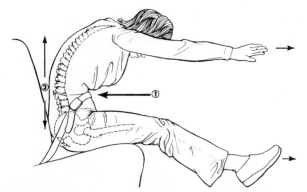

FIGURE 10–33. (*1*) An improperly placed safety belt can cause significant injury to the abdominal viscera and the spine. (*2*) Fractures are likely to occur where fixed vertebrae meet mobile vertebra, e.g., T10. (See Spinal Injury in Chapter 5.) (From Connolly JF: DePalma's The Management of Fractures and Dislocations: An Atlas. Philadelphia, WB Saunders, 1981, p. 76.)

ring itself. Instability of the ring requires a break in two places, which may be associated with significant blood loss. Compress the pubic symphysis gently to check for tenderness. Again, stop if there is pain or movement of the bone (Fig. 10–35).

EXTREMITIES. The extremities should be inspected for open wounds, deformities, swelling, discoloration, and other signs of fracture. With *gentle* palpation, note tenderness, swelling, deformity, and crepitus. It is important to compare one extremity with the other to note subtle differences in size. Be systematic and go from proximal to distal as you compare upper, then lower, extremities.

NEUROVASCULAR ASSESSMENT OF DISTAL EXTREMITIES

A neurovascular examination of parts distal to an injury should always be performed and documented. Distal pulses and capillary return should be noted, as well as the color and temperature of the skin. Again, compare the two limbs. Remember that hypovolemic shock can result in absent pulses, poor capillary return, and pallor and coolness of all extremities. Vascular compromise secondary to a fracture should cause findings in the affected limb only.

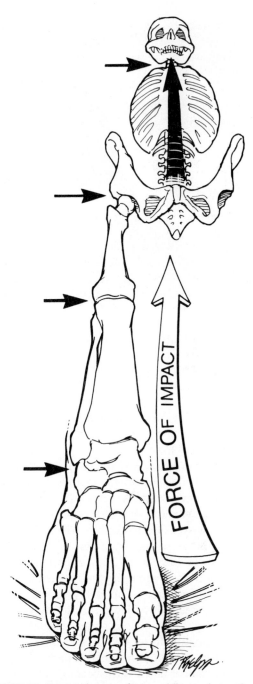

FIGURE 10–34. Mechanism of injury: fall onto feet with related fractures to the heel and spine. (From Cardona VD, Hurn PD, Mason PJB, et al: Trauma Nursing From Resuscitation Through Rehabilitation. Philadelphia, WB Saunders, 1988, p. 118.)

It is difficult to feel the dorsalis pedis pulse in some normal individuals (and less often, the posterior tibial pulse). Therefore, capillary return and the condition of the skin take on greater significance. Record these findings and relate them to the hospital staff.

Testing for neurologic function should be limited to checking for light sensation and movement. Elicit sensation on the medial and lateral aspects of both sides

TABLE 10–2. Mechanism of Injuries With Obvious and Associated Injuries

Mechanism of Injury	Obvious Injury	Associated Injury
Dashboard injuries	Anterior knee	Femur and hip
Fall from height	Calcaneus (heel), possibly hands	Spine, legs, pelvis
Fall on hand	Wrist	Shoulder, arm

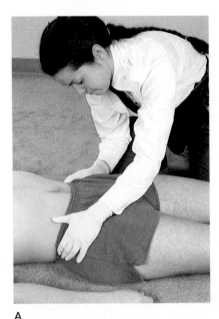
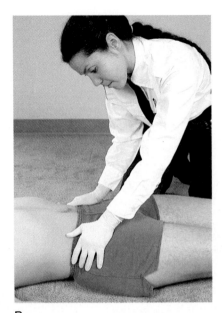
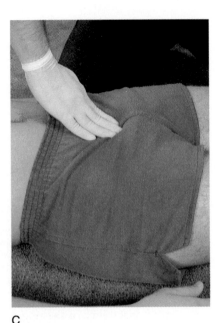

A   B   C

FIGURE 10–35. (*A*) Compress the iliac crests medially and (*B*) posteriorly, and (*C*) compress the symphysis pubis.

of the hands (palm and back) and feet (top and bottom) to check for skin areas innervated by separate peripheral nerves (Fig. 10–36).

Motor examination of the extremities must be undertaken with due consideration that there may be a fracture. Patients with obvious signs of fractures (such as deformity, crepitus, open fractures) should never be asked to move the affected limb or adjacent joints. Distal function can be checked by asking the patient to flex and extend the fingers and toes and wrists and ankles. It may be appropriate to restrict movement to the fingers and toes in some cases. The ability to flex and extend the phalanges is a good indicator that major nerves to the extremity are intact. No patient should be allowed to move an extremity or bear weight on a limb if there is a complaint of pain. Remember, impacted fractures still permit movement and weight-bearing with pain.

If a systematic routine is practiced, a reliable assessment of distal neurovascular function can be achieved in a few seconds.

Management

The goals of management for patients with extremity fractures are to reduce pain and prevent further injury by immobilizing the injured part. Minimizing any complications from fractures speeds healing. Immobilization prevents the further motion of bone fragments or dislocated joints and thereby minimizes pain and further damage to the surrounding soft tissues. It may also reduce blood loss. Without proper immobilization, bro-

ken bone fragments can cause further damage by tearing or pinching surrounding vessels, nerves, muscles, and other soft tissues. In extreme cases, a closed fracture might even be converted to an open fracture if sharp bone fragments move about and tear through overlying skin.

PRINCIPLES OF SPLINTING

There are many methods of immobilization and different types of splints. Certain principles of management should be adhered to regardless of the specific technique employed.

TREAT THE PATIENT AS A WHOLE. Saving the patient's life is the first priority. Assess and address life-threatening conditions before caring for extremity fractures. In some instances, the need for rapid transport may preclude splinting in the field, since the time taken to apply splints may delay treatment for life-threatening conditions.

ASSUME A FRACTURE UNTIL PROVEN OTHERWISE. There are many types of fractures, such as impacted or greenstick fractures, that may still allow function and normal motion of the extremity. However, if pain, tenderness, or the mechanism of injury suggests that a fracture is possible, treat it as such. Do not be misled by the absence of more obvious signs such as deformity, disability, or crepitus.

MINIMIZE MOVEMENT OF THE INJURED PART. Whenever possible, patients should be immobilized be-

FIGURE 10–36. Sensory nerves in the (*A*) upper and (*B*) lower extremities. (From Cardona VD, Hurn PD, Mason PJB, et al: Trauma Nursing From Resuscitation Through Rehabilitation. Philadelphia, WB Saunders, 1988, pp. 547 and 549.)

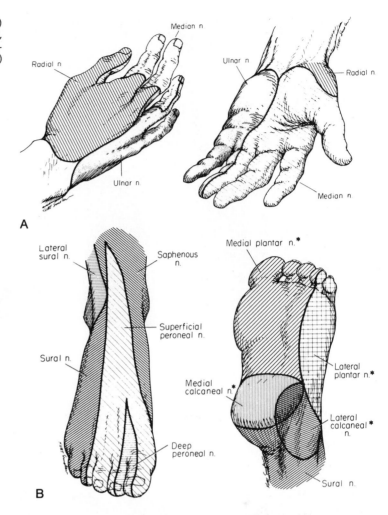

fore moving them. One should attempt to eliminate all unnecessary movement of the injured part. However, hazardous or life-threatening conditions may preclude splinting prior to movement.

PAD SPLINTS. The surface of the splint in contact with the patient should be well padded to avoid pressure points against soft tissues. Cut away clothing to expose the injured part so that folds of clothing do not act as pressure points beneath a splint.

SPLINT THE FRACTURE SITE AND ADJACENT JOINTS. To effectively immobilize a fracture, the joints above and below the fracture site should be immobilized. For example, when splinting fractures of the mid-forearm, the elbow and wrist should be immobilized. Likewise, to immobilize an injured joint, splint the bones above and below. For example, when splinting a fractured or dislocated elbow, include the humerus and the forearm.

CHECK AND RECHECK NEUROVASCULAR FUNCTION. Check distal pulses, capillary return, skin color and temperature, sensation, and motor function before and after splinting, and record your findings.

STRAIGHTEN ANGULATED FRACTURES. To facilitate splinting and provide proper immobilization, gently straighten angulated fractures. If resistance is encountered or the patient complains of pain, the extremity should be splinted in the position in which it is found. At times, straightening an angulation may restore blood flow by releasing entrapped vessels. Never forcefully attempt to straighten a locked extremity.

COVER OPEN WOUNDS. All open wounds over suspected fractures should be dressed and bandaged prior to splinting. If bone ends are protruding, do not attempt to reintroduce them back in through the wound by traction. Cover protruding bone fragments with a sterile moistened dressing covered by a dry dressing. In some cases, gentle straightening of a gross angulation may be necessary for splinting and movement of the patient, or to restore blood flow.

Types of Splints

There are several varieties of splints that are used to immobilize fractures. The EMT should be familiar with the advantages and disadvantages of each type.

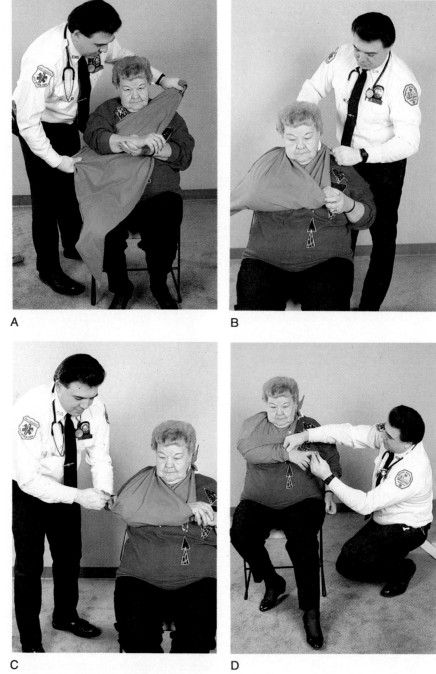

FIGURE 10–37. Applying a sling and swathe. (*A*) Place sling with the long end over the opposite shoulder and the apex toward the injured side. (*B*) Tie the sling at the side of the neck to avoid pressure. (*C*) Secure the end of the sling with a knot or twist. (*D*) Attach the swathe and check distal circulation.

RIGID SPLINTS.   Rigid splints are made of a rigid material such as cardboard, wood, metal, or plastic and should be well padded. They come in lengths of a few inches for fingers to 5 feet in length for fractures of the lower extremity not requiring traction. They are applied on either side of a fractured extremity and secured with roller bandages or cravats. These splints can be made

from readily available materials and also are commercially available. They are very versatile and can be adapted as needed to immobilize angulated fractures.

AIR SPLINTS.   Air splints are plastic splints that are filled with air to provide circumferential support to an injured extremity. They come in various lengths and configurations for use on distal upper and lower extremity fractures. The PASG can serve as an air splint for patients with lower extremity or pelvic fractures in the presence of shock. The air pressure within an air splint must be reevaluated with changes in environmental temperature.

WIRE LADDER SPLINTS. Wire ladder splints are constructed of thin metal rods. They are flexible and can be shaped and molded to conform to a fractured extremity. They should be well padded before application and attached with roller bandages or cravats.

PILLOW SPLINTS. A pillow can be used as a splint for an ankle or as an adjunct in the immobilization of dislocations. It can be attached with safety pins, bandages, or cravats.

SLING AND SWATHE SPLINTS. A sling is a triangle-shaped bandage that is used to support the weight of the arm, and a swathe is a folded triangular bandage or roller bandage used to bind the upper arm to the chest wall. The sling and swathe is used in the treatment of most upper extremity injuries as a primary method of immobilization or as an adjunct to splints. A sling and swathe can be bought commercially or improvised.

TRACTION SPLINTS. Traction splints are devices consisting of a metal frame and a pulley system to apply traction to the lower extremity. They range from a simple Thomas splint, consisting of a metal frame used with bandage materials to apply traction, to sophisticated devices such as the Hare or Sager splints with preattached Velcro fasteners and mechanical pulleys. Traction splints are used to immobilize fractures of the femur, and are an option for hip and tibia immobilization.

IMPROVISED SPLINTS. One may use blankets, magazines, cardboard, and other materials to accomplish the objectives of immobilization. The device is less important than the principles of treatment.

Methods of Splinting

UPPER EXTREMITY

APPLYING A SLING AND SWATHE. The sling and swathe is the primary immobilization technique for fractures to the clavicle, scapula, shoulder, and humerus. It is also useful for fractures of the elbow and forearm, treated with the elbow flexed. When applying the sling and swathe, care should be taken not to apply excessive pressure over the axillary region on the opposite side. The sling supports the weight of the arm and keeps the forearm elevated. The swathe serves to bind the upper extremity to the chest wall to prevent movement (Fig. 10–37).

P R O C E D U R E   1 0 – 1
APPLYING A SLING TO AN UPPER EXTREMITY

1. Carefully place a triangular bandage between the injured extremity and the chest wall, with the short point directed laterally.
2. Drape the superior portion of the long point over the shoulder on the noninjured side.
3. Bring the inferior long point over the shoulder on the injured side and tie a square knot, using the long points. The knot should be placed at the side of the neck for the comfort of the patient.
4. Wrap a cravat bandage (folded twice) around the injured arm, halfway between the elbow and shoulder. Tie the two ends of the cravat at the mid-clavicular line just above the nipple on the uninjured side.

Note: For further immobilization, a second cravat can be traversed across the elbow to the uninjured side.

Note: When applying a sling and swathe, the hand on the injured side should extend slightly from the sling so that circulation may be evaluated by examining the hand for pulse, color, temperature, and capillary refill.

APPLYING A RIGID SPLINT TO THE HUMERUS. Fractures to the shaft of the humerus should be immobilized with a rigid splint (Fig. 10–38A). The splint extends from the axilla to the elbow to provide additional support to the shaft of the humerus. Then a sling and swathe are applied over the rigid splint.

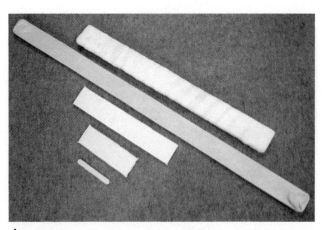

A

FIGURE 10–38. Applying a rigid splint to the humerus. (*A*) Different sized splints.

> ### PROCEDURE 10-2   APPLYING A RIGID SPLINT TO THE HUMERUS (TWO-EMT METHOD)
>
>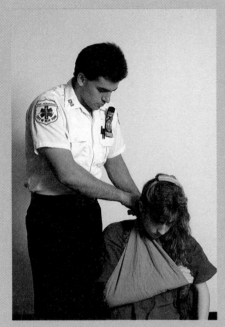
>
> B
>
> 1. EMT 1 maintains alignment to the extremity distal and proximal to the injury, while EMT 2 places a 9-inch splint on the medial aspect of the arm and attaches it with a roller bandage or cravats.
> 2. A sling is put in place by EMT 2, and a swathe attaches the arm to the chest wall (Fig. 10–38*B* and *C*).
> 3. Distal pulses are reassessed, and the fingernails are left exposed out of the sling to allow for evaluation of distal neurovascular function.
>
>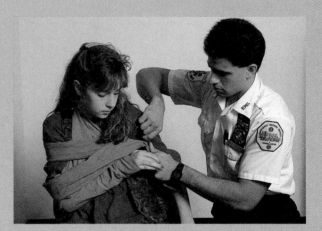
>
> C
>
> **FIGURE 10–38.** (*B*) The splint is applied to the inner humerus area (not seen in picture), and a sling is applied as described above. (*C*) A swathe is secured in place.

APPLYING A RIGID SPLINT TO THE FOREARM. To immobilize fractures of the mid-forearm, use a rigid 18-inch splint extending from the palm of the hand out past the medial aspect of the elbow (Fig. 10–39).

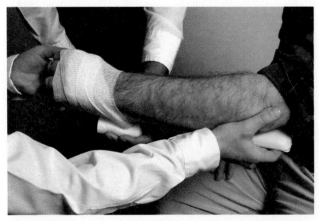

A

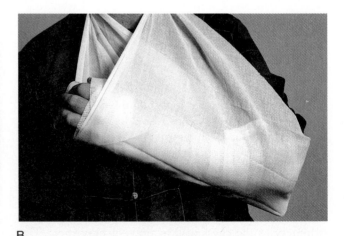

B

FIGURE 10–39. Applying a rigid splint to the forearm. (*A*) Maintain distal and proximal immobilization and attach the splint with a self-adherent bandage or cravats. (*B*) Attach a sling and elevate the extremity to reduce swelling.

PROCEDURE 10-3 APPLYING A RIGID SPLINT TO THE FOREARM (TWO-EMT METHOD)

1. EMT 1 maintains alignment with gentle traction distal and proximal to the site of injury.
2. EMT 2 places an 18-inch rigid splint along the anterior aspect of the forearm, extending from the proximal joint of the phalanges to the medial epicondyle of the humerus.
3. EMT 2 attaches the splint with a roller bandage or cravats at the elbow, mid-forearm, and hand.
4. EMT 2 then attaches a sling with the forearm flexed at the elbow. For injuries of the forearm and wrist, the forearm can be slightly elevated to minimize swelling and pain. Reassess the patient's neurovascular status.

SPLINTING THE ARM IN THE STRAIGHTENED POSITION. When the arm is found in a straightened position and a fracture of the forearm or elbow is suspected, the arm can be splinted in the extended position with a rigid splint.

PROCEDURE 10-4 SPLINTING AN ARM IN THE STRAIGHTENED POSITION (TWO-EMT METHOD)

1. EMT 1 maintains alignment distal and proximal to the injury with gentle traction (Fig. 10–40A).
2. EMT 2 places a rigid arm board from the proximal phalanges past the elbow along the anterior aspect of the arm (Fig. 10–40B).
3. Attach a swathe that binds the arm to the chest wall (Fig. 10–40C).

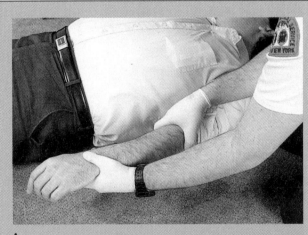

A

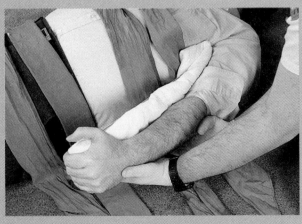

B

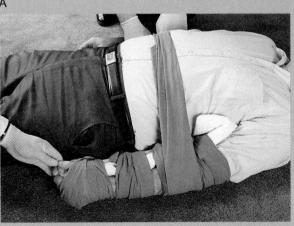

C

FIGURE 10–40. Splinting the arm in the straightened position. (A) Maintain distal and proximal immobilization. (B) Place cravats in approximate application locations and place the splint in place. (C) Attach the splint with cravats and secure the arm to the body.

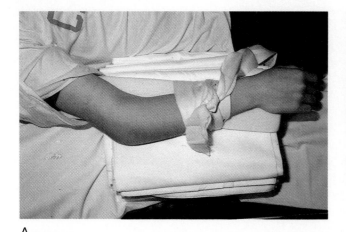
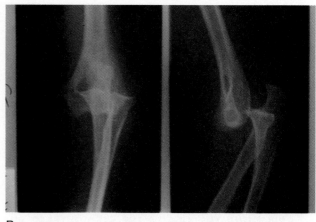

A

B

FIGURE 10–41. Applying a splint to the elbow in the angulated position. (*A*) Note deformity caused by dislocation of elbow and splint applied by prehospital personnel. (*B*) X-ray film of deformity shown in *A*.

APPLYING A SPLINT TO THE ELBOW IN THE ANGULATED POSITION. In the event that an elbow is angulated and locked due to a dislocation, it may be immobilized in the position found. A rigid splint can be bridged from the humerus to the distal forearm to prevent movement of the elbow (Fig. 10–41*A* and *B*).

PROCEDURE 10–5 **APPLYING A SPLINT TO AN ELBOW IN THE ANGULATED POSITION (TWO-EMT METHOD)**

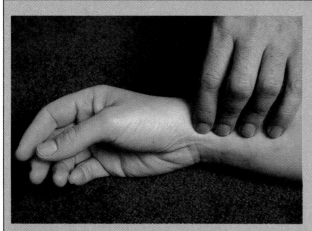

C

1. EMT 1 checks distal circulation (Fig. 10–41*C*).
2. EMT 1 maintains manual support to immobilize the elbow and EMT 2 places a splint from the medial aspect of the proximal upper arm to the distal forearm. The splint is attached with cravats or a roller bandage (Fig.10–41*D*).
3. Support the weight of the arm with a folded cravat attached to the wrist and secured around the neck (Fig. 10–41*E*).
4. Carefully reassess distal neurovascular function.

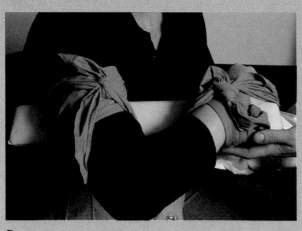
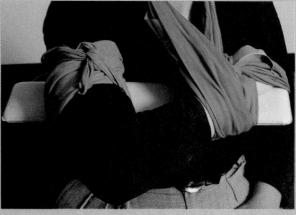

D

E

FIGURE 10–41. (*C*) Check distal circulation and nerve function. (*D*) Bridge humerus to forearm with an 18-inch splint and secure with cravats. (*E*) Use a cravat for a sling to avoid direct pressure on the elbow.

RIGID SPLINT TO THE WRIST. The wrist and hand region is simply immobilized by attachment of a 9-inch rigid splint that extends from the proximal joint of the phalanges to the mid-forearm. The forearm is then placed in a sling.

If the injury is proximal to the wrist, check radial and ulnar pulses as for all upper extremity injuries. If the injury is to the wrist and hand, use skin color and temperature and capillary return to gauge distal vascular function (Fig. 10–42A)

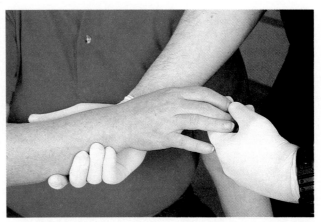

A

FIGURE 10–42. Applying a splint to the wrist. (*A*) Check distal circulation.

PROCEDURE 10-6 APPLYING A RIGID SPLINT TO THE WRIST (TWO-EMT METHOD)

1. EMT 1 maintains alignment by holding the extremity proximal and distal to the fracture site and applying gentle traction.
2. EMT 2 then places a wad of gauze or a roller bandage in the patient's palm to keep the hand and fingers in a position of function (Fig. 10–42B).
3. EMT 2 then places a 9-inch splint on the anterior aspect of the wrist and hand, extending from the proximal joint of the phalanges to the mid-forearm.
4. EMT 1 holds the splint in place while EMT 2 attaches it with a roller bandage and reevaluates distal circulation.
5. EMT 2 then attaches a sling and swathe (Fig. 10–42C and D) in place with the wrist elevated to reduce swelling (Fig. 10–42E).

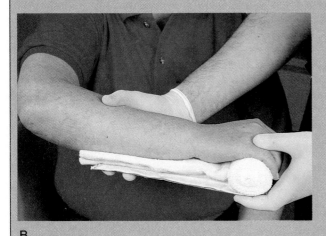

B

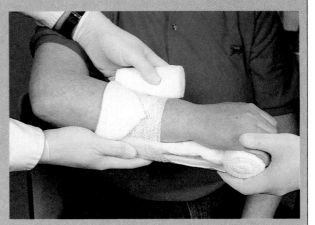

C

FIGURE 10–42. (*B*) Maintain distal and proximal immobilization and position the padded splint to extend from the fingertips to at least mid-arm. (*C*) A rolled bandage can be placed in the hand to maintain the position of function.

Continued

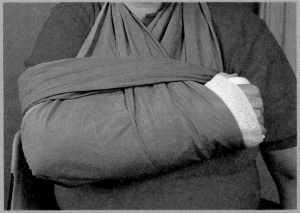
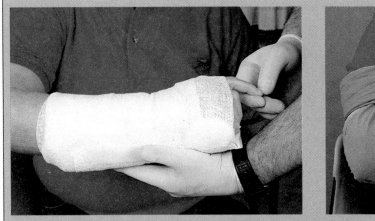

D

E

FIGURE 10–42. *Continued. (D)* Attach the splint with a self-adherent bandage or cravats. *(E)* Attach a sling and swathe (optional) to elevate the extremity and to reduce swelling.

APPLYING A SPLINT TO FINGERS. Fingers are splinted with a flexible aluminum splint or a tongue blade. The splint can be attached with $\frac{1}{2}$-inch tape or 2-inch roller gauze, taking care not to constrict distal blood flow. Multiple finger fractures might be immobilized with a rigid board splint or air splint (Fig. 10–43).

AIR SPLINT TO THE UPPER EXTREMITY. An air splint can be used in place of a rigid board splint for fractures of the upper extremity. The air splints are available in full-arm and partial-arm lengths.

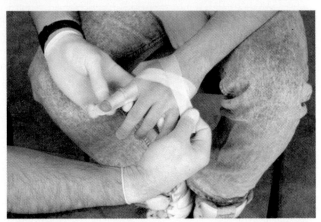

FIGURE 10–43. Applying a finger splint. Extend a tongue blade or commercial finger splint from the tip of the finger to the heel of the hand and tape in place.

PROCEDURE 10–7   **APPLYING AN AIR SPLINT TO THE UPPER EXTREMITY (TWO-EMT METHOD)**

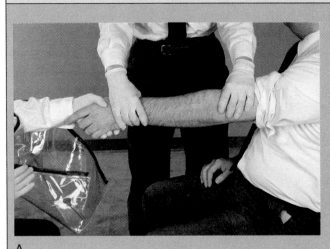

A

1. EMT 1 maintains immobilization with gentle traction.
2. EMT 2 slides the air splint around his or her own arm and then gently grasps the patient's hand (Fig. 10–44*A*).
3. The splint is then advanced up the patient's arm while EMT 1 maintains support (Fig. 10–44*B*).
4. Inflate the splint until thumb pressure results in a small indentation in the splint (Fig. 10–44*C*).
5. Reassess neurovascular function. Take care to reassess air pressure within the splint with changes in environmental temperature.

FIGURE 10–44. Applying an air splint. *(A)* While one EMT maintains distal and proximal immobilization, the other EMT slides the air splint around his or her own arm and grasps the patient's hand.

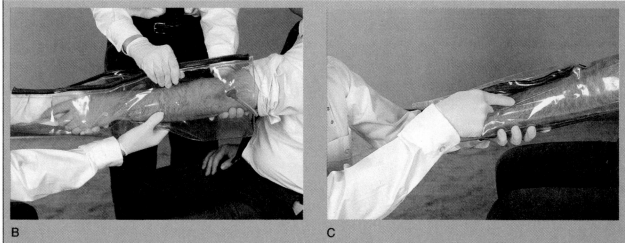

B   C

FIGURE 10-44. *Continued.* (*B*) While continuing to maintain immobilization, the splint is slid up the patient's arm. (*C*) The splint is inflated by blowing in the inflation tube and tested by compressing with your finger. The splint should experience a slight dent when full. (This splint is slightly underinflated.)

LOWER EXTREMITY INJURIES

IMMOBILIZATION OF PELVIC FRACTURES. The pelvis is best immobilized with a long spine board or the PASG. The PASG can be used to treat shock and to immobilize a pelvic fracture. It has been used even in hospitals for short-term treatment of these fractures, since it can help tamponade associated bleeding in some cases.

A spine board is used for all pelvic fractures. The patient should be securely attached with straps. The legs of the patient can be tied together after padding is placed between the legs to offer further immobilization (Fig. 10–45).

APPLYING A HARE TRACTION SPLINT. The Hare traction splint is an adjustable leg splint with a mechanical pulley to establish traction for fractures of the hip, femur, tibia, and fibula. The splint comes with various sized, padded ankle hitches, Velcro leg bands, and a Velcro groin strap to prevent the splint from slipping upward when traction is applied (Fig. 10–46A). Traction is achieved by fixing the splint against the ischial tuberosity of the pelvic bone (located at the base of each buttock).

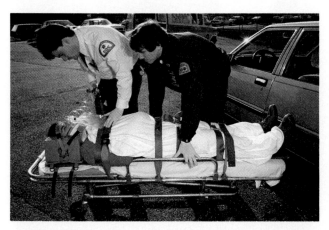

FIGURE 10-45. Spine board immobilization. A fully immobilized patient. This is discussed at length in Chapter 16, Lifting and Moving Patients.

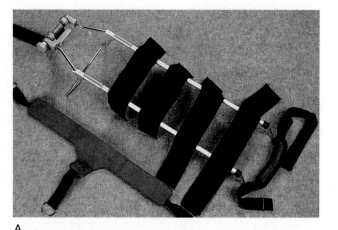

A

FIGURE 10-46. Applying a Hare traction splint. (*A*) The Hare traction splint with ankle hitch.

PROCEDURE 10–8   APPLYING A HARE TRACTION SPLINT (TWO-EMT METHOD)

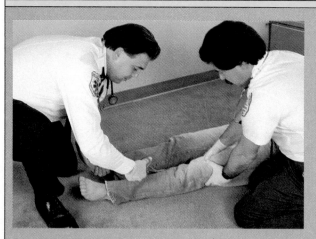

B

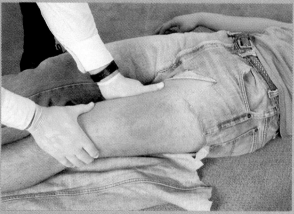

C

1. EMT 1 stabilizes the leg while EMT 2 cuts away the trousers and removes the shoe and sock from the foot on the affected side (Fig. 10–46*B* and *C*).
2. EMT 2 evaluates neurocirculatory function by checking the dorsalis pedis and/or posterior tibial pulse (Fig. 10–46*D* and *E*).
3. EMT 2 applies the ankle hitch and EMT 1 maintains traction with the ankle hitch while the splint is applied. The ankle hitch is positioned with the edge of the foam pad at the posterior of the heel bone. The other two straps are then crisscrossed over the ankle (Fig. 10–46*F* and *G*).
4. Adjust the splint so that the end is approximately 12 inches below the patient's foot and the Velcro straps are opened to receive the extremity (Fig. 10–46*H* and *I*).
5. Position the splint up against the ischial tuberosity (at the base of the buttock). EMT 1 may have to elevate the leg slightly to facilitate placement. The ischial strap is secured around the upper thigh (Fig. 10–46*J*).
6. Attach the rings of the ankle hitch to the hook of the pulley strap (the posterior hitch ring should be attached first). Traction is then established by rotating the adjustment knob of the pulley (Fig. 10–46*K*).
7. After firm, gentle traction has been established, attach two Velcro leg bands above the knee and two below the knee (Fig. 10–46*L*).
8. Monitor circulation to the extremity carefully, especially in older people. Color, temperature, capillary refill of the toes, and comparison of one foot to another can be used to determine adequate flow. Movement should be tested.

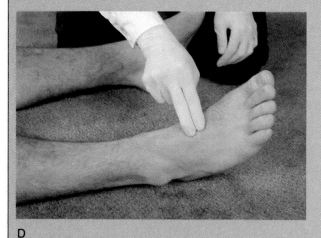

D   E

FIGURE 10–46. (*D* and *E*) Check distal circulation while maintaining immobilization of the knee. Check dorsalis pedis and posterior tibial pulses. (*F* and *G*) Attach ankle hitch while traction is maintained at knee (not shown). (*H* and *I*) Measure and adjust length of splint. (*J*) Place splint with ischial bar at the base of the buttocks with as little manipulation as possible. (*K*) Take up traction until the patient feels comfort or compare to the good leg. (*L*) Attach the Velcro leg bands and measure distal circulation. Other traction splints include (*M*) the Ferno traction splint,

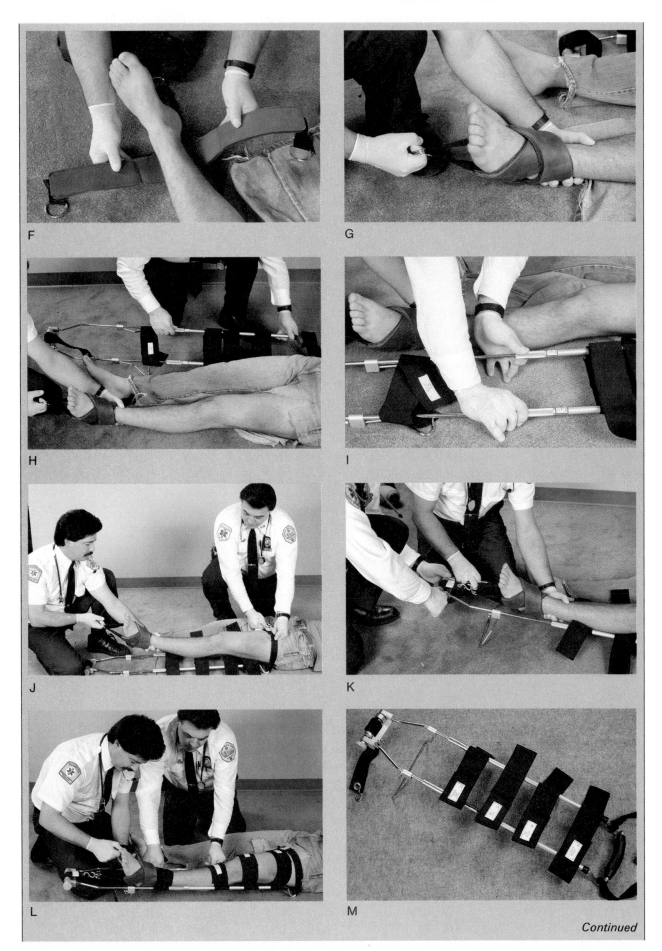

F

G

H

I

J

K

L

M

Continued

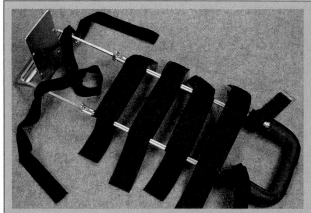
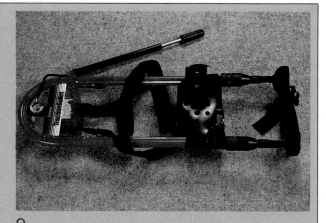

FIGURE 10–46 *Continued.* (*N*) Kipple traction splint, and (*O*) Donway traction splint, which has a pneumatic pump.

APPLYING A SAGER TRACTION SPLINT. The Sager traction splint is an adjustable leg splint with a mechanical pulley to establish traction for fractures of the hip, femur, tibia, and fibula. The Sager traction splint has a single adjustable bar that can be placed on the medial or lateral aspect of the leg (Fig. 10–47*A*). Traction is achieved by fixing the splint against the perineum.

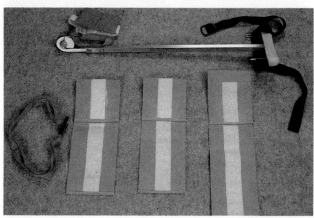

FIGURE 10–47. Applying a Sager traction splint. (*A*) The Sager traction splint with ankle hitch and straps. This application is being performed while immobilization is maintained, but the Sager splint can be applied without active immobilization due to the minimal movement needed to apply it.

PROCEDURE 10-9 APPLYING A SAGER TRACTION SPLINT (TWO-EMT METHOD)

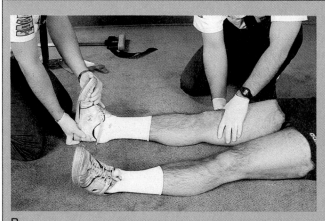

FIGURE 10–47. (*B*) Remove the shoe and sock.

1. EMT 1 stabilizes the leg while EMT 2 cuts away the trousers, and removes the shoe and sock from the foot on the affected side (Fig. 10–47*B*).
2. EMT 2 evaluates neurocirculatory function (Fig. 10–47*C*).
3. EMT 2 positions the splint on either the lateral or medial aspect of the leg and attaches the groin strap (Fig. 10–47*D*).
4. Attach the ankle hitch and apply traction (Fig. 10–47*E* and *F*).
5. Attach the elastic straps to the thigh, knee, and tibial area, and bind the ankles together to avoid lateral motion (Fig. 10–47*G* and *H*).
6. Monitor circulation to the extremity carefully, especially in older people. Color, temperature, and capillary refill of the toes, as well as comparison of one foot to another, can be used to determine adequate flow. Movement should be tested.

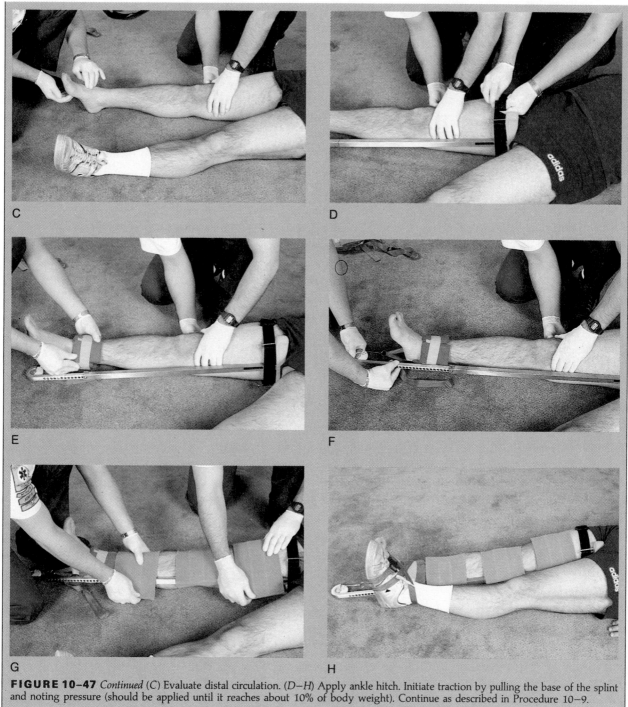

FIGURE 10–47 *Continued* (*C*) Evaluate distal circulation. (*D–H*) Apply ankle hitch. Initiate traction by pulling the base of the splint and noting pressure (should be applied until it reaches about 10% of body weight). Continue as described in Procedure 10–9.

ANTERIOR AND POSTERIOR DISLOCATIONS OF THE HIP. Dislocations of the hip are often locked and resist straightening. The patient should be placed on a long spine board and pillows should be placed between the knee area and the board to provide support. The legs can then be tied together for additional support. Traction splints are contraindicated for immobilization of hip dis-locations, due to the angulation and locking of the ex-tremity.

LONG BOARD RIGID LEG SPLINT. The long board splint can be used to immobilize fractures of the knee, tibia, and fibula in the straightened position.

PROCEDURE 10-10   *APPLYING LONG BOARD RIGID LEG SPLINT (TWO-EMT METHOD)*

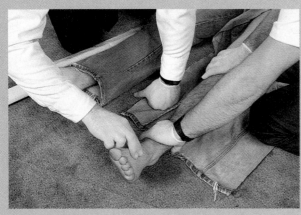

A

1. Assess distal circulation and function (Fig. 10–48*A*).
2. EMT 1 maintains gentle traction and support to the lower extremity.
3. EMT 2 places cravats in two locations above and below the knee and aligns the splints on the medial and lateral aspect of the leg. The groin should be padded (Fig. 10–48*B*).
4. Attach the cravats and tuck them into the splint on the medial side to avoid being caught during transport (Fig. 10–48*C*).

Note: Additional cravats can be attached at the chest and abdomen for further immobilization.

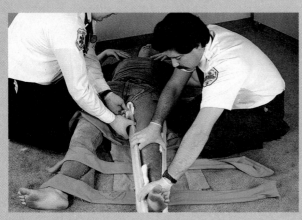

B

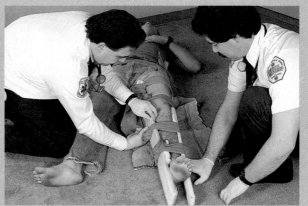

C

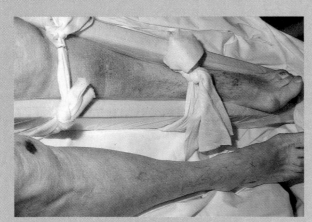

D

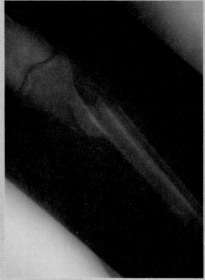

E

FIGURE 10–48. Applying a rigid leg splint. (*A*) Maintain immobilization, cut pants away, and check distal circulation. (*B*) Align splints and cravats along the length of the leg. (*C*) Attach cravats and elevate distal circulation. (*D*) Rigid splint applied to fractured tibia (note ecchymosis and indentation on anterior leg). (*E*) X-ray film of (*D*).

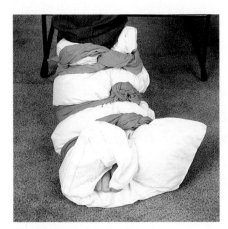

FIGURE 10–49. A pillow splint.

AIR SPLINT TO THE LOWER EXTREMITIES. To apply an air splint to the lower extremity, EMT 1 should hold the extremity immobile while EMT 2 slides the air splint around the affected leg, zippers the splint closed, and inflates it until a thumbprint is just visible. Again, monitor pressures during changes in environment.

PILLOW SPLINT. A pillow splint can be used to immobilize fractures of the ankle and foot and as an adjunct when immobilizing dislocations of the upper and lower extremities. The pillow can be wrapped around the ankle and foot and attached in place by safety pins, cravats, or roller bandages (Fig. 10–49).

UPPER EXTREMITY INJURIES

Recognition of Fractures, Dislocations, and Sprains

In the prehospital phase, recognition of extremity fractures and dislocations is based on knowledge of the mechanism of injury and the basic signs and symptoms of fractures such as pain, swelling, tenderness, and deformity. Additionally, certain types of fractures and dislocations are identified by their "classic" presentations. For example, fractures of the hip may result in external rotation and apparent shortening of the leg. Clavicle fractures often cause the patient to drop the affected shoulder and hold the arm on the affected side closely against the chest. Therefore, it is important for the EMT to have a concept of these essential diagnostic clues.

Additionally, many fractures are associated with other injuries. For example, fractures of the calcaneus (heel) are frequently accompanied by fracture of the spine and lower extremity. Identification of certain fractures is a cue for the EMT to search for common associated injuries that often are more serious than the primary fracture.

The following section addresses all these issues. Different fractures or joint injuries are discussed according to the common mechanism of injury, common sites and types of fractures and dislocations to that bone, the signs and symptoms special to the fracture that aid in recognition, associated injuries, and recommended prehospital treatment.

Clavicle

MECHANISM OF INJURY

The clavicle is a superficial bone and is susceptible to fracture by a direct blow to the anterior upper chest or from a fall on the lateral aspect of the shoulder. It is commonly fractured indirectly from falls on the outstretched hand, with the force being transmitted to the clavicle.

TYPES OF FRACTURES

Direct blows can cause fractures anywhere along the clavicle, whereas indirect forces tend to fracture the clavicle at the junction between the middle and lateral thirds of the bone.

Fractures of the middle third of the clavicle often result in characteristic deformity because of the pull of opposing muscles. The clavicle is tightly bound to the scapula over its lateral third by ligaments, and fractures to the lateral third of the bone are seldom displaced.

The clavicle can become dislocated from the sternum or the scapula. Dislocations of the sternoclavicular joint are usually anterior and are palpable. Rarely, the clavicle is dislocated posteriorly from the sternum, a position where it may compress vessels and cause airway compromise.

SIGNS AND SYMPTOMS

The patient with a clavicle fracture complains of pain in the shoulder and may hold the arm against the chest, with the opposite hand supporting the weight of the arm at the elbow. When fractures occur over the medial third of the bone, the sternocleidomastoid muscles elevate the medial fragment while the weight of the arm causes the unsupported lateral fragment to drop. The shoulder not only drops, but is also rotated inward because of the pull of the pectoralis major muscle. Thus, the affected shoulder drops downward and forward and is closer to the midline than is the opposite shoulder. The displacement of fragments causes a visible and palpable deformity and results in a characteristic drooping of the shoulder (see Fig. 10–26A).

Undisplaced fractures or fractures to the lateral aspect may cause pain with tenderness at the site.

ASSOCIATED INJURIES

Fractures of the clavicle may be associated with injuries to the rib cage, the underlying vessels (subclavian) and nerves to the arm, the lungs, and the pleura.

TREATMENT

The aim of treatment for a fractured clavicle is to immobilize the shoulder and support the weight of the upper arm. A sling and swathe accomplish both of these objectives.

Scapula

MECHANISMS OF INJURY

Because the scapula is well protected by overlying back muscles, a violent direct blow is usually necessary to cause a fracture to this bone. Fractures of the scapula therefore indicate that a great deal of force was absorbed by the patient and raise concern about damage to the underlying thorax.

TYPES OF FRACTURES

Fractures can occur over the spine, body, or other processes.

SIGNS AND SYMPTOMS

Since the scapula is so well protected by muscles, fractures are not usually displaced and may not be obvious. There may be some palpable irregularity, swelling, pain, and ecchymosis. The patient may hold the arm against the chest (adduction) and resist any attempts at abduction of the arm, since the scapula is used in initiating abduction.

ASSOCIATED INJURIES

Injuries to the ribs, spine, and lungs must be looked for when scapula fractures are suspected because of the violent forces necessary to fracture this bone.

TREATMENT

The sling and swathe are used to treat scapula fractures.

Dislocation of the Acromioclavicular Joint

The acromion process of the scapula is attached to the lateral aspect of the clavicle at the shoulder. The ligaments supporting this joint can be sprained to such a degree that dislocation results.

MECHANISM OF INJURY

Direct forces include a fall with the arm adducted to the side, or a force striking downward on the lateral aspect of the shoulder. Football players are prone to this injury. Falls on the outstretched arm during which the force is transmitted to this joint can cause dislocation as well.

TYPES OF DISLOCATIONS

A sprain to the ligaments holding the joint together may be so great that the ligaments tear and the joint separates.

SIGNS AND SYMPTOMS

The patient may complain of pain over the acromioclavicular joint that is aggravated by movement. With complete dislocation a deformity may be visible or palpable (Fig. 10–50).

TREATMENT

Support the weight of the arm with a sling and swathe.

Dislocations of the Shoulder

Dislocations of the shoulder involve displacement of the head of the humerus from the glenoid process of the scapula.

MECHANISMS OF INJURY

The humerus is usually displaced anteriorly, although posterior dislocations are infrequently encountered. An anterior dislocation usually results from a fall with the arm abducted and externally rotated. Or, for example, an anterior dislocation can occur in football

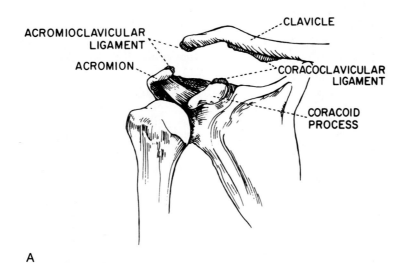

A

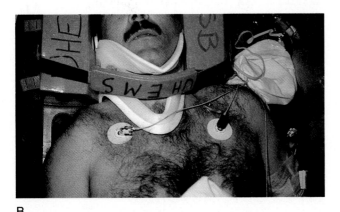

B

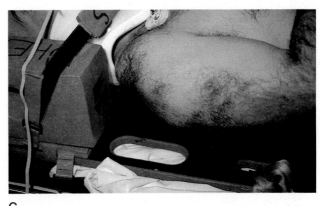

C

FIGURE 10–50. (*A*) Acromioclavicular joint separation. (*B* and *C*) Patient with injury shown in (*A*). (*A*, From Zuidema GD, Rutherford RB, Ballinger WF: The Management of Trauma, 4th ed. Philadelphia, WB Saunders, 1985, p. 684.)

when a tackler has his arm driven backward with forceful abduction and external rotation. It can also occur in a fall on the outstretched hand when the glenoid slides over the humerus. Posterior dislocation can result from a forceful blow delivered to the anterior humerus or from violent contractions of the deltoid during seizures, when the arms are internally rotated.

TYPES OF DISLOCATIONS AND FRACTURES

As noted, most dislocations are anterior; that is, the humeral head lies more anterior with respect to the scapula. The humerus can also be displaced posteriorly (5% of shoulder dislocations). Dislocations may be associated with fractures of the proximal humerus.

SIGNS AND SYMPTOMS

A good sign of anterior dislocation is the loss of the normal rounded contour of the shoulder, and the head of the humerus may be palpable anteriorly and

medially from its normal position. The patient may be able to abduct and externally rotate the shoulder but resists adduction and internal rotation (Fig. 10–51).

The posteriorly dislocated shoulder may cause the patient to hold the arm stiffly at the side in internal rotation.

ASSOCIATED INJURIES

Dislocated shoulders may be associated with fractures to the bones of the shoulders and tearing or overstretching of nerves and vessels. The axillary nerve, which provides sensation to part of the lateral aspect of the shoulder and activates the deltoid muscles, may be involved.

TREATMENT

The sling and swathe are the treatment of choice. However, when a patient presents with the arm locked in abduction or external rotation and resists movement, a pillow or blanket should be placed between the chest

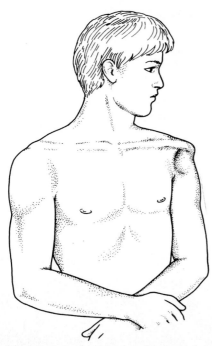

FIGURE 10–51. Deformity of anterior dislocation of the shoulder. (From Kitt S, Kaiser J: Emergency Nursing: A Physiologic and Clinical Perspective. Philadelphia, WB Saunders, 1990, p. 389.)

and arm for additional support. A sling and swathe can then be applied.

Proximal Humerus

MECHANISMS OF INJURY

Direct violence to the lateral aspect of the shoulder or indirect forces from falls on an outstretched arm with the elbow extended, as well as twisting forces, can cause fractures to the proximal humerus (Fig. 10–52).

TYPES OF FRACTURES

Fractures may be displaced or impacted. Displaced fragments may cause significant pain on attempted movement and limit or prevent use of the arm. Impacted fractures may permit motion and use of the arm, since the fragments are driven together and can function as a unit.

SIGNS AND SYMPTOMS

Displaced fractures may present with obvious deformity and other classic signs of fractures. Impacted fractures may cause less pain and ecchymosis, and the patient may still have the ability to use the arm. The ecchymosis may gravitate downward after a day or two. The EMT may encounter elderly patients with an im-

pacted fracture of the humerus who have fallen two days before and have pain with movement of an ecchymotic upper arm (Fig. 10–52B).

ASSOCIATED INJURIES

Injuries to the nerves of the upper arm as well as bleeding can result from these fractures.

TREATMENT

The treatment for fractures of the proximal humerus is the sling and swathe. If the patient is in the supine position, the arm can be bound to the side with swathes.

Shaft of the Humerus

MECHANISMS OF INJURY

The shaft of the humerus can be fractured from direct blows or indirect twisting forces secondary to falls on the elbow or outstretched hand. The shaft of the humerus is a common site for pathologic fractures in patients with cancer, since this is a common site for bony spread of cancer lesions (Fig. 10–52C). In these latter patients, little force is needed to cause a fracture.

TYPES OF FRACTURES

As with other long bones, angulation can occur. Deformities can be caused by displacement of the bone fragments by opposing muscles or by the overriding of fragments.

SIGNS AND SYMPTOMS

In addition to pain and swelling, different types of fractures may result in obvious deformity, abnormal mobility, crepitus, angulation, or shortening.

ASSOCIATED INJURIES

The classic injury associated with fractures of the humeral shaft is injury to the radial nerve, causing wrist drop. The radial nerve traverses the humerus and is occasionally severed or pinched, causing an inability to dorsiflex the wrist and hand. This may be obvious on examination for distal neurovascular function.

TREATMENT

Treatment may be provided by applying a 9-inch padded splint to the humerus and then using a sling and swathe to immobilize the elbow and shoulder. Place extra padding between the splint and the axilla. Attempt to gently straighten angulated fractures prior to splinting.

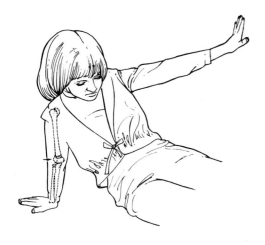

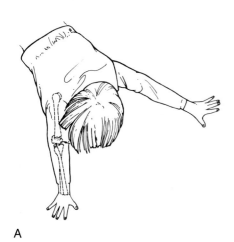

A

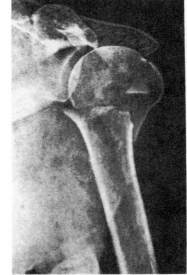

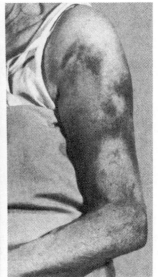

B

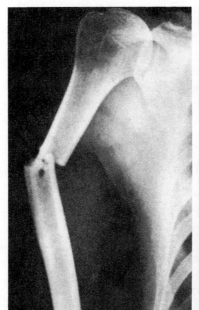

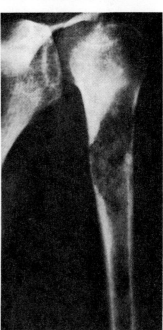

C

FIGURE 10–52. Falls (*A*) on an outstretched hand are the primary cause of fractures and dislocations in the upper extremity. (*B left*) A fracture of the neck of the humerus. (*B right*) Fractures of the humerus may present 1 or 2 days later with extensive bruising of the arm. (*C, left*) Angulation of humeral fracture. (*C, right*) The humerus is a common site for pathologic fractures resulting from cancer. Note the loss of bone density in the x-ray film shown. (*A,* from Connolly JF: DePalma's The Management of Fractures and Dislocations: An Atlas. Philadelphia, WB Saunders, 1981, p. 751; *B* and *C,* Adams JC: Outline of Fractures, 8th ed. New York, Churchill Livingstone, 1983, pp. 130 and 134.)

Distal Humerus

MECHANISMS OF INJURY

Fractures of the distal humerus are commonly seen in children and older adults. Direct blows over the olecranon or indirect forces from falls with the arm in various positions of flexion can cause these fractures. Other indirect forces involve twisting forces generated after falls on an extended arm.

TYPES OF FRACTURES

Because of the opposing forces of the forearm muscles, the biceps and the triceps, fractures of the distal humerus can result in grotesque deformities from overriding of fragments. Severe displacement can result in open fractures.

SIGNS AND SYMPTOMS

Deformity may be obvious with apparent shortening of the forearm and prominence of the end of the elbow. Ecchymosis and swelling from bleeding may be noted.

ASSOCIATED INJURIES

Injuries to nerves and vessels are encountered with fractures to the distal humerus because of their close proximity to the bones at the elbow joint.

Disruption of the arterial supply causing ischemia of the forearm muscles may result in a classic condition known as Volkmann's ischemic contracture. The arterial supply can be severed, occluded by thrombosis or spasm, or occluded by swelling of the surrounding soft tissues. The most classic sign of ischemic injury to the muscles is constant and increasing pain. The hand and wrist may assume a characteristic position, with the fingers and wrist flexed. Passive extension of the fingers is painful. The other signs of arterial injury in addition to pain are pulselessness, pallor, paresthesias (numbness, tingling, or prickling), paralysis, and external bleeding from an open wound.

TREATMENT

If a distal pulse and distal neurovascular function are present, the extremity can be splinted in the position in which it is found. One may use a rigid, padded arm board with a sling and swathe if the elbow is flexed or a rigid padded arm board for splinting in extension.

If these is no distal pulse or signs of distal neurovascular function and the arm is found in a flexed or grossly angulated position, one may attempt to straighten the extremity to restore the pulse prior to splinting. This may be necessary as well when the deformity is so gross as to prevent effective immobilization.

The distal neurovascular function should be rechecked after splinting and periodically thereafter. If there is loss of neurovascular function when the arm is splinted in the flexed position, check to make sure the splint is not constricting the extremity or reposition the limb in the straightened position.

Elbow

The elbow is formed by the humerus and the radius and ulna.

MECHANISMS OF INJURY

Falls on the elbow and direct blows can fracture the elbow, as can a fall on the outstretched hand with the elbow flexed. Hyperextension of the elbow joint as well as falls may result in dislocations.

TYPES OF FRACTURES AND DISLOCATIONS

Dislocations are usually posteriorly displaced and often associated with fractures. The olecranon is pushed posteriorly and is prominent, and the forearm may appear shortened (Fig. 10–53A).

Fractures without dislocations can occur to the olecranon and the radial head with marked local tenderness.

Children between 1 and 4 years of age are susceptible to slippage of the radial head from its ligaments after sudden traction on an outstretched arm. This condition, known as "nursemaid's elbow," occurs when one suddenly pulls a child's arm to keep the youngster from falling or the child is pulled up a stair with a sudden tug on the arm. It is most likely the cause of pain and disuse of an arm in a small child with no history of direct injury.

SIGNS AND SYMPTOMS

Signs of elbow fractures and dislocations include deformity with posterior protrusion of the olecranon and apparent shortening of the forearm, along with pain, swelling, and an inability to move the joint.

ASSOCIATED INJURIES

Dislocations of the elbow are frequently associated with fractures of the bones forming the joint. Fractures of the elbow run the same risks of associated injury as fractures of the distal humerus. These include nerve and vascular damage and Volkmann's contracture.

TREATMENT

If a pulse is present, splint the dislocated or fractured elbow in the position found. A splint can be bridged from the humerus to the forearm, thereby immobilizing

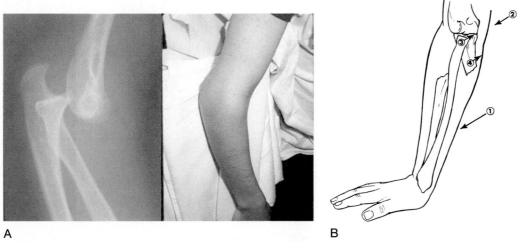

FIGURE 10–53. (*A*) Dislocation of elbow with result of deformity. (*B*) Mechanisms of injury of fractures in the forearm. (From Connolly JF: DePalma's The Management of Fractures and Dislocations: An Atlas. Philadelphia, WB Saunders, 1981, p. 899.)

the fracture site and the adjacent bones. A sling may be applied around the wrist to support the weight of the arm.

Flexion of a fractured elbow *may* compromise circulation. If the arm is flexed and there are signs of vascular compromise, you may try to restore circulation by gently attempting to straighten the elbow before splinting.

Forearm—Radius and Ulna

MECHANISMS OF INJURY

Direct blows to the forearm, as occur when the arm assumes a defensive posture in automobile accidents or fights, can cause fractures of the forearm, particularly of the ulnar bone. Indirect mechanisms again are usually the result of falls on the outstretched hand (Fig. 10–53*B*). The site of fracture depends on the position of the arm during the fall.

TYPES OF FRACTURES

The radius and ulna run parallel to each other, and often a fracture of one bone is associated with a fracture of the other. Displacement of fracture fragments can result from the force of the trauma or from the pull of muscles.

SIGNS AND SYMPTOMS

Both the ulna and the radius are relatively superficial bones, which aids in the identification of fractures. The ulna can be palpated along its entire length, as can much of the radius. Deformity is often obvious on inspection.

ASSOCIATED INJURIES

Displaced fractures are associated with nerve damage.

TREATMENT

The forearm should be splinted with a padded arm board that extends from the hand to the elbow. This immobilizes the wrist and forearm. A sling and swathe are then applied to support the weight of the arm, elevate the fracture site, and immobilize the elbow. Alternatively, a long arm board or air splint can be used to immobilize the forearm and both joints (wrist and elbow) in the extended position.

Wrist

MECHANISMS OF INJURY

The wrist is a common site of fractures that result from falls on the hand. The position of the hand on impact (flexed versus outstretched) often determines the type of fracture and position of the deformity. Punches with a flexed fist can also result in fractures, as can direct blows.

TYPES OF FRACTURES

Fractures of the distal radius with dorsal angulation of the distal fragment result from falls on the outstretched arm and are commonly known as Colles' fractures (Fig. 10–54). Less commonly, the reverse deformity (the distal segment displaced anteriorly) occurs from falls on the back of the hand with the wrist flexed. Either of the above fractures may occur with or without fracture of

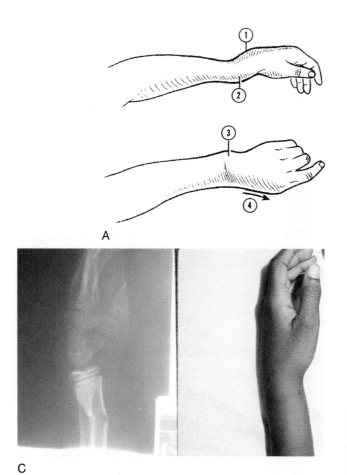

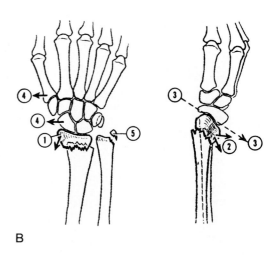

FIGURE 10–54. Colles' fracture of the wrist. (*A*) Note the dinner fork appearance due to (*B*) the displacement of the radial head. (*C*) Swelling of right wrist caused by fracture induced by fall on outstretched hand. (*A* and *B*, from Connolly JF: DePalma's The Management of Fractures and Dislocations: An Atlas. Philadelphia, WB Saunders, 1981, p. 1010.)

the distal ulna. Nondisplaced fractures of the distal radius and ulna or the carpal bones also occur.

SIGNS AND SYMPTOMS

Wrist fractures are recognized by pain and tenderness over the distal radius and carpal bones. Deformity of the distal radius makes some fractures obvious on inspection. Colles' fractures are said to have a "dinner fork" deformity (Fig. 10–54).

ASSOCIATED INJURIES

Nerve injuries affecting sensation and movement of the hand are associated with wrist fractures. Findings are related to the involvement of individual nerves to the hand. For example, injury to the ulnar nerve may cause sensory findings along the fourth and fifth fingers.

TREATMENT

Wrist fractures may be treated with a rigid splint or an air splint, after placing a bulky dressing in the hand. They are then elevated and supported with a sling.

Hands and Fingers

MECHANISMS OF INJURY

The hand is injured by direct blows. It is susceptible to crushing injuries from accidents in the home and workplace. These include crushing injuries from closing doors or industrial presses. Fractures from punching commonly occur at the fourth and fifth metacarpals and are known as "boxer's" fractures. Other injuries occur from the jamming of the fingers, as when a ball strikes the tips of extended fingers.

TYPES OF FRACTURES

Fractures of the shaft of the fingers can result in angulation and deformity. Dislocation of the fingers causes obvious deformity, with the locking of the fingers in a deformed position. If tendons are involved, there may be loss of movement at some joints.

Puncture marks made by teeth over a "boxer's fracture" can convert it into an open fracture.

SIGNS AND SYMPTOMS

Signs and symptoms of fractures include pain, swelling, loss of motion, and angulation of the fingers.

ASSOCIATED INJURIES

The hand is complex; nerves, tendons, and vessels are subject to injury. Early care is important to minimize complications and restore function.

TREATMENT

The hand should be splinted in the position of function or in a grasp position, as if the patient were holding a small ball in the palm. The fingers are slightly flexed at all joints, similar to the position the fingers assume when the hand is held relaxed at the side. Place a roll of gauze in the palm and then apply a rigid or air splint and sling. Isolated finger fractures can be splinted with a padded tongue blade or commercial finger splint or taped to the next finger with padding between the fingers.

LOWER EXTREMITY INJURIES

Pelvis

MECHANISMS OF INJURY

The pelvis can be fractured by direct compression forces or by direct blows or indirectly by forces transmitted from the femur or from vigorous muscle contraction (avulsion fracture). Compression forces can be applied from side to side, from anterior to posterior, or from superior to inferior, and result in different types of fractures. A pedestrian who is run over by a car tire could sustain a compression injury to the pelvis. Falls on the back are direct injuries that may cause fracture of the sacrum. The femur can indirectly transmit force to the pelvis during falls or automobile accidents. Avulsion fractures usually occur in adolescents who are engaged in vigorous muscular activity, with muscles tearing off their bony attachment.

A pelvic fracture usually indicates that a patient has sustained major violence.

TYPES OF FRACTURES

There are many types of pelvic fractures. They can involve an isolated segment of bone or more than one bone, with instability of the pelvic ring. (Ring structures require a break at two sites before separation or instability can occur.) Double breaks in the pelvic ring can occur

in different configurations. For example, fracture of the pubic rami on either side of the symphysis pubis will result in instability of the anterior portion of the pelvic ring. A break through the pubic rami and the sacroiliac joint results in instability of half of the pelvis and may be noted on examination when the iliac wings are compressed. Displacement of a section of the unstable pelvic ring can occur laterally, superiorly, or rotationally (Fig. 10–55).

Transmitted forces through the femur may cause pelvic fractures as well as dislocation of the hip and fracture of the acetabulum (hip socket). The type of dislocation often depends on the position of the leg upon impact, as well as on the direction of forces (see Hip Joint Dislocations later in this chapter). The presence of fractures and soft tissue injuries of the knee should raise suspicion of an associated pelvic or hip injury (Fig. 10–56).

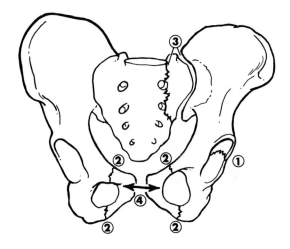

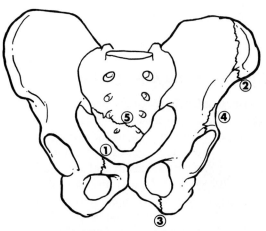

FIGURE 10–55. Examples of sites of fracture to the pelvic bones. (From Connolly JF: DePalma's The Management of Fractures and Dislocations: An Atlas. Philadelphia, WB Saunders, 1981, p. 463.)

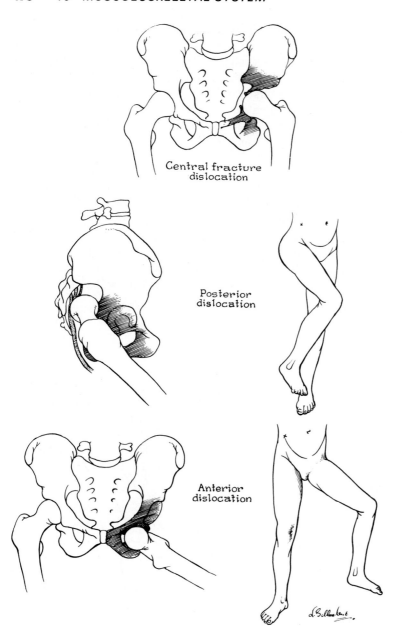

Central fracture
dislocation

Posterior
dislocation

Anterior
dislocation

FIGURE 10–56. Mechanisms of injury, types of fractures and dislocations, and classic positions of the hip. (From Zuidema GD, Rutherford RB, Ballinger WF: The Management of Trauma, 4th ed. Philadelphia, WB Saunders, 1985, p. 673.)

SIGNS AND SYMPTOMS

Suspect a pelvic fracture when there is pain in the pelvis or a violent mechanism of injury. Look for signs of bruising or deformity. Palpate the pelvic bones, noting tenderness, deformity, crepitus, or instability. Gently compress the iliac crests medially and posteriorly, looking for instability. Stop if there is any movement. Gently press the pubic symphysis, again noting tenderness or instability. Do not compress the pelvis if there are obvious signs of fracture such as deformity or open fractures.

ASSOCIATED INJURIES

Because of the violent trauma necessary to cause pelvic fractures, it is not surprising to note that over half the patients who sustain a pelvic fracture suffer other injuries. These other injuries involve the central nervous system, thorax, or abdomen, or fractures of other bones. Half the patients who suffer open fractures die as a result of bleeding or infection. For all pelvic fractures, the death rate exceeds 10%. Severe crushing injuries such as those sustained by pedestrians hit by automobiles or motorcyclists are the most lethal.

Rupture to the internal viscera in the pelvis can cause hemorrhage or perforation. Injury to the bladder, urethra, female genital tract, bowel, or nerves can occur. Bleeding from the penile urethra, the vagina, or rectum is possible. There are multiple large blood vessels that lie in the pelvic walls. These vessels can be lacerated by fractures, and brisk arterial internal bleeding can occur. It has been estimated that each pubic ramus that is fractured can cause a blood loss of 500 ml.

TREATMENT

Treatment consists of immobilization on a long spine board. The PASG should be applied if there are signs of hypovolemic shock. The PASG may help tamponade bleeding.

Hip Joint Dislocations

MECHANISMS OF INJURY AND TYPES OF FRACTURES

The hip can be dislocated in three general ways: posteriorly, centrally, or anteriorly. It generally requires a great deal of force, except for children under the age of 6 years. The position of the leg and hip at the time of impact is important in determining the type of dislocation that will occur.

POSTERIOR DISLOCATIONS. By far, posterior dislocations are the most common, usually resulting from dashboard injuries to the knee. Posterior dislocations are more apt to result when the hip is flexed, adducted, and internally rotated prior to a dashboard impact of the knee. The femoral head slips posteriorly out of the acetabulum, sometimes causing a fracture of the acetabulum or femoral head. The thigh can be locked in an abnormal position (Fig. 10–56).

CENTRAL DISLOCATION. A fall onto the side of the hip may force the head of the femur directly through the acetabulum, causing a central dislocation. The acetabulum fractures and the femoral head may protrude into the pelvis. This can also occur if force is applied to the knee and femur when the thigh is abducted and externally rotated.

ANTERIOR DISLOCATION. An anterior dislocation is much less common than a posterior dislocation. Anterior dislocation may occur when the thigh is abducted, flexed, and externally rotated and a force is applied to the back of the thigh, as in a fall. The femoral head is then forced forward out of the socket. The joint locks in an abnormal position.

SIGNS AND SYMPTOMS

Locking of the hip joint in an abnormal position is a key finding with hip dislocations, and the position of the leg gives the clue to the type of dislocation.

With posterior dislocation, the thigh and knee are flexed and internally rotated. There may be associated injuries to the knee and femur. If the sciatic nerve has been damaged, the patient may be unable to raise the foot or toes, and an area of abnormal sensation on the foot may be noted.

With anterior dislocation, the hip is flexed with the thigh widely abducted (lying flat) and externally rotated. The head of the femur may be palpable in the area of the femoral pulse, and the pressure of the overlying bone can even occlude this vessel.

Central dislocations may cause apparent shortening of the leg and limitation of motion if the femoral head has dislocated through the acetabulum and lies within the pelvis (Fig. 10–56).

ASSOCIATED INJURIES

Thirty percent of hip dislocations also have associated knee injuries. Sciatic nerve injuries are common and cause foot drop (inability to dorsiflex the foot) and sensory deficits of the foot. Because of the severity of the force necessary to dislocate the hip, there may be associated injuries to the spine and abdomen.

TREATMENT

The dislocated limb should be supported in the position in which it is found by placing rolled blankets or pillows beneath the extremity. Motion of the supported extremity is then restricted by use of long straps or bandages to attach one leg to the other. The patient is then secured to the long backboard for transport.

Hip Fracture

MECHANISMS OF INJURY

Hip fractures are common injuries in the elderly, usually occurring as a result of falls. Much greater violence is required to cause hip fractures in younger people.

TYPES OF FRACTURES

Hip fractures can occur at the femoral head, the femoral neck, or through the trochanters just below the femoral neck. The amount of twisting force applied to the femur during a fall may determine where the hip is fractured.

The fractured segments may be separated, the thigh

externally rotated, and the leg apparently shortened, resulting in loss or limitation of movement (Fig. 10–57). Or the fracture may be nondisplaced or impacted so that the leg appears normal and has some function, and the patient complains of pain on movement.

SIGNS AND SYMPTOMS

The classic finding of the fractured hip is external rotation and shortening of the leg. However, this does not always occur. In some patients with a hip fracture, pain on weight-bearing, movement, or palpation may be the only sign. Some patients are able to bear some weight after a fall and delay seeking care. In the field, pain in the hip in the elderly should be treated as a hip fracture.

TREATMENT

Application of a traction splint supports the fractured hip. An alternate method of immobilization is to tie the legs together after placing blankets or pillows between the legs. The PASG may be used when there are signs of hypovolemia.

Femur

MECHANISMS OF INJURY

Femur fractures are severe injuries and result from high-impact motor vehicle accidents, falls from heights, or gunshot wounds. They occur in a younger population more frequently than do hip fractures, and there are often other major associated injuries because of the great violence needed to fracture this strong bone.

Elderly patients with osteoporosis can sustain a fracture to the distal femur after a fall on a flexed knee.

TYPES OF FRACTURES

FEMORAL SHAFT. The femoral shaft is defined as the area from below the lesser trochanter to the junction of the middle and lower thirds of the femur. Femur fractures can be angulated, causing obvious distortion of the leg, and they can result in overriding of segments with deformity and shortening of the leg (Fig. 10–58).

DISTAL FEMUR. Fractures of the distal femur may involve the knee joint and run the risk of injury to the femoral or popliteal arteries and veins.

SIGNS AND SYMPTOMS

Fractures of the femur may be accompanied by marked swelling or deformity. The leg below the fracture site may be angulated or rotated, with evidence of open fractures.

ASSOCIATED INJURIES

Blood loss is significant with femur fractures, and a patient may show signs of hemorrhagic shock. Disruption of major vessels may impair circulation to the foot. Femur fractures are often open with the added risk of infection. Femur fractures also can cause fat embolism; although fat embolism usually occurs after 1 to 3 days, it may be the cause of unexplained dyspnea at the scene of the accident.

Because of the forces involved in femoral fractures,

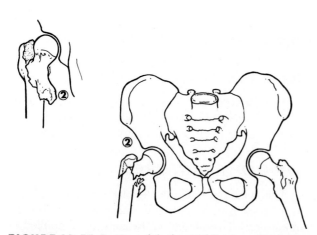
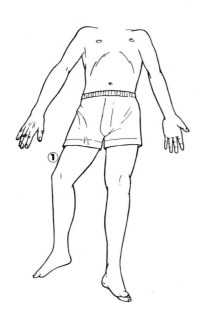

FIGURE 10–57. Position of the leg (*1*) following a hip fracture, and diagram of the hip fracture (*2*). (From Connolly JF: DePalma's The Management of Fractures and Dislocations: An Atlas. Philadelphia, WB Saunders, 1981, p. 1375.)

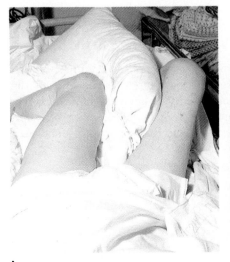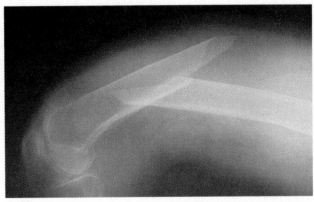

A   B

FIGURE 10–58. Femur fracture. (*A*) Note swelling of the left leg. (*B*) On x-ray film a displaced spiral fracture is identified.

there may also be significant trauma to other body organs and fractures in the hip and knee.

TREATMENT

The traction splint is used to stabilize and support the fractured femur and to counteract the tendency for fracture segments to override. It helps to reduce pain and counteract muscle spasm. Angulated fractures should be gently straightened before traction is applied. Patients with significant bleeding and hypovolemic shock can be treated with the PASG, which provides immobilization to the leg. Certain traction splints can be employed in combination with the PASG.

The potential for hypovolemic shock from femur fractures with or without signs of blood loss should not be underestimated. Swelling of the femur may give some clue as to the amount of blood loss, and continued swelling may indicate continuing bleeding within the thigh.

Patella

MECHANISMS OF INJURY

Fractures of the patella occur following direct blows, as when the knee strikes the dashboard of a car. They can also occur from violent contraction of the quadriceps muscle (whose strength the patella helps to maximize) when a person attempts to extend the flexed knee against resistance. Dislocations of the patella can occur following tangential blows to the edge of the patella, which pushes it laterally, or from sudden strong contraction of the quadriceps when a patient tries to recover balance after slipping.

TYPES OF FRACTURES

Direct blows may cause transverse or comminuted fractures. Often, the fragments remain nondisplaced within the broad fibrous structure of the quadriceps muscle that surrounds the patella. When the quadriceps muscle or its tendons are torn, displacement can occur.

The patella almost always dislocates laterally over the lateral femoral condyle.

SIGNS AND SYMPTOMS

Fracture fragments might be palpable following direct blows. Often, there is accompanying swelling and

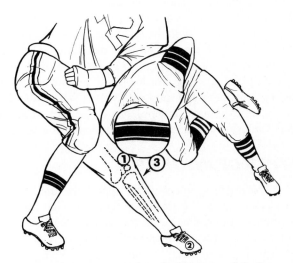

FIGURE 10–59. Injuries (*1*) to the ligaments of the knee can happen when the leg, in a normally immovable position (*2*), has an overpowering force (*3*) applied against it. (From Connolly JF: DePalma's The Management of Fractures and Dislocations: An Atlas. Philadelphia, WB Saunders, 1981, p. 1551.)

bruising, which is palpable over the patella or noticeable under and around it. Defects might be felt above or below the patella when the quadriceps muscle tears. The dislocated patella is palpable lateral from its normal position and the knee is usually flexed. The patient may inform you that he or she is subject to dislocations of the patella.

ASSOCIATED INJURIES

The patella protects the knee joint. Associated fractures in this area should be suspected.

TREATMENT

The treatment for fractures of the patella is to splint the knee in extension. Dislocations of the patella often reduce spontaneously when the knee is extended. The patient may have already extended the knee and may inform you that the "kneecap has popped back in." If a patient is unable to straighten the knee (attempts at gentle straightening are prevented by pain), it should be splinted in the position in which it is found. You may use rigid splints placed medially and laterally or a single rigid splint applied posteriorly to maintain extension of the splinted leg. A full leg air splint may also be used.

Knee Joint

MECHANISMS OF INJURY

Injuries to the ligaments of the knee may occur following stressful rotation (external or internal) of the knee, hyperextension injuries, and injuries to the flexed knee. The rotation injuries can result from rotation of a planted foot, as when a football runner plants his foot and is then tackled, with the resulting forces rotating the thigh and lower leg in opposite directions. The way hyperextension injuries occur can be illustrated by a football player getting struck on the anterior leg when the leg is planted and fully extended. Direct trauma to a knee, as from a car bumper, can cause both knee ligament injury and fractures of the bones of the knee.

TYPES OF INJURIES

The major ligaments that support the knee can be torn as a result of the above mechanisms. The collateral ligaments support the sides of the knee while the anterior and posterior cruciates limit motion anteriorly and posteriorly. The injury may involve overstretching of the ligaments or complete disruption of one or more sets. There may be associated fractures. Disruption of the ligaments results in instability and abnormal movement of the knee joint (Fig. 10–59 on p. 481).

SIGNS AND SYMPTOMS

Instability or abnormal position of the knee may be noted on the physical examination. A limitation of movement, laxity, or abnormal movement may be noted. Pain and swelling in the area are often present. The patient may state that a popping sound was heard.

TREATMENT

The leg should be straightened and splinted as is done for dislocations.

Dislocations of the Knee

MECHANISMS OF INJURY

Whenever the knee joint is carried through a greater than normal range of motion, tearing of the ligaments can occur. When these are accompanied by violent forces, severe tearing may result, with complete dislocation of the knee.

TYPES OF DISLOCATIONS

The knee may be dislocated in any direction.

SIGNS AND SYMPTOMS

The dislocated knee is a grotesque deformity. You should look for nerve and vascular damage, which is often associated with it.

ASSOCIATED INJURIES

Injuries to the vessels (particularly to the popliteal artery) and nerves are common with knee dislocations, and evaluation of distal function is important.

TREATMENT

After checking distal neurovascular function, the EMT should gently straighten a dislocated knee by applying manual traction to the tibia while realigning the joint. The leg should be immobilized with a traction splint *without traction* to help maintain the position. The traction splint avoids direct pressure on the knee. Traction itself is not applied since it may further displace the unstable joint, causing further injury to the ligaments. Other options include the rigid splint or long leg air splint. It is important to reassess distal neurovascular function after realigning the limb, after applying the splint, and periodically thereafter. It is important to remember not to forcefully straighten the limb if resistance is encountered or the patient complains of increased pain.

Dislocated knees are severe injuries and require early hospital intervention. If neurovascular deficits are encountered or the knee cannot be straightened, getting the patient to definitive care quickly is the highest priority.

Tibia and Fibula

MECHANISMS OF INJURY

Direct forces applied to the knee can cause fractures of the proximal tibia and fibula, with or without injury to the ligaments. Direct forces to the shaft of the tibia are illustrated in the case of the pedestrian struck in this area by a car bumper (Fig. 10–60). Twisting forces can cause spiral fractures of the shaft of the tibia or fractures of the distal tibia. Fatigue fractures, as encountered by joggers, often involve the tibia and fibula.

TYPES OF FRACTURES

Tibial and fibular shaft fractures from direct injuries can be transverse; oblique; and, with greater forces, comminuted and angulated. Because of the proximity of the tibia to the skin surface, open fractures are relatively common (see Fig. 10–60).

Rotational forces cause spiral type fractures and can cause fractures at different levels of the tibia and fibula (typically the distal tibia and proximal fibula). Patients with isolated fractures of the fibula may be able to bear weight, since this is not a weight-bearing bone.

SIGNS AND SYMPTOMS

The tibia, being superficial, lends itself to examination for the signs of fracture, and small deformities may be palpated.

ASSOCIATED INJURIES

Open fractures are common, and severe fractures are prone to compromise distal circulation. Bleeding into soft tissues and muscle compartments in the leg can compress arteries and cause a "compartment syndrome" (a condition in which increased tissue pressure in a confined anatomic space causes decreased blood flow, leading to ischemia and dysfunction) with pain and signs of poor distal circulation.

TREATMENT

Immobilization can be accomplished with the use of long leg rigid splints, full leg air splints, traction splints, or the PASG if there are signs of hypovolemic shock. Check distal circulation frequently and note that complaints of increasing pain may be a sign of vascular compromise. External compression of the vascular supply can occur from prolonged application of an air-filled splint, so give the time of application of the splint to emergency department personnel.

Ankle

MECHANISMS OF INJURY

Rotational injuries of the ankle cause fractures and sprains. Commonly encountered mechanisms causing ankle injuries include internal and external rotation and plantar flexion. However, it is difficult to distinguish a fracture from a sprain, and all the above mechanisms can result in either injury.

TYPES OF FRACTURES

Fractures and dislocations of the distal fibula and tibia usually occur from torsional forces (Fig. 10–61). Sprains involve the ligaments on the lateral and medial sides of the ankle and sometimes the ligaments anteriorly. Sprains result in pain, swelling, and possible instability.

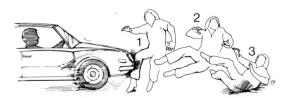

FIGURE 10–60. A bumper striking a pedestrian (*1*) is a common mechanism of injury for direct tibial shaft fractures (*2, 3*). (From Cardona VD, Hurn PD, Mason PJB, et al: Trauma Nursing From Resuscitation Through Rehabilitation. Philadelphia, WB Saunders, 1988, p. 107.)

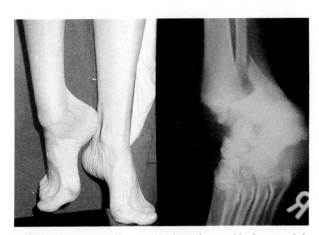

FIGURE 10–61. Deformity resulting from ankle fracture dislocation caused by a fall off the curb in an elderly woman.

SIGNS AND SYMPTOMS

Pain and swelling are common to both fractures and sprains. Dislocation occurs from severe injuries and presents as a rotated foot and grotesque ankle deformity.

ASSOCIATED INJURIES

Dislocations run the risk of causing neurovascular compromise.

TREATMENT

Gently straighten deformities after assessing distal neurovascular status. A pillow splint, air splint, or short leg rigid splint can be used for immobilization.

Foot

MECHANISMS OF INJURY AND TYPES OF FRACTURES

The talus bone transfers the weight from the tibia to the foot and can be fractured or dislocated by forced dorsiflexion and external rotation of the foot. Falls on the heel can cause fractures of the calcaneus. Twisting injuries can fracture the other bones in the foot. Direct trauma, as caused by dropping a heavy object onto the foot, is a common cause of foot and toe fractures.

SIGNS AND SYMPTOMS

Most bones of the foot are easily palpable. Be sure not to overlook a calcaneus fracture in a patient who has fallen and landed on the feet. The only sign of fracture may be pressure pain. Recognition of a calcaneus fracture is important, since it is associated with spinal injuries (Fig. 10–62).

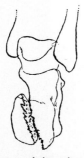

FIGURE 10–62. Fracture of the calcaneus. (From Connolly JF: DePalma's The Management of Fractures and Dislocations: An Atlas. Philadelphia, WB Saunders, 1981, p. 2007.)

ASSOCIATED INJURIES

Fractures of the calcaneus are associated with injuries to the vertebrae, other bones of the lower extremities (including the other calcaneus), and the wrist.

TREATMENT

The foot is best immobilized with an air splint or pillow splint. Preformed rigid splints applied posteriorly are commercially available. Isolated fractures of the toes can be taped to the neighboring toe.

REVIEW EXERCISES

1. List the major bones of the body.
2. Define the following:
   Ligaments   Tendons
   Cartilage   Appendicular versus axial skeleton
3. List the three types of muscle and describe their function.
4. List the major muscles of the upper and lower extremity and describe their function.
5. List three types of joints and explain their range of motion.
6. List four forces the cause musculoskeletal injury.
7. List four types of fractures and describe a related mechanism of injury for each.
8. List three common complications of fractures and dislocations.
9. Describe the assesment needed to identify nerve or blood vessel complications in the upper and lower extremities.
10. List the mechanisms of injury, types of fractures, associated injuries, and treatment for fractures and dislocations of the following bones and joints:
    Scapula   Humerus   Ulna   Radius
    Shoulder   Clavicle   Carpals Phalanges
    Pelvis   Hip   Femur   Patella
    Tibia   Fibula   Tarsals
11. List the steps of application for the following devices:
    Rigid splint for the forearm
    Sling and swathe
    Elbow splint in angulated and straightened positions
    Wrist and hand splint
    Finger splint
    Rigid splint for the lower extremity
    Pillow splint
    Sager traction splint
    Hare traction splint
    Air splint

REFERENCES

Adams JC: Outline of Fractures, 8th ed. New York, Churchill Livingstone, 1983.

Advanced First Aid, 3rd ed. American Red Cross.

American College of Surgeons, Walt A (ed): Early Care of the Injured Patient, 3rd ed. Philadelphia, WB Saunders, 1982.

Baxt WG: Trauma: The First Hour. Norwalk, CT, Appleton-Century-Crofts, 1985.

Chabner DE: The Language of Medicine, 4th ed. Philadelphia, WB Saunders, 1990.

Connolly JF: DePalma's The Management of Fractures and Dislocations: An Atlas, 3rd ed. Philadelphia, WB Saunders, 1981.

Dorland's Illustrated Medical Dictionary, 27th ed. Philadelphia, WB Saunders, 1988.

Hughes S: The Basis and Practice of Traumatology. Rockville, MD, Aspen, 1983.

Leonard PC: Building a Medical Vocabulary. Philadelphia, WB Saunders, 1983.

Nahum A, Melvin J: The Biomechanics of Trauma. Norwalk, CT, Appleton-Century-Crofts, 1985.

Passmore R, Robson JS (eds): A Companion to Medical Studies, Vol 1. Oxford, Blackwell Scientific Publications, 1969.

Raynor J: Anatomy and Physiology. New York, Harper & Row, 1977.

Simon R, Koenigsknecht S: Orthopedics in Emergency Medicine: The extremities. Norwalk, CT, Appleton-Century-Crofts, 1982.

Zuidema GD, Rutherford RB, Ballinger WF: The Management of Trauma, 4th ed. Philadelphia, WB Saunders, 1985.

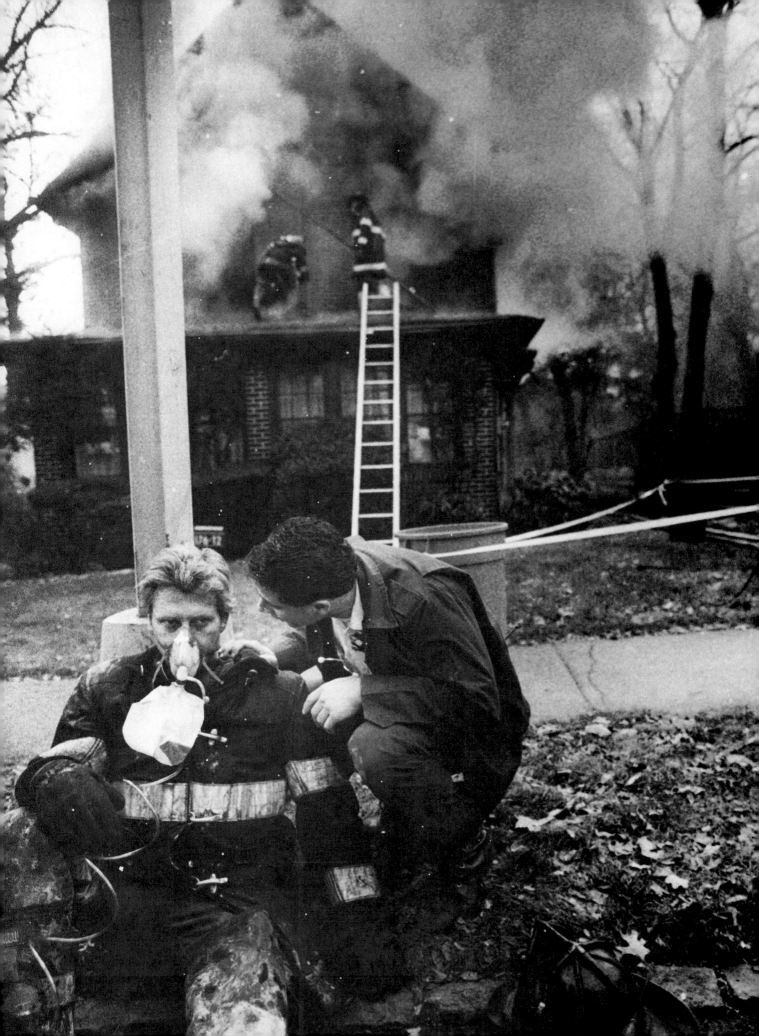

CHAPTER 11

ENVIRONMENTAL EMERGENCIES

OBJECTIVES

At the conclusion of this chapter the reader will be able to:

1. List two signs and symptoms of heat cramps.

2. List three signs and symptoms of heat exhaustion.

3. List three signs and symptoms of heat stroke.

4. Describe the treatment for hypothermia.

5. Define and list two characteristics each of first-degree, second-degree, and third-degree burns.

6. List three steps in the management of chemical burns.

7. Describe the precautions an EMT should take at the site where an electrical burn has occurred.

8. Describe the functions of a dosimeter and a survey instrument.

9. Explain the difference between irradiation and contamination.

10. Describe how to proceed after arriving at the hospital with a victim of a radiation accident.

11. Define decompression sickness.

12. Define air embolism.

13. Describe how to set up a staging area at a HAZMAT scene.

14. List three resources that can be consulted to help identify and provide information about hazardous materials.

15. Describe how to decontaminate a victim of a HAZMAT.

HEAT AND COLD EMERGENCIES

The body maintains a relatively constant temperature even when there are great fluctuations in the temperature of the outside environment. While we generally regard 98.6°F (Fahrenheit) or 37°C (Celsius) as the normal body temperature, there is some variation with daily activity. The range of normal deviation of the body's central core temperature is from 35.8 to 37.7°C (96.4 to 99.8°F). With strenuous exercise, the core body temperature can rise to 40°C. At night when the body is at rest the temperature may drop to 35.8°C (96.8°F) (Fig. 11–1). Variances from normal body temperature that are beyond this range are not well tolerated. If the temperature is too low or too high, the body can lose its ability to regulate temperature, causing extreme changes and death.

The body's maintenance of a normal temperature is a continuous process that is accomplished through the careful regulation of heat production and heat loss. The outside temperature in most parts of the world is less than the body's normal temperature. Therefore to maintain a temperature of 98.6°F or 37°C, heat must be generated internally. All metabolism within the body gives off heat as a byproduct. Increased metabolism, as with exercise, greatly increases heat production. Heat is distributed throughout the body by the cardiovascular system and lost primarily through the skin, the organ that is in greatest contact with the outside environment. The hypothalamus regulates the many factors involved with the production of heat as well as its loss or conservation (Fig. 11–2).

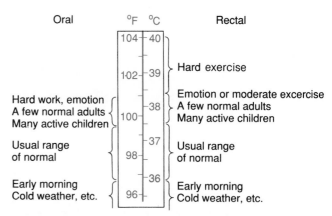

FIGURE 11–1. Range of normal temperatures in humans. (From DuBois: Fever. Courtesy of Charles C Thomas, Publisher, Springfield, Illinois.)

The body's core temperature is measured by oral or rectal thermometers, with the rectal temperature generally 1°F greater than the oral. An axillary temperature, obtained by holding a thermometer under the armpit, is generally 1°F lower than the oral temperature.

HEAT PRODUCTION

All metabolic processes within the body generate heat. The metabolism necessary to maintain cellular functions at rest is called the *basal metabolism*, and it provides a constant supply of heat. In comfortable environments, the basal metabolism generates more than enough heat to maintain the core temperature. The metabolic rate can be increased by hormones under the influence of the central nervous system. Muscular activity can greatly increase heat production. Shivering is a form of involuntary forced muscular activity that increases heat production when the body is exposed to cold. In fact, the

Heat Regulation

CORE TEMPERATURE

Most references to body temperature refer to the temperature of the body core, or the temperature within the skull, the thorax, and the abdominal-pelvic cavities. The body's regulatory processes maintain this core temperature within narrow limits. There is a greater variance in the temperatures within the body shell and the outer layers of the body, such as the skin and soft tissues, and the extremities. For example, at room temperature, there is a gradual reduction from the core temperature as one samples the temperature of the muscle, subcutaneous tissue, and skin. Also, various regions of the body's shell have different temperatures as the distance from the heat and trunk increases. For example, the skin of the arms and legs could be 31 to 32°C, the skin of the forehead 34°C, and the toes 27°C, while the core temperature is 37.1°C (Fig. 11–3).

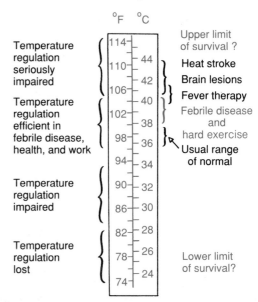

FIGURE 11–2. Body temperatures under different conditions. (From DuBois: Fever. Courtesy of Charles C Thomas, Publisher, Springfield, Illinois.)

FIGURE 11–3. Range of temperature in the forearm. *A* is under warm conditions, when the patient is comfortable. *B* is under cold conditions, which lead to shivering. (From Bazett and McGlone: Am. J. Physiol. 82:415, 1927.)

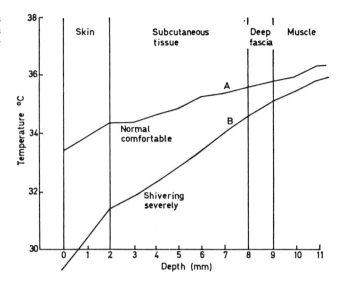

heat generated by basal metabolism and muscular activity could cause the core temperature to rise to dangerous levels if the excess heat is not released to the environment through the skin.

Heat is also gained from the environment when the temperature outside exceeds body temperature.

HEAT LOSS

There are five ways that heat can be lost from the body: *radiation, conduction, convection, evaporation,* and *respiration.*

RADIATION. Radiation is the *transfer of heat from a warmer environment to a cooler environment* that is not in direct contact with the body. The transfer of heat by radiation is in proportion to what is called the thermal gradient, or the difference between body and environmental temperatures. At 70°F, which is average room temperature, the body radiates heat to the environment. When the environmental temperature exceeds body temperature, heat is gained rather than lost.

CONDUCTION. Conduction is the *transfer of heat to objects in direct contact with the body.* Sitting on a chair that is cooler than body temperature results in the loss of body temperature to the chair. As the temperature of the chair becomes heated to body temperature, the transfer ceases.

The conduction of heat is influenced by the heat transfer properties of the materials in direct contact with the body. For example, water conducts heat much faster than air, and an increased transfer of heat occurs with wet clothing (five times greater) or immersion in cold water (25 times greater) as compared with air.

The air immediately surrounding the body is heated by conduction. However, air is a poor conductor of heat and once the air immediately surrounding the body is heated, it serves to insulate the body from further heat loss unless there is significant air movement—convection.

CONVECTION. Heat is first conducted to the air immediately surrounding the body. Heat is then convected, or *carried away by air currents, removing the warmed air and replacing it with cooler air.* Wind velocity influences heat loss via convection. The wind chill factor is a familiar reference to the chilling effects that wind can add to environmental temperatures. For example, on a day when the thermometer registers 50°F, a 20-mph wind makes the temperature feel like 32°F.

EVAPORATION. Evaporation is the loss of heat that occurs *when moisture vaporizes on the body's surface.* The rate of evaporation depends on the temperature, movement of air, and humidity (relative water content in the air for a given temperature). Air can hold more water vapor as the temperature rises. When the humidity is high, less perspiration evaporates. When perspiration runs off the body instead of evaporating, less cooling occurs. Air movement replaces the air immediately surrounding the skin, which has become more saturated with water vapor from evaporation, with "less humid" air.

The role of evaporation in heat loss needs special emphasis, because when the environmental temperature approaches or exceeds body temperature, evaporation is the only mechanism of heat loss.

RESPIRATION. Inhaled air is heated or cooled to body temperature. The body loses heat when inhaled air is cooler than body temperature because it gives off heat to the air as it passes through the respiratory tract on its way to the lungs. The body gains heat when the inhaled air is warmer than body temperature because the air is cooled by giving off heat to the respiratory tract on its way to the lungs. The respiratory tract is able to cool very hot dry air effectively because the moist respiratory tract is a much more potent conductor of heat than is air. This explains why the lungs are seldom burned by inhalation of hot dry air in fires but may be injured by inhalation of steam.

Under normal conditions, most heat loss occurs through radiation (60%). Evaporation accounts for approximately 22%, and conduction and convection to the air account for about 15%. Smaller amounts of heat are lost through direct conduction to objects, respiration, and the urine and feces (Fig. 11–4).

Obviously, environmental conditions have a great influence on how heat is lost. The environmental temperature, the wind velocity, and the humidity all affect the ability of the body to dissipate or conserve heat.

One feels comfortable on a hot day when the humidity is low, since it is easier for evaporation to occur. A fan or wind currents add to one's comfort by replacing the heated and moist air immediately around the body with cooler and dryer air, thereby promoting heat loss by conduction and evaporation. Conversely, high humidity and no wind velocity on a hot day constitute conditions that make the body more stressed to dissipate heat.

MECHANISMS OF CONTROL

BRAIN. The *hypothalamus* sets the body's thermostat and regulates temperature by influencing the *metabolic rate* (heat production), the *cardiovascular system* (heat distribution), and *the skin* (heat loss). When the hypothalamus senses a rise in body temperature, it will increase heat loss by inducing (1) vasodilation of skin vessels, thereby bringing heat to the surface of the body, where it can be lost by radiation, conduction, and convection; and (2) sweating, which speeds evaporation.

Cold body temperatures cause the hypothalamus to increase the metabolic rate and thereby the production of heat. Other receptors in the skin and spinal cord cause shivering (increase heat production), inhibit sweating, and induce vasoconstriction of skin vessels (to prevent heat loss).

CARDIOVASCULAR SYSTEM. The cardiovascular system brings heated blood from the body core to the skin and extremities. When more heat must be lost, the skin vessels dilate to allow more blood to be in contact with the skin so that heat can be lost through radiation, conduction, and convection. This vasodilation is accompanied by an increase in the cardiac output.

Conversely, when heat must be conserved, the skin vessels vasoconstrict to reduce heat loss to the environment.

Vasodilation and vasoconstriction of the skin's blood vessels can result in great changes in blood flow through the skin. Ordinarily, under resting conditions, about 5% of the cardiac output flows through the skin. For the 70-kg man with a cardiac output of about 5 liters per minute, this represents about 250 to 300 ml of blood flow per minute through the skin. The transfer of heat between the skin and the environment then takes place according to thermal gradients and the various mechanisms of heat exchange.

Under heat stress, when the skin vessels are dilated, the blood flow to the skin can increase to 3000 ml per minute, resulting in a large increase in cardiac output just to deal with heat loss. Additional demands such as those placed on the heart by muscular activity may lead to a feeling of exhaustion. Ordinarily, most individuals do not feel like undertaking strenuous activity on a hot humid day.

In cold conditions, when the vessels in the skin are vasoconstricted, blood flow can be reduced to 30 ml per minute, allowing less heat transfer to the cold environment.

SKIN. The skin, as the interface between the external and internal environments, has a primary role in heat regulation. In addition to its protective role as a barrier to infection and foreign elements, the skin insulates the body. The skin and its subcutaneous fat serve as a layer of insulation. Heat loss is also regulated by the skin through evaporation of perspiration and changes in the flow of blood to the skin. Evaporation is influenced by stimulation of sweat glands within the skin. Vasoconstriction and vasodilation of blood vessels within the skin influence the exchange of core body heat with the environment.

Heat Emergencies

There are three general types of heat emergencies. These are called *heat cramps, heat exhaustion,* and *heat stroke.* Heat cramps are muscular cramps that occur during strenuous exertion and excessive loss of body fluid through perspiration. Heat exhaustion occurs when the cardiovascular system cannot keep up with stresses imposed by a hot environment; rarely it can cause death. Heat stroke is a complete failure of the thermoregulatory system, which results in extreme rises in core body temperature and damage to cells. Heat stroke has a high mortality rate.

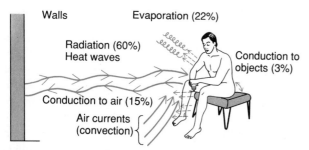

FIGURE 11–4. Mechanisms of heat loss. (From Guyton AC: Textbook of Medical Physiology, 8th ed. Philadelphia, WB Saunders, 1990, p. 887.)

PREDISPOSING FACTORS

Factors that predispose a person to suffer heat illnesses include climate, exercise and acclimation, age, preexisting illness, and drug and alcohol use.

CLIMATE. As previously mentioned, the temperature, humidity, and wind velocity all play a large role in heat illness. The outside temperature relative to the body temperature determines whether heat is lost by radiation and conduction or whether it is gained. High humidity decreases the rate of evaporation, since the air is already saturated with water. Mortality rates from heat emergencies increase threefold during heat waves.

EXERCISE AND TRAINING. Muscular activity greatly increases heat production. Athletes' temperatures may rise to 40°C. On hot humid days it is more difficult to dissipate this increased heat. Many heat emergencies occur among high school football players early in the season when the weather is still warm and among army recruits who are unaccustomed to strenuous exercise.

As one trains, sweating begins earlier and more sweating occurs. In fact, the amount of sweat can increase from 1 liter per hour to 3 liters per hour. From these figures it is clear that water replacement should be available on hot days during strenuous exercise (such as football practice or during marathon races). Otherwise, a person may become relatively hypovolemic. Sweat contains salt, and the amount of salt in sweat decreases as a person trains. Excessive loss of salt can cause heat cramps. Replacement of both water and salt can be accomplished by drinking balanced solutions such as Gatorade.

Awareness of the hazards of excessive exercise on hot, humid days has led to the institution of training programs that introduce gradual increases in the amount of daily exertion; supply a liberal amount of water; and encourage the wearing of loose, nonocclusive clothing, which promotes rather than inhibits evaporation.

AGE. The very old and the very young are at increased risk of heat emergencies. The tendency of some parents to wrap infants in occlusive clothing, even though the outside temperature is hot, places infants at increased risk. Neonates in particular are at great risk because they have a poor thermoregulatory mechanism and sweating capability during the first days of life.

Because the infant and some elderly patients lack mobility, they may remain in dangerous environments during heat waves. For example, an infant may be left in a car or a debilitated patient may be bedridden without air conditioning.

PREEXISTING ILLNESSES. Heart disease and dehydration compromise the cardiovascular response to heat. Obesity can inhibit heat loss because of the increased insulating effect of the excess subcutaneous fat. A febrile illness places an individual at increased risk, as

do fatigue and lack of sleep. Parkinson's disease, with its constant muscle tremors and increased heat production, is another condition that predisposes an individual to heat illness. The debilitated, retarded, or psychiatric patient may be at increased risk because of an inability to take appropriate precautions.

ALCOHOL AND DRUGS. Alcohol causes vasodilation and can cause a gain in heat when the environmental temperature is above body temperature. Amphetamines and cocaine can increase heat production, while certain other drugs (some tranquilizers and antihistamines) can affect the hypothalamus and inhibit sweating. Diuretics can result in dehydration and affect cardiovascular function. Drugs affecting mental function and judgment, such as narcotics, tranquilizers, and alcohol, can prevent people from taking appropriate precautions in hot environments.

SUMMARY

Basically, heat emergencies arise when (1) the environmental conditions overwhelm the body's ability to dissipate heat or (2) the body's thermoregulatory mechanisms are defective.

If environmental conditions are extreme, they can overwhelm a normal individual's capacity to dissipate heat. For example, a sauna or steamroom is not tolerated very long by even normal individuals. Normal individuals can also become victims of heat illness if they exercise too strenuously on a hot, humid day without acclimation, appropriate clothing, or adequate water intake. This is why football players and military recruits are sometimes victims of heat stroke.

Patients who are particularly susceptible to heat emergencies are those whose thermoregulatory functions are compromised. These individuals may suffer heat illness because of conditions that affect the hypothalamus, the cardiovascular system, or the skin; the inability to take appropriate measures under stress; or the use of alcohol or drugs.

HEAT CRAMPS

MECHANISM. Heat cramps are painful muscular contractions of heavily exercised muscles. It has been postulated that during excessive exercise or hard work cramps are caused by a disproportionate loss of fluid and sodium through excessive sweating, which is replaced with fluids that do not contain sodium (salt).

SIGNS AND SYMPTOMS. The diagnosis is made by a history of muscle cramping in *heavily used muscles*, either during or immediately following exertion. The individual usually experiences a period of excessive sweating.

TREATMENT. Treatment consists of moving the patient to a cooler environment and replacing fluid and salt losses with a dilute salt solution. A quarter teaspoon or less of salt in a quart of water or other balanced solution can be used. Immediate relief of cramping is best accomplished by stretching the cramped muscle.

HEAT EXHAUSTION

MECHANISMS. Heat exhaustion is caused by the cardiovascular system's inability to respond to the demands for increased blood flow to the skin while still maintaining flow to the muscles and other organs.

For the patient in a hot environment the blood vessels to the skin vasodilate and there is increased blood flow to the skin to dissipate the heat. In addition, if there has been a period of sweating and volume loss, the patient may be mildly hypovolemic. (*Note*: A previously dehydrated patient is more prone to this condition.) Some individuals may not be able to maintain cardiac output great enough to meet the simultaneous demands of the skin, skeletal muscles, and other body organs.

SIGNS AND SYMPTOMS. The patient is in a hot environment and may have had a period of recent exertion. The skin is usually moist. Because of inadequate blood flow to the skin, the body temperature may be elevated. Because of inadequate blood flow to the skeletal muscles, the patient may complain of weakness or exhaustion. Inadequate blood flow to other organs can result in multiple complaints such as dizziness, a feeling of faintness, nausea, and headache.

Because blood flow may be inadequate, the skin can appear gray or cold. However, it sometimes appears pink. Vital signs may be normal or there may be orthostatic hypotension and tachycardia. The body temperature may be normal or mildly elevated (to 102°F).

TREATMENT. When the patient is moved to a cooler environment (decreasing the demand for blood flow to the skin) and given modest amounts of fluids (1 to 2 liters), the condition is usually relieved. Therefore, treatment is directed toward reducing body temperature by placing the patient in a cooler environment and loosening or removing clothing that may be interfering with heat dissipation. A fan may speed the cooling process.

Place the patient in a supine (with legs elevated) position to ensure perfusion of vital organs. Fluid replacement can be accomplished with oral dilute salt solutions in patients with a good mental status. A balanced solution such as Gatorade or even plain water can be given to replace fluids.

HEAT STROKE

Heat stroke is a life-threatening emergency. The mortality rate for untreated heat stroke is 80%. The primary and most important measure is to lower the body temperature. The classic triad of signs and symptoms

of heat stroke is a patient with *altered mental status, elevated body temperature (> 104°F), and hot, dry skin.*

MECHANISMS. Heat stroke can occur in an individual of any age. It results from a failure of the heat regulatory mechanism in response to heat stress. Once the heat regulatory mechanisms are lost, the temperature rises quickly to dangerous levels. When the core body temperature rises to 107°F, direct damage to cells occurs, particularly to the cells in the brain and to those lining the blood vessels. As mentioned earlier, circumstances that can lead to heat stroke include the athlete running in a marathon race on a hot, humid day; the debilitated elderly patient with a febrile illness who is covered with blankets in bed in a hot environment; and patients who have preexisting conditions or who have taken drugs that retard sweating, increase metabolism, or affect cardiovascular performance and mental status.

Although some patients with heat stroke have moist skin, most are characterized by having hot, dry skin. The importance of evaporation as a heat loss mechanism is underscored by this common finding. On hot, humid days, evaporation may represent the major (and only) existing means to dissipate heat from the body. Once this mechanism is lost, the internal body temperature quickly rises to dangerous heights.

SIGNS AND SYMPTOMS. As mentioned earlier, heat stroke is characterized by an altered mental status, ranging from confusion to coma; high body temperatures (above 104°F), and hot, dry skin. However, the skin may be moist, particularly in younger individuals who have undertaken strenuous activities, and dry skin should never be an absolute criterion to make the diagnosis.

Because of the increased blood flow to the skin, due to vasodilation, the patient may appear pink or flushed. Most patients have this appearance. However, occasionally a patient doesn't have adequate cardiac output to meet the increased demands of the skin, and the skin may appear ashen. The heart rate can be increased, as can the respiratory rate. Some patients may be hypotensive. Seizures are not uncommon.

TREATMENT

Lowering the body temperature is the highest priority. With victims of heat stroke, efforts to reduce body temperature are more aggressive than are those with heat exhaustion victims. With the latter, more passive efforts are often adequate, such as fanning, moving the patient to a cooler area, and removing insulating clothing. With heat stroke, these efforts are supplemented by applying ice packs to areas where there are large superficial blood vessels such as the neck, armpits, and groin. Sheets or towels moistened with cool water can be applied and air can be circulated by fans or by fanning to promote evaporation. Oxygen should be provided,

TABLE 11–1. Heat Emergencies

Condition	Signs and Symptoms	Treatment
Heat cramps	Muscular cramps following exercise	Cool environment Fluid replacement with balanced salt solution Stretch affected muscle
Heat exhaustion	Weakness or exhaustion Dizziness, faintness Skin moist, pale (or pink), may be cool Vital signs normal or tachycardia, orthostatic hypotension, elevated temperature (<39°C)	Cooling efforts Cool environment Fanning Loosen or remove clothing Fluids Supine position (legs elevated)
Heat stroke	Altered mental state Hot, dry skin (may be moist) Elevated body temperature (usually >40°C)	Aggressive cooling measures (wet sheets, fanning, ice to vessels of neck, armpits, groin) Rapid transport Oxygen

and the patient should be transported quickly to the hospital (Table 11–1).

The application of ice to all parts of the body in the field is controversial, as is the application of ice water baths. While rapid lowering of body temperature is essential to successful treatment, it is important to follow local protocols, which may call for rapid transport to a hospital to apply therapy such as ice baths. In the field there is an additional problem with such aggressive measures. Patients with heat stroke have lost the thermoregulatory mechanisms and can become hypothermic if overcooled. In hospitals, active cooling is stopped when the temperature reaches 102°F to avoid this problem. This requires that a rectal temperature be taken with a special probe that gives an accurate core body temperature.

One technique that should *not* be used in cooling is the sponging of the skin with isopropyl alcohol. Children have absorbed this alcohol through the dilated superficial blood vessels in the skin and suffered toxic effects.

Cold Emergencies

Cold exposure can cause local injuries such as frostnip and frostbite as well as a lowered core body temperature, resulting in hypothermia and death.

Exposure to below-freezing environments for short time periods and to above-freezing environments for longer time periods can both result in local cold injury. Frostbite and frostnip involve freezing of the water between and within body cells, resulting in ice crystal formation. Trench foot is a localized cold injury that occurs without ice crystal formation.

Hypothermia is defined as a core body temperature below 35°C. When the body's ability to produce heat and regulate heat loss is unable to cope with the environment, hypothermia occurs. Severe stresses such as immersion in icy water can overwhelm the body's ability to produce heat and regulate heat loss and may result in death within minutes. On the other hand, patients with a compromised ability to generate heat or prevent heat loss may become hypothermic at room temperature.

The rewarming of patients with cold injuries is usually best done in the hospital setting. Prehospital care is directed toward preventing further heat loss, protecting the injured parts, and providing rapid transport.

PHYSIOLOGIC RESPONSE TO COLD

Ordinarily, the body produces more than sufficient heat to maintain body temperature. In temperate climates, more than 90% of the average body heat generated during daily activities must be lost. The mechanisms of heat production and heat loss have already been discussed.

Humans have learned to deal with extremes of cold by creating environments that insulate and warm them. Clothing, buildings, and heating systems make it much easier to live in temperate or cold climates.

When faced with cold, the body's thermoregulatory centers respond by increasing heat production and decreasing heat loss. Early responses to cold include an increase in the metabolic rate to generate more heat and vasoconstriction to reduce heat loss. Shivering occurs if these measures are inadequate.

Shivering is the involuntary contraction of small groups of muscles, which can generate great amounts of heat. It begins when the temperature of the body's central core is around 35°C (95°F). Shivering may continue for a few hours until the body's energy stores are depleted. Malnourished individuals and those with insulin shock may deplete their energy stores in a shorter period of time. While shivering commences involuntarily, it is abolished by physical activity and purposeful movements such as walking. Certain drugs such as phenothiazines, barbiturates, and alcohol may suppress or inhibit the shivering response. Shivering usually stops when the body temperature dips below 31°C (87.8°F) and muscle rigidity is noted. Once shivering stops, the body temperature may drop precipitously.

Signs that the central nervous system is affected may appear as early as 34°C (92°F), with amnesia and slurred speech. Alterations in mental status will progress

Street person, children, old people.

through irrational behavior, stupor, and coma as the temperature continues to drop.

A vicious cycle that inhibits escape from the cold develops with cold exposure. As the body temperature drops, mentation is affected and judgment may be disturbed. At the same time, the ability to effectively use the hands becomes impeded as the extremities (the shell) become subject to local cold injury. This begins as clumsiness of hand movements and progresses to stiffness of the limbs and muscular rigidity as the temperature drops. The inability to build a shelter or move to a safer environment leaves the victim subject to further exposure, more extensive freezing injuries to body surface parts and the extremities, and the lowering of the core body temperature. Once shivering stops, the body temperature drops more rapidly. Muscles become rigid and, eventually, the patient is unable to undertake voluntary movements and lapses into coma. Cold effects on the heart result in depression of the pacemaker, arrhythmia, and clinical death.

Cold has a direct effect on the rate of metabolism and, therefore, on oxygen needs. Metabolism decreases 6% for every centigrade degree that the body's temperature drops. The corresponding decrease in oxygen requirements increases the time from clinical to biological death, and patients have had full neurologic recovery following prolonged periods of cardiac arrest secondary to hypothermia. Therefore, resuscitation efforts should continue while attempts to raise the body temperature are made.

HYPOTHERMIA

Text

Depending on the type of exposure, cold injuries may take minutes or hours to occur. The temperature of the outside environment and the type of exposure, i.e., air or water immersion, are important variables.

ACUTE IMMERSION HYPOTHERMIA. Acute immersion in icy waters can result in death within 15 minutes, and rarely does one survive for more than 1 hour. At water temperatures of 15.5°C, exposure of 6 hours is the upper limit for most people. Since water is such a good conductor of heat, swimming instructors and others who spend prolonged periods in the water require water temperatures of 32°C to be comfortable.

SUBACUTE EXPOSURE. Exposure to cold air results in longer survival times than submersion in water of the same temperature. However, if clothing becomes soaked, it offers little insulation value, reducing the time until cold injury occurs. Likewise, the wind velocity plays a significant factor in tolerance (Table 11–2).

CHRONIC EXPOSURES. Hypothermia over a period of hours or days can occur, usually in compromised individuals. Factors such as disease and drug intoxication, which alter heat production, the ability to retain heat, or the ability to escape a dangerous environment, make an individual susceptible to hypothermia. Shock states can compromise heat production and compensatory actions and responses. Consider the following case.

• CASE HISTORY •

EMTs responded to a call about an "unconscious" patient in an apartment building. On arrival, they discovered an unresponsive 55-year-old man who was found by his neighbor, with a large scalp laceration and a pool of blood surrounding him on the floor. The laceration was not actively bleeding. The man was unresponsive to verbal and painful stimuli, had a blood pressure of 80/60, respirations of 12, a pulse of 80, and a smell of alcohol on his breath. The skin was pale, cool, and dry. A diagnosis of hypovolemic shock was made and PASG were applied, resulting in an improvement in blood pressure to 100/80, with no change in pulse or mental status.

Further assessment and treatment in the hospital confirmed the diagnosis of hypovolemic shock from a scalp laceration and revealed a core body temperature of 31°C. The EMTs noted that the apartment in which the patient was found was of normal temperature. Blood analysis showed that the patient had a significant blood alcohol level.

———

This case illustrates that extreme environmental temperatures are not necessary to cause hypothermia. The patient was intoxicated with alcohol (resulting in vasodilation and unconsciousness). Combined with the shock, this left him unable to maintain body temperature even though he was in a 70°F apartment. Radiation and conduction to both air and the floor exceeded the heat production from his metabolism, which was compromised by hypovolemic shock and malnutrition (from his alcoholism). The hypothermia explained why his pulse was "normal" in the face of hypovolemic shock.

PREDISPOSING FACTORS. Heat loss by radiation is proportional to the temperature difference between the environment and the body. Exposure of body parts, for example, a bare head, increases radiation losses. Conductive heat loss is increased by contact with water, ice, snow, metal, and other objects that conduct heat faster than does air. Convection heat losses are greater when the victim cannot find shelter from the wind or is improperly clothed. Wet clothing gives little insulation. Evaporation heat losses can occur with wet clothing or after sweating due to exertion

Age. Persons at the extremes of age are most susceptible because of their dependence on others and their relative immobility. The elderly may have difficulty in fleeing a cold environment, generating heat via mus-

TABLE 11–2. Wind Chill Chart

Wind Speed		Cooling Power of Wind Expressed as Equivalent Chill Temperature																				
Knots	Mph	Temperature (°F)																				
		40	35	30	25	20	15	10	5	0	−5	−10	−15	−20	−25	−30	−35	−40	−45	−50	−55	−60
		Equivalent Chill Temperature																				
Calm	Calm	40	35	30	25	20	15	10	5	0	−5	−10	−15	−20	−25	−30	−35	−40	−45	−50	−55	−60
3–6	5	35	30	25	20	15	10	5	0	−5	−10	−15	−20	−25	−30	−35	−40	−45	−50	−55	−60	−70
7–10	10	30	20	15	10	5	0	−10	−15	−20	−25	−35	−40	−45	−50	−60	−65	−70	−75	−80	−90	−95
11–15	15	25	15	10	0	−5	−10	−20	−25	−30	−40	−45	−50	−60	−65	−70	−80	−85	−90	−100	−105	−110
16–19	20	20	10	5	0	−10	−15	−25	−30	−35	−45	−50	−60	−65	−75	−80	−85	−95	−100	−110	−115	−120
20–23	25	15	10	0	−5	−15	−20	−30	−35	−45	−50	−60	−65	−75	−80	−90	−95	−105	−110	−120	−125	−135
24–28	30	10	5	0	−10	−20	−25	−30	−40	−50	−55	−65	−70	−80	−85	−95	−100	−110	−115	−125	−130	−140
29–32	35	10	5	−5	−10	−20	−30	−35	−40	−50	−60	−65	−75	−80	−90	−100	−105	−115	−120	−130	−135	−145
33–36	40	10	0	−5	−15	−20	−30	−35	−45	−55	−60	−70	−75	−85	−95	−100	−110	−115	−125	−130	−140	−150

Winds above 40 mph have little additional effect

Peripheral Cold Injury

Little danger	Increasing danger (flesh may freeze within 1 minute)	Great danger (flesh may freeze within 30 seconds)

Danger of Freezing Exposed Flesh for Properly Clothed Persons

Reprinted from the United States Air Force Survival Manual 64-3.

cular activity, and regulating body temperature. The neonate has less fat tissue for insulation, and inefficient shivering and thermoregulatory mechanisms. After a field delivery, the newborn must be kept warm.

Medical Conditions. Certain medical conditions can affect the ability to generate heat and regulate temperature. These include diseases causing malnutrition; infections of the blood; endocrine diseases, including diabetes and hypoglycemia; shock; and diseases of the brain. Conditions affecting the skin such as burns predispose the patient to hypothermia. Patients with spinal cord injuries may not be able to vasoconstrict vessels in large areas of skin, causing increased heat loss.

Drugs. Drugs or poisons that can predispose the patient to hypothermia include benzodiazepines, tricyclic antidepressants, general anesthetics, narcotics, organophosphates, carbon monoxide, glutethimide, barbiturates, and phenothiazines.

Alcohol. Alcohol causes vasodilation, which decreases the insulating property of the skin. It can also interfere with judgment, suppress shivering, and disturb central thermoregulation.

SIGNS AND SYMPTOMS. Patients with hypothermia can display various signs and symptoms depending on the core body temperature. Most standard thermometers measure ranges of temperature from 94° to 106°F and are not able to measure lower temperatures. There are hypothermic thermometers used in hospitals to measure the lower readings.

In general, the patient feels cold to the touch, has a decreased level of consciousness, has decreased motor ability, and tends to have depressed vital signs. Shivering, seen with mild stages, is lost as the temperature decreases below 88°F or 31°C and is replaced by muscular rigidity.

Mild Hypothermia—32 to 35°C

The earliest stages of hypothermia can be noted by cool skin, shivering, difficulty in speech and movement, and amnesia. The vital signs may be normal.

Moderate Hypothermia—26 to 32°C

As the body temperature drops, the patient becomes stuporous. Shivering stops and is replaced with muscular rigidity and the gradual loss of voluntary motion. Cardiac output drops, the pulse and respirations become depressed, and the pupils dilate. The pulse may become irregular, due to the development of arrhythmias. As the temperature approaches 28°C, ventricular fibrillation may develop.

Severe Hypothermia—Less than 26°C

With severe hypothermia, the cerebral flow is one-third of normal and the patient is unresponsive to pain.

Cardiac output is greatly depressed and significant hypotension is noted. Ventricular fibrillation and cardiac arrest are likely (Table 11–3).

TREATMENT

Treatment is largely determined by the time it will take to transport the patient and the degree of hypothermia. The goals of prehospital treatment are to reduce further heat loss and to transport the patient rapidly but gently to a medical facility where active rewarming can be initiated. Due to the risk of ventricular arrhythmias, gentle handling is required, modification of cardiopulmonary resuscitation techniques may be needed, and active external rewarming is usually not undertaken in the field.

Patients can sustain long periods of hypothermia and still make a full recovery. The greatest risk is from ventricular fibrillation, which is resistant to treatment until the body is rewarmed. Since a depressed pulse may be adequate to meet the reduced oxygen needs of the cold patient, care is taken to avoid maneuvers that may precipitate ventricular fibrillation. These maneuvers include rough handling, stimulation of the gag reflex, overventilation, unnecessary cardiac compressions, and active external rewarming. Once cardiopulmonary resuscitation is initiated, however, it should be continued until the patient is rewarmed. There are reports of full recovery after prolonged periods (longer than 3 hours) of CPR.

REDUCE FURTHER HEAT LOSS. In all instances, further heat loss must be avoided. This is accomplished by carefully replacing wet clothes with dry clothes or blankets, using sleeping bags or other insulating devices, and protecting the patient from the wind.

TABLE 11–3. Levels of Hypothermia

Temperature		Signs and Symptoms
(°C)	(°F)	
		Mild
35	95	Shivering begins
34	93.2	Amnesia
33	91.4	Poor muscular coordination
		Moderate
32	89.6	Stupor
31	87.8	Shivering stops
30	86	Irregular heart rhythms
29	85.2	Further loss of consciousness Pupils dilate
28	82.4	Ventricular fibrillation possible
27	80.6	Loss of voluntary motion
		Severe
26	78.8	Unresponsive to pain
24	75.2	Significant hypotension
22	71.6	Ventricular fibrillation likely

Adapted from Danze DF: Accidental hypothermia. In Rosen P (ed): Emergency Medicine: Concepts and Clinical Practice, 2nd ed. St Louise, CV Mosby, 1988, p. 667.

RESUSCITATION TECHNIQUES. The respiratory rate and pulse may be severely depressed. Supplemental oxygen, approximately 50%, should be given along with respiratory assistance. Respiratory rates of 2 to 3 breaths per minute have been observed. If respiratory assistance is needed, be careful not to hyperventilate the patient. Sudden hyperventilation can result in rapid changes in the acidity of the blood and lead to arrhythmias in the hypothermic patient.

Carefully insert any necessary airway devices to avoid stimulating a gag reflex, since this also may precipitate arrhythmias.

Careful assessment of pulses must be undertaken before initiating cardiac compressions. Peripheral pulses may be particularly difficult to palpate because of vasoconstriction and associated frostbite. The pupils may be dilated and unresponsive to light because of the hypothermia, and the blood pressure may not be measurable. Again, extra care must be taken because unnecessary cardiac compressions given to a hypothermic patient with a depressed, slow, and barely perceptible heartbeat may have the adverse effect of precipitating ventricular fibrillation.

ACTIVE REWARMING TECHNIQUES. Active rewarming techniques involve application of heat internally or externally. Generally, most active rewarming techniques are not recommended in the field. Internal techniques that are applied in the hospital setting include instillation of warmed intravenous fluids, peritoneal dialysis with warmed fluids, hemodialysis, instillation of heated fluids in the gastrointestinal tract, and administration of warmed humidified oxygen. In the hospital, rewarming procedures are guided by the patient's core temperature, with attention given to the critical temperatures, 28°C or 82.4°F, at which ventricular fibrillation is likely to occur.

In the field, such monitoring is not possible. Therefore, the recommended active rewarming techniques are limited to administration of warm humidified oxygen and application of local heat to the large superficial vessels. Warm fluids containing sugar can be given to the conscious patient who is capable of drinking.

In restricted circumstances, immersion in a tub of hot water (105°F) or application of warmed blankets or hot water bottles to the body's shell may be necessary. These techniques are not recommended for all patients because of the possibility of complications from "rewarming shock." Rewarming shock is a term used to describe the effects of extremity and shell rewarming before the core temperature can be raised, resulting in a sudden dilation of peripheral vessels and an increase in the size of the circulatory system before the heart has a chance to warm.

However, when one is far from a medical facility or trapped in a wilderness situation, active rewarming may be necessary.

TRANSPORT. Transport of the patient to a medical facility should be undertaken as soon as possible. The patient must be handled gently and a rough ride should be avoided. Again, sudden jolts or bumps may initiate arrhythmias. The patient can be placed in the head-down position.

PREVENTION OF HYPOTHERMIA

EMTs who attempt rescue missions in cold environments must be conscious of hazards and take appropriate precautions. These precautions are based upon principles of heat loss. Clothing must give adequate insulation and protection from wind and moisture, and layering is recommended to allow the rescuer to adapt to changes in environmental temperature and the production of heat from physical exertion. Wet clothing should be removed, since it gives little insulation and speeds heat loss from evaporation. Heat loss through radiation can be avoided by covering the body, particularly the head. Contact with conductors of heat such as metal, snow, and water should be avoided. Alcohol should be avoided because of its vasodilatory effect and its ability to suppress shivering.

Do not smoke when attempting a rescue mission in a cold environment because nicotine is a potent vasoconstrictor, and therefore it affects the thermoregulatory responses of blood vessels. Take along food that is high in carbohydrates to sustain heat production. Keep moving, which will also generate heat. Knowing your physical abilities is important, since the body temperature may drop rapidly after you become fatigued and you will be unable to continue rescue activities. Shelter must be sought before hypothermia clouds your judgment and hampers your motor abilities.

LOCAL INJURIES

Cold injuries tend to occur to the extremities and exposed ears, nose, chin, and cheeks, where there is a relatively large surface area for a small volume of tissue. These injuries tend to be localized and sharply demarcated, and they gradually progress from superficial to deep with continued exposure. The process is progressive. Vasoconstriction of the extremities in response to cold leaves less heat to warm the superficial parts. The water in the superficial tissues freezes and the vasoconstriction becomes more intense, which results in still less blood flow and freezing of deeper tissues. The entire area may become frozen. The ice crystals that form can cause damage to cellular structure, but in many cases recovery is possible following proper rewarming. Never rub or massage frostbitten parts because the movement of ice crystals can cause additional damage to the cells.

Upon rewarming, there is a marked vasodilation of the area, resulting in a change to marked flushed coloring. There is swelling from capillary leakage. If thrombosis

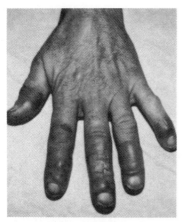

FIGURE 11-5. The appearance of superficial frostbite. (From Nelson RN, Rund DA, Keller MD: Environmental Emergencies. Philadelphia, WB Saunders, 1985, p. 33.)

forms in small vessels, it can affect the local circulation, cause areas to have stagnation of blood flow, and result in areas of different color (mottled appearance). For example, areas where venous blood flow is obstructed, causing poor capillary return, may appear bluish or purplish. These areas may alternate with areas of arterial vasoconstriction, which appear pale or gray, causing the mottled appearance.

FROSTNIP. Frostnip is a completely reversible cold injury secondary to intense vasoconstriction to cold exposure. Frostnipped areas first appear as a sudden blanching of the skin. There is a loss of feeling and a sensation of cold in the area, leaving the victim unaware of the process. The skin does not become hardened. The area can be warmed by applying firm pressure with a hand or other warm body part or by blowing warm breath on the area. Upon rewarming, the area may be red and a tingling sensation may be noted.

SUPERFICIAL FROSTBITE. If unrecognized, frostnip can lead to superficial frostbite, or the freezing of water within the upper layers of skin. The skin appears white and waxy and is firm to the touch, but the tissues beneath the skin are soft and resilient.

After thawing, the skin may appear flushed or mottled, with alternating patchy red-purple and blanched areas. There may be edema of the area, and blisters can form after 1 to 24 hours. The area is usually painful (Fig. 11-5).

DEEP FROSTBITE. With deep frostbite the freezing extends throughout the dermis and can involve subcutaneous tissues, muscle and tendons, neurovascular structures, and possibly even bone. The skin becomes white, feels frozen, and resists depression. It is difficult to gauge the extent of deep frostbite.

If an area of deep frostbite has been partially rethawed, the affected area may appear mottled and blue or gray. There is usually a line of demarcation separating injured from healthy tissue (Fig. 11-6).

TREATMENT OF FROSTBITE. Optimal treatment for frostbite requires well-controlled yet rapid rewarming, a technique that in most cases should not be undertaken in the field. Active rewarming, properly done, may be time consuming and can delay assessment of hypothermia and evacuation from the area, and the potential complications that follow thawing are best handled in the hospital. Furthermore, any part that is thawed has to be carefully protected from refreezing. It is worse for the part to thaw and refreeze than to remain frozen for the same period of time. The frostbitten part, whether frozen or thawed, must be carefully handled to avoid any further trauma.

The injured area should be protected from further heat loss, use, or traumatic injury. It should be dressed appropriately and protected from further cold injury by insulating the area with layers of clothing and blankets. Protect the area from moisture, and remove wet clothing.

If an area has thawed, do not break the blisters; rather, cover them with sterile dressings. If the hands or feet are involved, separate the fingers and toes with small

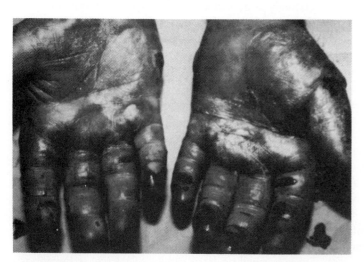

FIGURE 11-6. The appearance of deep frostbite. (From Nelson RN, Rund DA, Keller MD: Environmetal Emergencies. Philadelphia, WB Saunders, 1985, p. 34.)

folded dressings. Handle the area with care and do not allow the patient to walk on an affected lower extremity. Avoid exposure of the area to direct dry heat, as from a fire.

Oxygen should be administered and careful attention must be paid to assess the patient for hypothermia and other injuries, and to prepare for evacuation from the scene.

In wilderness situations or in other extraordinary circumstances where transport may be significantly delayed, the rapid rewarming technique may be advisable in the field. In rare instances in which transport may be delayed so long that slow rethawing would take place, rapid rethawing can be done if conditions permit and the part can be kept from refreezing.

In situations in which a victim must walk out of a wilderness or other area, it is best if the attempt is made on the frozen extremity and not on a thawed or partially rethawed one.

The following is used in the emergency department or when field transport is delayed and facilities permit. Be sure to know and follow your local protocols.

PROCEDURE 11-1
RAPID REWARMING*

1. Immerse the affected part into a basin of water large enough to accommodate the part without it touching the walls of the container.
2. Preheat and maintain the water temperature at about 40.6°C (105°F) and keep it between 37.8 and 43.3°C. Too warm a temperature may harm the part, and lower temperatures are not as effective. If no thermometer is available, water that is at 43.3°C can be estimated as the temperature that causes only slight discomfort. Water at 44.4°C is uncomfortable to most people.
3. Keep the water circulating to keep the temperature uniform. A whirlpool type tub is ideal; otherwise continuously stir the water as it is added.
4. Anticipate that the patient will feel pain on rethawing. The process is complete when the part is again soft and color and sensation are present.
5. Dress the area with sterile dressings. Do not break any blisters. Place folded sterile dressings between toes and fingers before covering a foot or hand.

Note: The thawed part must be protected from refreezing. The rapid rewarming process can take from 20 to 40 minutes.

---

* After Bangs C, Hamlet MP: Hypothermia and cold injuries. In Auerbach PS, Geehr EC (eds): Management of Wilderness and Environmental Emergencies. New York, Macmillan, 1983.

TRENCH FOOT OR IMMERSION FOOT. Prolonged exposure (10 to 12 hours) to above-freezing temperatures and dampness (generally below 10°C, 50°F) can result in cold injury to the extremities, particularly if they are wet. This condition is called trench foot or immersion foot and was a common cold injury in wartime when soldiers stood for long periods of time in cold, wet trenches. It causes damage to the small vessels and nerves and occurs in stages. The limb may have a different appearance, depending on when the EMT encounters the patient.

In response to the cold, the vessels in the extremity vasoconstrict, causing paleness or blueness and diminished pulses, and further lowering of the extremity's temperature. After a prolonged period of vasoconstriction, ischemic changes occur, including damage to small vessels and nerves with capillary leakage, associated edema, and decreased or absent sensation. Thus, early in the encounter the foot may appear cold, swollen, pale or blue, with diminished pulses and sensation.

This phase is followed by an increase in circulation to the area, as if to make up for the period of prolonged vasoconstriction and ischemia. This increased circulation makes the foot appear hot, red, and dry. Pulses may be bounding and the limb is extremely painful due to the cold and ischemic injury. The skin can atrophy or ulcers and gangrene can follow.

Patients who have experienced immersion foot injuries may suffer pain and discomfort in response to cold and weight-bearing for prolonged periods of time after the injury. As opposed to frostbite, injury results without ice crystal formation.

Treatment consists of keeping the extremity warm, dry, and protected from weight-bearing and further injury.

CHILBLAINS. Some individuals have an abnormal vascular response to mild cold that manifests as itching, redness, and swelling on the dorsal surfaces of the hands and feet following exposure to above-freezing temperatures. It most often affects women and children and persons with certain vascular and collagen diseases.

BURNS

Introduction

Burns can be caused by *thermal* (heat), *chemical*, or *electrical* injury. Thermal burns affect about 2 million individuals annually, and it is estimated that 3 to 5% of these burns are life-threatening. Most thermal burns occur in the home and are the result of flames or scalding water. For those under 3 years of age, hot liquids are the most common source of burns. Small children suffer scald burns when they reach for pots on a stove, spill hot liquids such as coffee or tea, or place their hands under hot water taps. From ages 3 to 14, burning clothing is the most common source of burns. Over age 60, complicating factors such as momentary blackouts or general debilitation may contribute to household accidents or impede the ability to escape.

The smoke produced by burning materials can contain a number of toxins, the most common of which is carbon monoxide. Carbon monoxide is a colorless, tasteless, odorless gas that impairs oxygen transport and contributes to over half the deaths from fires. In fact, many deaths from fires are the result of smoke inhalation alone, without any thermal burns. Because the inhalation of smoke has rapid and lethal effects, all victims require prompt removal from the toxic environment and administration of high-concentration oxygen to facilitate the removal of carbon monoxide.

Thermal Burns

The organ most commonly injured by burns is the skin, which accounts for about 15% of body weight in the adult. The skin serves as a protective barrier to infection, as a barrier to water loss, as a major thermoregulatory organ, and as a sensory organ for touch, pain, temperature, and pressure perception. The different layers of the skin contribute to these functions. The outer epidermis is relatively impermeable to water and bacteria. The dermis contains the blood vessels, nerves, and other structures such as hair follicles, sweat ducts, and sebaceous glands, which extend via ducts to the epidermis. Underneath the dermis is a layer of subcutaneous tissue that protects and insulates.

Problems that follow burns include loss of temperature control, loss of body fluids and water, and susceptibility to infection.

The scope of prehospital care is to stop the burning process, remove the patient from the smokey environment, provide supplemental oxygen to reverse the effects of carbon monoxide, treat the patient for shock, prevent infection, and transport the patient to the appropriate facility. The major emphasis must be given to assessing and treating life-threatening complications such as smoke inhalation, airway obstruction, and associated injuries or complicating medical conditions. Once the burning process has been stopped, the prehospital treatment of burns concentrates on preventing infection, maintaining body temperature, and minimizing pain. The ability to assess the depth and extent of burns is necessary to identify patients in need of transport to burn centers.

LIMITS OF HEAT TOLERANCE

The degree of heat and the length of exposure are critical variables in determining the extent of a burn injury. Contact with heat sufficient to raise the body temperature to 60°C results in cell death. If the temperature remains below 45°C, generally no cell damage occurs. Cells exposed to temperatures above 45°C may have various degrees of damage, depending on the duration of exposure to a given temperature. For example, a scalding burn resulting from spilled hot water is less severe than one resulting from immersion in water of the same temperature. Likewise, melted synthetic materials or substances such as tar, which adhere to the skin, continue to produce burn injury until the substance is removed or cooled. The effects of chemical burns depend on the type and concentration of the chemical and the duration of exposure. The effects of electrical burns depend on the voltage, the resistance of the tissues, and the length of contact.

CLASSIFICATION AND ASSESSMENT OF BURNS

Burn injuries can be classified by widely accepted criteria used to assess their severity. These criteria include the depth, extent, and location of burns, as well as complicating factors such as age, respiratory involvement, and associated medical or traumatic conditions.

Depth of Burns

The classification of burn depth is based on skin anatomy and is spoken of in terms of degrees (Fig. 11–7).

FIRST-DEGREE BURNS. First-degree burns involve the epidermis only and spare the deeper layers. Sunburn is a common example of first-degree burns. They can also occur as a result of minor flash injury or at the periphery of more severe burns. The skin appears reddened and is dry and warm to the touch. Generally, first-degree burns are painful, since the nerves in the deeper layers are left intact. The pain may not occur for several hours, as with sunburns. There may be slight edema due to congestion and dilation of the intradermal vessels.

First-degree burns heal spontaneously after small scales of the epidermis peel off. Since there is no loss of skin function, first-degree burns are not included in estimating the extent of burn injury, even though some individuals with extensive sunburns feel ill and may have a slightly elevated body temperature.

SECOND-DEGREE BURNS. Second-degree burns involve the epidermis and extend into but not through the entire dermis; hence they are referred to as partial-thickness burns. They are commonly caused by flash injuries or spill scalds.

Second-degree burns can have different appearances, depending on the extent of dermal injury. A common characteristic is edema and blister formation, due to tissue damage and accumulation of plasma from injured capillaries (Fig. 11–8A and B). The blisters and wound surface may be moist or weeping. Generally,

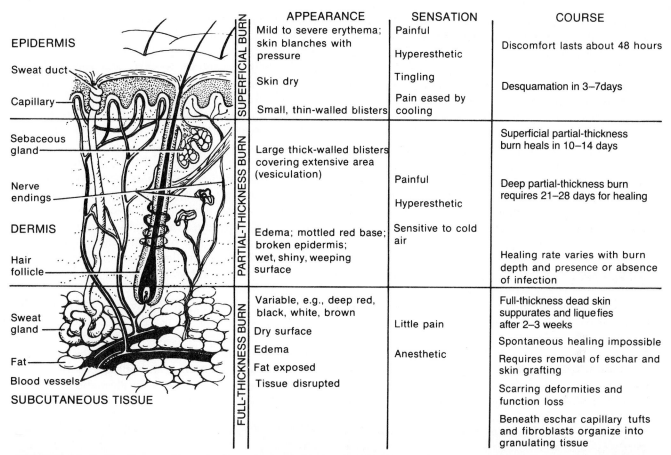

		APPEARANCE	SENSATION	COURSE
EPIDERMIS	SUPERFICIAL BURN	Mild to severe erythema; skin blanches with pressure	Painful	Discomfort lasts about 48 hours
Sweat duct			Hyperesthetic	
Capillary		Skin dry	Tingling	Desquamation in 3–7days
		Small, thin-walled blisters	Pain eased by cooling	
Sebaceous gland	PARTIAL-THICKNESS BURN	Large thick-walled blisters covering extensive area (vesiculation)	Painful	Superficial partial-thickness burn heals in 10–14 days
Nerve endings			Hyperesthetic	Deep partial-thickness burn requires 21–28 days for healing
DERMIS		Edema; mottled red base; broken epidermis; wet, shiny, weeping surface	Sensitive to cold air	
Hair follicle				Healing rate varies with burn depth and presence or absence of infection
Sweat gland	FULL-THICKNESS BURN	Variable, e.g., deep red, black, white, brown	Little pain	Full-thickness dead skin suppurates and liquefies after 2–3 weeks
		Dry surface		Spontaneous healing impossible
Fat		Edema	Anesthetic	Requires removal of eschar and skin grafting
Blood vessels		Fat exposed		Scarring deformities and function loss
SUBCUTANEOUS TISSUE		Tissue disrupted		Beneath eschar capillary tufts and fibroblasts organize into granulating tissue

FIGURE 11–7. Classification of burn depth in relation to the skin. First-degree (superficial), second-degree (partial thickness), and third-degree (full thickness). (From Luckmann J, Sorensen KC: Medical-Surgical Nursing: A Psychophysiologic Approach, 3rd ed. Philadelphia, WB Saunders, 1987, p. 1616.)

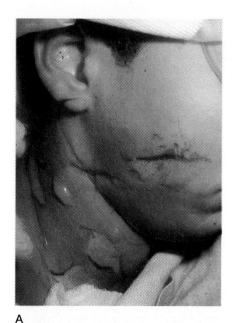

A

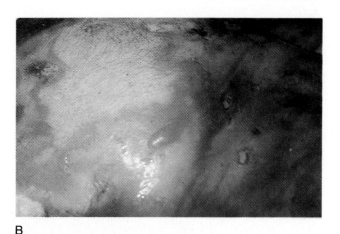

B

FIGURE 11–8. (*A*) Second-degree burns from brief exposure to flame. (*B*) Example of a deep second-degree burn with blistering surrounded by third-degree burn.

blisters should be left intact, since they provide a barrier to infection. The edema may restrict blood flow, particularly if it is circumferential (completely circles an extremity).

The color may vary, depending on the depth of the burn. The burn may appear pink or red and blotchy; deeper burns may be darker or pale and colorless.

Second-degree burns vary in their sensitivity, depending on the depth. More superficial second-degree burns can be extremely painful and sensitive to touch and air movements. Deeper second-degree burns may have normal or decreased sensation to touch. Very deep second-degree burns may have no sensation, and it is difficult to distinguish these from third-degree burns (and actually of no practical significance in the field). Skin functions are lost with second-degree burns, leading to fluid loss, body heat loss, and susceptibility to infection. However, second-degree burns can heal spontaneously, since some skin tissue and structures such as hair follicles or sweat glands, which can regenerate new skin, are spared.

THIRD-DEGREE BURNS. Third-degree burns involve the full thickness of the epidermis and dermis. They can be caused by extreme heat, prolonged exposure to flames, or immersion scalds. The skin can appear charred, yellow-brown, dark red, or white and translucent. Often, thrombosed veins are visible.

In marked contrast to first- and second-degree burns, there is no pain or sensation, since the nerves in the deeper layers of the dermis are destroyed.

The texture of the skin in full-thickness burns is leathery. Having lost its normal resilience, such skin can restrict movement and the expansion of underlying structures. This is particularly true if the burn extends over a large surface or circles a limb or the torso (circumferential). For example, third-degree burns of a large portion of the chest wall can limit lung expansion. Circumferential burns of the extremities can constrict blood flow. The constriction can progress over time, and in the hospital setting incisions are sometimes made through the leathery skin to allow chest wall expansion or distal blood flow to an extremity.

Third-degree burns heal only from the margins of the wound, since there are no cells left in the destroyed dermis capable of generating new skin tissue. Therefore, third-degree burns require skin grafting, which involves transplantation of skin from an unaffected body area to the burn site. See Figure 11–9 for illustrations of third- and fourth-degree burns.

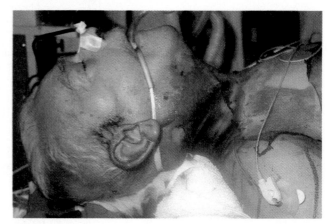

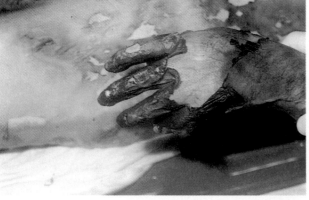

FIGURE 11–9. (*A*) Third-degree burns covering most of torso. Red and charred areas have a leathery feel. (*B*) Third-degree burns around neck. Circumferential burns can impair circulation (neck, extremities) and breathing (torso). (*C*) Third- and fourth-degree burns to hand. Note charring of fingers with sloughing of nails and skin.

A

B

C

FOURTH-DEGREE BURNS.   Burns can involve tissues beneath the skin as well, and include subcutaneous tissue, muscle, and even bone. This is sometimes called a fourth-degree burn. Electrical burns can cause damage to deeper underlying structures as the current travels through the body.

Extent of Burns

The amount of skin burned plays a large role in the severity of a burn injury. Calculations of the extent are made according to the rule of nines. For adults, the body is approximated into surface areas of 9% and 18% to facilitate estimates. The head and neck and each arm are considered as areas involving 9% of the body surface area. The front of the torso, the back of the torso, and each leg are considered to be areas involving 18% of the body surface area. The genitalia are considered to be 1% of the body surface area. Summation of all these areas accounts for 100% of the body. The palm is considered to represent about 1% of the body surface area and might be used to estimate and describe smaller areas of burn. An adjustment is made in the calculations for infants, who have a greater surface area on the head in comparison with the rest of the body. The head in children is said to account for 18% of the body surface area, and each lower limb for ~14%. Hence, one can remember by approximation differences between the adult and the infant or small child by the phrase "steal 9% from the legs and give to the head." The trunk and arms remain the same.

The body surface charts (Fig. 11–10) allow visualization of the rule of nines. While there are gradations between the infant and the adult, these two rules give useful approximations and should be committed to memory.

Always describe the depth and extent of areas burned in reports and communications, for example, second- and third-degree burns to the entire right arm (9%) and anterior trunk (18%). For reports you may want to distinguish second- and third-degree areas on a patient diagram by using different marking techniques.

Location of Burns

There are certain locations on the body where burns are more critical, due to their tendency to develop in-

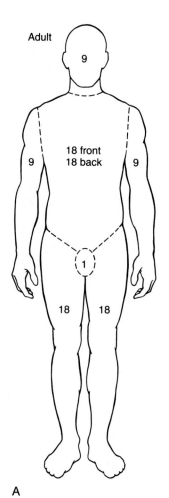

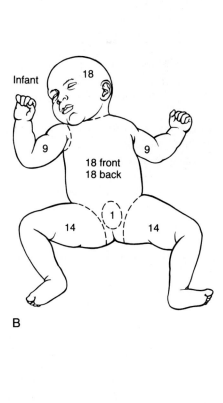

FIGURE 11–10. Body surface chart of the "rule of nines": (*A*) adult; (*B*) child.

fection, loss of function, or respiratory involvement. Critical areas include the face, perineum and genitalia, and the feet and hands.

Burns to the perineum and genital area are prone to infection due to contamination from fecal bacteria. Significant burns to the hands and feet require special handling to avoid contractures and scarring that will restrict future function. Facial burns are more severe because they can involve special structures and may be accompanied by respiratory tract involvement. If burns are circumferential, they are considered severe because the loss of elasticity or edema around an entire extremity or body cavity can compromise blood flow or breathing. Circumferential burns can involve the extremities, the neck, or the torso.

Complicating Factors

There are certain historical or physical factors that make recovery from a burn more difficult or even increase the likelihood of death. For example, age is such a factor. Elderly patients are much less likely to survive, regardless of the extent of a burn. Other factors include the presence of inhalation injuries, associated injuries or medical conditions, and certain preexisting conditions.

INHALATION INJURIES.   Inhaled steam or extremely hot air, smoke particles, and toxic gases can cause direct damage to the respiratory tract. This can result in airway compromise or damage to the lungs themselves.

Steam carries more heat than air and can overwhelm the ability of the upper respiratory tract to cool air to body temperature before it reaches the delicate alveoli. Particles of smoke carry heat, as well as toxic chemicals, deep into the respiratory tract. Being trapped in a closed space or unconsciousness increases the risk of inhalation injury. Physical signs that should raise suspicion of inhalation injury include singed nasal hairs, sputum with black particles (carbonaceous sputum), burns around the mouth and nose, hoarseness of the voice, and respiratory distress (Fig. 11–11).

AGE OF THE PATIENT.   The severity of a given burn is increased if patients are at extremes of age. Generally, adults over the age 60 years and children under the age 5 years are considered at increased risk.

ASSOCIATED CONDITIONS.   Associated traumatic injuries may take precedence over the burn injury as the greatest immediate threat to life and may complicate the treatment of the burns. Preexisting medical conditions that may hamper recovery may also raise the severity of a burn injury. Such conditions include lung disease, cardiac disease, diabetes, or any severe injury or illness.

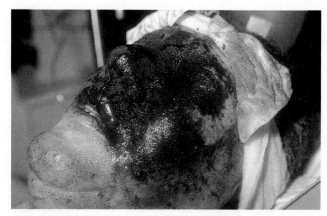

FIGURE 11–11. Signs of inhalation injury include burns around mouth and nose and singed nasal hairs. Carbon particles from gas burner explosion account for blackened appearance.

Burn Severity Classification

Burns are classified by severity for patient triage and transport decisions. Local protocols often use burn severity as the criterion for determining which facility should be selected. This decision is often made directly in the field. There are widely accepted national criteria that may be adjusted to reflect local resources (Tables 11–4 and 11–5).

The depth and extent of burns are the major determinants in classifying the severity of a burn. Only second- and third-degree burns are counted when assessing extent of the burn, since first-degree burns do not result in loss of skin function. Other factors, as discussed above, are also used in determining whether a patient should be considered as having sustained a minor, moderate, or major burn injury.

TREATMENT OF THERMAL BURNS

STOP THE BURNING PROCESS.   Remove the patient from the burning or smokey environment and extinguish the flames with blankets or water. The patient whose clothing is burning should be covered with a blanket, placed on the ground, and rolled slowly to extinguish the flames. Running in panic allows flames to spread and rise upward toward the face. Remove smoldering clothing if it is not adherent to the skin. Pour water over smoldering articles of clothing that are adherent to the skin to stop the burning process. Cool water applied with a face cloth or immersion may help limit the severity of certain burns such as scalds if applied shortly after the accident.

Caution should be used in applying cool compresses to extensive areas of burned skin because of the chance of inducing hypothermia. Generally, once smoldering has been stopped, cool compresses should not be left on more than 20% of the body surface area. Cool compresses

TABLE 11–4. Clinical Classification of Burn Depth

	First-Degree	Second-Degree (Partial Thickness) Superficial	Deep	Third-Degree (Full Thickness)
Color	Bright red	Red and mottled	Dark red or pale yellow to off-white	Very dark red in children; pearly white, charred; translucent and parchment-like. Bronzed—strong acid injury; dissolution of skin with exposed deep tissues—strong alkali injury
Surface	Dry with focal exfoliation	Blisters with copious exudate	Denuded surface with minimal exudate	Dry and leathery with thrombosed dermal and subdermal vessels visible. Smooth and silky—strong acid injury; liquefaction necrosis—strong alkali injury
Sensation	Painful	Painful	Diminished pinprick sensation; intact dermal sensation	Anesthetic except for deep pressure sensation in subdermal tissues
Time for healing	3–6 days	10–21 days	More than 3 weeks	Grafting always required
Cause	Sun or minor flash injury	Flash injury; spill scalds	Scalds of longer duration; flash of high intensity; brief exposure to flame	Flame burns; strong chemicals; contact with hot objects; electricity; prolonged scalds

From American College of Surgeons: Early Care of the Injuried Patient, 3rd ed. Philadelphia, WB Saunders, 1982, p. 88.

can be left on for a few minutes until the burned skin returns to normal body temperature.

TREAT LIFE-THREATENING CONDITIONS FIRST. Patients should be assessed carefully for the presence of airway compromise and respiratory distress. Look for stridor, hoarseness, use of accessory muscles, cyanosis,

TABLE 11–5. Burn Center Triage Criteria

I. Minor burn injury: Can be treated on outpatient basis and admitted for grafting of small full-thickness burns
  A. Second-degree burns
    1. Less than 15% total body surface in adult
    2. Less than 10% total body surface in child
  B. Third-degree burns: Less than 2% of total body surface
II. Moderate uncomplicated burn injury: Can be treated at a general hospital by personnel with experience in burn care or at a specialized burn treatment facility
  A. Second-degree burns
    1. 15–25% of total body surface in adult
    2. 10–20% of total body surface in child
  B. Third-degree burns: 2–10% of total body surface
III. Major burn injury: Best treated at burn unit or burn center
  A. Second-degree burns
    1. More than 25% of total body surface in adult
    2. More than 20% of total body surface in child
  B. Third-degree burns: More than 10% of total body surface
  C. Patients with lesser burns but with complicating features:
    1. Significant burns of hands, feet, face, or perineum
    2. Inhalation injury
    3. Significant fractures or other mechanical trauma
    4. Significant preexisting disease, e.g., diabetes
    5. Either extreme of age; less than 5 or more than 60

From American College of Surgeons: Early Care of the Injured Patient, 3rd ed. Philadelphia, WB Saunders, 1982, p. 100.

and other signs of respiratory distress, as well as for signs of inhalation injury. If there is evidence of smoke inhalation, shock, or extensive burns, administer high-concentration oxygen, humidified if possible. Patients suffering from smoke inhalation should be assumed to have inhaled carbon monoxide, for which high-concentration oxygen is the main treatment.

Assess the patient for associated trauma and shock caused by other injuries. Shock can be caused by hypovolemia resulting from fluid loss from the burns and sometimes from vasodilation secondary to pain. Usually the shock from burns is not severe within the first hour, and fluid replacement for burn fluid loss can be done in the hospital setting.

Obtain a history that includes the circumstances surrounding the burn and the source and duration of the thermal injury or smoke inhalation. Was the patient in a closed space or unconscious? Inquire about preexisting medical conditions that may complicate therapy.

COVER THE WOUND. The burn wound should be covered with sterile or clean dressings or sheets. Remove rings or bracelets that may become constricting. Never apply ointments or any other substance on the burn, since it will have to be removed in the hospital to allow for proper assessment, cleansing, and more definitive care. Leave blisters intact. Covering the wound often gives the patient some pain relief.

In cool environments, use blankets to insulate and maintain body temperature, since burn patients are susceptible to hypothermia. Transport according to local protocols (see Protocol: Burns [Thermal/Electrical]).

✦ P R O T O C O L ✦

BURNS (THERMAL/ELECTRICAL)

1. Ensure that the scene is safe for entry. If not, obtain assistance from trained firefighters as needed.

2. Extinguish burning clothing, and stop the burning process.

> *CAUTION!*
>
> MANUALLY STABILIZE THE HEAD AND CERVICAL SPINE IF TRAUMA OF THE HEAD AND NECK IS SUSPECTED!

3. Ensure that the patient's airway is open and that breathing and circulation are adequate.

4. Place the patient in a position of comfort *ONLY IF DOING SO DOES NOT COMPROMISE STABILIZATION OF THE HEAD AND CERVICAL SPINE!*

5. Administer high-concentration oxygen if respiratory burns are suspected and in all burns involving flames.

6. Assess for shock. IF SHOCK IS PRESENT, REFER IMMEDIATELY TO THE *SHOCK* PROTOCOL (Chapter 5).

7. Remove smoldering clothing not adhering to the patient and rings, bracelets, and other constricting items.

8. FOR ALL BURNS apply dry sterile dressings to the burned area.

NOTE: DO NOT PUNCTURE UNBROKEN BLISTERS!

9. Obtain and record the initial vital signs, and repeat en route as often as the situation indicates.

10. Transport, keeping the patient warm. THIS IS IMPORTANT SINCE THESE PATIENTS TEND TO LOSE HEAT AND BECOME HYPOTHERMIC!

11. Record all patient care information, including the patient's medical history and all treatment provided, on a Prehospital Care Report.

From Manual for Emergency Medical Technicians. Emergency Medical Services Program. Albany, New York State Department of Health, 1990.

Smoke Inhalation

Smoke inhalation is the most common cause of death in fires. Smoke is hot air containing noxious gases as well as small particles of various sizes to which toxic chemicals are attached. The type of gases given off during fires depends on the substance burned and varies with the heat of the fire. Specific toxic gases are covered under poisoning, Chapter 12.

DEATH FROM SMOKE INHALATION

Death from smoke inhalation results from lack of oxygen. There are four general ways that smoke interferes with oxygen delivery and utilization. First, fires consume oxygen, *lowering the percentage of oxygen in the air*. This is a particular problem if the fire is in a closed space.

Second, carbon monoxide, the most common toxic gas, is a byproduct of combustion. Carbon monoxide binds with hemoglobin and interferes with oxygen transport to the tissues. Small concentrations of this odorless, colorless, tasteless gas in the air breathed can result in lethal levels in the blood, since carbon monoxide has a 200 times greater affinity for hemoglobin than does oxygen. All smoke inhalation victims should be considered to have inhaled carbon monoxide and should be treated with oxygen.

Another way that smoke can cause death is by impairing the tissues' ability to use oxygen. For example, in some fires, cyanide gas is produced. Cyanide poisons the tissues and interferes with oxygen metabolism at the tissue level. Sources of cyanide include burning polyurethane, polyacrylonitrile, wool, and silk.

A fourth way that smoke can lead to hypoxia is from direct injury to the airways. Heat and irritant gases in smoke can lead to swelling of the airway, bronchospasm, and damage to the delicate alveoli. Heat injuries are usually the result of moist heat (steam or intense heat) that overwhelms the ability of the airways to cool air to body temperature.

Irritant gases such as hydrochloric acid, chlorine, or phosgene produce an inflammatory reaction and can damage capillaries and cause edema in the airways or alveoli. These irritant gases can be formed from burning plastics or from industrial fires. Small particles in smoke can carry heat as well as attached chemicals down into the lower airway.

ASSESSMENT

HISTORY. Important historical facts, including the duration of exposure and the type of burning materials producing the smoke, should be noted. Was the person found on a smoldering polyurethane couch, or was the source of smoke an electrical fire that melted insulating materials? Was the victim exposed to steam? Victims who are at higher risk include those who were unconscious in the burning environment or trapped in a closed space, since they had no chance to seek areas of better ventilation. Were firemen wearing self-contained breathing apparatus? Note the time the victim was removed from the burning environment and the duration and concentration of oxygen administered. These facts are necessary to accurately interpret the tests for carbon monoxide levels that are done in the hospital.

Symptoms of smoke inhalation include complaints of burning of the eyes, nose, and throat; tearing; coughing; tightness in the chest; and shortness of breath with moderate exertion. The symptoms vary considerably, depending on the substances burned, the duration of exposure, and so forth. Some patients may have no specific complaints even though they may have inhaled toxic levels of carbon monoxide.

PHYSICAL EXAMINATION. On physical examination, look for burns of the face, singed nasal hairs, hoarseness, and stridor. Erythema and particles in the oropharynx and carbonaceous (black particles) sputum may be noted. Wheezes and rales are not usually present initially. If they are present, they represent early evidence of lower airway tract involvement. Other signs of hypoxia, including cyanosis, tachypnea, and tachycardia, can be present in severe cases.

The cherry-red color that occurs with carbon monoxide poisoning comes from the color of carboxyhemoglobin (the carbon monoxide–hemoglobin complex), but is not a common finding (Fig. 11–12).

TREATMENT

Primary treatment includes removal of the patient from the environment and administration of high-concentration oxygen. Whenever possible, humidified oxygen should be used. If there are signs of airway compromise (stridor, hoarseness), early transport is important, since airway compromise can progress.

Chemical Burns

General Principles

Chemicals cause burns similar to thermal burns. The type and concentration of the product and the duration of exposure are the important variables in determining the severity. The key difference between chemical and thermal burns is that chemicals continue to burn until they are removed. Therefore, the cardinal principle to follow in managing chemical burns is to initiate immediate and thorough irrigation of the affected areas. Large amounts of water (gallons) should be used and irrigation should continue for 20 to 30 minutes. Splashes should be avoided, since they can contaminate unaffected areas as well as the rescuer. Garden hoses or showers are ideal for irrigation, since they provide a continuous stream that dilutes and washes away the caustic elements. The pressure from a hose should be adjusted to avoid high-pressure streams and resultant traumatic injury to injured tissues.

Acids and alkali (Fig. 11–13) are the most common chemicals that produce chemical burns. Alkalis tend to take longer to remove. In general, one should not use a neutralizing agent (such as a weak alkali) for an acid burn for two reasons. First, seeking out an appropriate neutralizing agent wastes time. It has been shown that there is a difference in severity with a delay of as little as 2 minutes. Patients should initiate removal on their own and not await the arrival of rescuers. Second, the chemical reaction resulting from use of a neutralizing agent may produce heat and add a thermal component to the injury.

DRIED CHEMICALS (LIME)

If powder or dried chemicals are involved, they should be brushed off, and contaminated clothing and shoes removed before irrigation. Dried chemicals may collect in pants cuffs and shoes. Lime is a good example of such a chemical. Lime or calcium oxide is converted

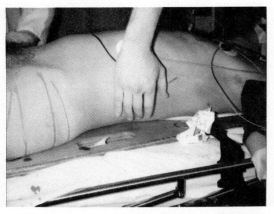

FIGURE 11–12. A patient with carbon monoxide poisoning causing poisoning of half the blood and resulting in cherry-red appearance to the skin. This patient, even though just resuscitated from cardiac arrest, has bright red appearance to the skin. This finding is attributed to the change in the hemoglobin color when it attaches to carbon monoxide. See the contrast of a normal hand against the skin. This cherry-red color is not always or even often seen in victims of carbon monoxide poisoning.

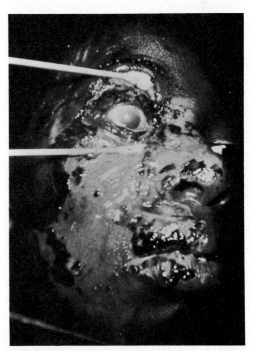

FIGURE 11–13. Alkali burn to the face. (From Zuidema GD, Rutherford RB, Ballinger WF: The Management of Trauma, 4th ed. Philadelphia, WB Saunders, 1985, p. 274.)

to a very caustic chemical, calcium hydroxide, with the addition of water. Large amounts of water, sufficient to provide a continuous and thorough irrigation, must be available, since small amounts can activate the chemical but not remove it.

SPECIAL CONSIDERATIONS

Although most chemicals encountered are handled with simple irrigation, there are certain substances that require special handling.

PHOSPHORUS. Yellow or white phosphorus is a chemical used in munitions and industries that make insecticides, poisons, and fertilizers. Phosphorus combusts spontaneously when exposed to air—therefore, affected parts should be kept submerged in water or covered with soaked dressings.

SODIUM AND POTASSIUM. Sodium and potassium metals also ignite spontaneously in air but also react with water to form more caustic products. Therefore, smoldering fragments of sodium or potassium that are imbedded in the skin should be extinguished with a fire extinguisher, smothered with sand, or covered with petroleum jelly.

HYDROFLUORIC ACID. Hydrofluoric acid is used in industry and is present in grout cleaners. It is caustic to the skin and also readily penetrates into the dermis, where it dissociates and continues to cause injury until it is deactivated. Water is used for irrigation, as with other acid burns. However, deactivation of the chemical that has penetrated the skin may require the application of dressings soaked in calcium chloride, calcium gluconate, or magnesium oxide paste. In the hospital calcium salts are at times injected into the skin to accomplish this purpose. Advanced EMT units carry calcium salt solutions.

PHENOLS. Phenols and related compounds such as cresol or creosol, which are used in industry and found in preservatives or disinfectants, can penetrate skin and be absorbed systemically. Since water may not penetrate skin damaged by phenols, the treatment of choice is a special solution of polyethylene glycol (PE) and methylated spirits in a 2:1 mixture. If this mixture or PE is available it should be applied prior to water irrigation. It is important to know that there are substances such as PE that facilitate removal of some caustic products such as phenol. They may be available at an industrial plant that commonly handles these toxic substances.

Usually water irrigation remains the treatment of choice and should be used immediately unless dealing with metallic sodium or potassium.

Once irrigation techniques are initiated, a call can be made to the regional poison center to elicit further instructions when appropriate. Caustic substances in the eye require continuous irrigation, with the eye held open by force if necessary for at least 20 minutes or until discontinued by hospital staff. The technique for eye irrigation has been covered in the section on eye injuries in Chapter 9.

Electrical Burns

Electricity is a fundamental entity of nature consisting of negative and positive forces. It is observable in the attractions and repulsions of bodies electrified by friction and in natural phenomena such as lightning or the aurora borealis.

In the United States, about 1,000 people die each year from electrical injuries. At high risk are workers involved in industrial accidents and children. Electrical accidents occur due to downed power lines, the malfunctioning of home appliances, children chewing through electrical lines, accidental contact with TV antennae by unskilled individuals, and contact with high-tension power lines (often by adolescent boys).

When electricity traverses the body, it is converted to heat that burns the tissues in its path. High-voltage arcs generate intense amounts of heat and can burn a person nearby. Death can result from the passage of current through vital organs, which causes respiratory or cardiac arrest.

The EMT must take due precautions to protect himself or herself and the victim from further injury. Knowing some basic properties of electricity may help guide you to take correct actions. Electricity is the movement of electrons from a point of higher concentration to a point of lower concentration. Electricity is often described in terms of three variables: amperage, voltage, and resistance. Amperage is the number or volume of electrons flowing. Voltage is the force with which movement occurs. Resistance is the degree of hindrance to electron flow. These three concepts are interrelated by the formula

$$A \text{ (amperage)} = V \text{ (voltage)}/R \text{ (resistance)}$$

Current can be direct or unidirectional in flow or it can alternate or switch the direction of electron flow at a given number of cycles per second. Flow from a battery is direct current, whereas household current is usually alternating current.

Generally, exposure to low voltage is less serious than to high voltage. However, fatalities have occurred with voltage as low as 45 to 60 cycles per second. Household current is capable of causing tetanic contraction of human muscle, preventing release of the electrified object by the victim. Amperage, which is not usually known, also does more damage as the milliamperes increase: from tingling, to tetanic contraction, to fatal organ damage. If current passes through the brain, it may cause respiratory arrest. If it passes through the heart, it may cause cardiac arrest.

Resistance is defined as a measure of the hindrance to electron flow through a given material. Materials vary tremendously in their resistance. For example, copper wires offer relatively low resistance and conduct electricity readily: they serve as good conductors. Rubber has a very high resistance to electrical flow: rubber serves as an insulator. Good conductors offer low resistance. Poor conductors offer high resistance. Lightning rods illustrate some of these properties, Lightning rods, made of metal, which is a good conductor, are used to direct electricity from the roof of a house along insulated wires to the ground. Since electricity seeks to flow along the path of least resistance from a higher to a lower potential, lightning rods prevent electricity from traveling through a highly resistant wooden roof, which would generate heat and fire. Instead the electricity is directed to the earth, which can absorb the current. In fact, *Webster's Dictionary* defines the term "ground" as a large conducting body, as the earth, used as a common return for an electrical circuit and an arbitrary zero of potential.

Cars are insulated from the ground by their rubber tires. Thus, a downed power line in contact with a car may leave the occupants unharmed as long as they avoid direct contact with the ground. However, if they step out of the car while holding onto the door, they will be part of the circuit consisting of the wire, the car, their bodies, and the ground, and they will suffer electrical injury.

When electrical current passes through the body as part of its circuit (usually to the ground), it follows an internal path of least resistance. Skin and bone offer high resistance to electrical current, muscle offers less, and the vessels and nerves offer the least resistance to electrical flow. Therefore, current passing from arm to arm tends to pass along the vessels and nerves in the arms and thorax. Even high current can enter and exit at relatively small surface areas and one cannot gauge the extent of internal injury from the external appearance.

Wet skin, offering less resistance, is more easily penetrated by electricity than dry skin. For example, even household current that penetrates wet skin can cause fatal ventricular fibrillation.

ELECTRICAL BURNS TO SKIN

Burns to the soft tissues, because of the heat generated from electric current, can extend from first-degree to fourth-degree burns. Third-degree and fourth-degree burns can vary from those that look gray-white to those that appear charred. Thermal burns can also be caused by the intense heat generated by electric arcs that are nearby but not in direct contact with the body. The longer the duration of contact, the greater the burn.

Remember that electrical burns tend to be more extensive than can be judged from their external marks.

TYPES OF ELECTRICAL BURNS

ARC BURNS. A high-voltage current traveling through the air can cause temperatures to reach 2,000 to 3,000°F, an intense heat (flash) that causes thermal injury. For example, clothing may ignite, adding to the burns.

SPECIFIC INJURIES. The most immediate life-threatening effects of electrical injuries are respiratory and cardiac arrest. Early resuscitation can salvage some victims. For example, respiratory arrest following a lightning injury can be prolonged, but victims who have received early respiratory support have recovered. Associated falls may cause fractures and other injuries.

ASSESSMENT AND TREATMENT

The first priority is to assess whether hazards continue to exist. Are there fallen wires? Any downed wire should be considered as charged until the appropriate authorities such as power company personnel confirm that the power is off. When encountering victims entrapped in a vehicle in contact with a downed wire, have them remain in the vehicle. Do not touch the vehicle yourself, since that will place you in a circuit from the vehicle to the ground. If there is a fire in the car, victims should jump out or throw small children to rescue personnel (making sure there is never a circuit from the car to the ground). After ensuring rescuer safety, perform the ABCs of life support with appropriate concern for the cervical spine if falls or violent contractions have occurred. Look closely for any fractures and splint appropriately. When assessing the skin, look for both entrance and exit wounds. Cover the wounds with sterile dressings and transport the patient to the hospital.

RADIATION INJURIES

Definitions

Due to the unique nature of radiation emergencies the following definitions are provided to guide you through this section. These and other terms are further clarified as the chapter progresses. Take a moment to become familiar with these important terms before reading further.

Radiation The process of emitting radiant energy (energy traveling as wave motions; specifically the energy of electromagnetic waves) in the form of waves or particles. The process by which energy is transmitted through space or matter not affected by it.

Ionizing radiation Any radiation that displaces electrons from atoms or molecules, thereby producing ions. Alterations in the molecules within cells can disrupt normal function.

Radioactive The ability of a substance to emit rays or particles from its nucleus.

Radioactivity The property possessed by some elements (such as uranium) of spontaneously emitting alpha and beta particles and gamma rays by the disintegration of the nuclei of its atoms.

Isotope One of two or more atoms with the same atomic number (the same chemical element) but with different atomic weights. (The nuclei of isotopes have the same number of protons but different numbers of neutrons.) Isotopes of an element have very nearly the same chemical properties but somewhat different physical properties. "Unstable" isotopes break down spontaneously to smaller atoms, and in the process they emit radioactive energy as particles of waves.

Irradiated Term used to describe a person or substance exposed to ionizing radiation. For example, someone who has been x-rayed is said to have been irradiated. These individuals represent no threat to others who come in contact with them.

Contamination Radioactive material is physically present on a person or object. Radiation can be spread to others.

Decontamination The process by which radioactive material is removed from a person or object.

Roentgen Special unit of exposure to radiation. Measured from the ionizing effect of radiation on air molecules within a chamber.

Rad Special unit of an absorbed dose of radiation. When ionizing radiation passes through matter, some of its energy is imparted to the matter. The amount absorbed per mass of material is called the absorbed dose.

Rem Special unit of dose equivalent. Equivalent to the absorbed dose in rads multiplied by the quality factor, the distribution factor, and other modifying factors.

Physical half-life The time required for a radioactive substance to lose 50% of its activity by decay.

Curie The special unit of activity (the number of nuclear transformations occurring in a given quantity of material per unit of time); 1 curie equals 3.7×10^{10} nuclear transformations per second.

Introduction

Radiation is a form of energy transmission, as in radiation from the sun. When we speak of radiation injuries, we are referring to the effects of ionizing radiation, or radiation with the potential to alter the function of the body's cells by altering or ionizing the molecules that make up the cell.

Ionizing radiation can cause instant biochemical changes in the cells. These biochemical alterations can affect immediate or future cell function. High doses of radiation sustained over a short time can lead to an *acute radiation syndrome* that can result in severe illness and death. Smaller doses may result in later genetic effects, an increased risk of cancer, and cataracts, or it may affect growth and development and life span.

Small amounts of radiation are not harmful. We all receive small doses of radiation each day from the sun, the earth, and other natural and manmade sources. Workers who are exposed to radioactive materials in the workplace may receive greater exposure. There are limits set on the amount of radiation to which they can safely be exposed.

Radiation cannot be perceived by our senses. We need special instruments to alert us to its presence. Workers who are exposed to radiation wear instruments to monitor the exposure encountered on the job.

Radiation injury calls to mind threats of nuclear war and disasters such as those that occurred at Chernobyl or Three Mile Island. Fortunately, radiation injuries are not part of everyday emergency care. Prior to Chernobyl, the Federal Emergency Management Agency (FEMA) noted that in 40 years, fewer than 1,000 persons in the world are known to have been involved in serious radiation accidents, with only about 450 receiving medically serious doses of radiation or contamination and with fewer than 21 resulting fatalities. According to FEMA, "rescuers, physicians and nurses who were monitored while providing emergency care and treatment to victims of radiation accidents in the past received radiation exposures less than or comparable to exposures received in medical diagnostic studies."

Most frequently, radiation accidents occur in the workplace, where expert help and advice are at hand to guide the actions of emergency personnel who must care for victims who may have combined radiation and traumatic injuries. Because of the special nature of radioactive materials, special precautions are taken and plans made in advance should an emergency occur. However, since radioactive wastes are transported along highways, an EMT might be called to the scene of a traffic accident that involves potential radiation injuries. In addition to knowing how to summon expert help and advice, EMTs should have an understanding of the basic principles regarding radiation hazards so they can initiate lifesaving interventions and emergency care while simultaneously taking precautions to prevent unnecessary radiation exposure to themselves, the public, and the accident victims.

Basic Biophysics

A simple understanding of radioactivity can be obtained by considering the atom. An atom is the smallest building block of an element. An atom consists of protons, neutrons, and electrons. Most atoms are stable, meaning the various components stay together in a given configuration with equal numbers of protons, neutrons, and electrons. However, some elements exist in more than one form, having in common the same number of protons but different numbers of neutrons. Therefore, they would have the same atomic number and similar chemical properties but different atomic weights and possibly different physical properties. The different forms of an element are called *isotopes*. Some isotopes are "unstable" in that they have a tendency to break down spontaneously to smaller atoms *while emitting energetic rays or particles* from the nucleus in the process. Such isotopes are called *radioactive* and the energy emitted is called *nuclear radiation*, since it emanates from the nucleus. When discussing radioactive material it is important to use terms that identify the particular isotope, such as U 238 or 238 Uranium.

Common units of measurement used to quantify the amount of radioactivity include the roentgen, rad, rem, and curie. Ionizing radiation can result in an electronically measurable charge in the air through which it passes. This charge is measured as a *Roentgen* (or R). *Rad* is a measurement of the amount of radiation absorbed by a material or the body. *Rem* is a unit equal to the absorbed dose in rads multiplied by modifying and quality factors, allowing for some comparison of the effects of different types of radiation. All these units are also expressed as the 1/1000 parts or milliroentgens (mR), millirad (mrad), and millirem (mrem)—1000 mrem = 1 rem. The unit of measurement used to express the radioactivity or nuclear transformations per second of a quantity of radioactive material is called the *curie*.

Types of Radiation

Classic types of radioactive emissions are alpha particles, beta particles, gamma rays, and neutrons. The first three are the most common, since neutron-type radiation injuries are found only in high-technology installations, such as nuclear reactors or linear accelerators (radiation generators or particle accelerators are also described as Van de Graaff, cyclotrons, synchrotrons, betatrons, or bevatrons; they accelerate the various charged particles that make up atoms to high energy levels). Again, it is important to remember when discussing radioactive material that there is a certain amount of natural radiation that we are exposed to every day from sources such as the atmosphere, earth, and foods. The average amount of annual exposure in the United States from these natural sources ranges from 100 to 400 mrem/year.

ALPHA RADIATION

An alpha particle is a positively charged particle consisting of two protons and two neurons (identical to a helium nucleus with a 2+ charge). It is the least penetrating form of radiation and travels only a few centimeters in the air. It can be stopped by a sheet of paper, clothing, and the epidermis of the skin. It is dangerous only if ingested, inhaled, or absorbed through broken skin. Within the body, alpha radiation can affect nearby tissues. Transuranic isotopes are the most common source of alpha particles involved in accidents.

BETA RADIATION

Beta particles are charged particles that have the mass of an electron. They have either a negative or a positive charge (called positrons). In air they can travel from less than 1 foot to several feet, depending on the energy. Beta particles travel somewhat deeper than alpha particles into the dermal layer of the skin, where they are stopped. They can cause burns similar to thermal burns if left in contact with the body for a length of time. They can be stopped by protective clothing. Like alpha particles, they usually are dangerous only if they cause internal contamination through ingestion, inhalation, or absorption through a break in the skin.

Because alpha and beta particles are matter, they can cling to the skin or clothing or contaminate a person. *Contamination* is a term defined as a radioactive substance dispersed in materials or places where it is undesirable. Like any other matter, these radioactive materials can be spread to other persons or things. Proper handling is required to contain the radioactive materials until they can be removed from places and people during *decontamination* procedures. In practice, measures used to handle victims contaminated by radiation accidents are similar to the precautions taken with victims of communicable diseases.

GAMMA RAYS

Gamma rays are high-energy electromagnetic radiation rays similar to x-rays but more energetic. They can penetrate the body and cause damage by ionizing molecules in their path. Biochemical transformation of ionized molecules is instantaneous and may lead to biologic effects manifesting at a later time. The gamma ray does not cause contamination of the victim and the victim is of no risk to others. The victim exposed to gamma rays is said to have been *irradiated*.

Gamma rays can travel long distances and penetrate most materials with ease. Dense materials such as lead are the best shielding against gamma rays.

NEUTRONS

Neutrons are uncharged particles found in the nucleus of an atom. Neutron emissions occur in nuclear reactors, along with other types of radioactivity. Neutrons are much more penetrating than alpha and beta particles and can cause considerable damage to underlying tissue. They can "activate" the body and materials in their path such as rings, belt buckles, coins, and tie pins. Because they are found only in special situations, they are mentioned here only for completeness. The remaining discussion focuses primarily on alpha, beta, and gamma radiation, which are more likely to be encountered.

CONTAMINATION VERSUS IRRADIATION

The EMT must make a clear conceptual distinction between the two main types of radiation injuries: contamination and irradiation. The former, *contamination*, is caused by radioactive *particles* that are physically present. The latter, *irradiation*, is caused by radioactive energy in wave or ray form and, similar to an x-ray, passes through but is not physically present on the body. *Thus, the contaminated victim can spread radioactive materials to others; the irradiated patient cannot.*

CONTAMINATION. Contamination may be external or internal. *External contamination* means that the presence of radioactive materials is limited to the skin and clothing. *Internal contamination* occurs when radioactive materials enter the body through ingestion, inhalation, or a break in the skin. Once within the body, radioactive materials can be *incorporated* as part of the body's structure. External contamination and internal contamination demand different responses. External contamination itself is rarely a medical emergency. The primary concern with the externally contaminated patient is proper handling to prevent unnecessary spread of radioactive materials to the patient, the rescuer, and others. The primary concern with internal contamination is prompt institution of appropriate medical measures to eliminate, dilute, bind up, or block the effects of the radioactive material before it becomes incorporated within the body.

As mentioned, alpha and beta particles *contaminate* the victim, behaving like any other matter. Fortunately, they are of limited danger when they remain external, on the skin, causing only external contamination. Although the beta particles may cause burns to the skin if

prolonged contact occurs, they usually do not constitute a severe threat to the victim or rescuer. The presence of external contamination should not interfere with the delivery of necessary emergency care to the acutely injured individual.

Radioactive particles are a hazard to the victim if they enter within the body, causing internal contamination. Internal contamination is a medical emergency, since the radioactive materials may be chemically incorporated within the body's molecules and organs, where they continue to give off radioactive emissions to nearby tissues until they are either eliminated from the body or completely decay. Internal contamination is no hazard to the rescuer who takes appropriate precautions such as use of a positive-pressure device rather than mouth-to-mouth ventilation.

IRRADIATION. Gamma rays, which irradiate a victim, are electromagnetic waves of energy and do not behave as particles. Hence, they pass through or penetrate the body but do not remain as radioactive materials either on or within it. The victim is said to have been *irradiated* and presents no more risk to another person than does the patient receiving radiation therapy for cancer. Any damage to the victim irradiated by gamma rays is a result of the biochemical transformations resulting from ionization of molecules during their penetration. *Risks to the rescuer exist if and when the source of gamma rays continues to emit radioactivity in the area surrounding victims, but never from the victims themselves (unless the source of the gamma ray is inside or on the victim).*

TYPES OF PATIENTS

It should be clear that irradiation and contamination are two different results of radiation injury. Since they can exist in combination, there are potentially four distinct types of injuries that you might encounter after responding to the site of a possible radiation injury. These are:

Irradiated with no contamination
External contamination
Internal contamination via inhalation, ingestion, or a break in the skin
Simple trauma

A patient may have a combination of any of the above conditions.

Patients with Radiation Injuries

IRRADIATED PATIENTS

The irradiated patient is one who has been exposed to gamma rays or x-rays. Like the patient who has received x-rays, he is no threat to others and is not radioactive. Thus, a radiation detection instrument does not detect radioactivity from a patient who has been irradiated.

Irradiation injuries result from overexposure of industrial workers to unshielded radioactive sources, such as occurs in industries that use sealed radioisotope sources for radiography or sterilization, or from injuries sustained at weapons research or reprocessing facilities.

EXTERNAL CONTAMINATION

The patient with external contamination has radioactive dust particles or solid, liquid, or gas materials on the skin or clothing. The material may emit alpha, beta, or gamma radiation.

External contamination can occur during laboratory and maintenance work in hospitals, universities, and many industries. Major accidents such as explosions, fires, apparatus breakage, or container ruptures might cause serious contamination problems. Transportation accidents involving trucks carrying nuclear products are another potential contamination hazard.

INTERNAL CONTAMINATION

As noted earlier, there are three main ways for internal contamination with radioactive materials to occur: by inhalation, ingestion, or absorption through the skin or wound. The radioactive materials continue to emit alpha, beta, or gamma rays (depending on the material) until they are either eliminated from the body or decay completely and cease emitting radiation. Certain types of radioactive materials may be incorporated within a specific organ. For example, radioactive iodine may be concentrated in the thyroid gland. To minimize or prevent incorporation, internal contamination must be treated as soon as possible. Treatment is dictated by the properties of the isotope(s) and the route of contamination.

INHALATION. Inhalation of radioactive dust, gaseous substances, or particles following fires or explosions can result in internal contamination through the respiratory tract. In situations where possible inhalation of radioactive materials is suspected, a common procedure is to obtain nasal swabs of accessible areas in each nasal passage for later identification of the presence and type of radioactive materials. This may be done by personnel at the site of the accident and is usually recommended before decontamination efforts commence. Moistened cotton-tipped applicators are used to swab each nostril and then placed in a sealed container for later laboratory analysis and labeled with the patient's name, the time, and the date.

INGESTION. Ingestion of radioactive materials can be caused by ingestion of accidentally contaminated foods or liquids, accidental touching of the lips with contaminated hands, or other accidental or suicidal ingestions of isotopes. Ingestion can also occur as the body clears inhaled radioactive materials and they pass through the pharynx. Internal contamination following inhalation or ingestion rarely constitutes a significant threat to the rescuer. Vomitus should be treated as external contamination.

There should be no smoking, eating, or drinking in a contaminated area.

ABSORPTION. Radioactive materials can enter the body through an open wound or burn and be absorbed. Likewise, during an explosion, solid particles or fragments may be imbedded in the skin. Some isotopes such as radioactive hydrogen (tritium) and radioactive iodine may pass through intact skin. It is important to ascertain the properties of the contaminant as soon as possible to be able to address special hazards dictated by the nature of the chemical properties of the isotope, i.e., corrosive, toxic, soluble, etc.

MEASURING INSTRUMENTS

Because we cannot see radioactivity, we need to measure it with instruments. There are two basic types of instruments that are required. One, the *dosimeter*, measures the total or accumulated dose of radiation absorbed at the site of measurement and is used as a personnel monitoring device. The other, the *survey instrument*, measures the amount of radiation exposure per minute at the site of measurement.

DOSIMETERS OR PERSONNEL MONITORING DEVICES. Dosimeters are radiation-measuring instruments used to monitor the total accumulation of radiation. Dosimeters are worn by individuals who work with radioactive particles or by rescue personnel. It is assumed that if the dosimeter is worn on the torso, the amount of radiation measured is similar to the total whole body radiation. The unit of measurement is called a Roentgen (R) or milliroentgen (mR) (1/1000 of a Roentgen).

Basic types of dosimeters include *film badges* or photographic film; thermoluminescent devices (TLD); and *pocket dosimeters*, which are pocket ionization devices worn like a pocket pencil. A permanent record can be obtained from film badges and TLDs, which document total exposure to beta and gamma radiation (and some can measure neutron capability). The pocket dosimeter, worn like a pocket pen, has a scale that can be read at the site to monitor total exposure at different times. Rescuers may use pocket dosimeters to ascertain whether it is safe for them to remain in the area of exposure after consultation with the radiation safety officer. Pocket dosimeters should be charged or zeroed prior to use to eliminate the need to subtract the recorded accumulated background radiation from environmental sources (Fig. 11–14*A*).

SURVEY INSTRUMENTS. Survey instruments measure the *rate of exposure* and calculate it in terms of Roentgens per hour or milliroentgens per hour. The Geiger-Müller counter is an example of a survey instrument. As nuclear radiation penetrates the enclosed chamber of a survey meter, electrically charged (ionized) particles are produced. As these particles are collected, they produce a small electrical current that is amplified and measured. The size of the current is related to the rate at which the ionized particles are produced in the chamber, and thus to the radiation exposure rate. Hence, the meter can be calibrated in Roentgens per hour (R/hr) or milliroentgens per hour (mR/hr). All civil defense survey meters are designed to measure gamma radiation, and some are able to detect the presence of beta radiation. Special instruments for alpha radiation detection are also available.

The usefulness of survey instruments is great. First, EMTs can determine whether there is still a significant risk of irradiation at an exposure site. Second, they can predict their exposure dose over time should they enter the area. They can use this information to make risk calculations prior to entering an area and make the necessary plans to reduce individual exposure. Third, the survey instrument is used to determine if a victim or rescuer has been contaminated and can be used to monitor the decontamination process (Fig. 11–14*B* and *C*).

USE OF INSTRUMENTS AT THE ACCIDENT SCENE

Both dosimeters and survey instruments have a role at the site of a radiation accident. The use of survey instruments is necessary to determine if victims are contaminated and if there are still significant exposure hazards in the area. Dosimeters, or personnel monitoring devices, are worn by EMTs and other medical and rescue personnel for their own safety.

Both types of instruments should be available in all places that work with radioactive materials and in hospitals. They should be brought by specially trained personnel to the scene of transportation accidents involving radioactive material, as part of the community response plan to nuclear accidents. Plants and laboratories working with radioactive materials are required to have an emergency plan that provides for experts and equipment to handle radiation accidents to be available.

Radiation safety officers, or radiologic monitors, should have the necessary expertise to use and interpret the results of survey and personnel monitoring devices and

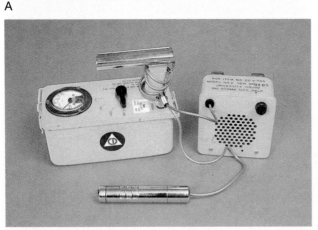

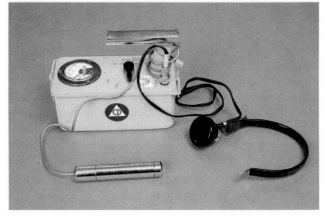

A

B

C

FIGURE 11–14. (*A*) Dosimeter with charging unit. Survey meter with (*B*) headset and (*C*) speaker.

to direct initial safety, rescue, and containment efforts. They are necessary to guide the decontamination process. EMTs should follow the advice of the radiation safety officers whenever they are available.

ACUTE RADIATION SYNDROME—FACTORS AFFECTING SEVERITY OF EXPOSURE

The severity of a radiation exposure is affected by the strength of the radioactive source, the type of radiation, the duration of exposure, the area of the body exposed, the distance from the radioactive source, the amount of shielding between the source and the victim, and the age and condition of the patient.

ACUTE RADIATION SYNDROME. When high doses of radiation are absorbed over a short period of time, e.g., minutes to hours, signs and symptoms known as "acute radiation syndrome" may be encountered. This syndrome results from damage to the bone marrow, gastrointestinal tract, central nervous system, and cardiovascular system as the dosage increases. For example, at an exposure of 50 rem, patients may have no visible effects, but a small percentage of persons who have been exposed may show a depression of white blood cells and platelets on blood testing. Physical signs and symptoms may first appear at a dose of 100 rem, with nausea and vomiting occurring in a small percentage of exposed persons. At 200 rem most patients show signs of nausea and vomiting, with more profound depression of the bone marrow. At 400 rem about 50% of the exposed individuals die within weeks. An exposure of 600 rem can result in a near 100% death rate if there is no medical intervention.

At doses of 1000 rem, gastrointestinal complications begin to appear as nausea, vomiting, and diarrhea of immediate onset. At doses of 3000 rem there are additional irreversible cardiovascular effects, resulting in irreversible hypotension and a central nervous system syndrome with rapid onset of drowsiness, uncoordination, and convulsions.

Genetic effects may occur at smaller doses. A 5- to 25-rem exposure is the minimal dose detectable by chromosome analysis. The sperm count is reduced in males at doses of 25 rad. Procreation should be avoided for a period of time following exposure. Pregnant women and women who may be pregnant should avoid any exposure to the site of a radiation accident.

Known long-term effects from radiation include cataracts, cancer, alterations in growth and development if the exposure occurs during fetal development, and possibly a shortened life span.

For comparison, note that exposure to natural radioactive sources results in an average of 125 mrem per year. Doses from x-rays vary with the examination, from 66 mrem from a chest x-ray to 10,000 mrem from a lumbar spine examination (four views).

The stronger the radioactive source, the greater is the dose received over a given unit of time for a patient at a fixed distance from the exposure.

TYPES OF RADIATION

As noted previously, gamma radiation and neutrons are the most penetrating forms of radiation. Like x-rays, they pass through all body tissues. Alpha and beta particles do not penetrate through intact skin, and damage is limited with careful decontamination.

Internal contamination with alpha and beta particles requires early medical attention to consider the use of agents to hasten the elimination of the isotope and to block toxic effects on the organs.

DURATION OF EXPOSURE

The duration of exposure is important. Rescuers can gauge the amount of time they have to enter an exposure area if they have knowledge of the exposure rate. For example, if the exposure rate is 100 R/hr, 15 minutes in the area may result in absorption of 25 R. Rescue workers can reduce individual exposure by sharing the time spent in the danger zone. The shorter the time spent in a radiation field, the less radiation the body absorbs.

AREA OF THE BODY EXPOSED

Penetrating radiation affects the cells through which it passes. Limitation of the exposure to an extremity, for example, may limit damage to this area and not result in the radiation syndrome.

Different parts of the body can tolerate different amounts of radiation. The maximal permissible occupational standards for the hands are several times the allowable limit for the gonads or the whole body. The shielding of parts of the body during medical or dental x-rays is an example of limiting body exposure.

DISTANCE FROM THE SOURCE

The greater the distance from the source of radiation, the less the radiation dose that is absorbed. If the source of radiation emanates from a single point, radioactivity falls inversely with the square of the distance. Thus, if one doubles the distance away from the source, the intensity falls off by a factor of four. If radiation sources are scattered, however, this inverse square rule does not apply. However, one always decreases radiation exposure significantly by increasing the distance from the material.

SHIELDING

EMTs may shield themselves from the source of exposure by use of lead aprons or other dense materials (such as keeping a vehicle between themselves and the source). At times, it may be more practical to shield the source itself. Protective clothing should be utilized to minimize exposure.

EMERGENCY CARE FOR RADIATION INJURIES

EMTs should know the scope of care expected of them in their area so that they can be adequately prepared. In most events, EMTs would be called if there was need for emergency medical attention for victims at a radiation accident site. Preplanning for radiation accidents is done by industries that use radioactive materials, all hospitals accredited by the Joint Commission on Accreditation of Health Care Organizations, and responsible government agencies. These plans include the establishment of responsibility for radiologic monitoring and decontamination, as well as transportation of uninjured victims. If EMTs are expected to participate in monitoring or rescue efforts, they should receive appropriate specialized training in each aspect of their expected performance, such as use of survey instruments, use of protective clothing, and familiarity with decontamination processes following local protocols.

Protection and Containment

When responding to the victims of radiation accidents, rescue and medical personnel also must think of preventing undue exposure to themselves and the public. Rescuers should not become victims themselves.

Early identification of the source and its activity helps guide subsequent actions. A safety zone should be established to prevent the public from entering a dangerous area. Both local and regional experts who are identified in the regional radiation emergency plan should be notified as early as possible to mobilize the needed expertise and resources to guide rescue and decontamination efforts. Protective gear should be utilized and radiation protection principles must be followed to limit radiation exposure as much as possible.

Identification of Source

The first question to ask when responding to the scene of a radiation accident is whether risks of irradiation or contamination are present. If there is a radiation safety officer present at an accident in the workplace, then invaluable advice is available.

Obtain information about the specific type of isotope(s) involved. This may be obtained from onsite personnel, labels on container vehicles (Fig. 11–15), or shipping papers. The Department of Transportation (DOT) guidebook gives a sample of the type of placard displayed on radioactive materials (Fig. 11–16). Materials shipped by interstate commerce display this placard and include information about the maximum external radiation at the surface and at 3 feet (Table 11–6).

Identifying information can also be gathered from contaminated patients. A patient who is suspected to have inhaled contaminants should have a sample taken from each nostril with a nasal swab before being decontaminated. The moistened swab should be gently rubbed against the nares, placed in a container, and sealed for later analysis. Body wastes of patients who may be contaminated can be saved for later analysis and monitoring. Do not forget to consider other characteristics of the contaminant once it is identified. It may have corrosive, soluble, or insoluble chemical properties that call for special handling.

Notification

Know the state or local agency responsible for responding to radiation accidents and make sure it is notified. Expert help is also available from the United States Department of Energy Regional Coordinating Office for Radiological Assistance. Another source is the Radiation Emergency Assistance Center/Training Site (REAC/TS), which provides a 24-hour consultation ser-

Text continued on page 520

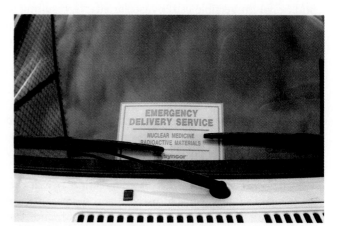

FIGURE 11–15. Medical agents containing radiation (usually low level) may be delivered by automobile with signs such as these displayed here.

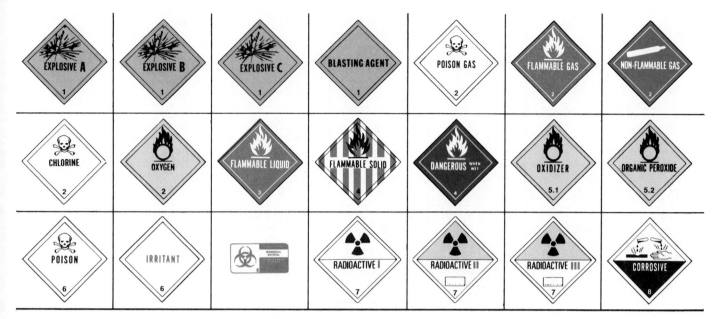

General Guidelines on Use of Labels
(CFR, Title 49, Transportation, Parts 100-177)

- Labels illustrated above are normally for *domestic shipments*. However, some air carriers *may* require the use of International Civil Aviation Organization (ICAO) labels.

- Domestic Warning Labels *may* display UN Class Number, Division Number (and Compatibility Group for Explosives only) [Sec. 172.407(g)].

- Any person who offers a hazardous material for transportation MUST label the package, if required [Sec. 172.400(a)].

- The Hazardous Materials Tables, Sec. 172.101 and 172.102, identify the proper label(s) for the hazardous materials listed.

- Label(s), when required, must be printed on or affixed to the surface of the package near the proper shipping name [Sec. 172.406(a)].

- When two or more different labels are required, display them next to each other [Sec. 172.406(c)].

- Labels may be affixed to packages (even when not required by regulations) provided each label represents a hazard of the material in the package [Sec. 172.401].

Check the Appropriate Regulations
Domestic or International Shipment

Additional Markings and Labels

HANDLING LABELS

Cargo Aircraft Only
172.402(b)

Bung Label
172.402(e)

ORM-E
172.316

INNER PACKAGES COMPLY WITH PRESCRIBED SPECIFICATIONS
173.25(a)(4)

172.312(a)(c)

Package Orientation Markings

Fumigation
173.9

EMPTY

173.427

Here are a few additional markings and labels pertaining to the transport of hazardous materials. The section number shown with each item refers to the appropriate section in the HMR. The Hazardous Materials Tables, Section 172.101 and 172.102, identify the proper shipping name, hazard class, identification number, required label(s) and packaging sections.

Poisonous Materials

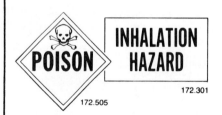

172.505

172.301

Materials which meet the inhalation toxicity criteria specified in Section 173.3a(b)(2), have additional "communication standards" prescribed by the HMR. First, the words "Poison-Inhalation Hazard" must be entered on the shipping paper, as required by Section 172.203(k)(4), for any primary capacity units with a capacity greater than one liter. Second, packages of 110 gallons or less capacity must be marked "Inhalation Hazard" in accordance with Section 172.301(a). Lastly, transport vehicles, freight containers and portable tanks subject to the shipping paper requirements contained in Section 172.203(k)(4) must be placarded with POISON placards in addition to the placards required by Section 172.504. For additional information and exceptions to these communication requirements, see the referenced sections in the HMR.

FIGURE 11–16. (*A*) Hazardous materials warning labels. *Illustration continued on following page*

DOMESTIC PLACARDING

Illustration numbers in each square refer to Tables 1 and 2 below.

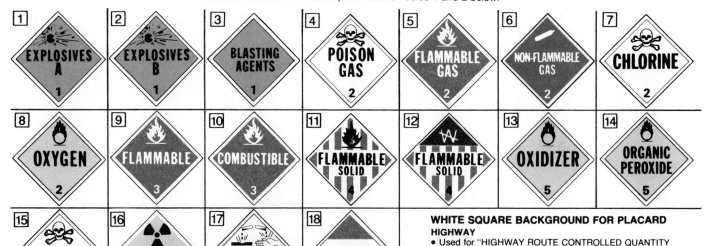

WHITE SQUARE BACKGROUND FOR PLACARD
HIGHWAY
• Used for "HIGHWAY ROUTE CONTROLLED QUANTITY OF RADIOACTIVE MATERIALS." (Sec. 172.507)
RAIL
• Used for RAIL SHIPMENTS "EXPLOSIVE A," "POISON GAS" and "POISON GAS RESIDUE" placards. (Sec. 172.510(a))

Guidelines

(CFR, Title 49, Transportation, Parts 100-177)

• Placard any transport vehicle, freight container, or rail car containing any quantity of material listed in Table 1.
• Materials which are shipped in portable tanks, cargo tanks, or tank cars must be placarded when they contain any quantity of Table 1 and/or Table 2 material.
• Motor vehicles or freight containers containing packages which are subject to the "Poison-Inhalation Hazard" shipping paper description of Section 172.203(k)(4), must be placarded POISON in addition to the placards required by Section 172.504 (see Section 172.505).
• When the gross weight of all hazardous material covered in TABLE 2 is less than 1000 pounds, no placard is required on a transport vehicle or freight container.
• Placard freight containers 640 cubic feet or more containing any quantity of hazardous material classes listed in TABLES 1 and/or 2 when offered for transportation by air or water (see Section 172.512(a)). Under 640 cubic feet see Section 172.512(b).

TABLE 1

Hazard Classes	No.
Class A explosives	1
Class B explosives	2
Poison A	4
Flammable solid (DANGEROUS WHEN WET label only)	12
Radioactive material (YELLOW III label)	16
Radioactive material:	
Uranium hexafluoride fissile (Containing more than 1.0% U^{235})	16 & 17
Uranium hexafluoride, low-specific activity (Containing 1.0% or less U^{235})	16 & 17

Note: For details on the use of Tables 1 and 2, see Sec. 172.504 (see footnotes at bottom of tables.)

TABLE 2

Hazard Classes	No.
Class C explosives	18
Blasting agent	3
Nonflammable gas	6
Nonflammable gas (Chlorine)	7
Nonflammable gas (Fluorine)	15
Nonflammable gas (Oxygen, cryogenic liquid)	8
Flammable gas	5
Combustible liquid	10
Flammable liquid	9
Flammable solid	11
Oxidizer	13
Organic peroxide	14
Poison B	15
Corrosive material	17
Irritating material	18

UN or NA Identification Numbers

MUST BE DISPLAYED ON TANK CARS, CARGO TANKS, PORTABLE TANKS AND BULK PACKAGINGS

PLACARDS OR ORANGE PANELS

1090 and

Appropriate Placard must be used.

• When hazardous materials are transported in Tank Cars (Section 172.330), Cargo Tanks (Section 172.328), Portable Tanks (Section 172.326) or Bulk Packagings (Section 172.331), UN or NA numbers must be displayed on placards, orange panels or, when authorized, plain white square-on-point configuration.
• UN (United Nations) or NA (North American) numbers are found in the Hazardous Materials Tables, Sections 172.101 and 172.102.
• Identification numbers may not be displayed on "POISON GAS," "RADIOACTIVE," or "EXPLOSIVE A," "EXPLOSIVE B," "BLASTING AGENTS," or "DANGEROUS" placards. (See Section 172.334.)
• In lieu of the orange panel, identification numbers may be placed on plain white square-on-point configuration when there is no placard specified for the hazard class (e.g., ORM-A, B, C, D, or E) or where the identification number may not be displayed on the placard. See Section 172.336(b) for additional provisions and specifications.
• When the identification number is displayed on a placard the UN hazard class number must be displayed in the lower corner of each placard (see Section 172.332 (c)(3)).
• Specifications of size and color of the Orange Panel can be found in Section 172.332(b).
• NA numbers are used only in the USA and Canada.

Additional Placarding Guidelines

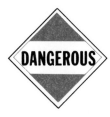

A transport vehicle or freight container containing two or more classes of material requiring different placards specified in Table 2 may be placarded DANGEROUS in place of the separate placards specified for each of those classes of material specified in Table 2. However, when 5000 pounds or more of one class of material is loaded therein at one loading facility, the placard specified for that class must be applied. This exception, provided in Section 172.504(b), does not apply to portable tanks, tank cars, or cargo tanks.

CAUTION: Check each shipment for compliance with the appropriate hazardous materials regulations — Proper Classification, Packaging, Marking, Labeling, Placarding, Documentation — prior to offering for shipment.

FIGURE 11–16 *Continued* (B) *Hazardous materials warning placards. Illustration continued on opposite page*

The shipment of hazardous materials internationally is governed by one or more regulatory bodies with regulations that may be similar to domestic regulations or radically different. Canada, for example, has adopted wordless placards and labels because their country is bilingual. Canada also requires cargo and rail tanks to use retro-reflective placarding. However, Canada and the United States have reciprocity regarding the use of wordless and worded placards and labels.

Several international organizations govern the transportation of hazardous materials according to the mode of transportation. If a shipment is going by water, the International Maritime Organization (IMO) has authority. The International Civil Aviation Organization (ICAO) is concerned about the safe shipment of dangerous goods

(*i.e.,* hazardous materials) by air. Transport Canada (TC) is the Canadian counterpart to the U.S. Department of Transportation (DOT).

The United Nations publishes "Recommendations for the Transport of Dangerous Goods," a publication that is used by many nations of the world when promulgating regulations. Since the safe transport of hazardous materials is of concern to people everywhere, the work done by the United Nations is of critical importance world-wide. Labels and placards used in the Canadian, IMO, and ICAO regulations are generally based on the U.N. Recomendations, although Canada has some labels and placard designs that vary from the U.N. White borders are optional on International Placards.

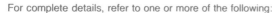

Flammable Solid — **Oxidizer** — **Non-flammable Gas**

Spontaneously Combustible — **Keep Away From Food** — **Corrosive Gas**

Flammable Gas — **Flammable Liquid** — **Dangerous When Wet**

Poison — **Miscellaneous Dangerous Substances** — **Infectious Substance**

Examples of Wordless Placards and Labels

Pictured here are typical wordless placards and labels required for use in Canada and many other countries around the world.

Examples of International and Canadian Placards and Labels

Spontaneously Combustible and Keep Away From Food placards and labels are used internationally and in Canada. The Corrosive Gas placard and label are used exclusively in Canada. Most placards and labels used internationally are similar (color and symbols) to those required by DOT regulations.

UN Class Numbers

Class 1: Explosives
Class 2: Gases (compressed, liquified or dissolved under pressure
Class 3: Flammable liquids
Class 4: Flammable solids or substances
Class 5: Oxidizing substances. Division 5.1, Oxidizing substances or agents. Division 5.2, Organic peroxides.
Class 6: Poisonous and infectious substances
Class 7: Radioactive substances
Class 8: Corrosives
Class 9: Misc. dangerous substances

Examples of Explosive Labels

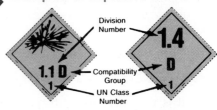

The Numerical Designation represents the Class or Division. Alphabetical Designation represents the Compatibility Group (for Explosives only). Division Numbers and Compatibility Group combinations can result in over 30 different "Explosives" labels (see IMDG Code/ICAO).

For complete details, refer to one or more of the following:
- Code of Federal Regulations, Title 49, Transportation. Parts 100-199. [All modes]
- International Civil Aviation Organization (ICAO) Technical Instructions for the Safe Transport of Dangerous Goods by Air [Air]
- International Maritime Organization (IMO) Dangerous Goods Code [Water]
- "Transportation of Dangerous Goods Regulations" of Transport Canada. [All Modes]

U.S. Department of Transportation
Research and Special Programs Administration
Copies of this Chart can be obtained by writing OHMT/DHM-51, Washington, D.C. 20590.

FIGURE 11-16 *Continued* (*C*) Examples of Canadian and international placards and labels. (US Department of Transportation, Research and Special Programs Administration, 1988.)

TABLE 11–6. Radiation Dose and Risks to Rescuer

Label	Dose Rate At Surface (mrem/hr)	Dose Rate At 3 feet (mrem/hr)
Radioactive White I	<0.5	—
Radioactive Yellow II	0.5–50	<1
Radioactive Yellow III	50–200	1–10

Adapted from Richter LL, Berk HW, Teates CD, et al: A systems approach to the management of radiation accidents. Ann Emerg Med 9:303–309, 1980.

vice to any person requesting advice on handling radiation accidents. REAC/TS can be contacted by

1. Calling (615) 576-3131 Monday through Friday (8:00 AM to 4:30 PM)
2. Calling (615) 481-1000 beeper 241, a 24-hour telephone service at Oak Ridge Hospital
3. Writing REAC/TS, Box 117, Oak Ridge, Tennessee 37830
4. Or one can call Chemtrex, (800) 424-9300, another source of information

If victims require hospital treatment, the hospital should be contacted as early as possible to prepare the necessary equipment and personnel for handling radioactive patients. Tell the hospital (1) a radiation accident has occurred, (2) the number of victims who are contaminated and not contaminated and the extent of the injuries, (3) the type of isotope(s), if known, or other identifying information, and (4) the latest updated information.

Protection Principles

It is your duty to try to prevent unnecessary radiation exposure of the public, rescuers, other medical personnel, and victims. This is done by following basic radiation protection principles, creating a safety zone, and using protective gear.

The basic principles used to minimize exposure to radiation include limiting the exposure to the smallest portion of the body possible and considering time, distance, and shielding.

- *Limit exposure to the smallest portion of the body possible*—Avoid touching radioactive materials directly. Use tongs or instruments instead.
- *Limit the time of exposure*—Minimizing time in the exposure zone should be accomplished by use of an efficient work plan. If exposure levels are high, the patient should be removed as quickly as possible to a safe area. As in the case of fires or poisonous

gases, removal of the patient to a safe environment takes priority over splinting and other aspects of emergency care. If extrication and removal are complicated, rescuers should consider sharing exposure time, which will reduce individual exposure.

- *Maintain the greatest possible distance from the source*—Small changes in distance can greatly reduce exposure.
- *Suitable shielding*—To protect against gamma rays, lead shielding is required. The source itself may be shielded to prevent exposure. Other methods used to place shields between the source and the victim include positioning a vehicle between them and using concrete walls or mounds of earth as shields.

Exposure Limits in Lifesaving Situations

If there is knowledge of the radiation levels, then rescuers are advised to consider the following advice from the National Council on Radiation Protection and Measurements (NCRP).

PLANNED OCCUPATIONAL EXPOSURES UNDER EMERGENCY CONDITIONS*

It is compatible with the risk concept to accept exposures leading to doses considerably in excess of those appropriate for lifetime use when recovery from an accident or major operational difficulty is necessary. Saving of life, measures to circumvent substantial exposures to population groups, or even preservation of valuable installations may all be sufficient cause for accepting above normal exposures. Dose limits cannot be specified. They should be commensurate with the significance of the objective and held to the lowest practicable level that the emergency permits. The following is offered as general guidance.

Lifesaving Action
This applies to search for and removal of injured persons or entry to prevent conditions that would probably injure numbers of people.

- Rescue personnel should be volunteers or professional rescue personnel (e.g., firemen who "volunteer" by choice of employment).
- Rescue personnel should be broadly familiar with the consequences of exposure.
- Women capable of reproduction should not take part in these actions.
- Other things being equal, volunteers above the age of 45 should be selected.
- Planned dose to the whole body should not exceed 100 rem.

---

* From NCRP Report no. 39, 1971, pp. 99–100.

- Hands and forearms may receive additional dose of up to 200 rem (i.e., a total of 300 rem).
- Internal exposure should be minimized by the use of the best available respiratory protection, and contamination should be controlled by the use of available protective clothing.
- Normally, exposure under these conditions shall be limited to once in a lifetime.
- Persons receiving exposures as indicated above should avoid procreation for a period of up to a few months.

Actions in Less Urgent Emergencies

This applies under less stressful circumstances where it is still desirable to enter a hazardous area to protect facilities, eliminate further escape of effluents, or control fires.

- Persons performing the planned actions should be volunteers broadly familiar with exposure consequences.
- Women capable of reproduction shall not take part.
- Planned whole body dose shall not exceed 25 rem.
- Planned dose of hands and forearms shall not exceed 100 rem (including the whole body component).
- Internal exposure shall be minimized by respiratory protection, and contamination controlled by the use of protective clothing.
- Normally, if the retrospective dose from these actions is a substantial fraction of the prospective limits, the actions should be limited to once in a lifetime.*

SAFETY ZONE

A safety zone should be maintained to prevent unnecessary exposure to responding rescuers and the public at large. Guide 63 from the DOT 1984 Emergency Response Guidebook advises that for certain radioactive materials, onlookers should be kept at least 150 feet upwind, that the hazardous area should be isolated, and that unauthorized personnel should be denied entry.

USE OF PROTECTIVE GEAR

To provide the greatest safety to the rescuers, protective clothing, including, at a minimum, gloves, masks, and surgical gowns, should be used. Shoe covers should also be used. If they are not readily available, paper bags can be secured over the shoes with tape; this offers protection if the area is not wet.

Following standard protocols, a film badge with the name of the rescuer should be attached to his or her street clothes. Large size surgical trousers and pullover shirts should be available to fit easily over street clothes. If available, waterproof shoe covers should be attached to the cuffs of the protective trousers with tape. A surgical gown is put on with a pair of surgical gloves, which can

be taped to the sleeves. A surgical hood and mask offer protection to the face and head. A second pair of surgical gloves can be put on, which will allow the top pair to be removed should they become contaminated. Finally, a second dosimeter should be attached to the neck of the gown so that it can be easily read, but be careful not to place it in an area where it can be easily contaminated.

Assessment

The first priority, as always, is the provision of life-saving emergency care. When exposure is continuing at life-threatening levels, rapid removal from the danger zone takes highest priority. After removal, the ABCs of life support should commence. The rescuer must determine the relative safety of entering the exposure area based on the recommendations of the NCRP, listed under Planned Occupational Exposures Under Emergency Conditions, above.

If contamination is the main hazard to the EMT, lifesaving care should be given to the victim after donning surgical gloves, gown, and mask. Avoid internal contamination from mouth-to-mouth ventilation by use of other appropriate positive-pressure ventilation devices. Removing the victim's clothing generally removes 80 to 90% of the contamination. Seal it in a plastic bag, label it, and leave it in the contaminated zone for later retrieval and disposition.

Rarely is the contaminated victim a threat to the rescuers. Precautions taken during the handling of contaminated victims are aimed at preventing the spread of radioactive materials and preventing or minimizing internal contamination. The patient should be removed to a safe zone, free from threats of irradiation, where the presence and extent of contamination can be determined if a radiologic monitor is available.

If the patient is contaminated, areas around wounds should be assessed and cleaned to prevent internal absorption. In addition, the nares should be assayed with a cotton swab, since it will be harder to detect if there was an inhalation hazard once decontamination efforts begin.

If there is a possibility of internal contamination, the time that will elapse before appropriate medications are given to limit or minimize absorption and incorporation becomes an important factor and the patient should be treated as a medical emergency.

Usually, acute symptoms that occur immediately after the accident are not due to irradiation, unless extremely high (lethal) doses have been absorbed. Therefore, it is important to look for another cause so as not to overlook an additional medical emergency (see Protocol: Approach to Patient Exposed to a Radiation Accident).

* From NCRP Report no. 39, 1971, pp. 99–100.

✠ P R O T O C O L ✠

APPROACH TO A PATIENT EXPOSED TO A RADIATION ACCIDENT

A. *Special Assessment Considerations*

The following guidelines should be followed when treating a patient exposed to a radiation accident:

1. ALWAYS DO A 10-SECOND SCENE SURVEY!

2. Protect yourself from the dangers of exposure.

3. Alert the dispatcher to notify the police, fire department, EMS HAZMAT Response team, EPA, and Department of Environmental Protection (DEP).

4. Before care can be administered, the patient must be decontaminated by a HAZMAT team.

5. Have the patient remove all jewelery, clothing, and shoes.

6. Administer appropriate patient care.

7. Before transporting the patient, cover the ambulance stretcher mattress with a blanket.

8. Wrap the patient in the blanket and fashion a head covering from a sheet.

9. Only the patient's face should show when ready to transport.

10. Make the necessary notification to the hospital that the patient is being transported prior to the arrival of the patient.

B. *Treatment*

After the patient has been decontaminated refer to the appropriate basic life support protocol for the treatment of each patient.

ALL PATIENTS ARE TO BE TREATED SYMPTOMATICALLY AND TRANSPORTED IN THE USUAL MANNER!

From Manual for Emergency Medical Technicians. Emergency Medical Services Program. Albany, New York State Department of Health, 1990.

ASSAYING FOR CONTAMINATION

EXTERNAL. The radiologic monitor assays, or tests, for beta and gamma emitters over the entire body with a Geiger-Müller survey meter. You should record the results, along with the areas of distribution on a body diagram as you would for a burn victim (see Fig. 11–10). Determine if wounds are contaminated by taking a survey directly over each wound or from samples of wound secretions. Wipes from the wounds may be saved as samples for later assay and identification.

INTERNAL. All nasal swabs and samples from wounds should be saved in separate, tightly lidded and labeled containers. In addition, it is appropriate to collect and label all urine, vomitus, and feces for later analysis to determine the extent of internal contamination and monitor the effectiveness of the decontamination effort.

Depending on the local protocol and the location, decontamination may be done entirely at the scene or take second priority after care for life-threatening injuries and be done at the hospital. The EMT's main role is always to provide emergency medical care. The extent of the EMT's duties regarding assaying and decontamination varies with local protocol and the location of the accident. Regardless, the EMT is expected to function within the general guidelines common to all radiation accidents.

Treatment

The main priority is the treatment of the medical emergency while minimizing the potential for the incorporation or spread of radioactive materials to others. The following decontamination procedures are adapted from general guidelines for hospital emergency medical services distributed by the Federal Emergency Management Agency. These principles apply regardless of the location where decontamination takes place. Some industries and hospitals have separate rooms and showers for decontamination purposes. Your responsibilities will vary depending on the area in which you practice. In most instances, you will not be involved in decontamination efforts; however, you may be called upon to assist.

DECONTAMINATION Decontamination has three purposes: first, to prevent or minimize transfer of contaminants to an internal site; second, to reduce the amount of radiation dosage from the contaminant; and third, to prevent the spread of contamination to other persons and areas.

ESTABLISH PRIORITIES. Care for contaminated wounds and body orifices first to minimize the amount of absorption. Then focus on areas on the intact skin with the highest levels of radioactivity. Take into consideration the chemical properties of the radioactive material. Is it corrosive, toxic, soluble, or insoluble? Do the guidelines for removal vary? This information may be available by consulting guides after a specific substance has been identified.

Gross decontamination may be accomplished by removing the clothes and covering the patient with a blanket. Contaminated clothing may be left at the site in labeled plastic bags for later retrieval and disposal.

REMOVAL FROM THE INTACT SKIN. Take care when removing contaminants from the intact skin surface to limit mechanical, thermal, or chemical irritation to the skin. When intact, the skin is an effective barrier against absorption. For example, a soft brush and gentle soap should be used to avoid skin irritation. Tepid (not hot) water should be used, since hot water may cause vasodilation. Scrub the area gently for 3 to 4 minutes, rinse for 2 to 3 minutes, then blot the area dry and remonitor. Repeated scrubs may be necessary. If contamination persists after 2 to 3 washes, lava soap or a mix of half Tide or similar type of laundry detergent and half cornmeal can be used. If still more decontamination is necessary, chlorine bleach can be used full strength to clear small areas and as a dilute solution for large areas. Decontamination stops when radioactivity cannot be reduced to a lower level after implementing the above measures. Hair may be problematic. It should not be shaved, as shaving may irritate the intact skin.

Ambulatory patients can shower or wash in a sink or basin. If repeated showers are necessary, use a clean towel following each shower. Avoid getting wash water into body orifices. Water should be saved if feasible.

P R O C E D U R E 1 1 – 2
DECONTAMINATING WOUNDS AND BODY ORIFICES*

1. Drape the area around the wound to limit spread of contaminants.
2. Irrigate the wound repeatedly with saline, water, or 3% hydrogen peroxide.

   Note: Drapes and dressings should be removed as they become contaminated. Use a forceps or other instrument to remove contaminated particles. Imbedded fragments may have to be removed surgically.

3. Monitor the irrigation fluid and remonitor the wound to judge the effectiveness of the decontamination procedures.
4. After the wound is decontaminated, cover it with a sterile waterproof dressing and decontaminate the surrounding area.

   Note: Contaminated burns are treated like any other burns.

   Note: Body orifices are decontaminated by irrigation, much as they would be if other hazardous substances were inhaled, ingested, or in the eyes and ears. Contamination of the oral and nasal cavities should be removed with gentle irrigation, turning the head to the side and using suctioning. The awake and alert patient may rinse and brush the teeth and spit out the fluid, avoiding swallowing. With ingestion, a nasogastric tube may be passed to remove contaminated stomach contents. When irrigating the eyes, use a gentle stream diverted away from the nasal area to avoid drainage into the lacrimal duct. The ear canals can be gently irrigated and suctioned.

---

* Adapted from Federal Emergency Management Agency: Hospital Emergency Department Management of Radiation Accidents. Washington, DC, 1984.

INTERNAL CONTAMINATION. If there is a possibility of internal contamination, the physical and chemical nature of the contaminant determines the speed and extent of incorporation within the body. The internally contaminated patient must be treated as a medical emergency, and expert advice must be obtained regarding the administration of medications to dilute, eliminate, bind, or block the effects of the radioactive material. For example, potassium iodide may be given to block the uptake of radioactive iodine (Iodine 131) by the thyroid gland. If given to a patient within 2 hours after contamination, it may reduce uptake of Iodine 131 by about 90%.*

ARRIVAL AT THE HOSPITAL

Nuclear power plants and some industries have prior arrangements with hospitals for the care of radiation victims, which may include separate entrances and areas for care of contaminated victims. Nearly all hospitals have plans for caring for patients with radiation injuries. The hospital plan is implemented upon notification and verification that a potential radiation accident has occurred. The hospital personnel need as much information as possible before your arrival in order to have staff and supplies ready. In addition to the possible use of special entrances for contaminated victims, hospitals establish contamination control procedures similar to strict isolation precautions for certain infectious diseases and "dirty" (infected) surgical cases. A decontamination room is designated and a path is formed to the ambulance reception area. The area and path are designated radioactive so as to keep out unnecessary personnel. The floor is covered with paper or plastic coverings, as are wall switches, doorknobs, and other equipment, to limit the spread of radioactive contamination and to facilitate the cleanup. A control person is assigned to limit access into the area. Follow this person's instructions.

The staff uses protective clothing and dosimeters and may provide these to ambulance personnel if they are needed as part of the team that implements the decontamination procedures noted above.

The emergency physician and the radiation officer meet the ambulance at the entrance to the emergency department. The physician assesses the patient for life-threatening injuries while the radiation safety officer determines whether the victim is contaminated. If the victim still has clothing on, a decision may be made to leave it in the ambulance.

An emergency cart should be brought out. The ambulance stretcher is placed on the covered floor and the patient can be transferred to a clean stretcher and wrapped in clean blankets by hospital personnel so that

---

* Adapted from Federal Emergency Management Agency: Hospital Emergency Department Management of Radiation Accidents. Washington, DC, 1984.

a noncontaminated stretcher enters the hospital. The EMTs may be asked to remain in the ambulance until they and their equipment can be monitored and decontaminated. A buffer zone is established between contaminated and clean areas within the hospital, which is staffed with a "floating" nurse or aide.

EMTs are monitored by the radiation safety officer. At the demarcation ("clean line") between potentially contaminated and clean areas they should remove protective clothing in the sequence outlined below, placing it in a plastic container marked "contaminated."

PROCEDURE 11-3
REMOVING CONTAMINATED CLOTHING

1. Remove outer gloves first, turning them inside out as they are pulled off.
2. Give the dosimeter to the radiation safety officer.
3. Remove all tape at trouser cuffs and sleeves.
4. Remove the outer surgical gown, turning it inside out; avoid shaking it.
5. Remove the surgical shirt.
6. Remove the head cover.
7. Pull the surgical trousers over the shoe covers.
8. Remove the shoe cover from the foot and let the radiation safety officer monitor the shoe; if it is clean, step over the line, remove the other shoe cover, and have the other shoe monitored.
9. Remove inner gloves.
10. Monitor feet and hands for the final time and take a shower.

Note: A complete body survey should be done of each staff member at the control line. The radiation safety officer's advice should be followed during the above procedure and during decontamination of the ambulance. If the EMT was contaminated, he or she should consult a physician for advice.

The Transportation Accident

Among the most challenging situations for EMTs are transportation accidents that involve radioactive materials and victims who require emergency care. The authors Mettler and Porter advise that it is very unlikely that medically significant amounts of radioactive material will be released because of stringent federal packaging regulations. Thus, they recommend that immediate medical care be delivered with the patient wrapped in blankets, and that any contamination of the EMTs' hands and clothing is of no medical urgency. The following recommendations are for the handling of transportation accidents in which one of the vehicles displays a radioactive material sign.

PROCEDURE 11-4
HANDLING TRANSPORTATION ACCIDENTS INVOLVING RADIOACTIVE MATERIAL*

1. Perform lifesaving functions, even if this involves mouth-to-mouth resuscitation. Manage trauma appropriately.
2. In addition to gloves, don protective clothing.
3. Place the patient directly on a stretcher. Do not put a blanket between the patient and the stretcher. The blanket may be placed over the patient.
4. Move the patient at least 20 yards from the vehicle involved in the accident if he or she will not be transported to the hospital immediately.
5. Instruct other people who are involved in the accident, and who are not seriously injured, to stay 20 yards away from the vehicle but not to leave the scene of the accident until it can be ascertained whether they have been contaminated.
6. Place a blanket under the stretcher, and wrap both the stretcher and the patient in the blanket. This prevents the spread of contamination in the ambulance and at the hospital. If the patient requires medical assistance while being transported in the ambulance, the blanket may be unwrapped.
7. If radio communication exists between the hospital and the ambulance, notify the hospital that a possibly contaminated and injured patient is en route. Ask whether the hospital has a specific area for handling such patients. Many hospitals do have a special emergency radiation area, which is distinct and often completely separate from the routine emergency department.
8. Inform the hospital of the nature of the patient's injury, so that special equipment can be prepared and taken to the radiation emergency area.
9. If possible while en route, notify the state police of the suspected radiation accident. The state police often have radiation equipment available or know where it can be obtained.
10. Upon arrival at the hospital, bring the patient (keeping the blanket wrapped as previously described) to the area designated by the hospital personnel.
11. Place the stretcher on the floor and unwrap the blanket.
12. Cut off the patient's clothing, but leave the clothing on the blanket. If surface contamination is present, taking off the clothing will remove at least 90% of it.
13. Lift the patient onto a clean hospital stretcher. The hospital staff should be gowned in regular operating room garb (shoe covers, surgeon's cap, mask, gloves, and gown).
14. Remove your outer clothing and place it either in a plastic bag or on the blanket, as discussed previously. The blanket should be wrapped up,

enclosing the stretcher, the patient's clothes, and the EMT's outer clothing.

Note: Although it has proved very difficult to suspend contamination in ambient air, care should be taken to avoid shaking the blanket or clothing.

15. Ask hospital personnel for soap, a washcloth, and a basin to wash both the patient's and the EMT's face and hands (in that order). Place the washcloths on the blanket.

Note: Do not leave the immediate area. If contamination is present, it may be on your shoes and can be spread to other parts of the hospital or emergency room.

16. Return to the ambulance the same way you entered the hospital and lock the back door. Other people should be kept away from it until someone with a radiation detector has confirmed that there is no contamination on you or in the ambulance.

17. If there are several patients involved in the accident, return to the scene and proceed as before.

Note: Borrow another clean blanket, surgeon's gloves, and gown.

---

* From Mettler FA, Porter SW: The emergency response to radiation accidents. In Auerbach PS, Geehr EC (eds): Management of Wilderness and Environmental Emengencies. New York, Macmillan, 1983, pp. 639–640.

Summary

Understanding basic principles of radiation injuries allows the EMT to function effectively as part of a team when responding to radiation accidents. In addition to providing emergency care, EMTs must act to protect themselves and others from unnecessary radiation exposure and contamination. Steps involved include identification of the substance, notification of authorities, establishment of a safety zone, and use of protective gear. Actions should be guided by radiation protection principles: namely, time, distance, shielding, and limitation of exposure to the smallest possible body part. The role of the radiation safety officer is key, since special instruments and expertise are necessary to detect the presence and evaluate the significance of ionizing radiation. The survey instrument allows evaluation of the amount of exposure from an unshielded source and determines whether victims are contaminated. The dosimeter allows measurement of accumulated exposure to the patient and rescuers. The irradiated patient presents no hazard to the EMT. The contaminated patient must be handled carefully, and decontamination may be started at the scene or in the hospital, depending on circumstances and the degree of injuries. Internal contamination is a medical emergency calling for expert advice and treatment to prevent incorporation of the radioactive

material within the body. While most radiation accidents have not resulted in any medically significant exposure to rescuers or field personnel, the EMT must be aware of the potential danger in high-technology areas, where high exposure levels may be encountered. The guidelines established by the National Council on Radiation Protection and Measurements should be followed. Transportation accidents present the greatest challenge, since the EMT may be the first respondent on the scene. Preplanning is the key to effective management of these infrequent situations. Know your role within the local protocols. Special training and equipment lists are available from the references cited at the end of this chapter.

DIVING ACCIDENTS

In 1984, there were approximately 2.8 million scuba divers in the United States, with an average accident rate of 5/100,000. The majority of the accidents involved decompression sickness (DCS) and air embolisms (AE). There is a significant increase in the number of people who are diving for recreation and as an EMT you may be called to evaluate or transport an individual suffering from dysbaric illness.

Divers have many ways of exploring the environment beneath the sea. These include skin diving that involves diving below the surface; breathing air from the surface through a tube or snorkel; and scuba diving, which involves the use of a self-contained underwater breathing apparatus that allows the diver to carry an air supply and breathe for varying lengths of time—depending on how deep the water and for how long the diver stays under water.

Physics and Gases

The following definitions provide a basic understanding of some of the terms connected with diving and its effects on the human body.

Pressure   The amount of pressure or force exerted by the earth's atmosphere, which varies with the elevation.

Gauge pressure   The pressure being measured above the atmospheric pressure (in diving due to the pressure of the water). Atmospheric pressure is not taken into account.

Absolute pressure   Gauge pressure plus atmospheric pressure.

Ambient pressure   The absolute pressure surrounding an object or diver.

Hydrostatic pressure   The pressure of a column of water above and acting on a body immersed in it.

Pressure and the Diver's Body

On the surface of the earth we are exposed to the pressure exerted by the atmosphere above us. The pressure becomes greater as we descend into the water, because water is heavier than air. One atmosphere of pressure represents 14.7 lb per square inch on the body at sea level. For each additional 33 feet of sea water, there is another one atmosphere of pressure exerted on the body. Gases in the body can be compressed under pressure. The solid and liquid parts of the body are not compressed; rather, the pressure is transmitted through them. At sea level, body tissue contains about 1 liter of gaseous nitrogen in solution. During descent into the water, because of the effects of increasing pressure, nitrogen gas molecules dissolve in the tissues and move from one area to another until the partial pressure of the gas is equal at each point.

While breathing ambient pressure gas from a scuba tank, more nitrogen is loaded into the tissues, since for a given volume of air in the lungs, more molecules of oxygen and nitrogen enter the lungs per given volume. The added "nitrogen load" dissolves in greater amounts into the tissues.

During ascent, as long as the pressure changes are gradual, this added "nitrogen load" reverses itself as the nitrogen molecules move from the tissues to the blood and out with exhaled air. Ordinarily, this process occurs without awareness or complications.

If a diver surfaces too rapidly, greater than 60 feet per minute, the gas within the body expands faster than it can be eliminated by transit through the bloodstream and out through the lungs. "Bubbles" of nitrogen form in tissues and the bloodstream and cause symptoms known as the "bends." Depth/duration (time) guidelines have been established to prevent the occurrence of these bubbles and the subsequent decompression sickness.

Because of the complications that result from waiting for a bubble to redissolve, the hyperbaric chamber (recompression therapy) has been used to speed up the gas elimination process. The application of pressure reduces the size of the bubbles and usually the symptoms of decompression sickness, and allows the slow return to atmospheric pressure. Recompression followed by slow decompression assists bubble resolution and is thus the basis for recompression treatment.

Decompression Sickness

Decompression sickness is known as the bends, or caisson's disease, because bridge and tunnel workers, who worked in airtight chambers (caissons) beneath rivers, experienced severe pain in the hips and lower extremities when they returned to the surface pressure without decompression. Divers who do not decompress properly or surface too rapidly also experience the bends or more lethal complications, depending on the speed of ascent.

Decompression sickness is caused by the release of gas bubbles into tissue and blood. The bubbles are carried by the bloodstream to the cardiopulmonary system, brain, spinal cord, joints, muscles and the inner ear. These bubbles cause circulation blockage (ischemia and infarction), as well as blood clot formation. As a result, mild or severe symptoms can occur.

Over 50% of the cases of decompression sickness develop within 1 hour of the dive, and 90% within 6 hours. Fewer than 1% will delay beyond 6 hours. Altitude exposure (especially after flying) can precipitate decompression sickness.

Fatigue, skin rash, and weakness are considered to be mild symptoms. Severe symptoms consist of pain or weakness in the extremities, paralysis, unstable walking, respiratory difficulties (chokes), or unconsciousness upon surfacing. The pain is usually localized and increases in severity with time. Divers usually describe it as deep and burning pain. It is often felt in the joints, because these areas can stand the least tissue displacement by the bubbles.

There is a form of decompression sickness that has gotten more recognition lately. It is called "spinal bends" and is caused by nitrogen bubbles forming in the spinal cord. Initial symptoms include a sharp back pain that eventually radiates to the front. Next, the diver experiences paresthesias of the extremities, which may progress to an unstable gait followed by paralysis.

When a diver surfaces from a dive and behaves in an unusual manner; appears confused; has loss of manual dexterity; experiences dizziness, vertigo, or a spinning sensation; has a skin rash; feels weakness and fatigue; or has a loss of memory, he or she may have early signs of decompression illness. Not all of these symptoms need be present, as a diver may show only one symptom or combinations of many symptoms.

When assessing a patient suspected of having decompression sickness, keep in mind that blood circulation is a vital factor in the elimination of excess nitrogen, and so older people with poor circulation tend to be more susceptible. Overweight people are also susceptible because of the high solubility characteristics of nitrogen in fat. Scar tissue from past injuries can be points where quantities of nitrogen build up. Other risk factors that predispose an individual to decompression illness are being in poor physical condition; being fatigued; diving with a hangover; performing hard work in deep, cold water; and making multiple dives per day over a period of 7 to 10 days.

The prognosis for decompression sickness is good for most people who are treated promptly.

Air Embolism

The most dangerous problem a diver can develop is an air embolism. If a scuba diver holds his or her breath and ascends from 33 feet, the air in the lungs expands to twice its volume, according to Boyle's Law. If the expanding air is not allowed to escape, the pressure in the lungs becomes greater than the pressure surrounding the chest area, and the alveoli burst, carrying the air through the pulmonary vein to the left side of the heart, into the aorta, and finally into the carotid arteries leading to the brain.

Symptoms of air embolism may be present when the victim reaches the surface or may begin a few minutes afterward. EMTs may find the patient with bloody froth at the mouth, dizziness, visual blurring, disorientation, numbness or paralysis in the extremities, convulsions, and possibly the cessation of breathing. All of these symptoms signal CNS injury. Whenever a diver is unconsciousness, you must suspect an air embolism and begin treatment immediately.

Because of the extensive heart, lung, and brain damage than can occur, a high fatality rate is prevalent with this particular accident.

History of a Diving Accident

In any situation suggesting an underwater diving accident, the primary question is "Did the victim breathe compressed air underwater?" The compressed air could be from a scuba tank, hose, bucket, or submerged car. If so, or if the victim is unconscious, consider that you are dealing with a diving accident until proved otherwise.

Take a complete history of the diving accident. It is imperative to obtain a complete dive profile for the whole day and not for just the final dive. Ask how many dives have been made; what was the depth and bottom time of each dive; what was the surface interval between dives; what type of equipment was used; what type of diving activity and environmental factors were involved. Ascertaining the type of entry into the water, if a buddy was present, and the kind of breathing gas that was used are all necessary information. The victim must be transported without delay to the nearest hyperbaric facility. The history may be obtained from the victim's buddy or other divers who were involved.

Emergency Care and Contact Information

Since the signs and symptoms of decompression and air embolism can develop many hours after diving,

---

PROCEDURE 11-5
TREATING UNDERWATER DIVING ACCIDENT VICTIMS

The following interventions are recommended for the immediate care of an underwater diving accident victim.

1. Perform basic life support.
2. Immediately place the victim on the left side with the head and chest inclined downward (Trendelenburg position) until he or she receives treatment in a recompression chamber. This position is thought to prevent "bubbles" from entering the left side of the heart.
3. Maintain an open airway and prevent aspiration of vomitus.
4. Administer oxygen at the highest possible concentration using a tight-fitting double seal mask. Use an endotracheal tube in an unconscious victim. The oxygen can begin to off-load bubbles and to deliver a greater supply to the areas deprived of oxygen.
5. Maintain the patient's body temperature.
6. Give the conscious victim nonalcoholic liquids such as a balanced salt solution (Gatorade). This replaces fluids that are lost during the dive from breathing dry dehumidified air plus the fluid that is lost from the bends (capillary leakage).
7. Start intravenous fluid replacement for unconscious victims (Ringer's lactate or normal saline).
8. Contact a physician specializing in diving accidents for consultation. The national divers' alert telephone network can be reached at 919-684-8111.

Note: If air evacuation is used, it is important that the victim not be exposed to decreased barometric pressure. Flight crews should maintain cabin pressure at sea level as much as possible to avoid causing bubbles that are already in the tissue and blood to expand further.

Note: It is important to note that recompression should never be attempted in water because it results in incomplete recompression and is extremely dangerous.

---

the victim may seek emergency help in the community. Emergency personnel must be able to recognize the symptoms, institute emergency measures, obtain a complete history, call the Divers' Alert Network to verify the correct diving accident procedure, and support the victim until he or she reaches the nearest hyperbaric trauma center.

Barotrauma

When the diver is unable to equalize the pressure differential in the body's air-filled cavities during descent, the result can be barotrauma, or "squeeze." The most commonly affected areas are the ears, but squeezes can occur in the sinuses, face, lungs, or the total body if the diver is wearing a dry diving suit.

Middle ear (otic) barotrauma is the most common complication of diving. It results from inadequate pressure equalization between the middle ear space and the external environment. This can be due to poor eustachian tube function, very rapid descent, or a structural abnormality. The negative middle ear pressure relative to the increasing ambient pressure (the absolute pressure surrounding the diver) results in fullness and pain in the involved ear and eventual tympanic membrane rupture if the change in pressure is too great for the eardrum to withstand. If a forceful Valsalva's maneuver (forced expiration against a closed mouth and pinched nostrils) is performed under these conditions, the inner ear pressure can increase sharply, and a rupture between the middle ear and inner ear may occur, with very serious consequences. Inner ear injury has the following symptoms: sustained ringing in the ears, dizziness or a sensation of spinning, and possible deafness. These patients should be transported in a semisitting position to the nearest medical facility.

The five cranial sinuses are potential sites for barotrauma upon descent or ascent. The condition usually occurs with descent, however, and causes intense pain over the involved sinus. Pain may be felt toward the back of the head, usually indicating sphenoidal sinus involvement. Sinus barotrauma is caused by blockage of the sinus opening (ostium) secondary to mucosal congestion, hypertrophy, or sinusitis. During descent, when there is subsequent reduction of air volume in the sinus cavity, there is transudation of fluid and blood into the sinus. During ascent, expansion of the enclosed air expels blood and mucus from the sinus ostium.

Treatment includes cessation of all diving activities and the correction of any predisposing factors. Divers with upper respiratory infections may require antibiotic therapy.

The teeth are also susceptible to varying degrees of barotrauma. The diver should be sure any dental work is completed before attempting to dive so that there will not be any spaces between the teeth, fillings, and gums.

HAZARDOUS MATERIALS

Overview

The first principle of medicine is to do no harm. When dealing with a hazardous material (HAZMAT) situation in the prehospital care setting this phrase takes on a special meaning. When the EMT responds to a call, there will be times when the presence of hazardous materials may not be obvious. When this happens, both patients and EMTs can unknowingly be in great danger. Hazardous materials can be deceiving because their effects may not be evident immediately. Therefore, it is essential for the EMT not to assume anything when dealing with a potential HAZMAT situation.

The most important thing for the EMT to remember when dealing with the HAZMAT is to secure the scene in such a way that he or she is not in danger and patient care can be done without further harm to the victim. Remember that emergency medical service is only part of the system required to bring a HAZMAT under control. The EMT requires assistance from the police, fire department, and other personnel who are trained to deal with hazardous materials.

Safety

Upon arrival on any scene where hazardous materials may be present, medical personnel should follow a number of rules. First, all EMTs responding to a potential hazardous material incident should wear full turnout gear, including a coat, a helmet, gloves, and, when appropriate, a self-contained breathing apparatus (SCBA). A special containment suit may be required just to enter the area for the purpose of providing emergency medical care. Remember, no emergency personnel should use SCBA or any other rescue equipment unless they have received appropriate training in its safe and effective use. The purpose of wearing this gear is to protect the EMT while he or she provides emergency medical care.

When the EMT arrives on the scene of a HAZMAT, his or her primary responsibility is to provide emergency medical care, not to act as part of the containment team. It is important to have all duties and tasks understood before an incident occurs, so that those responsible for providing patient care concentrate on that task exclusively. In those incidences when rescue, containment, and firefighting duties are required of the EMT, they should be performed only until the safety of victims and rescue personnel is ensured. The victims of a hazardous material incident deserve the full attention of the EMT whenever possible.

Remember, EMTs are of no help to their patients if they themselves are injured. Let those who are appropriately trained and who have the necessary equipment secure the scene.

The Scene

Upon arrival at a hazardous material incident, one's senses can provide extremely valuable information about the safety of the scene. Look at the scene from a distance whenever possible. Use binoculars if you cannot get close enough to see with the naked eye. You should observe if there is a cloud of smoke, indicating that the material was ignited. Listen for noises that might indicate that there is a leak. Use your sense of smell. If there is a strange odor, you should probably try to relocate upwind from the source.

Once this initial evaluation has been done, a final determination should be made concerning whether the scene is safe enough to initiate rescue efforts. Summon the appropriate emergency agency needed to secure the scene—the fire department or special HAZMAT units.

THE STAGING AREA. When responding to a HAZMAT incident, it is important to identify a staging area. The staging area must be a location where patient care can be rendered in a safe and efficient manner before the ill and injured are transported to the hospital.

When determining a location for a staging area, a number of factors need to be considered. First, is it safe? Is it far enough away and upwind from the scene so that fumes, run-off, or a secondary explosion will not further endanger those who have been rescued? Second, if decontamination is required, can it be done effectively, safely, and without secondary contamination occurring to patients and EMTs? Decontamination may have to be done in an area away from the staging area, depending on the contaminating material and the amount of exposure. Third, will the area allow for the flow of ambulances and other emergency vehicles required to bring in supplies and personnel and to take the ill and injured to a hospital? Try to prevent grid lock, the inability of vehicles to move in an expeditious fashion. The police or fire department should be given the responsibility for handling traffic control whenever possible. Fourth, is there enough room to provide the best and most appropriate care possible?

Space may be at a premium, but attempt to meet as many of these criteria as possible. The initial planning at the site can be very beneficial to both EMTs and patients, particularly if the number of ill or injured people is significant.

Identification of the Hazardous Materials

The EMT must always remember the importance of identifying hazardous materials promptly and correctly whenever a hazardous material situation exists. This information is important for a number of reasons. EMTs need to know what the potential hazard is so they can make the scene safe for themselves and the victims. Special equipment and precautions may be required for a safe and efficient rescue. The need for decontamination and how it can be carried out properly must be deter-

mined. Different hazardous materials have different effects on the human body. Therefore, it is imperative when identifying a hazardous material to find out what the health hazard is as well as any particular treatment that might be required.

There are many ways that this can be accomplished. The first method of identification is placards. Placards are signs that identify hazardous materials by color, symbols, category names, and numbers. Figure 11–16 illustrates domestic and international placard systems. It is important to be methodical and safe when trying to identify materials. Time can be a crucial factor. Make sure that the identification of all potentially hazardous materials is accurate. A number of pitfalls might be encountered when trying to do this. Some materials that are being transported are listed by their trade names. The components that make up the material may not be readily known. Many substances that are transported are made up of numerous materials that can be dangerous. In addition, these materials can be more hazardous when combined with other substances than when in their original state. The transport vehicle may not be marked or may be marked inappropriately.

The bill of lading, as required by law, is the second type of identification system (Fig. 11–17). However, it may not be with the vehicle. Vehicles may not be placarded or may be placarded incorrectly. These circumstances can lead to potentially dangerous situations. If you identify a substance incorrectly, the treatment provided and the precautions taken could be inappropriate. This could affect the safety of the emergency personnel as well as the outcome of patient care. As a final note, whenever working in a situation where hazardous materials are thought to be involved, caution should be taken. EMTs may not realize that there is a hazardous materials situation until they are in the middle of it. Be especially cautious when dealing with tractor trailers or railroad cars designed for the transport of bulk material.

A number of books are available that provide information on identifying hazardous materials as well as precautions and treatments for those who have been exposed. A very important book for the identification of hazardous materials is the *Emergency Response Guidebook for Initial Response to Hazardous Materials Incidents,* published by the United States Department of Transportation. This book lists the hazards and actions for the various classes of hazardous materials. It is organized in outline form for quick reference at the HAZMAT scene. Table 11–7 illustrates the information provided for chlorine.

It is important that the EMT have ready access to this resource when it is needed. Preplanning is essential. It should be decided before a hazardous materials incident occurs that this book will be available, for example, by contacting the dispatcher or by placing a copy of a resource book in every vehicle as part of the standard

EXAMPLE OF SHIPPING PAPER

The following shipping paper is only illustrative since it may be varied in format. However, all descriptions will be basically the same. You should look for this type of entry to determine the shipping name of the hazardous material, its classification and its ID number. With certain exceptions, shipping papers identifying hazardous materials are required:

- To be in the cab of the motor vehicle;
- To be in the possession of a train crew member;
- To be kept in a holder on the bridge of a vessel;
- To be in an aircraft pilot's possession.

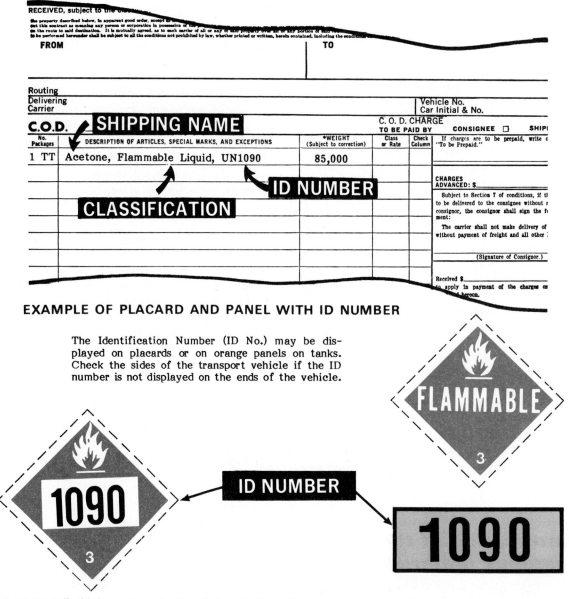

EXAMPLE OF PLACARD AND PANEL WITH ID NUMBER

The Identification Number (ID No.) may be displayed on placards or on orange panels on tanks. Check the sides of the transport vehicle if the ID number is not displayed on the ends of the vehicle.

FIGURE 11–17. Bill of lading with explanation of elements. (From Emergency Response Guidebook for Initial Response to Hazardous Materials Incidents. United States Department of Transportation.)

equipment. No matter what the approach, it should be understood by everyone and applied consistently.

The Chemical Transport Emergency Center CHEM-TREC is a 24-hours-a-day, 7-days-a-week resource service available to provide advice on how to handle chemical emergencies. The toll-free number to contact CHEM-TREC is 1-800-424-9300. CHEMTREC has the most extensive resources for identifying types of chemicals and their composition, and for locating the shipping source. When using CHEMTREC, it is important to make

TABLE 11–7. Hazardous Materials—Guide 20

Potential Hazards	Emergency Action (*Continued*)

Potential Hazards

Health Hazards
Poisonous; may be fatal if inhaled.
Contact may cause burns to skin and eyes.
Contact with liquid may cause frostbite.
Run-off from fire control or dilution water may cause pollution.

Fire or Explosion
May ignite other combustible materials (wood, paper, oil, etc.).
Mixture with fuels may explode.
Cylinder may explode in heat of fire.
Vapor explosion and poison hazard indoors, outdoors, or in sewers.

Emergency Action

Keep unnecessary people away; isolate hazard area and deny entry.
Stay upwind, out of low areas, and ventilate closed spaces before entering.
Self-contained breathing apparatus (SCBA) and structural firefighter's protective clothing will provide limited protection for short-term exposure to these materials.
Fully-encapsulated protective clothing should be worn for spills and leaks with no fire.
Evacuate the leak or spill area immediately for at least 50 feet in all directions.
CALL CHEMTREC AT 1-800-424-9300 FOR EMERGENCY ASSISTANCE. If water pollution occurs, notify the appropriate authorities.

Fire
Small Fires: Dry chemical, CO_2 or Halon.
Large Fires: Water spray, fog, or standard foam is recommended.
Move container from fire area if you can do it without risk.
Cool containers that are exposed to flames with water from the side until well after fire is out. Stay away from ends of tanks.
For massive fire in cargo area, use unmanned hose holder or monitor nozzles; if this is impossible, withdraw from area and let fire burn.

Spill or Leak
Keep combustibles (wood, paper, oil, etc.) away from spilled material.
Stop leak if you can do it without risk.
Use water spray to reduce vapor; do not put water directly on leak or spill area.
Isolate area until gas has dispersed.

Emergency Action (*Continued*)

First Aid
Move victim to fresh air and call emergency medical care; if not breathing, give artificial respiration; if breathing is difficult, give oxygen.
Remove and isolate contaminated clothing and shoes at the site.
In case of contact with material, immediately flush skin or eyes with running water for at least 15 minutes.
Keep victim quiet and maintain normal body temperature.
Effects may be delayed; keep victim under observation.

Potential Hazards

Fire or Explosion
Cannot catch fire.
Container may explode in heat of fire.

Health Hazards
Vapors may cause dizziness or suffocation.
Contact with liquid may cause frostbite.

Emergency Action

Keep unnecessary people away; isolate hazard area and deny entry.
Stay upwind, out of low areas, and ventilate closed spaces before entering.
Self-contained breathing apparatus (SCBA) and structural firefighter's protective clothing will provide limited protection.
CALL CHEMTREC AT 1-800-424-9300 AS SOON AS POSSIBLE, especially if there is no local hazardous materials team available.

Fire
Move container from fire area if you can do it without risk.
Cool containers that are exposed to flames with water from the side until well after fire is out. Stay away from ends of tanks.

Spill or Leak
Do not touch spilled material.
Stop leak if you can do it without risk.

First Aid
Move victim to fresh air and call emergency medical care; if not breathing, give artificial respiration; if breathing is difficult, give oxygen.
In case of frostbite, thaw frosted parts with water.
Keep victim quiet and maintain normal body temperature.

From Emergency Response Guidebook for Initial Response to Hazardous Materials Incidents. United States Department of Transportation.

sure that information from the scene can be easily transmitted. Therefore, if you are either going through dispatch or contacting CHEMTREC directly, it is essential to make sure that either the specific radio channel or telephone line is kept open and available for urgent and essential transmissions. You should have the following information available to provide to CHEMTREC before the initial call is made.

1. The identification number
2. The name of the product
3. The name of the manufacturer
4. The name of the shipper
5. The type of vehicle or container involved (if a vehicle is involved, a rail car number or truck number should be obtained)

6. The location of the incident
7. The weather conditions (wind and velocity)
8. The particulars of the site (rural or urban, landscape, and so forth)
9. The name of the designated contact and the telephone number where that individual can be reached.

There are other resources that should not be overlooked when dealing with a hazardous material incident. There are federal, state, and local agencies that have experts who deal with these types of emergencies. Some of these agencies have a legal obligation and authority to intervene in situations that impact on either the public health or the environment. These resources should be identified before you have a need to access them. The telephone numbers for agencies, listing a contact person for each, should be available for either the dispatcher or the incident commander whenever a HAZMAT situation is being handled. This list should be reviewed and updated on a regular basis. Finally, medical control may be helpful in assisting with the identification of hazardous materials.

COMMUNICATIONS

Communications is one of the most important elements for running and controlling the operation of a HAZMAT scene. All aspects of communications must be handled according to a set procedure that ensures that information flows in an orderly manner and that it is accurate. A number of different aspects of communications should be considered when dealing with a HAZMAT situation. From the onset of the call, all pertinent information concerning the call should be obtained by the dispatcher so that the responding units can be as informed as possible before arriving at the scene. Upon arriving at the scene, it is imperative that as much information as possible be relayed to the dispatcher. This information includes the following:

1. A concise overview of the situation
2. The estimated number of victims
3. The identification of the hazardous materials
4. The possibility of immediate dangers due to fire, explosion, downed electrical wires, etc.
5. The need for assistance and the type needed (fire, police, special HAZMAT unit, etc.)
6. The status of the scene, including the safety of the public, traffic (grid lock?), the weather (wind and direction), etc.

If it is determined that assistance is required from CHEMTREC, then as much of the information from the list presented in the section of this chapter entitled "Identification of the Hazardous Materials" as possible should be relayed to the dispatcher if he or she will be contacting CHEMTREC. CHEMTREC can always be contacted by cellular telephone directly from the scene. If CHEMTREC is contacted via the dispatcher, then it is very important to make sure that the frequency being used from the scene to the dispatcher will not get tied up with other transmissions, thereby making it difficult to relay information.

Besides the communications between the scene and a dispatcher there is also the communications on the scene. This is essential for good scene operation. It is important for agencies to communicate with each other. The need for help with personnel, sharing of information about the safety precautions needed with the hazardous material, and integration of services are just a few of the types of messages that may have to be communicated. This can be done by radio, which means that common radio frequencies have to be available. Arrangements concerning common frequencies and quick accessibility

to radios that have the appropriate frequencies must be planned out before an incident. Also, it is imperative that no special codes or identifiers be used unless everyone understands what they mean. When more than one agency is trying to communicate by radio, the use of short, everyday English phrases is probably the most efficient way to proceed. The other possibility is that runners can help to pass information between agencies and different areas of the HAZMAT scene. What is important is that information must be passed as quickly and accurately as possible. Communications is an essential part of the emergency scene. It is the most expedient way of helping to identify and initiate resources. Make sure that communications are established as early as possible at any HAZMAT scene. The use of a command center or a communication van may help to facilitate this.

INCIDENT COMMAND

The general principles of incident command should be applied, particularly if there are multiple casualties. Refer to Chapter 17, Disasters and Triage.

One of the most important aspects of a HAZMAT situation is the way all the agencies involved coordinate their activities. There are two levels to be considered. The first is the way the incident is handled by the medical personnel. The second is how the medical operation interacts with the other emergency response groups involved at a HAZMAT scene.

TRIAGE

How the EMT handles the triaging of victims of a hazardous material incident varies depending on the situation at hand. The safety of the patients and the EMTs is of the utmost importance. A decision needs to be made quickly before the triaging even begins. Is the area safe? If it is safe, then the standard principles of triaging can apply (see Chapter 17).

If the area is not safe, then a decision to evacuate must be made. There may not be time to make any decisions on the degrees of injury. If imminent danger exists, proper precautions should be taken to protect the rescuers, and patients should be removed to a safe area. The removal of the patients from the area of danger to a decontamination area or safe area should be done, as conditions permit, according to appropriate patient care techniques. This means that backboards and other proper extrication techniques should be used to minimize the possibility of aggravating existing injuries. Once patients are in a safe area, triage can commence. The EMT is obligated to make sure that triage and patient care take place. Only when immediate danger exists for the EMT or the victim should the process be delayed. Once the danger no longer exists, triage and appropriate patient care need to proceed as quickly as possible.

DECONTAMINATION

There is always the possibility that victims and rescuers involved in a hazardous material incident may require decontamination. Decontamination can be accomplished in many different ways; what becomes most important to the EMT is that it be done quickly and safely. The following principles should be applied when decontaminating victims of a HAZMAT incident.

PROCEDURE 11-6
DECONTAMINATING VICTIMS OF A HAZMAT INCIDENT

1. Take the victim to a safe area where all clothing can be removed and an initial washdown can take place.

   Note: This should not be the staging area where patient care is taking place. This area should be warm enough so that patients do not become hypothermic. Once clothing is removed it needs to be placed away from the decontamination area. Run-off from the washdown should flow away from all personnel.

2. Washdown of exposed areas must be done for a minimum of 10 to 15 minutes if the use of water or a water solution is the approach of choice.

   Note: Remember that some hazardous materials should not be washed away with water. Once the type of material to which the patient has been exposed is identified, a determination can be made from experts (medical control; federal, state, local health or environment experts; or CHEMTREC) on the amount of time required for a washdown.
   Note: Make sure that the run-off from the decontamination will not endanger other rescue personnel or other safe areas.
   Note: Rescue personnel should make sure that they do not become contaminated during the decontamination process. Protective clothing and self-contained breathing apparatus might be necessary for certain types of hazardous materials.

3. Move the victim to another area for a second washdown or definitive patient care.
4. Decontaminate any vehicle that has been exposed to any hazardous material before it is used again.
5. Place all clothing that is contaminated and removed from victims and rescuers in an appropriate container that is sealed and sent to an approved area.

   Note: The agency responsible for containment should be able to provide guidance on how to dispose of these items.

   Rescuers are apt to become contaminated. If this occurs, full decontamination procedures are to be followed for the rescuer before moving to the area for patient care.

PATIENT CARE

The principles for patient care are no different in the HAZMAT situation than they are for any other situation. Additional factors that you may have to consider are the safety of the environment, the need to decontaminate the patients, and special protective measures for yourself. Once these are overcome, patient care should be done according to existing standards of prehospital medical practice.

The ABCs come first. You must remember that protection of the cervical spine should always be done when the mechanism of injury mandates. Hazardous materials are poisons that can potentially affect any body system. As many hazardous material exposures affect the airway and breathing, high-flow, high-concentration oxygen should always be considered.

Hazardous materials may come in contact with the skin. If so, first remove the patient from the source of the contamination and start the decontamination process. Some hazardous materials that come in contact with the skin require that the affected area be flushed with copious amounts of water. Yet there are exceptions to this, and it is important for the rescuer to act quickly to identify the substances and determine the best method of treatment. If it is determined that special care is required, then consult medical control, state or local HAZMAT specialists, a hazardous material guide, or CHEMTREC. Care should NOT be delayed while determining whether special care is required.

The important thing to remember is that medical care should be applied according to the standard of care that is taught throughout this course. Your decision to deviate from this standard should be made only in order to ensure the safety of the patients, rescuers, or the public. It is recommended in all HAZMAT situations that the source of exposure be identified as quickly as possible so that resources such as medical control, federal, state, and local health officers, CHEMTREC, or reference guides can help guide your handling of the situation and ultimately ensure the best patient care. Carefully review the following hazardous material protocol.

⚕ PROTOCOL ⚕

APPROACH TO THE PATIENT EXPOSED TO A HAZARDOUS MATERIAL
HAZARDOUS MATERIAL ACTION GUIDE

All personnel regardless of training should follow the guidelines listed below in regard to calls involving a hazardous material spill/incident:

1. ALWAYS DO A 10-SECOND SURVEY!

2. Never underestimate the size of the spill or incident.

Continued

3. Establish and maintain proper communications with the borough or city-wide dispatcher.

4. Stay upwind and upgrade at all times. Monitor weather and wind changes.

5. Do not breathe any smoke, fumes, or vapors.

6. Do not touch or walk through any spilled materials. You will only increase the size of the incident.

7. Do not eat, drink, or smoke at the scene of the incident. These are all direct routes of entry into the body.

8. Do not touch your face, nose, mouth, or eyes.

9. Eliminate all sources of ignition such as flares, flames, sparks, smoking, flashes, flashlights, gas and diesel engines, and portable radios.

10. If your unit is the first on the scene, notify the dispatcher and give a 10-12 (condition in progress report). Request the assistance of the EPA, DEP, police and fire departments, and the EMS HAZ-MAT response team.

11. Do not drive through any spilled materials. You will only increase the size of the incident.

12. Identify the substance, if possible, using the DOT EMERGENCY RESPONSE GUIDEBOOK. Inform the dispatcher of your findings.

13. Observe all safety precautions and directions as set forth by the incident commander, police and fire departments, EPA, DEP.

14. ALL ORDERS SHOULD BE TAKEN .FACE TO FACE!

15. Remain clear of all restricted areas until declared safe by the incident commander.

From New York City Emergency Medical Services Basic Life Support Protocols, 1990.

REVIEW EXERCISES

1. List three types of burns.

2. List the three classifications of burn depth and describe the appearance of each.

3. List the percentage of body surface area for the head, chest and abdomen, genitals, and upper and lower extremities for the adult and child, using the "rule of nines."

4. List four regions of the body that when burned are considered critical.

5. List four complicating historical or physical factors that are considered when determining the severity of burns.

6. Describe burns as minor, moderate, or severe based on percentage of body surface area of second- and third-degree burns.

7. List three signs of inhalation injury.

8. Describe the management of thermal burns.

9. Describe the basic management of chemical burns.

10. Describe the special management considerations for the following types of chemical burns:
    Dried chemicals (lime)
    Phosphorus
    Sodium and potassium
    Hydrofluoric acid
    Phenols

11. Describe the basic management of electrical burns.

12. Define air embolism (from diving) and list its signs and symptoms.

13. Define decompression sickness and list its signs and symptoms.

14. List the general steps of management for a diving accident.

15. Explain the function of a hyperbaric chamber.

16. Describe the mechanism of barotrauma.

17. Define ionizing radiation.

18. Describe the purpose of a dosimeter and a survey instrument.

19. Describe the difference between irradiation and contamination.

20. Define external contamination, internal contamination, and incorporation.

21. Describe the penetrating ability and relative hazards of the four kinds of ionizing radiation.

22. List the factors affecting the severity of radiation injury.

23. Describe the role of the radiologic monitor or radiation safety officer.

24. List the four radiation protection principles and explain their use in reducing radiation exposure.

25. Describe the role of prehospital personnel in patient management and decontamination of radiation victims at the scene and at the hospital.

26. Discuss the maximum allowable exposures for rescue personnel performing lifesaving actions and in less urgent emergencies.

27. List two ways heat can normally be produced in the body.

28. List five ways that the body normally loses heat.

29. List four predisposing factors to heat-related illness.

30. List the mechanisms, signs and symptoms, and treatment of the following heat-related disorders:
    Heat cramps
    Heat exhaustion
    Heat stroke

31. Define hypothermia.

32. Describe the differences between the following types of hypothermia emergencies:
    Acute immersion
    Subacute exposure
    Chronic exposure

33. List four predisposing factors to hypothermia.

34. List the signs and symptoms associated with the following degrees of hypothermia:
    Mild hypothermia: 32 to 35°C
    Moderate hypothermia: 26 to 32°C
    Severe hypothermia: < 26°C

35. List the management steps for hypothermia.

36. List the signs and symptoms and management steps for the following types of local cold injuries:
    Frostnip
    Superficial frostbite
    Deep frostbite
    Trenchfoot or immersion foot
    Chilblains

37. Describe the significance and uses of placards, labels, and bills of lading in hazardous material accidents.

REFERENCES

American Medical Association: A guide to the hospital management of injuries arising from exposure to or involving ionizing radiation. Chicago, American Medical Association, 1984.

Bangs C, Hamlet MP: Hypothermia and cold injuries. In Auerbach PS, Geehr EC (eds): Management of wilderness and environmental emergencies. New York, Macmillan, 1983.

Budassi SA, Barber J: Mosby's manual of emergency care practices and procedures. St Louis, CV Mosby, 1984.

Callaham M: Heat illness. In Rosen P (ed): Emergency medicine: Concepts and clinical practice. St Louis, CV Mosby, 1983.

Danzl DF: Accidental hypothermia. In Rosen P (ed): Emergency medicine: Concepts and clinical practice. St Louis, CV Mosby, 1983.

Federal Emergency Management Agency (FEMA): Hospital emergency department management of radiation accidents: Instructor Guide (IG 80/May 1984). Washington, DC, Federal Emergency Management Agency, Emergency Management Institute, National Emergency Training Center, 1984.

Goldfrank LR, Kirstein R: Hypothermia. In Goldfrank LR (ed): Toxicological emergencies: A comprehensive handbook in problem solving, 2nd ed. Norwalk, CT, Appleton-Century-Crofts, 1982.

Goldfrank LR, Osborn H, Weisman RS: Heat stroke. In Goldfrank LR (ed): Toxicological emergencies: A comprehensive handbook in problem solving, 2nd ed. Norwalk, CT, Appleton-Century-Crofts, 1982.

Gordon D: After Chernobyl: Reassessing U.S. response plans. Emergency Medical Service 15(9):13, 1986.

Guyton AC: Textbook of medical physiology, 8th ed. Philadelphia, WB Saunders, 1990.

Knopp RK: Near-drowning. In Rosen P (ed): Emergency medicine: Concepts and clinical practice. St Louis, CV Mosby, 1983.

Leonard RB, Ricks RC: Emergency department radiation accident protocol. Ann Emerg Med 9(9):462–470, 1980.

McElroy C, Auerbach PS: Heat illness: Current perspectives. In Auerbach PS, Geehr EC (eds): Management of wilderness and environmental emergencies. New York, Macmillan, 1983.

Mettler FA, Porter SW: The emergency response to radiation accidents. In Auerbach PS, Geehr EC (eds): Management of wilderness and environmental emergencies. New York, Macmillan, 1983, pp. 606–646.

National Council on Radiation Protection and Measurements: Basic radiation protection criteria, NCRP Report No. 39. Washington, DC, NCRP Publications, 1971.

National Council on Radiation Protection and Measurements: Management of persons accidentally contaminated with radionuclides, NCRP Report No. 65. Washington, DC, NCRP Publications, 1980.

Passmore R, Robson JS: A companion to medical studies. Edinburgh, Blackwell Scientific Publications, 1969.

Rosen P: Emergency medicine: Concepts and clinical practice, 2nd ed. St Louis, CV Mosby, 1988.

Shaw JF: Frostbite. In Rosen P (ed): Emergency medicine: Concepts and clinical practice. St Louis, CV Mosby, 1983.

Stasiak RS, Stewart CE, Redwine RH: Symptoms and treatment of radiation exposure: An overview for EMS personnel. Emergency Medical Services 15(9):21–29.

United States Department of Transportation: 1984 Emergency response guidebook: Guidebook for hazardous materials incidents. Washington, DC, Department of Transportation, 1984.

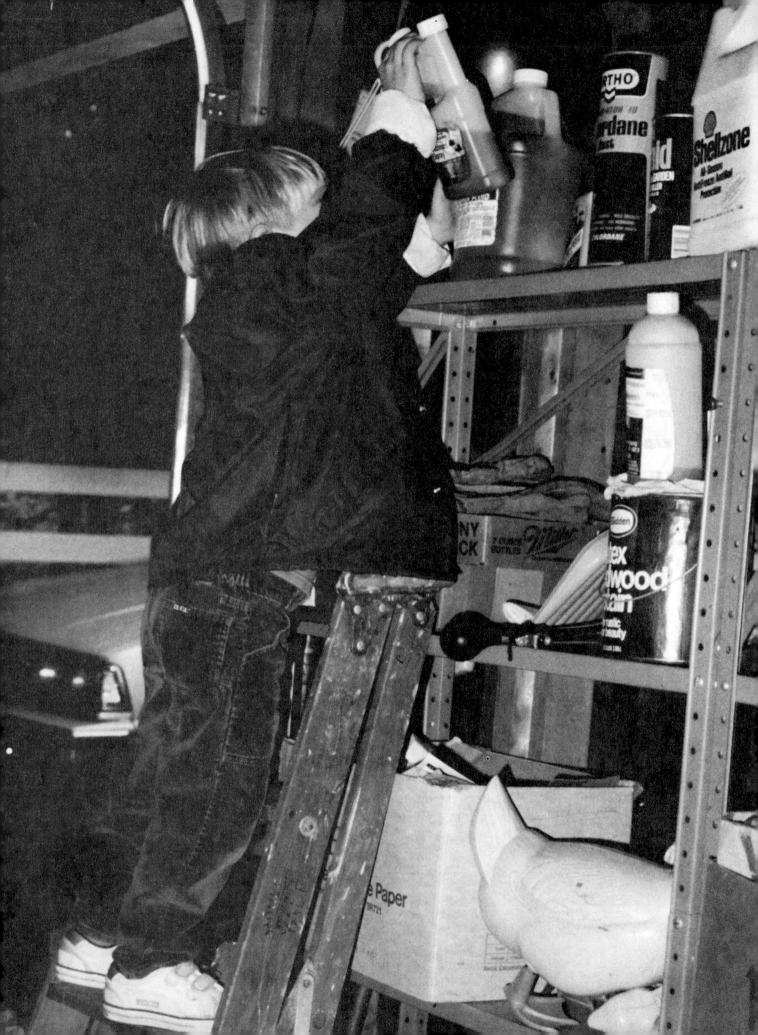

CHAPTER 12

MEDICAL EMERGENCIES

OBJECTIVES

At the conclusion of this chapter the reader will be able to:

1. Describe the purpose and function of insulin.

2. Describe the causes of insulin shock.

3. Describe the causes of diabetic coma.

4. Describe emergency care for a patient suffering an allergic reaction to an insect sting.

5. List four ways that poison can enter the body.

6. List three circumstances in which vomiting should not be induced in patients who have ingested poison.

7. Describe emergency care for a patient who has been bitten by:
   A pit viper
   A coral snake

8. Describe emergency care for a patient who has been stung by a marine animal.

9. Define *infectious disease*.

10. List four ways that infectious disease can be transmitted.

DIABETIC EMERGENCIES

Introduction

Diabetes is a disease caused by an inadequate secretion of the hormone insulin. Insulin helps regulate the utilization and storage of glucose. Glucose is a sugar molecule (a type of carbohydrate) used by the cells for energy. Glucose is absorbed into the bloodstream after a person eats food. As the blood glucose level rises, insulin is secreted and causes glucose to be moved into cells, where it is used for energy or stored for future use.

The body depends on glucose for its basic energy needs. While most cells also use other sources of fuel, such as fats, the brain depends almost exclusively on glucose. When deprived of glucose, the brain's function is altered and unconsciousness, seizures, and brain cell death can occur.

There are many complications of diabetes. These are related to a blood sugar that is too high or low, as well as complications from the abnormal metabolism that results from a lack of insulin. Two life-threatening conditions faced by diabetics that require emergency care are diabetic ketoacidosis (DKA) (diabetic coma) and hypoglycemia (low blood sugar or insulin shock).

Regulation of Glucose Metabolism

ACTIONS OF INSULIN

Insulin is produced within specialized cells in the pancreas, which are called the islets of Langerhans. As the glucose in the blood rises after a meal, the body secretes insulin to cause movement of the extra glucose and other food products into cells for immediate utilization as fuel and for storage for future needs. Some glucose is stored in the liver and muscle as a larger molecule called glycogen (composed of multiple glucose molecules). Some glucose is converted in adipose tissue to fat, where it is stored for future use. After transfer of glucose into the cells, the blood glucose level falls and insulin secretion is reduced.

The body uses both glucose and fats for fuel. After meals, glucose may be the main fuel used throughout the body. Between meals, fats are utilized. The brain, however, must continue to have an adequate supply of glucose, since it cannot burn fats for its energy needs.

ACTIONS OF GLUCAGON

To ensure an adequate supply of blood glucose between meals, the hormone glucagon causes stored forms of glucose to be released and glucose to be synthesized from other molecules. Glucagon is also secreted from the pancreas. Glucagon is secreted when the blood sugar level starts to fall. Glucagon causes glycogen to convert back to glucose molecules, which then enter the blood. It also can cause cells to make glucose from other molecules. The actions of insulin and glucagon maintain relatively constant blood concentration of glucose after eating and between meals.

Glucagon is released when there is increased utilization of glucose, such as during exercise or stress, or when there is reduced intake of glucose from meals (fasting). For example, during exercise, there is an increased and automatic uptake of glucose in the blood by muscle cells. (This uptake by actively exercising muscle does not depend on the presence of insulin.) As muscles consume the blood's glucose, the blood glucose level starts to fall, activating the release of glucagon. Glucagon in turn mobilizes stored glucose and makes glucose from other molecules to maintain the glucose needs of muscles and the brain.

Glucagon can be injected and is used to treat hypoglycemia (low blood sugar).

ACTIONS OF EPINEPHRINE

Epinephrine, released during stress or exercise, also has a glucagon-like effect. In hypoglycemia, or when there is low blood sugar, epinephrine causes further release of glucose from the liver. During stress, epinephrine increases the supply of both energy sources—glucose and fat (fatty acids)—to provide fuel for the fight-or-flight reaction.

Signs of epinephrine release can be noted in patients with hypoglycemia, such as pale, cool skin, tachycardia, sweating, and a normal or slightly elevated blood pressure.

Diabetes

Diabetics have a lack of insulin secretion by the pancreas. Untreated, they would have inappropriately high concentrations of blood glucose, with loss of glucose in the urine, and abnormal metabolism. Many people suffer from diabetes and call themselves diabetics. There are two general classifications of diabetics: type I and type II. The differences are based on severity of the disease, age of onset, and whether insulin is required as part of the treatment.

TYPE I—INSULIN-DEPENDENT DIABETES

Patients who have a severe or absolute lack of insulin are called type I, or insulin-dependent diabetics. Since the disease often develops early in life, it is also referred to as juvenile diabetes. Type I diabetics require

TABLE 12–1. Types of Insulin and Time of Action

Type	Onset	Peak	Duration
Regular	Early	4–6 hr	6–8 hr
Lente or NPH	Intermediate	8–12 hr	18–24 hr
Ultralente	Delayed	16–18 hr	>30 hr

TABLE 12–2. Oral Agents that Increase Secretion of Insulin from the Pancreas and have a Hypoglycemic Effect

Generic Name	Brand Name
Chlorpropamide	Diabinese, Glucamide
Glipizide	Glucotrol
Glyburide	Diabeta, Micronase
Tolazamide	Tolinase
Tolbutamide	Orinase

treatment with insulin, which must be injected intramuscularly on a daily basis. They must pay careful attention to their diet. There are different types of insulin. Insulin can be extracted from pork or beef pancreas and can also be made from human DNA. Insulin comes in different formulations, which vary according to time of onset, peak effect, and duration of action. Table 12–1 lists some common forms of insulin and their actions with respect to time of onset of action.

Different types of insulin can be given at different times during the day to manage predictable peaks of blood glucose following meals. Diabetics also receive careful dietary instructions. A patient's insulin intake and dietary regimen are individualized and adjusted according to the patient's life style, exercise patterns, and severity of disease.

Diabetics must be careful to balance their food intake with their medication. For example, if they take insulin and do not eat, their blood sugar level will drop too low. On the other hand, if they overeat or do not take insulin, their blood sugar level will rise too high. Other factors that can affect the balance between glucose and insulin are illness and exercise. Infections and fever may increase the body's insulin requirement. Exercise, with the automatic uptake of glucose by exercising muscles, increases the glucose requirements. Diabetics learn to adjust their food intake and insulin injections. They must test their urine or blood for glucose on a regular basis.

TYPE II—NON-INSULIN-DEPENDENT DIABETICS

Those diabetic patients who develop diabetes later in life may not require insulin injections. This type of diabetes is therefore referred to as non–insulin-dependent diabetes, type II, or maturity-onset diabetes. Some non-insulin-dependent diabetics can control their blood glucose by diet alone. Others require oral medications to stimulate the pancreas to secrete more insulin (Table 12–2). Some type II diabetics may eventually require insulin injections.

COMPLICATIONS OF DIABETES

Many complications of diabetes affect other organs in the body. Sometimes these effects are apparent only after several years. Generally, the younger the onset of

diabetes and the more severe the disease, the greater the chance of complications.

Diabetics are prone to accelerated atherosclerosis due to increased breakdown of fats that results in fatty deposits in the arteries. Complications from this narrowing of vessels include coronary artery disease, cerebrovascular disease, kidney disease, blindness, and ulcers on the distal lower extremities.

In addition, diabetics suffer from nerve damage. For example, they may have symmetrical (bilateral) loss of sensation, numbness, and pain and disagreeable sensations in the distal portions of the legs. The combination of impaired circulation and nerve damage in the legs can cause "diabetic foot." A diabetic is prone to repeated trauma to the foot because of the loss of sensation. Because the circulation is impaired, these minor injuries fail to heal and complications such as gangrene or necrosis of the toes and distal foot result.

Many diabetics suffer from a depletion of protein, weight loss, and weakness.

Diabetics are prone to infections. In turn, infections make the diabetes difficult to control, necessitate adjustments in daily insulin injections, and increase the chance of DKA or hypoglycemia. Infections are one of the major reasons that diabetics suffer diabetic ketoacidosis.

Diabetic Emergencies

There are two major problems encountered by EMTs: diabetic ketoacidosis and hypoglycemia (also called insulin shock).

DIABETIC KETOACIDOSIS

Diabetic ketoacidosis occurs when there is a relatively prolonged insulin deficiency, which causes the blood glucose to rise and fatty acids to be produced in the blood. Because of the complex complications that occur, DKA can be life-threatening.

DKA can occur in known diabetics who fail to properly balance their insulin intake with their diet and activity. It can occur in diabetics who are stressed by other illness, infections, and fever. In some diabetics it occurs despite proper management because they have such severe disease. It also can be the first symptom of diabetes to appear in someone who has no history of the disease.

The onset of DKA is gradual, and it may take hours to days for severe symptoms to appear.

SIGNS AND SYMPTOMS OF DIABETIC KETOACIDOSIS

Most signs and symptoms can be explained according to two major processes: dehydration caused by sugar loss in the urine and acidosis from the accumulation of fatty acids in the blood.

When there is a relative insufficiency of insulin, glucose cannot enter the cells and the concentration of glucose in the blood rises. As the blood passes through the kidneys, excess glucose is excreted in the urine and pulls water along with it by the process of osmosis. The water loss is great, with the patient urinating frequently to empty the bladder—a sign known as polyuria. As the patient loses body water and glucose, there are strong and frequent urges to replace fluids and foods—signs known as polydipsia (increased thirst) and polyphagia (increased appetite). Vomiting is a common complication, which worsens the fluid loss and prevents fluid replacement. Abdominal pain is frequently encountered, especially in children. If the condition is not corrected, the continued water loss leaves the patient dehydrated, hypovolemic, and, in late stages, hypotensive.

Despite the high blood glucose, the body senses a lack of glucose at the cellular level and increases the supply of both glucose and other energy sources. Glycogen breaks down, and glucose is made from other molecules, causing the blood glucose to rise still higher. However, without insulin, the glucose cannot be used effectively by the cells.

The body shifts to fat metabolism and breaks down fats to supply energy for the cells. The breakdown products from fats include fatty acids called ketoacids. In DKA, fatty acids are present in excess of the amount the body needs. These are real acids and cause the blood to become acidotic. Some fatty acids are converted to acetone. Acetone can vaporize easily, is expired in air, and gives a sweet, fruity odor to the breath—another sign seen in DKA.

To compensate for the buildup of acids in the blood, the diabetic person breathes faster and harder to blow off carbon dioxide. This deep and (usually) rapid pattern of respirations is known as Kussmaul's respirations. As the acidosis and blood derangements worsen, alterations in consciousness and coma occur. Progressive dehydration can lead to vascular collapse, and death can ensue if the condition is left untreated. The patient needs correction of the dehydration and acidosis and administration of insulin to shift the metabolism back to normal. DKA is a medical emergency. Review Table 12–3 to

TABLE 12–3. Signs and Symptoms of Diabetic Ketoacidosis

General Signs

Polyuria (frequent urination)
Polydipsia (excessive thirst)
Polyphagia (excessive hunger)
Vomiting
Abdominal pain (especially in children)
Fruity odor to the breath
Rapid and deep respirations (Kussmaul's respirations)
Altered mental status

Late Signs

Coma
Dehydration
Hypotension

reinforce the key signs and underlying pathophysiology related to diabetic ketoacidosis.

There are other metabolic disturbances that have signs similar to DKA. Some diabetic patients may have elevated blood sugar, dehydration, and an altered mental status without becoming acidotic or presenting with ketone breath and hyperventilation; this condition is referred to as hyperosmolar nonketotic coma.

Alcoholics, who tend to eat irregularly, can develop ketoacidosis without hyperglycemia because of the fasting and the breakdown of alcohol by the liver. They may even be hypoglycemic. They can have a ketone odor on the breath and experience hyperventilation.

Distinctions in the field are not important. These latter conditions are presented for your information, but the prehospital treatment for all of them is the same.

Hypoglycemia

Hypoglycemia, or abnormally low blood sugar, is the most common and treatable diabetic problem encountered in prehospital care. The major symptoms and signs are related to an altered mental status that is due to the brain's need for glucose and signs of epinephrine release.

Although hypoglycemia can occur for other reasons, the main cause is failure of diabetics to balance food intake with insulin administration (insulin shock). A typical patient might be a diabetic who took his or her insulin in the morning and then skipped meals. Depending on the onset of his or her insulin formulation, the patient is vulnerable to suffer hypoglycemia when the insulin action peaks. Other causes of hypoglycemia include insulin-secreting tumors, prolonged fasting, administration of hypoglycemic drugs, liver failure, and a combination of alcohol consumption and fasting. Never blindly attribute an altered mental status to alcohol use without considering the possibility of hypoglycemia as the cause.

Paradoxically, some individuals may secrete too much insulin after a meal and suffer a hypoglycemic reaction a few hours after eating.

SIGNS AND SYMPTOMS

ALTERED MENTAL STATUS. The signs of altered mental status are extremely variable. It is not uncommon for hypoglycemic patients to be mistaken as psychotic since they may display combativeness, hostility, and bizarre behavior.

The patient may progress from an agitated and excited state to a sleepier or more lethargic state with less spontaneous conversation, disturbances in judgment, and confusion. Further deterioration may result in seizures or coma. If untreated, severe hypoglycemia leads to brain death.

OTHER SIGNS OF HYPOGLYCEMIA. There are signs and symptoms that often precede alterations in mental status. Early signs may include hunger, nausea, uneasiness, weakness, and increased salivation. As the blood sugar level dips lower, the sympathetic nervous system and epinephrine responses are noted. Related signs include tachycardia; cold, pale, clammy skin; dilated pupils; and increased nervousness, trembling, and excitability. Review Table 12–4, which summarizes the essential signs of hypoglycemia.

TABLE 12–4. Signs and Symptoms Related to Hypoglycemia

Mental Changes

Lethargy
Less spontaneous speech
Bizarre behavior
Agitated, excitable, combative, or hostile behavior
Confusion
Seizures
Coma
(Can be confused with a psychiatric patient)

Early Signs (Not Always Elicited or Present)

Hunger
Nausea
Weakness
Uneasy feeling
Salivation

Sympathetic Nervous System Signs (with Lowered Blood Sugars)

Tachycardia
Pale, cool skin
Sweating
Dilated pupils
Trembling
Excitability

Note: In some cases only signs and symptoms of altered mental status may be present.

INDIVIDUAL VARIATION. Signs and symptoms vary from individual to individual. Some patients are prone to hypoglycemia. They often have the same symptoms with each event, which become known to family members and coworkers.

Many patients have general physical signs and symptoms before mental changes occur. Others may have no signs other than the altered mental status itself.

The onset of hypoglycemia is variable as well. An injection of rapidly acting insulin without eating causes early onset of hypoglycemia. Insulin-secreting tumors or long-acting insulin injected without eating may cause a gradual onset.

Often the signs of hypoglycemia are related to the blood glucose level. However, there are variations in the blood glucose level and related symptoms in different individuals. Since many diabetics test their blood glucose level at home, and some ambulance services use blood glucose tests in the field, the EMT should be forewarned that hypoglycemic reactions can occur with blood glucose in a "normal" range in insulin-dependent diabetics who have experienced a rapid fall in glucose.

ASSESSMENT OF THE DIABETIC PATIENT

The main distinction to make when encountering a diabetic emergency is whether the patient is hypoglycemic or in diabetic ketoacidosis. This is done by comparing the symptoms and signs encountered with the typical presentations of these two types of emergencies.

Either the history or the physical findings may alert you to these problems. During the history, you may first learn of diabetes during discussion of the chief complaint, history of present illness, medications, or past medical history. During the past medical history, EMTs routinely inquire about the presence of heart disease, hypertension, chronic obstructive pulmonary disease (COPD), or diabetes. During the primary survey, acetone breath and Kussmaul's respirations may be your first indication that there is a diabetic problem. Altered mental status should always cause the EMT to suspect a diabetic emergency.

CHIEF COMPLAINT. Often, diabetics or their family members offer the diabetic history as part of the chief complaint. Diabetics and family members are taught to recognize signs of hypoglycemia, and you may receive a call concerning a patient with "low blood sugar" or "insulin shock." Altered mental status, including bizarre behavior, seizures, or coma, should always raise the suspicion of hypoglycemia. Shortness of breath or abdominal pain may also be noted as the chief complaint in a patient with DKA.

HISTORY OF THE PRESENT ILLNESS. While taking the history of the present illness, you may discover that

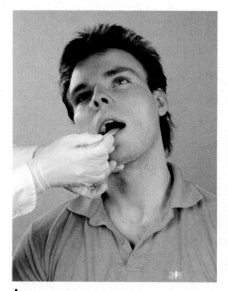
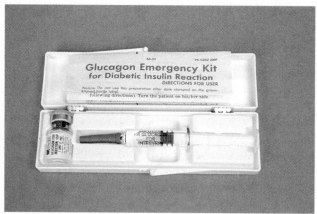

A   B

FIGURE 12–1. (*A*) Checking for a gag reflex. (*B*) A glucagon emergency kit.

a patient has taken insulin and not eaten or that the patient has not taken insulin. The patient may also report a history of frequent urination, thirst, and hunger.

PAST MEDICAL HISTORY.   As part of the past medical history, patients should be asked whether they have diabetes. During the medication history, they may indicate that they take insulin or a hypoglycemic drug. When this history is encountered, be sure to ask the following questions:

- When did you last take your medications?
- When did you last eat?
- When did you last measure your blood or urine glucose and what were the results?
- When did you last test your urine for acetone and what were the results?
- Have you experienced excessive urination and thirst?
- Did you have a recent infection or experience stress?
- Did you take additional sugar or glucagon before our arrival?
- Have you had similar episodes in the past? If so what was the problem?

PHYSICAL EXAMINATION.   The physical examination includes a search for a fruity odor on the breath, signs of dehydration, and evidence of adrenaline release. Review Tables 12–3 and 12–4 for common signs and symptoms.

TREATMENT OF DIABETIC PATIENTS

The treatment of hypoglycemia is straightforward, namely the administration of oral or intravenous glucose. An alternate method is to administer intramuscular glucagon. The administration of glucose or glucagon can

rapidly reverse a condition that otherwise could cause permanent brain damage. In fact, because of the simplicity and safety of therapy, administration of glucose or glucagon is performed routinely when hypoglycemia is suspected. It will not hurt the patient who has high glucose or even diabetic ketoacidosis.

CONSCIOUS VERSUS UNCONSCIOUS PATIENTS. In conscious patients, oral glucose solutions are preferred. One can give soda, juices, sugar water, or other glucose-rich solutions. Obviously, unconscious patients cannot be given oral fluids. Patients with an altered mental status should be tested by stimulating their posterior pharynx with a tongue blade to determine if a gag reflex is present (Fig. 12–1A). Give them small sips to drink to see if they can swallow without coughing or choking.

If there is no gag reflex, or if the patient is lethargic or does not have the ability to swallow, then other treatment may be necessary. Glucose, 50 ml of a 50% solution,* can be administered intravenously and a pretreatment blood sample can be drawn to test for glucose at the hospital (or in some systems in the field).

Glucagon is another drug carried by some diabetics that can be administered intramuscularly (Fig. 12–1B). A dose of 1 mg of glucagon can increase the blood sugar in 8 to 10 minutes. The patient usually responds in 5 to 20 minutes. It may not work in patients with low glycogen stores such as very young children, alcoholics, or malnourished individuals.

Some EMS systems may permit EMTs to administer glucagon or intravenous glucose to diabetics who are unable to swallow oral glucose. Figure 12–2 illustrates how to give an intramuscular injection of glucagon.

---

* In children, less concentrated solutions of glucose are given intravenously. Follow local protocols.

PROCEDURE 12-1 ADMINISTERING AN INTRAMUSCULAR MEDICATION

In this example, the medication is glucagon, which comes as dry powder (1 mg) and requires reconstitution (mixing) with 1 ml of diluting solution.

Note: Most emergency medications come already mixed. Always be familiar with the particular requirements of measuring and mixing any medication you administer. Confirm the medication, dose, and route of administration with your protocols or medical control physician (if appropriate).

1. Assemble necessary equipment (Fig. 12–2A).
2. Check for correct medication, correct dose, and expiration date, and determine that the patient is not allergic to this kind of medication (Fig. 12–2B).
3. Wipe the top of the diluting solution vial with alcohol (Fig. 12–2C).
4. Inject .5 cc of air into the vial and then withdraw all of the solution (1 ml) into the syringe (Fig. 12–2D).
5. Wipe the top of the medication vial with alcohol (Fig. 12–2E).

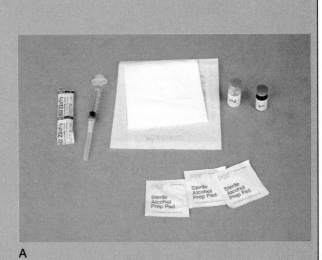

A

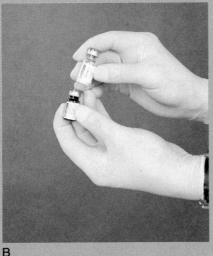

B

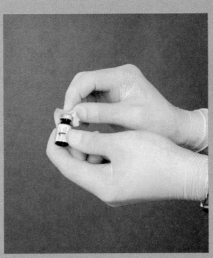

C

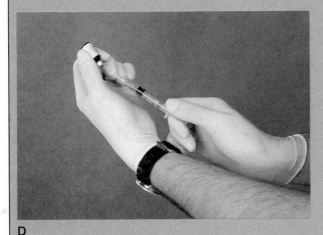

D

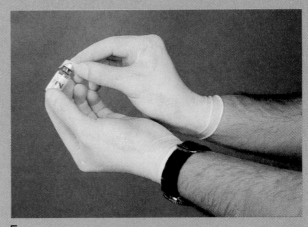

E

FIGURE 12–2A. Necessary equipment includes medication, diluting solution, proper-size syringe, proper-size needle (18- to 22-gauge, 1 to 1½ inches), sterile 4 × 4 pad, and alcohol wipes.

Continued on following page

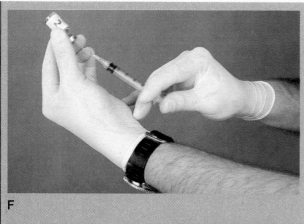

F

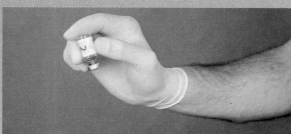

G

6. Inject the diluting solution into the medication vial (Fig. 12–2F).
7. Mix (by shaking) the water and medication. Then reinsert the syringe and withdraw the mixed contents into the syringe. Hold the syringe upright and clear air bubbles from the top of the syringe by tapping the syringe and expelling excess air (Fig. 12–2G).
8. Choose the correct injection site (mid-deltoid muscle) and prepare the patient for injection (Fig. 12–2H).
9. Clean the injection site with an alcohol wipe (Fig. 12–2I).
10. Properly insert the needle at a 90-degree angle, keeping the skin stretched (Fig. 12–2J and K).
11. Pull back on the plunger to check for blood. (If blood appears, withdraw the needle to avoid injecting directly into a blood vessel.) (Fig. 12–2L).
12. Inject the medication with a smooth, steady compression of the plunger (Fig. 12–2M).
13. Withdraw the needle in a quick, smooth motion, massage the injection site to aid in medication absorption, and properly dispose of the needle and syringe in an appropriate receptacle (e.g., sharps container) (Fig. 12–2N).

Note: Never recap a needle prior to disposal. This would increase the chances of a needle stick with a contaminated needle.

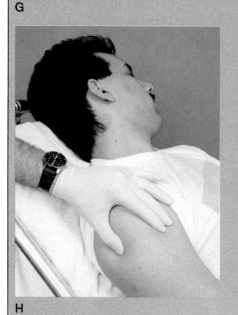

H

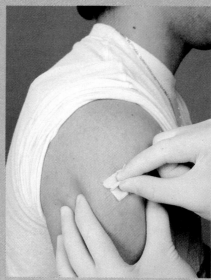

I

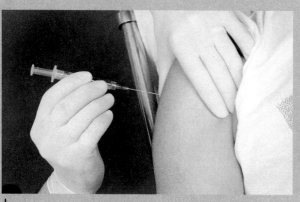

J

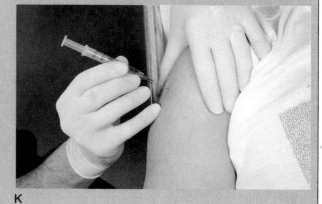

K

FIGURE 12–2. *Continued*

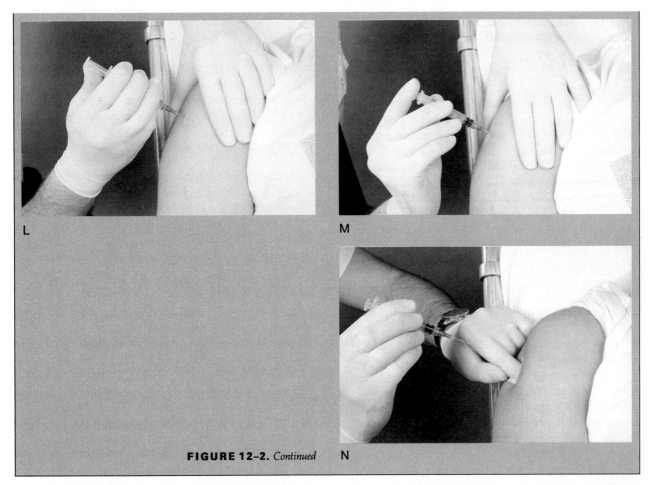

FIGURE 12–2. *Continued*

SUPPORTIVE CARE. Basic supportive care includes airway management, administration of supplemental oxygen, maintenance of body temperature, and proper positioning for shock or coma. Indications for these treatments should be obvious from the assessment of the patient. Patients with severe dehydration and hy-potension should be rapidly transported to the hospital. Carefully review the protocol for altered mental status, which summarizes the care of nontraumatic patients, including confused or unconscious diabetics who may have low blood sugar.

P R O T O C O L

ALTERED MENTAL STATUS (NONTRAUMATIC AND WITHOUT RESPIRATORY OR CARDIOVASCULAR COMPLICATIONS)*

1. Assure that the patient's airway is open and that breathing and circulation are adequate, and suction as necessary.

2. Administer high-concentration oxygen. In children, humidified oxygen is preferred.

3. Obtain and record the vital signs, including determining the patient's level of consciousness.

4. IF THE PATIENT IS UNRESPONSIVE OR RESPONDS ONLY TO PAINFUL STIMULI, transport immediately, keeping the patient warm.

   IF THE PATIENT IS CONSCIOUS, HAS A GAG REFLEX, AND IS ABLE TO DRINK WITHOUT ASSIST-ANCE, provide glucose or a sugar solution (if available) by mouth, then transport, keeping the patient warm.

5. Repeat and record the vital signs, including the level of consciousness and Glasgow Coma Scale, en route as often as the situation indicates.

6. Record all patient care information, including the patient's medical history and all treatment provided, on a prehospital care report.

Adapted from Manual for Emergency Medical Technicians. Emergency Medical Services Program. Albany, New York State Department of Health, 1990.

* Local protocols may include testing blood for glucose and/or administration of intravenous glucose or intramuscular glucagon.

ANAPHYLAXIS

Introduction

Anaphylaxis is an allergic condition in which an *antibody–antigen* reaction results in the release of substances that can cause shock, bronchoconstriction, and airway obstruction. The onset of this reaction can be extremely rapid and can result in death within minutes. These patients need immediate treatment to reverse the effects of the anaphylactic reaction, maintain their airway patency, and stabilize their cardiovascular condition.

Pathophysiology
ANTIBODY–ANTIGEN REACTIONS

An antigen is a substance that is recognized as foreign to the body. An antibody is a protein that combines with an antigen to neutralize toxins that enter the body or to fight infection. Normally, antibodies are helpful in fighting disease and toxins. Antibody–antigen reactions take place constantly and are part of the body's normal defense against foreign materials and infection. Anaphylaxis is an antibody–antigen reaction gone "haywire," in which the effects are detrimental rather than protective.

In anaphylaxis, the reaction of an antigen with an antibody causes the release of chemicals such as histamine. Histamine causes blood vessels to dilate and capillaries to leak. With profound dilation of blood vessels, the blood pressure falls, resulting in shock. With plasma leakage from the capillaries, swelling of the skin, face, mouth, tongue, and other airway structures can occur.

The most common manifestations of an anaphylactic reaction involve the skin, respiratory, circulatory, and gastrointestinal systems. This is in contrast to other common allergic reactions, such as hayfever, which cause mild or local symptoms.

COMMON AGENTS THAT CAUSE ANAPHYLAXIS

Although multiple agents can provoke anaphylaxis, the most common include certain drugs, foods, and insect bites.

The antibiotics penicillin, cephalosporins (Keflex, etc.), tetracycline, and nitrofurantoin and local anesthetics such as lidocaine and procaine have frequently been implicated in anaphylactic reactions. Some dyes used for x-ray contrast studies can cause an anaphylactoid ("anaphylactic-like" reaction) response, as can anti-inflammatory drugs such as aspirin and indomethacin (Indocin).

Foods that cause anaphylaxis in sensitized individuals include nuts, shellfish, eggs, chocolate, cottonseed oil, grains, and beans. Food preservatives such as sulfites have also been implicated.

Insect stings, especially from yellow jackets, honey bees, wasps, and hornets, have also been associated with anaphylaxis. Honey bees leave their stinger in the victim, which can cause continued exposure. Fire ants, seen in the South, have been known to cause anaphylaxis.

THE ANAPHYLACTIC REACTION

As mentioned, when antigens react with the preformed antibodies in an anaphylactic reaction, specialized cells are activated to release histamine and other chemical substances. The actions of agents like histamine explain many of the signs and symptoms seen in anaphylaxis. These actions include the following:

The constriction of bronchial smooth muscle results in bronchial constriction and constriction of smooth muscle in the gastrointestinal tract causes abdominal cramps, vomiting, and diarrhea.

Increased permeability of capillaries causes leakage of plasma and protein, resulting in edema and loss of blood volume.

Dilation of the arterial vessels results in decreased peripheral resistance and a fall in blood pressure.

Dilation of the venous system causes venous pooling of blood, which in turn causes decreased venous return and decreased cardiac output and hypotension.

Increased mucous secretions in the respiratory tree and gastrointestinal tract further contribute to respiratory and gastrointestinal problems, which explains some of the symptoms seen in more localized allergic reactions (nasal congestion, sneezing, etc.).

Upper airway edema and acute bronchospasm lead to respiratory failure. Vasodilation and hypovolemia cause circulatory collapse. These are the primary complications of an anaphylactic reaction and may cause death.

Anaphylactic reactions vary significantly from patient to patient and with the degree of hypersensitivity, the amount of antigen absorbed or injected, and the route of exposure (Table 12–5).

Patient Assessment
HISTORY

Some patients may be aware that they are hypersensitive to a particular substance and can help you with this history. Indeed, some patients may carry identification bands or medication to block the anaphylactic response. An anaphylactic kit contains epinephrine and antihistamine agents. Other patients may not be aware that they are hypersensitive. You may connect the onset of symptoms with the administration of a drug, ingestion

TABLE 12–5. Symptoms and Signs of Anaphylaxis

Symptoms

Anxiety
Itching
✓ Sneezing, coughing, wheezing
Cramping, abdominal pain, vomiting, diarrhea
Facial, pharyngeal, and laryngeal edema; hoarseness; loss of voice, fainting

Signs

Hives, angioedema
Hypotension, tachycardia
✓ Wheezing, dyspnea
Stridor
Cardiac or respiratory arrest

of a particular food, or an insect sting. Usually, anaphylactic symptoms occur almost immediately after antigen contact. However, the route of administration (injection versus ingestion) affects the speed of onset.

PHYSICAL ASSESSMENT

SKIN AND GENERAL SIGNS. Common signs of an impending anaphylactic reaction involve several body systems. A feeling of warmth often precedes the reaction. The patient may describe tingling of the face, extremities, and upper chest region. Itching and generalized flushing of the skin and urticaria or "hives" (raised, red patches of skin) may also be present (Fig. 12–3A and B). Angioedema, a condition that results from vasodilation and causes hives and swelling of the face (especially the lips)

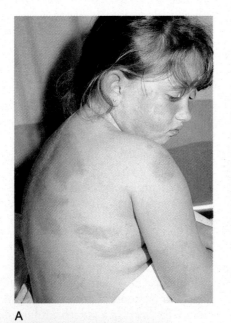

A

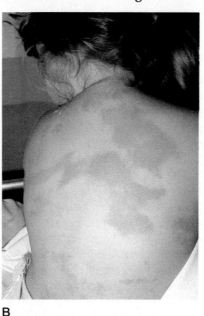

B

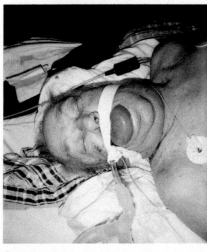

C

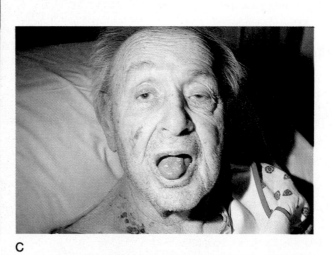

C

FIGURE 12–3. Urticaria. (A and B) Raised, red, itchy blotches on the skin are obvious on this young girl with an allergic reaction. Urticaria may be seen with anaphylaxis. However, it is most commonly seen without any signs of anaphylaxis. (C) This patient had an anaphylactic reaction, probably to a medication, with rapid swelling of the tongue and cardiac arrest from hypoxia. Intubation around the tongue and administration of epinephrine restored his airway and allowed for resuscitation. The patient later awoke and was discharged from the hospital in good health. (C, Courtesy of Lester Kallus, M.D.)

and airway, is also likely. The patient also may exhibit nasal congestion, sneezing, itching around the eyes, and abdominal pain. The patient may express a sense of impending doom (Fig. 12–3C).

RESPIRATORY SIGNS. As these reactions continue, the airway may become narrowed causing dyspnea, throat tightness, hoarseness, stridor, and other signs of respiratory distress, including cyanosis, use of accessory muscles of breathing, and suprasternal and intercostal retractions. Wheezing and rhonchi may be present, due to the narrowing of the bronchioles secondary to bronchoconstriction and mucus secretion. However, in the later stages, breath sounds may be absent or diminished due to hypoventilation. Ultimately, the patient may present with complete airway obstruction and respiratory failure. This can be the result of total airway closure or exhaustion due to the increased work of breathing.

CARDIOVASCULAR SIGNS. The cardiovascular signs associated with an anaphylactic reaction are primarily related to distributive and hypovolemic shock.

Diffuse vasodilation initially may cause a generalized "pink" appearance, due to increased blood flow to the skin. This phase may be short-lived as the cardiovascular system fights to maintain pressure and perfusion in an enlarging vascular space. Fluid loss, occurring through leakage of the capillaries, results in hypovolemic shock that is due to plasma loss to the cell and interstitial space; this further stresses the cardiovascular system.

As in most shock states, the early compensatory mechanism includes an increase in the pulse and respiratory rate. The skin becomes pale and diaphoretic as the patient decompensates. Ultimately, the patient becomes hypotensive and shows signs of decreased brain perfusion, including an altered mental state ranging from agitation to lethargy to coma.

Treatment

The extremis patient suffering an anaphylactic reaction requires the immediate administration of epi-

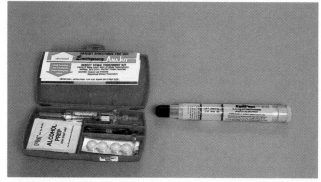

FIGURE 12–4. An AnaKit and EpiPen. Commercially available kits carried by persons with a history of anaphylaxis.

nephrine, which blocks the effects caused by the reaction. The primary goals of prehospital care of the anaphylactic patient include airway management, ventilation and oxygenation, support of circulation, and rapid transport.

LIFESAVING MEDICATIONS

The only definitive treatment for anaphylactic shock is the injection of epinephrine and other drugs to combat the reaction. The patient who carries the anaphylactic kit should self-administer the medications as quickly as possible. The EMT may assist patients to administer epinephrine according to state and local protocols.

Epinephrine is usually administered subcutaneously or intramuscularly at a dose of 0.3 mg (0.3 ml) of a 1:1000 solution. The pediatric dose is 0.01 mg/kg of a 1:1000 solution administered subcutaneously. In extreme circumstances, a more dilute (1:10,000) solution of epinephrine may be given intravenously or down an endotracheal tube. Some prescribed regimens also include the administration of an antihistamine, administered by mouth. Benadryl is a potent antihistamine that can block the effects of the reaction. However, once the reaction has taken place, antihistamines are of less value. If no medication is available at the scene, rapid transport is essential. See Figure 12–4 for examples of kits carried by patients with a history of anaphylaxis. Also, see Figure 12–5, which illustrates how to give a subcutaneous injection.

PROCEDURE 12–2 ADMINISTERING A SUBCUTANEOUS MEDICATION

In this example, the medication is epinephrine, or adrenaline, which is already mixed and in solution. Most emergency medications come already mixed. There is 1 mg of epinephrine in 1 ml of solution (1:1000 solution). Always be familiar with the particular requirements of measuring and/or mixing any medication you administer. Confirm the medication, dose, and route of administration with your protocols or medical control physician (if appropriate).
1. Assemble necessary equipment (Fig. 12–5A).

2. Check for correct medication, correct dose, and expiration date, and determine that the patient is not allergic to the medication (Fig. 12–5B).
3. Clear the top of the ampule of excess medication by tapping with your finger (Fig. 12–5C).
4. Carefully break off the top of the ampule at its neck using a 4 × 4 to prevent injury from the edges of glass (Fig. 12–5D and E).
5. Draw up the appropriate dose of medication into the syringe (0.3 to 0.5 ml) (Fig. 12–5F).

Continued

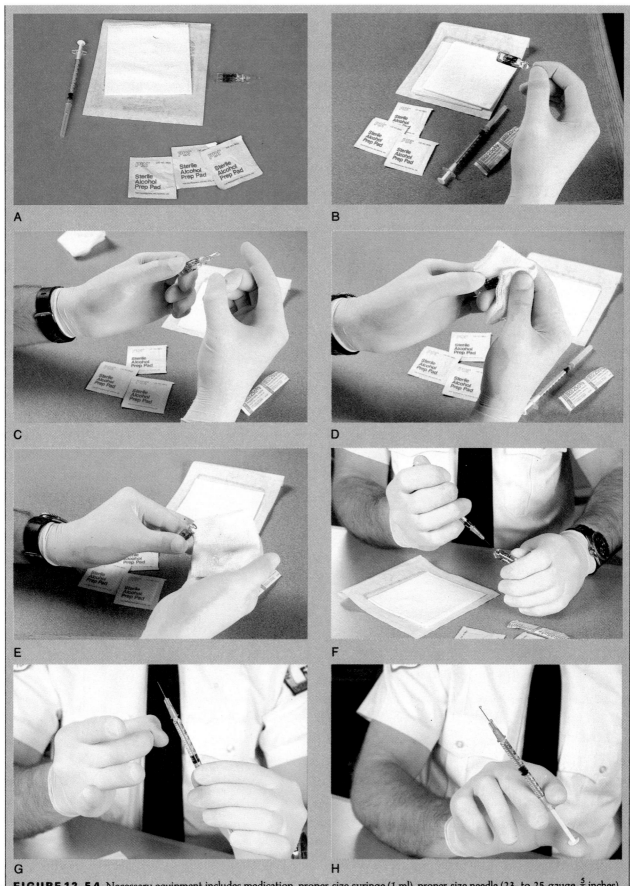

FIGURE 12–5A. Necessary equipment includes medication, proper-size syringe (1 ml), proper-size needle (23- to 25-gauge, $\frac{5}{8}$ inches), sterile 4 × 4 pad, and alcohol wipes.

Illustration continued on following page

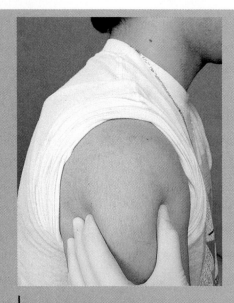

I

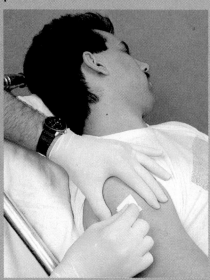

J

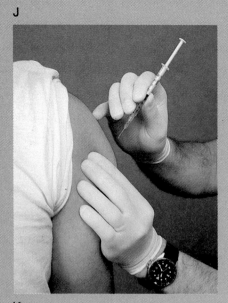

K

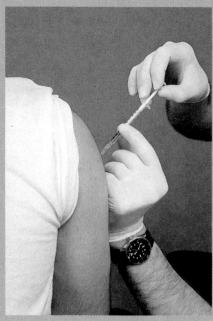

L

6. Hold the syringe upright and clear air bubbles from the top of the syringe by tapping the syringe and expelling excess air (Fig. 12–5*G* and *H*).
7. Choose the correct injection site (skin over mid-deltoid muscle) and prepare the patient for injection (Fig. 12–5*I*).
8. Clean the injection site with an alcohol wipe (Fig. 12–5*J*).
9. Properly insert the needle at a 45-degree angle, keeping the skin pinched to ensure injection into fatty tissue (Fig. 12–5*K*).
10. Pull back on the plunger to check for blood. (If blood appears, withdraw the needle to avoid injecting directly into a blood vessel.) (Fig. 12–5*L*).
11. Inject the medication with a smooth, steady compression of the plunger (Fig. 12–5*M*).
12. Withdraw the needle in a quick, smooth motion, massage the injection site to aid in medication absorption, and properly dispose of the needle and syringe in an appropriate receptacle (e.g., sharps container) (Fig. 12–5*N*).

Note: Never recap a needle prior to disposal. This would increase the changes of a needle stick with a contaminated needle.

13. With an epinephrine-loaded syringe from AnaKit (an insect sting emergency kit carried by people with a history of anaphylaxis) there is a rectangular plunger that allows for administration of two premeasured doses of 0.3 ml of a 1:1000 solution. After holding the syringe upright, push the plunger to clear out air. Then rotate the plunger one-quarter turn (clockwise) and inject as above, pushing the plunger until it stops (0.3 ml). By rotating the plunger another one-quarter turn to the right, a second dose can be given if indicated (Fig. 12–5*O* and *P*).

FIGURE 12–5. *Continued*

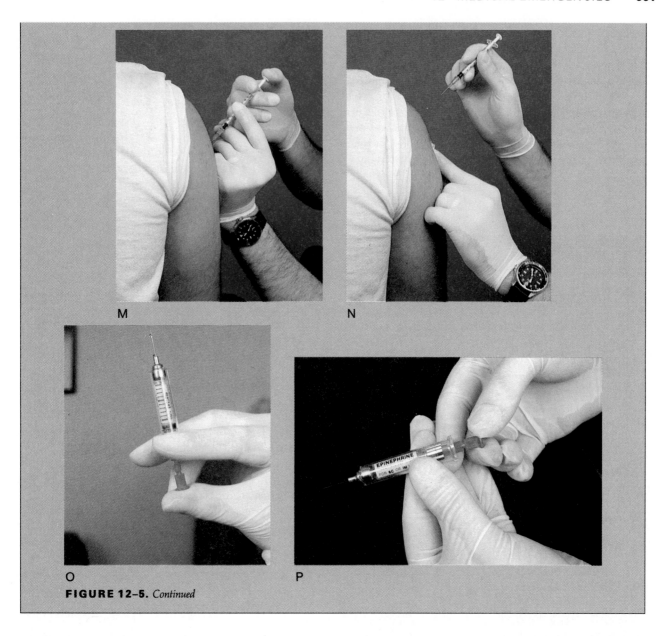

M   N

O   P

FIGURE 12–5. *Continued*

AIRWAY MANAGEMENT, VENTILATION, AND OXYGENATION

COMPLETE AIRWAY OBSTRUCTION. If the patient is exhibiting signs of complete airway obstruction, rapid transport is essential. Since airway obstruction procedures (abdominal and chest thrusts and finger sweeps) are of no value, rapid transport is the main priority. These patients require intubation, cricothyroidotomy, or tracheostomy to establish a patent airway.

During transport "forced positive pressure" with high-concentration oxygen should be attempted in the hope of delivering a minimal but lifesaving amount of air.

PATIENTS WITH RESPIRATORY DISTRESS OR FAILURE. High-concentration oxygen through a nonrebreather mask should be administered to all patients who are exhibiting signs of respiratory distress. Patients who are hypoventilating, as evidenced by respiratory rate, chest excursion, or altered mental status, should receive assisted ventilation with 100% oxygen.

CARDIOVASCULAR SUPPORT

Patients who are exhibiting signs of hypovolemic or distributive shock should be placed in the supine position with their legs elevated. The pneumatic antishock garment (PASG) should be applied according to the criteria of local protocols. The PASG can increase peripheral resistance and improve the circulatory status of the patient. All of these procedures should be performed while en route to the hospital, since the patient needs medication and may require invasive procedures to secure the airway or stabilize the cardiovascular condition.

Avoid rough handling, which can increase oxygen

consumption and further aggravate the patient's condition. As with all shock patients, prevent the loss of body heat so as to conserve energy and decrease the cardiovascular workload.

Vital signs should be recorded every 5 minutes when circumstances permit. Do not allow the patient to take anything by mouth except prescribed medications that may help reduce the effects of anaphylaxis. Review the following protocol for the treatment of anaphylaxis.

☤ P R O T O C O L ☤

ANAPHYLAXIS

1. Ensure that the patient's airway is open and that breathing and circulation are adequate, and suction as necessary.

2. Assist the patient in self-administration of prescribed epinephrine as necessary if the patient has an anaphylaxis (bee-sting) kit.

3. Transport the patient IMMEDIATELY in a position of comfort, while keeping the patient warm, reassuring the patient, and loosening tight clothing.

4. Administer high-concentration oxygen and assist ventilations if necessary.

5. IF VENTILATORY STATUS IS INADEQUATE, REFER IMMEDIATELY TO THE *RESPIRATORY ARREST (NONTRAUMATIC)* PROTOCOL.

6. Assess for shock. IF SHOCK IS PRESENT, REFER IMMEDIATELY TO THE *SHOCK* PROTOCOL.

7. IF CARDIAC ARREST OCCURS, PERFORM CPR ACCORDING TO AHA/ARC STANDARDS.

8. Obtain and record the initial vital signs, and repeat en route as often as the situation indicates. BE ALERT FOR CHANGES IN THE LEVEL OF CONSCIOUSNESS!

9. Record all patient care information, including the patient's medical history and all treatment provided, on a prehospital care report.

> If the patient is a child, maintain a calm approach to the parent and child. ALLOW the child to assume and maintain a position of comfort or to be held by the parent, preferably in an upright position.

> In children, avoid agitating the child. Administration of oxygen, preferably HUMIDIFIED, is best accomplished by allowing the parent to hold the face mask if tolerated, about 6 to 8 inches from the child's face.

Adapted from Manual for Emergency Medical Technicians. Emergency Medical Services Program. Albany, New York State Department of Health, 1990.

TREATMENT OF BITES AND STINGS

When an anaphylactic reaction occurs secondary to a bite or sting, additional measures are necessary to slow the absorption of the toxin.

Place a constricting band above an injury in an extremity. This band should be tight enough to reduce venous return but loose enough so as not to obstruct arterial flow. If it is present, carefully scrape the stinger or venom sack away. Place an ice pack over the bitten area to cause vasoconstriction and further reduce the rate of absorption.

POISONS AND OVERDOSES

Introduction
DEFINITIONS

A *poison* is defined by Webster's Dictionary as a substance that through its chemical action usually kills, injures, or impairs an organism. *Toxicology* is the study of poisons. The effects of a poison are said to be *toxic*, and poisons are often referred to as *toxins*.

An *overdose* is a term applied to self-administration of drugs, taken in excess or in combination with other agents, to the point where poisoning occurs. In this sense, poisoning can be seen to be a matter of degree. A substance that is beneficial in one dose can be detrimental or even lethal when taken in excess. An overdose can involve therapeutic drugs; alcohol; or illicit, or "recreational," drugs.

A poisoning may be *accidental*, for example when a child ingests household products or medications, thinking they are food or candy (Fig. 12–6). Or a poisoning can be *intentional*, as in a suicide attempt or murder. Poisoning can also occur from plants or from insect, snake, and arthropod venom. Poisoning that occurs by the latter means is referred to as *envenomation*.

Poisons can enter the body through the gastrointestinal tract (ingestion), airway (inhalation), or skin (absorption) or by injection (including envenomation).

An EMT might suspect a poisoning for several reasons. Signs of poisoning include nausea and vomiting, abdominal pain, diarrhea, dilation or constriction of the pupils, excessive salivation or sweating, abnormal respiration, unconsciousness, and convulsions. The history may indicate poisoning before signs or symptoms have occurred.

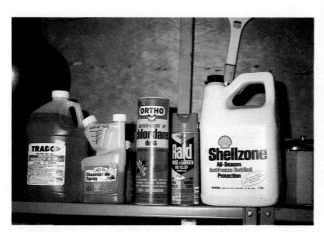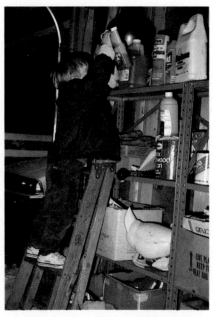

FIGURE 12–6. Hazardous household materials. Toxic substances commonly found in garages include antifreeze (ethylene glycol), insecticides, chlordane, organophosphate and organophosphate-type poisons, and windshield deicer containing methanol. Note the child who crawls up the ladder and thereby gets into toxic substances.

CARDINAL RULES IN DEALING WITH SUSPECTED POISONS

TREAT THE PATIENT, NOT THE POISON. The clinical condition of the patient, rather than the specifics of the overdose, is the first priority in almost all cases. Establish the need for cardiorespiratory support and maintain and protect the airway. There are exceptions to this rule, however, since a few toxins, such as cyanide or nitrites, may require rapid transportation of the patient to a hospital for administration of an antidote. However, most cases require supportive care. Even in cases for which rapid transport for antidote administration is the lifesaving step, patients benefit from ventilations with high-concentration oxygen en route.

PROTECT YOURSELF AND BYSTANDERS FROM INADVERTENT POISONING. Toxic gases and toxins absorbed through the skin can be as dangerous to the EMT as to the victim. EMTs must take precautions to ensure that they do not enter a toxic environment without protection. Likewise, they must be careful lest they inadvertently contaminate their skin with a toxin that can be absorbed. The EMT should take precautions so as not to become another victim.

LOOK FOR CLUES OF TRAUMA. Does an evaluation of the scene, physical findings, or the history indicate that the patient also suffered trauma? Overdoses can lead to falls, automobile accidents, and other traumatic injuries. This information is important for both field and hospital evaluation, particularly with patients who are unconscious or who have an altered mental status. Conversely, in clear-cut cases of trauma, do not overlook the possibility that the patient is also suffering from poisoning or, more likely, the effects of alcohol or drug overdose.

MAINTAIN A HIGH LEVEL OF SUSPICION. Poisons are not always obvious. This applies to individual cases and cases where several individuals suddenly become ill. Clues are available to EMTs that are not evident to emergency department staff.

Look for patterns of multiple exposures to help identify poison epidemics in a community. For example, many people in a building suffering from headaches, nausea or vomiting, and loss of consciousness suggests the possibility that carbon monoxide poisoning has occurred through a common ventilation system.

The fact that Tylenol had been contaminated with cyanide poison in Chicago several years ago was discovered in part by alert EMTs who overheard two ambulance radio transmissions that described young patients inexplicably struck down by what appeared to be central nervous system and cardiac problems after they had recently taken Tylenol.

Overview
INCIDENCE

There are over 5 million poisonings each year in the United States, accounting for over 10,000 deaths.

Most accidental poisonings occur in children under the age of 5 years. The toddler who puts everything into his or her mouth may accidentally ingest household products, unsecured pills, and other agents. In the adolescent and older groups, suicide is often attempted by poisoning, usually via ingestion. Recreational drug users and addicts may overdose by injecting drugs of unknown strength purchased illegally or by using combinations of different drugs. Industrial accidents account for a significant number of poisonings. Snakes, certain insects, arthropods, and sea creatures can cause poisoning through injection of their venom.

There are over 250,000 potentially poisonous drugs and commercial products.

Because of the number of poisonings that occur each year and the extensive number of potentially toxic products, poison control centers have been established in regions throughout the country.

POISON CONTROL CENTERS

Poison control centers provide information on toxins, management of poisoning victims, and antidotes. A regional poison control center is accessible by phone at all times to physicians, EMS personnel, and the public. Learn and remember the number of your regional poison control center. Often they have "handles" to aid recall. For example, the New York City Poison Control Center's telephone number is (212) P-O-I-S-O-N-S.

Poison control centers can do the following:

1. Provide access to experts in toxicology. Poison control centers have full-time staffs and part-time consultants who can be reached by phone.

2. Coordinate emergency response. Within a region, a poison control center can provide advice to patients at home, refer some to area hospitals with poisoning care capabilities, and advise EMTs, physicians, and nurses on immediate and long-term treatment.

TYPES OF EXPOSURE

INGESTION. The most common route of entry into the body for poisons is ingestion through the gastrointestinal tract. This type of ingestion includes the suicidal patient who takes all the pills in the medicine cabinet, the street alcoholic who drinks methanol (wood alcohol, windshield-washer solution) in place of ethanol, and the toddler who roams into a neighbor's garage and drinks from an open bottle of antifreeze (ethylene glycol).

INJECTION. Injected poisons that are self-administered (drugs injected intravenously) can include an overdose of opioids that a drug addict injects when "shooting up" or an overdose of insulin that a diabetic inadvertently administers. Bee stings and venomous snake bites are other examples of injected poisons. Poisons injected directly into the bloodstream have the fastest onset of action.

INHALATIONS. Carbon monoxide is the most commonly inhaled toxin. Other toxic gases such as cyanide, phosgene, and nitrous dioxides may be inhaled in industrial or agricultural accidents or with smoke from fires. When rescuing victims of poisoning by inhalation, EMTs must be particularly careful to take protective measures to avoid exposure to themselves and others. Glue sniffing, freebasing cocaine, and smoking crack are other examples of poisoning by inhalation.

ABSORBED—CUTANEOUS. Poisons can be absorbed through the skin. Common examples of these include insecticides such as organophosphates. Corrosives such as acid or alkali usually damage the skin itself; however, hydrofluoric acid (used in the cleaning of building surfaces and the manufacture of computer chips) can both chemically burn the skin and be absorbed into the circulation. Cocaine, snorted through the nose, is absorbed by the membranes in the nasopharynx.

MANAGEMENT

The range of services delivered by the EMT varies with the individual case—from supportive care and reassurance that an ingested product is not toxic (many ingestions are nontoxic—particularly with children) to cardiopulmonary resuscitation. Many patients who die from an overdose do so because of respiratory depression. By properly managing the airway and providing necessary ventilatory support and supplemental oxygen, the EMT offers lifesaving treatment to many victims of overdose. Most poisoned patients who arrive alive at a hospital that is capable of treating the poisoning will survive, even if they arrive comatose.

The EMTs provide critical historical information from the scene. Containers of toxic agents should be brought to the hospital when possible. Check for any noticeable odors that may give a clue to toxin identification (Table 12–6). Search for clues of trauma. Since there are so many potentially toxic agents, any information gathered from the scene is especially important in terms of hospital evaluation.

PROVIDE CARDIORESPIRATORY SUPPORT. Since most deaths occur from alterations in or depression of respiration, the first and most important measure is to assess the need for basic life support. There are hyperacute patients who are found in such distress that the first and most necessary measure is to institute artificial resuscitation. These patients range from the smoke inhalation victim retrieved by firefighters from a burning building to the overdose victim on the street who has slow, inadequate ventilations. Providing these patients with high-concentration oxygen through a bag-valve-

TABLE 12-6. Diagnostic Odors

Odor	Posssible Substance
Acetone (sweet, like russet apples)	Lacquer, alcohol, isopropyl alcohol, chloroform, ketoacidosis
Acrid (pear-like)	Paraldehyde, chloral hydrate
Alcohol (fruit-like)	Alcohol, isopropyl alcohol
Ammoniac	Urea
Bitter almonds	Cyanide (in choke cherry, apricot pits)
Carrots	Cicutoxin
Coal gas (stove gas)	Carbon monoxide (odorless but associated with coal gas)
Disinfectants	Phenol, creosote
Eggs (rotten)	Hydrogen sulfide, mercaptans, Antabuse
Fish or raw liver (musty)	Hepatic failure, zinc phosphide
Fruit-like	Amyl nitrite, alcohol, isopropyl alcohol
Garlic	Phosphorus, tellurium, arsenic (breath and perspiration), parathion, malathion, selenium, dimethyl sulfoxide (DMSO), thallium
Halitosis	Acute illness, poor oral hygiene
Mothballs	Camphor-containing products
Peanuts	RH-787 (Vacor)
Pungent, aromatic	Ethchlorvynol (Placidyl)
Shoe polish	Nitrobenzene
Tobacco (stale)	Nicotine
Violets	Urinary turpentine
Wintergreen	Methyl salicylate

(From Goldfrank LR: Toxicologic Emergencies, 2nd ed. New York, Appleton-Century-Crofts, 1982, p. 253. Used with permission.)

mask or pocket mask can be lifesaving. Circulatory support may be necessary as well.

Unconscious patients or patients with deteriorating mental status must be transported with precautions to protect their airway. They must be continuously assessed for the need for respiratory support. The left lateral recumbent position, with the head down, may be used during transport to protect the airway from vomitus or secretions. Consider the possibility of a cervical spine injury in any unconscious patient and, if indicated, protect and support the patient's cervical spine.

DECONTAMINATE THE VICTIM.
Ocular exposure and skin contamination call for immediate action to remove the toxin. Eyes should be flushed with lukewarm water for at least 20 minutes. Make sure the eyes are open and do not use the full force of a faucet, which may damage the eye. Contaminated clothing should be removed and contaminated skin flooded with water (or soap and water) as soon as possible to remove any remaining toxins and minimize contact with the body (see the section on absorbed toxins later in this chapter). Be gentle when washing the skin to avoid abrasions that will permit greater absorption. Wear protective clothing to avoid contamination by splashes or direct skin contact. If at all possible, decontaminate the patient before placing him or her in the ambulance for transport.

GATHER THE HISTORY OF THE POISONING.
Because there are so many types of poisons, the history taking is especially important. The EMT is at the scene. There may be clues available such as empty pill bottles or containers, which will be invaluable to hospital personnel and the poison control center when trying to identify the substances. The classic information that must be sought follows:

What is the posion?
How was it taken? Was it ingested, inhaled, absorbed, or injected?
When was it taken?
How much was taken?
What evidence supports the history? For example, are there any empty pill bottles, commercial products, plant samples, etc.?

These are critical questions that should be asked of the patient, family, or others present at the scene. In many cases, multiple agents might have been taken.

Note that in many cases the history may be unreliable. A suicidal patient may want to hide knowledge of the toxin to hinder treatment. A distraught patient who has taken multiple agents (e.g., everything in the medicine cabinet) may not have stopped to consider or read what the medications were. Household products not stored in their original containers could be difficult to identify.

PERFORM A FOCUSED PHYSICAL EXAMINATION.
Following the primary survey, your examination of the patient should take note of the vital signs, the pupils, the skin (for color, moisture, and temperature), breathing, the abdomen, and a brief neurologic examination. The neurologic examination should include the mental status, and, if the patient is unconscious, the use of the Glasgow Coma Score helps document the degree of coma. If a patient is awake but has an altered mental status, the gag reflex should be checked to see whether the patient can protect the airway should vomiting occur (see Fig. 12-1). *Vomiting is never induced in patients without a gag reflex since they may aspirate the stomach contents into their lungs.* Patients without a gag reflex must be transported with diligent attention given to protecting the airway and ensuring adequate ventilations.

Some poisons present a classic clinical picture that may be obvious on clinical examination. For example, the patient with an opioid ("narcotic") overdose often presents with altered mental status (lethargy to coma), shallow and slow respirations, and pinpoint pupils. There may be fresh or old needle marks over the veins ("tracks"), indicating intravenous drug use. An organophosphate poisoning victim displays evidence of secretions coming from many sites—sweating, drooling, urinating, defecating, vomiting, and tearing. The EMT gradually learns about different clinical effects of various poisons. It is important to document findings noted during the physical examination to (1) help time the onset of drug effects and (2) chart the progression of signs as the toxic agent is further absorbed or eliminated.

Always look for signs of injury as well. The poisoned patient may have suffered trauma from a fall or accident. Without this information, definitive treatment may be delayed.

INSTITUTE TREATMENT. Regardless of the type of poison or the route of exposure, poison treatment centers around three major goals. These are:

1. *Prevent further absorption*—remove any poison that is not yet absorbed into the body. Following poison ingestions, induction of vomiting is one means of removing toxins that are still in the stomach. However, the induction of vomiting may be disastrous for certain drugs or poisons (e.g., caustic agents, most hydrocarbons) or certain patients (e.g., infants or patients with coma or no gag reflex). Therefore, always call medical control or the poison control center before attempting to induce vomiting. Activated charcoal given orally as a slurry (watery mixture) binds most toxins still within the gastrointestinal tract and prevents absorption. There are very few contraindications to the use of charcoal.

2. *Hasten elimination*—speed up the elimination of toxin already absorbed so as to shorten the time that it acts on the body. For oral ingestions, a cathartic can be given to quicken the evacuation from the bowels. Certain toxins in the bloodstream may be removed by hemodialysis or charcoal hemoperfusion. (All of these elimination techniques are generally employed after arrival at the hospital.) Figure 12–7 shows examples of commercially available syrup of ipecac, charcoal, and a cathartic.

3. *Treat signs and symptoms*—certain signs and symptoms may respond to medical treatment. A remedy that counteracts a poison, called an *antidote*, may be available. Most antidotes are administered in the hospital

setting. Oxygen, the antidote for carbon monoxide poisoning, is routinely administered by EMTs. Naloxone, an antidote for opiates (heroin, morphine, methadone, etc.), is administered by many advanced EMTs and paramedics, either intravenously or intramuscularly.

Other patients may require drug therapy that counteracts the effects of a poison, but does not remove or eliminate the toxin itself. In fact, true antidotes are available for only a few drugs and poisons. The major treatment for the poisoned patient is supportive care, which is initiated, as indicated, by the EMT.

The methods to achieve these treatment goals vary with the type of poisoning. General principles for handling ingestions, inhalations, skin exposures, and injections are covered in the respective sections later in this chapter.

DEALING WITH THE POISONED PATIENT. Overdosed or poisoned patients may have many types of reactions. Patients may have altered mental status from the emotional events surrounding an overdose or from the physical effects of the drugs. They can be agitated, despondent, uncooperative, and difficult.

Suicidal patients may be extremely depressed and despondent. They may have left a note. They may have overdosed in an area where they are likely to be found. Other patients may purposely hide any toxic products to prevent discovery or take an overdose in an area where it is unlikely that they will be discovered.

Parents may feel extremely guilty about a child getting into toxic substances around the home.

EMTs themselves may experience feelings of hopelessness when dealing with a patient who has abused drugs. On the other hand, EMTs may feel a sense of identity with patients of similar age who have attempted suicide.

EMTs must maintain a professional approach in dealing with poisoned patients to minimize the potential for emotional responses that interfere with care. At all costs, avoid antagonizing the patient. Be careful not to label patients. Express to patients that your first and foremost priority is to deal with the poisoning. In this way you are more apt to gain the cooperation of the patient, family, and bystanders. Patients who are antagonized are less receptive to treatment and transportation to the hospital.

Psychiatric consultation is obtained in the hospital setting for patients who have intentionally poisoned themselves.

PROTECTIVE CUSTODY: PATIENTS REFUSING MEDICAL ATTENTION. Some patients may refuse medical care. They may insist that they want to die and be left alone. These patients must not be abandoned. Encourage them to accompany you to the hospital. Call police if necessary to place these patients in protective custody. Patients cannot be presumed to be acting in their best

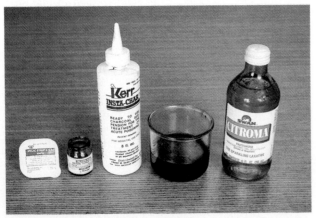

FIGURE 12–7. Examples of commercially available products: syrup of ipecac, charcoal, and a cathartic.

interest if they are suicidal or if the drug or poison has altered their mental status and judgment.

Ingested Poisons

GENERAL PRINCIPLES

In most cases, poisons are ingested. After assessing the need for basic life support, gather the history, perform a brief physical examination, and institute treatment.

HISTORY

Ask the patient or bystanders *what* the patient might have taken.

Establish the *time* that the ingestion occurred. Were all the pills taken at once, or did the patient take more and more of a substance at repeated intervals? Some patients may inadvertently take a toxic level of pain killers by repeatedly taking medication beyond the prescribed dosage, seeking relief from pain.

How much did the patient take? How many pills from each bottle? How many ounces of a liquid substance?

As *evidence*, bring along the containers of any substance ingested. Obtain the pill container or the bottle with any identifying marks and bring it to the hospital. Prescription bottles have identifying information that may help establish the amount and strength of any medication that was possibly ingested.

In the case of commercial products, it is most important to bring the container. Again, the possible amount ingested can be estimated. The contents on the label can be checked for toxic effects. And in cases where there is no listing of ingredients, the poison control center or manufacturer may be called to obtain information about ingredients. Obtaining the brand name alone is inadequate. Companies invest large sums of advertising dollars to get brand loyalty among customers. Ingredients may change but the company may continue to use well-selling labels. This is one reason why, whenever possible, the container should be brought to aid identification.

Has the patient *vomited or instituted home treatment* since the ingestion? Vomitus should be saved and brought to the hospital for possible analysis.

PHYSICAL EXAMINATION

Perform a brief physical examination. Note the vital signs, pupils, skin, breath sounds, abdomen, mental status, and neurologic findings and any peculiar odors (see Table 12–6). Always check for the presence of a gag reflex before you consider inducing vomiting or giving anything by mouth. Note that alterations in body temperature, both increased and decreased, are commonly encountered from both drug effects and exposure.

Is there evidence from the physical findings that a poisoning has occurred? Remember that it takes time with some substances for the effects of poisoning to become evident. The suicidal patient who has a change of heart and calls for help hours after taking a bottle of acetaminophen may have no symptoms when you arrive. Yet without hospital treatment, there may be delayed and fatal effects. Other patients may have alterations in consciousness or other physical complaints related to the onset of toxicity. As you perform the primary and secondary surveys, note pertinent positive and negative findings.

PREVENTION OF ABSORPTION

The main aspect of prehospital treatment for poison ingestions is to make sure the patient is medically stable and to try to maintain that state by preventing further absorption and hastening elimination. Prevention of absorption is accomplished by inducing vomiting, administering activated charcoal, or diluting the body's poisonous contents. These maneuvers are appropriate for the alert patient. The drowsy or unconscious patient must have other treatment rendered in the hospital setting, and the mainstay of treatment in the field is basic life support.

SYRUP OF IPECAC. Inducing vomiting is usually accomplished by giving syrup of ipecac. Syrup of ipecac is a standardized mixture of natural alkaloids that causes vomiting in about 60% of patients in 15 minutes and in nearly 90% of patients within 30 minutes. The dose for adults is 30 ml, or 2 tablespoons, and for children over age 1, it is 15 ml, or 1 tablespoon (Fig. 12–8). Infants

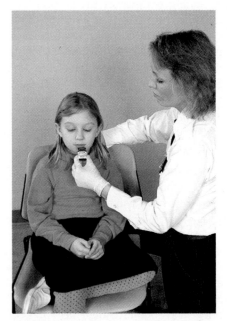

FIGURE 12–8. Administration of syrup of ipecac.

TABLE 12–7. Emesis with Syrup of Ipecac

Dose

Adult
  30 ml (2 tbsp)
Children
  6–12 months, 10 ml (2 tsp)
  1–5 years, 15 ml (1 tbsp)
  Over 5 years, 30 ml (2 tbsp)
  One additional dose (a second dose) may be given if the
    patient has not vomited within 30 min

Contraindications

Child younger than 6 months of age
Nontoxic ingestion
Comatose patient
Patient experiencing seizures
Any patient expected to deteriorate rapidly
Ingestion of a strong acid or alkali
When vomiting will delay administration of an oral antidote
Compromised gag reflex
Patient with a hemorrhagic diathesis (cirrhosis, varices,
    thrombocytopenia)
Concomitant ingestion of sharp, solid materials (thermometer,
    glass, nails, razor blades)
Evidence of significant vomiting prior to ipecac utilization
Any patient with an accidental "pure" petroleum distillate or
    turpentine ingestion, or any patient who is symptomatic
    (pulmonary, neurologic, cardiac) following a hydrocarbon
    ingestion.

(From Goldfrank LR, Flomenbaum NE, Lewis NA, Weisman RS, How-land MA: Goldfrank's Toxicologic Emergencies, 4th ed. New York, Appleton & Lange, 1990. Used with permission.)

less than 12 months of age should have vomiting induced only in a hospital setting or upon advice from the poison control center. (Table 12–7).

After giving the syrup of ipecac, give water or other available liquid (8 to 16 ounces to adults and 4 to 8 ounces to children). These additional fluids serve to dilute the contents and provide a liquid that can be "vomited," aiding removal of the poison. Do not give excessive fluids, as this tends to move the stomach contents into the intestine, reducing removal by vomiting.

Generally, patients vomit within 20 minutes. Again, they must be awake and have a gag reflex. If not, there is a danger that they will not protect their airway when vomiting occurs; they could aspirate the vomitus into the lungs, causing pneumonia.

There are a few contraindications to the induction of vomiting with ipecac.

- Unconscious or seizing patients
- Patients without a gag reflex
- Patients who have swallowed a corrosive substance such as an acid or alkali, which will damage the esophagus again when vomited
- Certain hydrocarbons that pose little chance for absorption but a high risk for aspiration pneumonia from vomiting. Some hydrocarbons with organophosphates, heavy metals, or halogen ions (fluoride, chloride, and iodine) should be vomited, but the issue is so complicated that the regional poison

control center should be consulted on a case-by-case basis.
- When the administration of ipecac may delay administration of an oral antidote

Dilution of a toxic substance by administering water or milk is indicated for corrosive ingestions such as acids or alkali (such as lye or drain pipe cleaner). Give 1 or 2 glasses of water or milk.

OTHER METHODS OF STOMACH EMPTYING. Gastric lavage is an alternate method of emptying the stomach. It is usually performed in the hospital setting. It is the method of choice for unconscious patients or patients without a gag reflex. The airway is usually protected by intubating the patient before passing the gastric tube. It may also be used when ipecac is contraindicated.

Gastric lavage is accomplished by insertion of a large oral gastric tube. This technique used to be referred to as "pumping the stomach." The advantage of gastric lavage is that removal is immediate, whereas ipecac takes several minutes to work. Secondly, after ipecac-induced vomiting, a patient usually continues to vomit for some time afterward, delaying administration of charcoal or other oral drugs or agents. With lavage, there is no protracted vomiting and charcoal can be given immediately.

Some urban hospitals may elect to bring alert patients to the emergency department for lavage of stomach contents rather than to have ipecac given in the field. Since ipecac takes 15 to 20 minutes to induce vomiting, transport and lavage may offer a more timely method of stomach emptying. Local protocols direct the preferred treatment.

ACTIVATED CHARCOAL. Activated charcoal is an absorbent material that binds most toxins. It keeps them within the gastrointestinal tract until they are eliminated, thereby preventing absorption into the body. The dose of charcoal is usually 1 g per kilogram of body weight (a minimum of 50 to 100 g for adults). It comes premixed as a thick liquid or as a powder that must be mixed with water to form a soup-like slurry. Sometimes sweeteners are added to make it more palatable to children. There is almost never any harm resulting from administering activated charcoal. (Some physicians choose to withhold its use after large acetaminophen [i.e., Tylenol] overdoses for fear that it will absorb the antidote [acetylcysteine, or Mucomyst] that they may choose to administer.)

Activated charcoal should not be confused with burnt toast, or "universal antidote," which does not have nearly the same absorbency potential. These other agents are generally not in use today (Table 12–8).

ENHANCE EXCRETION

Excretion through the gastrointestinal tract can be enhanced by administering a cathartic such as sorbitol

TABLE 12-8. Activated Charcoal

Dose

Adult and child
  Initial dose: 1 g/kg body weight or 10:1 ratio of activated charcoal:drug, whichever is greater. Following massive ingestions, 2 g/kg may be indicated; however, it may be difficult to administer doses in excess of 100 g.

Repetitive Doses

0.5 to 1 g/kg body weight every 2 to 6 hr tailored to the dose and dosage form of drug ingested (larger doses and shorter dosing intervals may occasionally be indicated).
Note: Do not use repetitive doses or cathartics routinely.

Procedure

1. Add 4–8 parts of water to chosen quantity of activated charcoal, if in powdered form. This will form a transiently stable slurry that the patient can drink or have placed down an orogastric hose.
2. The activated charcoal can be given in a mixture with the chosen cathartic.
3. If the patient vomits the dose, it should be repeated. Smaller, more frequent, or continuous nasogastric administration may be better tolerated. An antiemetic is sometimes needed.
4. Repetitive doses are useful for drugs with a small volume of distribution, low plasma protein binding, biliary or gastric secretion, or active metabolites that recirculate.

Contraindications

Caustic acids or alkalis (ineffective, and will accumulate in burned areas, making endoscopy difficult)
Ileus (for repetitive dosing)
Patients with a risk of aspiration and an unprotected airway

(From Goldfrank LR, Flomenbaum NE, Lewis NA, Weisman RS, Howland MA: Goldfrank's Toxicologic Emergencies, 4th ed. New York, Appleton & Lange, 1990. Used with permission.)

TABLE 12-9. Cathartics

Dose

Adults and children
  Magnesium citrate: 4 ml/kg to 300 ml per dose
  Magnesium sulfate: 250 mg/kg up to 30 g
  Sorbitol: 0.5–1 g/kg (0.5 g/kg in children, with a maximum 50 g of 35% concentrate in children over 1 year.)

Precautions

Not warranted in routine management of trivial ingestions in children
Do not use phospho-soda in children.
Do not use repetitive doses of magnesium-containing cathartics
Sorbitol administration in children should be used cautiously, with attention paid to fluid and electrolyte status.
Do not use repetitive doses of cathartics in children.
Oil-based cathartics should not be used because of the risks of aspiration and enhanced toxin absorption.

Contraindications

Adynamic ileus
Diarrhea
Abdominal trauma
Intestinal obstruction
Renal failure (magnesium sulfate or citrate)

(From Goldfrank LR, Flomenbaum NE, Lewis NA, Weisman RS, Howland MA: Goldfrank's Toxicologic Emergencies, 4th ed. New York, Appleton & Lange, 1990. Used with permission.)

or magnesium sulfate (Table 12–9). After removing the stomach contents, these agents are given to induce diarrhea, speeding transit time through the gastrointestinal tract, and thereby reducing the chance for absorption of the poisonous agent through the intestine. They may be given with charcoal or after charcoal is administered. Some liquid charcoal preparations are now premixed with sorbitol. Do not administer a cathartic to a patient who is dehydrated or who has kidney failure, except on instructions from medical control.

TYPES OF INGESTIONS

There are numerous agents that are encountered in accidental and intentional poisonings and overdoses. The most common drugs encountered in toxic ingestions include amphetamines; barbiturates; benzodiazepines; opioids, or narcotics; non-narcotic analgesics; sedative-hypnotics; antidepressants (especially "tricyclics"); and phenothiazines. Some general classifications of types are discussed, with examples of symptoms, types of agents, and unique considerations in management.

SEDATIVE-HYPNOTICS AND ANTIANXIETY AGENTS. Sedatives, which allay activity and excitement; hypnotics, which induce sleep; and antianxiety agents are commonly prescribed. In general, the most severe toxic effects are respiratory depression and alteration of mental status (from relaxation through stupor to coma). Deaths are usually secondary to respiratory depression. When used in combination with alcohol, the effects of the depressants on mental status and respiration are markedly increased.

Management considerations include assisting with ventilations, administering supplemental oxygen as necessary, and protecting the airway of the patient who has an altered mental status by transporting the patient in the left lateral recumbent position with the head down.

OPIOIDS (NARCOTICS). Opioids (narcotics) are a special class of depressants. They alter the perception of pain. A patient may feel pain but it does not "hurt." In excess, they cause depressed mental status and coma and slow or stop respirations. Most narcotics cause pinpoint pupils.

The patient with depressed respirations, a depressed mental status, and pinpoint pupils displays the classic signs of the opioid, or narcotic, overdose. Intravenous users of narcotics such as heroin may have track marks or scarring over veins from previous injections.

Examples of opioids include morphine, heroin, meperidine (Demerol), codeine, and oxycodone (Percodan and Percocet). The word "narcotic" should be reserved for opioids or opiates such as the drugs mentioned.

However, common usage of "narcotics" often refers inappropriately to most drugs of abuse, including such stimulants as cocaine and phencyclidine (PCP or angel dust).

Naloxone (Narcan) is an antidote to narcotics and rapidly reverses the respiratory and mental depression. Paramedics commonly use Narcan as an agent in the field.

PSYCHIATRIC MEDICATIONS.   Psychiatric patients are prescribed a range of medications. These include phenothiazine tranquilizers, tricyclic antidepressants, monoamine oxidase inhibitors, and benzodiazepines (such as Valium, Librium, and others). In the event of an overdose, a range of problems can be encountered. Findings include:

Muscle spasms
Dry skin
High or low body temperature
Hypotension or hypertension
Abnormal heart rhythms
Cardiac arrest
Fast or slow heart rates
Altered respirations—depressed
Altered mental status to coma
Seizures

Be particularly alert to depressed respirations, low blood pressure, seizures, and abnormally low or high temperatures. These drugs can cause a progression of changing signs over a short period of time.

Monoamine oxidase inhibitors can cause a hypertensive crisis when taken in combination with certain drugs and foods high in tyramine (such as beer, wines, and certain cheeses) or tryptophan (broad beans).

STIMULANTS.   Stimulants include amphetamines, methylphenidate (Ritalin), and cocaine. Illicit stimulant drugs include cocaine and its altered forms "crack" and "freebase" (usually smoked or inhaled), phencyclidine, and amphetamines. Cocaine overdose can occur from ingestion when drugs are swallowed to avoid detection during an arrest or when drug transporters swallow balloons or condoms filled with cocaine to avoid detection. In the latter instance, the condoms can burst and massive amounts of cocaine can be absorbed through the intestine, invariably killing the smuggler very rapidly.

Stimulant overdoses cause excitability and can induce seizures. Fast heart rates, hypertension, and chest pain can occur. Behaviorally, patients can be anxious, delirious, and paranoid. Psychotic and violent behavior is possible. Sudden death can result from acute cardiac arrhythmia.

PCP is usually smoked. Cocaine is often inhaled as "crack" or "freebase." Amphetamines may be taken as pills, injected, or smoked as "ice."

After assessing the need for cardiorespiratory support, be conservative. The major problems in the pre-

hospital setting may be behavioral and psychologic. To gain compliance, reassure the patient. Be nonthreatening, and offer as calm an environment as possible. Maintain verbal contact with the patient. Do not be judgmental. Avoid restraints if possible, since these patients are often in a hyperactive state and strain against restraints, which can cause elevations in body temperature and the breakdown of muscle tissue (rhabdomyolysis) from hyperactivity and severe muscle strain.

Stimulant overdose can cause myocardial infarction, bleeding in the brain, and convulsions with subsequent coma and respiratory depression.

ALCOHOL.   Alcohol is the most common drug abused in the United States. It has a depressant effect on mental status and respirations when taken in high doses. When taken in combination with depressant drugs, it adds to the respiratory and mental status depression. The mixture of alcohol with other drugs is responsible for a large number of severe overdoses and deaths.

Acute alcohol intoxication by itself can be lethal. It can cause coma and even respiratory failure. Some patients end up choking on their own vomit. Deaths occur in adolescents who are unfamiliar with alcohol and drink excessive amounts, causing extremely high blood alcohol levels.

PRESCRIPTION DRUGS FOR HEART AND LUNGS. Patients who are suicidal may take any available medications. Drugs prescribed for circulatory and respiratory ailments can cause a wide range of symptoms. Of particular concern are alterations in heart rate and rhythm, alterations in blood pressure, and arrhythmias.

ANALGESICS.   Over-the-counter analgesics (pain killers) can cause death from overdose. Salicylates (aspirin) and acetaminophen are commonly encountered. There are many brand names.

Early after the overdose, there may be few, if any, symptoms. Aspirin overdose can cause increased respiration rates early on. Later, coma can occur. Aspirin overdose may require hemodialysis. Acetaminophen causes no symptoms or mild gastrointestinal discomfort (including nausea and vomiting) and malaise during the first 24 hours. After 48 hours, with severe doses, evidence of liver damage can appear. It is important that all patients with acetaminophen or aspirin overdose receive evaluation by a physician to see if treatment is necessary.

COMMONLY INGESTED COMMERCIAL AND INDUSTRIAL PRODUCTS

Hydrocarbons, caustics, insecticides, and other household products are most commonly taken by children, particularly toddlers, or by particularly despondent or psychotic adults.

Caustics include both acids and alkalis. Acid products include toilet bowel cleaners, bleaches, metal cleaners, and battery acid. Alkalis are found in drain cleaners (lye, Drano) and Clinitest tablets (used by diabetics to test their urine for sugar). Chemistry labs and industrial sites are sources of caustic exposure (usually spills).

Caustics should be diluted by having the patient drink 1 or 2 glasses of water or milk. (Even though some containers may still advise trying to neutralize corrosives or caustics, poison control centers recommend dilution alone to avoid additional damage from the heat of neutralization.) Ingestion of acids or alkalis is one of the situations in which vomiting should not be induced so as to avoid reexposing the esophagus to a second passage of a substance that causes chemical burns.

METHANOL AND ETHYLENE GLYCOL. Two substances that can initially cause signs of mild inebriation (or no findings at all) but if left untreated can lead to coma and death are methanol and ethylene glycol. Methanol is found in "dry gas," windshield-washing solution, and as a fuel for warming food (Sterno). Ethylene glycol is most commonly found as antifreeze. Patients who ingest either of these substances suffer from severe acid formation ("metabolic acidosis") in the blood when these products are broken down by an enzyme. Formation of the acid breakdown products can be delayed by administering ethyl alcohol (i.e., "drinking alcohol"), which binds to the same enzyme preferentially.

In an attempt to blow off excess acid, the patient may hyperventilate.

Patients poisoned with methanol or ethylene glycol need hospital care and, in severe ingestions, dialysis. EMTs may be directed by the poison control center to administer alcohol to patients who are alert, particularly in rural areas, where time to the hospital is prolonged.

HYDROCARBONS. Hydrocarbons are molecules predominantly composed of carbon and hydrogen. Materials containing hydrocarbons include gasoline, kerosene, cleaning fluids (carbon tetrachloride), spot removers (trichloroethene, trichloroethylene), and rubber and plastic cements (toluene, acetone, benzene, etc.).

Hydrocarbons can cause central nervous system changes (euphoria, stupor, delirium, coma), cardiac arrhythmias, and severe pulmonary damage. Of particular concern is the ability of hydrocarbons to cause death by causing a terrible inflammatory reaction in the lungs when aspirated.

Vomiting is not induced with larger-size hydrocarbon ingestions such as mineral oil. They are usually not absorbed to a significant degree through the gastrointestinal tract, but if aspirated during vomiting, can cause severe pneumonia.

Ingestions of medium-size hydrocarbons, such as kerosene, gasoline, or turpentine, may benefit from induced vomiting if the quantity ingested was greater than 1 ml/kg.

Ingestions of smaller-size hydrocarbons and those containing benzene, toluene, halogen molecules (chlo-

ride, fluoride, etc.), heavy metals, insecticides, and camphor are indications to induce vomiting. The smaller the size, the more volatile the substance and the more easily it can be absorbed through the gastrointestinal tract.

Toddlers and suicidal patients are most often the victims of hydrocarbon poisoning. Occasionally, especially during fuel shortages, someone siphoning gasoline ingests small quantities.

It is often difficult to estimate the amount ingested. Toddlers in particular smell of hydrocarbons as they spill it over their clothes while drinking it. Contaminated clothing should be removed and the skin flushed with water.

The poison control center should be consulted on hydrocarbon ingestions to see if vomiting should be induced.

INSECTICIDES. Insecticides are ingested inadvertently by toddlers and deliberately by individuals making suicide attempts. One common class of insecticides is organophosphates.

Organophosphates cause an overstimulation of secretions, bronchoconstriction, and muscle weakness. In excess, they cause death by respiratory muscle paralysis or by pulmonary secretions and bronchoconstriction. In addition, there is an outpouring of secretions from most orifices, including vomiting, salivation, sweating, lacrimation (tearing), urination, and diarrhea: SLUD is an acronym used to help remember the latter four signs. There are usually small pupils and a slow heart rate. The slow heart rate is notable, since these patients often have respiratory distress, a situation in which one would expect the heart rate to increase in an attempt to compensate for the respiratory compromise. In severe cases, patients require antidotal therapy. Prehospital treatment centers on providing supplemental oxygen and ventilatory support. Rapid transport is indicated in severe cases since administration of atropine can be lifesaving.

Organophosphates may also be absorbed through the skin. When toddlers drink organophosphates they often spill them over their clothing. Their skin should be flushed with water and washed with soap and water. A garlicky odor may be noted but is often accompanied and masked by a hydrocarbon smell.

FOOD POISONING. Food poisoning can be caused by bacteria, toxins produced by bacteria, and viruses. It is caused by improperly cooked or canned foods and by contamination of food with fecal bacteria by food handlers. It is often suspected when two or more persons become ill after eating the same foods. Usually, the symptoms include nausea, vomiting, and diarrhea (sometimes bloody).

The most severe type of food poisoning is *botulism*, which may begin as a flu-like illness but then causes severe weakness, paralysis, and ventilatory arrest. Treatment requires respiratory support and artificial ventilations and use of an antitoxin.

Poisonous mushroom consumption can cause gastrointestinal disturbances, hallucinations, and delirium. One type of mushroom, *Amanita muscaria*, can cause excessive salivation, tearing, and bradycardia and may require drug treatment. Mushroom poisoning usually occurs when individuals looking for psychedelic effects or exotic edible mushrooms mistake toxic mushrooms for the edible varieties.

Care is supportive. It is extremely important to bring any available mushrooms or even mushroom fragments found at the scene with you to help with identification.

PLANTS. Many common household and wild plants can cause adverse effects. These include gastrointestinal, circulatory, and neurologic effects. In addition, they can cause severe skin and mucous membrane irritation. One common household plant, the dieffenbachia, can cause severe irritation and swelling in the mouth if ingested by toddlers. When chewed, the crystals in the leaf make it feel as if the patient has bitten into ground glass. Treatment in this latter case centers on keeping the airway open. In general, care is supportive and the plant should be brought along to aid in identification.

Table 12–10 lists agents found in poisoning and overdose and provides management considerations.

Inhaled Poisons

RESCUE CONSIDERATIONS AND PRECAUTIONS

Victims of toxic gas must always be approached with consideration for the safety of the rescuers. Rescuers are of no use to a victim if they become incapacitated as well. There have been many instances of EMTs and rescuers succumbing to the same toxic gases or fumes that claimed the initial victims. Rescuers should avoid inhalation of fumes. If entering a contaminated area or a closed space, they should wear a self-contained breathing apparatus.

Victims of inhalation should be removed from the toxic environment and given necessary ventilatory support and humidified supplemental oxygen.

The most commonly encountered poisonous gas is carbon monoxide. This gas is found in fires, charcoal burners, automobile exhaust fumes, and inadequately ventilated stoves and home heaters. Treatment for victims is administration of 100% oxygen. Severe cases may also require hyperbaric oxygen treatment if available.

POISONOUS GASES

The greatest concern in toxic gas exposure is asphyxiation, or death from lack of oxygen. Gases can cause asphyxiation by simply displacing the oxygen in the air, by causing chemical actions within the body, or by irritating the respiratory tract.

ASPHYXIANTS. Simple asphyxiants include carbon dioxide and small hydrocarbon molecules such as methane (cooking gas). When present in high quantities they can displace or dilute the oxygen in air and the victim becomes hypoxic.

Carbon dioxide is heavier than air. It collects in poorly ventilated areas such as mine shafts and in the holds of ships.

Methane, ethane, and propane are made up of small hydrocarbon molecules that have no color or odor to warn the victim. When used commercially, mercaptans are added to give a warning odor, as in gas stoves. These gases can collect in closed spaces where leaks are present. There is a great potential for explosion if there is a spark, which can even be caused by turning on an electric light switch in a room where these gases have collected.

Chemical asphyxiants include carbon monoxide, cyanide, and hydrogen sulfide. Carbon monoxide exposure is expected to be significant at all fires. The vast majority of victims who die in fires do so from smoke inhalation and carbon monoxide poisoning. Carbon monoxide is also present in engine exhaust. It is odorless and colorless. It binds to hemoglobin and affects its ability to transport and deliver oxygen to the tissues as well as the tissues' ability to use the oxygen. It gives little warning as to its lethal effect. Victims might early on feel headaches and nausea and often attribute this to a flu-like illness. Judgment is disturbed, coordination and motor ability are impaired, and victims may collapse on exertion. With judgment and movement impaired, victims become lost and disoriented or do not have the power to flee the toxic environment. If high concentrations are in the atmosphere, fatal inhalations can occur in less than a minute.

The treatment is administration of 100% concentration oxygen. Extreme cases might be referred to a hyperbaric chamber. See the section on smoke inhalation in Chapter 11.

Cyanide is found in industries such as electroplating, photography, metallurgy, and metal cleaning. It is used as a fumigant on cargo ships. It is also used as a chemical agent. Some fires, particularly those that involve burning polyurethanes, produce cyanide.

Cyanide is rapid acting and affects the ability of the body to utilize oxygen. Clinical symptoms are nonspecific. Initially, the patient may have increased heart and breathing rates. Later, the breathing may slow and the heart rate decrease. Treatment with high-concentration oxygen is necessary along with administration of an antidote.

Many industries have cyanide antidote kits available for use. The treatment is to administer nitrites to

Text continued on page 570

TABLE 12-10. Management of Drug Overdose and Poisoning

Drug/Substance	Trade or Street Name	Signs/Symptoms	EMT Management	Special Comments
Household Products Acids	Toilet bowl cleaners Rust removers Metal cleaners and polishes Tile and grout cleaners	Severe pain in mouth, stomach, chest (substernal)	NEVER INDUCE VOMITING Give patient Milk Milk of magnesia Egg whites (dilutes the acid)	Have patient sit up during transport
Alkalis	Automatic dishwasher detergent Drain cleaners Oven cleaners Washing soda Ammonia Bleach	Severe pains in mouth, stomach, chest (substernal) Burns in mouth and esophagus Associated difficulty with swallowing	NEVER INDUCE VOMITING Give milk or water	Have patient sit up during transport Watch airway closely for edema causing restricted ventilation
Hydrocarbons	Petroleum products Gasoline Fuel oils Paint thinners Paint solvents Kerosene Lighter fluid Furniture polish	Most common symptoms are respiratory distress with coughing and choking Patient may develop pulmonary edema Abdominal pain may be present Convulsions (seizures) Patient may be comatose Monitor for arrhythmias	NEVER INDUCE VOMITING Treat with up to 100% oxygen depending on severity of overdose Control secretions with suction as required	Have patient sit up during transport if possible
Cyanide	Laetrile overdose Contaminated fruit Seed crop fumigants Photochemicals Electroplating	Initial stage Confusion Rapid respirations Later stage Depressed respirations Vomiting Seizure Comatose	Some paramedic programs have cyanide antidote kits available. Support vital signs and respiration. If antidote kit is not available, transport patient to nearest medical facility having antidote	
Pesticides	Warfarin base: rat killer Strychnine base: rodenticides Arsenic base: insect sprays, ant and roach killers, liquid insect killers, DDT pesticides, organophosphates	Warfarin type Severe gastrointestinal symptoms Progressive lethargy/apathy Strychnine based Acute illness Severe nausea/vomiting Respiratory distress Tonic stiffening Arsenic based Acute gastrointestinal symptoms DDT Severe gastroenteritis	Warfarin poisoning: Patient must be seen at hospital for blood-clotting problems Patients who are conscious with gag reflex can be given ipecac Support ventilation as required Tonic stiffening requires antiseizure medicines	Illicit drugs, e.g., heroin, are sometimes cut with strychnine Some pesticides contain anticholinergic agents
Perfumes/Deodorizers	Products containing perfumes and deodorizers are too numerous to list here	Produce severe gastroenteritis Respiratory problems from aerosol products may be present	Give oxygen as required Support vital signs	

Table continued on following page

TABLE 12–10. Management of Drug Overdose and Poisoning *Continued*

Drug/Substance	Trade or Street Name	Signs/Symptoms	EMT Management	Special Comments
Plants Poisonous plants	Glycosides Foxglove Azalea Rhododendrons	Glycosides Nausea/vomiting Hypotension May have bradycardia (heart rate <55 per minute)	Support with oxygen as required Support hypotension as with hypovolemia Use cardiac monitor if available	Bring plant sample to hospital
	Alkaloidal toxins Hemlock Nightshade	Alkaloidal toxins Lethargy, which may progress to seizures and coma		
	GI irritants Philodendron Deiffenbachia Holly	GI irritants Severe nausea/vomiting Diarrhea Hypotension		
Poisonous mushrooms	*Amanita muscaria*	10–30 minutes after ingestion: severe nausea/vomiting followed rapidly by seizures; death may occur	Support with oxygen as required Support hypotension as with hypovolemia Use cardiac monitor if available	Bring plant sample to hospital
Hallucinogenic mushrooms	Psilocybin and psilocin	Severe mood disturbances Hyperventilation Nausea/vomiting Fever Reduced level of consciousness	Use ipecac if patient has gag reflex and is conscious Calm patient as necessary Support vital signs and ventilation as required	Onset 15–30 minutes after ingestion lasting up to 4–6 hours
Drugs, sedatives, hypnotics, tranquilizers *Barbiturates (long-acting)* Phenobarbital	Luminal (prescription); barbs, purple hearts (street)	Miotic pupils Respiratory depression to complete arrest Gradual onset of lethargy to coma Hypotension Hypothermia	Consult physician concerning ipecac, as drug may depress patient's gag reflex at the same time ipecac begins to work Support ventilations and blood pressure as per hypovolemia Check patient's gag reflex and level of consciousness frequently Use cardiac monitor if available	Most abused drug next to Valium and alcohol May be used to reduce effect of amphetamines causing mixed overdose Usual dose: 15–30 mg three times per day
Barbiturates (intermediate-acting) Amobarbital	Amytal (prescription); blue ice, blue lady, turquoise blue birds (street)	Faster onset but shorter duration than phenobarbital	Same as phenobarbital	
Secobarbital	Seconal (prescription); red birds, red devils, downers, laybacks, reds (street)	Level of consciousness from agitated to comatose		

Generic name	Trade/street names	Signs and symptoms	Treatment/Nursing actions	Comments
Pentobarbital	Nembutal (prescription); block busters, nemmies, nebbies (street)			Usual dose: 30 mg 3–4 times per day; 100 mg at bedtime
Pentobarbital/Amobarbital combination	Tuinal (prescription); Christmas tree, rainbows, tootsie (street)	Pupils may be small		
Other Sedatives Glutethimide	Doriden/CB,D	Rapid onset of coma (1 hour) Stupor or coma may alternate with alert or hyperactive behavior Pupils may be dilated/fixed Sudden apnea and hypotension may occur	Monitor vital signs and ventilation closely Avoid ipecac because coma may develop rapidly	Usual dose: 1 tablespoon at bedtime; repeat after 4 hours
Methaqualone	Quaalude (prescription); super/quads, soapers, roarers, ludes (street)	Sedative-hypnotic, action similar to that of short-acting barbiturates; coma and respiratory depression most common Possible hallucinations	Support ABCs as required	Abrupt withdrawal can cause serious side effects, including seizure, chills, general behavior change, anxiety If mixed with alcohol, drug can be fatal
Methaqualone hydrochloride	Parest, Soma			
Methyprylon	Noludar	Pulmonary edema Diaphoresis Drowsiness, nausea, vomiting		Usual dose: 400 mg at bedtime
Meprobamate	Miltown, Equanil, Mepriam, Saronil, Tranmep, Meprospan	Extreme drowsiness progressing to coma Possible hypotension Possible respiratory arrest	This drug is usually slow to produce severe effects; can use ipecac if given within 15–20 min after ingestion of drug Support ABCs as required	Large quantity of alcohol makes overdose possible with smaller dose Usual adult dose: 1200–1600 mg per day in divided doses
Ethchlorvynol	Placidyl	Onset of coma in 1 hour, which can be prolonged for days Seizures Depressed ventilation Absence of response to painful stimuli	Support vital signs and respiration Be prepared for seizure Avoid ipecac, as drug has rapid action in large quantities	Combination of Placidyl and amitriptyline can cause patient to be delirious Usual adult dose: 500–1000 mg
Diazepam	Valium	Unconsciousness from Valium, Ativan, and Tranxene is rapid (10–30 min) Unconsciousness from Librium, Dalmane, and Serax is slow (hours)	Do not use ipecac with Valium, Ativan, and Tranxene because of rapid action of drugs	Valium is the most widely prescribed and abused of all sedatives
Lorazepam Chlordiazepoxide Flurazepam Clorazepate Oxazepam	Ativan Librium Dalmane Tranxene Serax	Initially patient will be sleepy, confused; slurred speech with possible difficulty in controlling motor functions will progress to coma, respiratory depression, and/or respiratory arrest	Support vital signs and respiration as required	Alcohol is often used with these drugs; makes even small dose unpredictable Usual adult dose: 2–4 mg per day

Table continued on following page

TABLE 12–10. Management of Drug Overdose and Poisoning *Continued*

Drug/Substance	Trade or Street Name	Signs/Symptoms	EMT Management	Special Comments
Opiates and derivatives Opium Opium tincture Laudanum Morphine sulfate Codeine Diacetylmorphine Hydromorphone Oxycodone Meperidine	Numbers in parentheses indicate potency equal to 10 mg of morphine sulfate Paregoric (25 ml) Morphine Codeine (60–100 mg) Heroin (3 mg) Dilaudid (2 mg) Percodan (50 mg) Demerol (80–100 mg)	Pupils are small to pinpoint and are nonreactive Respiratory arrest is common, also shallow slow respirations Patients are stuporous to comatose but are often arousable to painful stimuli; will return to unconsciousness when stimulus is relaxed Patients may have pulmonary edema and/or atrial fibrillation Look for fresh injection sites in arms, legs, between fingers and toes, as well as tattoos near large veins to hide needle marks	Support vital signs and ventilation as required Patient may be talking but not have gag to protect airway Antidote is naloxone (Narcan), which is usually available from paramedics or most medical facilities These patients may have underlying communicable diseases from poor care of needles and poor living habits Treat pulmonary edema as required	Strychnine is often used to "cut" opiates; side effect is seizure and hypothermia Be alert; patients can be dangerous Do not relax vigilance in presence of patient or friends; stick to medical approach only Have police in attendance
Methadone	Dolophine (8 mg) Methadone Amidone			Methadone often used in detoxification of heroin addicts; withdrawal symptoms are slower and less severe
Oxycodone and acetaminophen Propoxyphene Propoxyphene and acetaminophen	Percocet Darvon Darvocet, Darvocet-N	Pupils may not be pinpoint Can produce all other effects of opiates Darvocet-N may present with symptoms of hypoglycemia	Same as opiates	Can be refined and injected
Etorphine hydrochloride	M99	Is a thousand times more potent than morphine with sedative and respiratory effects	Same as opiates	Used only by veterinarians to immobilize large animals
Stimulants Amphetamine	Benzedrine (prescription); benz, bennies (street)	Agitation, flushing, perspiration, tachycardia, hypertension	Support vital signs and ventilation as required	Barbiturates often used to control "high"; therefore patient may have combined symptoms Usual doses: 5–60 mg per day
Dextroamphetamine Methamphetamine	Dexedrine (prescription); dexies, copilots (street) Desoxyn, Methedrine, Obedrin-L (prescription); black beauties (street)	Patient may be hyperactive, with muscle twitching Anxiety with visual hallucinations may occur	Handle patient with caution—may have rapid mood changes May require restraints in best interest of patient	
Amphetamine and dextroamphetamine	Biphenamine	Nausea, vomiting, abdominal cramps Hyperventilation Moderately dilated pupils	Ipecac should be considered if patient has active gag reflex and is conscious	

Drug	Trade/Street names	Signs and symptoms	Treatment	Comments
Methylphenidate	Ritalin (prescription); ritlins (street)	When severe, can lead to seizure and coma		Ritalin used for hyperactive children to reduce hyperactivity; often injected, for street use, causing abscesses on skin and "cotton fever" from cotton ball fibers through which drug was strained for injection. Usual dose 10–60 mg per day, divided 2–3 times per day
Phenmetrazine Cocaine	Preludin (prescription); snow, coke (street)	Patient often combative		
Hallucinogens, psychedelics DMT (dimethyltryptamine) LSD Mescaline Peyote Psilocybin		Pupils are large. Patient is agitated, hot, flushed, delirious with hallucinations. Toxic level of LSD usually lasts 12–24 hours	Protect patient from injury to EMT(s) and themselves. Support vital signs and ventilation as required	Combination of hallucinogen and phenothiazines may cause cardiovascular failure, shock, and death
Phencyclidine	PCP, animal tranquilizer (prescription); angel dust, peace pill, angel fuzz, supergrass (with marijuana) (street)	Pupils may be mid-size to large. Combative behavior changing to depression. Respiratory arrest. Effect may last 2–4 days. Hallucinations	Same as above. This patient can be extremely dangerous; patients have been known to break their own limbs during restraint without acknowledging injury	PCP can be easily manufactured outside the lab in large quantity, with varied composition as a result. Patient may react differently to same-size dose. Is used in many forms
Tetrahydrocannabinol	Marijuana, grass, pot, weed, Colombian gold, Thai sticks, etc. (street)	Anxiety, agitation. Large pupils with "bloodshot" whites of eyes. Appears drunk. Hyperventilation secondary to surprising extra effect of "good" drug	Observation is usually sufficient. Occasional hypotension when used in conjunction with alcohol. Treat hyperventilation as usual	
Psychotropic agents Phenothiazines Chlorpromazine Trifluoperazine	Thorazine, Promapar, Chlor-PZ; Stelazine	Lethargy, which may progress to coma. Orthostatic (postural) hypotension to profound hypotension	Treat hypotension with elevated extremities. Support ventilation. Monitor cardiac arrhythmias if monitor is available	All phenothiazines lower the seizure threshold
Thioridazine Prochlorperazine	Mellaril Compazine	Pulmonary edema (Mellaril). Cardiac arrhythmias. Dystonic reactions (swollen tongue, rigid jaw with face distorted)	Be prepared for cardiac and/or respiratory arrest. High-flow oxygen or bag mask assist	
Haloperidol Perphenazine	Haldol Trilafon	Limbs tonic, respiratory distress. Seizures	These patients require immediate care to treat severe symptoms early	Patient can become extremely ill rapidly

Table continued on following page

TABLE 12–10. Management of Drug Overdose and Poisoning *Continued*

Drug/Substance	Trade or Street Name	Signs/Symptoms	EMT Management	Special Comments
Antidepressants				
Tricyclics				
Amitriptyline	Elavil, Endep	Patients are often excited but can progress rapidly to coma	Treat same as phenothiazines	Patient can become extremely ill rapidly
Imipranil	Tofranil	Tachycardia and arrhythmias are very common	Cardiac arrhythmias with sudden death are the greatest danger	
Desipramine	Norpramin	Hypertension or hypotension		
Nortriptyline	Aventyl	Seizures		
Doxepin	Sinequan	May have symptoms of phenothiazines and tricyclics		
Amitriptyline and perphenazine	Triavil, Etrafon			
MAO inhibitors	Parnate Marplan Niamid Nardil	Same as tricyclics		Foods such as cheese and wine may cause symptoms of toxicity
Atropinic anticholinergics				
Belladonna	Atropine, belladonna	Classic atropine intoxication Delirious ("mad as a hatter"), flushed ("red as a beet"), dilated pupils ("blind as a bat"), absent perspiration ("dry as a bone")	Control hypotension as required Control hyperthermia as required	Jimson weed and nightshade contain belladonna
Antihistamines				
Diphenhydramine	Benadryl	Sedative effect with low dosage	Same as anticholinergics	Commonly used by public as antinausea medicine
Dimenhydrinate	Dramamine	Symptoms the same as anticholinergics in high dosage		
Mild analgesics				
Salicylate	Aspirin and others (over 400 preparations contain salicylate)	Initial symptoms: headache, nausea, hyperventilation Later symptoms: lethargy to coma Seizures Increased perspiration, hyperthermia	Use ipecac as soon as possible if patient is conscious; aspirin tends to form hard "ball" in stomach if not removed	
Acetaminophen	Tylenol, Datril, often combined with mild opiates	Nausea, general ill feeling Liver damage may occur in large quantity overdoses after 24 hours	Use ipecac as soon as possible if patient is conscious Administer large quantities of fluid orally to cause excretion naturally	

Compound	Trade name	Signs and symptoms	Treatment	Comments
Other compounds				
Phenytoin	Dilantin	Slurred speech, hypotension; Occasional dystonic posturing (see phenothiazine); Coma is rare except with massive overdose; May develop AV block arrhythmia	Support vital signs and ventilation; Cardiac monitor if available; be prepared to assist heart block with CPR should hypotension occur	Overdose may be accidental, as each patient's ability to metabolize this drug varies
Lithium	Eskalith, Lithane	Muscle tremor, blackout spells, slurred speech, dizziness, blurred vision, dry mouth, fatigue, lethargy, confusion, stupor, coma; early signs of diarrhea, vomiting, dizziness	Support vital signs and ventilation	Lithium toxicity is closely related to serum lithium levels, and can occur at doses close to therapeutic levels; Treats manic-depressive patients only
Iron				
Ferrous gluconate	Fergon	Nausea, vomiting, diarrhea, stomach upset, weak/rapid pulse, decreased blood pressure	Induce vomiting with ipecac; Hospital must pump stomach within first hour, as stomach may perforate from treatment	
Ferrous sulfate	Feosol, Mol-Iron, others	Heavy dose can cause brisk bleeding in stomach/intestine and black tarry stools (from hemorrhage); Shock		
Ferrous fumarate	Feostat, others			
Alcohol compounds				
Ethanol	"Alcohol"	"Drunkenness"-like symptoms, coma, and respiratory depression with large quantities; Loss of gag reflex	Normally supportive; May require aggressive airway management with children and young adults (often first-time users)	Often used mixed with a variety of drugs
Methanol	Sterno	Dilated, slow-reacting pupils; Usually takes 8–36 hours to take effect: headache, blurred vision, seizures, nausea, vomiting, abdominal cramps, to coma	Main treatment is performed by hospital; Contact physician for ipecac in field	As little as 2 teaspoons can be toxic; 2–8 oz can be fatal
Ethylene glycol	Antifreeze	Hyperventilation; Coma occurs rapidly; may cause pulmonary edema seizures	Same as methanol	As little as 100 ml may cause coma

(Adapted from Copass MK, Soper RG, Eisenberg S: EMT Manual, 2nd ed. Philadelphia, WB Saunders, 1991.)

the victim. The kit contains an ampule of amyl nitrite, which can be administered at the scene. If directed to do so, break the amyl nitrite capsule and have the patient inhale fumes for 30 seconds every minute. Use a new ampule every 3 minutes. Cyanide victims need emergency transport to a hospital setting where more nitrites can be given intravenously.

Hydrogen sulfide is a gas that smells like rotten eggs. It is used in industries such as petroleum and rubber processing. It results from the decay of organic matter. Exposure can occur in sewers, animal rendering plants, tanneries, fertilizer plants, and farming. Because of the characteristic odor, victims usually flee from exposure. However, over time, the nose becomes insensitive to the smell, leaving workers exposed to increasing levels in the environment. Treatment includes administration of high-concentration oxygen.

IRRITANT GASES. Irritant gases cause inflammatory damage to the airway and bronchoconstriction. They react with water in the airway to cause toxic reactions to the mucosa.

The most soluble agents, such as ammonia, sulfur dioxide, and hydrogen chloride, react almost immediately, causing tearing, coughing, and an uncomfortable sensation in the nose and throat. Victims are impelled to flee. Unless the irritant gases are inhaled in extreme concentrations, in a closed space, or by an unconscious victim, damage is usually confined to the upper airway. Closure of the upper airway is of greatest immediate concern.

By contrast, irritating gases with low solubility such as phosgene and nitrous dioxides are less likely to react immediately in the upper airway. As a result, the warning irritation may not be present and victims often inhale these agents over a longer period of time. Likewise, because the gases are not consumed by reaction with the water in the upper airway, they enter the lower airway where damage can occur over hours to days. These patients develop severe symptoms some time after they have been removed from the smoke or gas exposure.

There are other agents that have effects on both the lower and upper airways. A table of these gases is included for your review (Table 12–11).

ORGANOPHOSPHATES. The spraying of fields and gardens with insecticides can result in inhalation of organophosphates. When these are inhaled, the patient may first experience bronchoconstriction and excessive pulmonary secretions before the onset of the other symptoms described previously.

Management

Principles of management are as follows:

1. Remove the victim from the source. Assess the need for basic life support.

2. Assess the upper airway. Look for hoarseness or stridor. Transport rapidly if there are signs of oral pharyngeal edema, since this presents the risk of airway closure.

3. Give humidified oxygen.

Note that some effects of exposure to poisonous gases can be delayed.

Absorbed Poisons

The skin is damaged by corrosive and caustic agents that can cause severe chemical burns. They should be flushed from the skin with copious amounts of water after contaminated clothing is removed. Eyes should be gently and thoroughly irrigated with water for at least 15 to 20 minutes. If the agent is a dry powder (e.g., dry lime), it should be brushed off the skin before flushing with water.

The skin is a large organ and many agents can be absorbed through the skin into the body. Insecticides are an example of a systemic toxin that can be absorbed. Toxic agents should be washed off the skin by flooding it with water and then washing with soap and water. Contaminated clothing must be removed and placed in a secure container for proper handling to prevent exposure to others. Call the poison control center to help identify the agent and the best course of management in the field.

The EMT must wear protective clothing to avoid contamination with the toxic substance by direct contact or splashes.

Injected Poisons
GENERAL PRINCIPLES

Injections cause the most rapid onset of drug effects. There is little to be done to eliminate injected drugs. Usually, injection emergencies are self-administered overdoses. However, bites and stings can result in injections of venom through the skin as well.

COMMONLY INJECTED DRUGS

Heroin, amphetamines, and cocaine are the most commonly injected drugs. Management is the same as if the drugs were ingested or inhaled, except there is no attempt made to prevent absorption.

INSECT BITES AND STINGS

The most severe reaction to stings is anaphylaxis. Other effects are usually local. Before swelling occurs, be sure to remove constricting clothing and jewelry.

The bites of the brown recluse spider (Fig. 12–9), which is primarily found in the South but can occur nationwide, can cause local necrosis about the bite. The

TABLE 12–11. Toxic Gases

GAS	SG*	Odor	Color	PHYSIOLOGIC EFFECT	TREATMENT	TYPES OF FIRE
		PROPERTIES				
Simple Asphyxiants						
Carbon dioxide (CO_2)	1.53	Odorless	Colorless	Simple asphyxiant; concentrations of 10% in atmosphere → unconsciousness	O_2	Combustion; blast furnace
Methane (CH_4)	0.55	Odorless	Colorless	Simple asphyxiant	O_2	Coal mines; marsh gas
Chemical Asphyxiants						
Carbon monoxide (CO)	0.97	Odorless	Colorless	Asphyxiation (COHb)	O_2	All fires
Cyanide (CN)	0.93	Bitter almonds		Chemical asphyxiant, cyanide, pink color may be seen	Lilly Cyanide Kit	Polyurethane, nitrogen-containing polymers, wool, silk, polyacrylonitrile
Hydrogen sulfide (H_2S)	1.19	Powerful nauseating smell (olfactory fatigue)	Colorless	Chemical asphyxiant like CN with irritant properties	Lilly Cyanide Kit	Sulfur and its components; decaying organic matter; industry
Irritant Gases (Irritation Proportional to Solubility)						
Sulfur dioxide (SO_2)	2.23	Rotten eggs	Colorless	Intensely irritating to eyes, nose, throat; usually upper airway effects	Supportive	Coal, oil, rubber, common oxidation product of sulfur
Ammonia (NH_3)	0.6	Noxious	Colorless	Intensely irritating to eyes, nose, throat; usually upper airway effects	Supportive	Melamine; used in industry to produce fertilizers, plastics, explosives; commercial refrigerant
Hydrogen chloride (HCl)	1.27	Chlorine	Colorless (anhydrous white mist hydrated)	Irritant; delayed effects reported; myocardial irritability in PVC exposure reported; may be secondary to CO	Supportive	Polyvinyl chloride and other plastics; products continue to be evolved after control of flames and dissipation of smoke (overhaul phase)
Chlorine (Cl_2)	2.5	Chlorine	Greenish yellow	Irritant; pulmonary edema	Supportive	Plastics
Irritants (Less Soluble than Above)						
Phosgene ($COCl_2$)	1.4	Mowed hay	Colorless	Irritant; poorly perceived in concentrations capable of producing toxic effects; pulmonary edema after latent period	Supportive	Polyvinyl chlorinated hydrocarbon; CCl_4 fire extinguishers (old); degreaser in welding, in poorly ventilated areas
Nitrogen dioxides (NO_2, N_2, O_4)		Pungent odor	Heavier than air, reddish brown	Only mild irritant to eye and respiratory tract; pulmonary edema; bronchiolitis	Supportive steroids might be considered	Celluloid, guncotton, dynamite, acetylene and electrical arc welding in enclosed and underventilated areas (silo filler's disease)
Nonirritant (Note Specific Pathologic Effect)						
Arsine (AsH_3)		Garlic	Colorless	Nonirritating; attaches to sulfhydryl groups of Hb; hemolysis, acute renal failure, jaundice	O_2, transfusion since arsine nondialyzable, and dialysis for acute renal failure	Hosing down hot dross containing arsenide metals; combustion of fossil fuels; coal mines, marsh gas

*SG = The weight of gas as compared with that of air. An SG greater than 1 will cause the gas to settle low in the environment and increase the potential for inhalation.

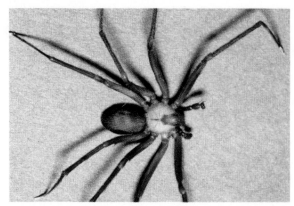

FIGURE 12–9. Brown recluse spider. (From Auerbach PS, Geehr EC (eds): Management of Wilderness and Environmental Emergencies, 2nd ed. St Louis, CV Mosby, 1988. Courtesy of Sherman Minton, M.D.)

brown recluse spider has a dark color band on its back that is shaped like a violin. The venom causes local pain, then spreads out from the bite site to the surrounding skin. Many patients are not aware that they have been bitten until they notice a painful red spot, sometimes with a central blister. The center darkens, the surrounding area blanches, and the outermost ring gets reddish, in some cases leading to a "patriotic bull's-eye" appearance. Very few individuals have systemic reactions, with fever, chills, and weakness, and, in the worst cases, problems with their breakdown of blood cells and clotting mechanisms. The treatment is hospital based.

The black widow spider is more common and is found throughout the United States. The female has a characteristic shiny black body with a red hourglass shape on the abdomen. The venom contains a neurotoxin, and in severe cases weakness and respiratory depression can occur. Most often the symptoms are pain at the site, abdominal pain, and lower extremity weakness. At the site of the bite, there may be slight swelling and faint bite marks. Rigidity and tenderness of the abdominal muscles occur, along with fever, chills, rigidity, and spasms of other large muscle groups. Antivenom is available for severe cases. The need for antivenom in all but the most extreme case has been questioned. Small children and debilitated adults are believed to be most susceptible to severe consequences. Treat black widow spider bites like snake bites. Immobilize the extremity as if it were fractured, and avoid unnecessary movement.

Fire ants, found in the southern parts of the United States, can inflict multiple stings if encountered in the loose mounds of dirt that they inhabit. Each sting can

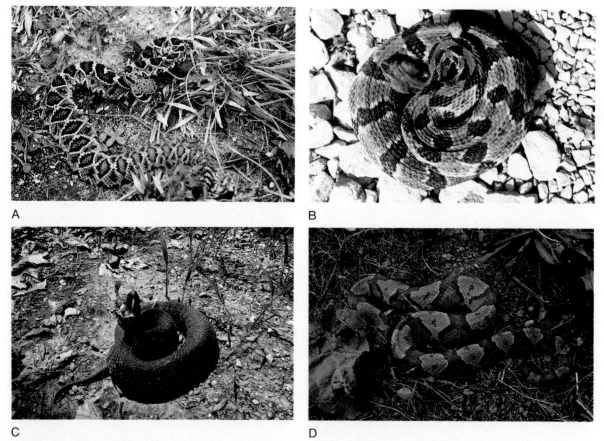

FIGURE 12–10. North American pit vipers. (*A*) Eastern diamondback rattlesnake. (*B*) Timber rattlesnake. (*C*) Cottonmouth. (*D*) Copperhead. (From Auerbach PS, Geehr EC (eds): Management of Wilderness and Environmental Emergencies, 2nd ed. St Louis, CV Mosby, 1988. Courtesy of Sherman Minton, M.D.)

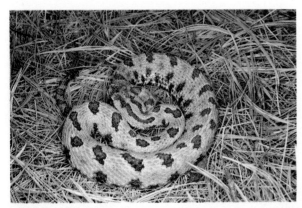

FIGURE 12–11. Pigmy rattlesnake. (From Auerbach PS, Geehr EC (eds): Management of Wilderness and Environmental Emergencies, 2nd ed. St Louis, CV Mosby, 1988. Courtesy of Sherman Minton, M.D.)

give rise to a raised papule, which develops pus in 6 to 24 hours. Care is supportive.

Scorpion and tarantula bites in the United States cause local pain but are not fatal.

SNAKE BITES

Venomous snakes in the United States include the pit vipers (rattlesnakes, cottonmouths, copperheads (Figs. 12–10 and 12–11) and coral snakes (Fig. 12–12).

The pit vipers cause local necrosis. With severe cases, systemic effects occur and death may result. Definitive care requires use of antivenom.

The coral snake causes no local necrosis. The nervous system is affected when the poison is absorbed. Onset of effects may be delayed up to 12 hours after envenomation.

Because of the different actions of the two types of venom, it is important to distinguish from the outset the type of snake, to determine whether envenomation took place, and to apply treatment accordingly.

Antivenom is available to treat severe envenomations. Controversy exists as to the best field therapy. It is generally agreed that since coral snakes kill by systemic effects and do not damage the tissues at the bite site, methods to delay absorption from the wound are a principal aim of treatment. Conversely, since pit viper bites are apt to cause local tissue damage but less likely to cause death if absorbed, many do not recommend attempts to delay systemic absorption from the wound. Concentration of pit viper venom in the extremity may cause loss of the entire limb.

HOW DO YOU RECOGNIZE A PIT VIPER BITE? Pit vipers can be distinguished from nonpoisonous snakes by their elliptical pupils, the pit (heat sensor) between the eyes and nostril, fangs (Fig. 12–13), and the single row of plates on the tail. The bite is noted by the presence of fang marks at the bite site (Fig. 12–14). The fangs are needle sharp and used by the snake to inject the

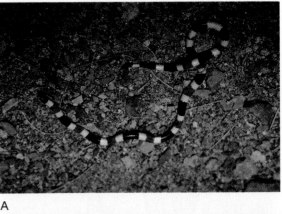

A

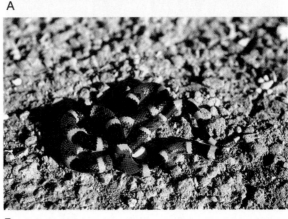

B

FIGURE 12–12. Coral snakes. (A) Sonoran coral snake. (B) North American coral snake. (From Auerbach PS, Geehr EC (eds): Management of Wilderness and Environmental Emergencies, 2nd ed. St. Louis, CV Mosby, 1988. Courtesy of Sherman Minton, M.D.)

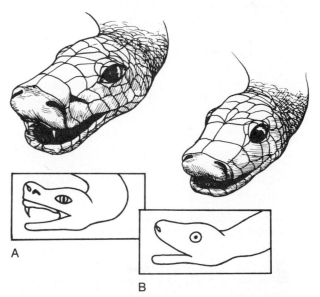

A

B

FIGURE 12–13. The characteristics of a poisonous snake contrasted with those of a nonpoisonous snake. (A) The head of a pit viper: note the elliptical eyes, heat-sensing pits on the sides of the head near the nostrils, fangs, and triangular head. (B) The head of a nonpoisonous snake: note the round eyes, no fangs, and rounded head. (From Wiener SL, Barrett J: Trauma Management for Civilian and Military Physicians. Philadelphia, WB Saunders, 1986, p. 468.)

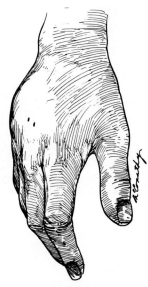

FIGURE 12–14. Illustration of a pit viper bite. (From Wiener SL, Barrett J: Trauma Management for Civilian and Military Physicians. Philadelphia, WB Saunders, 1986, p. 468.)

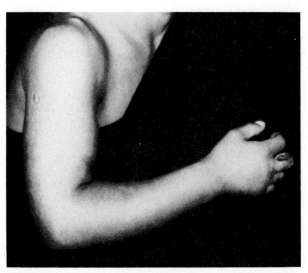

FIGURE 12–15. A swollen arm following a rattlesnake bite. (From Wiener SL, Barrett J: Trauma Management for Civilian and Military Physicians. Philadelphia, WB Saunders, 1986, p. 470.)

venom. Other common symptoms of a pit viper bite are swelling, pain, and redness at the site (Fig. 12–15).

MANAGEMENT OF PIT VIPER BITES. When approaching the snake bite victim, do the following:

1. Move out of range of the snake—generally less than the length of the snake.
2. Observe the approximate size of the snake, since the larger the snake, the larger the potential envenomation.

If possible, bring the dead snake (or have it brought) to the hospital for identification. Do not handle the dead snake directly, or even the decapitated head, since reflex actions of the snake can cause envenomation.

> ## PROCEDURE 12–1
> ## TREATING A SNAKE BITE
>
> 1. Have the victim rest and immobilize the extremity with a splint as you would for a fracture.
> 2. If swelling is present, make a small mark at its edge so any changes are evident on later evaluation.
> 3. Transport the victim to the closest hospital that is able to care for snake bites.
>
> *Note*: Follow local protocols for coral snake bites, which may call for application of a pressure bandage over the bite to decrease systemic absorption.
> *Note*: Be sure you know your local protocols for handling snake bites.
> *Note*: Do not use ice or cut the wound in an attempt to suck out the venom.

HOW DO YOU RECOGNIZE A CORAL SNAKE? Coral snakes are found in the southern United States. They are distinguished by their red, yellow, and black bands. The red and yellow bands on the coral snake are next to each other and there is a saying:

> "Red on yellow, kill a fellow,
> Red on black, venom lack."

This is useful to help distinguish the coral snake from nonvenomous look-alikes.

Coral snakes have very small fangs and their bite marks are more noteworthy than their fang marks. The fangs are tiny and close together. A drop of blood may be expressed after envenomation, confirming that fangs entered the skin. Often the coral snake holds on and "chews" the victim for a few seconds, and has to be pulled off. Victims have described this sensation as pulling off Velcro. Early signs and symptoms may be mild, and there is usually only minimal redness and swelling at the bite site. This is in contrast to pit viper bites, which are marked by early pain and swelling at the bite site.

MANAGEMENT OF CORAL SNAKE BITES. The approach to the patient is the same as for pit viper bites.

Treatment rests with early antivenom administration. Otherwise, treatment is the same as with pit viper bites, except that many experts recommend application of a "loose" elastic bandage above or around the bite site to slow systemic absorption until antivenom can be given. If a constricting bandage is applied proximal to the wound, it should allow one finger to enter beneath it and not obliterate distal pulsations (Fig. 12–16).

Most authorities recommend against the use of ice

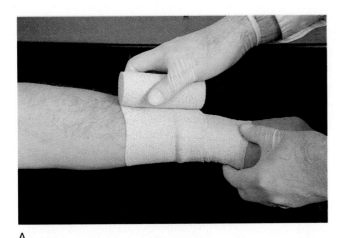

A

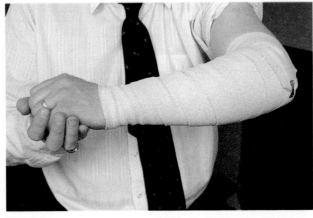

B

FIGURE 12–16. (*A* and *B*) Ace bandage wrap for a coral snake bite. Using a broad elastic bandage, roll it over the bite site and continue up the extremity as if treating a sprain.

and cutting and sucking out of venom. Learn and follow your local protocols.

Note that exotic poisonous snakes may be kept as pets. Often pet owners or friends are bitten when they are intoxicated and handle these snakes carelessly. Since keeping venomous snakes is illegal, persons bitten in this way may hide the true history.

Marine Animals

Certain sea animals cause stings and punctures with their spines.

Stinging animals include the jellyfish, Portuguese man-of-war, anemones, and corals. Treatment consists of flooding the affected area with sea water (never fresh water) and washing with alcohol if available. Alcohol deactivates the toxin. Apply shaving cream, sand, or talcum powder to the area and then scrape it off—in hopes of removing any remaining tentacles and nematocysts, which cause the stinging.

Avoid washing the area with fresh water, since this may precipitate the nematocysts to fire.

Punctures can occur from cone shells, urchins, stingrays, and spiny fish. Treatment consists of immobilizing the affected area and soaking it in water as hot as the patient can tolerate for 30 to 90 minutes. However, be careful to avoid water that is too hot—check it with your hand to be sure it will not cause heat injury. The toxin introduced into the wound should be inactivated by the hot water.

Drugs of Abuse

Drug abuse is one of the greatest problems in modern society. Both illicit and legal drugs can be abused.

Drug or substance abuse involves the repeated self-administration by ingestion, inhalation, or injection for a sense of well-being, or a "high." As a person continues to use a drug, he or she develops *tolerance* to the drug effects. Tolerance means that larger and larger doses are required to reach the same feeling of well-being. The drug abuser may begin to mix different substances to seek a unique or different "high," or sense of euphoria. A person becomes *dependent* on a drug when he or she cannot sustain the sense of well-being without drug administration. This dependency can be psychologic or physical. Physical and psychologic *withdrawal* symptoms can occur if the person stops using the drug. Ultimately, the person may become *addicted*, a condition manifested by compulsive behavior concentrated on obtaining the drug.

The most commonly abused drug in the United States is alcohol. Withdrawal from prolonged drinking can cause shakes, tremors, and seizures. In severe cases, *delirium tremens* can result, with the patient experiencing hyperactivity, increased respiratory and pulse rates, increased temperature, and hypertension. The patient may have hallucinations and commonly sees insects crawling around him or her. Delirium tremens is a medical emergency and can cause death if untreated.

Other drugs of abuse include heroin, cocaine, LSD, PCP, and many prescription drugs.

The EMT's contact with patients who are abusing drugs often occurs when they have taken an overdose, have a behavior emergency, or are experiencing trauma complicated or caused by a drug overdose. Many patients deny involvement, making it difficult to gather a reliable history. Often, the EMT has to treat psychologic and physical manifestations simultaneously. Table 12–12 lists some commonly abused drugs, their street names, how they are taken, and their associated signs and symptoms.

The following protocol summarizes the care of a victim of poisoning or overdose.

TABLE 12–12. Commonly Abused Drugs

Drug	Street Name	How Used	Symptoms and Signs
Marijuana Hashish	Pot, grass, reefer, weed, hash, sinsemilla, joint	Smoked Ingested	Loss of interest Recent memory loss Dry mouth and throat Mood changes Increased appetite
Alcohol	Booze, brew, hooch	Ingested	Impaired coordination Impaired judgment
Nicotine	Smoke, butt, coffin nail	Smoked Chewed	Tobacco smell Stained teeth
Amphetamines	Speed, uppers, pep pills, bennies, dexies, black beauties, meth, crystal	Ingested Injected Sniffed	Dilated pupils Increased energy Irritability Nervousness Needle marks
Cocaine	Coke, crack, snow, white lady, toot	Snorted Injected Ingested Smoked	Dilated pupils Increased energy Restlessness Intense anxiety Paranoid behavior Needle marks
Barbiturates	Downers, barbs, yellow jackets, red devils, blue devils, double trouble	Injected Ingested	Constricted pupils Confusion Impaired judgment Drowsiness Slurring of speech Needle marks
Methaqualone	Ludes, sopors, quaaludes	Ingested	Slurring of speech Drowsiness Impaired judgment Euphoria Seizures
Heroin Morphine	Junk, scag, dope, horse, smack, dreamer	Injected Smoked Sniffed Skin popped	Constricted pupils Needle marks Drowsiness Mental clouding
Codeine	School boy	Ingested Sniffed	Constricted pupils Drowsiness

Demerol
  Methadone
  Percodan
  Pentazocine
		Ingested
		Injected
			Constricted pupils
			Drowsiness
			Mental clouding
			Needle marks

PCP (phencyclidine)	Angel dust, hog, killer weed, supergrass	Smoked Snorted Injected Ingested	Dilated pupils Slurring of speech Hallucinations Blurring of vision Uncoordination Agitation Confusion Aggressive behavior
LSD (lysergic acid diethylamide)	Acid, cubes, purple haze	Ingested Injected	Dilated pupils Hallucinations Mood swings Increased alertness Acute panic reactions
Mescaline	Mesc, cactus	Ingested	Dilated pupils Hallucinations Mood swings
Psilocybin	Magic mushrooms	Ingested	Dilated pupils Hallucinations Mood swings
Airplane glue* Paint thinner*		Inhaled Sniffed	Poor motor coordination Impaired vision Violent behavior

TABLE 12–12. Commonly Abused Drugs *Continued*

Drug	Street Name	How Used	Symptoms and Signs
Nitrous oxide	Laughing gas, whippets	Inhaled Sniffed	Hilarity Euphoria Lightheadedness
Amyl nitrite	Poppers, rush, locker room, snappers, amies	Inhaled Sniffed	Hilarity Dizziness Headache Impaired thought

* The active agent in airplane glue and paint thinner is toluene. Naphtha, methyl ethyl ketone, and gasoline may produce similar symptoms.

(From the Department of Transportation Emergency Medical Technician National Standard Curriculum, 1985.)

 P R O T O C O L

APPROACH TO THE VICTIM OF POISONING OR DRUG OVERDOSE

1. *Special Assessment Considerations*

   A. Survey the scene, note especially:
      1. Hazardous situations
      2. Remnants of the poison or drug
      3. Containers and/or drug paraphernalia
      4. Vomitus

   B. Determine age and weight of patient.

   C. Attempt to determine the drug or poison:

      (1) How was it taken?
      (2) How long ago was it taken?
      (3) How much of the substance was taken?
      (4) Was it taken all at once or over a period of time?
      (5) Did the patient vomit?
      (6) Antidotes taken?
      (7) Previous contact to Poison Control?

   D. Determine the patient's present signs and symptoms such as urticaria, injection sites, skin color, breath odor, burns to mouth, etc.

   E. Determine the patient's medical history.

   F. If the patient is unconscious, perform a Glasgow Coma Scale and record the findings.

   G. Assess need for advanced life support (ALS) assistance, being mindful that ALS can assist with special poisonings such as narcotics and insecticides.

   H. If possible, bring the product or substance and container with the patient to the hospital.

   > *CAUTION!*
   >
   > TAKE PRECAUTIONS NOT TO CONTAMINATE SELF OR OTHERS!

2. *Treatment*
   Patients who are conscious:

   A. Remove the patient from any hazards.

   B. Maintain ABCs.

   C. Administer high-concentration oxygen.

   D. Assist ventilations as necessary by bag-valve-mask with supplemental oxygen or demand valve resuscitator.

   > *NOTE!*
   >
   > SUCH PATIENTS MAY DETERIORATE RAPIDLY. BE ESPECIALLY ALERT FOR RESPIRATORY INSUFFICIENCY OR ARREST.

SWALLOWED POISONS

   A. If possible, contact the Poison Control Center or EMS Telemetry Control for instructions on treatment, which may include the administration of milk, water, or ipecac, induction of vomiting, etc. DO NOT INDUCE VOMITING FOR HYDROCARBONS, ACIDS AND BASES, AND CAUSTIC SUBSTANCES.

   B. Transport, keeping the patient warm.

   C. Obtain and record the vital signs and repeat as necessary.

   > *CAUTION!*
   >
   > DO NOT ATTEMPT TO NEUTRALIZE POISONS OR DRUGS UNLESS DIRECTED TO DO SO BY POISON CONTROL OR EMS TELEMETRY CONTROL!

   > *CAUTION!*
   >
   > DILUTION OF POISONS OR INDUCTION OF VOMITING IS CONTRAINDICATED IN UNCONSCIOUS OR CONVULSIVE PATIENTS!

   > *NOTE!*
   >
   > DO NOT ATTEMPT TO INDUCE VOMITING UNLESS DIRECTED TO DO SO BY POISON CONTROL OR TELEMETRY CONTROL.

Continued

INHALED POISONS

A. Ensure that the scene is safe for entry. If danger of poisonous gases, vapors, or sprays or a low-oxygen environment is present, it may be necessary to obtain assistance from trained rescue personnel.

B. Remove the patient to fresh air.

C. Place the patient in a position of comfort.

D. Ensure that the patient's airway is open and that breathing and circulation are adequate.

E. Administer high-concentration oxygen.

F. Transport, keeping the patient warm.

G. Obtain and record vital signs, and repeat as necessary en route.

H. Record all patient care information, including the patient's medical history and all treatment provided, on the prehospital care report.

INJECTED SUBSTANCES

A. Attempt to calm the patient.

B. Remove jewelry from affected area if swelling begins.

C. Place injection site lower than the patient's heart if possible.

D. If the injury is from a snake, implement snake bite operating procedure.

SURFACE CONTACT SUBSTANCES

A. Remove patient from source as soon as this can be done *SAFELY*.

B. Remove all contaminated clothing.

C. Rinse affected area thoroughly with saline or sterile or plain water for 5 to 10 minutes.

D. Bandage any substance burns with a dry sterile dressing.

SKIN OR EYE(S) CONTAMINATION

A. Refer to the BURNS/CONTAMINATION (CHEMICAL/RADIATION) PROTOCOL IN CHAPTER 11.

PATIENTS WHO ARE UNCONSCIOUS OR HAVE ALTERED MENTAL STATUS

A. Ensure that the patient's airway is open and that breathing and circulation are adequate, and suction as necessary.

B. Administer high-concentration oxygen.

C. Transport, keeping the patient warm.

D. Obtain and record the vital signs, and repeat as necessary en route to the hospital.

E. Record all patient care information, including patient's medical history and all treatment provided, on the prehospital care report.

From Manual for Emergency Medical Technicians. Emergency Medical Services Program. Albany, New York State Department of Health, 1990 and New York City EMS Academy Training Protocols.

COMMUNICABLE DISEASES

Introduction

Communicable (infectious or contagious) or *infectious diseases* are capable of being spread from one person to another. The common cold is a communicable disease that is well known to everyone. Sneezing and coughing can spread the virus that causes the "cold" from an infected person to others. Not all infectious diseases are as benign as the cold. Some are life-threatening. The EMT must take precautions to prevent the spread of diseases from the EMT to patients, from patients to EMTs, and from the EMT and the patient to others.

The EMT cares for many patients who have infectious diseases requiring emergency care. At times, it may be obvious that a patient has signs of infection; at other times, this may not be obvious. This explains why EMTs should have a basic understanding of infectious diseases so they can take appropriate precautions for all patient contacts. The EMT should appreciate how infections are spread, the body's response to exposure to infectious agents, and the actions to take before, during, and following care of an infected patient. Armed with this knowledge, and following the guidelines in this text, the EMT can confidently provide the necessary care to sick patients and at the same time minimize the hazard to the EMT.

The precautions one takes to prevent the spread of infectious disease are called infection control. *Infection control* is the practice of common-sense actions to block the spread of infectious agents. Once learned, they become part of the EMT's everyday behavior.

Infection control practices are routinely followed in hospitals and all other health care settings. The Centers for Disease Control (CDC) publishes guidelines that help standardize infection control practices across the country. Recently, the CDC specifically addressed infection control guidelines for emergency workers in response to federal law. This document is entitled "Guidelines for Prevention of Transmission of Human Immunodeficiency Virus and Hepatitis B to Health-Care and Public-Safety Workers," and is published in the *Morbidity and Mortality Weekly Report* in 1989.

CDC guidelines are constantly updated in light of new knowledge about infectious diseases and are the basis for most of the recommendations in this text. EMTs should keep up with current guidelines by attending continuing medical education courses and following updates in local practices, protocols, and procedures.

INFECTIOUS AGENTS

Infections are caused by *microorganisms* (not visible to the naked eye) that are toxic to the body. These microorganisms include agents classified as bacteria, viruses, fungi, and parasites. Infectious agents multiply and can cause direct and indirect damage to the body. Microorganisms that are harmful to the body are said to be pathogenic.

Some infections can be treated with medications that inhibit or kill the microorganisms. For example, there are many antibiotics used to treat bacterial infections. Penicillin may be taken for a particular type of sore throat, or pharyngitis, caused by the streptococcus bacteria, commonly called "strep throat." There are some antiviral drugs, but for many viral infections there is no "cure." Most viral infections are successfully eliminated by the body's own immune system, without the need for medication. Athlete's foot, caused by the tinea fungus, can be treated with antifungal agents. There are a variety of drugs that are effective against many parasitic infections.

There are many severe infections for which there is no effective treatment once the infection begins. For some of these infections, such as polio, rubella ("German measles"), measles, diphtheria, tetanus ("lockjaw"), pertussis ("whooping cough"), and hepatitis B, vaccination or immunization can prevent the infection. If no immunization or cure is available, as is currently true for acquired immunodeficiency syndrome (AIDS), then preventing exposure is of the greatest importance.

Not all microorganisms are harmful. For example, certain bacteria inhabit the intestine, where they aid digestion. Other bacteria are found in the upper respiratory tract and on the skin surface. These bacteria can be harmful if they enter a part of the body where they are not normally found. Intestinal bacteria that spill into the peritoneal cavity—as can happen with a ruptured appendix or a stab wound to the abdomen—can cause a life-threatening infection. Bacteria that normally inhabit the mouth, if aspirated into the lung, can cause pneumonia.

THE SPREAD OF COMMUNICABLE DISEASES

Infectious agents spread from a source to a host. A *source* of infection may be a person, an insect, an object, or another substance that carries or is contaminated by an infectious agent. A *reservoir* is a source in which infectious agents can live and multiply, such as a sewer. For example, the cholera epidemic in London in the 1850s was traced to water supplied from a very polluted portion of the River Thames. During the Middle Ages, the bubonic plague, which killed one of every four people in the world, was carried by rats as well as spread from human to human. An outbreak of typhoid fever was once caused by a cook (Typhoid Mary) who unknowingly carried the disease-causing *Salmonella typhi*.

After a susceptible person or host is infected by a microorganism, the organisms can multiply until symptoms of the disease appear. The time between *contact* with an infectious agent and the onset of signs and symptoms is called the *incubation period*. During the incubation period the host may or may not be infectious to others, depending on the particular infection. The time period during which a person can transmit an infectious disease to others is called the *communicable period*. The communicable period may be before, during, and even after the symptoms of a particular disease occur. A *carrier* is a person who shows no signs of the disease yet harbors an infectious organism; this asymptomatic carrier may be a source of infection to others (as in the case of Typhoid Mary).

Exposure is a term used to signify one's coming in contact with, but not necessarily being infected by, a disease-causing agent. The type of exposure necessary to transmit disease varies for each infectious agent. Some, such as measles, are highly contagious and can be transmitted simply by being in a room with someone with the disease. Others, such as hepatitis B or HIV, the AIDS virus, are not spread through "casual" contact. Some organisms have a greater infective potential than others.

For example, hepatitis B virus has been found to be more likely than the HIV (AIDS virus) to cause infection if a health worker suffers a stick from a contaminated needle.

In general, the greater the number of microorganisms transmitted to the host, the more significant the exposure. For example, a person receiving a transfusion of contaminated blood has a greater exposure than one suffering a needlestick from the same source.

Not everyone who is exposed to a source of infection becomes sick. Health care workers are exposed to patients with infectious conditions as part of their work. Infectious diseases that are spread by health care workers or within a health care setting are given a special name—*nosocomial infections*. Understanding what factors and conditions of an exposure can lead to actual infection is part of infection control. These factors include mode of transmission, type and duration of contact, host susceptibility, and whether or not appropriate precautions were used.

MODES OF TRANSMISSION

The CDC Guideline for Infection Control in Hospital Personnel (Williams) lists four major ways that microorganisms can be transmitted: contact, vehicle, airborne, and vector-borne. The following description is adapted from that paper for the use of EMTs.

CONTACT TRANSMISSION

Contact transmission is the most important and frequent means of transmission of nosocomial infections. Contact transmission can be divided into three subgroups: direct contact, indirect contact, and droplet contact.

DIRECT CONTACT. This involves direct physical transfer between a susceptible host and an infected or colonized person. Examples of when this can occur include instances when EMTs move or lift patients, apply dressings, or perform other procedures requiring direct personal contact. Taking care of patients generally involves some direct contact. Direct contact can also occur between two patients, one serving as the source of the infection and the other as a susceptible host.

INDIRECT CONTACT. This involves personal contact of the susceptible host with a contaminated intermediate object, usually inanimate, such as instruments, dressings, or other infected material. If proper care is not taken, personnel can contaminate objects when assembling or handling critical equipment (such as respiratory therapy equipment) or during other procedures that involve inanimate objects.

DROPLET CONTACT. Infectious agents may come in contact with the conjunctivae, nose, or mouth of a susceptible person as a result of coughing, sneezing, or talking by an infected person. This is considered "contact" transmission rather than airborne, since droplets usually travel no more than about 3 feet. "Close contact" is used to refer to a distance within 3 feet of an infected person. Tuberculosis infection in the lungs is typically spread this way. Colds can be spread either this way, through direct contact, or through indirect contact.

There can be several steps involved in the contact transmission. For example, someone with an active eye infection (conjunctivitis) touches his hand to the infected eye and some time later shakes another person's hand. This second person now rubs his or her own eye, thus placing the infectious agent in the eye. This scenario actually occurred in one hospital, where some 200 hospital workers developed conjunctivitis. Many colds are also transmitted in this way (from the mouth or nose of an infected person to another's hand, and from this person's hand to the mouth or nose). Obviously, washing your hands between patient contacts is an essential common-sense step in infection control.

VEHICLE ROUTE

The vehicle route applies in diseases transmitted through contaminated substances, such as the transmission of non-A, non-B hepatitis by contaminated blood. In this example, blood is the vehicle for the spread of hepatitis.

AIRBORNE TRANSMISSION

Airborne transmission occurs by the dissemination of either droplet nuclei (residue of evaporated droplets that may remain suspended in the air for long periods of time) or dust particles in the air that contain the infectious agent. Organisms carried in this manner are then inhaled by or deposited on the susceptible host.

VECTOR-BORNE

Vector-borne transmission is of greater concern in developing countries; for example, malaria is transmitted by mosquitoes. Lyme disease, spread by the deer tick, is an example of a vector-borne disease that is endemic to many portions of the United States. The control of the disease is sometimes related to elimination of the vector.

TYPE AND DURATION OF CONTACT

The type and duration of contact are factors to consider when determining the relative risk from exposure. Much depends on how great a threat the exposure poses. For example, injecting an infectious agent into the bloodstream would represent a more serious exposure than spilling the same agent on the skin. An infected patient who coughs directly into the EMT's face is more likely to cause spread of infection than if the EMT were 5 feet away from the patient. Wearing clothing soaked with blood for an hour during patient care and transport represents a more significant exposure than a splash of blood on intact skin that is washed off minutes later.

It is important for EMTs who may be exposed to infectious agents to record the type and duration of contact when filing incidence or occurrence reports, or on the patient record. Part of infection control includes the identification and follow-up of exposed individuals, which may occur after the EMT has delivered the patient to the hospital. For instance, the EMT may deliver an unconscious patient to the hospital and the patient may later be found to have a contagious type of meningitis. Knowing precisely who cared for the patient, what was done to the patient, and what contact the EMT had with the patient allows infectious disease control to contact the EMT for proper follow-up evaluation and care.

HOST SUSCEPTIBILITY

Not everyone who comes in contact with an infectious agent develops an infectious disease. In fact, most do not.

RESISTANCE.   One's ability to fight off infection following exposure to infectious agents is called *resistance.*

The body has many means of warding off infection. Barriers such as the skin and mucous membranes prevent entry of harmful bacteria to other more susceptible tissues. The acidic pH in the stomach acts as a barrier to many organisms. White blood cells can consume infectious agents and produce antibodies that block and bind invading organisms and the toxins they produce. The lymph nodes filter out organisms brought through the lymphatic circulation.

IMMUNITY.   A person's immunity helps ward off infection. A person has immunity or protection against a specific disease when the body is able to mount its defenses so that the infection is quickly halted before the infecting agent can establish itself. A person's immune system is able to recognize a particular microorganism and rapidly neutralize its toxic effects and ability to multiply.

Beyond the ability of one's natural defense system, immunity can be achieved by several means. Infants have antibodies from the mother's blood that protect them against many common diseases. Since it is obtained at birth, it is called *congenital immunity.* These antibodies from the mother are not formed by the infant's own immune cells, and thus the protection is temporary.

Vaccination is a means of acquiring immunity. Vaccines contain microorganisms that are killed or weakened so that exposure to the vaccine is enough to stimulate the immune system but not enough to cause disease. This "primes" the immune system, so that the body can later respond to the infection with that particular microorganism. When reexposed, the vaccinated or immunized individual already has antibodies circulating in the blood that are ready to attack the microorganism. Also, the body has an enhanced ability to quickly produce more antibodies and white cells as needed to prevent infection. This is called *active immunity.*

Vaccination is a standard method used to control disease in the world today. For example, smallpox has been eliminated from the planet because of the vaccine against it. As is well known, there are standard vaccinations recommended for all individuals by the Centers for Disease Control. For example, recommended schedules for active immunization of infants and children in the United States include vaccinations for polio, diphtheria, tetanus, pertussis, measles, mumps, rubella, and *Haemophilus influenzae.* Other vaccinations exist and are recommended on a case-by-case basis. For example, emergency physicians, nurses, and EMTs are among those health care workers advised to receive immunization against hepatitis B.

A person can also acquire immunity to a particular infection from actually having that infection. For example, a person who has had rubella, or German measles, is usually immune and does not contract this disease again if reexposed. Thus, one can become immune to German measles, either through actually having experienced the disease itself or through vaccination against the disease; if you have had the infection, you do not need the vaccine. A person's immune status to diseases such as rubella can be checked by measuring the amount of circulating antibody to rubella in the blood.

Poliomyelitis is caused by any one of three different "strains" of the polio virus. Thus, someone who has had poliomyelitis is immune to only one of the three strains and could be reinfected unless vaccinated (which protects against all three strains). The reason there is no vaccine against the common cold is that several hundred different agents cause the common cold, and no vaccine yet developed would protect against all of them.

Passive immunity to certain disease can be conveyed to an exposed individual by injection of antibodies (called immune globulin) from others who have suffered the disease. In such cases, the injected antibodies, rather than the body's own antibodies, fight the infection. Passive immunity is offered if there has been a high-risk exposure to an unprotected individual. For example, tetanus and hepatitis B antibodies can be given to exposed and susceptible individuals. A person is considered to be susceptible if his or her tetanus shots (vaccine) are not up to date, or, in the second example, if he or she has not received the hepatitis vaccine.

HIGH-RISK INDIVIDUALS.   Some individuals are at high risk for infection because their general health status is poor, their immune system is compromised, natural barriers have been damaged (as in a burn patient), or they have had significant exposure.

For example, the influenza vaccine is recommended for the elderly and patients with respiratory and cardiac disease because these patients would be least likely to fend off complications of the flu. Although they may be at no more risk than a normal person in acquiring the infection, they are at greater risk of serious complications from the infection itself. Diabetic patients are more prone to infections for a variety of reasons and are at greater risk of getting an infection, as well as at greater risk for complications of an infection.

Patients with immune system deficiencies, such as patients with AIDS are at risk for opportunistic infections (from common organisms not usually infecting healthy individuals). Because of these patients' poor immune systems, these usually harmless organisms have the "opportunity" to infect them, something that would not occur in a person with a healthy immune system.

Health care providers are at risk for multiple and

more significant exposures than is the average person. For example, the emergency care professional is more apt to encounter blood contaminated with hepatitis than is the average person. Therefore, health care workers are considered to be at "high risk" for particular infections because of the work they must do in caring for sick patients. Before the days of antibiotics and vaccines (and EMTs), many physicians and nurses contracted diseases such as poliomyelitis, tuberculosis, smallpox, and diphtheria from patients with these diseases. Today, hepatitis B represents one of the most common serious diseases transmitted from patient to health care provider. Vaccination against hepatitis B serves as protection against this disease.

Health care workers must also take precautions not to spread disease to the patients for whom they care. For example, while the young healthy EMT may not be at high risk for complications of influenza, high-risk (elderly, debilitated) patients they care for could suffer fatal complications from influenza if they contract it from the EMT. Therefore, health workers are also advised to obtain the vaccine out of concern for their patients and are advised not to work when infected or infectious.

THE USE OF PRECAUTIONS

It is very important for EMTs and other health professionals to use precautions to minimize or prevent transmission of disease. EMTs can take several actions to prevent infecting their patients during patient care. For example, hand washing after patient contact is a simple and very important step to prevent the spread of disease from one patient to another. Dressings applied to open wounds should be sterile so that bacteria from the EMT's hands or an unsterile dressing do not enter the wound. Equipment used on one patient must be cleaned before it is used on another patient. Bed linen should be replaced with clean linen for the next patient.

Likewise, the prudent EMT takes actions to prevent significant exposure by following infection control guidelines. These include maintaining one's personal health status and immunizations; being aware of health and safety; and employing actions to block the spread of infection. The latter include hand washing; using sterile technique; cleaning, disinfecting, and sterilizing equipment after use; wearing personal protective gear; practicing universal precautions; and employing simple isolation procedures.

SPECIFIC COMMUNICABLE DISEASES

There are many infectious diseases that are of concern to the EMT. Diagnosing specific disease is beyond

the parameters of prehospital care. But it is important to understand some of the most frequently encountered conditions to appreciate the range of possible diseases, the importance of infection control, and the relative low risk of exposure to the EMT if safe practice patterns are followed.

General Signs of Infection

Fever and chills are a common response to infections. It is believed that fever has a therapeutic role in fighting infection by increasing the activity of the immune system. However, very high fevers (or sudden changes in temperture) can cause seizures in small children, and temperatures over 105°F can be very dangerous at any age. The absence of fever does not rule out infection. In fact, the notable absence of fever for infections that usually cause fever can sometimes suggest that the patient has an impaired immune system that prevents the patient from mounting a fever in response to the infection.

Rashes may be seen with many infectious diseases. Together with other clinical findings, they may aid in making a specific diagnosis. Some rashes, such as the vesicles seen in chickenpox, may be filled with infectious particles and can spread the disease by direct contact. Many viral infections that typically cause rashes are quite specific in the appearance and distribution of the rash, so much so that the specific infectious diagnosis can be immediately made visually.

Other localized findings are dependent upon the location and type of infection. Cough and sputum could signify either pneumonia or an upper respiratory infection. Fever and flank pain are typical of a kidney infection. A severe headache or a stiff neck with fever, with or without an altered mental status, suggests meningitis.

The body's response to infection often includes an increase of white blood cells circulating in the bloodstream. These cells may produce antibodies and may also directly ingest and destroy products of infection. Often the physician measures the white blood cell count to establish the diagnosis of infectious diseases. Bacterial infections typically cause a higher than normal white blood cell count, and viral infections typically cause the patient to have a lower than normal white blood cell count, although there are many exceptions to this. An extremely low white cell count, as is sometimes seen in cancer patients who have received chemotherapy, is sometimes very serious because the patient lacks an adequate number of white cells to battle against the infection.

Several diseases of concern are described below and in Table 12–13.

Text continued on page 586

TABLE 12–13. New York State Department of Health Infection Control Guidelines for Prehospital Care Services

Infection	Mode of Transmission	Recommended Precautions	Exposure Follow-up	Relative Risk in EMT Setting
AIDS/HIV (human immunodeficiency virus)	Needlestick, blood splash into mucous membranes (e.g., eyes, mouth), or blood contact of open wound	Universal precautions for prevention of blood-borne diseases	Scrub exposed area with soap and water. Contact infection control or infectious disease personnel at local hospital if exposure involved blood contact with broken skin, mucous membrane, or needlestick	Low—no cases reported (Risk among health care workers in general is very low)
Chickenpox	Respiratory secretions and contact with moist vesicles	Not a problem for persons who have had chickenpox. Careful hand washing after contact with moist lesions. Persons who are susceptible should avoid contact	Persons who are not immune (i.e., have not had chickenpox) should avoid contact with other susceptible persons who would be at risk for complications (e.g., cancer patients) from days 10–21 after exposure. There is no risk of spread to others (e.g., children at home) until the exposed, susceptible person develops chickenpox	None if immune. Significant if not immune
Common cold	Contact with respiratory secretions	Hand washing. Avoid contact of infectious materials with eyes, nose, or mouth	None	Unknown—probably significant if in early stages
Diarrhea Campylobactor Cryptosporidium Giardia Salmonella Shigella Viral Yersinia	Fecal/oral	Gloves for direct contact with stool (feces). Hand washing	Contact personal physician if symptoms develop	Unknown—probably low, providing hands are washed after contact with stool
Epiglottitis due to Haemophilus influenzae (usually seen in very young children)	Contact with respiratory secretions	Masks on crew where possible. Don't try to put a mask on a child	Contact infection control or infectious disease personnel at local hospital. Rifampin prophylaxis may be recommended if there has been intimate (e.g., mouth-to-mouth) contact with respiratory secretions	Unknown—probably low
German measles (rubella)	Respiratory droplets and contact with respiratory secretions	Rubella vaccine for nonimmune persons to eliminate risk from potential exposure. Masks for susceptibles	Susceptibles should avoid contact with other susceptible persons from days 7–21 after exposure. Pregnant women who are not immune to rubella should contact their obstetrician	Unknown—susceptible persons are at increased risk
Hepatitis A	Fecal/oral	Gloves for direct contact with stool (feces). Hand washing	Contact infection control or infectious disease personnel at local hospital regarding immune (gamma globulin prophylaxis)	Minimal

Table continued on following page

TABLE 12–13. New York State Department of Health Infection Control Guidelines for Prehospital Care Services *Continued*

Infection	Mode of Transmission	Recommended Precautions	Exposure Follow-up	Relative Risk in EMT Setting
Hepatitis B	Needlestick, blood splash into mucous membranes (e.g., eye or mouth), or blood contact of open wound. Possible exposure during mouth-to-mouth resuscitation	Universal precautions for prevention of blood-borne disease. Hepatitis B immunization	Hepatitis B immune globulin and hepatitis B vaccine for persons who have not previously received the vaccine or are otherwise immune	Significant (6–30% chance) if exposed to blood of a hepatitis B carrier and no pre- or postexposure prophylaxis is provided
Hepatitis non-A, non-B	As with hepatitis B	As with hepatitis B	Role of immune globulin not clear. CDC suggests one dose	Unknown—probably low
Herpes simplex (cold sores)	Contact of mucous membrane with moist lesions. Fingers are at particular risk for becoming infected	Gloves for contact with moist lesions. Hand washing	None	Unknown—probably significant if lesions are present (most people have antibodies)
Herpes zoster (shingles) localized, disseminated (see chickenpox)	Contact with moist lesions	Not a problem for persons who have had chickenpox. Hand washing after contact with moist lesions	Observe for symptoms if susceptible to chickenpox	Localized—very low and only if a person has not had chickenpox
Influenza	Airborne	Masks may help reduce exposure. Influenza vaccine	None	Unknown—probably significant during flu epidemics
Legionnaires' disease	No person-to-person transmission	None	None	None
Lice: head, body, pubic	Close head-to-head contact. Both body and pubic lice require intimate contact (usually sexual) or sharing of intimate clothing	Hand washing. Avoid head-to-head contact if head lice present. Body and pubic lice not a problem in this setting	Head lice: Observe for nits on hair shafts. Contact physician if significant exposure occurred for consideration of prophylactic shampoo. Body or pubic lice: None	Unknown—head may be significant. Body and pubic probably not a risk
Measles	Respiratory droplets and contact with nasal or throat secretions. Highly communicable	Measles vaccine if no prior history of disease. Masks are not likely to be of significant benefit. Persons susceptible to measles should avoid contact, if possible	Measles immunity should be checked. If susceptible, measles vaccine should be administered and contact with other susceptible persons from the 5th through the 21st day after exposure and/or 7 days after the rash appears should be avoided. Notify the health department	Unknown—probably significant if lesions are present (most people have antibodies)

Disease	Mode of transmission	Precautions for crew	Recommendation	Risk to personnel
Meningitis *Meningococcus*	Contact with respiratory secretions	Masks on crew for close contact	Rifampin prophylaxis for persons who have given mouth-to-mouth ventilation to a confirmed case	Unknown—probably low unless mouth-to-mouth ventilation is done
Haemophilus influenzae (usually seen in very young children)	Contact with respiratory secretions	Masks on crew where possible. Don't try to put a mask on a child	Contact infection control or infectious disease personnel at local hospital. Rifampin prophylaxis may be recommended if there has been intimate (e.g., mouth-to-mouth) contact with respiratory secretions	Unknown—probably low
Viral	Fecal/oral	Thorough hand washing after contact with feces	Contact personal physician if symptoms develop	Unknown—probably low
Mumps (infectious parotitis)	Respiratory droplets and contact with saliva	Mumps vaccine if no prior history of having disease	If susceptible to mumps, e.g., never had the disease or vaccine, avoid contact with other susceptible persons from the 12th to 26th day after exposure or until 9 days after development of mumps	Unknown—most adults are immune
Scabies	Close body contact	Wash hands and arms carefully after contact	Observe for symptoms (itching, tiny linear burrows or "tracks," vesicles—particularly around finger, wrists, elbows, and skin folds) and contact physician	Unknown—probably low
Tuberculosis, pulmonary	Airborne	Mask on patient if diagnosis of pulmonary tuberculosis is suspected	Baseline PPD for previously negative reactors with second PPD in 3 months. Converters to a positive reaction should be seen for medical follow-up	Unknown—depends on level of patient's infectivity and contact time. Most transmission occurs in household setting where duration of exposure is extended
Wounds, infected and draining	Contact—more of a concern for cross-contamination	Wear gloves for contact with infected areas. Hand washing	None	Probably none

(From A Prehospital Care Provider's Guide to AIDS. Albany, New York State Department of Health, January 1990.)

Blood-Borne Diseases of Great Concern

ACQUIRED IMMUNODEFICIENCY SYNDROME (AIDS)

The acquired immunodeficiency syndrome, or AIDS, was first described in 1982 as a disease of unknown etiology that resulted in a defect of cell-mediated immunity. Without getting into unnecessary details, immunity to many bacterial infections is mediated through the production of antibodies. Immunity to fungi, parasites, and other more unusual infections is mediated primarily through what is called cell-mediated immunity. Because of this particular type of impaired immunity, AIDS patients are susceptible to very unusual infections that are not seen in healthy individuals.

After an extensive search, a virus was isolated that was found to be the cause of AIDS. This virus lives in blood, lymph tissue, and certain other body fluids, and over time it causes the body to lose its natural defenses against disease. When this happens, the body is open to attack by a whole set of illnesses from mild to life-threatening infections, as well as to an increase in the occurrence of certain types of tumors.

A common type of pneumonia seen in AIDS patients that is virtually never seen in healthy individuals is *Pneumocystis carinii* pneumonia, or PCP.

The most common tumor seen in AIDS patients is called Kaposi's sarcoma, a cancer that affects the skin and the lining of blood vessels. This tumor typically spreads throughout the body.

The AIDS virus has also been found to infect the central nervous system, causing many different neurologic problems. Of course, because of the impaired immunity, many other infections can affect the central nervous system as well.

Of critical importance to the EMT is the fact that individuals who appear healthy may be infected with the AIDS virus (human immunodeficiency virus [HIV]) for many years without any clinical symptoms. Since there are no clues to the presence of infection during this phase, and because anyone may be infected with the virus, it is safest to assume that appropriate precautions must be used on all patients of all ages.

The term "AIDS" refers to those patients who are infected with the virus who have had a documented opportunistic infection. This stage, with which most people are familiar through the press, is really the final stage of infection with the AIDS virus. As noted above, the first stage of infection is generally asymptomatic and can continue for as long as a decade. In most patients infected with the virus, the disease progresses to the second stage, characterized by weight loss, fatigue, lethargy, swollen lymph nodes, and chronic diarrhea. Such patients are described as having AIDS-related complex, or ARC. This stage can last for quite some time, until the patient finally develops an opportunistic infection, at which point the patient is said to have AIDS. During all of these stages, the patient can transmit the virus to uninfected individuals.

The AIDS virus is transmitted by direct contact with body fluids. Common high-risk modes of transmission include sexual contact, either anal or vaginal and oral; needle sharing among intravenous drug abusers; needlesticks or transfusion of blood or blood products infected with the AIDS virus; and from mother to fetus. Blood transfusion as a cause of AIDS has now been virtually eliminated.

The AIDS virus is not transmitted by air or by casual contact. The sharing of food, utensils, and water; social contact; contact with nasal or oral secretions through kissing, coughing, or sneezing; sweat; and contact with tears, urine, vomitus, or feces have not been shown to transmit the disease. In addition, toilet seats, bathtubs, showers, handshakes, clothing, linens, and other inanimate objects (other than contaminated needles) are not sources of transmission. Where there has been no sexual contact, family members of patients infected with HIV have not become infected.

According to the Centers for Disease Control, 176,047 adult cases of AIDS have been reported as of May 1991; 111,815 of the individuals represented by that number have already died. There have also been 3,089 children under the age of 13 infected with the AIDS virus, of which 1,611 have died. AIDS has been reported in all areas of the United States. In addition to reported cases of AIDS, an estimated 1.2 million Americans are infected with the virus but have not yet developed AIDS; the majority of these individuals have no symptoms. Currently, there is no known cure for the disease, nor is there a vaccine. Some medications have been shown recently to slow the progression of the disease, particularly if taken during the asymptomatic or ARC stage. The treatment of patients with AIDS continues to be a rapidly evolving field.

In testing individuals for the AIDS virus, the antibody test usually shows the presence of antibodies 6 to 12 weeks following infection, although current tests may be negative for up to a year after exposure, in spite of active infection. Thus, no test can provide 100% certainty that an individual is not infected. This fact reemphasizes the need for the EMT to be ever cautious and to meticulously follow the proper precautions with all patients.

The AIDS virus, HIV, is actually associated with a low risk to the health care provider. *"Thus far there have been no confirmed reports of prehospital care workers acquiring*

*HIV during job-related activities."** In a large study of health care providers who sustained either a needlestick injury or mucous membrane contact with blood of an HIV-positive patient, 0.34% were positive for the virus on follow-up. Other studies have reported isolated cases of infection that appear to be work related, and these studies also confirm a low overall risk. *"In sum, while the risk of HIV transmission to health care workers is not zero, it is exceedingly low."**

Currently, a number of recommendations can be made to minimize the possibility of infection. It is recommended that all sexually active individuals practice safe sex. This includes the use of condoms during vaginal or oral sex, avoidance of anal sex with or without a condom, avoidance of vaginal or oral sex with someone who uses intravenous drugs or who engages in anal sex, and avoidance of sex with someone you do not know well or with someone you know has several sex partners. Obviously, unprotected sex (without a condom) as well as the sharing of intravenous drug needles with an infected person should be avoided.

For the health care provider, an awareness that the virus lives in blood dictates that protection should be directed against contact with blood and bodily fluids that contain blood. Contact can occur not only through needlestick exposure but also from blood spilled onto open wounds, abrasions, rashes on the skin, or mucous membranes, including the eyes and mouth.

The risk of infection from other bodily fluids in the health care setting is unknown. Therefore, precautions should be followed regarding exposure to spinal fluid, fluid from the chest cavity and abdomen, and fluids in the uterus or womb surrounding an unborn child. The risk through contact with feces, nasal secretions, saliva, sputum, sweat, tears, urine, and vomitus is extremely low or nonexistent. For example, the risk of getting AIDS from a human bite is thought to be extremely low or nonexistent. However, these body fluids may carry other organisms that cause disease. As such, common sense would dictate that appropriate precautions be taken, and all body fluids should be treated as potentially infectious.

Effective precautions mandate the use of universal precautions, barrier protections, and strict adherence to needle precautions. Gloves, goggles, gowns, and face masks should be routinely used in any situation in which there is potential for blood to be splashed. A change of clothing should always be available in case your clothing becomes blood soaked.

HEPATITIS

Hepatitis is an infection of the liver caused by one of three different types of viruses. Hepatitis A virus is spread by oral-fecal routes and is sometimes called infectious hepatitis. Hepatitis B, is contracted in the same manner that AIDS is; in addition, it can be contracted via saliva of an infected person through a bite. Non-A, non-B hepatitis is thought to be spread in a manner similar to hepatitis B. The virus that causes hepatitis B is called HBV.

Hepatitis B is of concern to health workers. About 25% of infected individuals develop acute hepatitis, and of these, 6 to 10% become HBV carriers. These carriers are at risk of developing active liver disease and are infectious to others. The Centers for Disease Control estimates that there are about 300,000 new HBV infections in the United States each year. Of these, 12,000 are health care workers, and 500 to 600 of them are hospitalized. Each year 200 to 300 health care workers who contract hepatitis caused by HBV die.*

To minimize the risk of infection with HBV, you should practice the same personal practices as you would to avoid HIV. In addition, you need to be more concerned about becoming infected through a bite from an infected person.

There is additional protection. A vaccination against HBV is available (90% effective for 7 years) and is recommended for all EMTs. Also, following a possible exposure, passive and active immunity is available that offers some protection against infection. Blood can be tested for antibodies against HBV.

Risk of infection after a needlestick is much greater for HBV (6 to 30%) than for HIV (0.5%).

Precautionary measures taken by EMTs to avoid HBV infection are the same as those taken to avoid HIV: universal precautions, barrier protections, strict adherence to needle precautions, and protective clothing and gear. A change of clothing should always be available in case your clothing becomes blood soaked. In addition, the availability of a vaccination against HBV allows EMTs to greatly reduce any risk of contracting hepatitis B.

Respiratory Secretions and Airborne Exposures

Several other diseases of concern to the EMT are spread by respiratory secretions or airborne contact.

MENINGITIS   Stiff Neck.

Meningitis, or infection of the meninges (the covering of the central nervous system), can be caused by a virus, bacteria, or other organisms. Meningitis can occur with or following a respiratory infection, and symptoms include fever, headache, a stiff neck, and an altered mental status. The *Meningococcus* and, to a lesser degree, *Haemophilus influenzae* are of some concern if there is very

* A Prehospital Care Provider's Guide to AIDS. Albany, New York State Department of Health, January 1990.

close contact with a patient's respiratory secretions, as occurs with mouth-to-mouth resuscitation. Follow up is recommended. An antibiotic, rifampin, may be prescribed if the exposure is significant. Certain viral meningitis can be spread by fecal-oral routes.

CHICKENPOX

Chickenpox is very contagious and is spread by respiratory secretions and contact with the moist vesicles (Fig. 12–17). The same virus causes shingles. Most adults have had chickenpox in their childhood since it is so contagious. If no prior exposure is known, the EMT should take precautions to avoid close contact with a known case, especially if an immune partner or other immune EMT is available to render patient care.

✓ MEASLES

Measles is spread by respiratory droplets and contact with nasal secretions. It is highly contagious (Fig. 12–18). A vaccine is available, but there was a recent outbreak of measles in several colleges that was thought to be due to inadequate immunization in the affected individuals when they were youngsters. Since "childhood" viruses are generally much worse in adulthood, EMTs should be immunized against them and avoid contact when possible if they have no immunity.

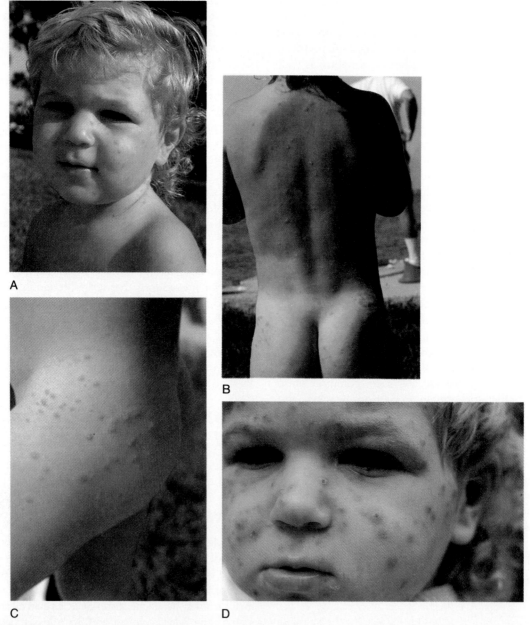

FIGURE 12–17. Four pictures of the same child on sequential days following onset of chickenpox. Note flat red lesions initially (*A*) progressing to distribution over trunk and extremities with vesicles or fluid-filled raised lesions (*B, C*) and then eventual scar formation on center of vesicles. (*D*) Chickenpox is a very contagious disease. Some patients have complications, such as shortness of breath from pneumonia, that require transport to a hospital.

FIGURE 12–18. (*A* and *B*) A patient with measles and complication of shortness of breath, which required hospitalization and supplemental oxygen.

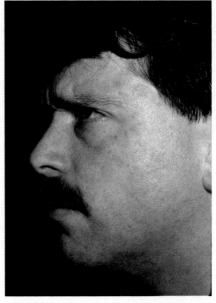 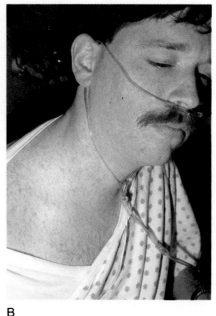

A   B

Rubella (German Measles)

Respiratory droplets and contact with secretions also spread rubella. Rubella should be avoided by women who are pregnant or who are not sure if they are pregnant. Health workers are urged to know whether they are immunized against rubella.

TUBERCULOSIS

The tuberculosis rate is increasing in many parts of the country, in part because of AIDS, and EMTs should be aware of its existence. It is spread by droplets. Patients with active tuberculosis can be given a mask to wear (an oxygen mask will also afford some protection) to block its spread. Checking for exposure to tuberculosis is often part of a physical examination for health workers, often with the purified protein derivative (PPD) skin test.

Close Contact

HERPES ZOSTER

Herpes zoster, or shingles, is a localized infection that first manifests as pain, then as pustules. The virus responsible is the same one that causes chickenpox. If a person has had chickenpox, then he or she is immune.

LICE AND SCABIES

Lice can infect the head, body, or pubic area (Fig. 12–19). Close contact is required. Scabies, usually first noted about the fingers, likewise is spread by close contact. While these two conditions are caused by separate agents, they both cause itching and are cured by the same treatment.

FECAL-ORAL ROUTE

Diarrhea, if infectious in origin, can be spread by the fecal-oral route. Hepatitis A can also be spread in this way. Routine use of gloves to avoid direct contact with stool and hand washing are key measures used to avoid exposure.

There are many infectious diseases. Those discussed above are only a few examples of diseases that are of concern to the EMT. Other infectious diseases are in-

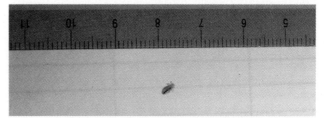

A

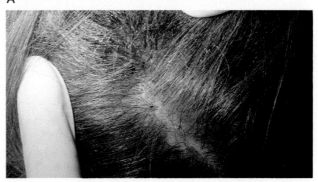

B

FIGURE 12–19. (*A*) *Pediculosis capitis*, or head louse, seen against a millimeter ruler and (*B*) visible in scalp of patient. Also note eggs, or nits, along the hair follicles. Nits are seen as small, white, oval objects along the shaft of the hair. *Pediculosis capitis* is very contagious and is caused by direct contact with hair, clothing, or combs of an affected person.

cluded in Table 12–13. Knowing about how infectious diseases are spread allows EMTs to better understand the need for practicing infection control.

Infection Control

PERSONAL HEALTH STATUS AND HEALTH EVALUATIONS

The first step in infection control is to ascertain your personal health status through physical examination and review of your immunization history and status. EMTs should be immunized in accord with current recommendations to minimize their chances of contracting and spreading infectious diseases.

An EMT's health status should be evaluated periodically. Good health and up-to-date immunizations minimize risks for both EMTs and their patients.

EMTs should not work if they have an illness that may be contagious to patients. They should check with their own physician or medical director if they have questions about the risk they may present to patients.

PERSONAL HEALTH AND SAFETY EDUCATION

An ongoing personal health and safety education program is an essential component of infection control. Knowledge about medical practices and updates keep EMTs aware of hazards and opportunities to reduce risk and improve care. Ongoing continuing medical education programs involve instruction from infection control experts from local hospitals.

IMMUNIZATIONS

Immunizations should be up-to-date. Records of immunizations and personal health status should be available to the medical director for protection of both EMTs and patients. These records, which should be confidential, are important sources of information should questions regarding exposure arise.

ACTIONS TO BLOCK THE SPREAD OF INFECTION

HAND WASHING.   Hand washing remains the most important measure to block the spread of infection. Hands and exposed skin should be washed immediately if contaminated with blood, body fluids, or potentially contaminated articles, and after gloves are removed. Always wash your hands after patient contact and before caring for another patient. Use ordinary soaps. Do not wash your hands in food preparation areas. Have a waterless antiseptic hand cleanser available on the ambulance for use when contamination occurs away from soap and water. Follow the manufacturer's instructions.

ASEPTIC TECHNIQUE.   Practice aseptic technique, especially when caring for open wounds or with instruments that enter the skin or touch normally sterile parts of the body.

Cleaning, Disinfection, and Sterilization.   Make sure that equipment and the ambulance are properly cleaned, disinfected, or sterilized. The level of cleaning required is dictated by the intended use of the equipment (Table 12–14). Note that HIV is destroyed by many chemical disinfectants such as 70% alcohol, hydrogen peroxide, glutaraldehyde, quaternary ammonium chlorides, formalin, lysol, iodine, chlorhexidine gluconate/ethanol mix, and household bleach (5.25% sodium hypochlorite) in dilutions between 1:100 and 1:10. These agents are capable of viral inactivation within 1 to 10 minutes. Soap and water also readily inactivate the virus, as does exposure to drying.

UNIVERSAL PRECAUTIONS.   Universal precautions refer to the approach to body substances and fluids that may carry the HIV or HBV virus. Since the EMT cannot tell from outward appearance who is carrying these viruses, it is wisest to apply precautions to every (universal) situation. Blood, semen, vaginal secretions, and body fluids that surround the lungs, heart, brain, joints, abdominal organs, and fetus are included. Breast milk has been linked to cases in infants, acquired through breast-feeding.

Other substances such as urine, feces, nasal secretions, sputum, sweat, tears, and vomitus are not likely to contribute to blood-borne infection. Universal precautions do not apply unless blood is visible. However, since other diseases can be spread through these fluids, it makes sense to use barrier precautions (gloves) and to handle these substances carefully.

The potential for HBV and HIV to be spread by saliva is also believed to be remote. Universal precautions are not necessary when in contact with saliva outside the mouth (e.g., wiping drool). But if the fingers have contact inside the mouth (as when inserting an airway or clearing the airway), universal precautions should be used. Mouth-to-mouth contact with saliva should be avoided.

PERSONAL PROTECTIVE GEAR.   Personal protective gear consists of barriers to prevent direct contact with blood or other fluids that may carry HBV or HIV. Such gear should be routinely available for EMTs.

Gloves.   Gloves must be standard equipment. Different gloves are required for different purposes. Use heavy gloves that meet Occupational Safety and Health Administration (OSHA) requirements for situations where there are sharp edges or broken glass. Use regular disposable medical gloves in most situations. Use sterile disposable medical gloves when delivering an infant or caring for burn wounds. Use utility gloves for cleaning.

TABLE 12–14. Reprocessing Methods for Equipment Used in the Prehospital Health Care Setting*

Sterilization:	Destroys:	All forms of microbial life including high numbers of bacterial spores
	Methods:	Steam under pressure (autoclave), gas (ethylene oxide), dry heat, or immersion in EPA-approved chemical "sterilant" for prolonged period of time, e.g., 6–10 hours or according to manufacturers' instructions. Note: liquid chemical "sterilants"should be used only on those instruments that are impossible to sterilize or disinfect with heat
	Use:	For those instruments or devices that penetrate skin or contact normally sterile areas of the body, e.g., scalpels, needles, etc. Disposable invasive equipment eliminates the need to reprocess these types of items. When indicated, however, arrangements should be made with a health care facility for reprocessing of reusable invasive instruments
High-level disinfection:	Destroys:	All forms of microbial life except high numbers of bacterial spores
	Methods:	Hot water pasteurization (80–100°C, 30 minutes) or exposure to an EPA-registered "sterilant" chemical as above, except for a short exposure time (10–45 minutes or as directed by the manufacturer)
	Use:	For reusable instruments or devices that come into contact with mucous membranes (e.g., laryngoscope blades, endotracheal tubes, etc.)
Intermediate-level disinfection:	Destroys:	*Mycobacterium tuberculosis*, vegetative bacteria, most viruses, and most fungi, but does not kill bacterial spores
	Methods:	EPA-registered "hospital disinfectant" chemical germicides that have a label claim for tuberculocidal activity; commercially available hard-surface germicides or solutions containing at least 500 ppm free available chlorine (a 1:100 dilution of common household bleach—approximately $\frac{1}{4}$ cup bleach per gallon of tap water)
	Use:	For those surfaces that come into contact only with intact skin, e.g., stethoscopes, blood pressure cuffs, splints, etc., and have been visibly contaminated with blood or bloody body fluids. Surfaces must be precleaned of visible material before the germicidal chemical is applied for disinfection
Low-level disinfection:	Destroys:	Most bacteria, some viruses, some fungi, but not *Mycobacterium tuberculosis* or bacterial spores
	Methods:	EPA-registered "hospital disinfectants" (no label claim for tuberculocidal activity)
	Use:	These agents are excellent cleaners and can be used for routine housekeeping or removal of soiling in the absence of visible blood contamination
Environmental disinfection:		Environmental surfaces that have become soiled should be cleaned and disinfected using any cleaner or disinfectant agent that is intended for environmental use. Such surfaces include floors, woodwork, ambulance seats, countertops, etc.
IMPORTANT:		To ensure the effectiveness of any sterilization or disinfection process, equipment and instruments must first be thoroughly cleaned of all visible soil

* Defined as setting where delivery of emergency health care takes place prior to arrival at hospital or other health care facility.
(Reported from Centers for Disease Control: Guidelines for prevention of human immunodeficiency virus and hepatitis B virus to health-care and public-safety workers. MMWR 38(S-6), 1989.)

TABLE 12–15. Examples of Recommended Personal Protective Equipment for Worker Protection Against HIV and HBV Transmission* in Prehospital† Settings

Task or Activity	Disposable Gloves	Gown	Mask‡	Protective Eyewear
Bleeding control with spurting blood	Yes	Yes	Yes	Yes
Bleeding control with minimal bleeding	Yes	No	No	No
Emergency childbirth	Yes	Yes	Yes, if splashing is likely	Yes, if splashing is likely
Blood drawing	At certain times	No	No	No
Starting an intravenous (IV) line	Yes	No	No	No
Endotracheal intubation, esophageal obturator use	Yes	No	No, unless splashing is likely	No, unless splashing is likely
Oral/nasal suctioning, manually cleaning airway	Yes§	No	No, unless splashing is likely	No, unless splashing is likely
Handling and cleaning instruments with microbial contamination	Yes	No, unless soiling is likely	No	No
Measuring blood pressure	No	No	No	No
Measuring temperature	No	No	No	No
Giving an injection	No	No	No	No

* The examples provided in this table are based on application of universal precautions. Universal precautions are intended to supplement rather than replace recommendations for routine infection control, such as hand washing and using gloves to prevent gross microbial contamination of hands (e.g., contact with urine or feces).
† Defined as setting where delivery of emergency health care takes place away from a hospital or other health care facility.
‡ Refers to protective masks to prevent exposure of mucous membranes to blood or other potentially contaminated body fluids.
§ While not clearly necessary to prevent HIV or HBV transmission unless blood is present, gloves are recommended to prevent transmission of other agents (e.g., Herpes simplex).
(Reprinted from Centers for Disease Control: Guidelines for prevention of human immunodeficiency virus and hepatitis B virus to health-care and public-safety workers. MMWR 38(S-6), 1989.)

Put gloves on when you anticipate the need for universal precautions. Table 12–15 indicates the appropriate situations in which to use different types of protective equipment. Change gloves between patients or whenever they are torn or soiled. Avoid touching personal items such as combs when wearing gloves.

If you use reusable gloves that become contaminated with body fluids, wash them with soap and water and then wipe them with disinfectant and hang them in an inverted position to air dry.

Masks, Goggles, and Gowns. When you anticipate that blood will be splashed, as with an arterial bleeder, or when heavy bleeding or discharge of body fluids is expected (childbirth, trauma with heavy bleeding), use barriers to protect your eyes, mucous membranes, and clothing. A face shield or mask (surgical mask) and goggles should be used. Impervious gowns should be used to protect clothes. An extra change of clothing should be available.

Use of these protective devices can be guided by the situation (see Table 12–15). If no bleeding or body fluids are present, the EMT should not routinely require use of these devices.

NEEDLES AND SHARPS. Since being stuck by a contaminated needle or other sharp object represents perhaps the highest risk of contracting HIV or HBV, proper handling of needles and sharps is of the utmost importance. Used needles should never be recapped, bent or broken by hand, removed from disposable syringes, or otherwise manipulated. Do not allow the tip to touch any part of your body. Instead, place the used needle (and any attached disposable syringe) in a puncture-resistant container for disposal at a later time. These puncture-resistant containers should be as close to the site where a needle is used as possible. For EMTs, it is important to have one in the ambulance in easy reach of the patient care area and another that can be brought to the patient's side whenever a needle is to be used in the course of care.

Care of the needle to avoid inadvertent sticks of the EMT or other caregivers is of the highest priority. Pay particular attention if you are handling a needle in a highly charged and active situation such as a resuscitation.

ISOLATION. If you know or suspect a patient has a contagious disease, prevent unnecessary exposure to others by isolating the patient or contaminated equipment. Knowledge of the mechanism of transmission guides practice. For example, if you know or suspect that a patient has measles, advise the triage nurse of the condition and bring the patient to the appropriate area within the emergency department. Do not allow others to have unnecessary contact with contaminated objects until they are cleaned.

DECONTAMINATION AND CLEANING. Blood spills are cleaned as soon as possible. Take protective precautions to prevent unnecessary contact by using gloves, boots over shoes, or protective face and eye gear as the situation dictates. After wiping up visible material with disposable towels, place soiled toweling in a plastic bag to prevent contamination with other surfaces. You may use a red plastic bag (common to hospital systems for handling "infectious waste") to mark the contents. Once the visible material is removed, clean the surface with a 1:100 solution of household bleach or other appropriate germicide. Let the area dry. First remove contaminated coverings and then your gloves, and place them in the plastic bag. Wash your hands after removing the gloves.

RECOMMENDATIONS FOR DECONTAMINATION AND CLEANING OF RESCUE VEHICLES

Clean-Up Kit

Household utility gloves
Plastic spray bottle with cleaning agent
Plastic spray bottle with disinfectant solution or bottle with concentrated household bleach to be diluted with water (1:100 dilution approximates 1/4 cup bleach per gallon of water)
Disposable toweling
Plastic bags (hospital red bags, household plastic bags)
Basket/carrier to hold cleaning supplies

Clean-Up Procedure for After Each Call

1. **Prepare vehicle for cleaning/decontamination.**
   a. Always wear utility gloves throughout clean-up procedure.
   b. Remove used or soiled linen and place in designated bag for laundering. Either leave laundry at the hospital or reprocess in the EMS laundry using warm water, detergent, and bleach as recommended on the product labels.
   c. Discard any soiled dressings, bloody materials, and other contaminated, non-sharps waste in a red bag and leave at the hospital.
   d. Place reusable equipment that needs reprocessing in plastic bag (any color other than red).
   e. Check the vehicle for any needles or other sharps that may have been left and carefully dispose in a sharps container.

2. **Check for areas soiled with blood and other visible body substances and remove.**
   a. Remove moist blood and other body substances with paper toweling and discard in a red bag.
   b. Spray cleaner on affected area and remove any remaining blood or body substance. Dispose of towels in red bag.

c. Spray disinfectant on affected area, wipe over the surface, and allow to air dry. Dispose of towels in red bag.

3. **Spray cleaner on remaining surfaces with which the patient had contact as well as surfaces that were used in the course of providing prehospital care. Wipe the surface with toweling and allow to air dry.**

Periodic Cleaning of Rescue Vehicles

On a regular basis (e.g., weekly, monthly), as determined by the frequency of vehicle use and obvious need, the floors, walls, interior and exterior of cabinets and drawers, benches, and other surfaces, should be thoroughly cleaned. The same cleaning agent used between cases can be used for this more extensive cleaning. A supply kit should be kept in a central location for this purpose (e.g., pail, reusable cleaning cloths that are laundered after use, supply of cleaning agents). Wipe with toweling and allow to air dry.

Since carpeting and permeable seat cover in the patient compartment of ambulances are more difficult to clean than nonpermeable surfaces, their use is not recommended.

NOTE: Bleach solution should be made up fresh at the time of use or daily.

A Prehospital Care Provider's Guide to AIDS. Albany, New York State Department of Health, January, 1990.

See Recommendations for Decontamination and Cleaning of Rescue Vehicles.

Linen and Clothing.   The risk of transmission from contaminated linen and clothing is negligible. Fold or roll soiled linen and place it in a plastic or cloth bag for laundering. Wash your hands after handling. Use gloves if it is heavily contaminated. If blood soaks through clothing, avoid direct contact with your skin by changing clothes and washing as soon as practically possible.

The following protocol summarizes the approach to a patient with a communicable disease.

P R O T O C O L

APPROACH TO THE PATIENT WITH A COMMUNICABLE OR INFECTIOUS DISEASE

1. *Control of Infection*

   A. It is the responsibility of all health care providers to limit the possibility of cross-infection among patients. Preventive procedures are a critical part of fulfilling this responsibility.

   B. The following procedures are to be followed at all times:

      (1) Wash hands thoroughly after any patient contact.
      (2) Do not use linen or disposable items on more than one patient.
      (3) Linens and items that are not designed for multiple use are to be appropriately disposed of as soon as possible after their use.
      (4) All equipment is to be maintained in a clean and sanitary condition.

2. *Handling Patients with Possible Communicable Disease*

   A. During the call:

      (1) Assess and treat the patient according to standard protocols.
      (2) Wash hands and forearms thoroughly after contact with the patient.
      (3) Wear appropriate protective clothes, according to the following categories:

      CATEGORY I—BLOOD/BODY FLUID PRECAUTIONS

      (Gloves only) With the high incidence of viral disease in our patient population, all blood/body fluids must be presumed to be infectious. Therefore, the EMTs should wear nonsterile, disposable gloves whenever they may contact blood/body fluids such as feces, urine, or skin infections.

      CATEGORY II—RESPIRATORY PRECAUTIONS

      (Mask) TB is on the rise in indigent and alcoholic patients and may be spread by close contact with respiratory secretions. EMTs should place a mask on any patient with a cough that has lasted more than 48 hours.

      CATEGORY III—SECRETION PRECAUTIONS

      (Mask and gloves) Such diseases as varicella (chickenpox), rubella (German measles), rubeola (measles), and meningococcal meningitis may be spread by close contact with respiratory secretions and/or skin rashes. As a general rule, EMTs should use gloves and mask if the patient has a skin rash and a fever.

      CATEGORY IV—CONTAMINATION PRECAUTIONS

      (Gloves, mask, gown) These precautions should be taken when the EMT identifies a patient who is grossly contaminated with infectious material, which would otherwise contaminate the EMT's uniform or when there is a chance of splattering of body fluids.

Continued

(4) Avoid direct contact with body fluids and secretions, including sputum, blood, urine, and feces.

(5) Note all personnel in contact with the patient.

B. At the receiving facility:

(1) Report appropriate information to the emergency room staff.

(2) Request that the facility notify the EMS office of operations as soon as a positive diagnosis is made.

C. After the call:

(1) Report incident to the supervisor on duty.
(2) Dispose of linens according to hospital protocols.
(3) Thoroughly clean and disinfect all parts of the ambulance compartment that were in contact with the patient.
(4) Change uniform if necessary.

Adapted from New York City EMS Academy Training Protocol.

Linen can be washed with detergent and bleach in accordance with laundering product recommendations. Clothing can be handled similarly. Detergent washing and drying render materials safe. Dry cleaning is also an effective decontamination method if clothing cannot be laundered.

DISPOSAL. Dispose of waste in accordance with local or state regulations.

POSTEXPOSURE FOLLOW-UP

If you are exposed to an infectious disease, file a report with your agency and inform your medical director, physician, or other designated individual according to policy. For some conditions it is important to have follow-up as soon as possible. Every EMT should know the policy of the agency for his or her own protection. Follow-up with the hospital is necessary in most cases to confirm the existence of an infectious condition. Assessment is made as to the extent of exposure and the risk to the EMT. This information aids the EMT's physician in guiding postexposure care.

Hospitals have infection control programs that track the contacts of patients who have certain infectious conditions. At times the diagnosis is made after the EMT has left the patient. Hospitals use the prehospital care record as one means to reach other people (including the EMTs) for follow-up and evaluation. Figure 12–20 provides an example of a letter used for such follow-up.

Summary of Communicable Diseases

Infection control practices are designed to block the spread of infectious disease among patients, EMTs, and the public at large. Infection control must be practiced until it becomes a habit. The EMT who understands methods of disease transmission and the facts about HBV, HIV, and other contagious diseases incorporates principles and techniques of infection control into his or her daily practice. Such practice lowers the risk to acceptable levels and makes the EMT a sophisticated partner in the care of patients who have infectious conditions. Continued updates in infection control are recommended.

Request for Infection Control Evaluation of Possible Communicable Disease Exposure

Dear (Emergency Room Medical Director, Infection Control Practitioner):

During a recent transport of a patient to your facility, one of our prehospital care providers was involved in an event that may have resulted in exposure to a communicable disease.

I am asking your assistance in the evaluation of the source patient who was transported to your facility and the circumstances surrounding this event to determine whether our prehospital care worker is at risk for infection and/or requires medical follow-up.

Attached is a "Request for Infection Control Evaluation of Possible Communicable Disease Exposure" form, which was initiated by the exposed worker. Please complete the patient evaluation section and communicate the findings to the designated medical provider.

The evaluation has been developed to provide confidentiality assurances for the patient and the exposed worker concerning the nature of the exposure. Any communication regarding the findings is to be handled at the medical provider level.

We understand that information relative to human immunodeficiency virus (HIV) and AIDS has specific protections under the law and cannot be disclosed or released without the written consent of the patient. It is further understood that disclosure obligates persons who receive such information to hold it confidential.

Thank you for your assistance in this very important matter.

Sincerely,

FIGURE 12–20. Sample letter used to obtain follow-up on a patient. (From A Prehospital Care Provider's Guide to AIDS. Albany, New York State Department of Health, January 1990.)

Summary of Medical Emergencies

Medical emergencies cover a broad spectrum of EMS work and present with a variety of signs and symptoms. Not all medical emergencies require diagnosis in the field. However, conditions such as diabetic ketoacidosis, hypoglycemia, and anaphylaxis require rapid recognition of life-threatening problems (i.e., airway obstruction) and administration of essential prehospital care. This includes airway management, oxygen therapy, actions to support circulation, and timely access to definitive care.

REVIEW EXERCISES

1. List two signs and symptoms of anaphylaxis for each of the following body systems:
   Skin and general signs
   Cardiovascular system
   Respiratory system
2. List three common agents that cause anaphylaxis.
3. State the prehospital emergency care for a patient suffering an anaphylactic reaction.
4. Define *diabetes*.
5. Describe the purpose and function of insulin.
6. List four signs or symptoms of diabetic ketoacidosis.
7. List four signs or symptoms of insulin shock (hypoglycemia).
8. Describe the predisposing causes of insulin shock.
9. Describe the predisposing causes of diabetic ketoacidosis.
10. Define infectious or communicable disease.
11. List four ways a communicable disease can be transmitted.
12. Describe universal precautions.
13. List steps EMTs must take in maintaining equipment and vehicle following exposure to a communicable disease.
14. List personal health measures an EMT can take to reduce personal risk.
15. Define *poison*.
16. List four ways a poison can enter the body and give two examples of each.
17. State how to contact the nearest poison control center.
18. List three circumstances when vomiting should not be induced in patients suffering from ingested poison.
19. State how to induce vomiting in adult and pediatric patients.
20. List the general steps of emergency care for victims of the following poisons:
   Inhaled   Injected
   Ingested   Absorbed
21. Describe the physical characteristics of a pit viper and those of a coral snake.
22. List four signs or symptoms manifested by a patient bitten by a pit viper.
23. List four signs or symptoms manifested by a patient bitten by a coral snake.
24. List emergency care for snake bites.
25. List three examples of stinging marine animals.
26. Describe emergency care for marine animal stings.
27. List six signs and symptoms of a patient who has abused chemical substances.
28. List the general treatment procedures to be followed when caring for substance-abuse patients.

REFERENCES

*ACIP: General recommendations on immunization. MMWR 38:205–227, 1989.

Cahill GF: Arky RA, Perlma AJ: Diabetes mellitus. In Rubenstein E, Federman DD (eds): Scientific American Medicine. New York, Scientific American, 1987.

Cahill GF: Hypoglycemia. In Rubenstein E, Federman DD (eds): Scientific American Medicine. New York, Scientific American, 1987.

*Centers for Disease Control: A curriculum guide for public-safety and emergency response workers: Prevention of transmission of human immunodeficiency virus and hepatitis B virus. Atlanta, Centers for Disease Control, 1989.

*Centers for Disease Control: Guidelines for prevention of transmission of human immunodeficiency virus and hepatitis B virus to health-care and public-safety workers: A response to P.L. 100-607, the health omnibus programs extension act of 1988. MMWR 38(S-6):1–37, 1989.

Guyton AC: Textbook of Medical Physiology, 8th ed. Philadelphia, WB Saunders, 1990.

Hunt G: Bites and stings of uncommon arthropods. Postgrad Med 70(2):91–113, 1981.

Kizer KW, McKinney HE, Auerbach PS: Scorpaenidae envenomation: A five-year poison center experience. JAMA 6:807–810, 1985.

Moss H, Binder L: A retrospective review of black widow spider envenomation. Ann Emerg Med 16:2, 1987.

Nelson RN, Rund DA, Keller MD: Environmental emergencies. Philadelphia, WB Saunders, 1985.

*A Prehospital Care Provider's Guide to AIDS. Albany, New York State Department of Health, January 1990.

Rabinowitz D, et al: Diabetes mellitus. In Harvey AM, et al (eds): The Principles and Practice of Medicine, 18th ed. New York, Appleton-Century-Crofts, 1972.

Schwartz GR (ed): Principles and Practice of Emergency Medicine, 2nd ed. Philadelphia, WB Saunders, 1986.

Sullivan JB, Jr, Wrangert WA: Reptile bites. In Auerbach PS, Geehr EC (eds): Management of Wilderness and Environmental Emergencies, 2nd ed. St. Louis, CV Mosby, 1989.

*Williams WW: CDC guideline for infection control in hospital personnel. Part of the manual entitled. Guidelines for prevention and control of nosocomial infections. Atlanta, Centers for Disease Control, Center for Infectious Diseases: Hospital Infections Program, reprinted February 1986.

* Especially recommended references for further review and understanding of infectious diseases and infection control.

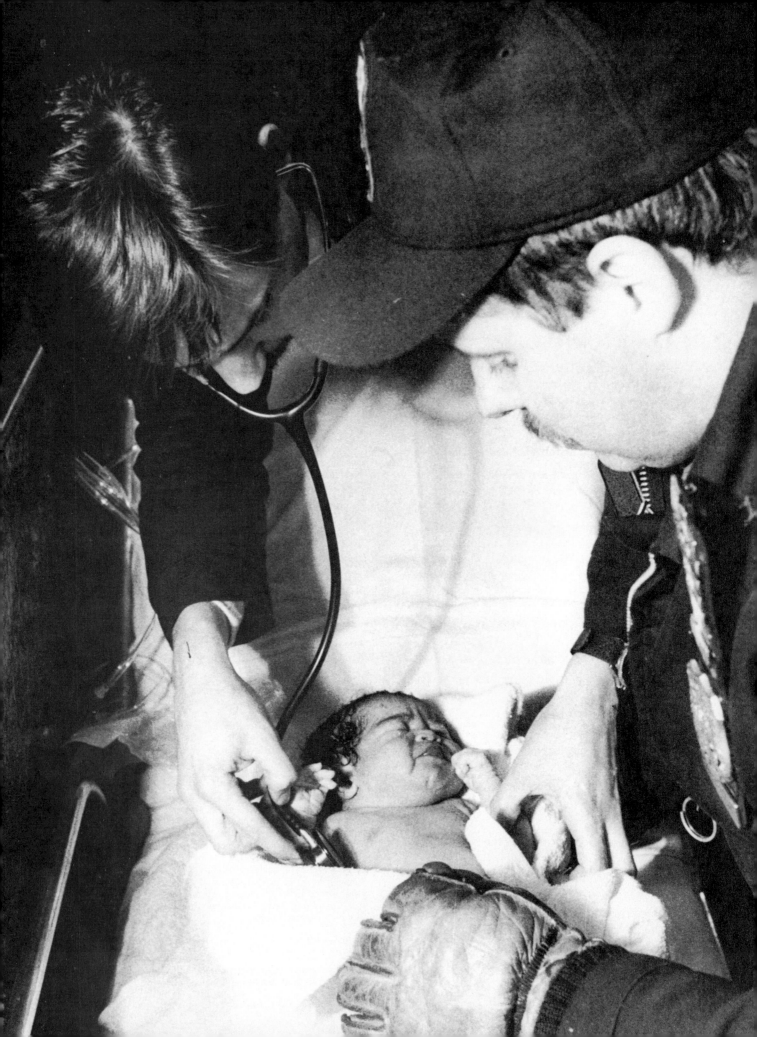

CHAPTER 13

OBSTETRIC AND GYNECOLOGIC EMERGENCIES

OBJECTIVES

At the conclusion of this chapter the reader will be able to:

1. Identify on a diagram the following:
Uterus	Umbilical cord
Cervix	Amniotic sac
Vagina	Perineum
Fetus	Ovaries
Placenta	Fallopian tubes

2. Define the following:
Spontaneous abortion	Presenting part
Bloody show	Eclampsia/preeclampsia
Crowning	Ectopic pregnancy
The three stages of labor	Pelvic inflammatory disease

3. List the contents and state the purpose of an emergency OB kit.

4. List three indications of imminent delivery.

5. Perform a newborn survey and demonstrate that you know how to proceed in the presence of a cleft palate, spinal cord defect, or other abnormality.

6. Demonstrate infant resuscitation procedures.

7. Describe how and when to cut the umbilical cord.

8. Describe how to help in the delivery of the placenta.

9. Describe postpartum care of the mother.

10. Define premature baby and postmature baby and list special considerations for the care of each.

11. Describe and demonstrate procedures for:
Breech delivery	Excessive bleeding in the mother
Prolapsed cord	
Arm or leg presentation	Care of the pregnant trauma victim

INTRODUCTION

Assisting at the birth of a baby is among the EMT's most rewarding professional experiences. By becoming knowledgeable about basic obstetric and gynecologic medicine you will be prepared to calmly assist with delivery of a baby or other emergencies that may arise.

ANATOMY AND PHYSIOLOGY OF THE FEMALE REPRODUCTIVE SYSTEM

The *uterus*, home for the fetus during the 280 or so days of pregnancy, is a hollow organ with thick, muscular walls. The widest part of this pear-shaped structure is the upper segment, called the *fundus* (Fig. 13–1A). The fundus is about 2 inches wide in the nonpregnant woman. The lowest segment of the uterus, which protrudes into the *vagina*, is the *cervix*. The opening from the cervix into the vagina is the *external os*. The opening at the other end of the cervix, into the body of the uterus, is the *internal os*. Glands in the cervix secrete an alkaline mucus that is thin during ovulation, which allows sperm to enter easily. In the days following *ovulation*, the mucus becomes increasingly viscous until it forms a mucus plug. This plug remains in place throughout pregnancy as a barrier to bacteria or is shed with the lining of the uterus during *menstruation* if pregnancy does not occur.

There are no glands in the vagina, but friendly bacteria normally found in the vagina produce lactic acid. This acid keeps the pH of the vagina low and serves as a barrier against infection. When something upsets the growth of this bacteria, such as taking a strong antibiotic that kills not only harmful bacteria but also the friendly bacteria, an infection in the vagina may accur. *Vaginitis*, an infection of the vagina, is usually signaled by a white or greenish discharge and itching. In very young girls and older women the vagina is less acidic, and vaginitis is more common.

Like the heart, the uterus is composed of three layers: the endometrium, myometrium, and perimetrium. The length of the entire uterus from top to bottom is about 3 inches. The body of the uterus lies in the pelvic cavity, posterior to the urinary bladder but tilted slightly forward over the top (Fig. 13–1B). The uterus is held in position by three ligaments: the *broad, uterosacral*, and *round* ligaments. Overstretching of these ligaments can cause the uterus to prolapse into the vagina.

Attached to the outer lateral walls of the uterus by the *ovarian ligaments* are the two *ovaries*. The ovaries are the sex glands of the female and are responsible for

housing and maturing the eggs and also for the production of the hormones *estrogen* and *progesterone*, which are vital to both menstruation and pregnancy. This function classifies these structures as endocrine glands. All of a woman's eggs are formed by the fifth or sixth month of fetal development, after which no new eggs can be created. At birth a female has about 200,000 eggs in each ovary, but they undergo a massive degeneration throughout life. By puberty there are an estimated 50,000 eggs in each of these almond-shaped organs, any one of which, when fertilized by a male sperm under the right conditions, can grow into a fetus. Only about 400 of these eggs ever actually mature during a normal female's life span.

Arising from the upper outer walls of the uterus above the ovaries are two trumpet-shaped structures called the *fallopian tubes*. The length of these tubes varies from about 3 to 6 inches, and they each contain, at the end proximal to the ovary, fringelike projections (called *fimbriae*) that help to sweep the mature egg upward into the tubes. Muscular contractions of the tubes and gently swaying cilia (hairs), which line the tubes, speed the egg on its way to the uterus.

The external surface of the female genitalia, which extends from the vaginal opening downward to the rectum, is the *perineum*. The urethral opening is anterior to the vaginal opening. During childbirth, the perineum is often torn as the baby is expelled. Lacerations around the urethra, vagina, and rectum are common in uncontrolled births. An incision into the perineum, called an *episiotomy*, is often made by an obstetrician to prevent a jagged tear.

The ovaries, uterus, and fallopian tubes receive their blood supply from two major bilateral arteries, the ovarian arteries and the uterine arteries (Fig. 13–2). The ovarian arteries arise directly from the aorta and eventually connect with the uterine arteries before sending branches to supply both the ovaries and the fallopian tubes. The uterine arteries are branches of the internal iliac (hypogastric) artery. The uterine arteries either supply blood to or give rise to other arteries that supply blood to the entire uterus, vagina, ovaries, and tubes. They ascend along the lateral uterine walls and are the major blood supply of the female genitalia. Since these vessels arise from such large and important arteries, you can appreciate the amount of blood that can be lost in damage to, or bleeding from, the uterus or ovaries.

About once a month in the normal adult female, one of the eggs contained in the ovaries matures and bursts out of its special casing. This release by the ovary of a mature egg is termed *ovulation*, and this generally occurs about 14 days before the onset of menstruation. As soon as ovulation occurs, the uterine lining becomes soft and spongy in preparation for receiving a fertilized egg. Fertilization by the male *sperm* occurs in the fallopian tube, and the fertilized egg then travels through the tube

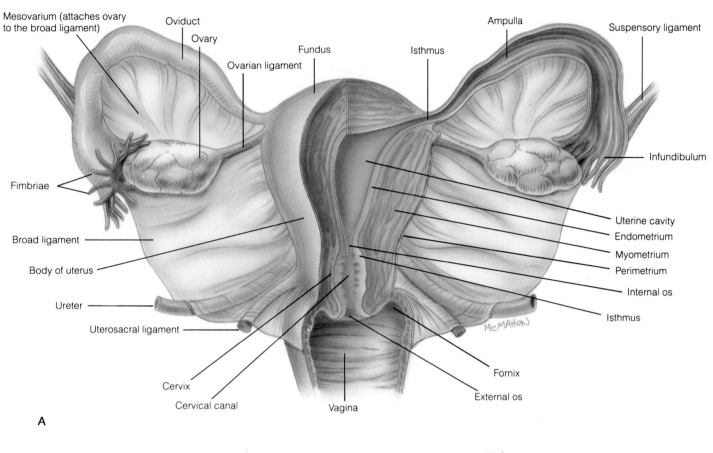

A

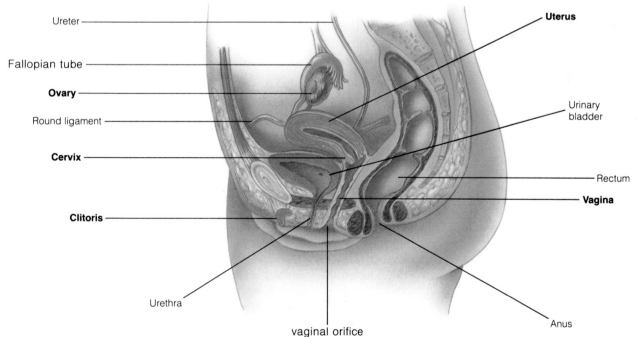

B

FIGURE 13–1. Anatomy of the female reproductive system. (*A*) Anterior view (*B*) Side view. (From Beischer NA, Mackay EV: Obstetrics and the Newborn: An Illustrated Textbook, 2nd ed. Philadelphia, WB Saunders (Formerly Holt-Saunders Pty Limited, Merrickville, Australia), 1986, pp. 709 and 712.)

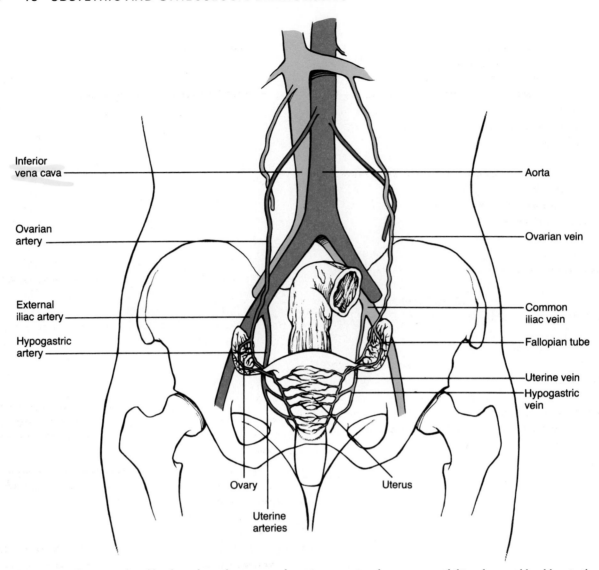

FIGURE 13–2. The tremendous blood supply to the uterus and ovaries presents a dangerous possibility of severe blood loss in the event of injury or hemorrhage. Notice that the uterine arteries descend directly off the aorta.

and enters the uterus. The resulting *embryo* implants itself into the thick, nourishing lining of the uterus and, if all goes well, grows into a *fetus*. If pregnancy does not occur, the rich lining is sloughed off and expelled, along with the ovum, through the vagina during the menstrual period.

Although some cramping may occur during the menstrual flow, severe pain is not normal. The color of the flow is darker than fresh bleeding from a wound would be and changes to a brownish discharge toward the end of menstruation. Menstruation usually lasts from 5 to 7 days. Some women may experience *spotting*, a very light vaginal bleeding, during ovulation, which occurs about 2 weeks prior to menstruation. Vaginal bleeding at any other time during the menstrual cycle is abnormal and suggests the need for medical attention.

PREGNANCY

Implantation of the embryo in a pregnant woman occurs about 7 days after fertilization, usually in the upper segment of the uterus. By this time, the single cell has multiplied into a sphere containing hundreds of cells. The outermost cells eventually develop into the *placenta*, an organ of pregnancy also referred to as the "afterbirth," since it is expelled after the baby is born. The placenta is a very vascular organ that serves as an exchange area. Here nutrients and oxygen from the mother's bloodstream are delivered to the fetus, and waste products such as carbon dioxide cross from the fetus to the mother's circulation. Growing from the fetal side of the placenta and completely encasing the baby is a membranous sac with two layers. The inner layer is the *amnion*. The membranes contain not only the developing fetus but also from 16 to 32 ounces (at term) of a clear, watery liquid known as *amniotic fluid*. The fetus floats in this fluid, which cushions it against injury and also helps it to maintain a constant body temperature. If, at any time during labor, the fetus is deprived of oxygen, the bowels of the fetus may empty into this fluid, giving the fluid a greenish tinge. Depending upon the severity of the lack of oxygen, the fluid color may range from yellow to "pea soup" green. Since the early feces of the newborn is called *meconium*, we say that this fluid is "meconium stained." Meconium-stained fluid alerts you that the baby is or has been stressed. If this fluid is aspirated by the baby at birth, there are often severe problems. Approximately 20% of the babies who pass meconium before delivery will have some type of respiratory distress.

Connecting the fetus to the placenta that nourishes it is the *umbilical cord*. About 1 inch wide and 22 inches long at term, this structure contains three blood vessels surrounded by a clear, gelatinous substance. The largest vessel is the *umbilical vein*, which carries oxygenated and nourishing blood to the baby. There are also two *umbilical arteries*, which carry waste products away from the baby to the placenta. This is one of two instances when oxygenated blood is carried by a vein and waste products are carried by an artery. The only other place this occurs is in the pulmonary circulation (see Chapter 4).

The life of the fetus is dependent upon uninterrupted two-way flow between the mother and the fetus via the umbilical cord. Occasionally, there are fewer than three vessels in the cord. This may mean that there are other defects in the baby.

The delivery of nutrients to and removal of waste products from the fetus occur in the placenta through the processes of osmosis and diffusion. Blood cells and larger molecules cannot cross this *placental barrier*, but there are many harmful substances that can. Many drugs can be harmful to the fetus and should not be taken by a pregnant women without the express consent of her physician.

The 40 weeks of pregnancy are divided into three equal periods called *trimesters*, each lasting about three months. Most of the fetal organs and features are formed by the end of the first trimester. Birth defects, either congenital or drug-induced, are often present by the end of the first trimester. The exceptions are cocaine-related problems, which have recently been shown to affect the fetus at any stage of development. The strong vasoconstricting action of cocaine cuts off the blood supply to the fetal brain, causing atrophy and death to certain areas of the brain. The head size of babies born to cocaine-addicted mothers has been found to be smaller than normal.

Maturation and growth continue throughout the second and third trimesters, with the largest weight gain occuring in the third trimester. It is in this last trimester that the fetus acquires subcutaneous body fat and the mature liver and lungs that make life outside the womb possible. The specific age of the fetus is the *gestation*. The gestation is referred to in weeks, e.g., 20 weeks' gestation or the 20th week of gestation.

Physiologic Changes of Pregnancy

Women undergo massive physiologic changes during pregnancy. Understanding the type and extent of these changes is essential when learning to care for these patients.

HEMATOLOGIC AND CARDIOVASCULAR CHANGES. Plasma volume during pregnancy is increased by up to 50%. This raises the cardiac output from 5 liters per minute to about 7 liters per minute. At the same time, the red blood cell (RBC) volume increases by only 18 to 32%. This dilution of the blood is often referred to as "anemia of pregnancy." The heart rate increases 15 to 20 beats per minute, while the blood pressure becomes lower than normal in the last two trimesters. Thus, the classic symptoms of shock—hypotension, tachycardia, along with low hemoglobin and hematocrit—are normal in pregnancy and may confuse the person treating this patient.

Because of the greatly increased blood volume, a pregnant patient can lose up to 35% of her blood volume before a change in her vital signs occurs. At the first sign of hypovolemia, a self-protective measure in the mother causes constriction of the uterine arteries, redirecting blood to her major organs. This compensatory mechanism, which severely affects the fetus, will occur long before an observer notes a change in the mother's vital signs. Once the traditional signs of hypovolemia appear in the mother, it may be too late to save the fetus. In fact, in a study of 103 cases of blunt maternal trauma done by Rothenberger, Quattlebaum, Pery, and associates, published in 1978 in the *Journal of Trauma*, it was shown that shock in a pregnant woman carries an 80% chance of fetal mortality.

Compression of the Vena Cava. The positioning of the mother can intensify the effects of hypovolemia. When the mother lies supine, the bulk of the fetus compresses the mother's vena cava against her spinal column (Fig. 13–3). In fact, at 36 weeks' gestation, 90% of mothers have *total occlusion* of the inferior vena cava when lying supine. Vena caval compression inhibits venous return of blood to the heart, causing an enormous decrease in cardiac output. This event magnifies the body's perception of hypovolemia and causes even greater constriction of the uterine arteries. The well-known method of treating shock by elevating the legs is ineffective because it does not relieve the compression of the vena

Inferior vena cava

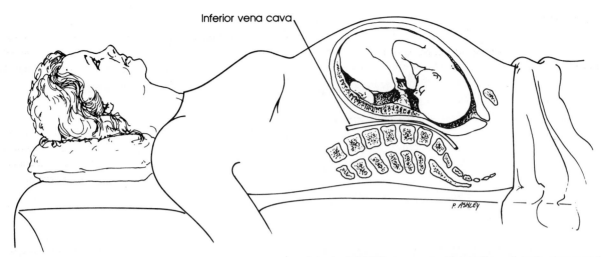

P. ASHLEY

FIGURE 13–3. Compression of the vena cava between the spine and the heavily pregnant uterus. Never allow a heavily pregnant patient to lie flat on her back. (This is not a factor in early pregnancy.) (From Burroughs A: Bleier's Maternity Nursing, 5th ed. Philadelphia, WB Saunders, 1986, p. 88.)

cava by the baby. A typical example of this syndrome is the pregnant woman who has her hair washed at a beauty parlor in a reclining chair. Shortly after reclining, the woman becomes unconscious. She is left supine in the chair while an ambulance is called, and thus remains unconscious. When an ambulance arrives, the simple act of lifting the woman to a stretcher and placing her on her left side relieves the vena caval compression, restoring cardiac return and cardiac output and thus consciousness to the patient.

Compression of the vena cava may be relieved somewhat during a labor contraction, since the muscular contractions of the uterus raise the fundus of the uterus, in effect lifting its weight from the vena cava. However, the contractions of the uterus also affect blood flow through the placenta, so the fetus really has no time to recover from the stress. Many pregnant women simply cannot tolerate lying supine without passing out or at least feeling dizzy, regardless of whether they are in labor or if blood loss has occurred. *It is essential to transport a pregnant patient on her left side* (Fig. 13–4). In severe trauma cases, where stability of the cervical spine and

airway management take precedence and you must keep the patient supine, place pillows or a wedge under the right side of the spine board (Fig. 13–5). The uterus can also be manually displaced to the left side by placing your hand firmly against the right side of the uterus and pushing firmly enough to lift the bulk of the baby off the vena cava.

PULMONARY CHANGES. The respiratory rate remains the same or may increase slightly during a normal pregnancy, but the tidal volume increases by 50%. Oxygen consumption is greatly increased because of the

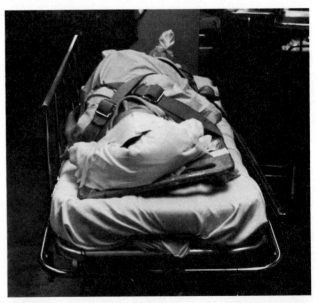

FIGURE 13–5. In cases of spinal injury, where the patient cannot be placed on her left side, place pillows, rolls, or wedges under the right side of the spineboard. The uterus can also be manually displaced to the left with the flat palm of your hand. Oxygen and, if available, IV Ringer's solution should be administered to the pregnant trauma victim. (From Cardona VD, Hurn PD, Mason PJB, et al: Trauma Nursing From Resuscitation Through Rehabilitation. Philadelphia, WB Saunders, 1988, p. 655.)

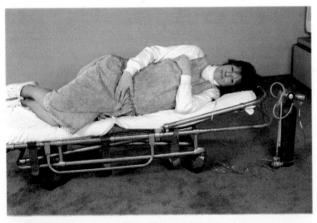

FIGURE 13–4. This is the position of choice for a pregnant patient.

high fetal demand for oxygen. At the same time, there is upward displacement of the diaphragm caused by the growing fetus, so dyspnea and shortness of breath are common, especially in the heavily pregnant woman. The elevation of the diaphragm reduces the residual capacity, making the pregnant patient more prone to hypoxia. This is even more exaggerated when she is supine. If a pregnant patient is having difficulty breathing while lying on her left side, she can be transported sitting up.

GASTROINTESTINAL CHANGES. *Progesterone*, the hormone of pregnancy, has a slowing effect upon the digestive tract. Well before the pregnant uterus begins to crowd the abdominal contents, gastric emptying is decreased. Even if the patient has not eaten for several hours, food remains in the stomach for a much longer period of time. *Always assume that the pregnant patient has a full stomach.* Progesterone also causes some relaxation of the sphincter between the stomach and the esophagus, so there is always an increased chance of vomiting by the pregnant patient. It follows that aspiration is a major concern if the patient is unconscious.

The appendix moves upward and laterally during pregnancy, so that by the fifth month, it is at the level of the iliac crest. The pain noted in appendicitis in pregnancy is therefore noted in the right upper quadrant instead of the right lower quadrant and is usually accompanied by fever, vomiting, and tachycardia.

GENITOURINARY CHANGES. The urinary bladder, formerly located within the bony pelvis, becomes an abdominal organ in the second and third trimesters of pregnancy (Fig. 13–6). Compression of the bladder between the uterus and the abdominal wall causes the

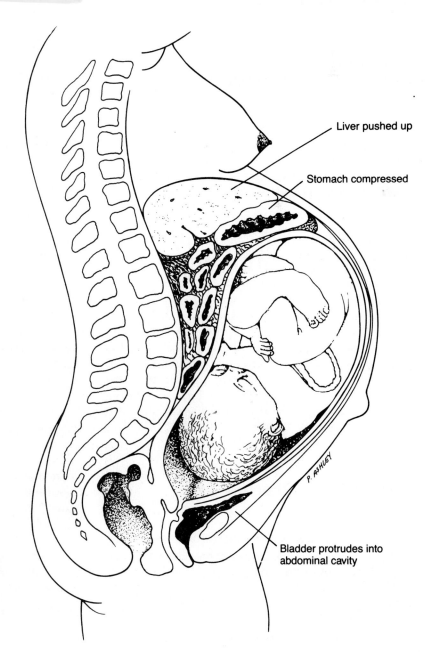

Liver pushed up

Stomach compressed

Bladder protrudes into abdominal cavity

FIGURE 13–6. Anatomic changes in pregnancy can confuse diagnosis, make treatment more difficult, and give rise to certain injuries that would be unusual in the nonpregnant patient. The bladder now protrudes into the abdominal cavity (compare with position of bladder in Fig. 13–1*B*), and there is crowding of the stomach, liver, and intestines. The diaphragm is pushed up, leading to a decreased residual capacity in the lungs. (From Burroughs A: Bleier's Maternity Nursing, 5th ed. Philadelphia, WB Saunders, 1986, p. 96.)

bladder to remain full most of the time, and the woman experiences an annoying need to urinate frequently. These changes make the bladder more susceptible to injury from both blunt and penetrating trauma. The bladder is no longer protected from injury by the bony pelvis. Furthermore, the fullness of the bladder and its poor ability to empty may cause the "burst balloon" type of rupture when blunt trauma occurs. Bladder infections during late pregnancy are fairly common and often mimic premature labor. The patient often experiences flank pain and a low-grade fever. The usual sign of a bladder infection—frequency of urination—is often left out of the history because the patient has probably felt this for a long time, and her chief complaint now is pain. Uterine contractions may be present, which are generally relieved by giving the patient a lot of fluids and treating the bladder infection.

The uterus itself, while shielding the abdominal contents from injury as it grows in size, becomes more susceptible to injury as it leaves the bony pelvis. In fact, as pregnancy progresses, a penetrating wound to the abdomen will almost always involve the uterus, with or without its contents. The uterus in turn acts as a protective barricade for other organs.

Blood flow to the uterus during pregnancy is greatly enhanced. This increased vascularity may be a cause of grave concern should the uterus be injured. Pelvic fractures, a severe cause of blood loss even in a nonpregnant patient, are especially dangerous at this time.

LABOR AND DELIVERY

The mature fetus weighs about 7 pounds and is most often found in a head-down flexed position. The bulk of the uterus is no longer a pelvic organ but rather occupies much of the abdominal cavity. The cervix has become shorter and thicker and contains a viscous mucus plug that helps to prevent bacteria from entering the uterus through the vagina. Labor, the process by which the baby is born and the afterbirth expelled, is divided into three stages.

The Three Stages of Labor

You should make every attempt to transport the mother to the hospital environment for delivery. Knowing the signs of approaching delivery enables you to make a decision about whether to transport or prepare for delivery at the scene.

THE FIRST STAGE OF LABOR

The first stage of labor is the period that begins with the first contraction and ends when the cervix has been fully stretched or dilated to a diameter of 10 cm, or about 4 inches. Before the cervix can be completely dilated, it must be *effaced*, or thinned (Fig. 13–7). The first stage of labor can be further divided into three phases: *early labor*, *active labor*, and *transition*. During each labor pain, the uterine muscles contract, plunging the baby's head against the inside of the cervical canal. Throughout *early labor* the major change is effacement, or thinning, of the cervix. The cervix dilates only to about 4 cm. The contractions are usually mild and often irregular. In the *active phase*, dilatation of the cervix progresses to 8 cm, and the mucus plug begins to come out. This is often tinged with blood and is therefore called the *bloody show*. The mucous discharge often becomes quite bloody toward the end of labor, which may be upsetting to the mother. You should explain that this is a normal part of labor. During *transition*, the cervix dilates fully, and the mother becomes quite uncomfortable.

When evaluating contractions, you will want to determine *how long the contractions last* and *how far apart they are*. A contraction is measured from the first tightening of the uterine muscle to complete relaxation. To find out how far apart the contractions are, time them from the beginning of one contraction to the beginning of the next contraction. The contractions of *early labor* are generally quite mild and come at irregular intervals. Typical of early labor are contractions that occur every 10 to 15 minutes and last a minute or less.

As a woman goes into *active labor*, the contractions become stronger and more painful; commonly, they are 5 minutes apart and last about a minute. As *transition* approaches, the contractions come at 2- to 3-minute intervals and last 60 to 90 seconds. She may be *diaphoretic* (perspiring heavily) and experiencing nausea and vomiting. Since the pregnant woman always has a full stomach, vomiting alone is not a sign of transition.

A woman who is about to have her first baby is called a *primigravida*. The first stage of her labor may last 14 hours or longer. Once the cervix has been softened and stretched by a delivery, later babies are usually born much more quickly. Knowledge of the phases of the first stage of labor and their characteristics can be useful in helping to calculate how far along the patient is in her labor. However, labor contractions do not always follow textbook rules. Early labor contractions can sometimes begin as strong, regular, and painful contractions and then fade away a few hours later. False labor, a condition in which labor pains occur with no dilatation of the cervix, may be identical in appearance to real labor and may last for hours. These patients are often quite em-

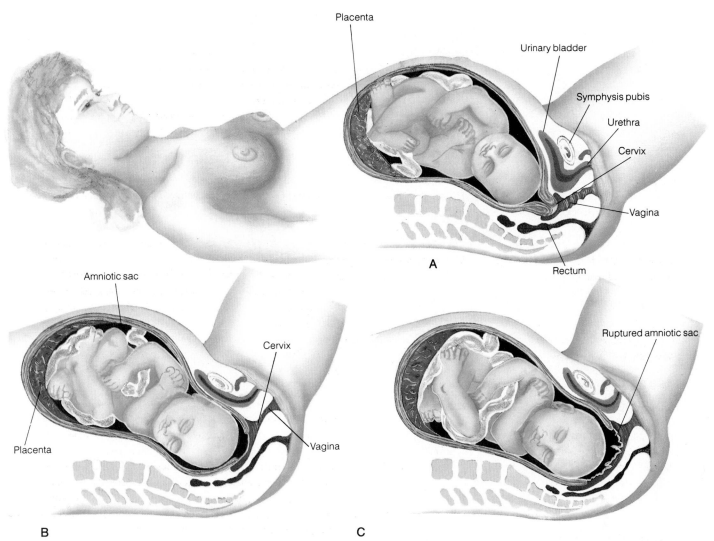

FIGURE 13–7. Effacement and dilatation of the cervix. (*A*) The cervix is long, closed, and thick. This patient is in early labor. (*B*) The cervix is now completely effaced and about 7 to 8 cm dilated. The baby's head is beginning to push into the vagina. This patient is entering the transition phase of the first stage of labor. (*C*) This is a fully dilated patient with ruptured membranes in the second stage of labor. (From Gaudin AJ, Jones KC: Human Anatomy and Physiology. Orlando, Harcourt Brace Jovanovich, 1989, p. 748.)

barrassed that they have rushed to the hospital when they were not in labor and must be reassured that even the obstetrician cannot be sure that labor is not false labor until actual dilatation of the cervix occurs from the contractions.

THE SECOND STAGE OF LABOR

The second stage of labor begins with full dilatation of the cervix and ends when the baby is delivered. During this time, the baby must travel through the pelvic cavity.

THE PELVIC CAVITY. The pelvic cavity is shaped rather like a bent tin can. The fact that humans walk upright is the major factor in the unusual shape of the human pelvis, and the result is that humans suffer a more difficult and painful labor than four-legged animals, who have a straight pelvis. The bones are welded together, giving the internal diameters little capability for expansion, and the birth canal is just barely large enough to allow passage of a normal-sized infant. There are only four joints in the pelvis, and none of them allows a great deal of expansion for labor. The two *sacroiliac* joints (the joints formed by the sacrum and ilium of the pelvis) and the *symphysis pubis* are nearly immobile. The *sacrococcygeal* joint (the joint formed by the sacrum and the coccyx) may allow the coccyx to move backward in childbirth, but this joint is often rigid, a condition that can cause uncomfortable back pain during labor.

The diameters of the pelvic inlet (Fig. 13–8), where the baby first enters the pelvis, and pelvic outlet (Fig. 13–9), from which the baby must emerge to be born, are markedly different. The transverse diameter is the largest diameter of the pelvic inlet, while the antero-

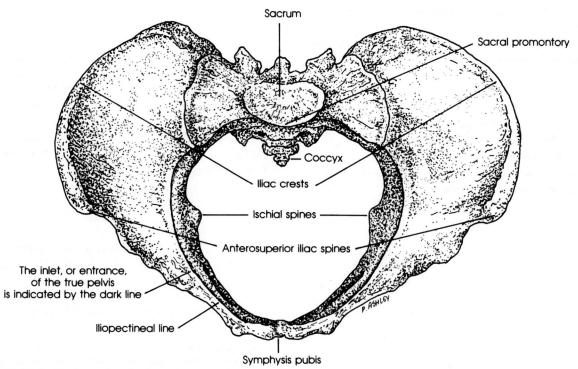

FIGURE 13–8. The heart-shaped pelvic inlet as seen from above. Because of the sacral promontory, the anteroposterior diameter (about 11 cm) is shorter than the transverse (13 cm) diameter. The baby's head usually enters the pelvis facing the mothers right or left side. (From Burroughs A: Bleier's Maternity Nursing, 5th ed. Philadelphia, WB Saunders, 1986, p. 20.)

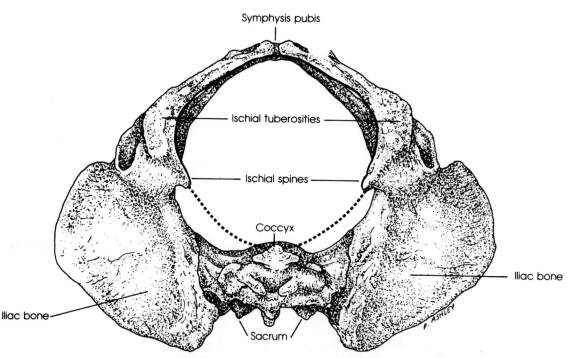

FIGURE 13–9. The diamond-shaped pelvic outlet through which the baby must emerge to be born is much different from the inlet. Because of the ischial tuberosities, the anteroposterior diameter (11.5 cm) is now greater than the transverse (11 cm) diameter. The baby must now turn its head and shoulders to the wider diameter, facing either the mother's public bone or anus. As the shoulders emerge, they must also be aligned with the anteroposterior diameter, so that the baby's sternum faces the mother's right or left leg. Any traction given during childbirth is always given with the largest (anteroposterior) diameter upward or downward. (From Burroughs A: Bleier's Maternity Nursing, 5th ed. Philadelphia, WB Saunders, 1986, p. 22.)

posterior diameter is the largest diameter of the pelvic outlet. This means that the baby's head and shoulders must twist as the baby descends into the pelvic cavity in order to be born.

Molding of the baby's head to suit the shape of the pelvis often occurs to accommodate this passage, giving the newborn an elongated and occasionally misshaped head (Fig. 13–10). You may assure the mother that this will subside spontaneously within a few days following birth. If the mother has an abnormally shaped pelvis that lessens the diameter of the pelvic canal, birth may be delayed or even impossible. Likewise, if the baby is oversized or has an unusually large head, it may have considerable difficulty negotiating the pelvic canal.

PRESENTATION. A third possible impediment to movement of the baby through the birth canal may be a wrong *presentation* (Fig. 13–11) of the baby. The *presenting part* of the baby is the lowermost part that first enters the pelvis. The presentation refers to this presenting part. For example, in a *vertex presentation*, the baby is sharply flexed with the chin on the chest and occipital, or vertex, portion of the head is the first portion of the body to enter the pelvis. This is the most desirable and most common presentation. In a *breech presentation*,

the breech, or buttocks, are lowermost in the pelvis. In a *frank breech* the buttocks are the presenting part. If one or more of the feet enters the pelvis first, it is termed a *footling breech*. When the baby is lying transverse in the uterus there may be a *shoulder presentation*, in which case the baby cannot be delivered vaginally even if the cervix is fully dilated. In a *chin presentation*, the baby cannot be delivered vaginally, since the neck is hyperextended and will break if extended more. A similar situation exists in a *brow presentation*, in which the baby's forehead is the presenting part.

As the presenting part descends into the pelvis, pressure is exerted on the rectum, and the mother has an intense urge to move her bowels. Indeed, as the presenting part fills the pelvic cavity, any fecal material in the rectum is expelled. *Never allow a laboring mother who feels an urge to move her bowels to go to a toilet.*

When the presenting part has traveled well down into the vagina, the perineum begins to bulge. The mother usually has an uncontrollable urge to bear down with each contraction and, as she pushes, the presenting part becomes more and more visible. Between contractions the presenting part may recede back into the vagina. When the widest part of the presenting part has advanced so far as to be bulging out of the vagina, and the baby

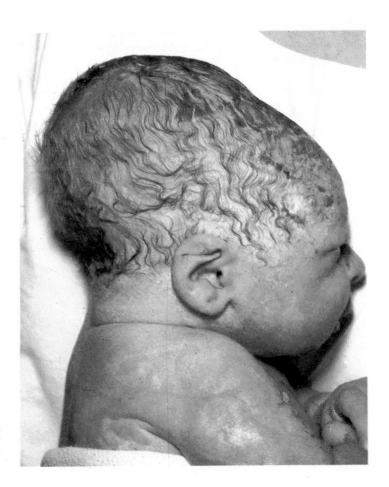

FIGURE 13–10. Openings and softness in the baby's skull allow molding of the baby's head to the shape of the mother's pelvis. The misshapen appearance of the baby's head disappears within a day or two. (From Beischer NA, Mackay EV: Obstetrics and the Newborn: An Illustrated Textbook, 2nd ed. Philadelphia, WB Saunders (Formerly Holt-Saunders Pty Limited, Merrickville, Australia), 1986, Color Plate 103.)

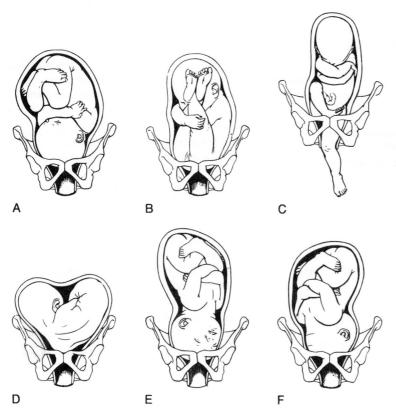

A   B   C

D   E   F

FIGURE 13–11. Various presentations. The safest and most common presentation is the vertex (*A*). Frank breech, (*B*) footling breech (*C*), or shoulder presentation (*D*) may lead to a prolapsed cord and usually requires prompt cesarean section delivery. Brow (*E*) or chin (*F*) presentation may harm the fetus through hyperextension of the neck and may also require a cesarean section. The mother may have all the signs of advanced labor but be undeliverable vaginally without causing grave harm to the baby. If the presenting part is not a visible vertex presentation, or if there is a partially delivered frank breech (as in Fig. 13–39), proceed to the hospital for delivery. (From Ross Laboratories, Clinical Education Aid No. 18, G-174, 1984.)

no longer recedes between contractions, *crowning* has occurred (Fig. 13–12). Once crowning has occurred, birth will follow shortly.

Mechanics of Childbirth

To be able to anticipate the events that occur after crowning and know how to best intercede for the mother and baby, you must first familiarize yourself with the mechanics of birth (Fig. 13–13). To simplify this discussion, it is assumed that the baby is in a normal vertex presentation.

FLEXION. The baby's head becomes *flexed* (chin on chest) as it meets resistance upon entering the pelvic

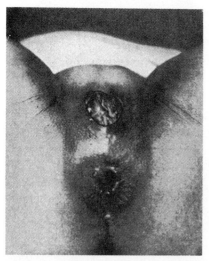

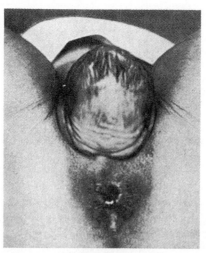

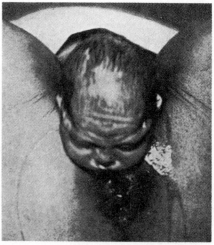

A   B   C

FIGURE 13–12. (*A*) Distention of the perineum with part of the baby's head visible during contraction. The head may recede between contractions, so the mother should be checked for crowning during a contraction. (*B*) Crowning is complete and the head has begun to extend upward toward the pubic bone. Once crowning has occurred, the presenting part no longer recedes between contractions. (*C*) The baby's head is born and drops down toward the mother's anus. (From Greenhill JP: Obstetrics, 14th ed. Philadelphia, WB Saunders, 1974.)

FIGURE 13–13. The mechanics of childbirth refers to the movements that the fetus must make in order to negotiate the changing diameters of the female pelvis. (*A*) As the head descends into the pelvis, it becomes flexed sharply onto the chest. The head is still in the pelvic inlet and faces the mother's side because the transverse measurement is the largest diameter of the pelvic *inlet*. (*B*) To enter the pelvic outlet, the head has turned to face the mother's anus. (The largest diameter of the *outlet* is the anteroposterior diameter.) (*C* and *D*) The head must extend to follow the plane of the birth canal. (*E* and *F*) The shoulders now move into the largest diameter of the pelvic outlet (anteroposterior), and the head rotates externally to stay in line with the shoulders. (*G*) Expulsion of the baby. (From Ross Laboratories, Clinical Education Aid No. 13, G-169, 1979.)

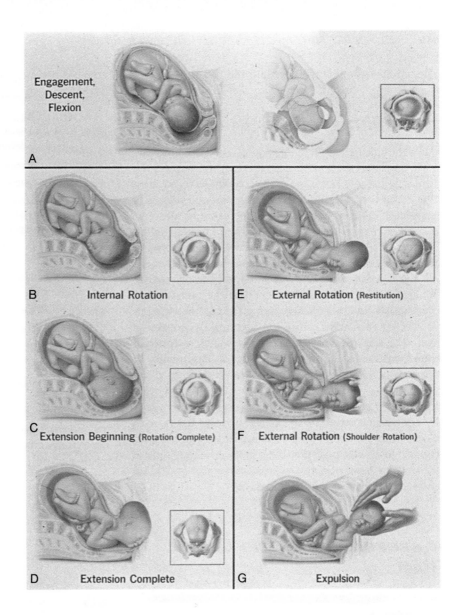

A — Engagement, Descent, Flexion

B — Internal Rotation

C — Extension Beginning (Rotation Complete)

D — Extension Complete

E — External Rotation (Restitution)

F — External Rotation (Shoulder Rotation)

G — Expulsion

canal. This presents the smallest possible diameter of the head to the pelvis. The smaller the mother's pelvis, the more the baby's head must flex to enter.

INTERNAL ROTATION. Remember that the pelvic outlet, from which the baby emerges to be born, is of a different shape than the pelvic inlet where the baby first enters the pelvis. The baby's head usually follows the path of least resistance. Therefore, while the head is usually facing one of the mother's sides when it first enters the pelvis, it must now turn 90 degrees as it descends into the pelvic outlet. By the time this *internal rotation* is completed, the baby is facing either the mother's anus (most common) or straight up ("sunny-side up"). The *sunny-side up* or posterior position often accompanies a longer and more painful labor because the wider diameter of the baby's skull is presenting to the mother's pelvis.

EXTENSION. Since the vagina is pointing upward, the baby's head, which was greatly flexed before internal

rotation occurred, must now extend under and then around the symphysis pubis as crowning occurs. The head rises upward in *extension* until it is completely born, after which it will drop down toward the mother's anus if not supported.

EXTERNAL ROTATION. After the head is born, it must realign with the shoulders (remember that the head is turned 90 degrees during internal rotation). It must now rotate either to the left or right, depending upon which position it was in before internal rotation. Since the shoulders follow the same route of internal rotation that the head has already completed, the head rotates even farther to one side to stay in line with the body. Finally, it is facing one of the mother's thighs. This is *external rotation*.

EXPULSION. After the head is born, the body usually follows rapidly. The *anterior* (uppermost) shoulder becomes fixed against the symphysis pubis so that the *posterior* (lower) shoulder can pivot upward and be born.

The anterior shoulder follows and the rest of the body is easily born, since it is much smaller in diameter.

THE THIRD STAGE OF LABOR

The third stage of labor begins when the baby has been born and ends with the delivery of the placenta. After the baby is born, the uterus continues to contract every 2 or 3 minutes, but the contractions are relatively painless. Now that the baby has been born, the uterus is greatly reduced in size, and the surface area for attachment of the placenta to the uterine wall is comparatively reduced in size. The placenta is literally squeezed off the uterine wall, and placental separation occurs. While the placenta is still attached to the uterine wall, the uterus is round and hard during the contractions but flat during relaxation. Once the placenta has separated from the uterine wall, the uterus assumes a constant round, hard shape. You will also note a lengthening of the umbilical cord as the placenta descends toward the vagina. After delivery of the placenta, the uterus becomes a solid wall of muscle below the level of the umbilicus. By contracting strongly upon itself it slows the flow of blood from the open blood vessels that were previously connected to the placenta. Even with excellent muscle contraction, however, you can expect from 50 to 200 ml of blood to be lost during this stage.

Assessment of the Labor Patient

The initial role of the EMT caring for a labor patient is assessment. Making a decision about whether to transport the mother to the hospital immediately or to deliver the baby at the scene can be determined by the following criteria.

HISTORY

Asking the patient the following questions should help you obtain a brief history.

IS THIS YOUR FIRST PREGNANCY?   Primigravidas may take an hour or more of hard pushing to deliver, even after the cervix has been fully dilated, whereas women who have given birth previously often have very short and unpredictable labors. If the woman has had other children, ask her if her previous deliveries were long or short. Make sure to ask if her previous deliveries were by cesarean section (surgical abdominal delivery) or normal vaginal delivery. Although most hospitals are now attempting to allow women to give birth vaginally even if they have had a previous cesarean section, there is more of a risk involved. Therefore, a laboring mother who has had a previous cesarean section should be transported immediately, if possible.

WHAT TIME DID YOUR CONTRACTIONS BEGIN AND HOW FAR APART ARE THEY?   Labor pains are irregular in early labor and may occur intermittently for days before real labor begins. Be sure to find out what time the patient began to feel regular contractions. The pains get closer together as labor progresses, until they are 2 to 3 minutes apart and regular. Remember, it generally takes an average of 14 hours for a primigravida to become fully dilated. A primigravida who has had irregular contractions or pains that are 10 minutes apart for 3 hours is probably in very early labor. Ask the patient where the pains are felt. Typical labor pains are felt in the suprapubic area. Some are felt as low back pain. Upper abdominal pain or flank pain is probably not labor.

HAS YOUR WATER BROKEN?   If the answer to this question is yes, ask what color the fluid was. Remember, if the fluid was meconium stained, there may be a problem with the baby. Do not be surprised if the patient is not sure whether or not her membranes have broken. Fullness and pressure on the bladder often causes urinary incontinence. Pregnant women are often unsure if they have voided or ruptured membranes. Rupture of membranes may occur with a huge gush of fluid or a tiny trickle, or a small amount of fluid may be expelled with each contraction. While the membranes often rupture as labor progresses, they may rupture before labor has begun or may need to be ruptured at the time of delivery. Rupture of the membranes alone is not a sign of active labor.

DO YOU HAVE AN URGE TO MOVE YOUR BOWELS?   As the presenting part moves well down into the pelvic canal and begins to put pressure on the nerves of the rectum, the mother experiences an intense urge to move her bowels. Delivery is usually quite near, although a first-time mother may have a strong urge to push for an hour or more before delivery. If the mother has had previous childbirths and now has a strong urge to push during the contractions, instruct her to pant-blow out of her mouth to avoid bearing down too hard. This may help to prevent an explosive delivery and excessive tearing of the perineum.

HAVE YOU HAD BLEEDING OR A BLOODY SHOW?   Bloody show is normal, especially toward the end of labor. If the bag of waters has ruptured, the bloody show may appear excessive as it mixes with the amniotic fluid. The mother should be reassured that this is normal. Excessive bleeding, however, or passing large clots of blood is abnormal and will be discussed later in this chapter.

WHEN IS YOUR DUE DATE?   This refers to the date that the doctor has estimated for delivery of the baby.

If the mother is more than 2 weeks early, radio ahead to the hospital so that the nursery can prepare for a possible premature baby. You will need to prepare for a special birth if the infant is premature.

An infant who weighs less than 5.5 pounds or is born before 38 weeks of gestation is considered *premature*. The younger the gestational age, the more likely it is that the baby will have respiratory and other problems. The respiratory problems occur because there is not enough *pulmonary surfactant* in the lungs of a premature infant to keep the lungs expanded. Remember that pulmonary surfactant prevents the small alveoli from collapsing on exhalation. Heat regulation is also underdeveloped in a premature infant, so special care must be taken to maintain a warm environment for this baby. Assemble newborn resuscitation equipment and turn on the ambulance heater. Even if the woman is not sure of her due date, the premature baby is not difficult to recognize (Fig. 13–14). The premature baby's ears are flatter from lack of cartilage and not fully defined as in a term baby, and the whorls on the soles of the feet, much like

fingerprints, are not well developed so that the feet appear smooth. The premature baby has very little body fat and appears scrawny and bony.

Special care should be given to the premature baby once it is breathing:

- Wrap it snugly in a warm blanket. As added protection, an outer layer of plastic wrap or aluminum foil can also be used. Be sure to keep the outer wrap away from the baby's face. Keeping the head covered will reduce heat loss.
- Provide 100% oxygen and positive-pressure ventilation as needed; these babies are prone to respiratory distress due to immature lungs.
- Do not allow very premature babies (less than 34 weeks) to nurse. They cannot coordinate sucking, breathing, and swallowing and are prone to aspiration.
- Handle very gently. Premature babies are more prone to intracranial hemorrhage and other injuries. The blood volume of a very premature infant is

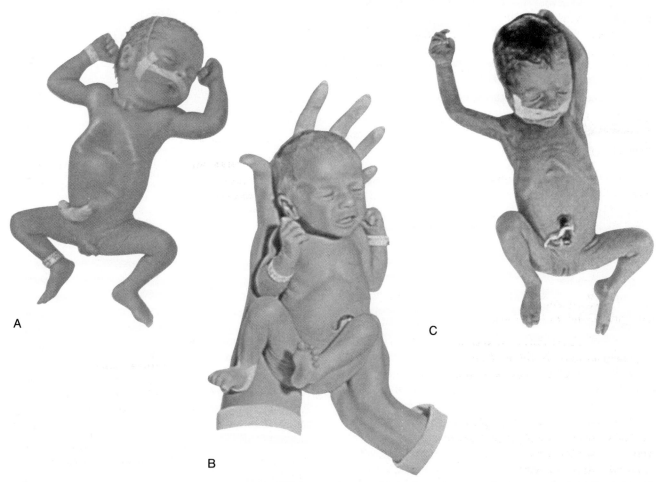

A

B

C

FIGURE 13–14. Sternal retraction (*A*) and cyanosis (*C*) are typical signs of respiratory distress in the premature infant. (*B*) A typical premature infant. Absence of body fat, underdeveloped ears, and lack of whorls on the soles of the feet are common before the 38th week of gestation. These infants have excessive amounts of vernix present at birth. (From Ross Laboratories Clinical Education Aid No. 5, 1985.)

only a few ounces, so even a slight loss of blood can lead to shock.

- Avoid subjecting the premature infant to infection.
- The baby should be transported in a prewarmed ambulance with a temperature of between 90°F and 100°F. The air-conditioning should be turned off in the warmer months.
- Radio ahead and advise the hospital that you are transporting a premature baby.

The premature baby is also covered with an unusually large amount of *vernix*. Vernix is a white, creamy substance, much like hand cream, that covers the baby. It protects the baby's skin within the watery confines of the uterus.

Occasionally, a woman may remain pregnant beyond the day when her baby should have been delivered. An infant beyond 42 weeks' gestation is *postmature*. When a baby remains in the womb more than 2 weeks past the optimal delivery time, the placenta may begin to deteriorate. The baby receives less nourishment as a result, and may suffer weight loss while in the uterus. This child is often born in an unhealthy state and appears scrawny, like the premature infant. Vernix has disappeared, so that the skin is often waterlogged and peeling, especially on the palms and the soles of the feet (Fig. 13–15). Unlike the premature baby, the postmature baby's ears are completely formed.

HAVE YOU HAD ANY PROBLEMS WITH THIS PREGNANCY? DO YOU HAVE ANY MEDICAL PROBLEMS? DO YOU TAKE ANY MEDICATIONS? These are all important questions to ask your patient. The patient may have a condition that would make vaginal delivery impossible, such as *placenta previa* (the placenta covers the cervix), which will be discussed later in this chapter. Mothers with a history of cardiac problems could experience grave difficulties, especially while pushing during the second stage of labor.

Diabetic mothers should be transported immediately, since rapid intervention is necessary for a good fetal outcome. When a diabetic becomes pregnant, she develops a resistance to insulin. As a result, her blood glucose levels are often very high, and large amounts of insulin are required to keep the mother's blood glucose level stable. Glucose crosses the placental barrier, but the larger insulin molecule does not. A baby born to a diabetic mother has been constantly exposed to unusually high levels of glucose. In response to the high levels of glucose thus introduced, the baby produces its own insulin in large amounts. Since insulin is a growth hormone, the infants of diabetic mothers are large, often exceeding 10 pounds (Fig. 13–16). It is unlikely that you could assist in the delivery of a baby this size without major complications. In addition to its size, the baby may be born with any of a number of birth defects that are more common in infants born to diabetic mothers.

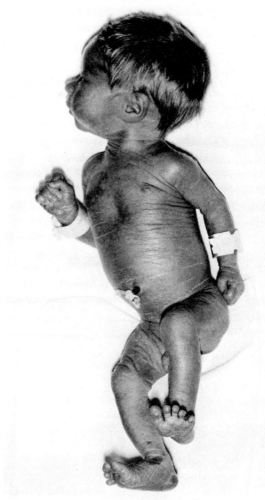

FIGURE 13–15. Like the premature infant, this postmature baby has no body fat but was born with little or no vernix and has wrinkled, peeling, water-logged skin. (From Beischer NA, Mackay EV: Obstetrics and the Newborn: An Illustrated Textbook, 2nd ed. Philadelphia, WB Saunders (Formerly Holt-Saunders Pty Limited, Merrickville, Australia), 1986, p. 182.)

Another problem associated with infants born to diabetic mothers is *hypoglycemia*. The huge supply of glucose to which this baby is accustomed ceases once the cord is cut, but the baby may still be producing abnormal insulin levels. This excess insulin quickly uses up the infant's available glucose reserve, causing the baby to become *hypoglycemic* shortly after birth. Since the brain is very dependent upon glucose to function, the baby's blood glucose must be monitored immediately after birth and corrected to prevent brain damage. The high-risk nature of diabetic deliveries makes it vital that you attempt to get the mother to the hospital to deliver.

PHYSICAL ASSESSMENT

If you have determined through the oral history that your patient is probably in early labor (irregular, mild pains with no urge to push; membranes not rup-

FIGURE 13–16. This 14-lb, 14-oz baby was born to a diabetic mother. Despite the healthy appearance of the apple-cheeked face, this baby is more prone to acidosis from chilling than a normal baby and can quickly become hypoglycemic after delivery. Because these babies are usually large, a history of diabetes should alert you to the fact that you may not be able to deliver this infant alone, even if the mother appears to be in very active labor. Shoulder dystocia (entrapment of the shoulders in the pelvis after the head has delivered) is also more common infants of this size. (From Beischer NA, Mackay EV: Obstetrics and the Newborn: An Illustrated Textbook, 2nd ed. Philadelphia, WB Saunders (Formerly Holt-Saunders Pty Limited, Merrickville, Australia), 1986, Color Plate 53.)

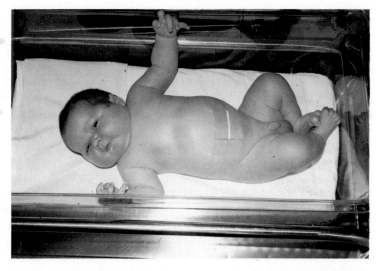

tured; and no bloody show), it is probably not necessary to subject your patient to the embarrassment of a physical examination. If a physical evaluation is necessary, you should make every attempt to provide privacy for the patient within a calm environment. You are more likely to gain her trust if you assume a soft-spoken, professional manner and inform the patient as to what you are about to do before you do it.

A brief physical assessment should allow you to complete your evaluation of the maternity patient. Take note if there is a bloody show and whether the show is heavy or just a slight pink staining. Note whether there is leaking of amniotic fluid and the color of the fluid. Check for bulging of the perineum and see if there is any part of the baby visible. Check during the contraction, since the presenting part recedes between contractions until crowning occurs, and the mother may be farther along in labor than it otherwise appears.

Your judgment is required when determining whether to transport immediately. If *crowning* has occurred (see Fig. 13–12), or if the presenting part is at all visible, prepare for delivery at the scene. Otherwise, simply attempt to calm the mother and transport, but be prepared for a delivery en route. If possible, place the stretcher on the ambulance in reverse, so the patient's head is toward the rear of the vehicle, and remember to turn on the heat. This makes things easier for you and provides a better environment if you have to deliver the baby while on the way to the hospital.

Management of Normal Labor and Delivery

The fact that the EMT who is about to deliver a baby probably does not have time to wash up is a graphic reminder of the importance of thorough hand washing between calls. Unwrap the OB (obstetric) kit (Fig. 13–17), being sure to keep sterile items sterile. The

OB kit usually contains three cord clamps plus surgical scissors or a scalpel to cut and clamp the cord. Kits with scissors are preferable, since they are safer and easier to use in the event of a tight cord around the baby's neck. The kit also includes a rubber bulb syringe for suctioning the baby, sterile gloves, an apron, at least four towels, a dozen 4 × 4 gauze sponges, a baby blanket, sanitary napkins, and two large plastic bags for waste materials and the placenta. While you are opening the OB kit, your partner should be offering encouragement and moral support to the mother. If it is a public place, your partner can assign a person to create as much privacy as possible. If at all possible, place the mother on the ambulance stretcher for delivery so that a quick departure can be made in event of an emergency. If there is time, put on the apron and a pair of plastic goggles for protection against communicable disease.

If Betadine scrub solution or Betadine and sterile water are available, pour a small amount of each on a pile of five or six 4 × 4 dressings. With the wet dressings, wash the perineum, always washing in one stroke from the top of the perineum to the bottom. This will avoid

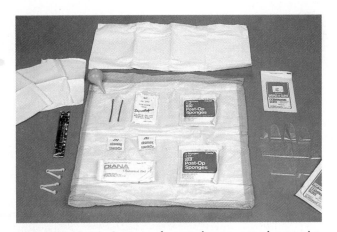

FIGURE 13–17. Contents of a typical emergency obstetrics kit.

contamination of the vaginal opening with fecal material. Discard each dressing after use.

After washing the perineum, put on a fresh pair of sterile gloves and set up a *sterile field*. A sterile field is an area in which you work that is sterile. If you are wearing sterile gloves, you may touch anything within that field. You can expand your sterile field by placing sterile drapes on the mother. When you have draped the mother, the sterile drapes, the washed perineum, and the inner contents of your OB kit are your sterile field.

Once you are wearing sterile gloves, it is essential to remember not to touch anything that is not sterile. You cannot touch the outside of your sterile glove with your other, ungloved hand. This is why the cuffs of sterile gloves are folded over. You can pick up and apply the first glove by the outside of the cuff, which will be against your skin anyway. The second glove is lifted by placing your sterile fingers *inside* the cuff, protecting your sterile hand from contamination by the ungloved hand. If you touch something outside of the sterile field, you are contaminated. If an unsterile object is placed on the sterile field, it is also contaminated. Practice is needed to master the skill of putting on sterile gloves and working in a sterile field.

The edge of the first drape is folded over your hands to prevent contamination of your sterile gloves and placed under the mother's buttocks. She is now supine with her knees bent and legs spread apart. Place a second drape across her abdomen, again being careful not to contaminate your gloves. Two more drapes are placed over her thighs.

Washing the perineum and preparing a sterile field are done in the ideal delivery but may not be possible in every case. Antibiotics can be given to the mother and baby at a later time if necessary, but a severely torn perineum or an injured baby is much more difficult to remedy. Control of the delivery should not be sacrificed in favor of setting up a sterile field and washing the perineum.

Delivery of the head should be controlled by gentle pressure on the back of the baby's head while the mother is asked to pant-blow during the contractions (Fig. 13–18). This prevents an explosive delivery, which would cause excessive tearing of the perineum and which can also harm the baby due to the sudden change of pressure to the head. If the membranes have not ruptured spontaneously by this time, break them and spread them away from the baby's face to minimize fluid aspiration and to create an airway. Once the head is born, give support to the head with one hand and palpate the baby's neck to see if there are one or more loops of cord around the neck. If there is a loose cord around the neck, you

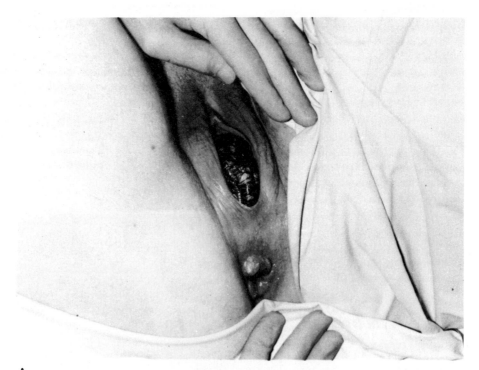

A

FIGURE 13–18. Vertex delivery (A) Part of the baby's head is visible, and the mother has been draped and positioned for delivery. (B) The head is crowning. Prepare to give slight counterpressure against the baby's head to prevent an explosive delivery. (C) Extension. Place a gauze over the anus to prevent contamination of the baby's face with fecal material, and begin to support the head. (D) The head rotates to the left or right as external rotation of the head begins.

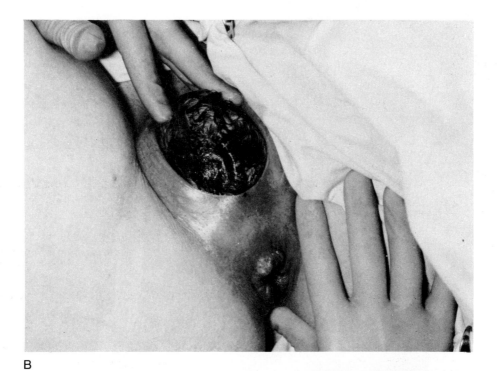

B

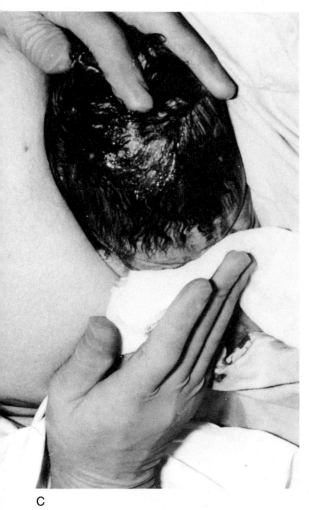

C

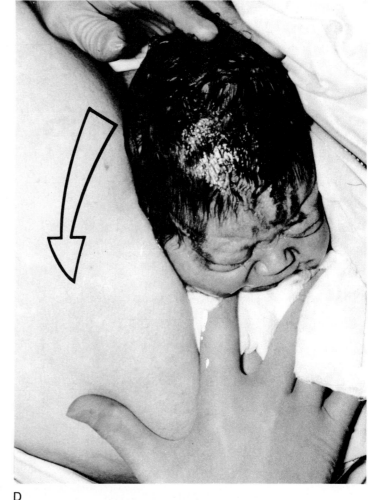

D

FIGURE 13–18 *Continued*

Illustration continued on following page

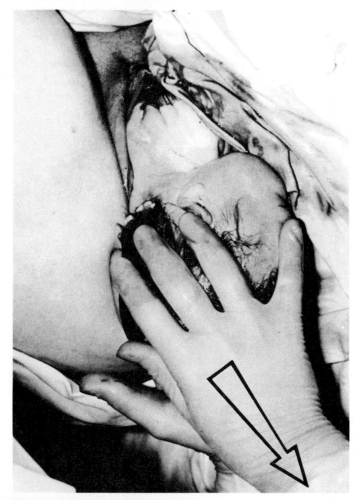

E

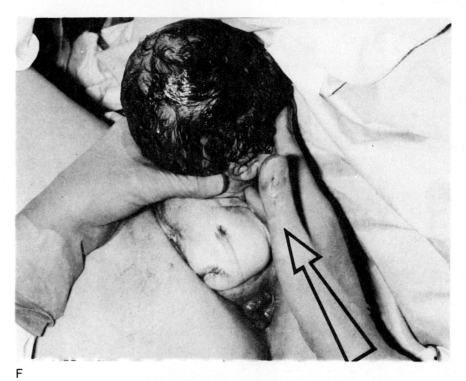

F

FIGURE 13–18 *Continued* (*E*) Apply gentle downward traction to deliver the anterior shoulder. (*F*) Apply upward traction to deliver the posterior shoulder. (*G*) Lift the rest of the body up and out of the birth canal, and prepare to grab the baby's feet. (From Beischer NA, Mackay EV: *Obstetrics and the Newborn: An Illustrated Textbook*, 2nd ed. Philadelphia, WB Saunders (Formerly Holt-Saunders Pty Limited, Merrickville, Australia), 1986, p. 374.)

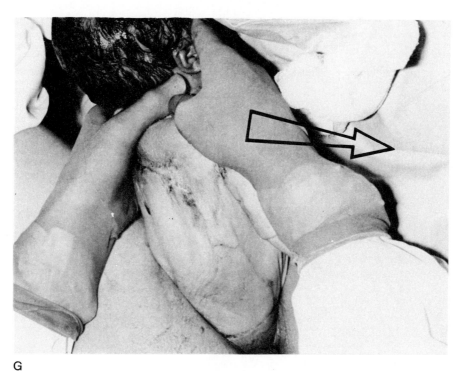

G

FIGURE 13–18 *Continued*

may attempt to slip it over the baby's head (Fig. 13–19). *Never pull or jerk the cord roughly, as it may tear.* If the cord is wrapped too tightly to slip free easily, the cord must be clamped and cut before delivery of the shoulders (Fig. 13–20). Place two clamps on the cord about an inch apart and cut the cord between the clamps. *Be sure that you make your cut between these clamps!* Then unwrap the loop or loops of cord from around the neck and proceed with the delivery. If there is meconium-stained fluid, the mouth should be suctioned now before continuing with the delivery.

As the head is born, it rotates externally to the left or right (see Fig. 13–18D), and delivery of the shoulders and then the body may follow easily. If the shoulders do not deliver spontaneously, it may be necessary to hold the baby's head in both hands and give gentle downward traction to guide the anterior shoulder under the symphysis pubis (see Fig. 13–18E). When the anterior shoulder is visible, lift the head upward to deliver the posterior shoulder (see Fig. 13–18F). Once the upper body is born, lower the body for drainage (see Fig. 13–18G) and prepare to catch the feet. These manipulations are always done gently and without twisting the baby's neck. Rough or improper handling can cause injury to the infant's clavicle or brachial plexus. If force is necessary for delivery, it is applied by the mother or by the use of *fundal pressure*. Fundal pressure is a downward, steady push on the fundus of the uterus to help expel the baby. You may push on top of the sterile abdominal drape or your partner can reach under the drape to give

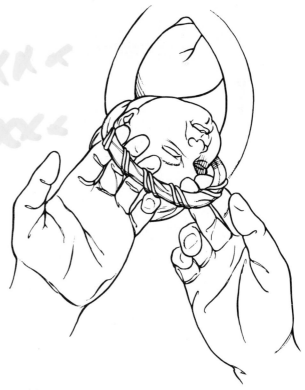

FIGURE 13–19. Loose cord around the neck. It is quite common to find the umbilical cord wrapped around the baby's neck. Ask the mother to pant-blow after the head has been delivered so that you can check for a cord around the neck. If it is loose, you may gently try to slip it over the baby's head. Rough handling of the cord may cause it to tear, with resultant bleeding through the cord.

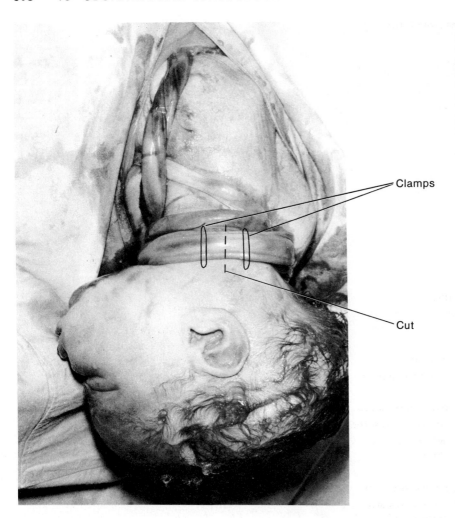

Clamps

Cut

FIGURE 13–20. Tight cord around the neck. If the cord is too tight to slip easily over the baby's head, it must be cut before the baby is born. Place two clamps *close together* on the cord and cut between the clamps. (From Beischer NA, Mackay EV: Obstetrics and the Newborn: An Illustrated Textbook, 2nd ed. Philadelphia, WB Saunders (Formerly Holt-Saunders Pty Limited, Merrickville, Australia), 1986, p. 485.)

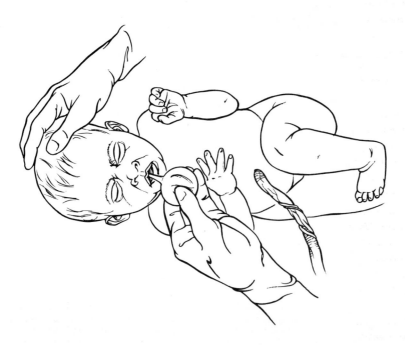

FIGURE 13–21. Suction the baby's airway thoroughly immediately after delivery. Be sure to compress the bulb *before* putting it into the baby's mouth to prevent blowing mucus further into the airway.

FIGURE 13–22. After suctioning, clamp the cord in two places and cut between the two clamps.

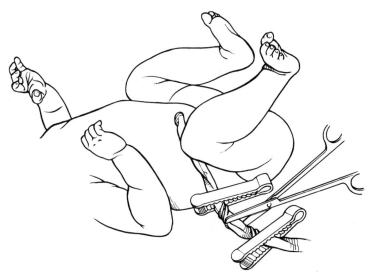

fundal pressure while you support the baby and the mother pushes. The mother can be asked to inhale deeply, hold her breath, and bear down as if moving her bowels. Her chin should be flexed on her chest while pushing and all pushes should be long and steady. The most effective pushing is done during a contraction, and each push should last 10 seconds.

Your partner should record the exact time of delivery while you remove blood and mucus from the baby's face and mouth with sterile gauze. While holding the baby slightly dependent, begin suctioning immediately after birth to clear the airway (Fig. 13–21). Compress the bulb syringe between two fingers and suction the baby's mouth and pharynx thoroughly, discarding the mucus each time. Take care to compress the bulb before putting it in the baby's mouth to prevent blowing mucus further into the baby's mouth.

Place the newborn on the sterile drapes that cover the mother's abdomen, and dry the baby vigorously with a clean towel. This helps to prevent heat loss and to stimulate respirations. If the mother wishes to, she may support her baby from the underside of the drapes on her abdomen. A brisk massage of the baby's back often brings forth a healthy cry.

The cord should now be clamped in two places and cut between the two clamps, about 6 to 8 inches from the baby (Fig. 13–22). Place the placental end of the cord on the mother's draped abdomen to prevent contamination from fecal material. Examine the stump of the cord to make sure that there is no bleeding (Fig. 13–23). Wrap the baby in a clean, dry towel, being sure to cover the head. The head is where the greatest heat loss can occur. Allowing the baby to become cold causes a dangerous increase in metabolic demands, thereby increasing the oxygen needs. In a baby who has not established good respirations, this becomes even more critical.

If the baby is breathing, administer high-concentration oxygen with a face mask held over the baby's mouth and nose until the infant turns a nice, healthy pink. Do not direct the oxygen at the baby's head or body, as this may cause further heat loss. Blasting oxygen right into a baby's face usually causes the infant to hold his or her breath. Observe the infant continuously for episodes of apnea or vomiting, and suction, stimulate, and resuscitate as necessary.

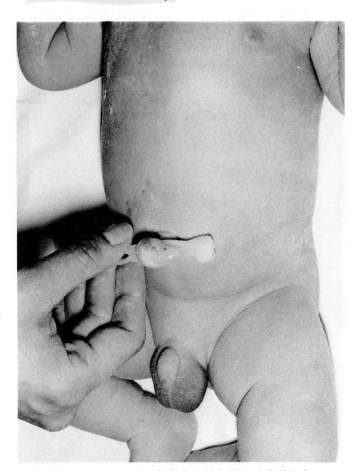

FIGURE 13–23. Be sure to check the umbilical stump for bleeding. Cord clamps may be defective or you may have cut too close to the clamp. (From Beischer NA, Mackay EV: Obstetrics and the Newborn: An Illustrated Textbook, 2nd ed. Philadelphia, WB Saunders (Formerly Holt-Saunders Pty Limited, Merrickville, Australia), 1986, p. 548.)

PROCEDURE 13-1
NORMAL CHILDBIRTH

1. Wash hands if there is time, then position and drape the mother, and prepare sterile field. *Do not leave the mother unattended to perform any of these acts.* The second EMT should lay out clean towels and infant resuscitation equipment in a warm area nearby.
2. Apply gentle counterpressure to the crown of the baby's head to prevent an explosive delivery. Ask the mother to pant like a puppy so that pushing is controlled.
3. Once the head is delivered, tell the mother not to push while you check for a cord around the baby's neck. If a tight cord is found (one that cannot be easily slipped around the baby's head), place two clamps very close together on the cord and cut the cord now.
4. If there is meconium-stained fluid, quickly wipe the baby's face with gauze to remove excess meconium; then suction the baby's mouth and nose with a bulb syringe before proceeding with the delivery. The mouth is always suctioned first because suction of the nose could elicit a gasp and the baby would aspirate the meconium inside the mouth.
5. Ask the mother to push as you give gentle traction if necessary to deliver the shoulders (downward traction for the anterior shoulder and upward traction for the posterior shoulder).
6. Suction with a bulb syringe when the infant is delivered.
7. Clamp and cut the cord if it has not already been cut. Examine the stump of the cord to make sure there is no bleeding.
8. Place the infant on towels for resuscitation.
9. When the placenta has separated, the uterus will form in a hard ball and there will be lengthening of the cord. Ask the mother to bear down while the placenta is delivered. Do not pull on the cord.
10. Place a warm blanket on the mother and observe the fundus of her uterus while transporting her to the hospital. Massage the uterus when necessary to prevent hemorrhage.

Resuscitation of the Newborn

Some infants require resuscitation immediately after birth. The longer you wait to resuscitate, the longer it will take to have the infant breathing on his own. For this reason, the need for resuscitation should be anticipated in all deliveries, with the appropriate equipment assembled and within reach before the delivery. A prolonged resuscitation involves drugs, intubation, and IV therapy. For this reason, any resuscitation started by the EMT that lasts longer than 1 minute should be continued en route to the hospital.

It is best if a second EMT takes over care of the baby immediately after the cord is clamped and cut. The EMT who delivered the baby should attend to the mother, and both patients now require the full attention of a caregiver.

The initial evaluation of the infant, which determines the amount and type of resuscitation required, is based on three criteria: respiration, heart rate, and color, in that order.

There should be at least two towels, one on top of the other, in the area where the newborn is placed. As soon as the baby is placed on the towel by the delivering EMT, the second EMT should quickly dry the baby's entire body. This should not take longer than 1 or 2 seconds. Discard the towel used to dry the infant and place him on the clean towel with the head only slightly extended. Hyperextension is avoided in infants because the delicate trachea is too pliable. Hyperextension may cause the trachea to kink or close off like a plastic straw.

The newborn should now be suctioned and the respirations evaluated. If the infant is not breathing, rub the infant's back vigorously or slap the feet *twice*. If the infant does not cry with this stimulation, inflate the infant's lungs, since further attempts to stimulate the infant would be a waste of time and would prolong the time of resuscitation.

If the infant remains apneic, inflate the lungs once or twice with a pediatric bag-valve-mask. An oxygen reservoir should be attached to provide 100% oxygen. The mask should fit tightly, covering the infant's mouth and nose but not touching the eyes. Clear masks are best since they allow you to observe secretions. For prolonged resuscitation, you may wish to insert an oropharyngeal airway (Fig. 13–24), but the time for this should not be wasted in the initial resuscitation. For the first few breaths, simply lift the jaw forward as you maintain a tight seal (Fig. 13–25).

The alveoli of a fetus are filled with fluid. Much of this fluid is squeezed out of the lungs during the birthing process, but some of the fluid remains. The rest of this fluid must be forced through the walls of the alveoli and into the general circulation. This requires many times the pressure of a normal infant breath. When an infant cries or breathes on his own at birth, he takes a huge breath. The pressure of this first great breath of life forces the fluid through the walls of the alveoli. If the infant does not take this first huge breath, fluid remains in the lungs and blocks a good oxygen exchange in the alveoli, even if the baby seems to be breathing on his own. As the baby is deprived of oxygen, the heart rate slows.

The second observation you make in a newborn is the heart rate. If the heart rate is less than 100 per minute, there is probably poor air exchange. Ventilate for 15 to

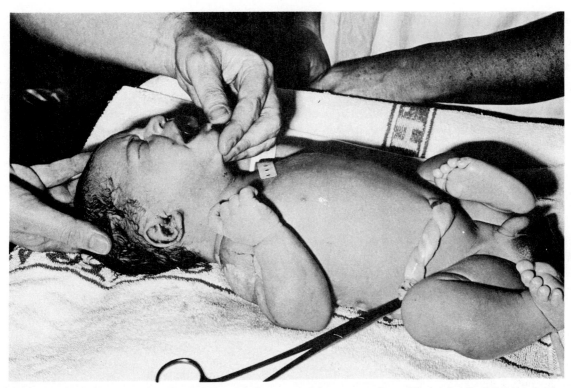

FIGURE 13–24. Placement of an oropharyngeal airway before positive-pressure ventilation. Notice that the baby's head is kept aligned with the body. Hyperextension of the neck is not recommended in infant resuscitation. (From Beischer NA, Mackay EV: Obstetrics and the Newborn: An Illustrated Textbook, 2nd ed. Philadelphia, WB Saunders (Formerly Holt-Saunders Pty Limited, Merrickville, Australia), 1986, p. 582.)

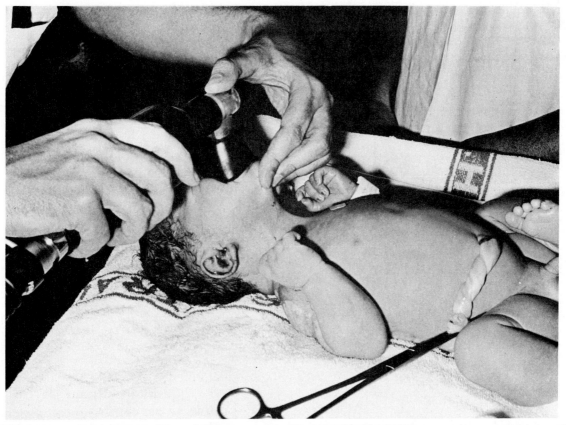

FIGURE 13–25. Positive-pressure ventilation. A tight seal is made and the jaw is lifted forward. (From Beischer NA, Mackay EV: Obstetrics and the Newborn: An Illustrated Textbook, 2nd ed. Philadelphia, WB Saunders (Formerly Holt-Saunders Pty Limited, Merrickville, Australia), 1986, p. 583.)

30 seconds with a bag-valve-mask with an oxygen reservoir; then re-evaluate the infant. The first few ventilations should move about 30 to 35 cc, a higher pressure than normal for an infant, to simulate the first big breaths of life. Subsequent ventilations should deliver 15 to 20 cc, with only the fingertips compressing the ventilating bag. A short period of positive-pressure ventilation is often enough to raise the heart rate to normal. If after 15 to 30 seconds of positive-pressure ventilation the heart rate remains either less than 60 per minute or between 60 and 80 per minute but not rising, chest compressions must be started. To begin chest compressions, an imaginary line is drawn between the infant's nipples. Two fingers are placed on the sternum below this line and the sternum is compressed $\frac{1}{2}$ to $\frac{3}{4}$ of an inch at a rate of 120 beats per minute (Fig. 13–26).

After 30 seconds of cardiac compressions, a 6-second evaluation of the heart rate is done. If the heart rate remains below 80, compressions are continued. If the heart rate is above 80 and the baby is breathing well, the third evaluation—color—is done.

The newborn's color should be pink except for a slight, normal cyanosis of the hands and feet. Cyanosis of the face with a pink body and an otherwise healthy-looking, crying baby is a pressure face. This is caused by the rupture of blood vessels in the face during the delivery. Poor air exchange or cooling of the baby results in a baby with bluish or very pale color. Black babies appear gray when cyanotic.

If the newborn is pale or cyanotic, oxygen should be delivered as close to 100% as possible until the infant

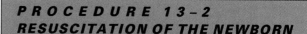

PROCEDURE 13-2
RESUSCITATION OF THE NEWBORN

1. Dry the infant and place on a clean towel in a warm place.
2. Position the infant with the neck only slightly extended.
3. Suction the mouth and then the nose with a bulb syringe.
4. Stimulate by rubbing the infant's back or slapping the feet.
5. Evaluate breathing.
6. Repeat step 4 twice only if the infant is apneic at this point.
7. If the infant is still not breathing, give positive-pressure ventilation with bag-valve-mask and 100% oxygen.
8. Evaluate the heart rate after 15 to 30 seconds of positive-pressure ventilation.
9. If the heart rate is less than 60 or between 60 and 80 but not increasing, begin chest compressions $\frac{1}{2}$ to $\frac{3}{4}$ of an inch at 120 compressions per minute.
10. After 30 seconds of chest compressions, check the heart rate for 6 seconds. If below 80, continue both chest compressions and positive-pressure ventilation. If heart rate is greater than 80, proceed to step 11.
11. Evaluate color. If the infant is now pink, continue to observe. If cyanotic, give as close to 100% oxygen as you can. Continue to evaluate breathing, heart rate and color during transportation to the hospital.

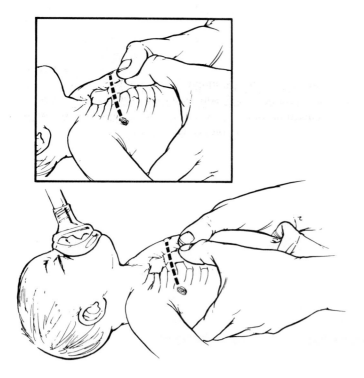

FIGURE 13–26. Cardiac compressions on the newborn. Compressions should be given in the *midsternum* area. (Reproduced with permission. © *Textbook of Pediatric Advanced Life Support,* 1988. Copyright American Heart Association.)

is pink. This is done through a tight-fitting face mask or by holding the oxygen tubing $\frac{1}{2}$ inch from the baby's nose. (This will deliver 80% oxygen if you do not wave the tubing or move it further than $\frac{1}{2}$ inch from the baby.) Oxygen cannot be delivered through a bag-valve-mask device unless you are actually ventilating the patient.

The skin color should be continuously observed en route to the hospital. If the baby turns pink and remains pink, the oxygen can be slowly withdrawn. Color is the major indicator of respiratory distress in the newborn, but you should look for other signs of respiratory distress, such as nasal flaring, sternal retractions (Fig. 13–14), and respiratory grunting. A respiratory grunt sounds like a weak, complaining cry during exhalation.

The Apgar Scoring System

The Apgar score (Table 13–1) is a system used to quickly evaluate a newborn in five specific areas. Although it reveals nothing about specific birth defects or injuries the baby may have suffered during the birthing process, it can give a general idea to the person receiving your report about how well the baby did at birth. The score is done at 1 minute after birth and repeated at 5 minutes after birth. As shown in Table 13–1, the areas to be evaluated are heart rate, respiratory effort, muscle tone, reflex irritability, and color. Most healthy newborns have a 1-minute Apgar score of 9, with 1 point deducted for cyanosis in the extremities only. Babies usually "pink up" by the time 5 minutes have passed so that the 5-minute Apgar score is often 10. Nonwhite babies should have pink gums. If the skin is gray, a poor color rating is given, and resuscitation is needed. A score below 7 is poor and means that the baby required some type of resuscitation effort. A baby with a score of 8 to 10 was crying spontaneously soon after birth and needed very little assistance of any kind from you. Scoring of the baby is often a retrospective event, and treatment or transport is never delayed so that you can score a baby.

Newborn Survey

Once you have established that the airway, breathing, and circulation of the newborn infant are adequate, you can perform a quick newborn survey before handing the baby over to the mother. The survey should not take more than 1 or 2 minutes and is only done to ensure that the baby is fit enough for handling or nursing by the mother.

To calm the mother, you should be aware of the common appearance of a newborn baby. The baby is slippery and, especially if premature, may be covered with vernix. There may be tiny white dots on the baby's nose and chin called *milia* (Fig. 13–27). They appear much like an infection, and your patient may be concerned about them. You can assure the mother that they are both common and normal and will recede within a week or two. Fine hair may cover not only the head but also the shoulders, forehead, or back, and this also disappears, as the baby matures. This extra hair is more prevalent in a premature baby and almost nonexistent in a postmature infant. A bluish discoloration of the entire face after the body has pinked up may occur after a difficult or explosive delivery and is called *pressure face*. Pressure face is caused by widespread rupturing of tiny surface blood vessels in the baby's face and heals within a few days. This is not to be confused with cyanosis around the mouth, a more ominous sign that the baby's respiratory efforts are inadequate.

The baby's head may be swollen or elongated because the head has actually molded itself into the shape of the mother's pelvis (see Fig. 13–10). This, as well as a flattening or sideways displacement of the nose, chin, or ears, may be upsetting to first-time parents, and you can confidently reassure them that this is only temporary. Occasionally, an infant suffers enough trauma at birth to develop a hematoma between one of the cranial bones and the overlying periosteum. This condition, *cephalhematoma*, is different and more serious than either molding or swelling of the soft tissues of the scalp. A cephalhematoma does not cross the suture lines of the skull (Fig. 13–28). The blood loss, which might be small for

TABLE 13–1. Apgar Scoring Chart

Sign	0	1	2
Heart rate	Absent	Slow (below 100)	Over 100
Respiratory effort	Absent	Weak cry, hypoventilation	Good strong cry
Muscle tone	Limp	Some flexion of extremities	Well flexed
Reflex response (foot slap)	No response	Grimace	Cry and withdrawal of foot
Color	Blue pale	Body pink Extremities blue	Completely pink

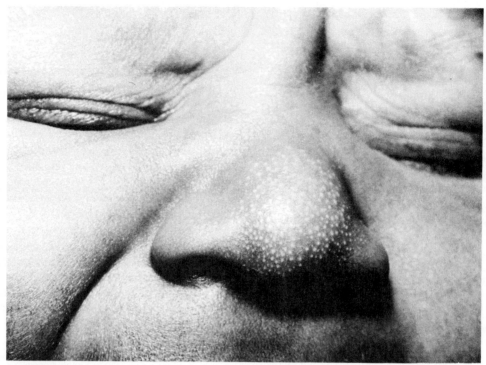

FIGURE 13–27. Milia, found on the nose and chin of many newborns, will disappear within a few weeks. (From Beischer NA, Mackay EV: Obstetrics and the Newborn: An Illustrated Textbook, 2nd ed. Philadelphia, WB Saunders (Formerly Holt-Saunders Pty Limited, Merrickville, Australia), 1986, p. 554.)

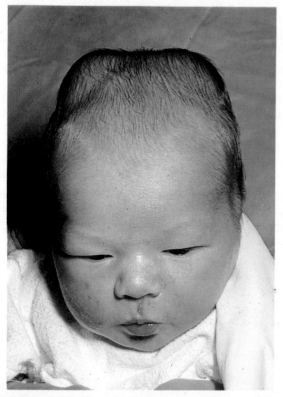

FIGURE 13–28. Bilateral cephalhematomas. These are different and more serious than either swelling of the soft tissue or molding. Notice that the hematomas do not cross the suture lines of the skull. This is because the hematoma is contained between the bone and the overlying periosteum. (From Beischer NA, Mackay EV: Obstetrics and the Newborn: An Illustrated Textbook, 2nd ed. Philadelphia, WB Saunders (Formerly Holt-Saunders Pty Limited, Merrickville, Australia), 1986, Color Plate 142.)

an adult, may be a large amount for a baby. The baby's immature liver may have difficulty handling the by-products of the destroyed red blood cells and the baby may become jaundiced. Rarely, a blood transfusion is required. If you notice this particular type of swelling, be extra cautious in handling the baby to prevent further injury.

Carefully place a finger in the baby's mouth to check for completeness of the palate (Fig. 13–29). A hole or separation in the palate is termed *cleft palate* and may be confined to inside the mouth or may extend to the upper lip or even involve the nose. While a cleft lip (Fig. 13–30) is an obvious defect, a cleft palate may not be noticed without this careful examination of the roof of the mouth. If you should discover a cleft palate or if the baby has a cleft lip, do not allow the mother to nurse. Babies with this defect may require more suctioning and may be more prone to aspiration.

Examine the baby's back for any opening in the spinal column. Spinal cord defects, in which the spinal cord or membranes may protrude from the back, are serious and often cause paralysis (Fig. 13–31). The opening must be protected from injury. Keep the baby in a prone position and minimize movement. The opening may be covered by loose sterile gauze moistened with warm sterile saline. Do not secure the dressing with tape. Use a loosely wrapped dressing or hold the sterile pad in place with the baby's blanket alone.

Take note at this time if the anus is patent. Passage

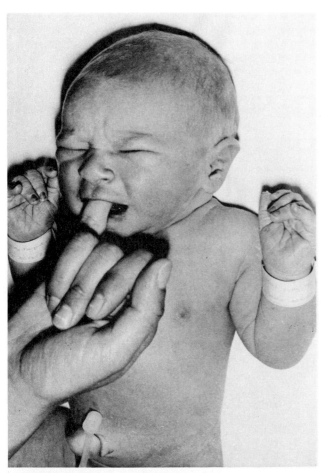

FIGURE 13–29. Cleft palate, a defective opening in the palate, should be checked for before the mother is allowed to nurse the baby. (From Beischer NA, Mackay EV: Obstetrics and the Newborn: An Illustrated Textbook, 2nd ed. Philadelphia, WB Saunders (Formerly Holt-Saunders Pty Limited, Merrickville, Australia), 1986, p. 547.)

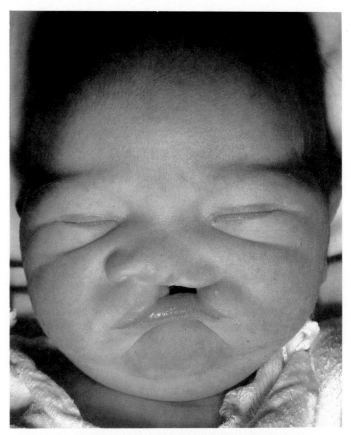

FIGURE 13–30. This baby suffers from both cleft palate and cleft lip. Airway management may be more difficult in this infant and the baby should be continuously observed while en route to the hospital. (From Beischer NA, Mackay EV: Obstetrics and the Newborn: An Illustrated Textbook, 2nd ed. Philadelphia, WB Saunders (Formerly Holt-Saunders Pty Limited, Merrickville, Australia), 1986, Color Plate 112A.)

of meconium or urine signifies that the kidneys and gastrointestinal tract are functioning, which is helpful information to pass on to nursery personnel.

A healthy baby should cry vigorously, and the baby's face and trunk should be a healthy pink. Some cyanosis in the extremities is normal. The arms and legs should move independently and flex spontaneously if you gently extend them and then let go. A limp arm could mean damage to the brachial plexus (the peripheral nerve supply to the upper extremity) and should be noted, along with any other obvious one-sided weakness of any body part. Brachial plexus damage (Fig. 13–32) is a fairly common birth injury that often resolves if treated properly. The baby presents with a limp, internally rotated arm with the fist closed. The arm should be immobilized in the blanket and not stretched or aggravated while en route to the hospital. Another birth injury is a fracture of the clavicle. The bone can sometimes be heard snapping during delivery, and the baby usually continues to cry even after he or she has been wrapped and cuddled. The infant should be handled gently and the information reported to nursery personnel.

Maintaining a Warm Environment

When a baby is allowed to become chilled, he or she must speed up the rate of metabolism to increase heat production. This requires the use of a great deal of both oxygen and glucose. The newborn's supply of glucose is limited compared to an adult or even an older baby. As the supply of glucose becomes exhausted, the blood sugar drops rapidly and the baby becomes *hypoglycemic*. In this state, brain damage may occur since brain tissue is very dependent upon glucose to function. At the same time, oxygen is quickly burned and exhausted by the excessive metabolic effort exerted to keep warm. Once the oxygen has been exhausted, *anaerobic metabolism, metabolism without oxygen,* occurs with the production of lactic acid as a byproduct, and the baby can quickly descend into a state of metabolic acidosis, a disturbance in which the acid–base status of the body shifts toward the acid side.

The three main objectives of the EMT caring for a newborn are:

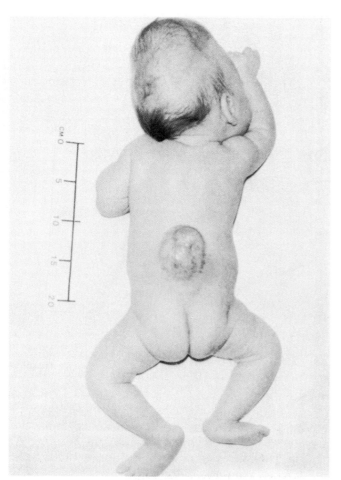

FIGURE 13–31. Spinal cord defect. Spinal defects may be much smaller than this and should be checked for during the newborn survey. Even a dime-sized defect can lead to later paralysis if roughly handled. If detected, a spinal defect should be covered with a sterile dressing moistened with sterile saline. Do not secure the dressing with tape. Keep it loosely in place under the infant's blanket while maintaining the baby in a prone position. (From Beischer NA, Mackay EV: Obstetrics and the Newborn: An Illustrated Textbook, 2nd ed. Philadelphia, WB Saunders (Formerly Holt-Saunders Pty Limited, Merrickville, Australia), 1986, p. 449.)

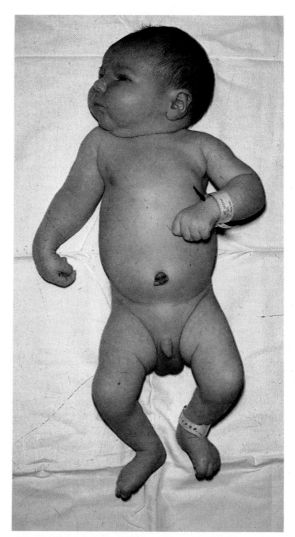

FIGURE 13–32. Damage to the right brachial plexus. Notice the typical position of this infant's limp right arm. The left arm is normal. Traction given during delivery should be gentle and controlled to prevent this type of birth injury. If you notice this type of injury, immobilize the arm within the blanket and minimize handling of the baby. (From Beischer NA, Mackay EV: Obstetrics and the Newborn: An Illustrated Textbook, 2nd ed. Philadelphia, WB Saunders (Formerly Holt-Saunders Pty Limited, Merrickville, Australia), 1986, Color Plate 140.)

1. Provide adequate ventilation through stimulation and oxygen administration, with intermittent suction, if required, to clear the airway.

2. Provide cardiac resuscitation if the newborn's heart rate is inadequate or nonexistent.

3. Keep the baby warm.

Third Stage of Labor and Care of the Mother

As soon as the infant has been stabilized and wrapped for warmth, he or she can be handed to the mother and the EMT can attend to her. If prolonged resuscitation of the baby seems necessary and there is a sufficient number of personnel, you may transfer re-

sponsibility for the baby to someone else while you attend to the mother. Be sure to keep your gloves sterile while handing over the baby.

As you note signs that the placenta has separated from the wall of the uterus (lengthening of the umbilical cord and contraction of the uterus into a raised globular shape), you should ask the mother to bear down. If the placenta does not begin to emerge with one or two pushes, place your hand on the sterile drape you have previously placed on the mother's abdomen and give gentle fundal pressure while she pushes (Fig. 13–33). Have a basin ready to receive the placenta and expect a gush of blood after the placenta is expelled. The weight of the placenta as it is expelled should be enough to extract the membranes. Do not pull on the placenta or you may tear the membranes and cause some of the

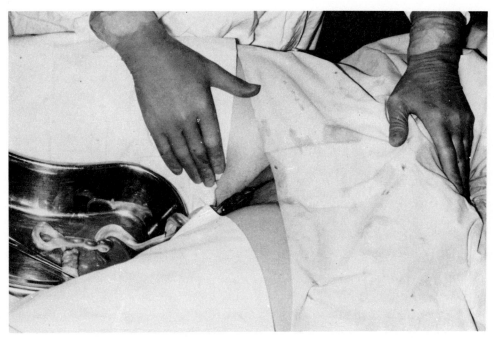

FIGURE 13–33. Delivery of the placenta with fundal pressure while the mother is asked to bear down. If the placenta does not deliver spontaneously within 20 minutes of birth, proceed to the hospital. (From Beischer NA, Mackay EV: Obstetrics and the Newborn: An Illustrated Textbook, 2nd ed. Philadelphia, WB Saunders (Formerly Holt-Saunders Pty Limited, Merrickville, Australia), 1986, p. 383.)

tissue to be retained inside the uterus. Not all placentas are formed normally. Occasionally there is more than one lobe to the placenta (Fig. 13–34), or the cord may not be well implanted into the placenta (Fig. 13–35). The retained placenta or the torn cord could cause a hemorrhage if you pulled strongly on the cord. Save the placenta in the bag provided in the OB kit, since the obstetrician or emergency physician may wish to examine it. Gently massage the uterus to ensure good contraction and prevent bleeding.

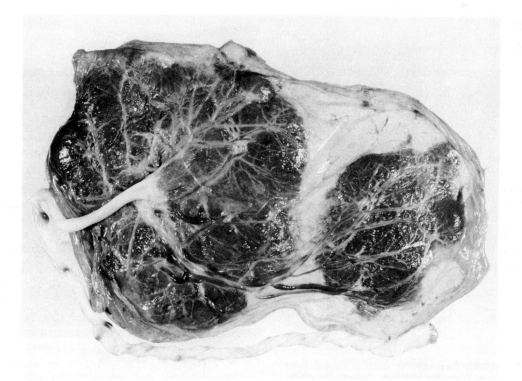

FIGURE 13–34. Extra lobe of placenta. Notice that the cord is divided between the lobes and that the cord to the smaller lobe is further divided into several vessels before it implants within the lobe. Pulling on the cord to deliver this placenta would probably result in tearing of the cord and hemorrhage. (From Beischer NA, Mackay EV: Obstetrics and the Newborn: An Illustrated Textbook, 2nd ed. Philadelphia, WB Saunders (Formerly Holt-Saunders Pty Limited, Merrickville, Australia), 1986, p. 384.)

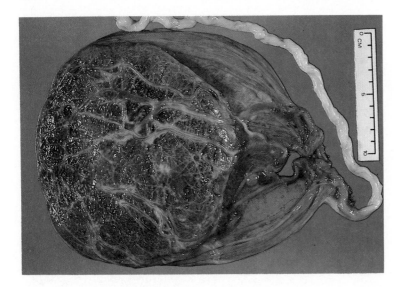

FIGURE 13–35. Single placenta with abnormal implantation of the cord. (From Beischer NA, Mackay EV: Obstetrics and the Newborn: An Illustrated Textbook, 2nd ed. Philadelphia, WB Saunders (Formerly Holt-Saunders Pty Limited, Merrickville, Australia), 1986, Color Plate 85.)

If the placenta does not deliver within 20 minutes, or if there are any complications with either the baby or the mother, transport immediately. Never delay transport for delivery of the placenta if there is any problem with either the mother or the baby.

If the placenta delivers, massage the fundus firmly until you can feel it contracted into a hard ball below the umbilicus (Fig. 13–36). As you massage the fundus you may see some blood expelled from the vagina. This is normal, but large clots or a large amount of blood indicates that the mother is bleeding abnormally. Continue to massage the uterus until the bleeding is minimal

and the uterus is firm. If the bleeding appears to be controlled and the fundus remains firm, remove the soiled drapes from the mother and place a sterile sanitary pad on the perineum. Do not directly touch any perineal lacerations, as they may be very painful. Ask the patient to straighten out her legs and bring them together. Keeping the knees bent for a longer time than is necessary increases the risk of clot formation in the legs.

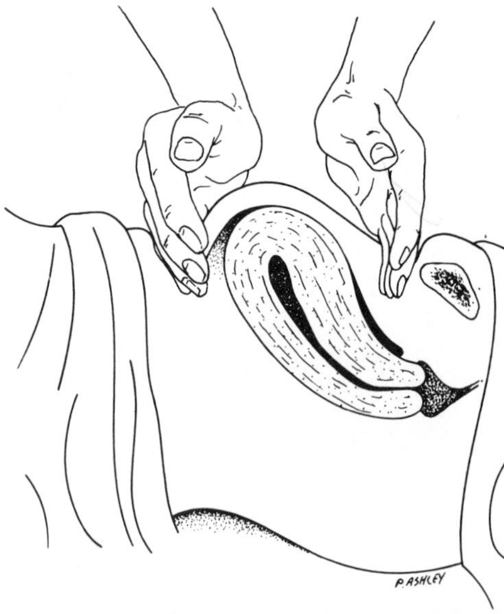

It is normal for women to shake in the immediate postdelivery period. This is a physiologic response to the shock her body has been through and the tremendous amount of energy expended during childbirth. Cover her with a warm blanket and proceed to the hospital. If the mother is planning to breast-feed, encourage her to nurse the baby at this time. An important hormone, *oxytocin*, is released into the mother's circulation when the baby suckles. Oxytocin aids in contracting the uterus and may prevent postpartum bleeding.

Never leave the mother alone at this time, with or without the baby. She is weak and tired from blood loss and the strain of delivery, and postpartum hemorrhage is most likely to occur in the first hour after delivery of the baby. If the hospital is some distance away, continue to check the fundus at least every half hour during the trip to make sure that the uterus stays contracted and that bleeding is minimal. Also, the baby should be continuously observed for apnea or aspiration of mucus.

COMPLICATIONS OF LABOR AND DELIVERY

Prolapsed Cord

Occasionally, the umbilical cord slips down past the presenting part of the fetus into the vagina. This complication, termed a *prolapsed cord* (Fig. 13–37), occurs

FIGURE 13–36. Massage the postpartum uterus to maintain tight contraction of the uterus below the umbilicus. Support the uterus above the pubic bone with one hand while massaging with the other to prevent prolapse of the uterus. (From Burroughs A: Bleier's Maternity Nursing, 5th ed. Philadelphia, WB Saunders, 1986, p. 306.)

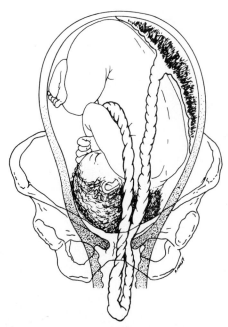

FIGURE 13–37. A prolapsed cord can be compressed between the baby's head and the pelvic bone or vaginal wall, cutting off the baby's circulation. (From Burroughs A: Bleier's Maternity Nursing, 5th ed. Philadelphia, WB Saunders, 1986, p. 254.)

most often in abnormal presentations such as breech or shoulder presentations. It may also happen when the membranes rupture early in labor before the baby's head is fully descended into the pelvis, in which case the cord may block the opening. Once the cord prolapses, the presenting part may compress the cord against the pelvic bones or the vaginal wall, thereby cutting off all or part of the fetal blood supply.

If a prolapsed cord is obvious, elevate the mother's hips with pillows or place her in a knee–chest position. Then, attempt to elevate the presenting part (NOT THE CORD!) manually by applying pressure to it with a gloved hand (Fig. 13–38). This position and elevation of the presenting part are maintained as you proceed to the hospital. Administer oxygen in high concentration and displace the uterus to the left to minimize vena cava compression. Rapid transport is vital, as is notifying the hospital so that preparations for an emergency cesarean section can be made.

Breech Delivery

Rarely, you may have to assist in delivery of a breech presentation. Unless the buttocks are clearly visible and about to emerge, every effort should be made to transport this patient quickly, since there are several adverse events that may complicate a breech delivery. Breech labors are usually longer than vertex labors as the buttocks do not make as good a wedge to dilate the cervix. Also, since the buttocks are not as large as the head, they may emerge before the cervix has fully dilated, leaving the head entrapped within the uterus. This is most common in premature babies, since the premature head is proportionately much larger than the body. As the fetus matures, the body becomes proportionately closer to the head in size, but even at full term the head has the largest diameter.

Large amounts of thick meconium are common in a breech delivery (Fig. 13–39), but the meconium is often expelled because of the pressure on the baby's abdomen.

FIGURE 13–38. If a prolapsed cord is detected, put gloves on and place your fingers within the vagina to elevate the presenting part; maintain this elevation on the way to the hospital. If possible, place the mother on her left side or in knee–chest position.

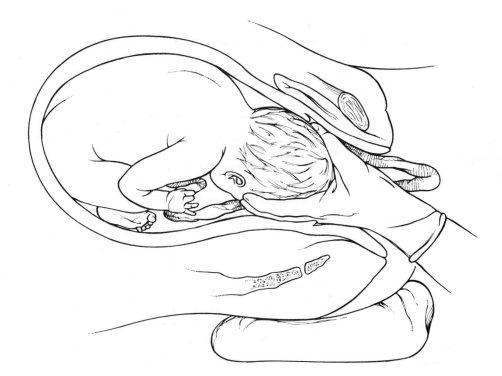

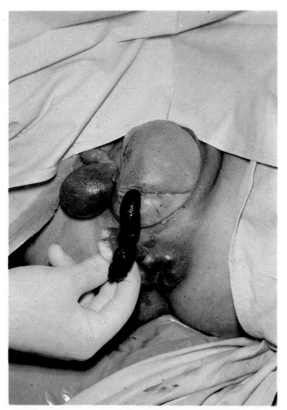

FIGURE 13–39. If a breech delivery has progressed this far spontaneously, you may prepare for delivery on the scene. Otherwise, rush the patient to the hospital for delivery. Note that meconium has been squeezed out by pressure on the infant's abdomen. (From Beischer NA, Mackay EV: Obstetrics and the Newborn: An Illustrated Textbook, 2nd ed. Philadelphia, WB Saunders (Formerly Holt-Saunders Pty Limited, Merrickville, Australia), 1986, Color Plate 29.)

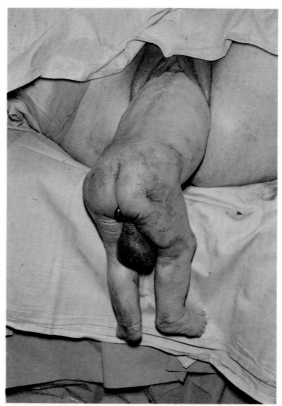

FIGURE 13–40. Allow the infant in a breech delivery to deliver by its own weight up to the nipple line. External rotation has not yet occurred. (From Beischer NA, Mackay EV: Obstetrics and the Newborn: An Illustrated Textbook, 2nd ed. Philadelphia, WB Saunders (Formerly Holt-Saunders Pty Limited, Merrickville, Australia), 1986, Color Plate 30.)

There is less cause for concern here than in a vertex delivery, where meconium is a much more ominous sign of hypoxia. Regardless of the cause, meconium aspiration is still a danger.

Prolapse of the umbilical cord is also a common complication in a breech presentation. Once the uterus has been partially emptied of the baby's body in a frank breech (see Fig, 13–11B), the placenta may separate prematurely from the contracted uterus before the head has been expelled, cutting off the baby's oxygen supply.

It is almost always necessary to assist somewhat in the delivery of a breech presentation. It is easiest if the mother scoots down to the very edge of the stretcher so that her buttocks are almost hanging off the end and her legs are flexed sharply. This assistance is given only after the body has partially delivered, since any other breech situation should be rushed to the hospital. The weight of the baby's body is often sufficient to allow delivery up to the scapula (Fig. 13–40). Once the baby's body is born to the level of the umbilicus, hook your finger between the umbilical cord and the baby's abdomen. Then pull out a loop of cord. This will prevent the cord from tearing. You may grasp the legs or feet

and pull down gently until the lower scapulas are visible. All deliveries should be slow and controlled. External rotation of the shoulders must occur for the shoulders and arms to be born. Once one of the baby's axillae appears, the body should either be lifted or pulled down to deliver the arms in whatever sequence they appear (Fig. 13–41). To deliver the anterior arm, apply downward traction, and to deliver the posterior arm, lift up the body. You may reach in with a finger to gently deliver the arm if it does not deliver spontaneously. After the shoulders and arms have delivered, the body should rotate so that the back is again facing upward. If the baby's head does not deliver spontaneously at this point, you must flex the baby's chin onto the chest before you can move the head through the curved plane of the pelvis (Fig. 13–42). Otherwise you could cause a severe neck injury or head trauma. While supporting the baby's body on your forearm, place the fingers of your left hand into the vagina and locate the baby's mouth; then place your fingers into the baby's mouth and pull gently to flex his or her chin onto his or her chest. At the same time, apply slight pressure on the back of the baby's head with the fingers of your other hand. Once the baby's

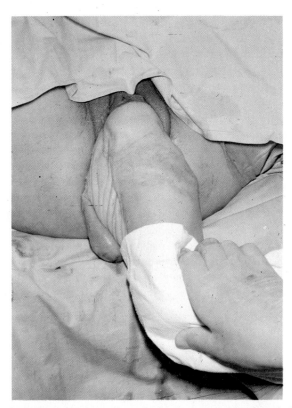

FIGURE 13–41. Meconium, almost always present in breech deliveries, will make the baby slippery and harder to handle. A towel has been placed over the baby's lower body to make the infant easier to handle. External rotation has occurred and upward traction was given to deliver the posterior shoulder. Downward traction is now delivering the anterior shoulder. (From Beischer NA, Mackay EV: Obstetrics and the Newborn: An Illustrated Textbook, 2nd ed. Philadelphia, WB Saunders (Formerly Holt-Saunders Pty Limited, Merrickville, Australia), 1986, Color Plate 31.)

head is flexed, you can apply gentle downward traction to complete delivery of the head. It is usually helpful at this time if your assistant gives gentle suprapubic pressure to keep the baby's head flexed. At this point the body should be lifted upward until the face and the rest of the head are born.

If you are unable to deliver a breech within 3 minutes, the mother should be transported to the hospital while you provide an airway for the baby. Exposure of the baby's body to the cooler outside environment as well as the forces of delivery may stimulate spontaneous respirations while the baby's face is still pressed up against the vaginal wall. To provide an airway, place your hand in the vagina with your palm facing the baby's face and form a "V" under the nose, pushing the vaginal wall away from the face. This maneuver alone may provoke delivery of the head. If not, elevate the mother's buttocks to relieve pressure on the umbilical cord, upon which the baby's body is resting. Administer oxygen in high concentration to the mother, and notify the hospital so that an obstetrician will be standing by.

Complications that may affect a breech-delivered infant include a prolapsed cord, premature separation of the placenta, meconium aspiration, a fractured clavicle, damage to the brachial plexus, and head and neck injuries such as a fractured skull or intracranial hemorrhage. Other abnormal presentations, such as a shoulder presentation or a footling breech (see Fig. 13–11C and D), are not deliverable vaginally, and the mother should be rushed to the hospital for an emergency cesarean section. Position the mother on her left side with her hips elevated, and administer high concentrations of oxygen.

FIGURE 13–42. Place your fingers inside the baby's mouth to flex the chin upon the chest before delivering the head in a breech delivery. Apply downward pressure with the fingers of your other hand against the back of the baby's head to aid in flexion. Suprapubic pressure can be given at the same time by your partner. If there is still difficulty, maintain an airway for the baby by forming a V with your fingers over the mouth and nose, pressing the vaginal wall away from the baby's face, and proceed immediately to the hospital.

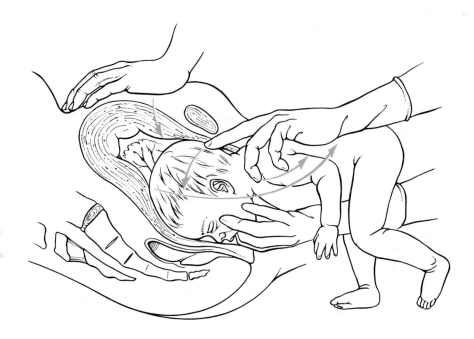

Shoulder Dystocia

Occasionally, the head delivers spontaneously but the shoulders become wedged in the mother's pelvis. If gentle downward traction combined with firm fundal pressure fails to expel the baby, then McRoberts maneuver may be attempted. McRoberts maneuver is a simple noninvasive method for easing delivery and consists solely of repositioning the mother. The mother should lie flat with her legs spread widely apart and flexed sharply on either side of her abdomen. This straightens out the normally curved sacrum and rotates the symphysis pubis. This may free the baby's impacted shoulder. If this fails, suction the baby's mouth and transport immediately, while supporting the head. This complication illustrates why the mother should deliver on the ambulance stretcher instead of on her own bed or a couch, since it is extremely difficult to move the patient while the baby's head is protruding.

Abruptio Placentae

Premature separation of the placenta from the uterine wall is an *abruptio placentae*. This abruption may be partial and may hardly affect the fetus, or it may be severe enough to cause fetal death. Mothers with hypertension or a history of an abruption in a previous pregnancy are at greater than average risk, since there is a 25% recurrence rate.

If the margin of the placenta separates (Fig. 13–43*A*), the resultant bleeding is evidenced by a flow of blood from the vagina. This blood is typically dark, menstrual-type bleeding, darker in color than the blood noted in placenta previa, since the blood may be older and may have traveled from a higher spot on the uterus. However, the abruption may be concealed, with the blood remaining trapped between the placenta and the uterine wall (Fig. 13–43*B*).

Symptoms of abruption include severe abdominal, pelvic, or back pain and a hard, rigid uterus. This can be distinguished from a normal uterine contraction in that there is no relaxation between labor pains. Cessation of contractions often means that complete abruption has occurred.

With concealed abruption, the blood collecting inside the uterus may cause the uterus to increase in size over a period of time. If abruptio placentae is suspected, measure and mark the fundus of the uterus with a felt-tip marker (Fig. 13–44). By the time you reach the hospital, it may be obvious that the uterus has increased in size and your initial diagnosis may be confirmed. Locate the fundus of the uterus by placing your fingers below the sternal notch and palpating downward until you feel a hard mass. This is where you would place a mark. In abruptio placentae you must transport quickly with the mother in a left lateral recumbent position with oxygen being administered.

Placenta Previa

In *placenta previa*, the placenta has been abnormally implanted so that it covers all or part of the cervical opening (Fig. 13–45). When labor begins and the cervix begins to dilate, the placenta is ripped from the uterine wall, causing a potentially life-threatening hemorrhage. The baby cannot be delivered vaginally and delaying a cesarean section in placenta previa where labor contractions are present puts both mother and baby in severe danger.

The symptoms of placenta previa differ from those of abruptio placentae in that the vaginal bleeding noted in placenta previa is bright red and the uterus relaxes between contractions if the patient is in labor. Other than normal labor pains, which may or may not be present, there is no pain associated with placenta previa.

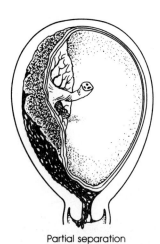
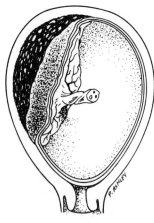

Partial separation   Complete separation

A   B

FIGURE 13–43. Abruptio placentae. (*A*) The edge of the placenta has separated and there is dark vaginal bleeding. (*B*) A concealed abruption with no vaginal bleeding. (From Burroughs A: Bleier's Maternity Nursing, 5th ed. Philadelphia, WB Saunders, 1986, p. 140.)

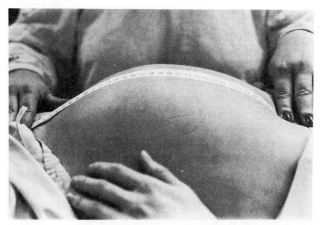

FIGURE 13–44. If abruption is suspected, measure the uterus from the pubic bone to the fundus and record the results, or mark the fundus with a felt-tipped marker. (From Cardona VD, Hurn PD, Mason PJB, et al: Trauma Nursing from Resuscitation through Rehabilitation. Philadelphia, WB Saunders, 1988, p. 655.)

With the current availability of *sonograms* (a test using sound waves to detect structures within the body) for pregnant women, dangerous conditions such as placenta previa can now be diagnosed long before a woman goes into labor. In such a case a cesarean section can be planned ahead of time so that the risk of the mother and baby bleeding to death is minimized. If you see in a pregnant woman bright bleeding that seems to be more than a bloody show, ask her if she has had a sonogram. Your patient may already know that she has either a low-lying placenta or a placenta previa. If you suspect a placenta previa, transport quickly with the patient in a left lateral recumbent position, administer oxygen and, if blood loss is severe, apply the pneumatic antishock garment (PASG) en route.

Ruptured Uterus

According to an article by Drs. Smith and Wynn in the July 1985 issue of *Topics in Emergency Medicine,* uterine rupture accounts for 5% of all maternal deaths. It occurs when a weakening of the uterine wall causes the uterus to split open. Women with a previous cesarean section or an aging uterus from multiple births are at the greatest risk. The current popularity of home births plus attempts made at vaginal delivery after a previous cesarean section may cause a rise in this grave complication.

The abdominal pain caused by a ruptured uterus is acute, and the patient describes it as a feeling that something has just given way. Once the uterus has ruptured, contractions cease entirely because the torn uterus cannot contract. You may actually be able to palpate the fetus beneath the thin abdominal wall. Vaginal bleeding is usually present, and this complication is most often confused with abruptio placentae. Signs of shock are soon present. The mortality rate for both fetus and mother is high. The mother may suffer an amniotic fluid embolism when amniotic fluid is released into the maternal circulation through the rupture in the uterus. This serious complication resembles a pulmonary embolism, with the major symptoms of dyspnea, chest pain, cyanosis, and shock.

Rapid transport for immediate surgery is the only hope for both the fetus and mother in the case of a ruptured uterus. Again, place the mother in the left lateral recumbent position and administer high-concentration oxygen and the PASG according to local shock protocols, but the abdominal compartment is never inflated in a pregnant patient.

Premature Rupture of Membranes

A pregnant woman in whom the membranes have ruptured should be hospitalized within 24 hours, even if labor has not begun. She is now at risk for a prolapsed cord until the physician can verify that the baby is in a

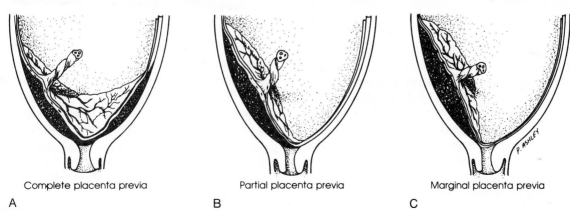

Complete placenta previa   Partial placenta previa   Marginal placenta previa

A   B   C

FIGURE 13–45. Three degrees of placenta previa. (*A*) Complete placenta previa. Bleeding will begin before or during early labor, and cesarean section must be performed to save mother and baby. (*B*) Partial placenta previa. (*C*) Marginal placenta previa. The placenta is near, but does not cover, the internal os of the cervix. (From Burroughs A: Bleier's Maternity Nursing, 5th ed. Philadelphia, WB Saunders, 1986, p. 138.)

vertex position with the head well down in the pelvis. Also, the pathway for bacteria to travel up to the baby is now open. Infection of the amniotic fluid by bacteria is called *amnionitis*. It produces a fever and *tachycardia* (rapid heart rate) in both the mother and the fetus, and the leaking fluid is usually cloudy and foul smelling.

Postpartum Hemorrhage

The term *postpartum* refers to the post delivery period. *Postpartum hemorrhage* is defined as a blood loss of greater than 500 ml following delivery and can be divided into two categories—early and late.

Early postpartum hemorrhage occurs within the first 24 hours after delivery and is most commonly caused by uterine atony (a failure of the uterus to contract after delivery). This may be brought on by retention of placental tissue. Early hemorrhage may also be caused by genital lacerations, although these are usually self-controlled or managed easily with pressure applied by a gauze pad. Uterine rupture, coagulation defects (blood-clotting problems), or, rarely, *placenta accreta* may be responsible. This is a condition in which the placenta has grown into the uterine wall and will not separate. In some cases, it can be managed only through *hysterectomy*, the surgical removal of the uterus. *Uterine inversion*, where the uterus actually turns inside out, and *prolapsed uterus*, a condition in which the supporting structures of the uterus fail so that the uterus dips out of the vagina, can both cause massive blood loss. Uterine prolapse occurs more often in older women who have had multiple births, where the structures that normally hold the uterus in place have become abnormally stretched and weakened. Uterine inversion may be precipitated by excessive traction on the cord while delivering the placenta or by bearing down too hard during the second stage of labor. This is one of the reasons that you are reminded never to pull on the cord and to be gentle in all maneuvers. A delivery where the mother is standing upright and there is no one to "catch" the baby can also cause this serious complication.

Following delivery, the normal uterus contracts firmly into a hard ball at or just below the level of the umbilicus. This strong contraction of the uterus is necessary to stop the bleeding from the raw placental site. When part of the placenta or any other matter such as part of the membranes is retained within the uterus, there may be a failure of the uterus to contract and it fills with blood. The larger the uterus becomes as it fills with blood, the less able it is to contract and thus stem the flow of blood, so the condition worsens.

Massive bleeding from the vagina is the classic symptom of postpartum hemorrhage, and signs of shock quickly follow. Upon palpation, the uterus is either poorly defined or feels like a soft, boggy mass, often above the level of the umbilicus. The uterus should be pressed several times to expel the blood and clots and then massaged until it becomes firm and hard. Notice that the uterus is supported with one hand to prevent prolapse as it is massaged by the other hand (see Fig. 13–36). The mother may complain that this causes an uncomfortable feeling in her bladder, in which case you should tell her to go ahead and void, since a full bladder interferes with uterine contraction. If the mother is able and agreeable, she can now attempt to nurse the baby. This releases oxytocin, which aids in contracting the uterus. If bleeding is severe, treat the patient for shock.

In the case of uterine inversion, you must attempt to replace the uterus immediately. Place your gloved fist into the inverted fundus of the uterus and attempt to reinsert the uterus. When the uterus is back in place, apply counterpressure to the fundus with your other hand by pushing on the mother's abdomen. This should control the bleeding. Elevate the mother's hips with a pillow to keep the uterus inside as you transport her quickly to the hospital.

Late postpartum hemorrhage usually occurs 6 to 10 days after delivery, and the most common cause is retained placental tissue. It may also be caused by infection, *coital* (sexual) trauma, or the *episiotomy* wound breaking open. The episiotomy is an incision made in the perineum by the doctor to make delivery of the baby easier and to prevent a jagged laceration, which is much more difficult to repair.

Treat all cases of postpartum hemorrhage with uterine massage and PASG. If you are IV certified, a large-bore (16- or 18-gauge) catheter should be inserted and a large amount of lactated Ringer's solution run in quickly.

Preeclampsia and Eclampsia

Preeclampsia is a toxemia (blood poisoning) of unknown cause that occurs during pregnancy. As many as one of 10 pregnancies is affected by preeclampsia, and it is the second leading cause of maternal death in the United States. The three main symptoms of preeclampsia are *elevated blood pressure* (defined as >140 mm Hg systolic or >90 mm Hg diastolic), *protein in the urine*, and progressively more severe *edema*. Possessing any two of these three symptoms classifies a patient as having preeclampsia, but all three are often present. To be distinguished from a person who had hypertension to begin with, a preeclamptic patient develops high blood pressure after 20 weeks of gestation. This patient has a typical puffy look (Fig. 13–46) and may complain of headache and dizziness (from the elevated blood pressure), blurred vision (from retinal edema), and epigastric pain (caused by hemorrhages beneath the liver). If edema

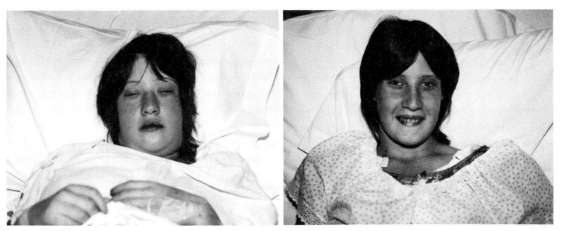

FIGURE 13–46. The typical puffy look (*left*) of the preeclamptic patient. Four days postpartum (*right*), the patient has resumed a normal appearance. (From Knuppel RA, Brukker J: High Risk Pregnancy: A Team Approach. Philadelphia, WB Saunders, 1986, p. 365. Photographs courtesy of Dr. Gary Cohen, University of South Florida College of Medicine, Tampa, FL.)

is severe, there may be signs of pulmonary edema. As the condition worsens, cerebral edema and the rupture of swollen cerebral blood vessels cause a severe headache. Ultimately, seizures occur. *The occurrence of a seizure classifies the patient as eclamptic.* While there are many theories as to what causes this grave condition, the exact cause remains unknown.

As preeclampsia worsens, the patient may suffer from *photophobia* (sensitivity to light). This is a grave symptom and often a warning that a seizure may be imminent. As the blood pressure rises, the potential for stroke, renal failure, and abruptio placentae increases. Although this patient has severe edema, she is actually hypovolemic because so much fluid has moved out of the blood vessels into the interstitial spaces.

Preeclampsia is much more common in primigravidas than in women who have already had children. The tendency may be inherited; however, it usually does not recur in subsequent pregnancies. According to an article entitled "Preeclampsia and Eclampsia," published by Drs. Greene and Keene in the July 1985 issue of *Topics in Emergency Medicine,* even having a previous 3-month pregnancy that ended in abortion may confer some protection against this condition. Other conditions that may contribute to a patient's developing preeclampsia include obesity, multiple pregnancy (more than one fetus), preexisting vascular disease such as chronic hypertension or diabetes, and malnutrition.

The only "cure" for eclampsia and preeclampsia is delivery of the baby, and the condition may remain for as long as 72 hours after the birth of the baby.

During interhospital transports, you may be accompanied by physicians or nurses who institute drug treatment. The following discussion may help you better appreciate and assist, since if the delivery occurs there will be two patients. Magnesium sulfate (MgSo₄) is often administered to these patients. They are often transferred from the hospital to which they were initially admitted and sent to a "high-risk" hospital. Since you may be in the position of having to transport a high-risk patient who is receiving magnesium sulfate en route, you should be aware of its properties and dangers.

The preeclamptic patient is both hypertensive and hyperreflexive. As magnesium sulfate is administered, the blood pressure should drop and the patient should become calmer and less hyperreflexive. Magnesium sulfate also has the ability to reduce or even stop labor contractions. For this reason it is also used to stop premature labor. Again, you may encounter its use in the transfer of a high-risk patient in premature labor. While magnesium sulfate has many benefits, use of this drug also carries a risk that the patient may develop magnesium toxicity, in which case the reflexes become severely depressed or absent, the level of consciousness and respiratory rate are decreased, and there is altered speech, poor swallowing ability, and a lowered response to command. Magnesium sulfate inhibits parathyroid hormone secretion and therefore may cause *hypocalcemia.*

Hypocalcemia is a dangerous lowering of calcium in the bloodstream. Calcium is essential to normal muscle contraction, especially of the heart muscle. In severe hypocalcemia, cardiac asystole or hypocalcemic tetany (a condition where the ankles and wrists may uncontrollably flex, along with other muscular effects, i.e., convulsions) may occur. These can be reversed with the administration of 1.0 gram of calcium gluconate IV. If you suspect that the patient is developing magnesium toxicity, stop the IV that is infusing the magnesium sulfate and prepare to assist in ventilating the patient.

Care of the preeclamptic patient includes providing a quiet, dark environment to avoid stimulating seizures. Sirens and lights should be avoided, and you should speak in a soft voice, avoiding any unnecessary jostling or noise. An airway and suction should be at hand in case the patient begins to seize. If seizures do occur, oxygen should be administered, since the fetal oxygen supply is cut off during the seizure. The blood pressure, respiratory rate, and hand-grasp reflex should be checked as transport begins and monitored every 15 minutes thereafter so that any changes can be recognized early. If signs of magnesium toxicity appear and the patient becomes progressively depressed in reflexes, speech, and respiratory rate, the magnesium sulfate should be discontinued until you arrive at the hospital and a physician can check the patient. Like any pregnant patient, this patient should be transported in the left lateral recumbent position. If pulmonary edema is present, the patient may be more comfortable in the full upright position with oxygen.

Babies born to a mother taking magnesium sulfate may also exhibit signs of magnesium toxicity. These may include general flaccidity, tremors from hypocalcemia, or respiratory depression or arrest. You should be prepared to resuscitate the infant if it becomes obvious that you are going to have a delivery in transit.

Disseminated Intravascular Coagulation

Where there has been widespread destruction of tissue, clotting factors are released into the bloodstream from the damaged cells, and serious complications can follow. In *disseminated intravascular coagulation* (DIC), a severe blood disorder, the blood components become disorganized and clots form spontaneously inside the blood vessels. As widespread clotting occurs, a large supply of platelets are used up so that the patient becomes platelet-deficient. Therefore, a situation occurs in which there is both hemorrhage and massive embolism formation at the same time.

This condition may be caused by abruptio placentae; amniotic fluid embolism, as may be seen in a ruptured uterus; *eclampsia*; or a septic or missed abortion, especially in the second trimester when the fetus has been dead for 6 weeks or longer. Symptoms might include bruising if the onset is gradual or massive hemorrhage as might be observed in a ruptured uterus. Signs of pulmonary embolism or other embolisms may also be present. The patient should be transported quickly with oxygen administered and each symptom treated as it occurs.

Vaginal Bleeding

Vaginal bleeding may be present in the pregnant or nonpregnant patient and has several possible causes. Abruptio placentae, placenta previa, and several other causes have already been discussed. Others, including rape, abortion, ectopic pregnancy, ruptured ovarian cyst, and pelvic inflammatory disease (PID) are discussed separately in the following section, but treatment of severe vaginal bleeding, regardless of the cause, is similar and

focuses on the prevention of shock. The patient should be placed in the supine position with the legs elevated. If the patient is more than 6 months pregnant, she should be placed on her left side (see Figs. 13–4 and 13–5). PASG should be used, but the abdominal compartment is never inflated in a pregnant patient. Oxygen should be administered if the patient is pregnant or if air hunger is apparent.

If possible, attempt to control the bleeding. As discussed previously, in postpartum hemorrhage this can sometimes be accomplished through uterine massage (see Fig. 13–36). In cases of perineal trauma or postdelivery wound separation, direct pressure with a soft sterile dressing or sanitary paid may help.

Evaluating the amount of bleeding strictly by the patient history may be difficult. The fear experienced by the patient when she notes the bleeding and perhaps feels she is losing her baby may make the amount of bleeding appear much larger to her than is actually the case. The patient may also have noted the bleeding while going to the bathroom and, when mixed with the water in the toilet bowl, the amount of blood may seem enormous. This is an instance when your communication skills are of great importance. Try to get the patient to describe the amount and type of bleeding in real terms, e.g., the number of pads, size of stain on each pad, size of clots, etc. Some modern sanitary napkin products hold a great deal of blood compared to the older products, and there is, in fact, a large difference in the amount of blood that each of the many different products available today hold. Because of this disparity, the amount of vaginal bleeding can be estimated more accurately by weight than by an actual pad count, which was formerly the accepted method of assessing vaginal bleeding. For example, one woman may say she has used 5 pads but actually each paid was changed when it held only a small amount of blood. Another woman may say she has used only 2 pads but each may have been soaked with blood.

When assessing vaginal bleeding, be sure to describe the *color* of the blood (dark, menstrual type blood or bright red blood), determine the absence or presence of *clots*, and try to be specific about the *amount* of blood. An example would be to write "scant pink stain noted on pad," or "soaked 2 pads with bright red blood and several dark clots noted."

Abortions

Abortions are categorized as follows.

INDUCED ABORTION. A voluntary termination of a pregnancy performed by a physician at the mother's request.

SPONTANEOUS ABORTION (MISCARRIAGE). Passing of the fetus before 20 weeks' gestation. After 20 weeks' gestation the delivery of a dead fetus would be called a *stillbirth*.

COMPLETE ABORTION. Passing all of the products of conception.

INCOMPLETE ABORTION. Passing some but not all of the products of conception. (This usually means that the fetus has been passed but the placenta has been retained.)

MISSED ABORTION. Retention of the fetus for 6 or more weeks after fetal death has occurred.

SEPTIC ABORTION. An abortion with pelvic or peritoneal infection. This is usually precipitated by the retention of the products of conception, as in a missed or incomplete abortion. It may also result from a lacerated or perforated uterus following an induced abortion, or in a patient who had an intrauterine device (IUD) (a device inserted into the uterus by a gynecologist, to prevent conception). In areas where abortions are illegal, septic abortions may result from poorly managed abortions performed without sterile technique and probably with makeshift instruments. In septic abortion the patient usually passes a foul-smelling fetus, and there will be fever, tachycardia, and abdominal tenderness. There may be shock present from blood loss or *toxic shock* (contamination of the blood with toxins from the bacteria that has infected the pelvis). There is usually a foul-smelling vaginal discharge. The patient may also exhibit signs of DIC.

THREATENED ABORTION. Vaginal bleeding in a pregnant patient with no dilatation of the cervix. There may be suprapubic cramping or pain referred to the lower back, similar in nature either to menstrual cramps or labor pains.

INEVITABLE ABORTION. Profuse vaginal bleeding with dilatation of the cervix. Once the cervix has dilated, there is no way to save the pregnancy.

MANAGEMENT OF THREATENED ABORTION OR STILLBIRTH

You may not be able to differentiate between a threatened abortion and an inevitable abortion, although the loss of a great deal of blood or leaking of amniotic fluid in the first trimester is nearly always a sure sign of imminent loss of the fetus. In the absence of amniotic fluid leaking, you may be able to aid the patient somewhat by elevating her hips. This may reduce stress on the cervix.

In the event of a stillbirth or abortion, you should respect any religious-related requests by the parents. Be sensitive to their individual needs. In deference to the parents' feelings, you should treat the body of a stillborn

baby with the same gentle care you would provide to a living infant. Wrapping the baby in a blanket and offering it to the parents to see and hold may help them to work through their grief at having lost a child. You can distinguish a stillborn from a baby whom you should resuscitate because the body of the stillborn is often macerated and sometimes foul-smelling. The skull has less substance than that of a normal newborn baby, and there is often pooling of blood.

Ectopic Pregnancy

According to Dr. John Patrick in his article "Ectopic Pregnancy," published in the July 1985 edition of *Topics in Emergency Medicine*, the leading cause of first-trimester death in nonwhite women and the cause of more than 11% of all maternal deaths in the United States is ectopic pregnancy. Ectopic pregnancy is a pregnancy that occurs outside of the uterine cavity. Ectopic pregnancies may occur in the cervix, ovaries, or abdominal cavity (Fig. 13–47), but 90% of all ectopic pregnancies occur within the fallopian tubes and are called tubal pregnancies. As the tubal pregnancy expands, the tube eventually ruptures and bleeding occurs into the abdominal cavity; the resulting damage to the fallopian tubes is a major cause of *infertility* (inability to conceive). Symptoms of ectopic pregnancy usually begin when the patient is 4 to 6 weeks pregnant.

Thirty percent of the patients who experience tubal pregnancies have a history of *pelvic inflammatory disease*, a condition that is discussed later in this chapter. The scarring caused by this disease makes the fertilized egg move too slowly or become entrapped within the tube.

Occasionally, tissue from the endometrium or lining of the uterus will grow outside of the uterus. This condition, *endometriosis*, can cause a blockage in the fallopian tube. The blockage prevents the egg from entering the uterus and a tubal pregnancy may occur. Abnormally narrow tubes caused by a genetic defect may have the same result.

Adhesions, which are thick internal scar tissues formed from previous abdominal surgery or infection, can be a contributing factor. Contraceptive use does not eliminate the possibility of ectopic pregnancy. One example of this is failed use of an IUD. Another example is a failed *tubal ligation*, a surgical procedure in which the fallopian tubes are severed, again to prevent pregnancy. A previous ectopic pregnancy also raises the chances for again incurring this serious condition, since it is likely to recur.

The symptoms of ectopic pregnancy include a history of *amenorrhea* (the patient has missed or stopped having menstrual periods) and a positive pregnancy test, even though the pregnancy is not in the uterus. There may be swelling in the abdomen, and the patient may

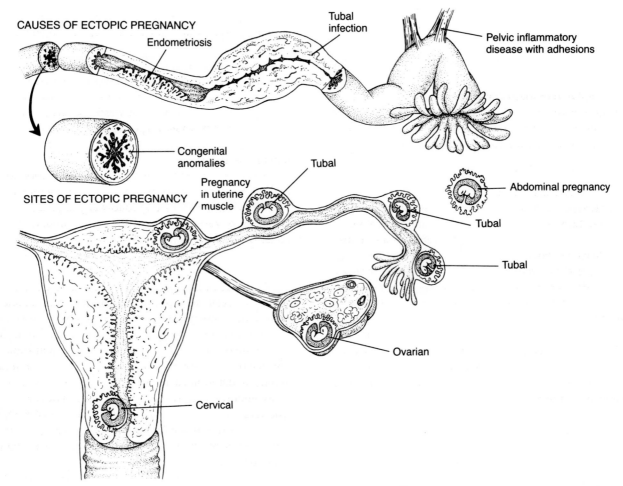

FIGURE 13–47. Common causes and sites of ectopic pregnancy. Ectopic pregnancy may occur in any of the above sites, but the most common site is the fallopian tube. Bleeding and rupture occur early in pregnancy, causing severe, sudden shoulder pain and abdominal tenderness. Vaginal bleeding may be present. (From Reeder SJ, Martin LL: Maternity Nursing, 16th ed. Philadelphia, JB Lippincott, 1987, p. 739.)

or may not tell you that she suspects or even knows that she is pregnant. Vaginal bleeding is often profuse and untypical of a menstrual type bleeding, since it is bright red. There is a *sudden onset* of poorly localized lower abdominal pain that may radiate to, or be felt solely in, the shoulder area. The severe shoulder pain is referred pain caused by bleeding into the peritoneal cavity, which irritates the diaphragm. There may also be some vaginal or rectal pain. Occasionally, nausea and vomiting may be present, and ectopic pregnancy is often mistaken for appendicitis. A patient with an ectopic pregnancy may have lost a great deal of blood and should be treated for shock.

Occasionally a cyst on one of the ovaries ruptures, causing symptoms similar to a ruptured ectopic pregnancy, although the vaginal bleeding may be absent. Severe shoulder pain in a woman of childbearing age who has no history of injury to the shoulder should alert you to the possibility of an ectopic pregnancy or a ruptured ovarian cyst. Both conditions can be life threatening because of blood loss.

Pelvic Inflammatory Disease

Pelvic inflammatory disease (PID) is a sexually acquired ascending infection of the uterus, fallopian tubes, and adjacent structures. It usually follows sexual contact but may occur after procedures that dilate the cervix, such as a suction abortion, insertion of an IUD, or an operation known as a *D and C*, which involves dilation of the cervix and *curettage* (scraping) of the uterine lining. The usual causative organism is either gonorrhea or chlamydia, both contagious venereal diseases, but PID may also be caused by *Staphylococcus* or *Streptococcus*.

PID is most common in sexually active young women between the ages of 15 and 24. Women using intrauterine devices (IUDs) are more susceptible, but the disease is virtually nonexistent in pregnant women, perhaps because of the thick mucus plug that forms in the cervix and prevents the travel of microorganisms into the uterus.

Painful intercourse may be the first early symptom of PID, but this is not likely to be the chief complaint when the EMT is interviewing the patient. The complaint is usually of a dull, aching abdominal pain. This pain is bilateral and continuous. There is usually a foul-smelling vaginal discharge, and more than half of these patients have vaginal bleeding and fever. In severe cases where the bowels have become involved, there may be nausea and vomiting. There may be evidence of toxic shock, in which case the patient should be treated as any patient with signs of shock.

Toxic shock syndrome, caused by *Staphylococcus,* is a life-threatening disease. *Staphylococcus* is often found on the skin and becomes dangerous when it enters the bloodstream. This may occur when a tampon or any surgical packing is left in too long, when a mosquito bite becomes infected, or when a boil is left untreated. Typical symptoms are flu-like, with fever, joint pain, watery diarrhea, and a typical sunburn-like flushed appearance on the face.

As mentioned earlier in this chapter, the incidence of PID creates a higher subsequent risk of a patient suffering from ectopic pregnancy and infertility. The patient should be transported to the hospital in whatever position is most comfortable for her.

TRAUMA IN PREGNANCY

As with all other patients, motor vehicle accidents are responsible for the majority of traumatic injuries in pregnant women. In general, if the damage to the vehicle appears to be minor, then the injury tends to be correspondingly minor also.

The injury is less severe if the mother is wearing a seat belt, especially one with a shoulder restraint. A lap belt alone is better than no seat belt at all, but it cannot prevent the violent flexion of the body that can greatly increase intrauterine pressure. This sudden increase in pressure can cause a burst-balloon type of uterine rupture. Even without an actual uterine rupture, the change in the shape of the uterus caused by the flexion can cause placental separation and fetal death. What is often not made clear to pregnant women, however, is the fact that a collision severe enough to cause this type of injury when the woman is wearing a seat belt is likely to do far greater harm, including the possibility of fatal ejection from the car, if no seat belt is worn at all. Since fetal survival is dependent upon ma-

ternal survival, it is essential that all pregnant women continue to wear seat belts, preferably of the shoulder-lap combination.

Pelvic fractures and blunt and penetrating wounds to the abdomen are serious injuries generally, but they are even more dangerous to the pregnant patient. Broken ribs or pelvic bones may cause uterine lacerations (Fig. 13–48), which can cause a great deal of blood loss.

Premature labor is a common complication of trauma in pregnancy. The uterine stimulation caused by blunt trauma to the abdomen may precipitate labor contractions and premature rupture of the membranes. Abruptio placentae is likely to follow any severe trauma, whether it is caused by motor vehicle injury, blunt trauma, or a fall. The extent of the abruption, rapidity of treatment, and age of the fetus determine the fetal outcome.

When treating the pregnant trauma victim, it is essential to recall the physiologic changes of pregnancy and how they affect your particular patient. Remember to assume that the stomach is full. This means that an emesis basin or suction for an unconscious patient should be at hand. You are treating two patients, and fetal outcome is determined by maternal outcome. It is especially important to prevent shock, which is devastating to the fetus. Controlling hemorrhage, the use of PASG (minus inflation of the abdominal compartment), and the administration of oxygen take priority over everything except, of course, spinal precautions and your initial ABCs. The pregnant transport position, which can be lifesaving for the fetus, should be implemented (see Fig. 13–4).

Because of the high incidence of trauma-induced premature labor, you should be prepared for the delivery of a premature infant en route, especially if the mother begins to have labor contractions. If delivery of a premature infant seems imminent, turn on the heat in the ambulance so that a warm environment is available for the baby, and radio ahead to the hospital so they will be prepared. In a triage situation, remember that this is a priority patient. Thermal injuries are managed in the same way that they would be for a nonpregnant patient.

RAPE

Extreme sensitivity must be used with the rape victim. You must always remember that rape is a crime of violence and not merely a sexual act. In an effort to preserve evidence, these patients should be encouraged not to bathe, shower, urinate, defecate, douche, brush their teeth, or change their clothes until they have been examined in a hospital. Victims may not be very receptive to this advice, since they feel dirty and violated and generally want to clean away any trace of the violation.

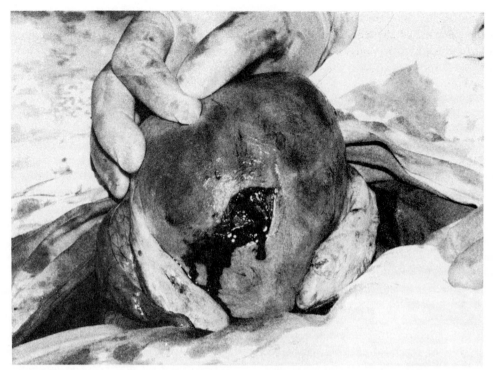

FIGURE 13–48. Uterine rupture and laceration due to trauma. This 20-year-old primigravida was a passenger in a motor vehicle during an accident. She was 36 weeks pregnant and was wearing a seatbelt that broke during the collision. She suffered broken ribs with a pneumothorax and abdominal bruises. Cesarean section was performed 4 hours after the accident, and a concealed partial abruption of the placenta was discovered, but both mother and baby survived. Uterine rupture is responsible for 5% of all maternal deaths. (From Beischer NA, Mackay EV: Obstetrics and the Newborn: An Illustrated Textbook, 2nd ed. Philadelphia, WB Saunders (Formerly Holt-Saunders Pty Limited, Merrickville, Australia), 1986, p. 201.)

The patient may reject treatment by a male EMT. If this is the case and a female is available, she could care for the patient. On the other hand, gentle, accepting care given by a male EMT may be beneficial to the patient and ease her post-traumatic adjustment period.

Rape victims often have injuries other than the psychologic trauma. If the victim has been assaulted, a complete physical assessment should be carried out and wounds treated accordingly, with the added reminder to preserve evidence if possible. However, patient welfare should never be jeopardized for this reason.

PERINEAL INJURIES

The perineum is one of the most vascular areas of the body, and injuries to the perineum can be both painful and involve quite a large loss of blood. They may result from a wide range of causes from rape to straddling a boy's bicycle. Snow skiing and the popular sport of gymnastics are also responsible for perineal injuries in girls and women of all ages. Vulvar lacerations or hematomas may occur, and there is often associated bladder or urethral injury with a painful spilling of urine onto the injured site. Bleeding should be controlled, if nec-

essary, with direct pressure; also, an ice pack applied to the site may slow the bleeding and provide some pain relief.

SUMMARY

Treating patients with obstetric or gynecologic problems entails special considerations. First and foremost is the need to recall the huge blood supply to the female organs and the possible consequences to patient outcome if bleeding is present. Second, you must try in every situation to maintain the patient's privacy. The anxiety of being exposed in public can contribute toward the creation of an uncooperative patient. Even though you are wearing a uniform, you must recall that you are a stranger to this patient, and she may be hesitant to allow you to treat her. Providing privacy from a crowd, if one is present, helps. If a husband is present in the case of a delivery or abortion, and if he is calm, his presence may be a great help to you. He can assume the task of holding his wife's hand, calming her, and helping her to breathe properly.

Many fine lines are drawn in the diagnosis of obstetric and gynecologic problems. Try not to get hung up on diagnosis, but rather treat symptomatically, as in controlling bleeding when possible and treating the patient for shock. If you are ever in doubt about whether you can manage a situation, proceed to the hospital while giving whatever support you can provide to the patient.

In the case of a stillborn or deformed infant, the parents may feel guilt and might even question you as to what they did to cause this condition. You may need to assure the parents repeatedly that they have not contributed to this situation and should not blame themselves. Emotional support in crisis situations may have as much of an effect on patient outcome as any other treatment you may provide.

REVIEW EXERCISES

1. List the location and function of the following anatomic structures:
    Uterus
    Cervix
    Vagina
    Fetus
    Placenta
    Umbilical cord
    Amniotic sac
    Perineum
    Ovaries
    Fallopian tubes

2. Define the following terms:
    Miscarriage/abortion
    Bloody show
    Crowning
    Presenting part

3. Define the three stages of labor.

4. List four physiologic changes that occur during pregnancy.

5. Describe the pathophysiology, signs and symptoms, and prehospital treatment of the following conditions:
    Eclampsia/preeclampsia
    Ruptured ovarian cyst
    Ectopic pregnancy
    Pelvic inflammatory disease

6. List three indications of imminent delivery.

7. List steps involved in predelivery preparation of the mother.

8. List the steps of care in a normal delivery.

9. Describe the postpartum care of the baby.

10. Describe how and when to cut the cord.

11. Describe the postpartum care of the mother.

12. List special considerations for multiple births.

13. Define a premature baby and list the special considerations for care.

14. Describe the procedures for:
    Breech delivery
    Prolapsed cord
    Arm/leg presentation
    Excessive bleeding in the mother
    Care of the pregnant trauma victim

15. Describe care of the rape victim.

REFERENCES

American Heart Association: Textbook of advanced cardiac life support. Dallas, American Heart Association, 1988.

American Heart Association: Textbook of pediatric advanced life support. Dallas, American Heart Association, 1988.

American Heart Association and American Academy of Pediatrics: Textbook of Neonatal Resuscitation. Dallas, American Heart Association and American Academy of Pediatrics, 1989.

Beischer N, Mackay E: Obstetrics and the newborn, 2nd ed. Philadelphia, WB Saunders, 1986.

Blake, Wright, Waechter: Nursing care of children. Philadelphia, JB Lippincott, 1970.

Burroughs A: Bleier's maternity nursing, 5th ed. Philadelphia, WB Saunders, 1986.

Cardona VD, Hurn PD, Mason PJB, et al: Trauma Nursing from Resuscitation to Rehabilitation. Philadelphia, WB Saunders, 1988.

Franaszek JB: Trauma in pregnancy. Topics in Emergency Medicine, July, 1985.

Greene CS, Keene M: Preeclampsia. Topics in Emergency Medicine, July, 1985.

Jacobs L, Bennett B: Shock. Emerg Care Q 1(2), 1985.

Klaus MH, Fanaroff AA: Care of the high risk neonate, 3rd ed. Philadelphia, WB Saunders, 1986.

Knuppel RA, Drukker Dauphinee JE: High risk pregnancy: A team approach. Philadelphia, WB Saunders, 1986.

Moore ML: Realities in childbearing, 2nd ed. Philadelphia, WB Saunders, 1983.

Patrick J: Ectopic pregnancy. Topics in Emergency Medicine, July, 1985.

Rothenberger D, Quattlebaum FW, Perry JF, et al: Blunt maternal trauma: A review of 103 cases. J Trauma 18(3):173–179, 1978.

Smith K, Wynn B: Complications in pregnancy. Topics in Emergency Medicine, July, 1985.

Sweet B: Mayes' midwifery: A textbook for midwives. London, Balliere Tindall, 1982.

Vestal KW, McKenzie CAM (eds): The American Association of Critical-Care Nurses: High risk perinatal nursing. Philadelphia, WB Saunders, 1983.

Ziegal, Van Blarcom: Obstetric nursing. New York, Macmillan, 1972.

Zuidema GD; Rutherford RB, Ballinger WF: The management of trauma, 4th ed. Philadelphia, WB Saunders, 1985.

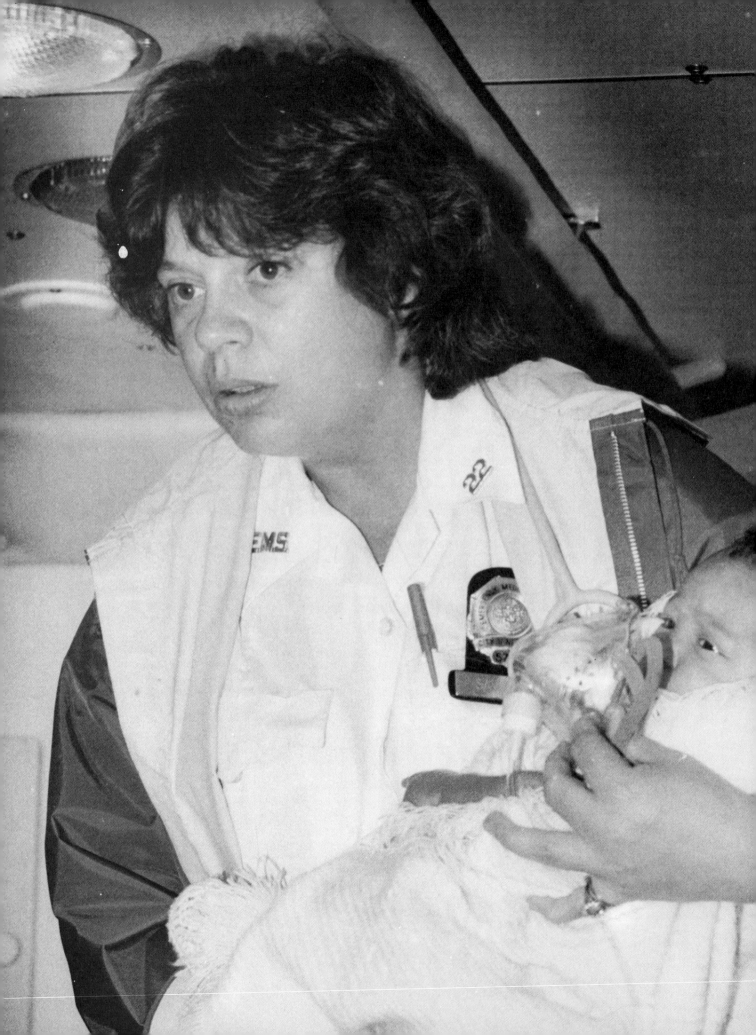

CHAPTER 14

PEDIATRIC EMERGENCIES

OBJECTIVES

At the conclusion of this chapter the reader will be able to:

1. Discuss the developmental differences for the following ages of children and how these differences alter the approach to the patient:
   Infant
   Toddler: 15 months to 3 years
   Small child: 4 to 8 years
   Preadolescent: 9 to 12 years
   Adolescent

2. Discuss the differences in anatomy and physiology of infants and children with respect to the following:
   Respiratory function
   Respiratory rate
   Pulse rate
   Blood pressure
   Metabolic considerations
   Neurologic differences
   Response to hypovolemia and shock

3. Demonstrate the steps of the primary and secondary survey for a pediatric patient.

4. List three signs and symptoms and the prehospital treatment for the following disorders in children:
   Croup
   Epiglottitis
   Foreign body obstruction of the upper airway
   Bronchiolitis
   Asthma
   Pneumonia
   Foreign bodies in the lower airway
   Near-drowning
   Sudden infant death syndrome
   High fever
   Seizures

5. List signs associated with child abuse.

6. Discuss the approach to the pediatric trauma patient.

INTRODUCTION

This text has covered physiology, anatomy, disease entities, and injuries as they apply to adults. Much of this information also applies to children and infants. However, in this chapter some important differences are discussed.

The call to help a child presents several challenges to the EMT. The pediatric emergency is usually more emotionally charged for all concerned: the child, the parents, the bystanders, and the EMTs. The EMT must remember the key differences between adult, child, and infant patients. Depending on the child's age, the EMT uses different approaches to obtain historical and physical information and to provide treatment.

As pediatricians say, "Children are not small adults." The EMT must develop the knowledge and skills to recognize the developmental, anatomic, and physiologic differences between children and adults. The range of emergencies and the response to illness in the child vary somewhat from the adult patient.

Epidemiology

COMMON CAUSES OF DEATH

The causes of most deaths in children are different from the causes of death in adults. After the first year of life, accidents and respiratory conditions account for the majority of deaths. There are approximately 23,000 deaths in children each year from accidents caused by motor vehicles (50%), falls (25 to 30%), drowning (10%), and poisoning and assaults (15%).

Causes of respiratory arrests in children include asthma, trauma, drug ingestion, drowning, smoke inhalation, sudden infant death syndrome (SIDS), infection (e.g., sepsis, meningitis, pulmonary croup, epiglottitis), and foreign body aspiration.

In children, cardiac arrest is rarely due to heart disease. Children do not suffer from the ravages of coronary artery disease and have strong hearts, except for the rare child with congenital heart disease or acquired cardiomyopathy. Pediatric cardiopulmonary arrests usually follow a respiratory insult. Since the child's heart is "strong," cardiac arrest usually implies that the heart has suffered a severe and *prolonged* period of hypoxia. The heart becomes oxygen depleted until it has such slow and weak beats that no pulse is conducted and eventually there is no activity at all (*asystole*). Figure 14–1 illustrates the downward spiral in the infant's condition that leads to cardiopulmonary arrest.

However, if children are resuscitated from respiratory or cardiopulmonary arrest, they have a better chance of brain recovery than does an adult suffering the same period of oxygen deprivation.

DIFFERENCES BETWEEN CHILDREN AND ADULTS

Sick or injured children cannot always fully understand what is happening to them. Pain and fear often cause children to be uncooperative and more difficult to evaluate.

Realize also that you have two patients, the child and the parent. Obviously, your primary attention is focused on the child, but you must consider the parent or parents as well. Parents may feel anxious, fearful, and impatient as they seek help and medical attention for their child. Not having medical backgrounds and having considerable emotional investment in the patient, they may overreact, since they may anticipate the worst possible condition or result from the emergency problem. In the face of their own panic they may not act rationally or in the child's best interest. It is important to mobilize the parents' energies into constructive activities to gather necessary history and to calm the child. To elicit their cooperation and support, you must gain their confidence. You can accomplish this by acting in a calm and professional manner. The parents want to believe you can help them and their child.

It is also important for you to understand and face your own emotional reactions to a sick child. We are all capable of both minimizing or overestimating the seriousness of an emergency situation. Our own reactions can be influenced by the behavior and atmosphere encountered at the scene. We all tend to see children as innocent and vulnerable (Fig. 14–2).

Once you understand your own and others' reactions to the sick or injured child, you can influence rather than get caught up in the emotional turmoil. With a calm, objective approach coupled with an understanding of pediatric prehospital care, you can create a positive impact.

Developmental Differences

You need to recognize that children pass through developmental stages from newborn, to infant, to toddler, to small child, to preadolescent, and to adolescent. Your approach, evaluation, and treatment must take into account the patient's developmental stage.

THE INFANT

The infant (to 1 year of age) has minimal language capability but responds to facial expressions and tone of voice. Infants are used to interacting with their parents and, beginning at about 8 months, may demonstrate

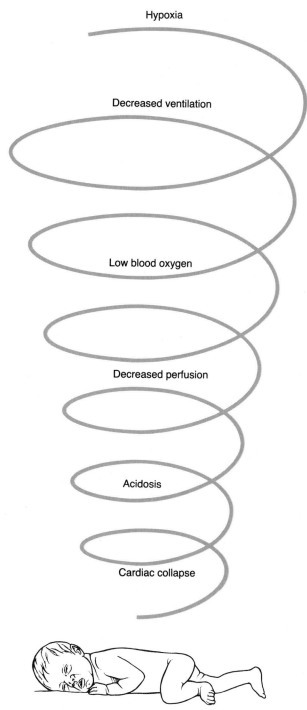

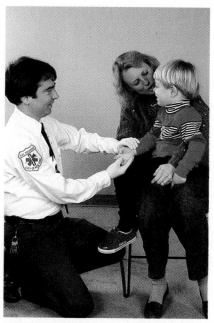

FIGURE 14–2. The EMT who is confident and exercises emotional control can become a positive force in an emotionally charged scene of a pediatric emergency. When possible, allow the infant or small child to remain with the parent. Approach in a nonthreatening manner.

FIGURE 14–1. The pediatric patient rarely suffers a cardiac arrest as a primary event. Cardiac arrest usually follows a respiratory problem and a sustained period of hypoxia.

anxiety when approached by strangers. The history comes from the parents, and you should examine the infant in sight of the parents or even while the baby is in their arms. Try to provide a warm environment, both emotionally and physically. For example, warm your hands and stethoscope (rub them together) before placing them on the infant.

Infants, particularly ill infants, may cry when touched by a stranger. Try to gather information such as respiratory rate and quality of breathing before you touch the baby. The baby may feel more secure and be less likely to cry if held in one of the parent's arms. Listen to the lungs first. Then perform your secondary survey in a *toe to head* fashion. This approach is utilized because examination around the face is most threatening to the infant.

THE TODDLER: AGE 15 MONTHS TO 3 YEARS

Age 15 months to 3 years includes the so-called terrible twos. No matter how charming you are, a child in this age range may refuse to cooperate with your examination and treatments. Fortunately, toddlers are easily distracted. Developmentally, they see themselves as individuals and are assertive, yet they fear pain and separation from their parents. You cannot really explain things to a toddler, but you can talk in a soothing tone of voice, examine the child on the parent's lap, and approach the child at eye level. Often, you can distract the child with a colorful toy or puppet and listen quickly to the lungs before the child reacts. Then examine the child from toe to head, leaving the more threatening head examination for last. If possible, do not undress the child all at once. Do not let the child see scissors or instruments unnecessarily. Do let the child play with your stethoscope and blood pressure cuffs.

THE YOUNG CHILD: AGE 4 TO 7 YEARS

Children from 4 to 7 years of age are in a period of intensive learning and have varied levels of ability to express their thoughts and feelings. These children are curious and communicative. They live in a world of intense play fantasy with imaginary friends and merge fantasy with reality. This means they have "magical thinking" and believe what they hear. These children may have a strong fear of pain and separation, especially under the circumstances of an emergency. However, if they are not in pain and you take a few moments to play with them, they can be very cooperative. You should be friendly and talk to the parents first. This way the child is more likely to perceive you as a friend. Approach the child at eye level in a nonthreatening manner, perhaps offering a toy and explaining things simply. Again, do not show sharp objects, but if the child sees scissors, explain their purpose in order to relieve any anxiety. Children in this age group are very interested in your stethoscope and blood pressure cuff. Should you have to perform a procedure, wait until the last minute to explain it and then do it immediately. Do not lie. If a procedure might be painful, tell the child "This may hurt a bit but it is necessary to help you." Do not overexplain or give the child too much time to fantasize about what terrible thing you are going to do.

THE PREADOLESCENT: AGE 9 TO 12 YEARS

Preadolescents are fighting between their desire to be treated as a child and their desire to be adults. They also have many personal fears and a strong fear of disfigurement. Talk to preadolescents first to demonstrate that you consider their opinion as being important. Explain what you are doing during your examination and treatment.

THE ADOLESCENT

What is true for the preadolescent is also true for the adolescent. Adolescents, having undergone the changes of puberty, want to see themselves as adults. However, under the stress of injury or sickness they may feel helpless and childlike. Respect their "space," answer their questions, respect their pubertal shyness, and allow them to retain as much control as possible. When talking to an adolescent, do not be confrontational.

GENERAL CONSIDERATIONS

Keep the child and parent together whenever possible. Separation causes anxiety, especially in a situation where several people are hurt. An emergency places the child in a frightening environment, and you are a stranger. The last thing children want is to be separated from their parents. Their imagination of what has happened to them and their parents can be much worse than the truth. This obviously does not apply if you must perform resuscitative procedures.

Be calm at all times. Calming the parents is also important, since children pick up signals from their parents.

Be honest. Again, do not say, "This won't hurt," when it will. Once you lose a child's trust, you lose whatever cooperation you may have gained.

Anatomy and Physiology

In general, the pediatric patient has a better ability to compensate physiologically in the early phases of severe illness and injury because the main compensatory mechanisms, the cardiovascular and respiratory systems, are young and healthy. However, when the child's compensatory mechanisms fail, his or her condition deteriorates rapidly and time is of the essence to reach definitive care. Therefore, the EMT must recognize early signs of stress, offer emergency care to help sustain the compensated state, and expedite treatment and transport to provide timely access to definitive care.

AIRWAY

The airway in infants and children differs in some very important ways from that in the adult. Infants and small children have small-caliber airways at all levels, including the nasopharynx, oropharynx, larynx, trachea, bronchi, and bronchioles. The tongue is large in relation to the airway and has a greater potential for obstruction. The *glottis* (opening of the larynx) lies anterior and superior compared to the adult airway and is protected by a relatively large, U-shaped epiglottis. The *cricoid* ring, at the base of the larynx, is the narrowest part of the upper airway (Fig. 14–3). In the adult airway, the vocal cords are the narrowest part of the airway. Imagine the infant's airway as a membranous tube rather than one supported by firm cartilage.

The anatomic differences at various ages become meaningful when managing the airway. For example, the position for opening the airway varies with age. For infants (less than 1 year old), place the head in the sniffing or neutral position to avoid bending or kinking the more membranous trachea. For toddlers and small children (1 to 8 years of age), extend the neck slightly but do not hyperextend. The relatively large tongue in the child makes maneuvers to lift the tongue off the airway especially important. When inserting an oropharyngeal airway, use a tongue blade to displace the tongue, since rotating the airway in the usual manner may inadvertently damage the soft tissues of the palate.

COMPARISON OF AIRWAY ANATOMY

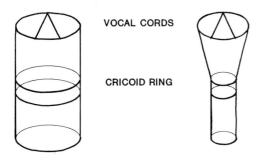

ADULT AIRWAY   PEDIATRIC AIRWAY

FIGURE 14–3. The narrowest portion of the child's airway is at the cricoid ring. The adult's airway is narrowest at the vocal cords. In the child, the epiglottis and tongue are relatively larger in proportion to the airway than in the adult.

Given the small-caliber airway of infants, small obstructions such as swelling or mucus can result in a significant blockage of airflow (Fig. 14–4). Whereas 1 to 2 mm of airway edema in an adult is inconsequential, it becomes a significant obstruction to an infant. Therefore, disease processes that affect the upper airway of an infant have the potential of significantly compromising the airway.

Infants prefer to breathe through the nose. In fact, infants are considered obligate nose breathers. Blockage of the nasal passages from mucus or swelling can significantly narrow the airway and increase a baby's work of breathing. Often an infant may have an upper respiratory infection such as the common cold. If the infant also has a disease of the lower airway, this blockage in the nasal pharynx may be all that is necessary to cause the baby to decompensate. Suctioning out the baby's nasal passages with a DeLee suction can significantly improve the clinical picture. Humidification of oxygen that the child breathes can also help by loosening any encrusted mucus or secretions.

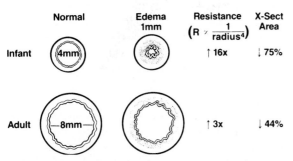

FIGURE 14–4. Small changes in the diameter of the infant's airway can have a great effect on airflow. This increases the likelihood of obstruction from foreign objects or mucus plugs. (From Coté CJ, Todres ID: The pediatric airway. In Ryan JF, Todres ID, Coté CJ, Goudsouzian N (eds): A Practice of Anesthesia for Infants and Children. New York, Grune & Stratton, 1986, p. 39.)

RESPIRATORY FUNCTION

The respiratory rate in children is much faster than in the adult, and it gradually decreases with age. Newborns have a respiratory rate of above 40. Infants (up to 1 year) have an average respiratory rate of 24 to 30 breaths/minute, younger children have a rate of 20 to 25 breaths/minute, and older children have a rate of 15 to 20 breaths/minute. You should be generally familiar with the range of variations in order to evaluate the patient's respiratory status properly (Table 14–1).

As with the adult, the rate of breathing alone is not the measure of adequate ventilation. Depth of breathing or tidal volume must also be considered. The evaluation of depth is done by observing for chest rise and listening and feeling for the movement of air. When positive-pressure ventilation is necessary, care must be taken not to overventilate, since the respiratory volumes of infants and children also vary with age. During ventilation you must be careful to observe chest rise closely to determine the end-point of ventilation. Infants and small children are more subject to gastric distention because of their small lung capacity and the tendency for excessive volumes and pressure of air to "overflow" into the esophagus.

Infants have very compliant chest walls. When they work harder at breathing and use their accessory muscles of respiration, supraclavicular, substernal, and intercostal retractions are noted along the supple chest wall. Retractions and nasal flaring, which are signs of increased work of breathing, are obvious on inspection. Infants and children can mount a vigorous respiratory and cardiovascular response to compensate for illness. However, since their energy stores are less, children can quite easily decompensate because any significant pathophysiology rapidly tires the muscles of respiration.

RESPIRATORY EFFORT AND FATIGUE

When they need to work to breathe, infants and children experience respiratory muscle fatigue more rapidly than adults. When this occurs they may experience a sudden *deterioration* (downhill course) in their condition. For example, children with asthma may be at home for extended periods while the parents attempt to break the attack and avoid hospitalization. During this time, the children experience increased work at breathing and may be unable to sleep. They become exhausted. The EMT

TABLE 14–1. Respiratory Rates in Infants and Children

Newborn—40 breaths/min
1 year—24 breaths/min
18 years—18 breaths/min

(Adapted from the American Heart Association: Textbook of Pediatric Advanced Life Support. Dallas, American Heart Association, 1988.)

must remember that the child may tire to the point where respiratory efforts are inadequate and assistance via positive-pressure ventilation is necessary. Beware when the child who has been working to breathe becomes tired and wants to sleep or lie down. Also, remember that anxiety and anxious behavior may be a sign of hypoxia, which appears before the patient becomes cyanotic.

Simple interventions such as administering high-concentration humidified oxygen and keeping the infant warm extend the *compensatory* or grace period. By adding oxygen you may decrease the need to work so hard at breathing. Except during the newborn period, there is absolutely no contraindication to using high-concentration oxygen. (For newborns, see Chapter 13.) Oxygen toxicity is not a consideration in prehospital transport. Humidifying the oxygen is important, since dried secretions might obstruct airflow and increase airway resistance. Therefore, give humidified oxygen when possible.

PULSE RATE AND BLOOD PRESSURE

The average pulse rate of the child decreases with age. For example, an infant's average pulse rate is 130 with a range from 100 to 190. Thereafter the average values decrease toward adult values (Table 14–2). When evaluating traumatized infants and children, you must be able to appreciate these values in determining the extent of blood loss and the severity of shock.

The blood pressure increases with age. Use the cuff size appropriate for an infant or child to prevent false readings. As a general rule, the width of the cuff should cover approximately two thirds of the length of the upper arm, and the bladder should cover approximately 75% of the arm's circumference. If the cuff is too small, readings are falsely high, and if it is too large, readings are falsely low. Tables 14–2 and 14–3 show the normal values for pulse and blood pressure from infancy through adolescence.

With the greater range and variability in normal vital signs, it is sometimes more difficult to interpret the significance of changes in blood pressure in the child. The American College of Surgeons considers a systolic

TABLE 14–2. Pulse Rates in Normal Children

Age	Range	Mean
Newborn to 3 mo	85–205	140
3 mo to 2 yr	100–190	130
2 yr to 10 yr	60–140	80
> 10 yr	50–100	75

(Reproduced with permission. © Textbook of Pediatric Advanced Life Support, 1988. Copyright American Heart Association.)

TABLE 14–3. Blood Pressure Values for Infants and Children

Formula for approximating the 50th percentile for systolic blood pressure of children over two years of age:

$$90 + (2 \times \text{age in years})$$

Formula for approximating lower limit for systolic blood pressure for children over two years of age:

$$70 + (2 \times \text{age in years})$$

(Adapted from the American Heart Association: Textbook of Pediatric Advanced Life Support. Dallas, American Heart Association, 1988.)

blood pressure of less than 70 mm Hg with tachycardia and cool skin an indicator of shock in children.

METABOLIC CONSIDERATIONS

Keeping the child warm is a simple and valuable measure that should not be underestimated. Infants and children have a higher baseline metabolic rate than adults. Their engine (so to speak) runs at higher rpms. This means that for their size, they need more fuel, which in humans is oxygen and glucose. To accomplish this they have a faster normal respiratory rate to capture the oxygen and a faster normal heart rate to deliver it to the tissues. They also consume more calories per unit weight than do adults, as any bleary-eyed new parent can attest to after nighttime feedings.

Part of the reason infants have a higher basal metabolic rate is that they are busy growing. Another explanation is that they need to expend more energy to remain warm. Notice that infants have proportionately larger heads and a greater skin surface area relative to body weight than do adults. This means they lose heat and moisture through the skin more easily. Their higher respiratory rate also adds to the amount of heat and water lost through the lungs.

The intake of food and water usually decreases in the sick or injured child. This can exhaust the *glycogen* (stored form of glucose) supply during the course of the illness. Since the metabolic rate is higher and because there are smaller reserves of glucose, children quickly use up their energy supplies. Fever will further increase the metabolic rate and complicate this situation.

It is important to keep the sick infant warm; otherwise the infant may consume his or her energy stores just to stay warm. The glycogen stored in the liver is then rapidly depleted and unavailable for other metabolic needs. *Remember, when the metabolic needs on a cellular level are not met, shock results.* A further problem is that infants less than 6 months of age cannot shiver in response to cold and therefore cannot generate heat through muscular contraction. By keeping the child warm and well-oxygenated, you help the infant conserve his or her energy reserves.

NEUROLOGIC DIFFERENCES

The very young pediatric patient's head is large in relation to the body. Thus, this patient is more likely to suffer head injury. The infant is capable of suffering blood loss within the cranium sufficient to cause shock. This is in contrast to the adult and child patient, in whom significant blood loss and hypovolemic shock are not possible with closed head injuries. Both infants and children are also more prone to *apneic* (absence of breathing) episodes with head trauma.

It is important to remember that the infant and child have a greater chance of recovering from brain hypoxia or head trauma than does an adult suffering a similar insult.

RESPONSE TO HYPOVOLEMIA AND SHOCK STATES

Hypovolemic shock is the most common type of shock in childhood. Acute dehydration and hemorrhage are the two causes of hypovolemia most often encountered by EMTs.

Hypovolemia from *dehydration* (not enough water) is likely in any sick child with increased metabolic needs and poor intake. Vomiting and diarrhea hasten fluid loss. The smaller the child, the more vulnerable that child is to dehydration.

The child tolerates a gradual loss of fluids during acute illness because fluid shifts from the cells and interstitial fluid to maintain the plasma volume. As this occurs, there is a progression of *signs of dehydration*. Initially, the small child or infant has tachycardia, less urine output, and dry mucosal membranes. This progresses to lack of tears, a sunken fontanelle, and sunken eyes. Late signs are skin tenting, delayed capillary refill, hyperventilation, an altered mental status (which includes irritability and lethargy), and a thready pulse. Hypotension is a very late sign (Table 14–4).

With acute blood or fluid loss, as occurs with in hemorrhage, the pediatric patient exhibits the same signs of shock as an adult. Remember that the total blood volume of children is significantly less than in adults. The average blood volume is 80 ml/kg. This means an average 10-kg 1-year-old infant would have 800 ml of total blood volume. What might be an insignificant 200-ml blood loss in an adult is 25% of the 10-kg baby's blood volume.

With healthy compensatory mechanisms, children can maintain their blood pressure until nearly 40% of the blood volume is lost. The drop in blood pressure in

TABLE 14–4. Signs of Dehydration

Time	Sign
Early	Tachycardia Less urine output Dry mucosal membranes
Intermediate	Lack of tears Sunken fontanelle Sunken eyes

Late	Skin tenting
	Delayed capillary refill
	Hyperventilation
	Altered mental status
	  Irritability
	  Lethargy
	Thready pulse
	Hypotension (very late sign)

the child is even a later finding than in adults. By the time children are hypotensive they are in deep shock.

Children and infants are also susceptible to other less common causes of shock. Distributive shock is seen with sepsis, anaphylaxis, and spinal cord shock, as well as in response to certain drugs. Following trauma, the pediatric patient can suffer obstructive shock from tension pneumothorax and cardiac temponade. Rarely will a child suffer cardiogenic shock. Possible causes of cardiogenic shock in a child include a myocardial contusion, previous congenital heart disease, or an acute *cardiomyopathy* (infection of the myocardium).

ASSESSMENT OF THE PEDIATRIC PATIENT

The general components of assessment of the pediatric patient are the same as for the adult: dispatch review, scene survey, primary survey, and secondary survey (history and physical examination). Variations in the specific approach relate primarily to the developmental and physiologic issues discussed previously. For example, the head-to-toe survey becomes the toe-to-head survey in infants and small children. Airway maneuvers used during assessment also change according to age, as does the evaluation and interpretation of vital signs. This section addresses the special considerations associated with the evaluation of infants and children who have acute medical problems and provides helpful tips on "what to look for" and "how to look." The time spent on the scene should be limited to gathering information needed to provide the immediate and necessary treatments to the infant or child. Additional information can be gathered while transporting the child and parents to the hospital.

Primary Survey

As part of the primary survey, the respiratory status and level of responsiveness are evaluated as you approach the patient. Pediatricians have described their ability to conduct this initial evaluation "from the doorway" as they approach a child. Their initial question, "Is this child significantly ill?" is followed by the question, "Am I dealing with a respiratory problem?" Answers may be apparent by general observation and initial handling of the child. Look for activity and playfulness, color, respiratory effort, and temperature.

A common scenario you may encounter is a screaming 3-year-old child, acting like the world is coming to an end, who is running about and is combative and uncooperative; the parents are hysterical and upset.

Standing in the doorway you assess the following: The child's airway is patent and functional, since the youngster is pink and screaming. The circulatory function is adequate since the child is upright and moving about. The youngster does not have meningitis, appendicitis, or other severe infectious processes or the child would be lying very still or showing evidence of distress. This child does not have an immediate life-threatening problem. By being calm and observant, you gather useful information before actually approaching the child. You can reassure yourself and the parents that you have time for evaluation, intervention, and transportation.

PHYSICAL SIGNS

Physical signs of illness are related to the age and development of the child. Careful observation along with recognition of the broad age categories represented by the designations infant, small child, large child simplify your observations. Since the respiratory system is the most important to evaluate in your initial assessment and the most important to control en route to the hospital, the discussion here of the physical examination includes both the general evaluation and the respiratory evaluation. Observation enables you to assess activity, color, some signs of dehydration, general nutritional status, and respiratory effort.

GENERAL SIGNS

On initial observation, note the general level of activity. Is the child

- Limp?
- Anxious/agitated?
- Drowsy?
- Normal?

When observing infants, look for eye contact with the parent or note whether the infant follows a toy with his or her eyes. The small child should be aware of and interacting with the environment. The infant or small child has no reason to be interested in your examination and should be appropriately upset. Be wary of a child who is "too good" or quiet during your examination.

Note the child's weight and nutritional status. Does the child appear too thin or wasted or is there evidence of adequate nutritional and fluid intake? Does the child feel warm? Is there a history of fever? Regardless of the underlying disease, children quickly become dehydrated. Are signs of dehydration present? Poor skin turgor, sunken eyes, and dry mucous membranes are common to all age groups. Look for a sunken fontanelle in the infant (see Table 14–4).

Look at the skin color. Signs include pallor, jaundice, flushing, and cyanosis. Cyanosis is of immediate concern. Before you approach the child, ask the parents to remove or lift the child's shirt. Look for mottling of the trunk in the infant. This is a large blotchy pattern of mixed pale and reddish to reddish blue areas evident on the skin, which may be evidence of inadequate perfusion. A cold environment can also result in mottling in the normotensive infant, especially in the extremities.

RESPIRATORY SIGNS

Evaluation of quality and quantity of breathing can likewise be done "from the doorway." Keeping the normal values for the age group in mind, note the respiratory rate. Notice whether the child is breathing easily or working hard to breathe, as demonstrated by the use of neck and other accessory muscles of breathing and supraclavicular, intercostal, or substernal retractions (Fig. 14–5). Look at the position the child assumes if there is respiratory distress. Children with respiratory distress may prefer to remain sitting. With obstruction of the upper airway, they may be found leaning forward, with the neck slightly extended and chin forward (sniffing position) and with the mouth open and tongue slightly protruding. How hard a child is working to breathe is as important as the rate of breathing. Look for nasal flaring, seen predominantly in infancy, a sign of respiratory distress. Notice also if there is nasal congestion. Listen for obvious stridor, grunting, wheezing, or cough. Stridor is a crowing sound made on inspiration, suggestive of upper airway obstruction. Stridor with retractions is of concern. Grunting is a rhythmic sound heard at the end of exhalation that may be mistaken for whining. This is a sure sign of significant respiratory compromise and is rarely noted past 3 years of age. Loud wheezing and cough can be heard without a stethoscope.

KEY RESPIRATORY FINDINGS TO NOTE IN CHILDREN

RETRACTIONS. *Retractions* are often visible on children because of the compliance or flexibility of the chest wall. Retractions are the inward depression of mus-

FIGURE 14–5. Nasal flaring and retractions are important indicators of significant respiratory distress in infants and children.

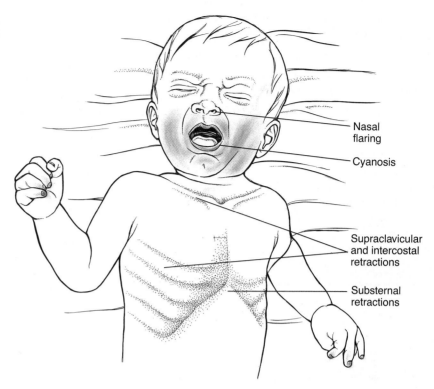

Nasal flaring

Cyanosis

Supraclavicular and intercostal retractions

Substernal retractions

cular areas and their attached ribs, which are drawn inward and reflect an increased work at breathing caused by obstruction to airflow. Retractions may be seen in different muscular areas. In croup, for example, nasal flaring and supraclavicular retractions may be seen with moderate distress, and intercostal and substernal retractions are evident as the distress becomes more severe.

STRIDOR. *Stridor* is the high-pitched noise usually heard at inspiration caused by obstruction to airflow in the upper airway. Severe airway obstruction may result in stridor at inspiration and expiration. Stridor is audible without a stethoscope.

WHEEZING. *Wheezing* is the high-pitched "musical" sound caused by the narrowing of the lower airways, obstructing airflow. This narrowing can be caused by edema encroaching on the airway or direct constriction of the small bronchioles. With asthma, wheezing is heard during exhalation. The exhalation is prolonged to allow time for air to exit from the narrowed airways. The wheezing is created by turbulence generated from increased expiratory pressures forcing air through narrow airways. There are many other causes of wheezing. See Table 14–5 for the causes of wheezing in pediatric patients that are of importance to EMTs.

COUGH. *Cough* is a protective reflex mechanism used to remove foreign material from the airway. Coughing is termed productive and nonproductive depending on whether there is any mucus or phlegm removed during the process. It is a general sign seen with many conditions.

CYANOSIS. As with adults, central *cyanosis* is a sign of low oxygen saturation of the hemoglobin in the blood. It is not an early sign of hypoxia, and other indications such as altered mental status may appear before cyanosis is present. Because cyanosis appears when a certain concentration of the hemoglobin in the blood is unsaturated with oxygen, it may be very late or absent in children with hemorrhage or anemia. Table 14–6 summarizes the signs of respiratory disorders in children.

Secondary Survey

TAKING A HISTORY

Obtaining a history in the child follows the same format as in the adult. After hearing the chief complaint, obtain the history of present illness, past medical history, medications, and allergies. For the infant, inquire about any problems during pregnancy or birth. Was the baby premature or kept in the hospital for an extra length of time? The younger the child, the more you must rely on the parents for the history. When speaking with

TABLE 14–5. Causes of Wheezing in Children

—Asthma
—Bronchiolitis
—Airway obstruction
—Pneumonia
—Upper airway congestion

TABLE 14–6. Summary of Signs of Respiratory Distress

Early Signs

Tachypnea (rapid breathing)
Tachycardia (rapid pulse)
Mottling of skin
Nasal flaring

Increasing Distress

Retractions and/or grunting (signifying increased work of breathing)
Increased tachycardia
Altered mental status
Poor peripheral perfusion

Prerespiratory Arrest

Cyanosis or grayish hue to skin
Bradycardia (a very ominous sign)
Shallow breathing or apnea

children, remember to use terms appropriate for their age and vocabulary.

PHYSICAL EXAMINATION

The primary survey is the same as for adults. The awake but sick child requires a different approach from an adult patient. Many children react with alarm if approached immediately, making elicitation of physical findings more difficult. The following considerations will help you obtain vital information.

On approaching the small child or infant you should initially listen to the lungs, as you do not know how long the child will remain quiet. When listening to the lungs (with a warm stethoscope), listen for quality of air movement and note any abnormal breath sounds, keeping in mind that normal respiratory and heart rates are faster in children.

Here are some tricks to help you assess the child's respiratory status. If the child is old enough to understand, ask the child to blow at your pen as if it were a birthday candle. The child takes a deep breath prior to blowing. Place your stethoscope near the nose to determine air movement and to ascertain whether the rhonchi heard during lung auscultation are transmitted upper airway sounds.

Often the child is crying and you are unable to adequately assess lung sounds. However, you already know that a strong cry is a good sign—a sick child is too busy working to breathe to put up a fight.

OTHER CONSIDERATIONS

The infant's skull bones are not fully fused until the baby is well into the second year of life. The anterior fontanelle, between the frontal and parietal bones, is the largest space between these bony plates. The average size is 3 cm × 3 cm at birth, which slowly decreases as the baby gets older. The level of the *fontanelle* (soft spot) relative to the skull is significant. In the normal infant, while sitting up, the soft spot should be level with the bones of the skull or only slightly depressed. In the dehydrated infant the fontanelle is depressed even when the baby is lying down. On the other hand, a bulging fontanelle may be reflective of increased intracranial pressure. The most common concern is meningitis; however, other causes such as subdural hematomas are possible. The strain of crying can also cause the fontanelle to bulge.

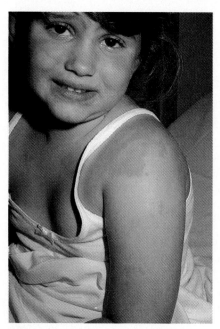

A

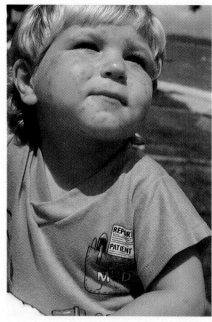

B

FIGURE 14–6. Two rashes commonly encountered in children. (*A*) Urticaria associated with an allergic reaction. (*B*) Chickenpox.

A stiff neck is an important physical finding. As discussed in Chapter 7, nuchal (back of the neck) rigidity is a key indicator of meningitis. The irritable infant or small child may be difficult to assess. Try to get the child to follow a toy or your keys by turning his or her head to an extent where the child has to flex the neck. Be aware that infants and small children younger than 18 months of age can have meningitis without either stiff neck or bulging fontanelles. Rather, they may be listless. The only presenting sign of a severely sick infant may be that in the parent's opinion the child is "just not acting right." Infants who were born prematurely are even more susceptible to serious infections in the first two months of life.

In a child with respiratory distress, especially stridor, you must specifically avoid examining the oropharynx. The only exception would be a direct visualization of a foreign body, which is discussed later in this chapter.

Rashes are common in children. They are associated with allergic reactions and common viral illness, such as measles, *rubella* (German measles), *varicella* (chickenpox), and a variety of nonspecific viral illness (Fig. 14–6). Rashes are also seen with bacterial illness such as *meningococcemia*. Making a specific diagnosis of children with rashes is often difficult. To complete the secondary

TABLE 14–7. Summary of Initial Evaluation

1. Initial evaluation "from the doorway"
   Evaluate overall appearance and color
     Cyanosis?
     Mottling (spotting with patches of color)?
     Pale?
   Evaluate respiratory rate
   Evaluate respiratory effort
     Stridor?
     Retractions (supraclavicular, intercostal, substernal)?
     Audible wheezing or crowing?
     Grunting?
2. Approach child
   Nasal flaring?
   Grunting?
   Flacid or agitated?
3. Hands-on examination
   Air movement at nares?
   Peripheral perfusion adequate?
   Quality of air movement?

survey, follow the same physical examination guidelines as for adults, remembering that in the very young child, you should do your complete head-to-toe survey in the reverse order. Review Table 14–7 to reinforce the key elements of pediatric assessment and review the protocol on the approach to the pediatric patient that summarizes the assessment process.

PROTOCOL

APPROACH TO THE PEDIATRIC PATIENT

1. *Initial Scene Assessment:*

   A. Assess the scene for safety.

   B. Note the number of patients, the mechanism(s) of injury, environmental hazards, and so forth.

   C. Call for additional personnel and/or equipment if needed.

2. *Expanded Primary Assessment/Resuscitation*

   A. AIRWAY
      —Is the airway open?
      —Will it stay open?
      —Jaw thrust/manually stabilize the head/neck.
      —Suction the patient's pharynx if necessary.
      —Insert oral/nasal airway as necessary.

   Identify and *correct* any existing or potential airway obstruction while protecting the cervical spine.

   B. BREATHING
      —Is breathing present?
      —Is it adequate?
      —Does anything endanger the patient's breathing?
      —How is the patient talking?
      —Can the patient take a deep breath?

      —How is the patient crying?
      —Assess the chest.
      —Inspect.
      —Palpate.
      —Auscultate.
      —Seal holes.
      —Stabilize flail segments.
      —Administer high-concentration oxygen.
      —Ventilate as necessary.

   Identify and *correct* any existing or potentially compromising factors.

   C. CIRCULATION
      —Is a pulse present?
      —Are peripheral and central pulses present?
      —Is obvious, serious internal/external bleeding present?
      —Is the patient in shock?
      —Note the skin color.
      —Note capillary refill.

   Identify and *correct* any existing or potentially compromising factors.

   D. *Disability.* What is the patient's level of consciousness? Consider the developmental age of the child

Continued

and assess the patient's level of consciousness as follows:

Alert—patient knows:
(1) His/her name
(2) Where he/she is
(3) Day of the week

Verbal—patient responds to verbal stimuli but does not respond appropriately to the above three questions.

Painful—patient responds to pain only. Is it an appropriate response?

Unresponsive—The patient does not respond verbally or react to pain.

Assess the patient's pupils.

Assess, quickly, the patient's ability to move his or her extremities. If indicated, apply a rigid collar (if appropriate size is available) and stabilize the head/neck.

E. *Expose* the patient as appropriate to locate life-threatening problems.

> **IMMEDIATE TRANSPORT DECISION**
>
> *IF THE PATIENT'S CONDITION DICTATES, THE VITAL SIGNS, SECONDARY SURVEY, AND TREATMENT SHOULD BE DONE EN ROUTE TO THE HOSPITAL.*

3. *Vital Signs*: Obtain and record the following on every patient initially, and repeat as often as the situation indicates.

A. Pulse: rate and quality

B. Respirations: rate and quality

C. Blood pressure: systolic and diastolic blood pressure

D. Skin: color, temperature, and moisture

4. *Secondary Survey*: Complete as indicated by the patient's condition.

A. Reassure and inform the patient and parent about the treatment.

B. Obtain and record any pertinent medical information from the patient, family, and bystanders. Check for medical identification.

C. Perform a head-to-toe assessment as indicated. Perform a toe-to-head examination in infants and small children.

5. *Field Treatment*: Administer appropriate treatment in order of priority. Refer to specific treatment protocols.

6. *Standby/Notifications*: If there is a need to notify the hospital of the arrival of a seriously ill or injured patient, the following information should be relayed to the dispatcher or Emergency department.

A. Patient information:

(1) Age and sex

(2) Chief complaint

(3) Subjective and objective patient assessment findings

(4) Level of consciousness and vital signs

(5) Pertinent history as needed to clarify the problem (mechanism of injury, previous illnesses, allergies, medications)

(6) Treatment given and patient's response, if any

(7) Other pertinent information as necessary

B. Notification of any delay in transport or any unusual circumstances

C. Estimated time of arrival (ETA)

7. *Arrival at the hospital*: Upon arrival at the hospital emergency department, submit a verbal report summarizing the above information to the *responsible* medical personnel. Submit the hospital copy of the prehospital care report to the *responsible* emergency department personnel after all crew members have had the opportunity to review it.

Adapted from New York State Basic Life Suport Protocols and New York City EMS Academy training protocols.

COMMON PEDIATRIC DISORDERS

Your primary concern as a provider of prehospital care is to quickly decide whether emergency intervention is necessary. Therefore, it is invaluable to learn the most common childhood diseases and gain confidence in evaluating and dealing with children.

Respiratory Disorders

A failing or failed respiratory system is the single most important cause of death in the pediatric age group.

Control of the airway, ventilation, and oxygenation are the most important elements of pediatric resuscitation. Except for the child with congenital heart disease or acquired cardiac disease, children normally have strong hearts. Therefore, as a general rule, *control or treat the respiratory system, and the heart will follow.*

When evaluating an infant or child with respiratory distress, it is important to differentiate between upper airway (at or above the trachea) and lower airway disease. Upper airway problems, which include croup, epiglottitis, foreign bodies, and trauma, obstruct airflow going into the lungs and can cause complete obstruction.

Lower airway diseases, affecting the middle and lower bronchioles and alveoli, may impede air movement out of the lungs and hinder oxygen exchange. This can cause air trapping and impaired oxygenation and can progress to generalized respiratory failure. Asthma, bronchiolitis, and foreign body obstruction are lower airway conditions that are encountered in prehospital care. Although lower airway diseases may ultimately progress to respiratory failure and arrest, they usually do so over a longer period of time as compared to upper airway processes such as epiglottitis.

UPPER AIRWAY DISEASE

The major upper airway diseases requiring EMT attention are croup, epiglottitis, and a foreign body in the airway. All run the risk of causing complete obstruction. The distinction has to be made between the infectious causes (croup and epiglottitis) and the presence of a foreign body, since the management differs. The obstructed airway maneuvers used to remove a foreign body are of no value for croup and epiglottitis. In addition, stimulation of the pharynx and epiglottis must be avoided if a patient has epiglottitis, since it can cause severe spasm and closing of the airway.

CROUP   Seal bark - Cool Air helps

1/2 - 3 yrs

Infection accounts for the majority of stridor in childhood. Within this group, *croup* is very common and epiglottitis is uncommon.

Croup is a viral infection affecting the larynx, trachea, and bronchi. It causes airway narrowing, especially at the level of the cricoid ring (Fig. 14–7) and produces stridor. The classic course begins with an *upper respiratory infection*, or cold. The child may be hoarse, have a low-grade fever and a cough that sounds like a barking seal, and then develop varying degrees of inspiratory stridor. Croup is often worse at night or upon awakening. Croup is most common from ages 6 months to 6 years, with the majority of cases occurring at less than 3 years of age. Keys to effective management are humidification, hydration, and oxygenation. Croup may appear to be cured by humidification or by the cool night air. In fact, many cases are asymptomatic by the time they reach the hospital or the physician's office. However, severe cases of croup can result in complete airway obstruction.

EPIGLOTTITIS   *don't look in mouth*

3-7 yrs
swelling, bending over .

Acute epiglottitis is an infectious swelling of the epiglottis (caused by a bacterial infection) that has a rapid onset of approximately 10 to 12 hours (Fig. 14–8). The major signs and symptoms include a high fever, a sore throat and *dysphagia* (difficulty in swallowing), and sometimes inspiratory stridor. The child frequently is sitting upright and leaning forward with his or her weight distributed on the hands, the mouth open, the tongue pro-

will not swallow .

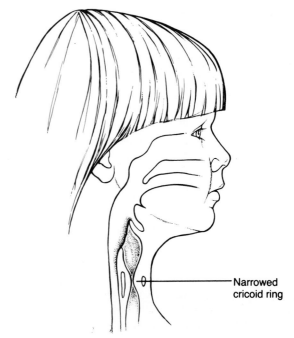

FIGURE 14–7. Croup can cause significant narrowing of the airway due to inflammation and mucus, especially at the level of the cricoid ring.

Narrowed cricoid ring

truding, and the chin thrust forward (tripod position). This maximizes the airway diameter and improves ventilation. Other key signs include restlessness, drooling, a flushed face, and signs of dehydration. Epiglottitis is handled as a potentially life-threatening emergency. Of

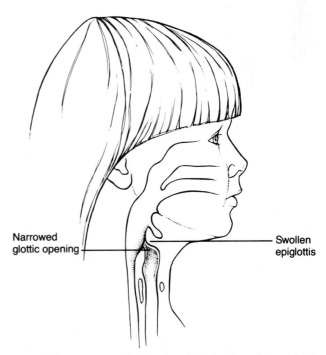

Narrowed glottic opening

Swollen epiglottis

FIGURE 14–8. In epiglottitis the inflamed and swollen epiglottis can obstruct the opening to the larynx. The EMT should avoid any manipulation of the posterior pharynx or attempt to "see" the epiglottis, since complete obstruction due to spasm can result.

additional concern is the fact that stimulation of the pharynx, as with examination using a tongue blade, can cause reflex spasm of the epiglottis, resulting in a total airway obstruction. Classically, the child has a mild upper airway infection and then becomes suddenly ill.

The child is showing you the key to management. He or she sits relatively still, holding the head in a particular position, which is keeping what little airway there is open, and he or she appears somewhat pale and ashen. The approach to management is gentle, calm handling, staying away from the child's airway. Let the child stay in the parent's arms even during transport so as to decrease the chance of oxygen consumption that may result from anxiety. Offer humidified oxygen, but if the child is alert and resists, leave the child be. In these circumstances, you or the parent may try to hold the mask near the child's airway. If cyanosis and lethargy become evident, you should attempt positive-pressure ventilation. Studies have found that ventilations with a bag-valve-mask can be effective in most patients with epiglottitis. Epiglottitis usually affects children from 2 to 6 years of age but also can occur in older children and adults. The following protocol summarizes the management of croup and epiglottitis.

PROTOCOL

CROUP/EPIGLOTTITIS—PEDIATRIC

IF THE CHILD PRESENTS WITH RESPIRATORY DISTRESS AND INSPIRATORY STRIDOR AND HAS A HISTORY OF UPPER RESPIRATORY INFECTION, SUSPECT:

CROUP IF ONE OR MORE OF THE FOLLOWING ARE PRESENT: LOW-GRADE FEVER, BARKING COUGH, AND STERNAL RETRACTIONS.

EPIGLOTTITIS IF ONE OR MORE OF THE FOLLOWING ARE PRESENT: HIGH-GRADE FEVER, MUFFLED VOICE, INABILITY TO SWALLOW, AND DROOLING.

A. IF THE CHILD IS CONSCIOUS:

1. MAINTAIN A CALM APPROACH TO THE PARENT AND CHILD. *ALLOW THE CHILD TO ASSUME AND MAINTAIN A POSITION OF COMFORT OR TO BE HELD BY THE PARENT, PREFERABLY IN AN UPRIGHT POSITION.*

2. Administer high-concentration oxygen (preferably humidified) by a face mask IF TOLERATED. *AVOID AGITATING THE CHILD!* Administration of oxygen may best be accomplished by allowing the parent to hold the face mask about 6 to 8 inches from the child's face.

3. Transport the child CALMLY in an upright position (in the parent's lap if necessary to avoid further agitation of the child), keeping the child warm. DO NOT FORCE THE CHILD TO LIE DOWN!

4. Obtain and record the initial vital signs, including capillary refill, IF TOLERATED WITHOUT AGITATION, and repeat en route as often as the situation indicates.

5. Record all patient care information, including the patient's medical history and all treatment provided, on a prehospital care report.

> *CAUTION!*
>
> *DO NOT ATTEMPT TO VISUALIZE THE CHILD'S OROPHARYNX!* DO NOT INSERT ANYTHING INTO THE MOUTH OR PERFORM STRESSFUL PROCEDURES THAT COULD CAUSE SUDDEN, COMPLETE AIRWAY OBSTRUCTION IN THESE CHILDREN!

B. IF THE CHILD IS UNCONSCIOUS OR BECOMES UNCONSCIOUS AND IS NOT BREATHING:

1. Open the child's airway with the head tilt–chin lift maneuver.

2. Ventilate the child at a rate appropriate for the child's age, using mouth-to-mouth or mouth-to-nose, pocket mask, or bag-valve-mask. ASSURE THAT THE CHEST RISES WITH EACH VENTILATION.

> ADEQUATE VENTILATION MAY REQUIRE DISABLING THE POP-OFF VALVE IF THE BAG-VALVE-MASK UNIT IS SO EQUIPPED!

3. Supplement ventilations with high-concentration oxygen.

4. Transport, keeping the child warm.

5. Obtain and record the initial vital signs, including capillary refill, and repeat en route as often as the situation indicates.

6. Record all patient care information, including the patient's medical history and all treatment provided, on a prehospital care report.

Adapted from Manual for Emergency Medical Technicians. Emergency Medical Services Program. Albany, New York State Department of Health, 1990.

FOREIGN BODY AIRWAY OBSTRUCTION

The child or infant with foreign body aspiration usually is a previously healthy child with a history of choking on something who now exhibits signs of upper airway obstruction, i.e., stridor, tachypnea, and difficulty moving air. For the purposes of treatment, an infant is defined as someone less than 1 year of age, and a child as someone between the ages of 1 and 8 years of age. These age parameters relate to average size at these ages. In other words, a small 13-month-old child may be treated as an infant, and a large 11-month-old infant may be treated as a child.

The following are the main considerations in the patient with upper airway obstruction: (1) Is the obstruction partial or complete? (2) Is immediate intervention needed or can the patient wait? (3) Is the obstruction caused by an infectious process or a foreign body?

To form a working assessment, it is important to perform a primary survey and gather key historical facts. First, to determine whether the obstruction is partial or complete, assess for level of consciousness, air exchange, and ability to speak or cry. Taking a brief history regarding recent upper respiratory infections, fever, and barking cough, or a history of choking after eating or playing with objects in the mouth helps clarify the cause of obstruction.

Treat all suspected infectious causes as if they are epiglottitis, that is, do not manipulate or attempt to examine the airway. Review the summary of croup, epiglottitis, and foreign body obstruction in Table 14–8 to clarify the major differences.

THE ALERT CHILD. If the child is alert, even with severe stridor and a rapid respiratory rate, keep your management to a minimum. Keep the child and parents calm and allow the child to remain in the parent's arms in the position of comfort that the child chooses. Supply humidified oxygen without agitating the child (from a face mask or nasal cannula or by holding a mask near the nose and mouth) and transport quickly. This holds true regardless of whether you suspect croup, epiglottitis, or a foreign body obstruction. *Even if you suspect a foreign body, if the child is alert and moving air, do not intervene.*

THE NONBREATHING (COMPLETE OBSTRUCTION) CHILD OR THE CHILD WITH A PARTIAL OBSTRUCTION WITH POOR AIR EXCHANGE. If the condition of an infant or child begins to deteriorate, with decreasing mental status, severe retractions without air movement, a rapid respiratory rate and pulse, and especially a very slow pulse, intervention becomes necessary. If you suspect an *infectious cause*, assist breathing with positive-pressure ventilation. If you suspect a foreign body obstruction, proceed with the foreign body airway obstruction protocol.

If the child cannot speak or cry or is exhibiting a weak, ineffective cough, stridor, and cyanosis (partial obstruction with poor air exchange), the child should be treated for a complete airway obstruction.

THE CHILD WITH COMPLETE FOREIGN BODY OBSTRUCTION (CONSCIOUS INFANT). The infant should be supported on your arm and thigh, face down with the head toward your palm and slightly dependent. Four back blows should be administered between the scapula, each given with the intent of removing the object (Fig. 14–9). The combination of back blows and gravity often removes the obstruction.

TABLE 14–8. Signs of Croup, Epiglottitis, and Foreign Body Obstructions

Croup	Epiglottitis	Foreign Body Obstructions
6 months–4 years	2 years–7 years	Any age (especially 3 months–5 years)
Slow onset	Sudden onset (hours)	Sudden onset (history of choking)
Low-grade fever	High fever	No fever
Sick, not toxic	Toxic	Not toxic
Cough (barking seal)	Muffled or quiet	Coughing initially
Hoarse	Dysphagia	Difficulty talking
Usually not drooling	Drooling	May drool
Agitated, moving	Quiet, classic tripod position	Either quiet or agitated

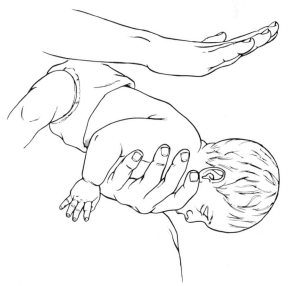

FIGURE 14–9. When back blows are being administered, the infant should be supported on your arm and thigh. The infant's head can rest across your palm to give further support to the head.

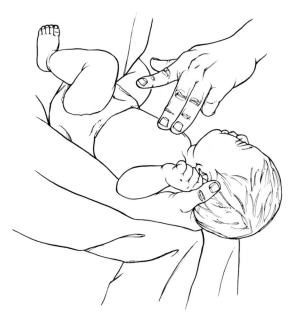

FIGURE 14–10. Chest thrusts are administered in the same position as cardiac compressions. The infant should be placed on a firm surface in order to deliver the most effective thrust.

If the obstruction is not removed, hold the baby between both arms along the long axis of the body, turn the infant to a supine position, and administer four chest thrusts in the same position as a cardiac compression, 1 fingerbreadth below the nipple line (Fig. 14–10). Continue to alternate back blows and chest thrusts until the obstruction is removed or the infant becomes unconscious.

PROCEDURE 14–1   **TREATING THE INFANT WITH COMPLETE AIRWAY OBSTRUCTION WHO BECOMES UNCONSCIOUS**

1. Perform a tongue-jaw lift (Fig. 14–11).
2. Look at the airway and perform a finger sweep (only if you see the foreign body).

(*Note*: If you cannot see the obstruction, do not perform a blind finger sweep.)

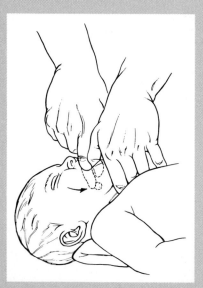

FIGURE 14–11. The finger sweep in the infant should be done while maintaining a jaw lift. The finger sweep is performed only after visualizing the foreign body.

3. After the finger sweep, attempt to ventilate (Fig. 14-12). If you cannot ventilate, repeat the series of back blows and chest thrusts, followed by a finger sweep (when object is visualized), and then reattempt ventilations. Repeat the cycle until you can ventilate the infant or during transport to the hospital.

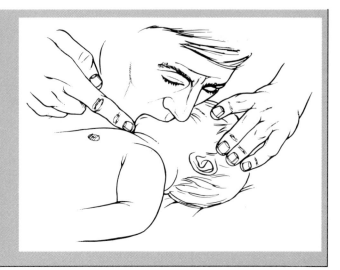

FIGURE 14-12. The infant is ventilated after performing a head tilt–chin lift procedure. The head is placed in the "sniffing" or neutral position. At times a folded sheet or towel placed under the shoulder blades will help maintain this position. This is particularly important when performing cardiopulmonary resuscitation. Mouth-to-mouth and mouth-to-nose ventilation methods are used in infants.

PROCEDURE 14-2
TREATING AN INFANT FOUND UNCONSCIOUS WITH A COMPLETE AIRWAY OBSTRUCTION

1. If the infant is unable to ventilate, try to reopen the airway and attempt a second ventilation.
2. If you are still unable to ventilate, administer four back blows, four chest thrusts, and a finger sweep in the same manner described in Procedure 14-1.
3. Attempt to ventilate the infant at the end of each sequence. If you are unable to clear the airway after several attempts, rapid transport is essential to obtain surgical intervention.
4. If the airway is cleared, check the pulse and respirations and proceed accordingly. If there is a pulse with no respirations, provide positive-pressure ventilation at the recommended rate.
5. If the infant has no pulse, perform CPR.

Note: Management of the child with a complete airway obstruction is the same as for the adult, with one exception. *The finger sweep procedure is done only when the object is visualized.*

✠ PROTOCOL ✠

OBSTRUCTED AIRWAY—PEDIATRIC

A. IF THE CHILD IS CONSCIOUS AND CAN BREATHE, COUGH, CRY, OR SPEAK:

1. DO NOT INTERFERE, AND DO NOT PERFORM BASIC LIFE SUPPORT AIRWAY MANEUVERS! *ALLOW THE CHILD TO ASSUME AND MAINTAIN A POSITION OF COMFORT OR TO BE HELD BY THE PARENT, PREFERABLY IN AN UPRIGHT POSITION.*

2. Administer high-concentration oxygen (preferably humidified) by a face mask IF TOLERATED. AVOID AGITATING THE CHILD! Administration of oxygen may best be accomplished by allowing the parent to hold the face mask about 6 to 8 inches from the child's face.

3. Transport immediately, keeping the child warm.

4. Obtain and record the initial vital signs IF TOLERATED, and repeat en route as often as the situation indicates without agitating the child.

5. Record all child care information, including the patient's medical history and all treatment provided, on a prehospital care report.

> REMEMBER: AGITATING A CHILD WITH PARTIAL AIRWAY BLOCKAGE COULD CAUSE COMPLETE OBSTRUCTION! AS LONG AS THE CHILD CAN BREATHE, COUGH, CRY, OR SPEAK, DO NOT UPSET THE CHILD WITH UNNECESSARY PROCEDURES (E.G., BLOOD PRESSURE DETERMINATION)! USE A CALM, REASSURING APPROACH, TRANSPORTING THE PARENT AND CHILD AS A UNIT.

Review the following protocol to summarize the management of airway obstruction.

Continued

B. IF THE CHILD IS UNCONSCIOUS AND NOT BREATHING

AND

IF FOREIGN BODY ASPIRATION WAS *NOT* WITNESSED:

> IF FOREIGN BODY ASPIRATION WAS WIT-NESSED, GO DIRECTLY TO STEP *1 AND AT-TEMPT TO CLEAR AIRWAY OBSTRUCTION.

1. Attempt to establish airway control using BLS tech-niques. Open the child's mouth, and remove any **VISIBLE** foreign body.

2. Administer two breaths using mouth-to-mouth or mouth-to-nose or pocket mask, observing the child for adequate chest rise.

3–I. IF THE CHILD'S *CHEST DOES NOT RISE:*

a. Check basic life support airway techniques. Re-open the child's airway using the head tilt-chin lift or jaw-thrust maneuver. (Grasping the child's tongue during the chin-lift maneuver may im-prove the success of opening the airway.)

b. Re-attempt ventilations using mouth-to-mouth or mouth-to-nose or pocket mask.

c. **IF THE CHILD IS YOUNGER THAN 1 YEAR OF AGE (INFANT) AND THE CHEST STILL DOES NOT RISE:**

   (*1) Position the infant in a head-down position.

   (2) Administer back blows and chest thrusts according to American Heart Association/American Red Cross (AHA/ARC) standards.

   (3) Open the infant's mouth, and remove any **VISIBLE** foreign body.

> DO NOT PROBE FOR SUSPECTED FOR-EIGN BODY WITH BLIND FINGER SWEEPS. THIS TECHNIQUE COULD IN-ADVERTENTLY FORCE THE OBSTRUC-TION FURTHER DOWN THE INFANT'S AIRWAY.

d. Re-attempt ventilations using mouth-to-mouth or mouth-to-nose or pocket mask.

e. **IF THE INFANT'S CHEST STILL DOES NOT RISE**, repeat the sequence of reopening the air-way, attempting ventilations, delivering back blows and chest thrusts, removing any **VISIBLE** foreign body, and re-attempting ventilations **ONLY ONCE!**

f. **TRANSPORT IMMEDIATELY IF UNSUC-CESSFUL**, repeating Step e throughout transport if needed, and keeping the infant warm.

g. Record all patient care information, including the patient's medical history and all treatment pro-vided, on a prehospital care report.

OR

C. IF THE CHILD IS 1 YEAR OF AGE OR OLDER AND THE CHEST STILL DOES NOT RISE:

(*1) Kneel at the child's feet or straddle the larger child.

(2) Perform abdominal thrusts according to AHA/ARC standards.

> DIRECT THE THRUSTS UPWARD IN THE MID-LINE. AVOID DIRECTING THE THRUSTS TO EITHER SIDE OF MIDLINE.

(3) Open the child's mouth, and remove any **VISIBLE** foreign body.

D. RE-ATTEMPT VENTILATIONS USING MOUTH-TO-MOUTH OR MOUTH-TO-NOSE OR POCKET MASK.

E. IF THE CHILD'S CHEST *STILL DOES NOT RISE*, repeat the sequence of reopening the airway, attempt-ing ventilations, delivering abdominal thrusts, remov-ing any **VISIBLE** foreign body, and re-attempting ventilations ONLY ONCE!

F. TRANSPORT IMMEDIATELY IF UNSUCCESS-FUL, repeating Step E throughout transport if needed, and keeping the child warm.

G. Record all patient care information, including the pa-tient's medical history and all treatment provided, on a prehospital care report.

3–II. *IMMEDIATELY UPON REMOVAL OF THE FOREIGN BODY AND/OR ESTABLISHMENT OF CHEST RISE IN A CHILD OF ANY AGE (INCLUDING INFANTS), ASSESS THE CHILD'S VENTILATORY STATUS!*

IF THE VENTILATORY STATUS IS ADE-QUATE, SKIP STEPS 4 THROUGH 8 BELOW AND PROCEED TO THE ADEQUATE VEN-TILATION SECTION.

IF THE VENTILATORY STATUS IS INADE-QUATE (THE CHILD IS CYANOTIC, THE RES-PIRATORY RATE IS LOW FOR THE CHILD'S AGE, OR CAPILLARY REFILL IS GREATER THAN 2 SECONDS):

4. Ventilate at the rate appropriate for the child's age using mouth-to-mouth or mouth-to-nose, pocket mask, or bag-valve-mask. **ASSURE THAT THE CHEST RISES WITH EACH VENTILATION.**

> *CAUTION!*
>
> ADEQUATE VENTILATION REQUIRES DIS-ABLING THE POP-OFF VALVE IF THE BAG-VALVE-MASK UNIT IS SO EQUIPPED!

5. Supplement ventilations with high-concentration oxygen.

6. Transport, keeping the child warm.

7. Obtain and record the initial vital signs, and repeat en route as often as the situation indicates.

8. Record all patient care information, including the patient's medical history and all treatment provided, on a prehospital care report.

> **IF THE VENTILATORY STATUS IS ADE-
> QUATE (THE CHILD IS BREATHING SPON-
> TANEOUSLY, THE RESPIRATORY RATE IS
> APPROPRIATE FOR THE CHILD'S AGE, CY-
> ANOSIS IS ABSENT, AND CAPILLARY REFILL
> IS LESS THAN 2 SECONDS):**
>
> 4. Administer high-concentration oxygen (prefer-
>   ably humidified) by a face mask IF TOLERATED.
>   **AVOID AGITATING THE CHILD!** Admin-
>   istration of oxygen may best be accomplished
>   by allowing the parent to hold the face mask
>   about 6 to 8 inches from the child's face.
>
> 5. Transport, keeping the child warm.
>
> 6. Obtain and record the initial vital signs, and
>   repeat en route as often as the situation indicates.
>
> 7. Record all patient care information, including the
>   patient's medical history and all treatment pro-
>   vided, on a prehospital care report.
>
> _____
>
> Adapted from Manual for Emergency Medical Technicians. Emergency
>   Medical Services Program. Albany, New York State Department of
>   Health, 1990.

OTHER UPPER RESPIRATORY PROBLEMS

It is common for children to develop upper respiratory infections. Most of these are the common "cold"
or sore throat with inflammation of the pharynx and
tonsils. From the EMT's perspective three points deserve
mention.

First, as noted above, secretions in the nasal passage
can narrow the infant's and child's airway. Second, the
upper respiratory problem may precede more severe
problems such as croup and epiglottitis or even severe
tonsillitis. Third, a call for help when the child "has a
cold" should prompt a search for complicating factors
such as dehydration, exhaustion, or early, but not yet
obvious, onset of more severe complications.

LOWER AIRWAY DISEASE ✗✗✗

The primary diseases affecting the lower airways
in pediatric patients are bronchiolitis (less than 1 year
of age), asthma, pneumonia, and other infectious processes, and foreign bodies that are small enough to
pass through the trachea and lodge in the smaller lower
airways. While it is possible to differentiate among
these conditions in the field, the therapy is the same. Basically, the patient with difficulty breathing without upper respiratory problems is treated by reducing stress
and exertion, administering humidified oxygen, and
transporting with monitoring to a hospital.

BRONCHIOLITIS.   Bronchiolitis is a viral illness affecting infants (usually 2 to 6 months of age but up to
2 years) that causes edema and mucus production in the
lower and smaller airways. This follows an upper respiratory infection and often occurs in the winter. The
narrowing of the airways results in turbulence and
impeded air flow. Wheezing, rhonchi, and rales can be
heard. O^2

ASTHMA.   Asthma is a common and recurrent condition that affects children and adults. Asthma causes
bronchospasm with mucus and edema production, resulting in the narrowing and obstruction of lower airways. This causes an increased resistance to airflow,
primarily during expiration. Wheezing is heard, usually
bilaterally, and expiration is prolonged.

Patients can die from asthma when the obstruction
is so complete that no effective air exchange takes place
or when they become exhausted. When this occurs, there
may be no wheezing whatsoever and the patient may
be unable to speak. With severe bronchospasm, increased
resistance is encountered during positive-pressure ventilation as well.

Asthma can be triggered by different conditions in
different patients. Some triggering events are infections
of the respiratory tract, allergies, and the withdrawal of
some medications (such as stopping steroids). Patients
with asthma often have treatment at home in the form
of nebulizers, which release a mist of bronchodilator
drugs such as alupent, epinephrine, and bronchosol.
Theophylline and steroids are other drugs that are taken
orally for asthma.

Again, be wary of the child with an altered mental
status or one who becomes lethargic and wants to lie
down.

Should an asthmatic patient require positive-pressure ventilation, high resistance to flow should be anticipated. Be sure to maintain an effective seal and use
proper technique when ventilating this patient. Note that
in some cases, ventilation cannot be adequately accomplished without drugs to relax the airway constriction.
In these cases, rapid transport may be lifesaving.

PNEUMONIA.   Children, like adults, can suffer from
both viral and bacterial infections of the lower airways
and alveoli. Pneumonia often follows a simple upper
respiratory infection; this may be viral or bacterial. Usually the patient has a complaint or history of fever and
cough. Dehydration as well as signs of a recent upper
respiratory infection may be present. Children often have
a hard time describing the symptoms of pneumonia. It
is not unusual for pneumonia to present with complaints
of abdominal pain, since irritation of the diaphragm may
be interpreted by the child as abdominal in nature. Also,
signs of pneumonia such as rales may become apparent
a day or more after the onset of fever and cough. When
rales are present, they may be heard with or without

wheezing and on one or both sides. Pleuritic pain may be noted.

The key to management is appropriate attention to the signs of respiratory distress and application of humidified oxygen and ventilatory support as needed.

The protocol for respiratory distress summarizes the care of children with shortness of breath.

✻ P R O T O C O L ✻

RESPIRATORY DISTRESS (SHORTNESS OF BREATH, DIFFICULTY BREATHING, ASTHMA)

> BE PREPARED TO DEAL WITH RESPIRATORY AND CARDIAC ARREST! MONITOR THE RESPIRATORY STATUS CONTINUOUSLY. IN CHILDREN, BE ALERT FOR SIGNS OF INCREASING RESPIRATORY DISTRESS. THESE MAY INCLUDE DECREASED RESPIRATORY RATE AND/OR DEPTH, DECREASED BREATH SOUNDS, CYANOSIS, VISIBLE SOFT TISSUE RETRACTIONS, AND DECREASED LEVEL OF CONSCIOUSNESS. BE PREPARED TO VENTILATE A SLEEPY, ASTHMATIC CHILD WHO HAS A SILENT CHEST!

1. Ensure that the patient's airway is open. IF THE AIRWAY IS OBSTRUCTED, perform obstructed airway maneuvers according to AHA/ARC standards.

> *NOTE!*
>
> IF THE PATIENT IS A CHILD, MAINTAIN A CALM APPROACH TO THE PARENT AND CHILD. ALLOW THE CHILD TO ASSUME AND MAINTAIN A POSITION OF COMFORT OR TO BE HELD BY THE PARENT, PREFERABLY IN AN UPRIGHT POSITION.

2. Administer high-concentration oxygen.

> *NOTE!*
>
> In children, avoid agitating the child. Administration of oxygen, preferably HUMIDIFIED, is best accomplished by allowing the parent to hold the face mask, if tolerated, about 6 to 8 inches from the child's face

> *AND*
> Assist the patient's ventilations as necessary.

3. Place the patient in a position of comfort.

4. Obtain and record the vital signs, and repeat en route as often as the situation indicates.

5. Transport, keeping the patient warm.

6. Record all patient care information, including the patient's medical history and all treatment provided, on a prehospital care report.

From Manual for Emergency Medical Technicians. Emergency Medical Services Program. Albany, New York State Department of Health, 1990.

FOREIGN BODIES IN THE LOWER AIRWAY

Foreign bodies such as peanuts, food, plastic, metal, and teeth can be inhaled past the upper airway only to lodge in the lower airways. A cough is usually noted. The cough is initially nagging and unproductive in nature. Wheezing may be heard on one side, reflecting the bronchospasm initiated by the presence of the foreign body in the airway. Sometimes the problem is not diagnosed for a period of time after the foreign body is inhaled. In these cases, the child may develop fever and mucus production as part of a generalized inflammatory response. Anatomically, the foreign body is more likely to lodge on the right side since the right mainstem bronchus offers the more direct pathway at the division of the trachea. These foreign bodies cannot be removed by the complete airway obstruction technique but rather by *bronchoscopy* (visualization with an instrument) or surgical intervention. Treatment in the field is directed at respiratory support.

In all cases of lower airway disease, treatment is based on the provision of humidified oxygen, the reduction of exertion and emotional stress, and transport in the upright position (or position of comfort). Careful attention is paid to signs of respiratory failure and the need for positive-pressure breathing.

RESPIRATORY FAILURE AND ARREST

When faced with a child with respiratory failure or arrest, immediate intervention is necessary. Essential lifesaving steps are performed as you look for the underlying cause.

Establishing an Airway

HEAD TILT–CHIN LIFT. As in the adult, the head tilt–chin lift is the preferred method for opening the airway of an infant and child; it is modified by the degree of neck extension relative to the age of the patient. For infants up to age 1 year, do not hyperextend the neck. Rather, leave it in a neutral or slightly extended ("sniffing") position by elevating the back of the head with your fingers or a towel (Fig. 14–13). With children up to age 8, slight extension of the neck may be useful, with care taken not to "hyperextend" so as to avoid any kinking of the membranous airway. Of course the ultimate test of effectiveness for all techniques is the demonstration of air movement by chest excursion or audible exhalation.

Figure 14–14 demonstrates the jaw thrust-without head tilt for the infant and child. As with the adult, this procedure is used for suspected spinal injury victims.

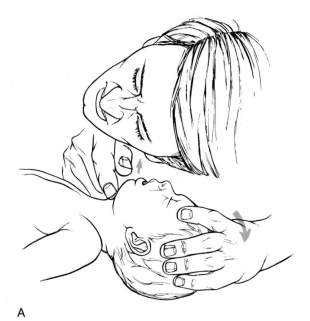

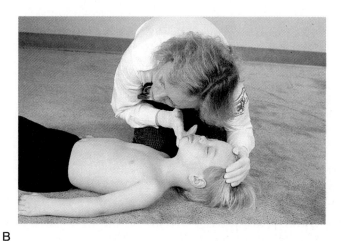

A   B

FIGURE 14–13. Using the head tilt–chin lift. (*A*) In the infant, keep the head in the sniffing or neutral position. (*B*) In the child, extend the neck back slightly.

Breathing

If the need for positive-pressure ventilation is established, provide two initial breaths and perform rescue breathing as in the adult with the following modifications.

VARY THE RATE OF VENTILATIONS ACCORDING TO THE AGE OF THE CHILD. Give one breath every 3 seconds for the infant, one breath every 4 seconds for the child up to age 8, and one breath every 5 seconds for the older child. *Use volumes in proportion to the size of* the patient. *Breaths should be gentle and given smoothly over a 1- to 1.5-second period* to avoid overinflation, gastric distention, and pressure-related injury such as pneumothorax.

A bag-valve-mask can be used to administer positive-pressure ventilation and afford the EMT a feeling of lung compliance during each ventilation (Fig. 14–15). Care should be taken when the device has a pop-off valve (pressure–release valve), since the airway resistance may exceed the pop-off valve setting, causing air leakage at the valve.

The pop-off valve is designed to avoid barotrauma. However, in cases where there is high airway resistance (e.g., resuscitation, asthma, near-drowning, etc.), the pop-off valve may release before adequate volumes of air can be delivered to cause chest rise. Pop-off valves can be closed shut with a finger or tape or in some cases by twisting.

Oxygen-powered breathing devices are not recommended for pediatric patients because high airway pressures may develop and cause tension pneumothorax or gastric distention.

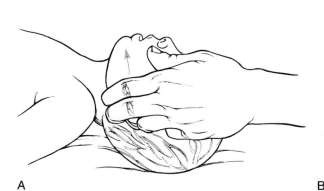

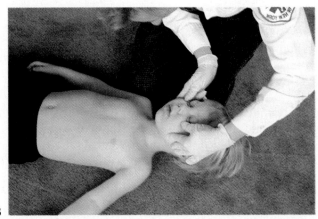

A   B

FIGURE 14–14. With suspected cervical spine injury, use the jaw thrust without head tilt. Place the fingers under the angle of the jaw and lift the lower jaw upward. (*A*) Infant and (*B*) child.

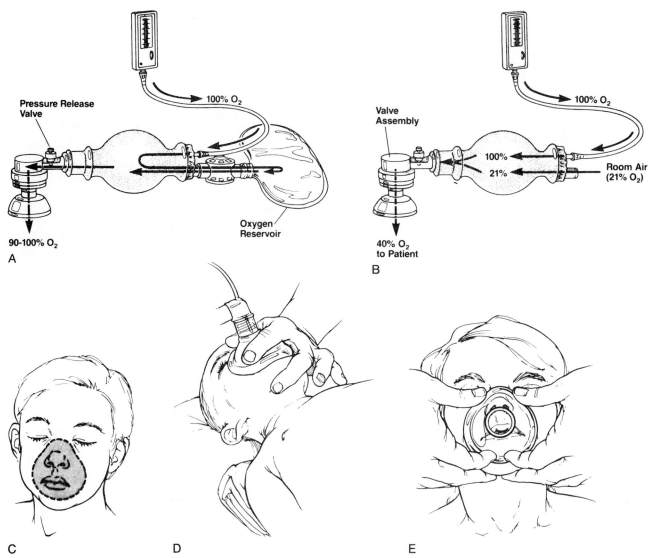

FIGURE 14–15. Pediatric bag-valve-mask technique. (*A* and *B*) Pediatric bag-valve-mask with and without oxygen reservoir (note "pop-off" or pressure-release valve). (*C*) Position of face mask. (*D*) One-handed technique for bag-valve-mask. (*E*) Two-handed technique for sealing mask. (Reproduced with permission. © *Textbook of Pediatric Advanced Life Support*, 1988. Copyright American Heart Association.)

Gentle pressure may be applied on the cricoid cartilage (Sellick maneuver) to help prevent gastric distention during positive-pressure breathing if the number of personnel permits this action. (Fig. 14–16). Place one finger over the cricoid cartilage (the ring right beneath the thyroid cartilage or Adam's apple) and press down gently. Gentle pressure is enough to help close off the esophagus and airflow into the stomach. Excessive pressure must be avoided, especially in infants, to avoid collapsing the trachea itself.

The mask and oropharyngeal airway should be selected according to the size of the patient. To measure the oropharyngeal airway, place the end with the flange next to the corner of the mouth. The tip of the airway should extend to the ear lobe. The mask should cover the nose without pressing on the eyeballs, and its lower end should rest on the chin just below the lower lip. Care should be taken not to press on the eyeballs, which could result in increased vagal stimulation and slowing of the pulse. Also, pressure on the soft tissues of the neck should be avoided, as this may result in obstruction of the airway. Again, when determining the volume to be delivered, chest excursion is the best indicator of effectiveness.

When rescue breathing is used, cover the infant's nose and mouth to establish an effective seal to avoid air leaks during positive-pressure ventilation. The child is ventilated with the mouth-to-mouth technique (Fig.

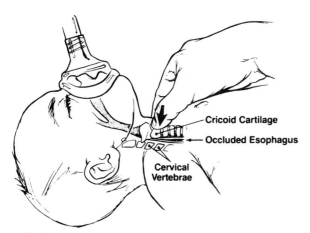

FIGURE 14–16. The Sellick maneuver is used with positive-pressure ventilation to avoid air flowing into the esophagus, thus preventing gastric distention. (Reproduced with permission. © *Textbook of Pediatric Advanced Life Support*, 1988. Copyright American Heart Association.)

14–17). If the chest rises, assess the heart rate, institute CPR, and follow the basic life support protocol. If adequate ventilation can be maintained by bag-valve-mask, pocket mask, or mouth-to-mouth or mouth-to-nose resuscitation, the patient should be transported in this manner with administration of high-concentration oxygen and suctioning as necessary. The DeLee suction is a practical method for removing liquid secretions from infants and very small children.

WHEN TO VENTILATE AN INFANT OR CHILD. You may arrive and find a child with respiratory distress and impending respiratory failure. Key signs of respiratory failure include cyanosis or mottling, very fast or slow respiratory rates relative to the age of the patient, little or no air movements, and labored breathing and retractions. Look for evidence of inadequate oxygenation such as altered mental status and dilation of the pupils, and also assess the heart rate and pulse strength. Hypoxia initially results in a rapid pulse as the heart tries to compensate but later leads to a slow pulse as the heart muscle becomes hypoxic. *The child who does not resist positive-pressure ventilation most likely needs it.* The child who resists your intervention is demonstrating a degree of oxygenation through his or her responsiveness and skeletal muscle exertion. Remember, of course, that hypoxic patients can become combative and make interventions difficult. When in doubt, ventilate and look for signs of responsiveness. If the infant is breathing inadequately, remember to time ventilations with the child's efforts to breathe. Otherwise, you are competing with normal chest expansion and therefore delivering smaller volumes of air.

Children who are fully responsive but experiencing respiratory distress should receive humidified, high-flow oxygen. The rapid addition of humidified oxygen at the highest concentration available can provide a small but crucial margin of safety and increase the likelihood of continued adequate oxygenation of brain and heart.

Again, children with signs of respiratory distress who are alert should be allowed to remain with their parents and be approached gently. Gently does not imply slowly, but avoid increasing this child's anxiety, which may increase the work of breathing and critical oxygen consumption.

Carefully review the following protocol to reinforce the management of respiratory arrest and respiratory failure.

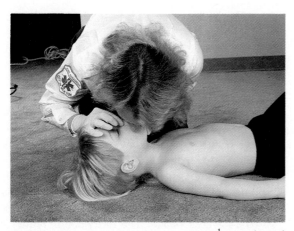

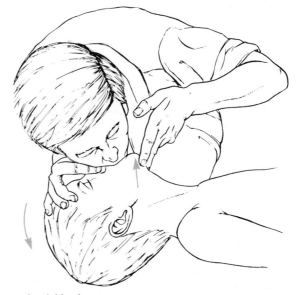

FIGURE 14–17. Use gentle breaths over 1 to $1\frac{1}{2}$ seconds until you see the child's chest rise.

✸ P R O T O C O L ✸

RESPIRATORY ARREST OR IMMINENT RESPIRATORY ARREST—PEDIATRIC

1. Establish airway control and ventilation using basic life support techniques according to AHA/ARC standards.

   a. Open the airway using the head tilt-chin lift or jaw-thrust maneuver.

   > USE THE JAW-THRUST MANEUVER IF TRAUMA IS PRESENT OR IF THE MECHANISM OF INJURY SUGGESTS THE POSSIBILITY OF SPINAL INJURY.

   b. Remove any VISIBLE airway obstruction by hand, and clear airway of any accumulated secretions or fluids by suctioning.

   > BE PREPARED TO PERFORM AIRWAY SUCTIONING WITH SUITABLE EQUIPMENT AS PART OF THE PRIMARY SURVEY!

2. IMMEDIATELY determine if the child is breathing adequately. IF THE VENTILATORY STATUS IS INADEQUATE (THE CHILD IS CYANOTIC, THE RESPIRATORY RATE IS LOW FOR THE CHILD'S AGE, OR CAPILLARY REFILL IS GREATER THAN 2 SECONDS):

   a. Ventilate at a rate appropriate for the child's age, using mouth-to-mouth or mouth-to-nose, pocket mask, or bag-valve-mask. ENSURE THAT THE CHEST RISES WITH EACH VENTILATION!
   AND

   b. Supplement ventilations with high-concentration oxygen.

   c. Insert a proper-sized oropharyngeal airway if the gag reflex is absent. If it is present, insert a nasopharyngeal airway.

3. Identify and correct any remaining life-threatening conditions noted during the primary survey.

4. Transport, keeping the child warm.

5. Obtain and record the initial vital signs, and repeat en route as often as the situation indicates.

6. Record all patient care information, including the patient's medical history and all treatment provided, on a prehospital care report.

From Manual for Emergency Medical Technicians. Emergency Medical Services Program. Albany, New York State Department of Health, 1990.

Near-Drowning

Over 5,000 children die each year of drowning. Logically, this occurs more commonly in the warmer areas of the country. Children aged 18 months to 3 years make up the most vulnerable population. In addition to drowning by falling into swimming pools, the inquisitive, fearless toddler also may drown in a bathtub, laundry pail, well, and rain barrel. Adolescents are another population that is over-represented statistically. This may be due to a combination of factors, including decreased supervision, increased risk-taking behavior, and coexisting alcohol and drug use.

Children fare much better following a near-drowning than do adults. This is especially true with a cold water immersion. There are numerous case reports in the literature of infants and children who survived prolonged ice water immersions. A few of these children had no signs of life when they were pulled out of the water and went on to full recovery. Overall, however, survival in the water is better when the water is warmer. But if there is prolonged submersion, freezing cold water may contribute to cell preservation and survival. The pathophysiology of drowning is the same for children as for adults. An important difference is that infants and children have an exaggerated mammalian diving reflex that shunts blood to the body core and slows down metabolism in response to sudden immersion in icy water.

All children found immersed in water should be immediately transported while the EMT performs CPR. In instances where the child is found in shallow water, you should consider the possibility of cervical spine injury and the need for in-line immobilization of the spine. A spine board can be used during the removal of such patients. When conditions permit, rescue breathing should be started in the water. At the first possible opportunity, high-concentration oxygen can be added. It is also important to maintain the patient's body temperature.

Sudden Infant Death Syndrome

The leading cause of death from age 1 month to 1 year is sudden infant death syndrome (SIDS). Each year about 8,000 infants die from SIDS in the United States. The incidence of SIDS in this country is *2 per 1,000* live births. The vast majority of children die while asleep and are found by their parents. This explains why the large majority of ambulance calls for SIDS patients occur in the early morning. Many of the children are in perfect health or might have had a minor respiratory infection prior to death.

SIDS is not an event associated with newborns, as it occurs beyond the first two weeks of life. The majority of cases occur before 6 months of age, with a peak at 10 to 14 weeks of life. The incidence is higher in late fall and winter (Table 14–9).

TABLE 14–9. SIDS Statistics

7,000 deaths per year (2 out of 1,000 live births/year)
Age range: 1–12 months; 90% less than 6 months
60% male
Appearance of SIDS babies
  Lividity (mottling in dependent areas)
  Cooling/rigor mortis occurs quickly (3 hours)
  Frothy drainage from mouth/nose
  Small marks (e.g., diaper rash) look more severe
  Appears well developed

SIDS can occur in any family, but the following are significant risk factors:

- Low socioeconomic group
- Adolescent mother
- Crowded living conditions
- Drug use during pregnancy (for example, a mother on methadone poses a 25-fold increase in risk)
- Black mother (poses a three-fold increase in risk)
- Native American mother (poses a five-fold increase in risk)

Risk factors associated with the birth are the following:

- Prematurity, especially if the baby had pulmonary complications and was on a respirator
- Multiple birth grouping (twins, triplets, etc.)
- Sibling of SIDS victim, risk increases from 5 to 10 times
- Near SIDS event, defined as any baby who has had an unexplained apneic event

There does not appear to be one cause of SIDS. Various theories offered relate to the immaturity of the neurologic system, poor control of the respiratory system, and airway compromise resulting in prolonged apnea. Whatever the contributing abnormalities, the result is cessation of respiration during sleep.

EMT AT THE SCENE

The scene of a SIDS death or near death is emotionally charged. There are two circumstances you may encounter. One is an infant who has been found by the parents in respiratory and cardiac arrest after a length of time, and the second is one in which the parents observed a period of apnea that was transient and now the baby appears fine. If the infant is not breathing, perform CPR and transport. If the infant is breathing, you should observe the baby for key signs associated with a postresuscitation or a thwarted sleep apnea experience. The child may have been resuscitated by a bystander or the parents by the time you arrive. The following observations obtained by your examination or the history given by the parents would indicate that the child has suffered a significant event:

- Is or was the child cyanotic?
- Was there evidence of shallow respirations?
- Was there evidence of respiratory or cardiac arrest?

Assess the child for the continued need for CPR and continue to monitor the infant en route to the hospital while administering humidified oxygen and keeping the infant warm. Additional observations that may prove useful to the physician to help judge the significance of the breathless period and events surrounding the illness include:

- Is the infant responsive or dazed?
- Is the infant's breathing labored or irregular?
- Is the infant's color pale, blue, flushed, or mottled?
- Is the infant limp, *hypertonic* (muscle spasm) or exhibiting jerking movements?
- Is there blood or vomitus on the bed sheet?

Unless the baby has clear signs of death (e.g., rigor mortis) and the parents are clearly aware of this, initiate resuscitation and transport. Avoid any delay at the scene. In the following months, the parents will relive this tragic event over and over again. They will feel better knowing everything possible was done that could have been done.

Parents may be experiencing denial, grief, and sometimes guilt. It is not unusual for victims of SIDS to have mottling in the dependent areas of the body, which may be confused as bruises associated with child abuse. Never be judgmental in these circumstances. If you suspect child abuse, report it to the physician at the emergency department. *Do not question the parents in a suspicious manner.* Your professional and tactful behavior in this situation is very important in helping the parents cope with the loss of their child. It is critical for them to feel that everything possible was done to save the child.

Twin siblings of SIDS victims may have an increased risk of SIDS or near SIDS. Therefore, a twin child should be evaluated and transported, and the history of a twin should be given to the emergency department staff.

The Febrile Child *take clothes off wet - normal water* ✓

Fever is common in children. In fact, a minor illness associated with a fever is the most common complaint that pediatricians encounter. Common misconceptions are that the fever itself is dangerous and that the higher the fever the more risk of causing a seizure. About 5% of children experience a simple febrile fit (see seizures, later in this chapter). However, it is not the increase in temperature that seems to trigger the seizure but rather the rapid rise of temperature. Therefore, the actual degree of the fever is not overly significant.

Children can mount a high fever with a simple viral illness or a fever can accompany a serious infection. In the absence of serious infection, children can tolerate high fevers quite well. Any febrile child should be transported with the final disposition and diagnosis left to the emergency department physician. The point is that it is not the fever itself but rather the cause of the fever that is worrisome.

It is common practice and a natural desire to cool down a febrile child. However, it is probably not necessary and may actually be dangerous. EMTs are not allowed to dispense or suggest use of medication; however, it should be noted on the call report if the parents have administered acetaminophen or aspirin. Aspirin use is now discouraged for children with fever because of the association of its use with *Reye's syndrome*. Reye's syndrome is a poorly understood syndrome involving the liver and brain, marked by coma and profound hypoglycemia. It seems to follow one week after chickenpox or influenza, and it has been linked to aspirin use in children.

A commonly taught practice to cool a febrile child is to cover the child with a cloth soaked with tepid water. It is important not to use alcohol or cold water because this only causes shivering and extremity vasoconstriction. The child is then at risk of an actual increase of core temperature due to peripheral vasoconstriction or, on the other hand, hypothermia that may occur during transport.

This same problem may also occur with use of tepid water soaks. The towels or sheets can quickly cool from the effects of the environment and become cold soaks. Given the high risk of hypothermia at the scene or en route, you should weigh carefully the use of this option. When transporting, remember that even a febrile child is at risk of hypothermia. The prehospital evaluation of temperature is done by simple tactile assessment. Actual measurement of temperature with a thermometer is not necessary and would only increase the time on the scene and act to disturb the infant or child.

Seizures

A seizure in a child is a common and usually controllable medical emergency. However, the sight of a seizing child is very frightening to parents and results in an emotional response that may interfere with optimal management. The seizure itself is usually not life threatening unless it occurs while a child is swimming, climbing or engaging in other such activities. As long as the airway is maintained, a child can tolerate a grand mal seizure in excess of 20 minutes without permanent damage.

Following is a review of the common definitions of terms associated with seizure disorders:

Seizure: an isolated event from an abnormal electrical discharge in the brain

Epilepsy: the tendency to have recurrent seizures

Convulsions: a seizure with a change in muscle or motor activity

Generalized convulsions: convulsions involving the entire body that are associated with the loss of consciousness

Focal seizure: involving one area of the body; not necessarily associated with an altered mental state

Petit mal seizures: extremely brief periods of loss of consciousness without loss of muscle tone, which are more common in children

The most common seizure that you are likely to encounter with pediatric patients is a simple febrile seizure. Approximately 3 to 4% of children between the ages of 6 months to 6 years with a febrile illness experience a febrile seizure. Often the seizure is the first sign of an illness. A simple febrile seizure is brief, lasting less than 5 minutes, and is associated with fever and a tonic-clonic (contraction and relaxation of skeletal muscles) generalized convulsion. The child is most likely to be in the *postictal* phase (lethargic, confused state following the tonic-clonic movements) of the seizure when you arrive on the scene, but the mental status is likely to improve during transport to the hospital.

A febrile seizure is considered complex if it is greater than 15 minutes in duration, if there is focality (localized to a part of the body), or if there are multiple episodes within 24 hours. Five percent of children with febrile seizures will present in status epilepticus. *Status epilepticus* is defined as a persistent generalized seizure lasting more than 20 minutes or a series of recurrent seizures without regaining consciousness.

Usually when you are called for a seizing child, the brief febrile seizure is over by the time you arrive. It is important to transport every child who has had a seizure, as there may be a serious underlying cause. Ten percent of children with meningitis have seizures, and in children less than 18 months of age, meningeal signs such as a stiff neck may not be present.

Causes of seizures in children are listed below:

Infections: encephalitis, meningitis, roseola, shigella

Metabolic disorder: hypoglycemia, hypoxia, fever, hyponatremia, hypocalcemia

Toxic substances: lead, aminophylline, lidocaine, cocaine, nicotine, phenothiazine, drug withdrawal, especially from prescribed anticonvulsants

Structural problems: trauma, bleeding, mass lesion, or scar in the brain

As opposed to adults, in whom vascular problems and tumors cause 47% of seizures, children have only a

3% incidence by these causes. On the other hand, infections, toxins, and metabolic causes are more common in children than in adults.

The mortality rate associated with status epilepticus is from 8 to 15%. Consider any patient who is actively seizing when you arrive as being in status epilepticus.

COMPLICATIONS OF SEIZURES. The complications associated with seizures are caused by their effect on many organ systems.

Respiratory problems encountered include decreased respiratory drive, airway obstruction by the tongue, risk of aspiration during the unconscious period, and ineffective respiratory muscles during seizure activity. All of the above can contribute to low oxygenation and retention of carbon dioxide.

Metabolic problems include rise of body temperature from persistent muscular activity, depletion of glycogen stores and blood glucose, and cell damage.

The central nervous system can be affected from prolonged electrical activity of the brain as well as from respiratory and metabolic complications.

Review the following protocol, which summarizes the management of children with seizures.

PROCEDURE 14-3
MANAGING A SEIZING CHILD

1. Protect the patient from self-injury and maintain the airway with the jaw thrust maneuver, if necessary.
2. Supplement oxygen delivery with a mask over the mouth and nose of the breathing patient or with a bag-valve-mask when necessary.

   Note: Do not force any objects into the mouth.

3. Try to cool the child with tepid water if he or she is febrile.
4. Ascertain if there is a history of previous seizures or other medical problems and if the patient is taking any medications. It is important to determine if any witnesses noticed the onset of the seizure. Did the seizure begin with a single body part (focal)? Inquire into the possibility of a toxic ingestion and try to determine the duration of the seizure and the time of onset.
5. On physical examination, assess the ABCs, the type of seizure, and the level of consciousness, and look for evidence of trauma, abuse, or dehydration.

P R O T O C O L

SEIZURE—PEDIATRIC

1. *Special Assessment Considerations*

   A. Establish and maintain airway control using basic life support techniques according to ARC/AHA standards.

   B. Use caution when opening the airway of a pediatric patient. Do not hyperextend the infant's neck!

   C. Protect the child from hurting himself or herself during the seizure.

2. *Treatment*

   IF THE CHILD IS HAVING A GENERALIZED TONIC-CLONIC SEIZURE:

   A. If the seizure is post-traumatic, use cervical spine precautions.

   IF THE SEIZURE IS NOT POST-TRAUMATIC:

   B. Place the child in the coma position unless airway or ventilatory maneuvers take priority.

   C. Open the airway using the headtilt-chinlift or jaw-thrust maneuver if possible.

   CAUTION:

   DO NOT FORCE ORAL AIRWAYS OR OTHER DEVICES INTO THE CHILD'S MOUTH IF THE TEETH ARE TIGHTLY CLENCHED. USE A NASOPHARYNGEAL AIRWAY IN THIS SITUATION IF NEEDED.

   D. Suction the airway as needed. AVOID STIMULATION OF THE POSTERIOR PHARYNX DURING SUCTIONING, AS THIS MAY CAUSE VOMITING.

   NOTE!

   BE PREPARED TO PERFORM AIRWAY SUCTIONING WITH SUITABLE EQUIPMENT AS PART OF THE EXPANDED PRIMARY SURVEY.

   E. Administer high-concentration oxygen (preferably humidified) by a face mask.

   IF VENTILATORY STATUS IS INADEQUATE (THE CHILD IS CYANOTIC, THE RESPIRATORY RATE IS LOW FOR THE CHILD'S AGE, OR CAPILLARY REFILL IS GREATER THAN 2 SECONDS), INITIATE THE RESPIRATORY DISTRESS OR ARREST PROTOCOL.

   F. Transport, keeping the child warm.

   G. Obtain and record the initial vital signs, and repeat as necessary en route as often as needed.

   H. Record all patient care information, including the patient's medical history and all treatment provided, on the prehospital care report.

Adapted from New York State Basic Life Support Protocols and New York City EMS Academy training protocols.

Trauma

Trauma is the number one cause of death of children from 1 year to 14 years of age, and the number two cause of death of infants. Many more children suffer debilitating injuries. A significant number of these deaths are preventable.

PREVENTION

The use of infant and child car seats, seat belts, and bicycle helmets is likely to significantly reduce morbidity and mortality. Educating the public on pedestrian and bicycle safety, the dangers of drunk driving, and child awareness is also important. Other environmental issues of importance are window guards, especially in urban areas; water safety; smoke detectors; fire prevention; and supervision of children at home. The use of childproof caps on medication containers has been shown to have significantly decreased the death rate from toxic ingestions in toddlers. Simple measures such as adjusting the temperature of household water heaters to safe levels (should not be greater than 130°F) could prevent serious scald injuries. EMTs should play an active role in community health education and prevention to reduce death and injury rates.

MECHANISMS OF PEDIATRIC INJURY

Children are less protected than are adults when subjected to blunt trauma. Their bones are more resilient, and forces are more easily transmitted to internal organs. Because of the resilience of the child's skeleton, clues to internal damage may be less obvious than in an adult. In addition, because of the child's small size, more vital organs are located within a small space and transmitted force can affect many organs before the force dissipates. This is important, because it increases the chances of multisystem injury and, therefore, the chances of dying. Due to the young and vital cardiopulmonary system, the child responds dynamically with initial compensatory mechanisms that can mask signs of blood loss. Serial examinations of the vital signs are necessary before vital signs can be felt to be stable in the traumatized child.

MOTOR VEHICLE ACCIDENTS

Statistically, for a variety of reasons, the youngest individual in a car is the most vulnerable to injury and death. As the car decelerates, the child or infant who is unrestrained or held in the parent's arms literally becomes a missile that smashes into dashboards and windshields. Ordinary car seats are not built to restrain a child, although there are some special car seats on the market that do this very effectively.

Children are also commonly victims of pedestrian accidents. Because of their size, children are more likely to experience direct injury to the vital organs from the bumper of a car. Most of these accidents occur in urban areas, where children often play in the streets. Male children from 4 to 12 years of age represent the largest group of pedestrian victims.

BICYCLE INJURIES

Children are often reckless on bicycles, underestimate their chance of injuries, and rarely wear helmets. In addition, they are often struck by motorists while playing near traffic. Common injuries from bicycle spills are abrasions, fractures, and head injuries. Children can strike the abdomen on the bicycle handle when they fly forward over the handlebar. Such injuries can damage internal organs such as the liver or spleen. The presence of tenderness or guarding is worrisome, but the absence of symptoms does not rule out a significant injury. These children should be transported immediately, with attention given to their vital signs and keeping them warm.

HEAD TRAUMA

Head trauma is a leading cause of death in children. However, with early attention, a greater number of children can be saved than can adults with similar Glasgow Coma Scores. Prevention of secondary brain damage is just as important as in the adult. Hypoxia and hypotension must be prevented and treated aggressively when encountered. Evidence of internal bleeding dictates rapid hospital intervention. Early diagnosis is important to prevent or treat increased intracranial pressure, and brief and serial neurologic examinations must be done to detect progression or deterioration. The Glasgow Coma Score is modified for age (Table 14–10). Pupil and motor

TABLE 14–10. Modified Coma Score for Infants

Activity	Best Response	Score
Eye opening	Spontaneous	4
	To speech	3
	To pain	2
	None	1
Verbal	Coos, babbles	5
	Irritable cries	4
	Cries to pain	3
	Moans to pain	2
	None	1
Motor	Normal spontaneous movements	6
	Withdraws to touch	5
	Withdraws to pain	4
	Abnormal flexion	3
	Abnormal extension	2
	None	1

(From Pediatric Annals 15(1):17, 1986.)

reactions are important findings that can be elicited rapidly and repeatedly.

NECK INJURIES

Infants have relatively large heads with small necks and weak cervical musculature. The head easily snaps forward on the frail neck musculature, which can result in devastating injury. As with adults, children with evidence of a head injury or violent force to the neck should receive immobilization of the neck. In general, the best immobilization is accomplished with the combined use of a high-cut rigid or firm cervical collar and a rigid back board. Infants and small children are apt to suffer from high cervical spine injuries (above C5), which can result in total loss of respiratory effort.

HEAD AND MULTISYSTEM TRAUMA

Children with head trauma also have a high rate of other organ or multisystem trauma. Accordingly, all children found with a head injury following a motor vehicle accident or fall should be evaluated and treated as a victim of multisystem trauma. The presence of head injury may make it difficult to assess other organs, so a high level of suspicion is necessary.

CHEST TRAUMA

The child's compliant chest wall allows damaging levels of trauma to be transmitted to intrathoracic structures without causing rib fractures. For example, there can be an underlying cardiac or pulmonary contusion without obvious external evidence. With healthy, pliable blood vessels, transsection of the aorta is rare in childhood. However, the compliance of structures within the chest and the relatively low pulmonary reserve volume (less ability to expand lung volume) make other conditions worse. For example, with tension pneumothorax the soft and mobile mediastinum shifts markedly and causes compression of the vessels, poor venous return to the heart, and obstructive shock. At the same time, pulmonary function is compromised. Hemothorax likewise can cause compression of thoracic contents. The child, like the adult, can lose a sufficient amount of blood in the thorax to bleed to death.

Rupture of the diaphragm occurs in children from severe motor vehicle accidents and falls, with the high abdominal pressure bursting the diaphragm and thrusting abdominal organs into the left side (usually) of the chest cavity. Pneumothorax from penetrating injuries or air from a rupture in the trachea, bronchus, or esophagus can result in respiratory compromise. Gastric distention, not uncommonly seen in trauma, causes elevation of the diaphragm and adversely affects the child in the same manner. All these conditions that displace organs in the chest cavity are more significant to the child because there is less pulmonary reserve volume.

A child may have none of these injuries but still be at risk for respiratory compromise from pulmonary contusions. Pulmonary contusions may cause slight edema or extravasation of blood and fluid into the alveoli. Initially, symptoms of respiratory distress may not be severe, but they can progress over a short time, resulting in an inability to oxygenate the victim. Therefore, careful continued evaluation of the child en route to the hospital, looking for a change in respiratory status, is warranted.

ABDOMINAL TRAUMA

Children have thin abdominal walls that provide little protection, and the organs that are subject to hemorrhage from trauma are relatively large. Force is easily transmitted across the abdomen and can affect multiple organs since they are packed closely together. Distention of the abdomen may be noted with severe hemorrhage. Since the hemorrhage from an abdominal organ can be rapid, and the child's condition can suddenly deteriorate after a period of compensation, the child with suspected abdominal trauma should be transported as soon as possible to the hospital, with the monitoring of vital signs and treatment of shock done en route. The most common internal injury in childhood is rupture of the spleen. An injury that is slightly less common but far more fatal is rupture of the liver. Injury to other hollow structures is also possible.

MUSCULOSKELETAL TRAUMA

The pliable bones of children break in different places than adult bones and often bend rather than break. However, the basic approach to injuries to their musculoskeletal system is the same as to an adult's. One difference is that traction may further injure the pediatric growth plate. Accordingly, traction is sometimes not used for femur fractures. Check local protocols for further clarification. Remember that a child also can bleed severely from a pelvic or femur fracture.

If hypotension develops, you may use the pneumatic antishock garment (PASG or MAST). The garment comes in pediatric sizes, and models are available down to 20 kg. Some pediatric surgeons maintain that the abdominal compartment should not be inflated because this might hinder the child's diaphragm from taking a full excursion. Follow your local protocols.

The following protocols review the overall management of the traumatized child and the management of shock states. Critical pediatric vital signs are also provided.

P R O T O C O L

MAJOR TRAUMA (INCLUDING TRAUMATIC CARDIAC ARREST)—PEDIATRIC

A. Establish and maintain airway control while manually stabilizing the cervical spine.

B. Assess the child's ventilatory status, including exposing the chest to locate and identify injuries.

   1. IF THE VENTILATORY STATUS IS INADEQUATE (THE CHILD IS CYANOTIC, THE RESPIRATORY RATE IS LOW FOR THE CHILD'S AGE, OR CAPILLARY REFILL IS GREATER THAN 2 SECONDS):

      a. Ventilate the child at a rate appropriate for the child's age using mouth-to-mouth or mouth-to-nose, pocket mask, or bag-valve-mask. ENSURE THAT THE CHEST RISES WITH EACH VENTILATION.

      b. Seal any open chest wounds.

      c. Supplement ventilations with high-concentration oxygen.

> *CAUTION!*
>
> ADEQUATE VENTILATION MAY REQUIRE DISABLING THE POP-OFF VALVE IF THE BAG-VALVE-MASK UNIT IS SO EQUIPPED!

   2. IF THE VENTILATORY STATUS IS ADEQUATE (THE CHILD IS BREATHING SPONTANEOUSLY AT A RESPIRATORY RATE APPROPRIATE FOR THE CHILD'S AGE, CYANOSIS IS ABSENT, AND CAPILLARY REFILL IS LESS THAN 2 SECONDS), administer high-concentration oxygen (preferably humidified) by a face mask as soon as possible.

C. Assess the child's circulatory status by palpating the brachial pulse in infants and the carotid pulse in children.

   1. IF THE PULSE IS ABSENT (TRAUMATIC CARDIAC ARREST):

      a. Initiate transport *IMMEDIATELY* while performing CPR according to AHA/ARC standards.

      b. Take appropriate steps to control hemorrhage.

      c. (1) Apply and inflate the leg compartments of an appropriate sized MAST, *OR*

         (2) Elevate the foot of the backboard 30 degrees if MAST is not available.

> *NOTE!*
>
> APPLICATION OF MAST SHOULD NOT DELAY TRANSPORT!

      d. Record all patient care information, including the patient's medical history and all treatment provided, on a prehospital care report.

   2. IF THE PULSE IS PRESENT:

      a. Search for any life-threatening hemorrhage and test capillary refill. If shock is suspected, go to step 3.

      b. Initiate transport IMMEDIATELY while assessing the circulatory status.

      IF CLINICAL PICTURE OF SHOCK IS PRESENT (TACHYCARDIA, CAPILLARY REFILL GREATER THAN 2 SECONDS, COLD CLAMMY SKIN, THIRST, RESTLESSNESS, AND/OR HYPOTENSION):

         (1) Apply and inflate appropriate sized MAST, according to the criteria for inflation, *OR*

         (2) Elevate the foot of the backboard 30 degrees if MAST is not available.

      c. Keep the child warm en route.

      d. Obtain and record the initial vital signs, including capillary refill, and repeat en route as often as the situation indicates.

      e. Record all patient care information, including the patient's medical history and all treatment provided, on a prehospital care report.

   3. IF LIFE-THREATENING HEMORRHAGE IS PRESENT:

      a. Initiate transport IMMEDIATELY while taking appropriate steps to control hemorrhage.

> RELATIVELY SMALL AMOUNTS OF BLOOD LOSS MAY BE LIFE-THREATENING IN SMALL CHILDREN!

      b. Assess for shock en route.

      IF CLINICAL PICTURE OF SHOCK IS PRESENT (TACHYCARDIA, CAPILLARY REFILL GREATER THAN 2 SECONDS, COLD CLAMMY SKIN, THIRST, RESTLESSNESS, AND/OR HYPOTENSION):

         (1) Apply and inflate appropriate sized MAST, according to the criteria for inflation, *OR*

         (2) Elevate the foot of the backboard 30 degrees if MAST is not available.

c. Keep the child warm en route.

d. Obtain and record the initial vital signs, including capillary refill, and repeat en route as often as the situation indicates.

e. Record all patient care information, including the patient's medical history and all treatment provided, on a prehospital care report.

> IF HEAD INJURY IS SUSPECTED, THE CHILD IS NOT ALERT, THE ARMS AND LEGS ARE ABNORMALLY FLEXED AND/OR EXTENDED (NEUROLOGIC POSTURING), OR THE CHILD IS SEIZING OR HAS A GLASGOW COMA SCALE LESS THAN 8, HYPERVENTILATE THE CHILD WITH HIGH-CONCENTRATION OXYGEN.

From Manual for Emergency Medical Technicians. Emergency Medical Services Program. Albany, New York State Department of Health, 1990.

P R O T O C O L

SHOCK—PEDIATRIC (OTHER THAN CARDIOGENIC)

NOTE!

FOR THE PURPOSE OF THIS PROTOCOL, PEDIATRIC SHOCK IS DEFINED AS SIGNS OF INADEQUATE PERFUSION SUCH AS:

1. ALTERED MENTAL STATE (RESTLESSNESS, INATTENTION, CONFUSION, AGITATION)
2. TACHYCARDIA
3. WEAK OR ABSENT DISTAL PULSES
4. CAPILLARY REFILL GREATER THAN 2 SECONDS
5. PALLOR
6. COLD, CLAMMY, OR MOTTLED SKIN

THIS PROTOCOL SHOULD BE USED EVEN IF THE SYSTOLIC BLOOD PRESSURE IS NORMAL OR IS DIFFICULT TO OBTAIN.

A LOW SYSTOLIC BLOOD PRESSURE (see Protocol: Critical Pediatric Vital Signs) MEANS THAT THE SHOCK IS SEVERE.

A CARDIAC CAUSE FOR SHOCK IN CHILDREN IS RARE.

1. Ensure that the patient's airway is open and that breathing and circulation are adequate.

> MANUALLY STABILIZE THE HEAD AND CERVICAL SPINE IF TRAUMA OF THE HEAD AND NECK IS SUSPECTED!

2. Administer high-concentration oxygen, and BE PREPARED TO VENTILATE THE PATIENT!

3. Place the patient in a face-up position.
AND
Elevate the patient's legs 30 degrees.

4. If available, apply and inflate appropriate size MAST according to criteria for inflation. (See Protocol: Critical Pediatric Vital Signs.) Inflate the leg compartments until the pop-off valves pop open.

DO NOT DELAY PATIENT TRANSPORT TO APPLY AND INFLATE MAST!

> IF THE PATIENT HAS AN EVISCERATION OR AN IMPALED OBJECT IN THE ABDOMEN OR LEGS, INFLATE ONLY THE MAST COMPARTMENTS NOT OVERLYING THE EVISCERATION OR IMPALED OBJECT!

5. Obtain and record the vital signs, and repeat en route as often as the situation indicates.

6. Transport, keeping the patient warm.

7. Record all patient care information, including the patient's medical history and all treatment provided, on a prehospital care report.

Adapted from Manual for Emergency Medical Technicians. Emergency Medical Services Program. Albany, New York State Department of Health, 1990.

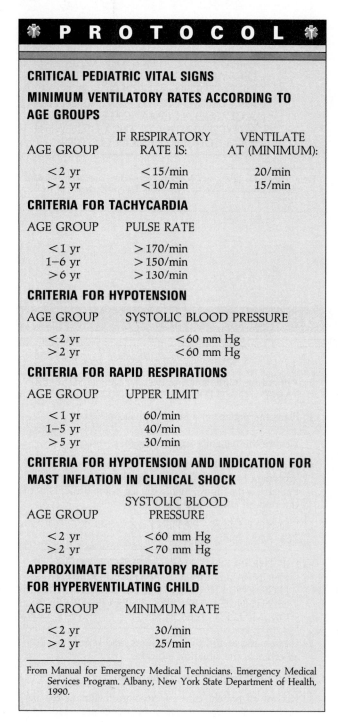

✠ P R O T O C O L ✠

CRITICAL PEDIATRIC VITAL SIGNS

MINIMUM VENTILATORY RATES ACCORDING TO AGE GROUPS

AGE GROUP	IF RESPIRATORY RATE IS:	VENTILATE AT (MINIMUM):
<2 yr	<15/min	20/min
>2 yr	<10/min	15/min

CRITERIA FOR TACHYCARDIA

AGE GROUP	PULSE RATE
<1 yr	>170/min
1–6 yr	>150/min
>6 yr	>130/min

CRITERIA FOR HYPOTENSION

AGE GROUP	SYSTOLIC BLOOD PRESSURE
<2 yr	<60 mm Hg
>2 yr	<60 mm Hg

CRITERIA FOR RAPID RESPIRATIONS

AGE GROUP	UPPER LIMIT
<1 yr	60/min
1–5 yr	40/min
>5 yr	30/min

CRITERIA FOR HYPOTENSION AND INDICATION FOR MAST INFLATION IN CLINICAL SHOCK

AGE GROUP	SYSTOLIC BLOOD PRESSURE
<2 yr	<60 mm Hg
>2 yr	<70 mm Hg

APPROXIMATE RESPIRATORY RATE FOR HYPERVENTILATING CHILD

AGE GROUP	MINIMUM RATE
<2 yr	30/min
>2 yr	25/min

From Manual for Emergency Medical Technicians. Emergency Medical Services Program. Albany, New York State Department of Health, 1990.

Child Abuse

Child abuse is a major problem. Only SIDS and accidents are responsible for more pediatric deaths. More than 100,000 children a year suffer permanent disability. This epidemic seems to be on the increase, with more and more reported cases each year. However, it is unclear whether the problem is worsening or whether there is increased awareness by health professionals, resulting in increased reporting. What is clear is that most children who suffer death or disability from child abuse have a previous history of a suspicious injury or suspected child neglect.

The majority of children suffering abuse are under 3 years of age. The younger the child, the higher the risk for abuse. Unfortunately, the most vulnerable are also most frequently the victims. Abused children and their siblings are often subjected to recurrent beatings. Unfortunately, we are probably underestimating and missing many cases of child abuse. This is certainly an area where prehospital personnel can play an important role. Only with early recognition can the morbidity and mortality of nonaccidental injury be reduced.

Abuse of children falls into categories of physical, sexual, and emotional mistreatment, and neglect. Most common is physical abuse, accounting for 80% of reported cases. This includes intentional trauma to soft tissues, the skeleton, the central nervous system, the viscera, the teeth, and the sensory organs, as well as intentional poisoning. One physician talks of the four Bs of active physical abuse: *Battered, Bruised, Broken, Burned* child. Most often you will see soft tissue injuries. Nonaccidental bruises and contusions are inflicted on all parts of the head and neck area and the trunk, including the flanks, buttocks, and extremities. With normal activity, children usually bruise themselves over bony prominences such as the forearm and anterior portion of the leg. Therefore, bruising over meaty areas is suspicious. Any injury with a pattern such as marks left by belts, bite marks, and electric cord marks are suspicious, as are multiple bruises in various states of healing (Fig. 14–18).

Unusual patterns of burns should also trigger the suspicion of abuse. Sharp demarcations are rarely seen in accidental burns. Note burns that have a shape or pattern. Any burn of the genitalia, or in fact any injury to that area, should be noted.

Intentional injury to the central nervous system (CNS) carries a particularly grave prognosis. CNS injuries account for only 15% of reported cases of child abuse but are the number one cause of mortality and permanent morbidity following intentional injury. An infant can suffer significant acute subdural hematomas from just being shaken vigorously without any external signs of injury. These babies can present with vomiting, agitation, seizures, and coma but may initially have nonspecific findings like poor feeding. Infants and children can also have chronic CNS injury that is usually associated with other systemic evidence of child abuse. Any fracture in an infant is suspicious, as are multiple fractures, especially when in various states of healing.

SEXUAL ABUSE

Harder to diagnose and harder to accept is the all too common problem of sexual abuse of children. This is a chronic problem, with the abuser usually being some-

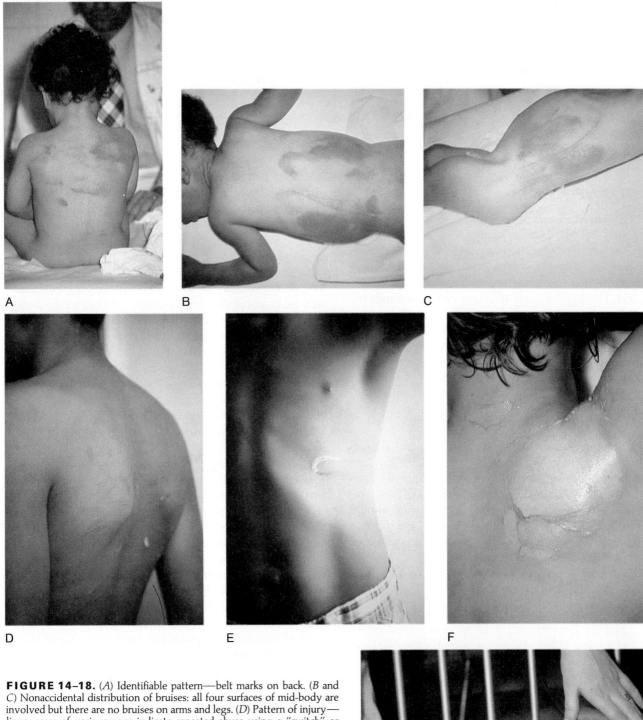

FIGURE 14–18. (*A*) Identifiable pattern—belt marks on back. (*B* and *C*) Nonaccidental distribution of bruises: all four surfaces of mid-body are involved but there are no bruises on arms and legs. (*D*) Pattern of injury— linear scars of various ages indicate repeated abuse using a "switch" or "whip." (*E*) Same patient as in part *D*. Loop pattern is consistent with a looped electric cord used as a whip. (*F*) Scald burn of shoulder and neck is typical distribution in "the toddler scald," which occurs when a toddler pulls a cup of coffee or a pan of water off a stove. This child was 7 years old and reported his mother threw a cup of tea at him. Perhaps not all "toddler scalds" are accidental. (*G*) Nonaccidental immersion scald—involvement of virtually the entire posterior surface of the legs indicates the legs were held under water, since even an infant this young would flex the knees to avoid the hot water. (Courtesy of Barbara Tenney, M.D.)

one known and close to the child. It crosses all socio-economic lines. Physical findings are often scant, but suspicion is raised by signs of external genital trauma or a child having difficulty walking. Frequently, children are reluctant to admit anything out of fear, guilt, and an unwillingness to break up the family. What is important for you to know is that you should take seriously a child's statement that someone is bothering him or her. Children cannot usually make up details about sexual advances.

CHILD NEGLECT

Children can also be subjected to more subtle forms of abuse. All children are entitled to adequate food, clothing, shelter, education, medical care, dental care, emotional nurturing, and appropriate supervision. Failure to provide this to a child is abusive and is considered neglect. These children are at risk for various self-inflicted injuries such as the unsupervised small child who accidentally sets the apartment on fire while playing with matches. These children are at as high a risk of growing up with severe emotional and development problems as is a child who is being physically abused.

OBTAINING THE HISTORY

The information you gather surrounding the occurrence of an injury is extremely important, but it would be unwise to undertake an investigation. Careful observation without accusation or confrontation allows you to transport the child to a hospital with the least amount of delay. This is in the child's best interest, and, once at the hospital, you can relay your suspicions and observations to the emergency physician.

As you obtain the child's history, the following should alert you to possible abuse:

- The parents' story is not consistent with the injury, e.g., the 9-month-old with an obvious deformity of a lower extremity, whose parents claim the child fell off the couch.
- The history changes, depending on who is giving the history.
- Witnesses give contradictory histories.
- The parent is reluctant to give a history.
- There was delay in obtaining medical attention.
- Timing of the injury is not consistent with clinical findings, e.g., "My child fell down two steps," but bruises are at various stages of healing and are scattered over the child's body (Table 14–11).
- Parents' response is not appropriate to the severity of the injury.
- The child is exhibiting inappropriate agitation with you or the family.
- There is obvious alcohol or drug use by the parents.

TABLE 14–11. Appearance of Bruises in Various States of Healing

Age of Bruise	Appearance
1–3 days	Red/blue
3–7 days	Purple
Greater than 7 days	Yellow/brown
Greater than 3 weeks	Brown to clearing

Pay particular attention to the environment, the sanitary state of the home, and any evidence of a struggle. Determine particularly the time of the incident, any witnesses, the history of recent illness, and the condition of the child's clothing (for example, the presence of blood or dried secretions).

The abused child may respond in various ways. The youngster may be overly friendly or withdrawn or may be inappropriate in responses, for instance, to pain. Be concerned about the child who is too good.

Be aware of your emotional response and be extra cautious to not ask questions in an accusatory tone. Try not to be judgmental. It may be helpful to realize that abusive parents usually want help and may themselves be victims of complex psychosocial situations. Often abused children grow up to be abusive parents.

Reporting laws vary from state to state. In your local area, you may not be legally mandated to report child abuse. However, you are morally and professionally responsible to set an investigation in motion if you suspect child abuse. All the laws are written so that one can report suspicions and be protected from litigation for false accusations. Those who are mandated to report suspected child abuse such as physicians and nurses, however, would be held legally responsible for failure to report on suspicion and can be subject to prosecution for failure to report. By careful, objective documentation of your findings at the scene and documentation of all subsequent conversations with health professionals regarding your findings, you are doing a great deal to help alleviate the problem of child abuse.

Summary

In the management of pediatric emergencies, the EMT must deal with an emotionally charged environment. The feelings of the patient, the parents, and the EMT must all be acknowledged. A professional and caring attitude that instills calm and confidence is required to enlist the support of the parents and the trust of the child. Approach children with respect and consideration for their developmental age.

Infants and children are not small adults. The differences in anatomy and physiology are of the utmost importance in both assessment and treatment. Children are dependent on others for basic needs. Although their hearts are strong and can compensate for severe insults, their small size leaves them vulnerable to sudden decompensation. Careful search for early signs of shock is critical to prevent collapse.

Control of the airway is most critical. Remember: control the airway and the heart will follow. Anatomic differences must be kept in mind in order to apply correct airway and ventilation therapy. A child's small airway is easily obstructed. Humidification, suction, and administration of supplemental oxygen can make a significant difference. A youngster's store of glucose is easily depleted, and maintenance of body temperature is important to conserve the child's energy stores.

REVIEW EXERCISES

1. List two developmental differences for the following ages of children and two ways this alters your approach to the patient:
   Infant
   Toddler: 15 months to 3 years
   Small child: 4 to 8 years
   Preadolescent: 9 to 12 years
   Adolescent
2. List one of the differences in anatomy and physiology of infants and children with respect to the following:
   Respiratory function
   Respiratory rate
   Pulse rate
   Blood pressure
   Metabolic considerations
   Neurologic differences
   Response to hypovolemia and shock
3. List the steps of the primary survey and the secondary survey for a pediatric patient.
4. List three signs and symptoms and the prehospital treatment for each of the following conditions:
   Croup
   Epiglottitis
   Foreign body obstruction of the upper airway
   Bronchiolitis
   Asthma
   Pneumonia
   Foreign bodies in the lower airway
   Near-drowning
   SIDS
   Febrile child
   Seizures
5. List five findings associated with child abuse.
6. List the steps of the approach to the pediatric trauma patient.

REFERENCES

American College of Surgeons Committee on Trauma: Advanced trauma life support: Instructor's manual. American College of Surgeons, 1985.

Glicklich M, et al: Steroids and bag valve mask ventilation in the treatment of acute epiglottitis. J Pediatr Surg 14(3):247, 1979.

Huerta C, Griffith R, Joyce SM: Cervical spine stabilization in pediatric patients: Evaluation of current techniques. Ann Emerg Med 16(10):1121–1126, 1987.

Ludwig, Fleisher: Surgical emergencies. In Textbook of Pediatric Emergency Medicine. Baltimore, Williams & Wilkins, p. 773.

Nelson KG: An index of severity for acute pediatric illness. Am. J. Public Health 70(8):804, 1980.

Schwartz GR, Safar P, Stone JH, et al: Pediatric trauma. In Principles and Practice of Emergency Medicine, 2nd ed. Philadelphia, WB Saunders, 1986.

Standards and guidelines for cardiopulmonary resuscitation and emergency cardiac care. JAMA 255:2954–2955, 1986.

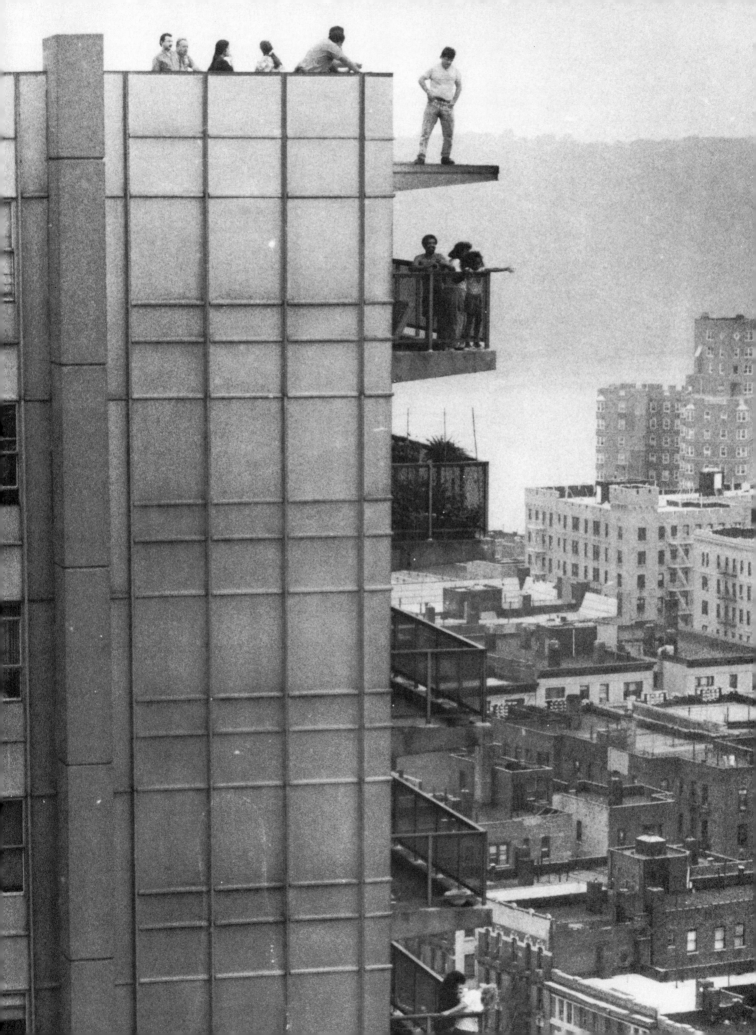

CHAPTER 15

PSYCHOLOGICAL ASPECTS OF EMERGENCY CARE

OBJECTIVES

At the conclusion of this chapter the reader will be able to:

---

1. Describe the scope of behavioral problems in the United States today.

---

2. List six guidelines for communicating with patients and their families.

---

3. Describe how to cope with a patient who has a personality disorder.

---

4. List five symptoms that a suicidal person may display.

---

5. Describe what an EMT should do when arriving at the home of a terminally ill patient who is nearing death.

INTRODUCTION

The Emergency Medical Services Act of 1973 outlined seven disease-specific categories around which EMS systems would be designed. Because the government recognized the seriousness of behavioral emergencies, they were included as one of the categories. Caring for patients with behavioral disorders is an area of medicine that is highly subjective, especially for those not specifically trained in psychiatry. Therefore, the standards and guidelines for prehospital care are necessarily general in nature.

There is probably no other area of medicine where the need for careful judgment and experience is more valuable or where there is a greater danger of displaying an inappropriate bias or reacting negatively to patients. This chapter serves as an introduction to one of the most complex areas an EMT will encounter.

Behavioral emergencies can be generally categorized by the type of behavior displayed, such as rage, anxiety, or an attempt at suicide, or by the cause of the behavior, for example, psychosis, hypoglycemia, or head trauma. Behavioral emergencies do not always occur in isolation; many times there will be an emotional component superimposed on an acute organic illness. This chapter covers the magnitude of the problem, types of behavior, their causes, and evaluation and treatment.

THE SCOPE OF THE PROBLEM

The medical profession often focuses its greatest attention on diseases and conditions that are understandable, measurable, and treatable, such as heart attacks and pneumonia. EMTs also receive most of their training on medical and traumatic conditions. It is easy for EMTs to get the impression that heart attacks are "real" problems and that behavioral problems are not as important. However, this is not true; behavioral emergencies present a great challenge and require a great deal of professionalism and compassion.

Morbidity and mortality statistics suggest that behavioral disorders are of major significance. Depression is said to be present in at least 5% of the population in the United States, with 10 to 20% of adults experiencing at least one episode of clinical depression at some time during their lives. It is estimated that 60% of patients seen by health professionals have underlying emotional disturbances that either cause or contribute to the reason for their visit. Depression is the most common mental disorder in elderly patients. Suicide is the tenth leading cause of death in the United States. About 25,000 people kill themselves each year. The rate of suicide in men over age 65 is at least three times that of the general population; more than 10,000 persons over age 60 kill

themselves each year. A young person attempts suicide every 90 seconds in the United States, and another is successful every 90 minutes. From 1950 to 1980, the suicide rate in the adolescent age group tripled. In fact, the death rate for the 15- to 24-year-old age group was the only one in which the overall death rate increased from 1950 to 1980, in large part because of suicide. Significantly, a large percentage of these suicide victims sought medical attention prior to the suicide. In many people, suicidal intentions and depression can be readily treated—if the diagnosis is made.

Medical professionals tend to discount symptoms in people who are difficult, demanding, angry, hysterical, intoxicated, or "crazy." This is an ordinary human reaction, but one that leads to dangerous medical judgment. It is unquestionable that many physical diseases present with behavioral manifestations and that many behavioral problems present with physical complaints. It must remain the goal of all health care personnel to diagnose and treat, and not to judge, discount the potential seriousness of a complaint, or (easier said than done!) become angry with a difficult patient. Remember that it is a natural tendency to discredit the importance of symptoms in people who are emotionally distraught. The interaction between the EMT and the patient often occurs in a highly charged atmosphere, where a person is intensely concerned about his or her well being, anxiety levels are high, and multiple distractions in the environment can interfere with successful care of the patient.

PRINCIPLES OF COMMUNICATION

General Guidelines

Although individual situations demand different types of interaction, and each EMT has a unique style, there are some general guidelines for communicating with patients and families that are useful.

FOCUS. Focus your attention directly on the patient, and maintain eye contact. Conversation between EMTs that is directed away from the patient may upset some patients and anger others.

DEVELOP CONTACT WITH THE PATIENT. Introduce yourself, informing the patient that you are an EMT and explaining your function.

TELL THE TRUTH. Although you may wish to limit what you say, speak truthfully and do not falsely reassure the patient. If you do not know the answer to a question, admit "I don't know."

COMMUNICATE EFFECTIVELY. Do not use medical terminology the patient may not understand, but on the other hand, do not talk down to the patient.

USE EFFECTIVE BODY LANGUAGE. The EMT's body posture and gestures should be calm and non-threatening. An aggressive "body language" can be frightening to the patient.

SPEAK CLEARLY. Speak slowly, clearly, and distinctly. With the patient who is hard of hearing, this may require a louder voice; however, avoid shouting, which may frighten the patient.

EXPLAIN TREATMENTS. Explain to the patient what you are going to do prior to doing it.

USE THE PATIENT'S NAME. Use the patient's proper name. Do not refer to a patient as "mom" or "dear." Referring to patients who are your seniors by the first name can be interpreted as being disrespectful. Also, trying to be the patient's "pal" or to "be cool" with the patient is inappropriate and phony. The novice EMT may believe such an approach may be more persuasive with the patient or may make it easier to enlist the patient's cooperation. However, professional demeanor will be much more effective and much less likely to precipitate a scene in which the patient refuses to cooperate.

ALLOW FOR RESPONSE. The patient should be allowed ample time to respond to questions and not be rushed. This requires expert judgment by the EMT, who must balance the time allowed for the patient to talk against the urgent need to stabilize the patient.

BE HELPFUL AND CONSIDERATE. Be aware of the patient's comfort. Is the patient cold? Is he or she in a comfortable position (if it is safe to reposition the patient)? Should a friend or family member accompany the patient?

LOOK BENEATH THE SURFACE. Try to sense the concerns and meanings beneath the patient's words. People call for an ambulance for a reason. A patient who states that he just needs his cardiac medications renewed may have been suffering from chest pain all night but may not tell the EMT this. Patients may deny their symptoms, but be alert when they have a sudden interest in keeping a clinic appointment, refilling medications, or wanting a "checkup."

BE PROFESSIONAL. Maintain a professional and calm demeanor at all times. Do not show anger or personalize a patient's negative remarks. Many people deal with stress and illness by becoming angry, making inappropriate remarks, or hurling insults. This is really just as much a part of the patient's "illness" as is the chest pain or shortness of breath. During times of stress, patients may not have the emotional strength or maturity to show appreciation for the EMT's efforts. Thus, do not be disappointed by the patient who is hostile toward you while you are putting forth your best efforts. The EMT must always be at his or her professional best, even when the job is a "thankless" one.

ANTICIPATE PROBLEMS WITH COMMUNICATION. Is the patient oriented, angered, hard of hearing, scared? What does the patient expect to happen? If there is resistance to your efforts, why?

ASSUME UNDERSTANDING. Always assume that the patient can understand what you are saying, even if it appears that he or she cannot. Avoid inappropriate remarks, and do not talk about the patient as if he or she is not there. It is common, for example, for stroke victims to be unable to speak but to be able to understand everything that is being said (Table 15-1).

Special Problems in Communication

ELDERLY AND CHILDREN

Be particularly careful to treat elderly patients with respect. Moving the patient must be done with extra care and a gentle touch. Be sensitive to the spouse's concerns, and allow the spouse to travel with the patient if possible. Again, remember not to address the patient by his or her first name.

When caring for a sick or injured child, allow the parent to accompany the child if at all possible. Objects such as a doll or special blanket will help make the child feel more secure. Interact with both the parent and child. If the child sees his or her parent accept the EMT, the child will be less fearful. As with adults, be honest with the child; do not make promises that cannot be kept. For instance, do not tell the child that he or she will not get a "needle" at the hospital when you do not know that for a fact.

DEAF AND BLIND PATIENTS

Deaf patients should be treated as having normal intelligence. The EMT should always look directly at the patient when speaking and should determine if the patient can lip read. If the patient cannot lip read, communication can be accomplished with short, written questions. It is important that the EMT not become impatient with the slow pace sometimes necessary for this type of communication. While performing procedures on the patient, the EMT should call attention to what is being done and, if necessary, write down an explanation. Incidentally, learning the alphabet in sign language, as well as simple signs for pain, time, and so on, can be accomplished quickly and is worth the small effort involved. Obviously, when a patient is deaf, the EMT should not attempt to communicate with the patient by shouting.

TABLE 15–1. Special Problems in Communication

Elderly patients
 Treat with special respect
 Move patient with extra care
 Be sensitive to the spouse's concerns

The sick or injured child
 Allow the parent to accompany the child
 Bring other objects that help make the child feel more secure
 Interact with both the parent and child
 Be honest with the child

Deaf patients
 When speaking to a person able to lip read, look directly at the patient's face and speak in a normal, slow voice
 Use short, written questions, if necessary
 Be patient
 Explain what you are doing to the patient

Blind patients
 Maintain physical contact
 Describe in detail what you are doing
 If patient has a Seeing Eye dog, bring dog with the patient or arrange for care of the dog

Patients who speak another language
 Use a translator if patient either does not speak English or if the EMT is unsure of whether or not the patient understands questions

Confused patients
 Use simple terms
 Give simple explanations
 Reinforce orientation and simple explanations
 Allow patient ample time to respond
 Assume that the patient can understand what you say

Mentally retarded patients
 Give simple explanations and reinforcement
 Determine capability of patient to understand
 Distinguish mental from physical disability
 Assume that the patient can understand what you say

Remember that blind patients have heightened senses of hearing, touch, and smell. The EMT should maintain physical contact with the patient and explain in detail what is being done or where the patient is being moved. If the patient has a Seeing Eye dog, the dog should either be brought with the patient or arrangements should be made for the care of the dog. During transport, the patient should be periodically informed as to what is happening.

NON–ENGLISH-SPEAKING PATIENTS

Patients who speak in another language or who speak minimal English should be interviewed through a translator. Speaking loudly in a language not understood by the patient is obviously ineffective. Some EMTs carry a manual of simple phrases in other languages for communication with such patients. In attempts to communicate with a patient who speaks minimal English, the

EMT and patient will often misinterpret and not understand each other; the patient may answer a question that is different from the one the EMT asked. If the EMT finds that the patient is having any difficulty in understanding, the interview should proceed in the patient's native language. Use visual clues to assist in translating questions and answers.

CONFUSED AND MENTALLY RETARDED PATIENTS

In approaching the confused or disoriented patient, the EMT should communicate in simple terms and try to understand what is causing the confusion. Avoid giving detailed explanations, and repeat several times where the patient is and what is being done. If the patient can respond, do not rush him or her; allow ample time for the patient to focus and respond to your questions.

As with confused patients, mentally retarded patients should be assisted by giving them simple explanations and reinforcement. The EMT should determine the level of communication appropriate for the patient, since some mentally retarded patients are quite capable of unsophisticated communication. It is important to distinguish mental from physical abnormalities. Although some patients may have physical malformations that give them the appearance of a mentally retarded patient, they may have quite normal mental faculties. As discussed before, always assume that the patient can understand what you are saying, and be careful not to say something that could insult the patient. Table 15–1 summarizes special problems in communication.

TYPES OF BEHAVIORAL DISORDERS

Situational Reactions

Situational reactions or emotional responses to circumstances such as a sudden illness, a death in the family, or some other difficult personal experience take many forms. These include the following:

- Anger
- Anxiety
- Paranoia
- Hysteria
- Denial
- Withdrawal

A great deal of sensitivity on the part of the EMT is required to successfully communicate with a patient experiencing such emotional stress.

Anxiety manifests itself as increased nervousness,

tension, pacing, hand wringing, and trembling. The patient may actually express this feeling to the EMT by saying "I'm scared." With *paranoia*, one sees a person who feels threatened by his or her environment and who may believe that someone is "out to get him"; such a patient might suspect that the oxygen administered by the EMT is a gas that is going to put him or her to sleep, or that the EMT is going to steal the patient's wallet. A person who is crying or screaming, refuses to communicate, and is obviously agitated and upset, is behaving in a *hysterical* fashion. The EMT might observe the patient crying uncontrollably and beating his or her fists repeatedly against a wall or throwing himself or herself to the ground. A person may manifest *denial* in a number of ways. For example, "He can't be dead" or "I just had a little chest pain; nothing's wrong with me" are expressions of denial. The EMT may arrive at an accident scene where someone has been killed and find the victim's friend sitting there, refusing to talk or interact with the EMT; this is *withdrawal*.

Personality Disorders

Personality disorders are character traits that interfere with a person's ability to function successfully in work or personal relationships. Such individuals are characteristically very manipulative and like to shift the responsibility and blame for events onto other people. The individual with a personality disorder will typically not perceive that he or she has a problem, although those around such a person certainly will. Such patients tend to be very self-centered and selfish. They are "takers" rather than "givers"; they demand attention; and they view themselves as kind, generous, and receptive. An EMT may encounter this type of person, for example, at the scene of a car accident. Having sustained only minor injuries, such a patient will still demand the EMT's time and attention and remain indifferent to the EMT's attempt to stabilize a more seriously injured person.

These patients can be quite trying and difficult to satisfy. There is no simple "trick" to dealing with them. It is important not to become angered by their behavior. Ignoring or belittling a patient's demands will only anger him or her. Be positive with the patient, but establish limits in a positive and professional manner. For example, saying "There's nothing seriously wrong with you; we have to take care of the other patient" will be interpreted by the patient as "We don't care about you; leave us alone." Instead, try saying something like "I see that you've hurt your ankle; we will try to take care of it as soon as we've made sure that the other patient will be OK." This shows that you are aware of the patient's injury and concerned about it, even if you cannot focus on it immediately.

Depression and Suicide

Individuals suffering from depression experience a variety of symptoms:

- Loss of sleep
- Loss of appetite
- Loss of sex drive
- Loss of pleasure in normally satisfying activities
- Feelings of sadness
- Feelings of guilt
- Feelings of hopelessness
- Physical symptoms

The depressed patient may describe feelings of sadness and sometimes profound feelings of guilt. Such an individual may express hopelessness, a key complaint that points to a significant risk for suicide. The person may hide his or her feelings quite effectively. Truly suicidal patients frequently seek medical attention for physical symptoms prior to taking their lives but do not express their depression directly. If the EMT sees a patient whose symptoms are difficult to attribute to an organic cause, suicide or depression should be considered as a possible explanation.

According to statistics, successful suicide attempts are more likely to be made by patients who have some of the following qualities:

- Single
- Socially isolated
- Unemployed
- Prior psychiatric history
- Recent loss of loved one
- Alcoholism or drug abuse
- Male
- Impulsive behavior
- Chronic or terminal illness
- Loss of job or status

Other characteristics displayed by those at risk for suicide would include impulsive behavior, chronic or terminal illness, and loss of a job or status. Although women attempt suicide more frequently than men, men are more often successful.

A person about to commit suicide will not always show signs of sadness or depression. In fact, a severely depressed patient who decides to end his or her life will often feel better once the decision is made because he or she knows that the period of suffering is going to end. Be very careful with the patient who says, "Nobody cares for me," or "I'll never be better." Be suspicious of "accidents" that could have actually occurred on purpose.

Sometimes a patient will make a suicide gesture (where the patient does not really intend to kill himself or herself) to get attention or for other motives. It is very difficult to distinguish between a gesture and a real attempt, and the EMT should always assume the attempt was real. Also, patients who make a suicide gesture will sometimes accidentally take enough drugs or other substances to actually kill themselves.

P R O C E D U R E   1 5 – 1
MANAGING THE SUICIDAL
PATIENT

1. When suspecting a potential suicide attempt, be sure to protect the patient from himself or herself.
2. Remove harmful objects from the vicinity of the patient.
3. Keep constant watch on the patient and *do not* leave him or her alone at any time.
4. Bring any pills, containers, or other materials that may assist in the diagnosis or treatment of the patient to the hospital.
5. If appropriate, have police accompany the patient in the ambulance.

Psychosis

The psychotic patient has disordered thoughts, distorted perceptions of reality, hallucinations, and inappropriate responses to the environment. Such a person will generally be oriented to time and place but may hear voices commanding him or her to perform certain acts, or he or she may have bizarre thoughts, for example, that the president of the United States has sent him or her on a secret mission or that the devil has captured his or her family. The EMT will have difficulty communicating with such a patient, who is often out of control and speaks incoherently or in a rambling manner that makes very little sense. Often the patient history will have to be obtained from bystanders, friends, or family members.

Organic Brain Syndromes

A person with an organic brain syndrome will also have disordered thoughts but, in addition, will be disoriented to place and time, manifest confusion, have difficulty with attention, experience varying levels of alertness, and may be incontinent. Asking the patient where he or she is, what day it is, and simple questions such as the name of the president of the United States will help clarify if the patient is oriented.

A patient who displays confusion and agitation would be referred to as delirious. Auditory hallucinations, in which the patient hears voices (often the voices tell the patient to do certain things, such as kill himself) are common both with organic brain syndromes and psy-

choses. Visual, tactile (touch), or olfactory (smell) hallucinations almost always have organic causes. An example of a visual hallucination would be a patient who sees a monster in front of him; an example of a tactile hallucination would be the person who is having a "bad trip" from LSD and feels spiders crawling under the skin.

The causes of organic brain syndrome are numerous. They include primary problems with the brain, such as tumor, trama, infections, or degeneration (e.g., senile dementia). They can also be caused by problems that are secondary to such conditions as low blood sugar, shock, or drug intoxication. Often, it is quite difficult to make the distinction between a person with psychosis and a person with an organic brain syndrome. It is generally safer to assume that the patient has an organic cause until it is proved otherwise.

Violent Behavior

A type of behavior that may overlap with any of those discussed above is violent or disruptive behavior. A variety of medical and psychological problems can ultimately manifest themselves in violent behavior, where a patient loses control and strikes out at the environment, endangering self and others. In general, violent behavior occurs in response to a person's overwhelming inner fear or frustration about his or her surroundings. It can often be averted by helping to prevent or deal with whatever is causing the sense of frustration and helplessness.

It is vital that the EMT recognize impending violence, first to ensure that he or she is not in jeopardy and then to assess what can be done to prevent an outburst. The EMT may recognize such a patient by the following signs:

- Angry voice
- Pressured speech
- Pacing
- Expressions of violence
- Psychiatric patients
- Drug intoxication
- Situational frustration

Psychiatric patients can easily become violent if threatened or subjected to prolonged questioning that they may perceive as inappropriate; a drug-intoxicated individual may suddenly and unexpectedly become violent; a patient subjected to delays in treatment or unsupportive remarks or who is scared by illness may react with anger or violence. Remember that a variety of toxins, drugs, alcohol, and metabolic abnormalities (e.g., low blood sugar or thyroid problems) can manifest themselves as violent behavior. Therefore, the EMT should look for clues in the environment, such as syringes, empty bottles of pills, fire (possible inhalation of carbon monoxide), or signs of trauma.

EVALUATION AND TREATMENT OF BEHAVIORAL DISORDERS

General Guidelines

The following guidlines are helpful when approaching patients who may be violent or uncooperative.

BE THE PATIENT'S ADVOCATE. Be helpful within reasonable and appropriate limits. Many health professionals have "their way" of doing things and refuse input from the patient. Anticipate which patients might present difficulties and offer them alternatives; allow them to make some choices in their treatment. For example, if a patient needs oxygen but is likely to refuse it, the EMT may offer the patient a choice between a face mask or nasal prongs. In this way, the patient feels that he or she is making a choice about the treatment, and the EMT accomplishes his or her desired objective. Also, there is no reason not to offer to help dress the patient or to help perform some other simple task. Although this is not in any "job description," it is helpful and often necessary to obtain the patient's cooperation.

COLLECT A HISTORY. Get as much history as possible regarding the patient's state. Is the behavioral disorder chronic or acute? If acute, when did it occur? What events occurred at about the same time? Might the patient have been exposed to toxins, taken drugs, or sustained trauma? Is there any past medical history? Is the patient wearing a medical alert tag? Was there a recent family event or other situation that could have caused emotional distress?

BE ACUTELY AWARE OF CIRCUMSTANCES. Detect the potential for violence in the patient's posture and attitude. Beware of a patient who is making menacing gestures or verbal threats of physical violence. Obtain police assistance if necessary.

KEEP COOL AND CALM. A patient who is deeply frustrated can be provoked by inappropriate remarks, hasty actions, or indifference to his or her concerns. If you radiate a sense of control and calmness, the patient will feel more secure and may be less prone to violence.

BE UNDERSTANDING. Try to understand the problem from the patient's point of view. The patient should be encouraged to ventilate his or her anger. Do not accuse or return anger or lecture the patient.

DESIGNATE ONE PERSON TO COMMUNICATE. Having one person as the primary communicator will keep the patient from feeling confused or threatened and can help him or her regain emotional control.

USE MINIMAL FORCE. In circumstances where all else fails, the patient may have to be subdued and restrained by appropriate personnel. Sometimes, if there are enough people to overwhelm the patient, the mere presence of a group will allow the violent patient to "give up" and cease resisting. In such a case, observation without restraints may be adequate. Often, particularly when it is extremely difficult to examine the patient, taking frequent vital signs will help the patient quiet down. If restraints are necessary, the straps should be padded and the patient should be positioned to allow for treatment of any medical problems.

STRESS AND CRISIS EVENTS

Death

When approaching the family of a person who has died, the EMT should be prepared for a variety of emotional responses, including denial, guilt, grief, anger, hysteria, withdrawal, or physical reactions. Of course, when arriving on the scene, treatment of the patient is of first priority, and CPR should be initiated unless specifically contraindicated by local or state guidelines. The EMT should be honest and straightforward and keep the family informed. Encourage emotional responses such as crying.

The EMT should adhere to the family's wishes to be alone or to see the body of the deceased. If the body is mutilated, the mutilated parts should be covered. Suggest that the family members seek follow-up counseling with a family physician, minister, or other resource person who can help them through the grieving process.

Particularly with unexpected deaths, as in cases of suicide or the death of younger patients who have been in good health, the family's emotional reaction can be very strong. The family is often in a state of disbelief or may manifest tremendous feelings of guilt or want to blame others for the death. It is absolutely essential that the EMT be supportive and make no judgmental comments, such as, "You should have brought him to the hospital" or "If only you had called earlier . . . ." In the face of any expressions of guilt by the family, the EMT should be supportive and avoid any comments that imply they were responsible for wrongdoing.

A family will often call for an ambulance long after the patient has died. The patient might be found dead in bed or might have been left alone for some time. As stated earlier, if there is any question as to the time of death, CPR should be initiated. Signs of rigor mortis or dependent lividity would indicate irreversibility. In these circumstances, the EMT must compassionately inform the family of the patient's death.

Terminal Illness

When treating a terminally ill patient, the EMT must allow the patient to express his or her feelings of denial, acceptance, peace, anger, depression, or relief. Acting in a calm, supportive manner will greatly benefit such patients. Since the patient and family have had time to adapt to the approaching death, emotions tend to be less charged. Of course, the EMT must medically act within appropriate protocols on the patient's behalf.

The EMT should not make denials if the patient indicates that he or she is dying. Often the patient will be looking for human warmth and communication and wish for his or her last minutes of life to be honest and direct. Such a desire should be met with compassion and an acknowledgment of what the patient is saying. It is inappropriate to offer false assurances.

The patient or family may want the patient transported to the hospital, which can provide comfort, pain relief, and support to terminally ill patients. Treatment of secondary complications, such as infection, may substantially prolong life or make the patient more comfortable.

When arriving on the scene, the EMT should assess the patient's and family's knowledge of the patient's condition. For instance, the family may know that the patient has terminal lung cancer, but the patient himself or herself may not be aware of this. Under this circumstance, it is not wise for the EMT to inform the patient of the diagnosis. However, should the patient know his or her diagnosis and want to discuss it, the EMT should not hesitate to use words that the patient uses, such as "cancer" or "death." If death is imminent, as manifested by hypotension or agonal respirations, it is appropriate to alert the family. The EMT could say "The patient has very weak vital signs" or "The signs of life are very weak."

The family should be allowed to be with the patient and to travel with the patient in the ambulance. If the patient or patient's family refuses treatment, it is best to contact medical control for guidance. The medical control physician can advise on the appropriateness of withholding treatment and allowing the patient to die based on local and state guidelines and laws regarding living wills (in which the patient has determined that particular types of treatment should not be initiated). If there is any doubt about withholding treatment, full effort should be directed toward resuscitating the patient.

The EMT should record the patient's final words (the "dying declaration") about his or her medical condition or statements to others. These pronouncements may be very meaningful to family members.

Victims of Crimes

Victims of crimes (e.g., rape, assault, attempted murder) and victims of abuse (e.g., child abuse, spouse abuse, parent abuse, family abuse) can provoke great sympathy, disgust, or anger in the EMT. It is most important to be calm, supportive, and nonjudgmental toward the patient and his or her family or friends. As always, the first priority is to dispense appropriate medical care to the patient. The EMT also cooperates with law enforcement officials to collect evidence, insofar as it does not interfere with the patient's care or rights.

Although many patients may display anger, violence, disbelief, hysteria, or extreme agitation in response to the event, others may be quiet and withdrawn, feel severely depressed, and experience shame and a profound sense of guilt ("I brought this on myself").

Particularly in cases of rape, but also in other cases of abuse, the patient has had control taken away; it is important to let the patient regain control. Allow the patient to ventilate his or her feelings, but do not push the patient to reveal specific details not related to prehospital treatment. Remember, particularly with rape cases, that the patient might be quite embarrassed. Although the EMT needs to determine if any significant injuries are present, more specific questioning is best done by medical personnel in the hospital.

To cooperate with law enforcement personnel, the EMT should not move or touch things in the patient's environment, except what is necessary to evaluate and treat the patient. If clothing must be cut, the EMT should note whether it was previously torn. List all injuries, and try to note the patient's comments word for word. The EMT may be called on to testify at a later date, so good record keeping is vital. Again, the EMT's first duty is to the patient, and care should not be delayed for legal reasons.

When managing a victim of crime, remember the following points:

- Administer appropriate medical care.
- Cooperate with law enforcement officials.
- Be calm, supportive, nonjudgmental.
- Help the patient to regain control.
- Help the patient to ventilate feelings.
- Obtain those details necessary for the management of the patient.
- Keep careful records.

The EMT's Response to Death

Dealing with death is quite difficult for anyone in the health field, because it represents the ultimate failure in caring for patients. It is common to feel helpless and inadequate or even embarrassed at being unable to save a patient. Sometimes EMTs may try to avoid interacting with the patient's family because of a sense of failure or guilt. Some will become hyperclinical, make inappropriate remarks, or try to relieve tension with humor.

The EMT must have an outlet for dealing with his or her inner feelings. This can be accomplished by talking about them with colleagues, a close friend or spouse, or a professional counselor. These feelings should *not* be dealt with in front of patients and their families. Each EMT's reaction is dependent on his or her personality, sense of stability, sense of duty, understanding of personal limitations, and philosophical and religious beliefs.

Many situations are overwhelming, such as the death of a child or a patient with whom the EMT identifies because of a similarity in background, age, or profession. Disasters with multiple deaths can be quite traumatic for the medical personnel caring for the victims; the panic, chaos, sights of mutilation, and feelings of being overwhelmed leave their emotional imprint. It has even been recommended recently that all medical personnel participating in disaster relief undergo a "debriefing," where feelings can be discussed and, hopefully, resolved.

Some EMTs will deny any significant emotional reaction to their work and will bury their feelings inside themselves. There are key symptoms, however, that often indicate the need to seek help. These include:

- Nightmares
- Inability to control one's temper
- Feelings of sadness
- Feelings of guilt
- Loss of appetite
- Loss of sex drive
- Loss of sleep
- Loss of pleasure in activities normally satisfying
- Sense of hopelessness
- Accusatory behavior
- Desire to leave the scene quickly
- Feelings of not being appreciated
- Apathy toward work
- Unable to accept criticism
- Wishing to quit work
- Physical symptoms
- Alcohol or drug misuse

It is vital that every EMT learn to recognize and admit his or her reactions and feelings and be willing to discuss them with a coworker, medical director, or counselor.

REVIEW EXERCISES

1. List six factors in effective communication with patients.

2. List three special considerations in dealing with each of the following patients:

Elderly patients
Sick or injured child
Deaf patients
Blind patients
Confused patients
Mentally retarded patients

3. Provide three examples of situational reactions.

4. List six symptoms of depression.

5. List seven risk factors of suicide.

6. Describe the basic management of the suicidal patient.

7. List five symptoms of the potentially violent patient.

8. List six general guidelines in the evaluation and treatment of behavioral disorders.

9. List the steps of management of the potentially violent patient.

10. Describe four typical negative responses to death that may be exhibited by the EMT.

11. List seven symptoms of job-related stress.

REFERENCES

Barry M: Therapeutic experience with patients referred for "prolonged grief reaction"—Some second thoughts. Mayo Clin Proc 56:744, 1981.

Bauer B, Hill S: Essentials of Mental Health Care: Planning and Interventions. Philadelphia, WB Saunders, 1986.

Burnum J: Diagnosis of depression in a general medical practice: Observations on "lack of pizzazz," the "blahs," and other complaints. Postgrad Med 72(3):71, 1982.

Edwards FJ: Psychiatric emergencies. EMS 14(3):46, 1985.

Gold M, Pottash C: Depression: Diagnosis and treatment with tricyclic antidepressants. Postgrad Med 69(6):104, 1981.

Guze SB: Early recognition of depression. Hosp Pract 16(9):87, 1981.

Judd R, Peszke M (eds): Psychological and behavioral emergencies. Top Emerg Med 4(4), 1983.

Kiely W: Psychiatric syndromes in critically ill patients. JAMA 235:2759, 1976.

Melson S, Rynearson EK: Unresolved bereavement: Medical reenactment of a loved one's terminal illness. Postgrad Med 72:172, 1982.

Motto J: Identifying and treating suicidal patients in a general medical setting. Res Staff Phys 3/83/79.

Osgood N: Suicide in the elderly: Are we heeding the warnings? Postgrad Med 72(2):123, 1982.

Osgood N: Identifying and counseling the suicidal geriatric patient. Geriatr Med Today 4(3):83, 1985.

Perry S, Gilmore M: The disruptive patient or visitor. JAMA 245:755, 1981.

Rabin P, et al: Crisis intervention in an emergency setting. Ann Emerg Med 12:300, 1983.

Twerski A: Over the edge. Emerg Med 15:169, 1979.

Wise M: Posttraumatic stress disorder: The human reaction to catastrophe. Drug Ther 3/83/97.

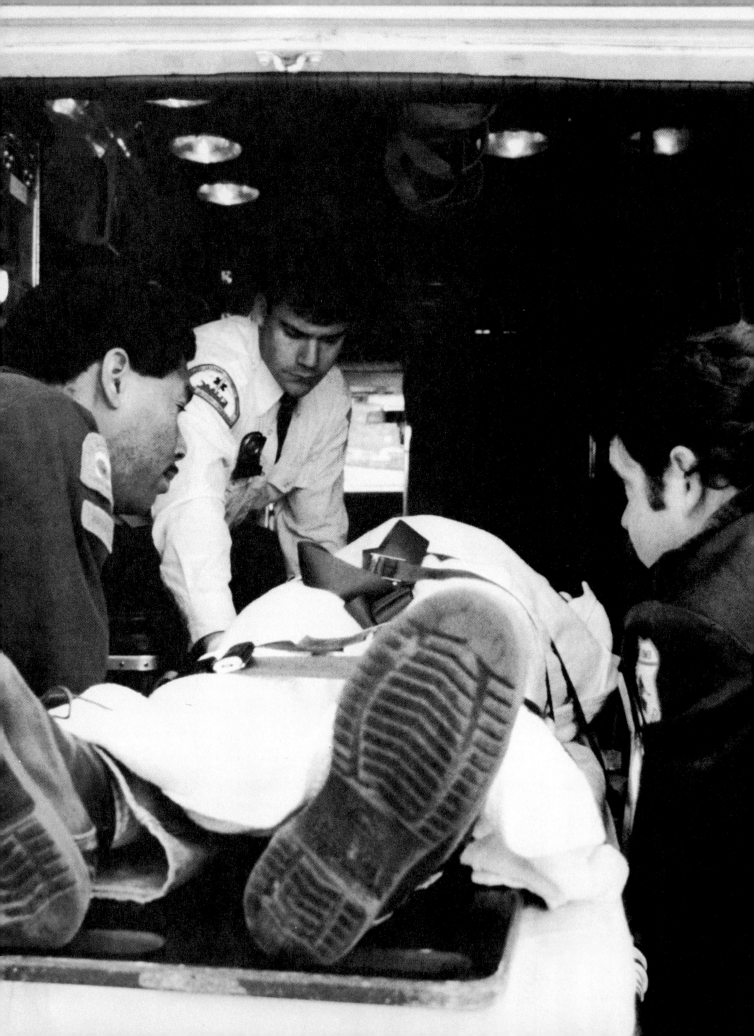

CHAPTER 16

LIFTING AND MOVING PATIENTS

OBJECTIVES

At the conclusion of this chapter the reader will be able to:

1. Perform direct two-rescuer lift of a patient from the ground and then position him or her on a stretcher.

2. Immobilize the neck and spine of a patient using a short board.

3. Immobilize the patient on a long board and move the patient to a stretcher.

4. Properly position a patient on a stretcher and load and unload the stretcher from all carrying positions in the ambulance.

OVERVIEW

The Purpose of Lifts and Carries

Each situation requires its own unique strategy for lifting and moving the patient. Factors including available personnel, terrain, hazards, and, most important, the condition of the patient influence the manner in which you remove and transport the patient from the scene. Optimally, a patient should not be moved until he or she has been splinted and prepared for transport. There are, of course, exceptions to this rule. If remaining on the scene will endanger the patient, you naturally must remove the patient from the area first and deal with specific injuries later. The selection of the appropriate lift and carry technique is as much a part of your patient care as splinting, bandaging, or administering oxygen therapy. In the case of the spinal injury victim, the appropriate lift and carry is often the most important aspect of treatment.

Improper lifting and carrying of the patient is not hazardous to only your patient. A back injury can last a lifetime, and guarding yourself against this possibility should be a major concern to you. Learning and practicing the proper scientific techniques for lifting and carrying patients as described in this chapter can help minimize the chance that you will sustain an injury.

Decision to Transport

It is not always possible to stabilize the patient before moving him or her. When a fire threatens to engulf the patient or the rescuers, the risk of staying to splint or bandage the patient far outweighs the benefits. If you must move a patient quickly, there are methods that minimize the chances of aggravating existing injuries. In each situation, you must weigh the potential hazards to the patient and others against the need for specific interventions. A person who is bleeding internally may exsanguinate if rapid surgical intervention is not obtained in a timely fashion. In this instance, you cannot take the time to apply a short spine board but must rapidly extricate the victim and transport him or her to a trauma center while performing essential life support measures en route. A patient with a complete airway obstruction that cannot be relieved by basic life support procedures also requires rapid transport. In highway accidents you may be unable to safely secure the scene, and caring for a patient in such a setting places you and the patient in jeopardy. Other circumstances that call for moving the patient rapidly from the scene include radiation accidents, the possibility of exposure to hazardous materials, the presence of toxic gases, or other situations in which environmental hazards exist.

As an EMT, you must integrate the time to transport into your overall treatment strategy for the patient.

Body Mechanics

The scientific use of specific, predetermined methods of efficiently lifting large weights so as not to injure oneself is known as body mechanics. The human body is composed of a system of levers and support structures that, if used correctly, can support a great deal of weight. However, if used incorrectly, severe and permanent injury can result. Know your physical capabilities and limitations, seek help when needed, and do not attempt to move a patient if you feel you cannot lift him or her.

CORRECT TECHNIQUE. The long bones of the body are the strongest bones. The largest of these is the femur, which also is surrounded by the largest and strongest muscle group in the body. Therefore, these are the support units you should use when attempting to lift heavy objects. Never lift with your back, as the back muscles that support the spinal column are relatively small and weak, which makes them prone to injury. The legs are used by bending them prior to lifting while maintaining the back as straight as possible. When lifting a patient from the ground, squat and place one foot in front of the other. Always get as close as possible to the person you are lifting, and keep your arms close to your body as you lift. This places your center of gravity closer to the patient, giving you more leverage and, in effect, making the patient lighter. At the same time, this helps you to maintain your balance. A see-saw illustrates the value of this closeness. When you are sitting toward the center of the see-saw, it is easier for your partner to raise you. As you move toward the very edge, it becomes much more difficult.

When holding or moving a stretcher, keep your back straight and tighten the muscles of your abdomen and buttocks, which provide the main support for your back. Maintain a firm grip on the device or patient and lift and move it slowly and smoothly and in unison with your partner (Fig. 16–1). Twisting or using sharp, jerky movements is more likely to result in an injury to you and discomfort to the patient. Always maintain firm footing and try not to keep your muscles contracted for too long a period of time, as this induces fatigue and increases the possibility of muscle strain or injury.

EMERGENCY EVACUATION TECHNIQUES

There are several methods of removing patients from a scene quickly. The one you choose for each

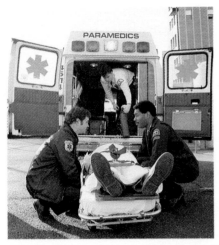

FIGURE 16-1. Proper body mechanics during lifting.

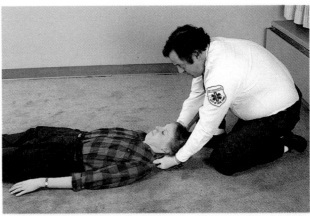

FIGURE 16-2. Grasp the patient's shirt or coat at the shoulder region and support the patient's head in your arms while dragging him or her to a safe location.

situation depends upon the number of rescue personnel available, the terrain over which you must move the patient, and the size of the patient. You should never attempt to lift a patient who you cannot fully support.

One-Rescuer Techniques

CLOTHES DRAG.   The simplest technique, which is also readily available for quickly moving a patient in almost all situations, is the clothes drag technique. In this technique, you grasp the shirt, sweater, or jacket of the patient and drag him or her, always along the long axis of the body (Fig. 16–2). An alternate technique for the clothes drag is the foot drag (Fig. 16–3).

BLANKET DRAG.   If a blanket is available, the blanket drag is preferable to the clothes or foot drag. It permits a long axis pull without dragging the patient's clothes or skin on the ground, and is therefore gentler on the patient.

FIREFIGHTER'S DRAG.   With the firefighter's drag, you drag the patient along the long axis of the body while keeping a low profile. This is used in a smoke-filled room, since smoke rises toward the ceiling and the safest place in the room is near the floor. To perform the firefighter's drag, tie the victim's hands together, place them around your neck, straddle the victim, and crawl along the floor.

FIREFIGHTER'S CARRY.   The firefighter's carry, which is also intended for use in a smoke-filled room, permits the fastest potential exit but is more likely to aggravate fractures or spinal injuries should they exist. To perform the firefighter's carry, stand at the victim's feet, toe to toe (Fig. 16–4A and B). Hold the patient's wrists and pull the patient toward you while you bend

your knees and waist, catching the victim across your shoulder (Fig. 16–4C and D). Holding the patient's arms and legs, stand to an upright position and hold the patient's wrists with one hand across the thigh. This permits you to have a free hand so that you can hold onto railings as you exit the building.

Two-Rescuer Techniques

EXTREMITY CARRY.   When two rescuers are available, the extremity carry is a practical way to remove a victim quickly. One EMT is positioned at the victim's head, supporting the victim under the arms. The second straddles the victim's knees, grasps the victim's wrists, and pulls the victim to a sitting position while the first EMT lifts under the arms (Fig. 16–5A). This should always be done in unison. The first EMT then grasps the patient under the armpits and supports the patient's

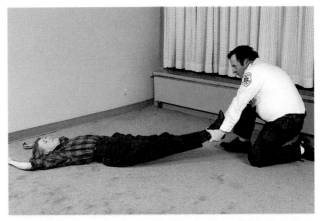

FIGURE 16-3. Grasp the ankles of the patient and drag the patient to a safe location.

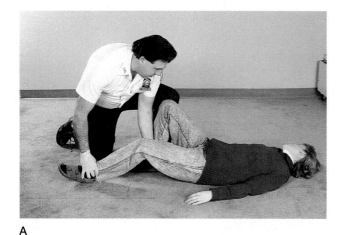

A

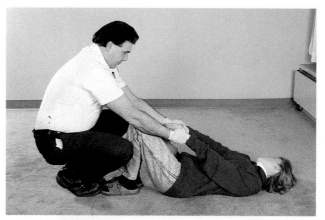

B

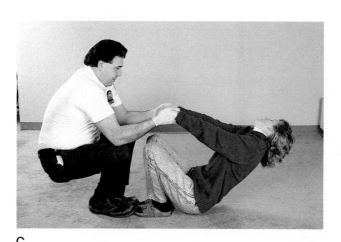

C

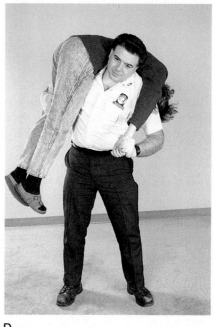

D

FIGURE 16–4. (*A*) Position yourself toe to toe with the patient; (*B*) hold the patient's wrists and tighten your back and abdominal muscles; (*C*) use your body weight to lift the patient toward you; (*D*) in one smooth motion pull the patient toward you, bend your legs, and catch the patient on your shoulder. This procedure must be done smoothly to avoid back injury.

wrist. The second rescuer supports the patient with one hand around each knee (Fig. 16–5*B*). Both EMTs rise smoothly to an upright position (Fig. 16–5*C*). The EMT holding the legs can then turn 180 degrees to facilitate forward movement of the patient (Fig. 16–5*D*).

ASSISTING AN AMBULATORY PATIENT. If the patient is able to walk or hobble, one or two EMTs can provide support while ambulating the patient to the ambulance. One rescuer can support the patient around the waist while wrapping the patient's arm around the rescuer's shoulder and holding the patient's wrist (Fig. 16–6*A*). Two rescuers can move the patient by placing their hands behind the patient while each holds the

patient's opposite wrist over his or her shoulder (Fig. 16–6*B*). This technique should never be used when ambulation may antagonize the patient's condition (i.e., fractures, heart attack, and so forth).

DEVICES FOR LIFTING AND CARRYING

Upon deciding to transport, you must select the device that is best suited to provide a safe and comfortable ride for the patient. Medical patients most often require a wheeled cot stretcher, which can be adjusted

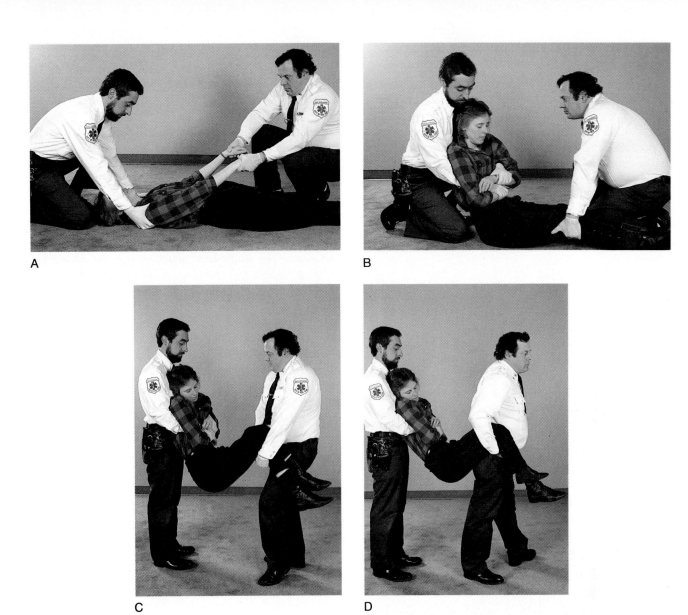

FIGURE 16–5. (*A*) Lift the patient with one rescuer supporting the armpits and one rescuer supporting the wrists. (*B*) The rescuer behind the patient should support the wrist with his arms through the armpits and the other person holds the patient beneath the knees. (*C*) Lift the patient up in unison in one smooth motion. (*D*) The rescuer at the legs turns 180 degrees, and the patient is evacuated

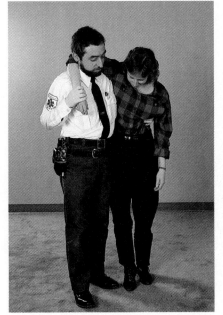

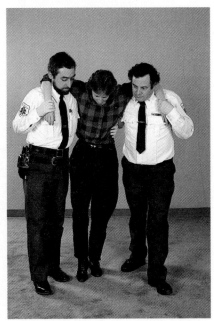

FIGURE 16–6. (*A*) One-rescuer assist. (*B*) Two-rescuer assist.

for sitting or lying in the supine or lateral recumbent position. Trauma patients, on the other hand, may require the use of several possible devices to effect a safe rescue. These devices are primarily designed to ensure proper immobilization of the spine to prevent spinal cord injury that might result from the twisting or bending of the spinal column. The major danger connected with moving a patient quickly in an emergency is the possibility of aggravating an existing spinal injury. Extremities are protected by splinting prior to transport, but if time does not permit, the patient may be splinted to the long spine board.

Stretchers

Stretchers are the most commonly used devices in prehospital care. There are several varieties of stretchers, including the basic wheeled cot stretcher (Fig. 16–7A); the folding stretcher, which may be canvas or vinyl with aluminum or wooden frames; the pole stretcher; and the scoop stretcher (Fig. 16–7B).

WHEELED COT

The wheeled cot stretcher is the preferred method for transporting patients along smooth terrain. It permits the movement of the patient along level ground without unduly fatiguing the EMTs. Since the stretcher becomes top heavy in the upright position, care should be taken in rougher terrain to avoid tipping it. Because of its weight and bulkiness, the wheeled cot stretcher is the least effective device when moving a patient over rough

terrain or down stairs. In these circumstances, the folding stretcher, the scoop stretcher, or the Stokes basket is preferred.

There are three basic types of wheeled cot stretchers; the multilevel, the two-level, and the single-level. The multilevel cot permits the adjustment of height to facilitate certain activities such as cardiopulmonary resuscitation, ventilation techniques, and movement of the stretcher along level ground. Both the multilevel and two-level stretchers permit the easy transfer of the patient from a bed to the stretcher and back to another bed again. The single-level stretcher has the advantage of being lighter and therefore more mobile.

There are other features to be found on certain wheeled cot stretchers. Most permit adjustment of the head of the stretcher at several angles, ranging from completely supine to sitting upright at 90 degrees. Additionally, some stretchers allow for elevation of the legs, knees, or the full Trendelenburg position. There is adjunctive equipment that may be attached to the wheeled cot such as IV poles, oxygen-carrying devices, and devices that carry monitor-defibrillators.

LOADING A WHEELED COT STRETCHER

Although there are many techniques for transferring a patient from a bed to a wheeled cot stretcher, the two most commonly used methods are the direct carry method and the draw sheet method. For lifting a patient from the ground to a wheeled cot stretcher, you would use the direct carry technique from floor level.

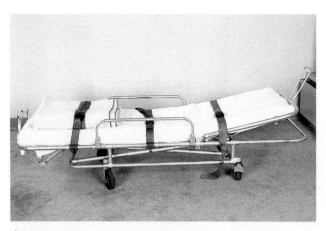

A

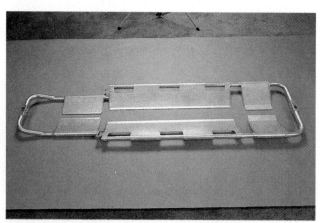

B

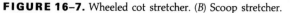
FIGURE 16–7. Wheeled cot stretcher. (*B*) Scoop stretcher.

PROCEDURE 16-1
LOADING A WHEELED COT STRETCHER (DIRECT CARRY TECHNIQUE)

1. Position the cot so that the head of the cot is at the foot of the bed, at a 90-degree angle to the bed.
2. Unfold the straps, lower the siderails, and open the sheets and blankets to prepare the stretcher for receiving the patient.
3. The EMTs stand together at the side of the bed, with the patient in a supine position.
4. The EMT at the patient's head reaches below the neck and supports the patient's shoulder with one arm and the lumbar region with the other arm.
5. The EMT at the patient's thigh supports the patient in the upper portion of the buttocks region and just below the level of the patient's knees.
6. Lift the patient up toward your chest.
7. The EMTs then rotate simultaneously at a 90-degree angle and gently place the patient on the stretcher.
8. Wrap the patient in blankets and sheets and secured with straps and siderails prior to movement.

PROCEDURE 16-2
LOADING A WHEELED COT STRETCHER (DRAW SHEET METHOD)

1. Place the draw sheet under the patient and lift the patient into the stretcher.
2. An EMT stands on each side of the patient and one EMT log rolls the patient, so that the patient is on his or her side and close to the edge of the bed. At this point, the other EMT places a folded draw sheet under the patient, tucking a sufficient amount of sheet under the patient.
3. The first EMT lowers the patient onto the draw sheet and the second EMT log rolls the patient to himself.
4. The first EMT can now unfold the draw sheet, after which the patient can be released to a supine position. The patient is now lying supine with a draw sheet spread out neatly beneath him or her.
5. Place the prepared cot directly alongside the bed, slightly lower than the bed to facilitate movement of the patient.
6. The EMTs can then grasp the top and bottom corners and gently transfer the patient to the stretcher by sliding the sheet.

Note: The EMT at the head should provide support to the patient's head with his or her arm and shoulder.

PROCEDURE 16-3
LOADING A WHEELED COT STRETCHER (DIRECT CARRY AT FLOOR LEVEL)

1. Both rescuers drop to one knee on the same side and close to the patient. (To maintain balance, both rescuers should be kneeling on the same knee.
2. Fold the victim's arms across the chest.
3. The head EMT places one arm under the patient's neck and shoulder and cradles the patient's head while placing the other arm under the patient's lower back.
4. The second EMT places one arm under the buttock region and the other arm just below the patient's knees. (Note that this is the same as in a direct carry at bed level.)
5. On command, both EMTs smoothly lift the patient onto their elevated thighs. In unison, they then stand to the upright position and rotate until they are directly adjacent to the stretcher, which has already been prepared to receive the patient. If the stretcher is elevated, they can place the patient directly onto the stretcher. If the stretcher is lowered, they should first drop to one knee and then load the patient onto the stretcher.

Note: This technique can work for both cot stretchers and folding stretchers. For noninjured patients, the extremity lift, which will be discussed later, can also be used.

MOVING THE STRETCHER

There are certain standard procedures in the movement of stretchers that help to ensure a smooth and safe transfer of the patient. The foot end of the stretcher should always go first, except when loading the patient into the ambulance. This is particularly important when going down stairs, since the stretcher is heavier at the head end, and the bottom EMT already carries a greater load because that end of the stretcher must be elevated. Roll the stretcher along the ground with one EMT at each end of the stretcher (Fig. 16-8). This facilitates the negotiation of narrow or crowded passages and allows smooth, natural movement. While rolling the stretcher along ground level, each EMT should maintain a firm grip, since the top-heavy stretcher may tilt and fall when a crack, crevice, or bump is encountered (Fig. 16-9). On moderately rough terrain, it may be necessary to carry the stretcher end to end, with the EMTs facing each other. This procedure, known as the end carry, is easily unbalanced but preferable in narrow spaces. If the terrain is very rough, the side carry method, where two EMTs are on each side of the stretcher, is the most stable method of carrying the stretcher. The disadvantage of this technique is that it requires more personnel.

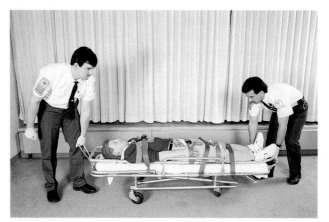

FIGURE 16–8. EMTs should be positioned at each end of the stretcher facing each other and moving the stretcher toward the patient's feet.

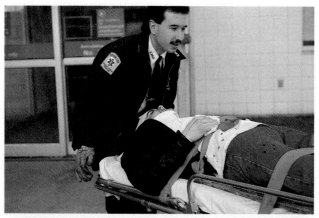

FIGURE 16–9. While moving over rough terrain or moving the stretcher over bumps or curbs, securely hold the stretcher at both ends.

PROCEDURE 16–4 LOADING THE AMBULANCE (SIDE CARRY METHOD)

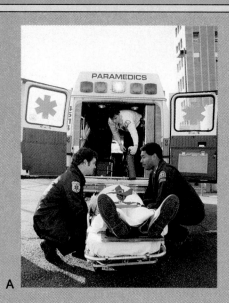

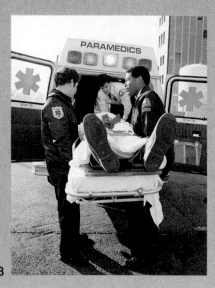

1. EMTs stand on opposite sides of the stretcher, bend their knees, and grasp the lower bar of the stretcher (Fig. 16–10A).
2. Position your hands at each end of the lower bar, with one hand palm-down and the other hand palm-up.
3. Upon command, both EMTs rise to the upright position and move the front wheels onto the floor of the passenger compartment (Fig. 16–10B and C).
4. Roll the stretcher forward until all wheels are on the passenger floor and the stretcher is guided into the sidebar to lock it in place.

   Note: If hanging stretchers are also used to carry additional patients, they should be loaded and secured prior to loading the wheeled cot stretcher.

5. Load the head of the stretcher first so that the EMT can attend to the patient.

   Note: The one exception to this is the active obstetric patient, since delivery of a baby en route, if necessary, is easier if the stretcher is loaded into the ambulance foot-first.

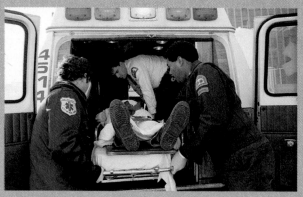

FIGURE 16–10. (*A*) Bend at the knees and straighten your back. (*B* and *C*) Lift smoothly to the upright position; rest the stretcher on the back of the ambulance, and lock it in place.

PROCEDURE 16–5   UNLOADING THE AMBULANCE

1. Unlatch the lock on the side of the stretcher and roll the stretcher so that the wheels are at the end of the floor.
2. With each EMT holding the bottom bar of the stretcher, as described previously, it is lifted from the back of the vehicle (Fig. 16–11A and B).
3. Lower the stretcher to the ground while keeping your back straight and bending at the knees.

   Note: To lift the cot stretcher, one EMT must pull on the lock release bar (Fig. 16–11C). This usually located on the side and lower corner of the stretcher.

4. Both EMTs then lift the stretcher to an upright position while holding the top bar of the stretcher (Fig. 16–11D).

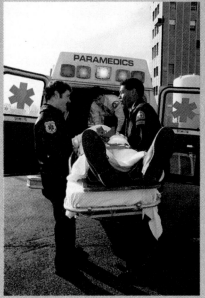

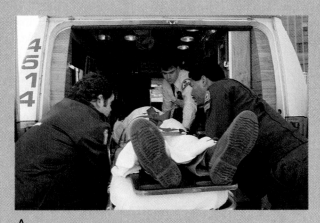

A

B

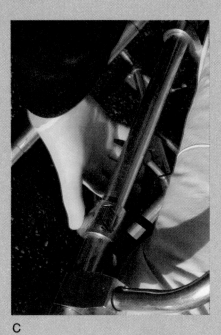

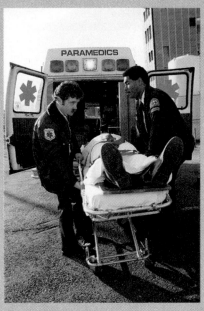

C

D

FIGURE 16–11. (A and B) Bring the stretcher to the back edge of the ambulance and lift it out holding the bottom bar of the stretcher. Carefully lower to the ground, maintaining alignment of the back. To raise the stretcher to the upright position, (C) grasp the release bar and (D) raise the stretcher to the upright position.

PORTABLE STRETCHERS

Portable stretchers are lightweight devices that can be folded and stored. They permit easy transfer of a patient down stairs and over rough terrain, unlike the bulky wheeled cot stretcher. They also give the ambulance more carrying power for use in multiple injury situations, since they can be removed from the storage cabinet and hung from the ceiling on specialized brackets or placed on the floor or on the squad bench. Like wheeled cot stretchers, portable stretchers should be carried end to end. Unlike the wheeled cot, they can also be loaded from that position.

SCOOP STRETCHER

The scoop stretcher is a specialized device that facilitates the easy lifting of supine patients. The aluminum frame consists of a rectangular tube with shovel-type flaps for sliding under the patient. The stretcher splits lengthwise into two equal halves, so that the patient can be "scooped" off the ground without changing the patient's position. Although this stretcher is an excellent means for the initial lifting off the ground of spine injury victims, they should be immediately transferred onto a long spine board to provide the support necessary for immobilization. Before sliding the halves of the stretcher under the patient, the scoop stretcher should be adjusted to a length just longer than the patient (Fig. 16–12A). Each half should then be positioned under the patient,

carefully guiding the edges of the stretcher one side at a time (Fig. 16–12B). The head end of the stretcher is connected first, after which the hips must be lifted slightly to allow connection of the bottom half to avoid pinching the patient (Fig. 16–12C). For spinal injury victims, cervical immobilization should be maintained throughout this procedure. The patient can then be placed on a cot stretcher and should be secured with straps prior to moving (Fig. 16–12D).

Cervical Collars

Cervical collars play an important role in spinal immobilization. They limit flexion and extension of the neck and to some extent lateral movement. There are several varieties of cervical collars, ranging from soft foam-filled types to rigid plastic collars. The foam-filled cervical collars are not suitable for spinal immobilization, since they allow more cervical motion.

Although cervical collars can contribute to immobilization, they are by no means capable of complete spinal immobilization. Cervical collars are an adjunct to more definitive immobilization devices, such as short and long spine boards with attachment straps for the torso and head.

When applying a cervical collar, the first concern is proper sizing of the collar. Collars come in sizes ranging from infant through extra large adult (Fig. 16–13A). A simple method for sizing cervical collars is to place the

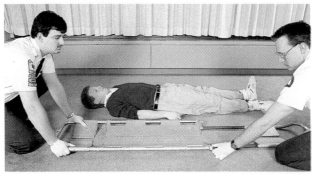

A

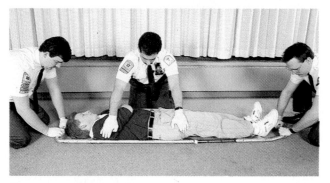

B

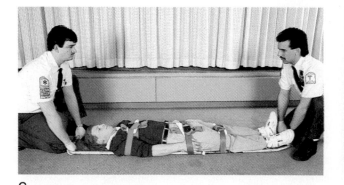

C

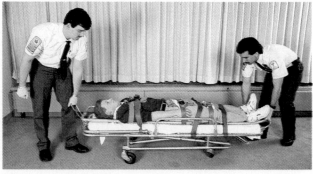

D

FIGURE 16–12. (*A*) Measure the length of the device next to the patient. (*B*) Carefully slide under both sides of the patient. (*C*) Lock the head and the feet sections of the scoop stretcher. (*D*) Place on the secondary device and secure in place.

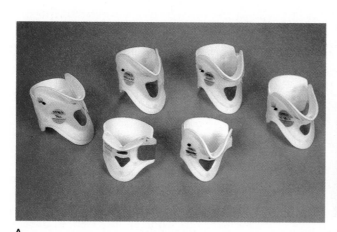
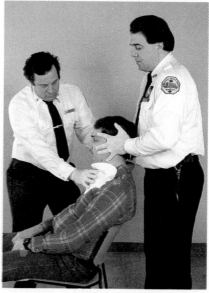

A   B

FIGURE 16–13. (*A*) Various sizes of cervical collars. (*B*) Sizing of cervical collar by noting the relationship of the chin groove to the base of the chin.

collar against the anterior neck and note the relationship of the chin groove to the base of the chin (Fig. 16–13*B*). Other techniques are recommended by the manufacturers.

Spine Boards

Spine boards are essential for lifting and moving patients with suspected spinal injuries. There are several varieties of spine boards (Fig. 16–14), but all provide

essentially the same function—rigid support for the spinal column to prevent further injury.

THE LONG SPINE BOARD

The long spine board is used as the primary device for removing patients who are lying in a supine or laterally recumbent. It is also used to facilitate a rapid extrication for an automobile accident victim. Additionally, the long spine board is used as a secondary support device for patients removed with a short spine board.

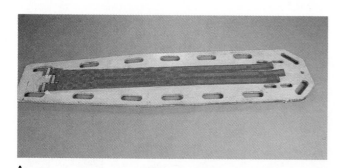
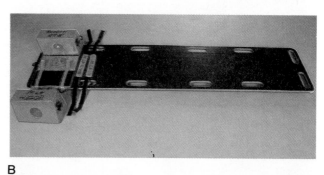

A   B

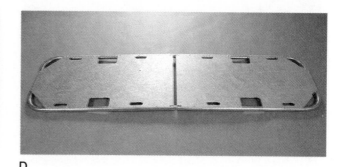

C   D

FIGURE 16–14. (*A*) Wooden spine board with narrowed end for use in helicopters. (*B*) Ferno board with head immobilizer. (*C*) Miller body splint. (*D*) Aluminum spine board.

PROCEDURE 16–6 **PLACING A PATIENT IN SUPINE POSITION ON A LONG SPINE BOARD USING THE LOG ROLL**

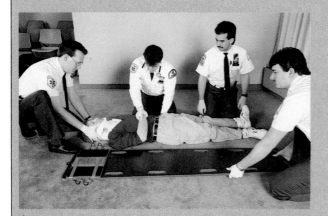

A

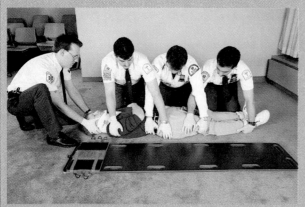

B

1. Apply cervical collar and place the patient's arms by his or her side.

   Note: One EMT maintains cervical immobilization manually throughout the procedure.

2. Three EMTs can be positioned at the side of the patient at the level of the chest, hips, and lower extremities while the long spine board is positioned on the other side of the patient.

3. Check the patient's arm on the side of the EMTs for injury prior to log rolling the patient.

4. Align the lower extremities (Fig. 16–15A).

   Note: The EMT at the lower extremities holds the patient's lower leg and the thigh region. The EMT at the hip holds the patient's lower legs and places the other hand on the top of the patient's buttocks. The EMT at the chest holds the patient's arms against the body and at the level of the lower buttocks, with the palms facing medially (Fig. 16–15B).

5. Upon command from the EMT at the head, all EMTs should rotate the patient toward themselves, keeping the body in alignment.

6. The EMTs then reach across with one hand and pull the board beneath the patient's arm (Fig. 16–15C and D).

7. Upon command from the EMT at the head, they gently roll the patient onto the board, then roll the board to the ground.

8. Strap the patient's torso and extremities securely to the board (Fig. 16–15E and F).

9. Immobilize the head with a head immobilizer or tape (Fig. 16–15G and H).

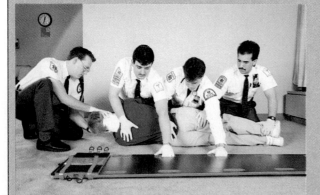

C

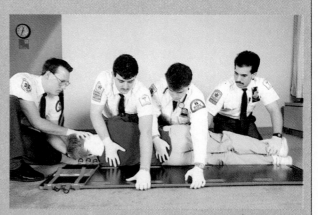

D

FIGURE 16–15. (*A*) Maintaining in-line immobilization, attach the collar and position the board. (*B*) Position rescuers at the patient's chest, hip, and lower extremity. (*C* and *D*) Rotate the patient and place board under his side. (*E*) Rotate the patient on to board. (*F*) Secure the torso at the chest, pelvic region, and legs. (*G* and *H*) Secure the patient's head with immobilizer or blankets and tape.

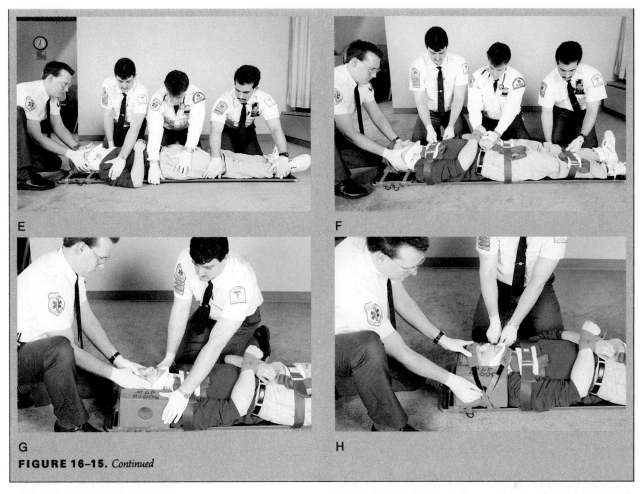

FIGURE 16–15. *Continued*

RAPID EXTRICATION

Patients who must be removed quickly from an automobile can be evacuated directly onto the long spine board by using the rapid extrication procedure. This particular technique is also recommended through the Prehospital Trauma Life Support (PHTLS) program and requires a minimum of three rescuers.

PROCEDURE 16–7   PERFORMING RAPID EXTRICATION

1. The first EMT positions himself behind the patient and maintains immobilization of the cervical spine and a second EMT performs a primary survey (Fig. 16–16*A*). Apply a rigid cervical collar (Fig. 16–16*B*).

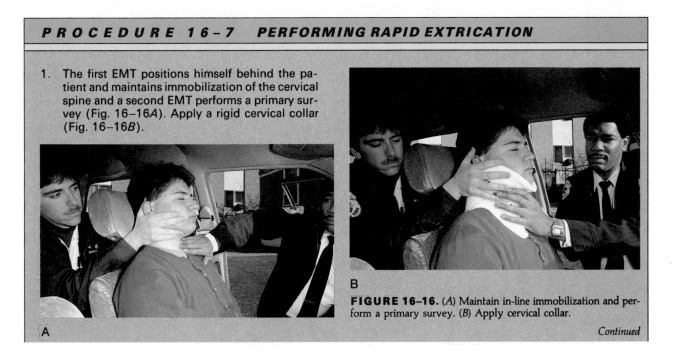

FIGURE 16–16. (*A*) Maintain in-line immobilization and perform a primary survey. (*B*) Apply cervical collar.

Continued

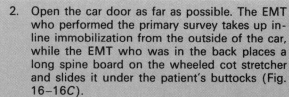

2. Open the car door as far as possible. The EMT who performed the primary survey takes up in-line immobilization from the outside of the car, while the EMT who was in the back places a long spine board on the wheeled cot stretcher and slides it under the patient's buttocks (Fig. 16–16*C*).
3. One EMT positions himself in the seat next to the patient on the opposite side of the EMT who is now holding immobilization and places his hands under the patient's thighs just proximal to the knees. A third EMT positions himself at the same side of the car as the EMT holding immobilization and grasps the patient under the armpit with one hand and in the mid-posterior thorax with the other hand (Fig. 16–16*D*). A fourth rescuer can steady the stretcher.
4. Upon command, the patient is rotated with the patient's back toward the board, so that the legs come in contact with the front of the seat. Upon a second command, the patient is then lowered to the board, with the EMT at the leg lifting, the EMT at the chest supporting and lowering, and the EMT maintaining cervical spine immobilization maintaining alignment and lowering to one knee (Fig. 16–16*E*, *F*, and *G*).
5. Once the patient is supine, the EMT holding the chest positions both hands in opposite armpits and on command slides the patient at 6 to 12-inch increments until the patient is properly positioned on the board (Fig. 16–16*H* and *I*).
6. The EMT in the car then comes out of the car and the board is properly positioned on the wheeled cot stretcher and secured (Fig. 16–16*J*).

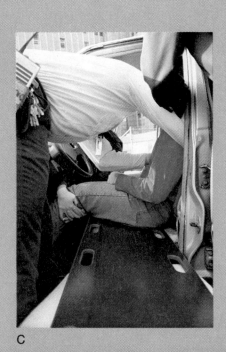

C

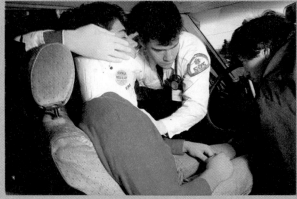

D

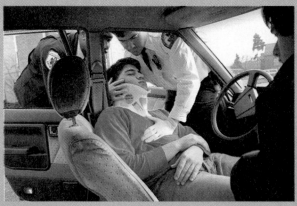

E

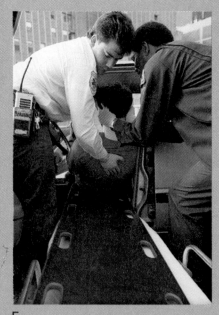

F

FIGURE 16–16. *Continued.* (*C*) The EMT takes over in-line immobilization from outside of the car, and the board is positioned under the patient. (*D*) The EMTs hold the patient's chest and legs and rotate, the patient with the back toward the door. (*E* and *F*) The patient is lowered to the board. (*G* to *I*) The patient is slid up the board. (*J*) The patient is secured to the board.

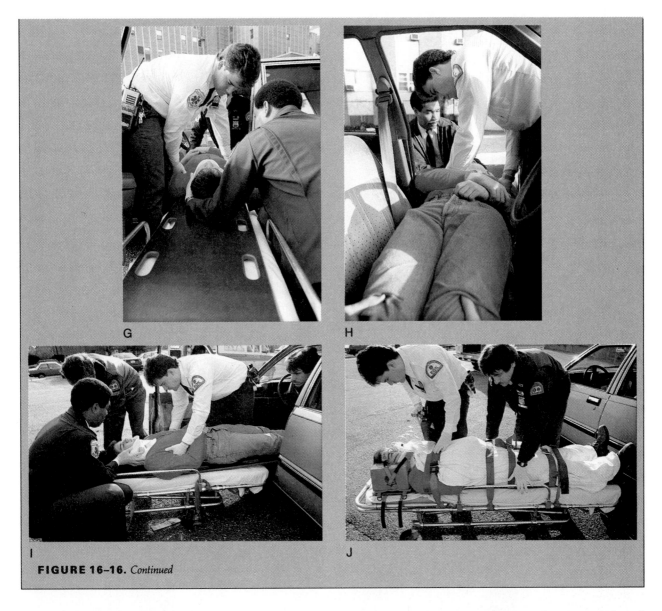

FIGURE 16–16. *Continued*

SHORT SPINE BOARD

The short spine board is used to immobilize and extricate victims of automobile accidents who are found in the sitting position. The short spine board may be wooden (Fig. 16–17A and B) or aluminum and is designed to extend from the base of the buttocks to just above the head. It is attached to the patient using straps and/or cravat bandages, while maintaining cervical immobilization.

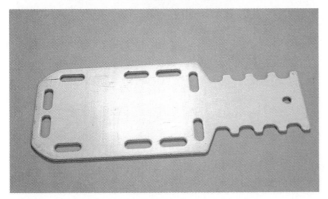

A

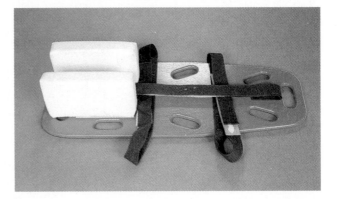

B

FIGURE 16–17. (A) Wooden short spine board. (B) Kansas spine board.

PROCEDURE 16-8   APPLYING THE SHORT SPINE BOARD

1. One EMT positions himself directly behind the patient and assumes cervical spine immobilization (Fig. 16–18*A*).
2. A second EMT applies a rigid cervical collar and prepares the board for insertion behind the patient.

    Place the board behind the patient by sliding the top half up between the other EMT's arms (Fig. 16–18*B*). The board should be adjusted so that it is positioned evenly.

    Note: In the technique demonstrated in Fig. 16–18, the EMT uses one long strap to secure the patient's torso in place. The lower torso strap is threaded through the board in the following manner (Fig. 16–18*C* to *F*): starting at the waist through the bottom hole in the side of the board; up through the hole in the side of the board, under the armpit, and over the shoulder; and around the back of the board, over the top of the shoulder, under the armpit, and out through the hole in the top of the board. The strap is then threaded through the lower hole and connected to the other end at the waist. The head is then secured with tape or Velcro attachment devices (Fig. 16–18*G* to *I*). As an option, pads can be placed behind the head prior to attaching the tape to fill in the occipital void.

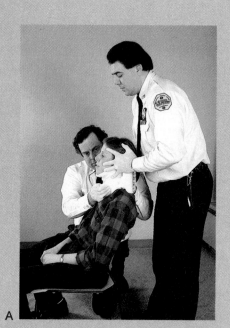

A

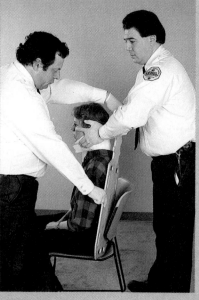

B

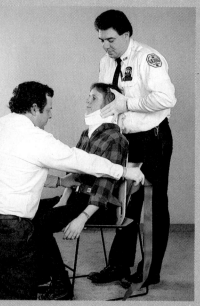

C

FIGURE 16–18. (*A*) Maintain in-line immobilization. (*B*) Position the board behind the patient. (*C*) Strap across the waist and through the lower opening, (*D*) up through the top opening, under the armpit, and over the shoulder, then (*E*) over the shoulder, through the armpit, and (*F*) around the waist, and secure strap. (*G* and *H*) Secure the head. (*I*) Padding optional.

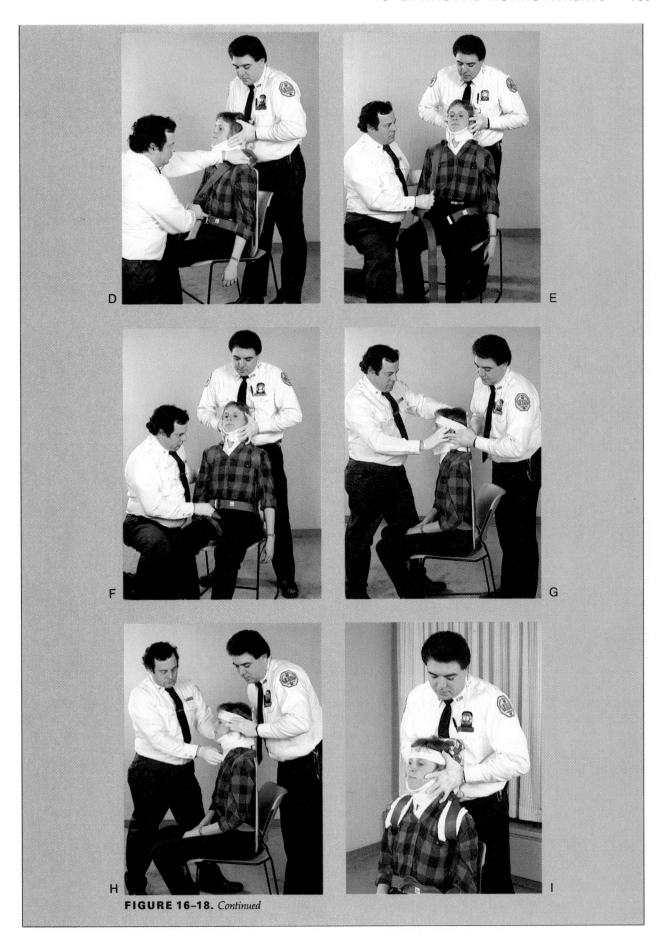

FIGURE 16–18. *Continued*

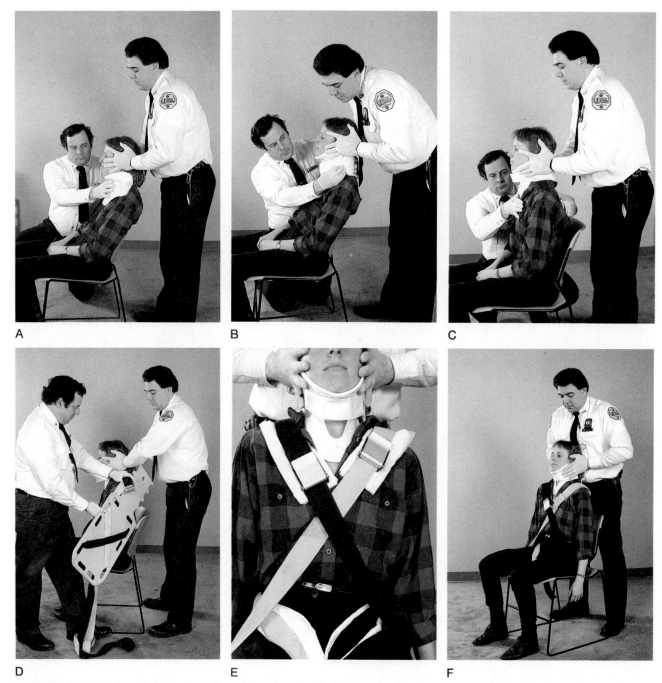

A

B

C

D

E

F

FIGURE 16–19. (*A* to *D*) Apply the collar and board as described previously. (*E* and *F*) Straps are criss-crossed in back of board prior to insertion. Torso straps are brought across the thigh, under the thigh, and up to the chest strap and buckle. Pad pressure areas as needed. Apply head immobilization as described previously.

Figure 16–19A to F demonstrates an alterate technique using two straps and a criss-crossed approach to strapping.

KENDRICK EXTRICATION DEVICE

The Kendrick extrication device, also known as K.E.D., represents a relatively recent evolution of the short spine board (Fig. 16–20). Its semirigid form permits easy and speedy application and provides effective immobilization of the spine.

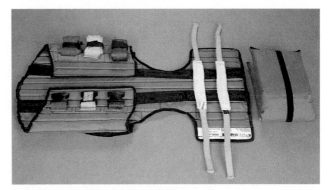

FIGURE 16–20. Kendrick extrication device.

PROCEDURE 16–9   APPLYING THE KENDRICK EXTRICATION DEVICE

1. One EMT maintains cervical spine immobilization from behind the patient.
2. Apply rigid cervical collar and position the K.E.D. behind the patient in the same manner as the short spine board (Fig. 16–21A to D).

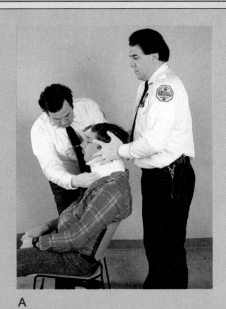

A

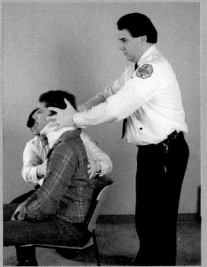

B

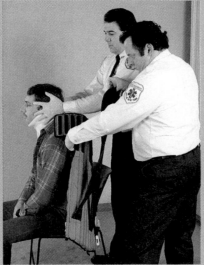

C

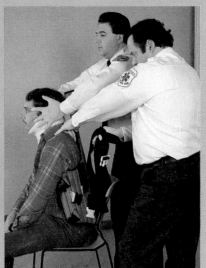

D

FIGURE 16–21. (A) Maintain in-line immobilization. (B to D) Position the device behind the patient.

Continued

3. Pull up the K.E.D. securely into the axillary region (Fig. 16–21*E*).
4. Attach the chest and abdominal straps, followed by the groin straps. (Care should be taken not to pinch the patient and padding may be necessary (Fig. 16–21*F* and *G*).
5. Secure the head, using the Velcro fasteners (Fig. 16–21*H* to *J*). As an option, the hands can be tied together to prevent the patient from grabbing fixed objects during movement (Fig. 16–21*K*).

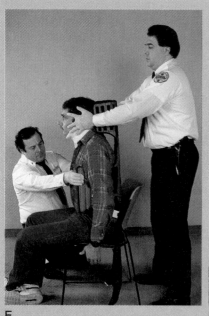

E

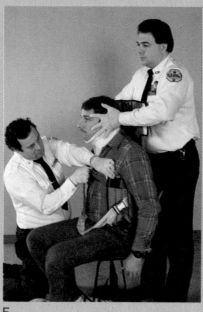

F

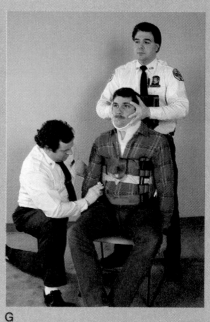

G

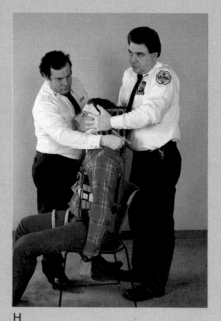

H

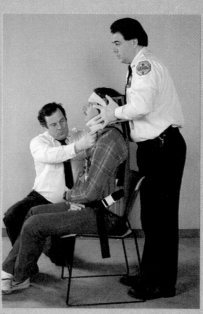

I

FIGURE 16–21. *Continued.* (*E*) Pull the device up under the patient's armpits. (*F* and *G*) Secure the chest and abdominal straps. (*H* and *J*) Secure the patient's head. (*K*) Optionally, secure the patient's hands.

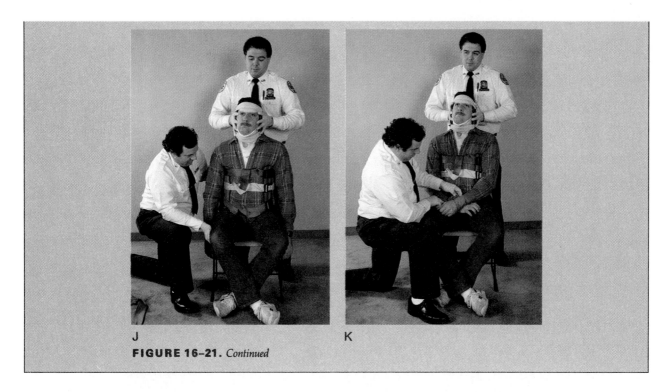

J   K

FIGURE 16–21. *Continued*

Stokes Basket

The Stokes Basket is an extrication device that is ideal for removing patients on rough terrain or during high-angle rescues, in which a patient must either be lowered from a height or lifted, as from a ditch or well. The Stokes basket is constructed of hard plastic or wire mesh with a metal frame. Before placing a patient in a Stokes basket, it must be well padded to prevent further injury to the patient (Fig. 16–22).

Stair Chair

The stair chair is a device designed to remove patients who are able to assume the sitting position to the ambulance. It is a primary lifting and carrying device in urban EMS systems, where a proliferation of narrow stairways make the use of a cot stretcher difficult and sometimes dangerous. It should never be used for patients with a suspected spinal injury or for patients who are or who may become unconscious. The patient should always be transferred to a wheeled cot stretcher as soon as you reach the ambulance, since the stair chair is not intended for transport purposes.

The extremity carry method, discussed previously in this chapter, is the preferred method for loading a patient into the stair chair (Fig. 16–23A). Prior to movement, the patient should be instructed not to grasp for the handrails, since this may cause the EMT to lose balance. To avoid accidents, it may be appropriate to secure the patient's hands if the patient is disoriented or a child (Fig. 16–23B).

The chair can be tilted back and rolled along smooth, level terrain (Fig. 16–23C). When descending stairs, the EMT at the patient's head should support the chair firmly with his or her hands at the outermost portion of the bar. The EMT at the foot may have to elevate the lower portion of the chair to prevent the wheel from hitting the stairs. Whenever possible, a spotter, such as a police officer, should be positioned below the EMT at the foot for extra support in the event that one of the EMTs trip (Fig. 16–23D).

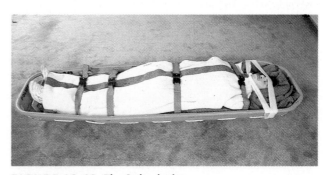

FIGURE 16–22. The Stokes basket.

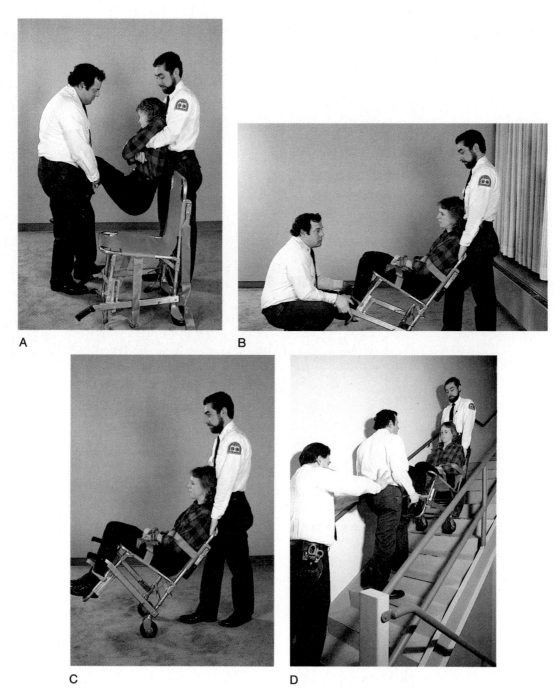

A   B

C   D

FIGURE 16–23. (*A*) Lift with the extremity carry. (*B*) Optionally secure the patient's hands and tilt the device. (*C*) Tilt to move along ground level. (*D*) Use spotter to move down stairs.

Rapid Takedown Procedure

The rapid takedown procedure is used when a victim with a suspected spinal injury is found upright at the scene of an accident. If the mechanism of injury is sufficient to cause spinal injury, this procedure should be used to secure the patient to a spine board. This procedure is adapted from the New York State Department of Health Critical Trauma Care Program.

P R O C E D U R E 1 6 – 1 0   PERFORMING RAPID TAKEDOWN PROCEDURE

1. Position the tallest crew member behind the patient and have him or her manually stabilize the patient's neck (Fig. 16–24*A*). This person's hands will not leave the patient's head and neck until the entire procedure is complete and the head is taped down to the board.
2. A second rescuer applies a rigid extrication collar to the patient (Fig. 16–24*B*).

Note: The purpose of applying the collar is to provide support to the neck as a back-up for the manual stabilization, not to replace the manual stabilization. It is important to note that the literature suggests that even the best collars still allow approximately 30% range of motion, which is certainly ample movement to displace a fractured vertebra, possibly transecting the cord (Fig. 16–14*B*).

3. The second rescuer carefully positions the long board behind the patient, working around the EMT who is applying manual stabilization. It is often useful to stand directly behind the patient with elbows spread to facilitate the placement of the backboard by a second rescuer (Fig. 16–24*C*).

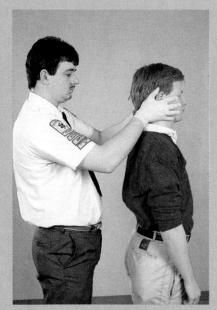

A

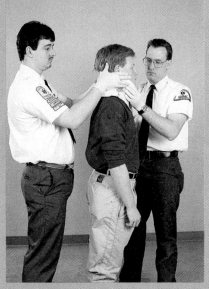

B

C

FIGURE 16–24. (*A*) In-line immobilization from behind. (*B*) Apply collar. (*C*) Place the board behind the patient and line up properly.

Continued

4. The second rescuer then looks at the backboard from the front of the patient to do any necessary repositioning in order to ensure that the long board is centered behind the patient.
5. The second and third rescuers, standing on either side of and facing the patient, reach under the patient's arm on their respective sides with the hand that is closest to the board and grab the backboard at a hole near the patient's armpit or higher (Fig. 16–24*D*). This will keep the patient from sliding off the board while being laid down.

Note: Actually, once the board is tilted back, the patient will be suspended temporarily by the armpits. To keep the patient's arm secure, the EMTs should grasp the arms at the elbow level with their other hand and hold the arm next to the patient's body.

6. Slowly lay the board down, tilting it backward so the head end begins to be lowered (Fig. 16–24*E* and *F*).

Note: It is important to first let the patient know what you are going to do so as not to make the patient any more anxious than he or she probably already is.
Note: The EMT who is stabilizing the patient's head and neck is to walk backward and squat down, keeping up with the speed at which the board is being lowered.

7. As the patient is lowered to the ground, the EMT near the head must allow the head to move slowly back to the neutral position against the board (Fig. 16–24*G*).

Note: Figure 16–24*H* demonstrates the same technique using two rescuers.

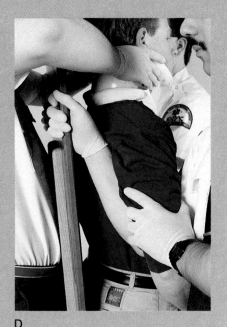

D

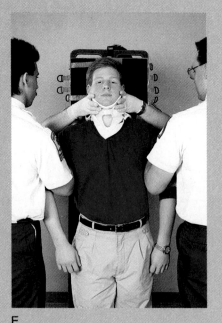

E

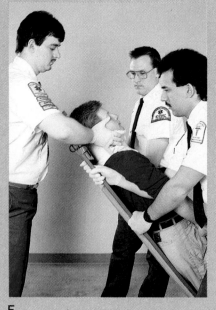

F

FIGURE 16–24. *Continued.* (*D*) Grab the board through the patient's armpits to next highest hole. (*E* to *G*) Lower to ground. (*H*) Alternate position for two rescuers.

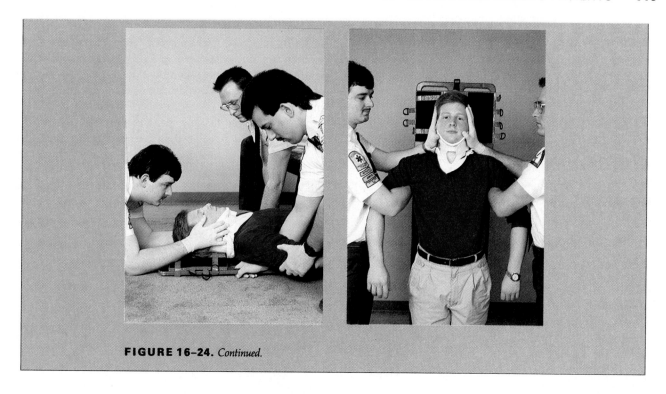

FIGURE 16–24. *Continued.*

SELECTING THE APPROPRIATE MODE OF TRANSPORT

The patient's condition is the main consideration when selecting the appropriate moving device. Factors such as airway maintenance, patient comfort, suspected spinal injury, shock states, and injured extremities dictate the device you choose and the position of the patient.

Medical Patients

Medical patients are most often transported on the wheeled cot stretcher, since it provides both comfort and can be adjusted to a variety of positions.

PATIENTS WITH DYSPNEA OR CHEST PAIN

Patients complaining of dyspnea or chest pain are generally transported in a semi-reclining or fully upright position on a wheeled cot stretcher. You should be guided by the patient, who is able to define for you his or her position of comfort. Patients with shortness of breath usually prefer the full upright position, since it allows maximum use of the diaphragm and chest muscles. In the supine position, the abdominal contents press upward against the diaphragm, making lung expansion a greater chore. Cardiac patients who are in shock require a supine position with their legs elevated to ensure optimal brain perfusion.

THE UNCONSCIOUS MEDICAL PATIENT

The primary concern for unconscious medical patients is airway management. They are generally placed in the left lateral recumbent position on a wheeled cot stretcher (Fig. 16–25). This helps to prevent aspiration if the patient vomits. Patients in need of resuscitation must naturally be placed in the supine position on a spine board or cardiac resuscitation board.

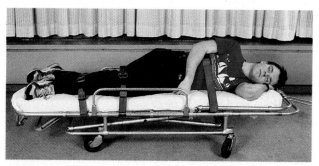

FIGURE 16–25. Left lateral recumbent position.

PATIENTS COMPLAINING OF ABDOMINAL PAIN

Patients in acute abdominal distress usually are most comfortable in the supine or lateral recumbent position with their knees bent. Some wheeled cot stretchers permit elevation of the knees to facilitate this position.

Trauma Patients

PATIENTS WITH EXTREMITY FRACTURES

Patients with isolated fractures of the upper extremities can be transported in the stair chair to the ambulance and then placed on a wheeled cot in a semi-Fowler's position. If lower extremity injuries exist, the patient must be transported on a portable or wheeled cot stretcher to provide proper immobilization and to elevate the injured part. When traction splints are applied, care should be taken to properly secure the splint prior to transport.

PATIENTS WITH A HEAD INJURY

Patients with isolated head injuries in the absence of spinal injury can be transported in a semi-reclining (45° angle) position. This reduces intracranial pressure and can decrease the potential of cerebral edema. If the patient has an altered mental state or is unconscious, he or she should be transported in the lateral recumbent position. If spinal injury is possible, the patient should be kept supine with careful attention paid to airway maintenance.

THE PATIENT WITH MULTIPLE INJURIES

Patients who have multiple injuries should be transferred on a long spine board to provide full body immobilization. As previously mentioned, the initial method of immobilization may vary. Patients found in the sitting position are usually removed on a short spine board or K.E.D. and then transferred to a long spine board. Patients who are found supine or who are in need of rapid extrication should be removed with a long spine board. The long spine board is then placed directly on the wheeled cot stretcher.

PREGNANT PATIENTS

Heavily pregnant women who are injured or in shock secondary to hemorrhage should not be placed flat on their backs if at all possible. This position causes the bulk of the fetus to compress the vena cava, thereby seriously affecting cardiac return. Most heavily pregnant women are uncomfortable in this position even if uninjured. The left lateral recumbent position is the position of choice, but a semi-reclining position is appropriate if the patient is very uncomfortable in the left lateral recumbent position. If the patient is about to deliver, the stretcher should be placed in the ambulance foot first and the patient placed in a supine or semi-reclining position with knees bent and spread apart. If you suspect a threatened abortion, the hips or foot of the cot should be elevated to prevent undue strain against the cervix.

REVIEW EXERCISES

1. Describe effective body mechanics during lifting.
2. List the steps of performance for the following emergency evacuation techniques:
   - One rescuer
   - Clothes drag
   - Blanket drag
   - Firefighter's drag
   - Firefighter's carry
   - Two rescuer
   - Extremity carry
   - Assisting an ambulatory patient
3. Describe the common uses and basic transfer procedures for each of the following devices:
   - Wheeeled cot stretcher
   - Portable stretcher
   - Scoop stretcher
   - Spine boards
   - Long spine board
   - Kendrick extrication device
   - Short spine board
   - Stokes basket
   - Stair chair
4. List the steps of performance for the following techniques:
   - Log roll
   - Rapid extrication procedure
5. In general, describe the ideal transport approach for the following patients:
   - Patients with dyspnea or chest pain
   - The unconscious medical patient
   - Patients complaining of abdominal pain
   - Automobile accident victims
   - Injured pedestrians
   - Patients with a head injury
   - Pregnant patients

REFERENCES

American Academy of Orthopaedic Surgeons, Committee on Allied Health: Emergency care and transportation of the sick and injured, 4th ed. Chicago, American Academy of Orthopaedic Surgeons, 1986.

American Red Cross: Advanced first aid and emergency care. Garden City, NY, Doubleday, 1982.

Butman A, Paturas J: Pre-hospital trauma life support. Akron, OH, Emergency Training, 1986.

Grant H, Murray R: Emergency care, 4th ed. Bowie, MD, Brady/Prentice-Hall, 1986.

Hafen B, Karen K: Prehospital emergency care and crisis intervention, 2nd ed. Englewood, CO, Morton, 1986.

United States Department of Transportation: EMT—A patient handling manual. Washington, DC, Department of Transportation Traffic Safety Administration, 1976.

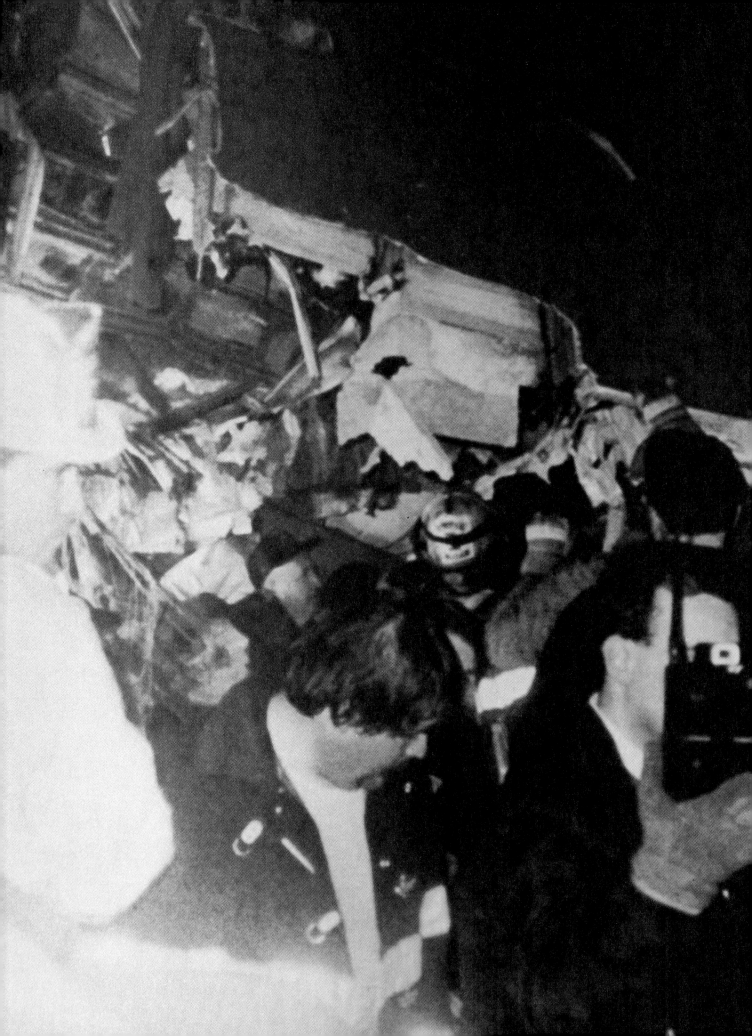

CHAPTER 17

DISASTERS AND TRIAGE

OBJECTIVES

At the conclusion of this chapter the reader will be able to:

1. Describe the difference between a closed and an open disaster scene.

2. Describe the difference between an active and a contained disaster situation.

3. List the four colors used to designate triage patients and explain what each color signifies.

4. List five things the first EMTs arriving on a disaster scene should try to ascertain.

SCENARIO

While responding to a call for an automobile accident, the dispatcher advises that he is receiving multiple calls and that apparently a school bus is involved in the accident. Upon turning the corner at the scene, you observe a large school bus on its side. The other vehicle involved is on fire. People are running past you, some with injuries. A police officer informs you that at least 25 children are in the bus and he is not sure of the severity or extent of their injuries.

What is your overall plan of action? How would you activate your disaster plan? What resources are needed? With whom do you need to communicate? What roles would you and your partner assume as the first responders on the scene? What steps can you take to prevent further injury, reduce the number of deaths, and transport the patients in a timely manner?

This chapter addresses these questions. Its function is to familiarize the EMT with the role of emergency medical services within the context of a community disaster plan.

DEFINITIONS

Disaster

The *American Heritage Dictionary on the English Language* defines a disaster as an occurrence inflicting widespread destruction and distress, a grave misfortune, or a total failure.

From the EMT's perspective, a disaster is any situation that totally overwhelms the resources available. For example, an ambulance capable of transporting two patients arrives at a scene where there are five injured people.

EMTs may often encounter situations where there are more casualties than their vehicle can accommodate. As part of an early scene assessment, the EMT routinely decides whether it is necessary to call for additional resources. A major disaster, however, requires a multiagency response to limit death and destruction.

Closed versus Open

A disaster scene can be classified as closed or open. An open situation allows easy access to victims from different directions. An open situation could also be spread over a large area, placing additional demands on the rescuers to search a large territory. For example, a group of injured people in a field is an open situation.

A closed incident has physical or geographic boundaries that prevent speedy access to or evacuation of patients. Examples include victims who are pinned in a bus accident, a high-rise fire in which victims are trapped on the top floor, a construction accident or building collapse with victims trapped beneath debris (Fig. 17–1), or an airplane crash in a wooded area where there are no accessible roads (Fig. 17–2).

To gain access to a closed incident, specialized resources are required. These resources may include helicopters, search and rescue teams, self-contained breathing apparatus, and specialized extrication equipment.

Active versus Contained

An active situation exists when the forces that contributed to or were associated with the disaster are still active, evolving, and ongoing. An active situation poses an ongoing threat to the rescuers, public, and victims. A contained situation implies that the likelihood of further injury is low, since the forces responsible for the disaster are exhausted or contained.

An ongoing fire is an active situation. Once the fire is extinguished or under control, it is considered contained.

Mutual Aid

Mutual aid is a predetermined response system that is established with neighboring communities to ensure a large-scale response of emergency personnel and vehicles, including police, firefighters, and ambulances, during a catastrophic incident. Even when faced with a disaster, the regular needs of the community must still be met. Often the outside units cover the normal response load of the area during a disaster.

EMS Command

The response to a disaster requires a systematic approach, with a central authority, or command, responsible for overall emergency operations. EMS command provides an essential function that is critical to success. The EMS command function represents one component of the overall command structure in a community disaster plan. The EMT may assume the responsibility of EMS command and other nonpatient care functions in the initial stages of a disaster (Fig. 17–3).

Triage

Triage means to sort casualties of a war or other disaster to determine the priority of need and proper

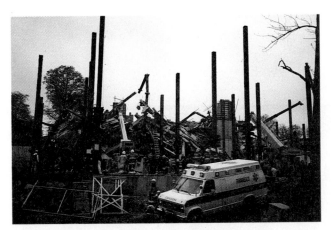

FIGURE 17–1. The building collapse in Bridgeport, Connecticut, represented a closed incident, since many of the victims were trapped beneath tons of debris.

Transport

Transport encompasses more than the movement of patients. The EMT in charge of transport may be responsible for the coordination of several areas. These include movement of vehicles and supplies into the disaster site, selection of traffic routes for rapid access and removal, traffic control to ensure that these routes remain open to emergency vehicles, selection of staging areas for arriving emergency vehicles and supplies, and communication coordination.

The role of the transport officer is pivotal to the outcome of the disaster operation (Fig. 17–4).

ESSENTIAL COMPONENTS OF DISASTER MANAGEMENT

place of treatment. Disasters require a change in the EMT's thinking about priority of care. *A cardinal rule in disaster triage is to protect and save the most people possible.* For example, a victim in cardiac arrest would have the lowest priority in a true disaster setting.

The three essential EMS components of disaster management are *command,* or *control; triage;* and *transportation.* These three functions constitute the basic nucleus around which all other activities are organized.

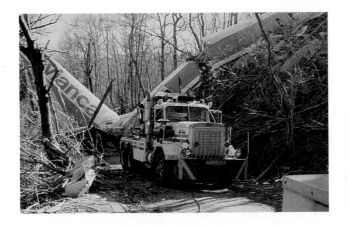

FIGURE 17–2. The Avianca plane crash, which occurred in January, 1990, evolved into a closed incident when the single access road became clogged with onlookers, cars, and rescue vehicles.

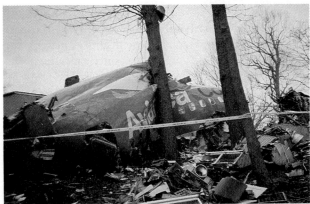

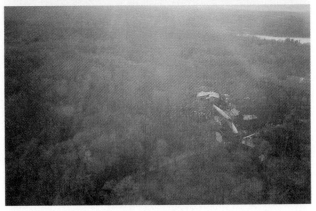

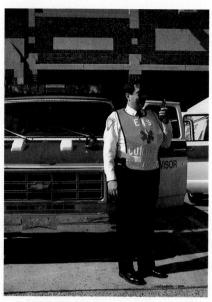

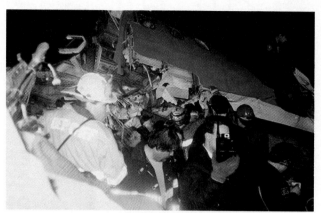

FIGURE 17–3. The EMS command plays an important role in the management of a disaster scene. The initial responding EMT must often assume this role until more senior command personnel arrive.

Each of these components should have an individual assigned to it, an area identified, and a function described.

Command

Command signifies the person ultimately in charge of the disaster response. It may be the fire or police chief, the EMS chief, the mayor, or the county executive. Who ultimately assumes command depends on the type of incident and the political structure within that region.

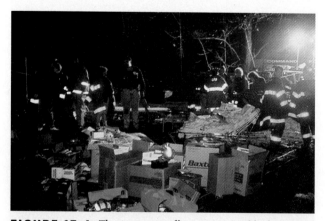

FIGURE 17–4. The transport officer is responsible for several functions, including movement of equipment and supplies, traffic route selection, staging of vehicles, removal of patients from the scene, and determination of hospital destination. The EMTs initially arriving on the scene must assume this role along with command functions until senior administrative personnel arrive.

For example, if there is a riot, police may be the primary command, with other public agencies assisting. On the fire scene, the fire chief heads overall operations, with other agencies assisting. If a situation occurs where the focus is primarily patient treatment, then the command is assumed by the EMS chief.

At any disaster, multiple agencies are likely to respond and make up a command structure. The medical personnel report to the EMS command officer or his or her representative. It is important for the responding EMT to be familiar with the command structure within local plans.

The EMS command officer is responsible for coordinating the emergency medical response with other agencies involved in the disaster. This individual is ultimately responsible for emergency medical operations and supervises the triage and transport areas.

Figure 17–5 illustrates a plan for organization of a disaster response as well as the various areas of responsibility and the chain of command. Local plans may have different tables of organization. Figure 17–6 specifically indicates the EMS responsibilities on the scene of a disaster.

Roles and Interagency Relationships

Effective disaster management requires cooperation among a large number of agencies and personnel. An understanding of the basic roles and responsibilities of

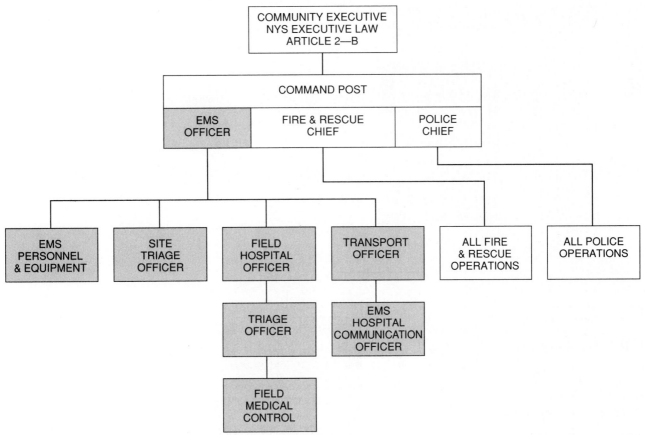

FIGURE 17–5. Multiple casualty incident community agency organization. No attempt is made here to provide the full scope of police or fire operational plans since these agencies have their own plans describing their responsibilities and the implementation of a "disaster" plan. In some cases, an agency has dual responsibilities (fire and EMS, police and EMS, and so on), but for the purposes of this model, the functions of EMS are separately emphasized. (Adapted from the New York State Department of Health MCI Manual.)

all involved helps avoid any duplication of efforts and conflicts at the disaster scene. These roles differ from community to community but there are some universal components within most systems.

POLICE. The primary function of police is to protect and serve. In a disaster, the police role may include scene security, traffic control, investigation, identification of the dead (Fig. 17–7), and notification of families.

FIRE. The primary function of the fire service is the protection of life and property. In a disaster, the fire role includes rescue and extrication (Fig. 17–8), fire suppression, hazard elimination, and scene safety.

OTHER AGENCIES. Other agencies included in disaster plans are public works, the Red Cross, the Salvation Army, social agencies, hospitals, and the military. These organizations operate within the sphere of their expertise, providing services as needed in coordination with the command post. Each of these agencies has its own command structure.

Communications

Communications represents one of the most essential elements of disaster management. Many disasters have had poor outcomes as a result of inadequate communications.

Within an overall plan, EMS communications should be separated from other disaster communications. Local disaster plans should identify specific communication channels for various participating agencies. The coordination of EMS communications is a function unto itself.

An individual must be identified as the coordinator of communications. This individual may be the dispatcher or someone at the scene. EMS command assumes this function or delegates it. All communications must go through this designated individual to avoid duplication, promote centralized record keeping, and maximize resource allocation.

Radiofrequency allocation is an option available to some EMS systems. A rule of thumb to effective

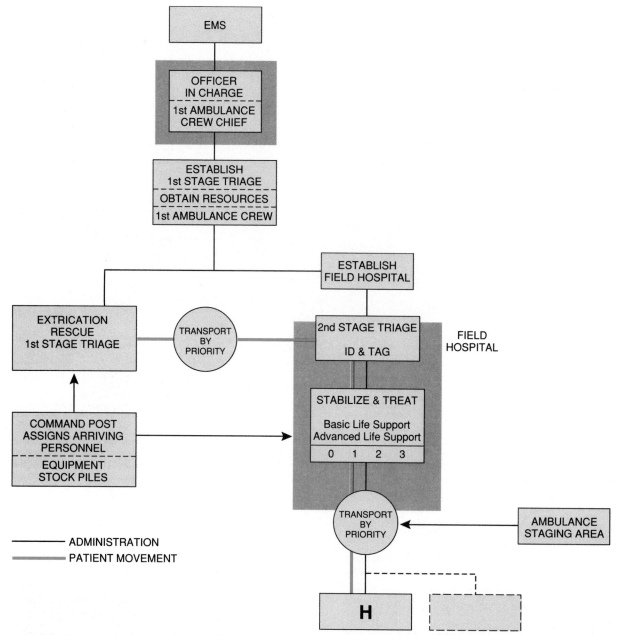

FIGURE 17–6. Field triage flow model. (Adapted from the New York State Department of Health MCI Manual.)

communications is to maintain radio silence unless information is requested of you or communications are necessary in the course of carrying out your assigned responsibility.

Communications may also include conveying necessary information to the public and media. Initially, this is a command post function that may be delegated by the command officer. EMTs should maintain patient confidentiality.

Documentation

Record keeping is an essential component of disaster management. It is used to maintain information about individual patients, key events, and the progress of the incident. Specific records that need to be kept on the disaster site are a major event log, the number of patients, conditions and triage categories, vehicles on the scene, personnel on the scene, hospital availability,

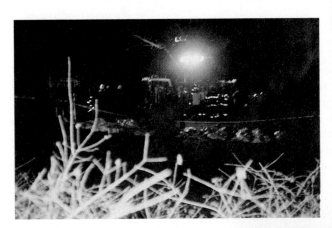

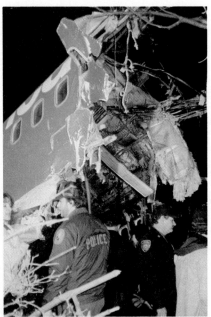

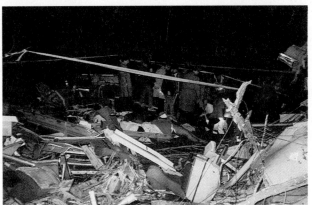

FIGURE 17–7. Police duties include identifying the dead, securing the disaster area, setting up a temporary morgue, investigating the incident, and securing valuables.

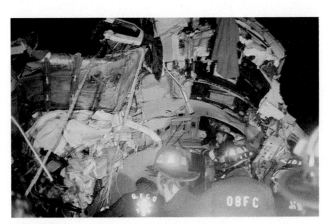

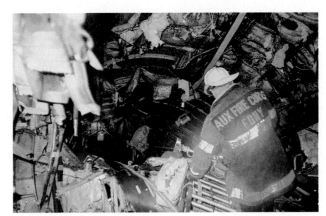

FIGURE 17–8. Firemen assist with gaining access, extrication, and rescue of plane crash victims.

the number of individuals transported, and hospital disposition and mode of transport. Figure 17–9 shows a patient destination log.

Safety

EMS command should oversee scene safety as it relates to EMS personnel. Scene safety is the responsibility of all rescuers involved in operations. Safety concerns are prioritized in the following order: (1) rescuer, (2) public, and (3) victim. A primary concern is not to add to the number of victims. Sometimes difficult decisions must be made not to commit personnel to insurmountable or potentially life-threatening situations.

Some injuries may be prevented through the use of protective clothing, fire suppression, lighting, crowd control, and traffic control.

Resource Recruitment and Allocation

As the disaster response evolves, EMS command relays the need for additional resources (including specialized equipment or personnel) through the dispatch center. In addition, the transport officer is notified by command of the impending arrival of personnel, equipment, and vehicles.

Traffic Control

In coordination with the police department, traffic routes should be established to ensure rapid access to and from the site.

The EMTs arriving first at the scene may have the ability to identify routes in and out for subsequent re-

MCI — PATIENT DESTINATION LOG

Location _____ Date _____

Dispatch No.	Patient Tag No.	Priority	Destination Hospital	Ambulance Agency Vehicle I.D.	Time Out

FIGURE 17–9. Multiple casualty incident patient destination log. (From the New York State Department of Health MCI Manual.)

sponders. This information should be transmitted to the dispatch center and to the first responding police units. Traffic control is critical from the start.

TRIAGE

There are three stages of triage. During the first stage of triage, no treatment is rendered. Victims are tagged with colored surveyor's tape and/or tags by category of injury and likelihood of survival (Fig. 17–10). The second stage of triage begins after patients have been removed to a safe area where more thorough assessment and medical care can be given. During the second stage, patients may be recategorized by priority. The second stage of triage is a collection point for all patients to ensure appropriate priority and transport. These functions are directed by a triage officer. The following charts explain the functions of the triage officer and triage support personnel.

TRIAGE SECTOR OFFICER

Located	TRIAGE AREAS
Radio ID	TRIAGE

Appointed by EMS Command Officer

- Establishes first-stage triage procedures (as dictated by incident type)
- Establishes second-stage triage procedures (prior to treatment or transport)
- Appoints triage support personnel, as needed
- Coordinates EMS activities including equipment and personnel needs within the triage (rescue/extrication) sector
- Coordinates actions with fire officers
- Coordinates patient movement through second-stage triage to treatment or transportation sectors

From New York State Department of Health, Emergency Medical Services Program: Field Manual for Multiple Casualty Incident Management. Albany, New York.

TRIAGE SUPPORT PERSONNEL

Located	ESTABLISHED TRIAGE AREAS
Radio ID	NONE ASSIGNED

Appointed by Triage Sector Officer

- Perform first-stage triage procedures, if established
- Perform second-stage triage procedures including prioritizing and tagging each patient

From New York State Department of Health, Emergency Medical Services Program: Field Manual for Multiple Casualty Incident Management. Albany, New York.

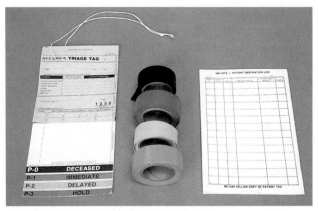

FIGURE 17–10. A triage tag, surveyor's tape, and patient log.

In certain circumstances, a third stage of triage, or field hospital, may be developed on site. This occurs if there are extraordinary delays in securing hospital care (e.g., because of isolation, weather conditions, earthquakes, floods) or in communities that mobilize field hospitals as part of their disaster plan.

Advanced life support occurs during the second and third stages of triage. Situations occur where multiple secondary triage sites are necessary. This requires the designation of additional triage officers.

In disasters, one must set priorities so that the greatest number survive.

Disaster Triage

A universal system of color coding is used to categorize patients at disasters. The colors used are red, yellow, green, and black.

RED

Red is used for critical patients with life-threatening conditions (hypotension or hypoxia) who have a chance to survive with early stabilization and transport. These patients require hospital care within 1 hour. Some systems use an emergent subclassification to identify critical patients in need of immediate physician or hospital intervention. Red-coded patients are critical patients who have a good chance of recovery after immediate definitive care. They may have conditions such as readily controllable hemorrhage, compound fractures, or mechanical respiratory problems.

YELLOW

Yellow is used for patients with potentially life-threatening injuries who must be treated within the next few hours. These patients do not have systemic signs of shock. However, their injuries can potentially cause death if not cared for.

In some systems, patients without life-threatening injuries are coded yellow if they are unable to walk. This is used to help estimate stretcher and transportation requirements. Of course, these patients would be transferred after the yellow-coded patients with potentially life-threatening injuries.

GREEN

Green-coded patients have no life-threatening injuries and generally are ambulatory. In some systems disaster victims are asked if they can walk as a means of rapidly assessing the number of victims who are ambulatory. These patients should be directed to the secondary triage area for further and closer triage. If the situation warrants, they may be asked to assist with removal of other victims.

It is amazing that in severe disasters such as plane crashes, injuries can range from minimal to those that cause sudden death. However, since all passengers suffered the same enormous force, constant reevaluation is necessary to ensure that internal injuries are not overlooked even in ambulatory cases.

BLACK

The patient found without signs of life or with obvious mortal injuries is classified as black and moved to the side or removed after the living are evacuated. In some circumstances, such as a plane crash, they may have to be removed to gain access to the living. In certain situations, where leaving the dead does not impede access to other victims, investigative personnel may prefer that the dead be left in place for accident investigation purposes.

Figure 17–11 provides an example of a triage protocol. Some systems have used a quick method to assess the major organ systems (respiratory, circulatory, and neurologic) to help separate mortally injured patients between black and red categories.

Sequence of Triage

Initial triage takes place at the accident site. Victims are moved to a separate area for stabilization and reevaluation. The secondary triage area should be the central collection point for all victims removed from the debris. Proximity to the transport area is essential. This area should be hazard-free and, when possible, protected from the weather.

At the secondary triage stage, patients are reevaluated with the intent to stabilize critical injuries and begin treatment. After secondary triage, patients should be sorted and grouped together. Signs or flags can be posted to identify separate areas (Fig. 17–12). The secondary triage area is the site where arriving medical personnel and medical supplies are gathered and more advanced treatment is initiated. Triage tags may be filled out at this time and identifying information elicited. Figure 17–13 describes how to use a triage tag.

Information about the number and classes of victims is relayed to the triage officer, and a decision is made as to whether a "field hospital" should be established. This decision depends on multiple factors, including the number of ambulances in relation to the number of vic-

PRIORITY	HANDLING	COLOR CODE	DESCRIPTION	PATIENT DIAGNOSIS
P-1	Immediate	Red	Life- or limb-threatening situations requiring immediate care	Airway or respiratory difficulties, severe burns, cardiac problems, uncontrollable or severe hemorrhage, open chest or abdominal wounds, severe head injury, severe medical problems, shock
P-2	Delayed	Yellow	Patients requiring care but will not worsen with delay	Burns, multiple or major fractures, spinal cord injuries, uncomplicated head injuries
P-3	Hold	Green	Patients with minor injuries and those of an ambulatory nature	Minor fractures and wounds, minor burns of less than 10% body surface area and no respiratory involvement, psychological problems
P-0	Deceased	Black	Patients with absence of vital signs	Casualties that have expired or those with injuries that are obviously incompatible with survival

FIGURE 17–11. Triage protocol. (Adapted from New York State Department of Health MCI Manual.)

FIGURE 17–12. Signs can be placed at the key operation areas of the disaster site to regulate the flow of patients and identify the disaster coordinators. These four signs are used to locate patients after secondary triage (P-1, P-2, P-3) and to define the area used for the command post (CP). (From New York State Department of Health MCI kit.)

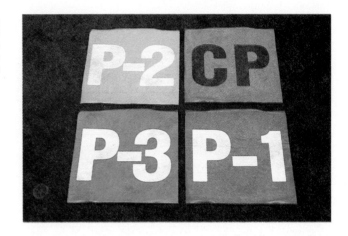

tims, weather conditions, availability of space, and the potential for advanced treatment on site.

By second-stage triage, all patients with potential spine injuries should be immobilized on a rigid stretcher and have a cervical collar placed. This may be done during the initial triage, but conditions can exist in which this is impossible. Oxygen is administered, major fractures are splinted, and shock treatment is begun, as the need indicates. Local protocols and plans dictate the level of care to be given at the scene of an accident.

Special Considerations for Triage

Special considerations during triage must be given to children, rescuers, and panicky or hysterical patients. Children should be kept with their parents when possible. Rescuers, when injured on site, must be removed from the scene immediately so as not to divert undue attention from the general rescue effort. Panic usually occurs when a victim fears death, perceives limited means of escape, and has no information about what happened. It is the responsibility of the EMT to reduce panic by providing information, giving stable and calm direction, and initiating care. Hysterical patients who cannot be calmed should be separated from other victims and removed from the scene. Of course, a careful medical evaluation of all hysterical patients is indicated to ensure they are not hypoxic or otherwise medically impaired.

TRANSPORT

The primary function of the transport officer is ambulance staging and dispatch. In communications with the EMS command or triage officer, decisions are made to deploy personnel and vehicles and ensure smooth traffic flow. Additional supplies and personnel arriving on the scene are stockpiled by the transport officer. Drivers should remain with their vehicles in the event that traffic routes or staging areas are changed. The ambulance without a driver constitutes a potential obstruction at a disaster site.

When an ambulance leaves the site with patients, the transport officer notifies the receiving hospital. In order to keep the air waves clear, only the basic patient condition is relayed. Ambulances transporting patients should be advised not to communicate with hospitals unless requested to do so by the communications coordinator.

Helicopters

When available, a landing area for helicopters should be established. Conditions permitting, helicopters can provide rapid evacuation of critical patients and expand the number of hospitals available for receipt of patients (Fig. 17–14). Systems with helicopter capability have specific protocols about landing area requirements and coordination with ground units and other helicopters (Fig. 17–15). These should be strictly adhered to because of the potential for accidents. Many helicopters have their own crews who pick up and attend to patients from the scene. EMTs should stay clear with their patients until advised to approach the helicopter by the pilot or a helicopter crew member.

Hospital Selection

Hospital selection is performed according to local protocol. In some cases, the closest hospitals become overloaded or are incapable of handling critically injured trauma or burn victims. In these situations, it may be necessary to transfer patients to other facilities.

Text continued on page 730

How to Use the NYS-EMS Triage Tag

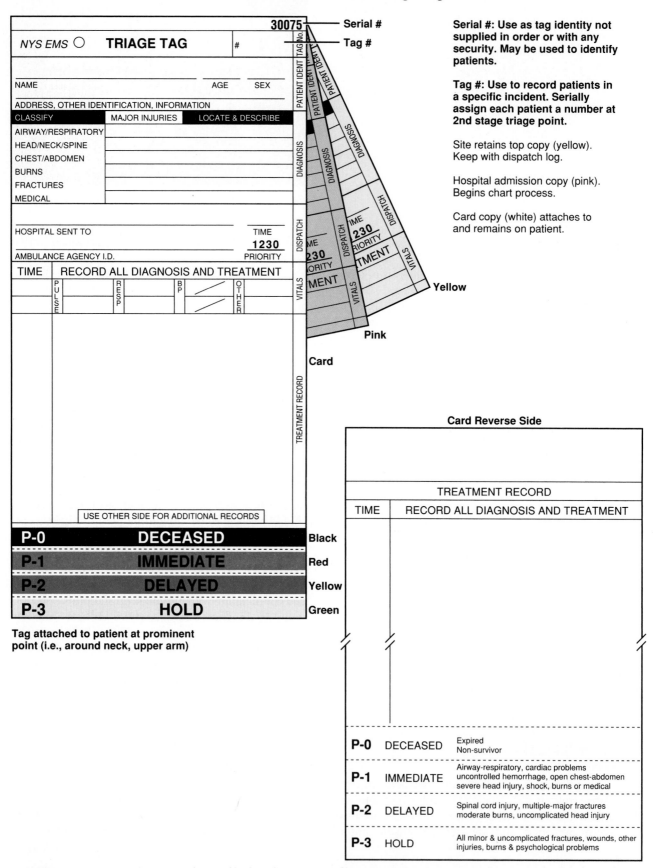

Serial #: Use as tag identity not supplied in order or with any security. May be used to identify patients.

Tag #: Use to record patients in a specific incident. Serially assign each patient a number at 2nd stage triage point.

Site retains top copy (yellow). Keep with dispatch log.

Hospital admission copy (pink). Begins chart process.

Card copy (white) attaches to and remains on patient.

Tag attached to patient at prominent point (i.e., around neck, upper arm)

Card Reverse Side

		TREATMENT RECORD	
	TIME	RECORD ALL DIAGNOSIS AND TREATMENT	
P-0	DECEASED	Expired Non-survivor	
P-1	IMMEDIATE	Airway-respiratory, cardiac problems uncontrolled hemorrhage, open chest-abdomen severe head injury, shock, burns or medical	
P-2	DELAYED	Spinal cord injury, multiple-major fractures moderate burns, uncomplicated head injury	
P-3	HOLD	All minor & uncomplicated fractures, wounds, other injuries, burns & psychological problems	

FIGURE 17–13. A typical triage tag (front and back) and explanation of how to complete the triage tag. (From New York State Department of Health MCI kit.)

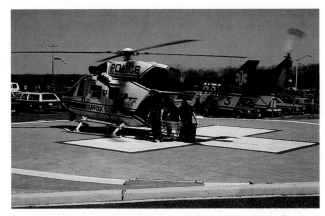 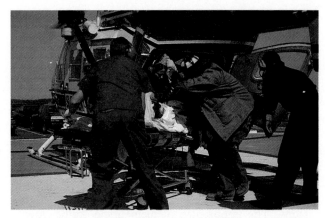

FIGURE 17–14. Helicopters can provide rapid access to critical patients and expand the number of hospitals available to receive patients.

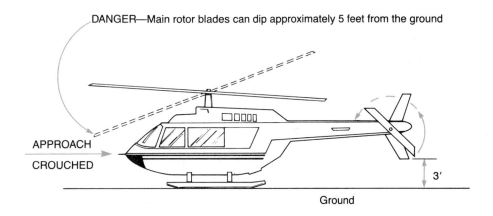

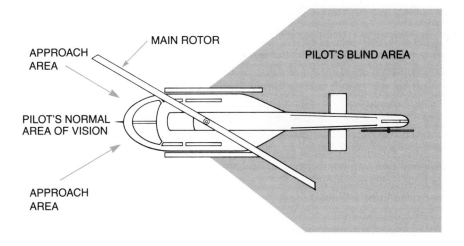

FIGURE 17–15. Helicopter safety protocol. When approaching a helicopter, you must remain in eye contact with the pilot by accessing from the zone defined in the illustration. (Redrawn from New York City Emergency Services Operations Manual.)

Convergence

Convergence is the rapid gathering of onlookers, rescuers, and members of the press at the scene of a disaster. This must be anticipated and dealt with quickly to ensure that incoming and outgoing traffic routes remain clear. Traffic control keeps back bystanders and onlookers and, at times, rescue personnel, who are asked to wait for instructions from the command post. The establishment of staging areas for the various types of responding vehicles is essential to prevent a convergence of rescue vehicles in one place. An ambulance blocked by a fire truck or other rescue vehicle is of no use at the scene. The importance of maintaining traffic flow cannot be overstressed.

The transport officer works with police to maintain traffic control.

STEPS OF DISASTER MANAGEMENT

1. *Planning* is essential to coordinate the many resources and personnel on the scene. Without planning, the success of disaster management is limited.

2. Depending on the type of disaster, *warning and evacuation* may or may not occur. Warning and evacuation are best exemplified by smoke alarms, hurricane warning systems, and the emergency broadcast system. Situations occur where no warning is possible, as in an explosion or transportation accident.

3. The *event* is the actual disaster that occurs—a bus slides off the road with 35 children on board, a plane crashes in a rural community, an earthquake strikes a major city.

The events that take place prior to the arrival of emergency personnel are beyond the rescuer's control. For example, survivors from an airplane crash at night may be lost in the woods and scattered over a large area. The victims capable of walking may run from the scene. There may be unfavorable traffic conditions because of the convergence of curious onlookers and neighbors, preventing a speedy response. The latter is such a common event that traffic and crowd control are essential elements in any disaster plan. The EMT must anticipate that these conditions will exist.

4. Following notification, the organized, dispatched *response* of emergency personnel and services to the scene begins. This response may last from hours to days.

5. *Recovery* is the process of demobilizing response vehicles and apparatus for the purpose of returning to normal operations in the community.

6. *Restoration* involves the rebuilding of the community in a physical and emotional sense. This includes critical incident stress debriefing, reconstruction, and the restoration of services (water, electricity, etc.) to the area.

ROLES AND RESPONSIBILITIES OF THE EMT

It is important for EMTs to have an overall sense of their regional disaster plan so they can assume the functions required at different points in time. If EMTs arrive on the scene first, they must assume many functions beyond that of normal patient care. These functions may play a greater role in the survival of victims than direct medical care and could include triage, transport, interhospital transfer, helicopter operations, extrication, or communications. In New York State, each ambulance is provided with a kit that provides some equipment often needed in a disaster (see the following chart).

Depending on when the first EMTs arrive at the disaster scene, they should be prepared to assume any or all of the following functions: command, triage, and transport. The following discussion assumes that two EMTs are the first responders at a disaster site. If there are more than two people, some functions can be delegated to speed operations.

Scene Assessment

Upon arrival at the disaster scene, perform a quick survey from your vehicle to obtain basic information about the type of equipment and resources needed. In a disaster, this is critical for rapid mobilization of additional resources.

Type of Incident

1. Establish the type of incident (fire, airplane crash, building collapse) and then determine if further injuries may occur. Is there fire or the presence of hazardous materials? Is the vehicle positioned safely relative to traffic, smoke, gas from spills, and so forth? Is this incident open or closed, active or contained?

2. Determine the specific location of the incident and identify the best access routes.

3. One EMT should leave the vehicle and walk to the scene. This EMT will estimate the patient numbers and injury types. He or she will also determine if the incident is open or closed, active or contained.

4. The second EMT stays with the ambulance, identifying possible staging areas and traffic routes into the site. It may be necessary early on to move the ambulance

THE NEW YORK STATE EMS MULTIPLE CASUALTY INCIDENT FIELD MANAGEMENT KIT CONTAINS THE FOLLOWING ITEMS:

- Field manuals
- Command officer identification vests
- Command post and area identification signs
- Plastic ribbon for triage & area marking
- Armbands for ancillary personnel
- Pencils (#2) and grease pencil

There are other items that may be useful resources for your agency's response plan. You need to consider the following:

Equipment and Supplies

1. Equipment

All equipment must be boldy marked, identifying the agency of ownership.

All cots/stretchers should be boldly marked to identify the agency and specific vehicle they are assigned to.

2. Agency Disaster Supplies:

Additional medical patient handling and administrative supplies need to be stored and made available. Typically these supplies include:

- 10 6' × 16"wooden spine boards
- Bandages, dressings
- Splints
- Oxygen and resuscitation equipment
- Pencils, clipboards, and felt tips or indelible markers

- Flashlights and lanterns
- Blankets
- Ground cover/tarps (conveniently colored red/yellow/green)
- Tape
- Advanced life support equipment
- Plastic resealable bags
- Masking or duct tape
- Pylons
- Stapler
- Morgue bag
- Boundary marking tape
- Rope or perimeter

3. Replenishment of Supplies:

- At scene
- After incident
- Special supplies (advanced life support)

Although the kit provided is intended for one time use, the intentional use of individual components in training can enhance multiple casualty incident preparation and education. Using triage tags on specific days, patient types, or multiple accident patients will familiarize ambulance personnel and hospitals with them. Staging, patient prioritizing, and patient handling are good drills for the education of all agency members. Management and incident command concepts should be applied at many incidents and events occurring almost daily.

From New York State Department of Health MCI Manual.

---

to expedite traffic control. Contact should be made with the communications center, informing them of the incident and relaying preliminary information.

5. As soon as the first EMT returns, the EMTs should try to ascertain the following information:

- Number of victims
- Specific location of incident
- Whether the incident is open or closed
- Whether the incident is active (continuing) or contained
- The need for special resources (e.g., lights, cranes, boats)
- Number of additional ambulances required
- Any other relevant information

6. Once these questions are addressed, this information should be immediately relayed to the communications center.

Communications

The two EMTs again separate and initiate the three primary functions of disaster management. One EMT approaches the disaster and initiates first triage. The second EMT remains with the ambulance and assumes command and transport functions. A major event log should be initiated. Similarly, a transportation log should be established with a record of all patients removed from the scene. A resource list should be developed that specifies personnel already available on the scene, requested resources yet to arrive, and hospital availability. The EMT in the command function must contact the supervising police officer and fire chief to establish a centralized command post. The ambulance, with its lights, radio, and shelter, serves as a good temporary command post.

By activating the community disaster plan, the local hospitals should be notified about the potential for incoming patients. Mutual aid plans are implemented, initiating a response to the disaster and back-up coverage for the community.

In coordination with the police department, an incoming and outgoing traffic pattern is established. A site for ambulance staging is selected and the next personnel to arrive at the scene are recruited to direct vehicles to this staging area and control their release for transport. Drivers should remain with their assigned vehicles.

In coordination with the fire department, a scene safety plan should be developed to minimize injuries to rescuers. This may involve the placement of lights, fire suppression, the placement of ladders, and initiation of safe extrication and rescue maneuvers.

The second EMT's primary function is the coordination of communications and the flow of information back to the dispatch center to ensure a proper response. Until relieved, this person represents the EMS command officer on the scene.

The first EMT must communicate with the second EMT regarding resource requirements. When available, identifying vests (Fig. 17–16) and helmets should be used.

As other units arrive on the scene, they are directed to the ambulance staging area to await instructions. EMTs carrying supplies from these vehicles respond to the scene and drivers remain with their vehicles. Until relieved, the driver is identified as the transport officer, whose function is to control traffic flow, gather supplies, stage additional vehicles, and communicate ambulance availability to the command post.

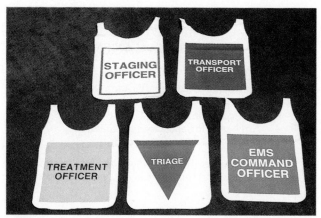

FIGURE 17–16. Vests that identify the key players at the disaster site help decrease the amount of confusion. (From New York State Department of Health MCI kit.)

Psychological Aspect

A disaster presents a situation of extreme duress for all participants—victims, families, rescuers, and the community.

The EMTs are faced with an enormous challenge. Not only are they administering psychologic first aid to the victims, but they themselves are affected by the enormity of the situation. To function effectively, EMTs must keep their own emotions in check.

It is important to acknowledge your own emotional response as you participate in the rescue. Natural empathy with the victims is normal. However, the EMT must be wary not to identify with the victims. The victims need the professional skills of the rescuers to maximize their chances of survival. Victims look to the EMT for signs (spoken and unspoken) of reassurance. Since panic is easy to spread in a disaster situation, the EMT should offer positive and encouraging feedback whenever possible.

After disasters, it is standard practice for rescuers to participate in *debriefing* exercises. These exercises serve many purposes, among which are the venting of emo-

tions and the sharing of common human reactions to the experience. Professional counselors may be available and rescuers should avail themselves of their services. Rescuers should feel free to share their emotions with fellow EMTs. Failure to acknowledge this type of stress can result in an EMT being unable to perform in the future.

Another valuable benefit that arises from debriefing is the opportunity to learn from the disaster experience. This knowledge can be used in future disaster planning and shared with other systems.

In debriefing settings, it is important to maintain patient confidentiality.

Disaster Drills

Disaster drills represent a method of training EMTs in the steps outlined in the local disaster plan. There are five types of drills.

Orientation. This is where the disaster plan is presented.
Discussion. This is a discussion of hypothetical situations in relation to the plan. Feedback is encouraged to analyze the overall approach.
Tabletop exercise. During the tabletop exercise, the participants try to solve a problem in a roundtable forum.
Emergency coordination simulation. This type of exercise requires the use of communications equipment and the physical movement of personnel and vehicles. No role-playing victims are used.
Full-scale field simulation. During the full-scale field simulation, role-playing victims are used for realism and are transported to hospitals. This may be a surprise exercise. It is recommended, however, that all participants be notified of the fact that it is a drill.

Each EMS organization handles the issue of disaster drills differently. EMTs should participate in this valuable experience.

CONCLUSION

No one looks forward to having a disaster; however, it is necessary to be prepared to respond should one occur in your community. It is the responsibility of each EMT to be knowledgeable about the disaster plan in his or her community and to be familiar with all the elements of successful disaster management. The first EMT at the scene of a disaster sets the tone for the future outcome of the operation.

REVIEW EXERCISES

1. Define the following terms:
   Disaster
   Multiple casualty incident (MCI)
   Triage
   Command post
   Mutual aid
2. List three important initial steps that EMS personnel should take upon arrival at the disaster scene.
3. Describe the roles of the following participants in a disaster:
   Triage officer
   Transport officer
   EMS command
   Communications officer
   Police
   Fire
4. Describe the function of the following areas within a disaster plan:
   Command post
   First-stage triage area
   Second-stage triage area
   Third-stage triage (field hospital)
5. Describe the proper use of triage tags.
6. Define convergence and discuss its importance at the disaster scene.
7. Describe the phases of a disaster.
8. Explain debriefing and its importance after a disaster.

REFERENCES

Nassau County Disaster Control Procedure (Revised). Nassau County, NY, Police Department and Fire Commission, January, 1988.

New York State Department of Health EMS Program: Field manual for multiple casualty incident field response. Albany, New York State Department of Health, 1988.

New York State Department of Health EMS Program: MCI: Emergency medical services management model for multiple casualty incidents. Albany, New York State Department of Health, 1983.

New York State Department of Health EMS Program: Operational update, number 87-41, Management kits for MCI field response. Albany, New York State Department of Health, 1988.

Pascarelli E: Hospital based ambulatory care. Norwalk, CT, Appleton-Century-Crofts, 1983.

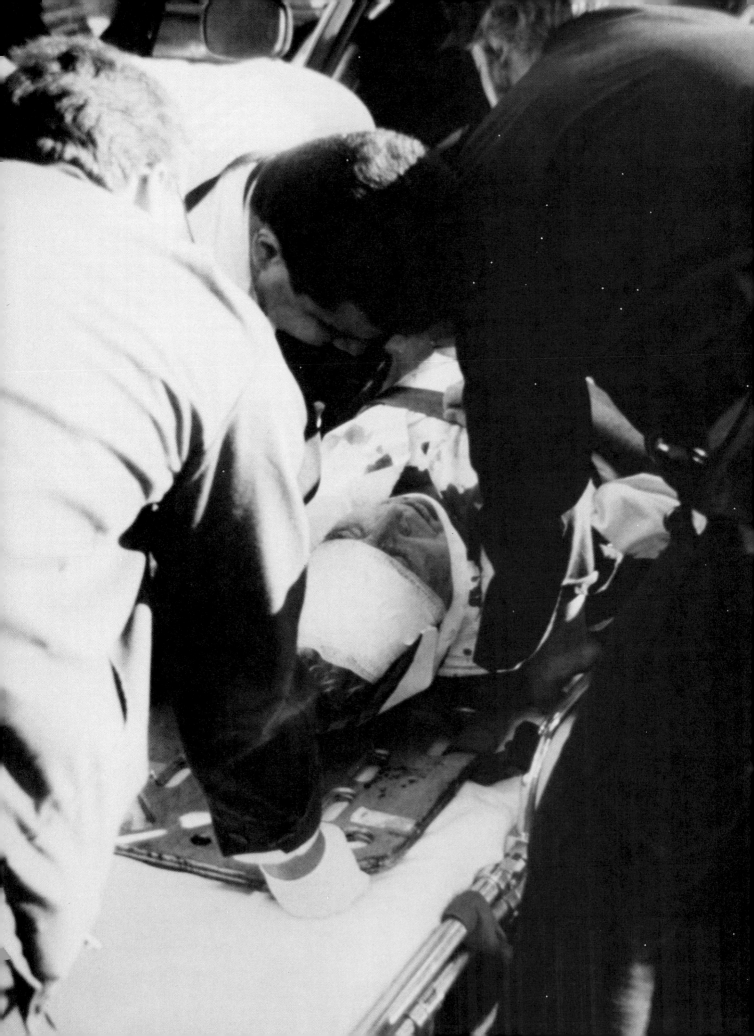

CHAPTER 18

EXTRICATION

OBJECTIVES

At the conclusion of this chapter the reader will be able to:

1. Describe the proper methods and appropriate times to use the following extrication equipment:
    Reflectors
    Hacksaw
    Vise grip pliers
    Fire ax
    Bolt cutters
    Blankets
    Pruning saw
    Bale hooks
    Jacks
    Air chisel
    Wrench (12-inch adjustable crescent)
    Screwdrivers (12-inch flat-head, 8-inch Phillips)
    Hammer
    Wrecking bar and crowbar
    Shovel
    Ropes
    Mastic knife
    Spring-loaded center punch
    Cold chisels
    Hand winch (or come along)

2. Describe how to cut a roof flap.

3. Describe how to immobilize, package, and remove a victim of an automobile accident.

You respond to an automobile accident in which there are injured occupants. The questions that should go through your mind as you approach the scene include the following: How many casualties will there be? How did the accident occur? Will assistance be needed? Is the victim trapped? Upon your arrival, you find two vehicles. One victim is pinned by the steering wheel in vehicle number one and two victims are in vehicle number two. The arm of the driver of vehicle number two is trapped in the space between his seat and the door post, and his feet are caught beneath the pedals. The head of the passenger in vehicle number two has been thrust through the windshield and is stuck. These situations present problems that have relatively simple solutions. However, unless you learn the skills of extrication and how to apply them, this scenario could result in unnecessary tragedy (Fig. 18–1).

Rescue of the entrapped victim is a specialized field. However, it is important for the EMT to be familiar with the use of basic hand tools and the principles of extrication.

INTRODUCTION

Freeing the trapped accident victim represents a challenging aspect of prehospital care. The stressful combination of a confined working environment; the trapped, unstable patient; and the surrounding chaos tests the nerves and stamina of the EMT. Early after your arrival you should determine whether additional resources are needed to attend to the multiple tasks required to save the victims. Fortunately, many EMS systems provide a separate division of rescue personnel to support the EMT in his or her extrication efforts (Fig. 18–2).

ROLE OF THE EMT

At the accident scene, the EMT's primary role is evaluation and emergency care. Proper assessment and treatment along with careful packaging of the patient for removal should be foremost in your mind. However, if rescue crews are not available, you should be sufficiently confident to carry out an efficient and safe extrication.

The availability of specialized crews for rescue varies from one locale to another. In cities, there are often separate rescue teams who specialize in extrication and rescue. EMTs must know how to rapidly access this needed support. The EMT in such an area does not have to maintain as high a degree of proficiency in rescue operations as does an EMT located in a place where such support does not exist. EMTs in rural or suburban areas may be required to be more proficient in extrication skills. In some locales, the EMTs may also function as the specialists in rescue and extrication—skills obtained from training beyond the EMT curriculum.

Regardless of where you work, it is desirable for all EMTs to have a basic knowledge of extrication and be proficient in the use of light extrication tools. The EMT's ability to make the distinction between light and heavy rescue circumstances is critical.

A light rescue situation is one in which an extrication can be accomplished through the use of hand tools and basic skills such as sliding the seat back, applying a short spine board, and removing the patient. A heavy rescue situation is one in which power tools and additional resources and personnel are required. The EMT must be able to quickly determine if light or heavy rescue services are needed as well as to assess if he or she is capable of handling the situation.

If rescue personnel are available, your role is to ensure proper assessment, treatment, and removal of the patient. EMTs should coordinate their efforts with rescue personnel.

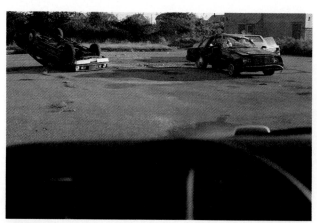

FIGURE 18–1. Look through the windshield to ascertain how many victims are inside the car. Are any victims trapped? What resources will you need?

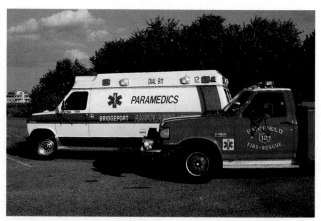

FIGURE 18–2. The EMS and the rescue team must work cooperatively to achieve the best possible patient outcomes. The key to success is cooperation.

Scene Safety

One of the most basic principles of rescue operations is that the scene must be assessed for potential danger to rescuers, the public, and the patient. It is important to recognize that not all patients who are in need of rescue can be rescued. There are certain situations that present such significant hazards to both rescuers and the public that an effort to effect the rescue may be both futile and costly (in terms of lives). The need to do a risk–benefit analysis is essential. The rescuer who runs into a burning building without assessing the safety of the scene and loses his or her life becomes an additional victim unnecessarily.

A classic example of a failure to assess hazards occurred several years ago. An EMT crew responding to a report of a child who had fallen into a pit entered a toxic environment without regard for their personal safety. They also failed to don their protective clothing and breathing apparatus. It is very difficult to critique the actions of individuals who have given their lives in an effort to effect a rescue; however, it is important to analyze and learn from past mistakes to prevent future loss of life.

In the case mentioned above, when the ambulance arrived, a father stated that his child had fallen into a pit that was used to store grass clippings. The EMTs entered this environment without the benefit of self-contained breathing apparatus. The first EMT entered the pit and found the child but was overcome by toxic fumes. The second EMT, seeing his partner in need of help, tried to rescue him and was overcome as well. Upon arrival of the volunteer fire department, one of the firefighters who knew the EMTs also entered the pit without benefit of a self-contained breathing apparatus. This individual also succumbed to the toxic fumes. The child for whom the original rescue had been initiated was subsequently retrieved and resuscitated. The lives of the three individuals who attempted the rescue were lost.

Your protective "envelope" represents the single most important factor in reducing EMT injury. A complete protective envelope consists of headgear, eye protection, respiratory protection (if required), gloves, boots, and coat (Fig. 18–3). In dealing with a rescue situation, it is essential to remember that patient care always precedes the rescue effort *unless a life safety hazard exists.* A life safety hazard is any situation in which the rescuers are risking serious injury or death as the result of entering the rescue area. A life safety hazard is encountered, for example, every time an EMT stops to assist an injured motorist on a dark, unmarked roadway. Remember, your value to the patient is lost if you are injured or killed.

The greatest and most common hazard encountered by EMTs is the traffic surrounding auto accidents. The wearing of dark clothing, the failure to don reflective vests, and the inappropriate use of traffic delineation

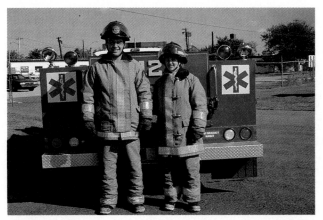

FIGURE 18–3. EMTs wearing the proper protective clothing to perform a rescue.

devices, all present unnecessary risks to EMTs. Traffic cones, flares, and the lights on the ambulance should be used to alert oncoming traffic that there is a hazard ahead and to protect those operating at the scene. While traffic control is usually a police function, situations occur that require EMTs to be knowledgeable about traffic hazards. Many EMTs have been badly injured and killed in traffic situations. The EMT must be alert to traffic hazards at all times.

Once the hazards are eliminated and you are wearing your protective clothing, the medical treatment for the entrapped patient becomes your priority. In this type of operation, your rapid assessment and treatment abilities are put to the test. The need for an accurate, focused approach is paramount because of the distractions of the environment.

Since most auto accidents involve more than one patient, it is important that the EMTs involved in the rescue effort perform triage prior to treatment. The ability to skillfully triage patients in an auto extrication situation may be hampered by limited access to the trapped victims. Additionally, the extrication time necessary to remove a patient may change the triage status of the patient. For instance, a patient who is a yellow priority (e.g., an individual with long bone fractures who is experiencing significant internal bleeding) might have to be recategorized as a red if the estimated extrication time is prolonged.

Time on the Scene

Since the trauma patient often requires surgical intervention in order to stabilize his or her condition, time is an important consideration in every rescue. As soon as possible, the patient must be evaluated to determine the need for lifesaving management, including rapid transport to a trauma center. The concept of time must be foremost in the mind of the rescuer, especially when several victims are entrapped and priorities must be established.

Patient care should include attention to life-threatening injuries; immobilization; and, when possible, rapid extrication. All patients should be immobilized to prevent further injury during the rescue effort.

EXTRICATION EQUIPMENT

The Basic Tools

The basic tools that EMTs use are essentially hand tools. The following list of tools is compiled from recommendations of the Committee on Trauma of the American College of Surgeons and the Department of Transportation National EMT Curriculum.

REFLECTORS. Traffic delineation devices are essential in maintaining the safety of the scene. Reflectors, flares, traffic cones, and battery-operated lights are recommended.

All traffic delineation devices have merit—the EMT must decide which device best fits the needs of a particular situation. The benefits and hazards of particular devices must be considered.

For example, flares, although clearly visible at night, are of less benefit in the daytime. In addition, if gasoline has spilled at the scene, flares represent a fire hazard and add to the risks already present.

A primary hazard to be wary of when caring for patients at an accident scene is the drunk or sleeping driver coming down the road. These individuals are operating their vehicles on muscle memory; they seem to be driving on "automatic pilot." The use of traffic cones is significantly effective with regard to these hazardous drivers. When an automobile hits and runs over a traffic cone, the cone makes a sound at the time of impact that continues as it is dragged beneath the undercarriage of the car. This may alert sleepy or drunken drivers and jog them back to a level of consciousness that enables them to react to the oncoming accident and keeps them from swerving into the accident site.

The placement of traffic delineation devices such as cones, flares, or reflectors should take into account the posted speed limit. A good rule of thumb is to place traffic devices at least three times the distance (in feet) of the posted speed limit. For example, if the speed limit is 55 miles per hour, the first delineation device should be placed approximately no closer than 165 feet from the accident site. Another technique is to place devices one and a half times the average stopping distance of oncoming traffic behind the accident site (see Chapter 19 for stopping distances). This allows all individuals approaching the scene to stop and react in an appropriate amount of time. Blind turns represent another type of problem. Quite obviously, devices must be placed before the turn begins and throughout the entire turn to alert

drivers passing through this area that a hazard exists ahead. Use as many devices as possible to alert traffic to the upcoming hazard.

WRENCH—12-INCH ADJUSTABLE CRESCENT. The 12-inch adjustable crescent wrench is useful for opening the nuts and bolts of most vehicles. To keep the rescue operation simple, it is usually easier to disengage a piece of metal than to distort or displace it from the vehicle (Fig. 18–4).

SCREWDRIVERS—12-INCH FLAT-HEAD, 8-INCH PHILLIPS. Screwdrivers are used to disengage car parts and as a blade to cut through metal. They can also be used as a prying tool to open windows when using lock-opening devices (Fig. 18–4).

HACKSAW. A hacksaw is an invaluable device used to cut through steering wheels, window posts, brake pedals, and other metal obstacles. Extra blades are essential in the event of breakage or tearing of the saw's teeth (see Fig. 18–4).

VISE GRIP PLIERS. Vise grip pliers are useful for the removal of nuts and bolts, as well as for stripping away the plastic covering from steering wheels (see Fig. 18–4).

HAMMER. A hammer can be used as a striking device to drive shearing instruments through metal (Fig. 18–5).

FIRE AX (FLAT HEAD). The fire ax is used to bend metal or to strike through glass (see Fig. 18–10). Figure 18–6 illustrates a flat head ax.

WRECKING BAR AND CROWBAR. The wrecking bar is a device used for prying metal and for leverage in moving objects in coordination with a crowbar (Fig. 18–7). A good wrecking bar is the Haligan tool. It can also be used for a variety of other purposes.

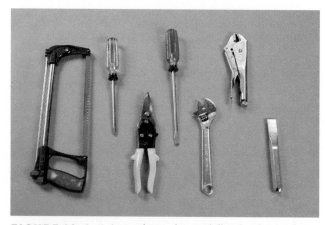

FIGURE 18–4. (*Left to right*) Hacksaw, Phillips-head screwdriver, tin snips, flat-head screwdriver, crescent wrench, vise grip pliers, and chisel.

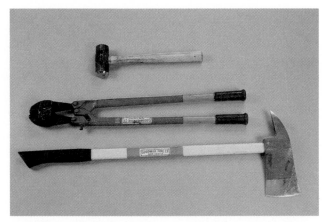

FIGURE 18-5. (*Top to bottom*) Hammer, bolt cutters, and ax.

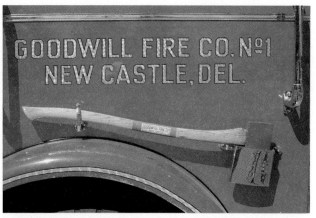

FIGURE 18-6. Flat-head ax.

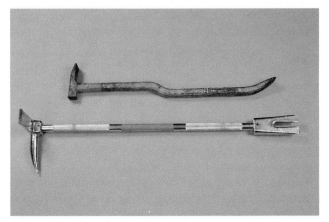

FIGURE 18-7. Wrecking bar and Haligan tool.

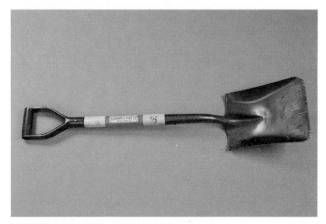

FIGURE 18-8. Shovel.

BOLT CUTTERS. Bolt cutters enable the EMT to cut through metal objects such as the steering wheel quickly and with minimal effort (see Fig. 18-5).

SHOVEL. A shovel is useful to move dirt or snow that blocks the rescue effort. Additionally, it may be used to create dikes of dirt to contain any spills. This prevents run-off and ignition of gasoline or other flammable liquids (Fig. 18-8).

TIRE IRON. The tire iron is available in most vehicles and can be used to cut through sheet metal, such as roofs or door panels.

ROPES. Ropes can be used to provide hand-holds on steep hills, to execute rescues from ditches, and to be thrown out to people who must be rescued from water. Care should be taken in the selection of ropes to ensure that the tensile strength is appropriate for the task at hand. Ropes require significant maintenance and protection (they should be stored in bags). Failure to do so can result in fraying and breaking, with possible tragic consequences (Fig. 18-9).

BLANKETS. Blankets used for the purpose of rescue should be thick, fire retardant, and capable of pro-

tecting the victims from glass shards and other objects. Normal ambulance blankets sometimes do not meet this requirement and therefore a specific rescue blanket should be acquired and maintained.

MASTIC KNIFE. The mastic knife and carpet cutters are useful tools for the removal of windshields and seat belts. A mastic knife's curved blade helps ensure patient protection when cutting is required (Fig. 18-10).

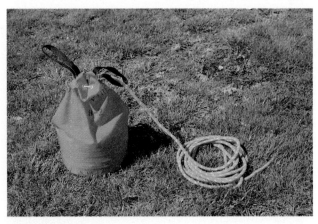

FIGURE 18-9. Rope.

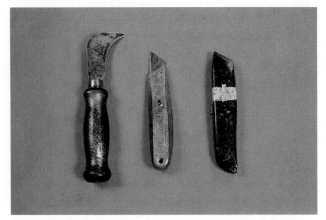

FIGURE 18-10. Mastic knife and carpet cutters.

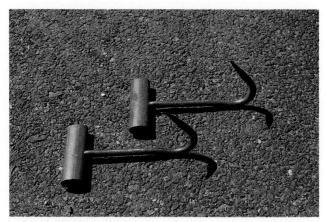

FIGURE 18-11. Bale hooks.

SPRING-LOADED CENTER PUNCH. The spring-loaded center punch is normally a device carried by the individual EMT. It should also be maintained in the ambulance rescue kit. This device effectively breaks window glass (with the exception of the windshield) while minimizing the risk of injury to the patient. The center punch initiates force at a focal point that shatters the glass without forcing it to fall. In other words, if properly applied, the entire glass should shatter but remain in the window frame for slow removal by the rescuer (see Fig. 18–28).

PRUNING SAW. The pruning saw is useful in cutting wooden objects that may present obstacles.

BALE HOOKS. Bale hooks are used during operations that require pulling and tearing. They can be useful in the removal of windshields (Fig. 18–11).

COLD CHISELS. The cold chisel is used in conjunction with a sledge hammer and can distort and sever objects with surprising accuracy. The availability of cold chisels in the tool box adds versatility to rescue techniques (see Fig. 18–4).

JACKS. The jacks that accompany most cars are capable of assisting in many rescue operations. They can lift, stabilize, and distort effectively. It is important to state that jacks should be used with cribbing.

STORAGE AND MAINTENANCE. Keep all rescue tools in their place and in good repair. A tool box should be dry and all tools should be kept in a neat and clean condition. Tools should be checked periodically. Total familiarity with their use is essential in order for you to be effective in those situations where minutes count. A periodic extrication drill on a junk vehicle is an effective way to allow all members of the EMS crew to reinforce the proper use of the various rescue tools. Tools that are rusty, dented, or dirty or that have loose bolts, as well as an improper knowledge of how to use them, are the most critical factors leading to ineffective rescue techniques.

Specialized Tools

The tools listed below are useful and basic to light rescue; however, the need for formal hands-on training and practice is essential in order to protect both you and the patient.

HYDRAULIC JACK SPREADER AND CUTTER. The hydraulic jack spreader and cutter is available in most

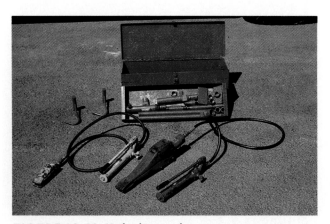

FIGURE 18-12. Hydraulic spreaders.

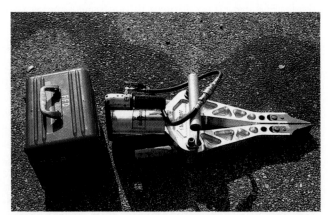

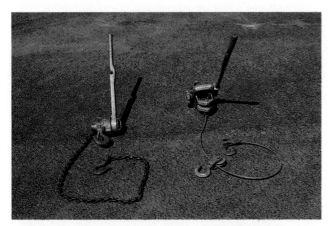

FIGURE 18–13. The hand winch (come along).

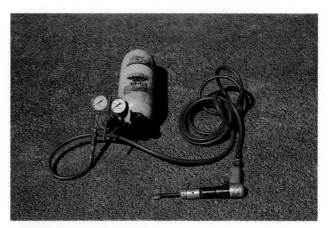

FIGURE 18–14. Air chisel.

communities. This device provides the ambulance crew with lifting, spreading, and pulling capability that would not be possible otherwise. This device is sometimes available through the local fire department or rescue squad (Fig. 18–12).

HAND WINCH (COME ALONG). This tool can be used to pull steering wheels, displace seats, and stabilize vehicles. This device should have a 5-ton capacity and a breakaway handle. The breakaway handle ensures that you cannot pull or lift more than 5 tons. If the breakaway handle breaks or bends, the hand winch should not release the load to which it is presently attached. The hand winch assists greatly during pulling and distorting operations (Fig. 18–13).

AIR CHISEL. The air chisel is a quick and prudent assistant. It should have a minimum generating pressure of 90 pounds per square inch (psi). The ambulance should carry additional air cylinders and chisels. The air chisel can cut panels of metal, glass, and plastic almost effortlessly. This device is a valuable piece of extrication equipment (Fig. 18–14).

Additional Rescue Equipment

The following additional equipment should be available either on the primary response vehicle or a heavy rescue vehicle with a maximum response time of 10 minutes (Fig. 18–15).

15-foot chain with a grab hook or running hook
2 × 4 inch wood cribbing sufficient to stabilize vehicles (various lengths may be required)

The following equipment should not be used unless the EMT has had specialized training:

Two ropes, 150-foot length, 5/8-inch Kernmantle construction with a maximum 2% stretch factor and an 11,000-lb minimum tensile strength (must be carried

in protective bags). Ropes must be kept clean and dry and periodically inspected.
Swiss seat or other type of rappelling harness
Carabiniers, locking type, minimum rod stock 10 mm (minimum of 10)
Stokes basket with lowering harness
Additional hand winch (minimum 5-ton with breakaway handle)
Self-contained breathing apparatus (SCUBA)
Hydraulic truck jack (minimum 4 tons)
Local extrication needs may necessitate additional equipment (e.g., scuba gear, aerial rescue equipment for tall buildings, mountain rescue equipment, etc.).

STAGES OF EXTRICATION

The extrication process can be divided into five distinct phases:

- Scene safety and gaining access
- Essential emergency care (rapid extrication)
- Disentanglement
- Immobilization and packaging
- Removal

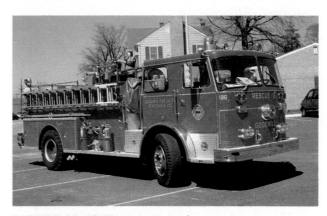

FIGURE 18–15. Heavy rescue truck.

Scene Safety

Upon arrival to the emergency rescue scene, the EMT has a responsibility to gain immediate access to the patient and provide lifesaving intervention. Part of this process involves assessing the need for additional assistance and specialized help and establishing scene safety.

Just as it is your responsibility to be familiar with the inventory of bandages and oxygen in the ambulance, it is also your responsibility to ensure that the vehicle is capable of responding and that all hand tools are functional. Make sure that the scene is safe. It is essential that prior to attempting a rescue you evaluate the need for respiratory protection, make sure the vehicle is stabilized, and evaluate all traffic and other life safety hazards.

PROTECTIVE ENVELOPE. Having the appropriate protective clothing is essential. Protective clothing should include, but not be limited to, headgear, eye protection, body protection, and foot protection. Unfortunately, protective clothing is bulky, hot, and generally not conducive to providing effective and timely treatment.

The decision to remove any component of protective gear is an individual one; however, with the removal of any component or piece, the potential for injury is expanded. For example, a cut on the hand from windshield glass could be avoided by wearing gloves; an object could be kept from entering the eye by wearing goggles, and injury from a direct blow to the head could be prevented by wearing a helmet.

In general, your uniform should be flame resistant and retardant. As discussed previously, the greatest threat to your safety is from traffic hazards. Does your clothing have a reflective capability?

Choose clothing that is conducive to safety in your work environment. The National Fire Protection Association created standards for protective clothing for firefighters. The federal Occupational Safety and Health Administration (OSHA) also has developed standards. These agencies are appropriate sources for information on this topic.

Remember, the areas of the body you are trying to protect are head, eyes, hands, torso, legs, and feet. The primary hazards that you face are from traffic, fire, debris, cuts, and toxic contamination. Your protective gear should provide sufficient protection against these threats. Your level of involvement in a particular rescue process also determines the type of protective clothing that you require (Fig. 18–16).

RESPIRATORY PROTECTION. A frequent area of concern to EMTs is respiratory protection. The use of self-contained breathing apparatus (SCUBA) should be restricted to those individuals who have specific hands-

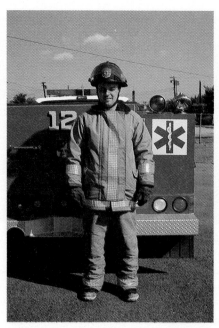

FIGURE 18–16. The EMT in protective clothing. Note the reflective stripes on the protective clothing that makes the EMT visible on the accident scene.

on training with this equipment. If you feel that you require such training, the local fire service can probably provide it (Fig. 18–17). EMTs should be able to recognize possible toxic environments and recognize the need for SCUBA use.

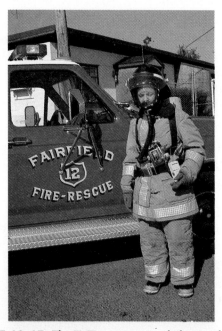

FIGURE 18–17. The EMT in protective clothing with self-contained breathing apparatus. Note the yellow personal distress device on the belt. If the EMT is motionless for a set period of time this device will activate. In addition, if in trouble, the EMT can activate the device manually and alert others involved in the operation. The helmet is tipped back to fully see the face piece; in a normal operation the helmet would be square on the head.

APPROACH TO THE SCENE.   The decisions you make while approaching the accident scene determine the effectiveness of the patient's rescue. You have the capability of making a rescue safe and efficient or a disaster. When approaching the scene, stop (ideally 100 feet away, uphill, and upwind), look, and listen. Observe what is happening (Fig. 18–18). How many cars? How many victims? What resources do you need? Are the resources presently with you or available to you in a timely fashion? When assessing a scene do a risk–benefit analysis. Determine whether a rescue attempt will pose an undue risk of injury to you or other rescuers. If the risk is greater than the benefit, it would be logical to take actions that would reduce the risk. For example, if a car is fully enveloped in flames upon your arrival, you would not initially place your hands in the car in an attempt to rescue the occupants but rather would attempt to extinguish the fire. Being capable of making risk–benefit analyses makes you an effective member of the rescue team.

Upon approaching the car, do a windshield survey (Fig. 18–19). Are the victims moving? Are they conscious? Are they attempting to exit the vehicle? During your approach to the car, make a quick check for downed electrical wires in the immediate vicinity. If wires are down, *do not touch anything*, retreat to a position of safety, protect all bystanders by establishing a hazard zone, and advise the occupants of the car not to attempt to exit. Contact the appropriate support service (local utility) and have them shut the power off and move the wires.

Evaluate the stability of the vehicle and determine whether it can be entered safely. Will the vehicle turn over? Is it on its side? On its wheels? Is it secure? Does the vehicle rock? Could the movement of the vehicle or a rescue attempt injure the patient because the vehicle still has the capability of moving? If this is the case, it is necessary to block the frame of the vehicle by using cribbing to prevent any movement and ensure stabilization. A vehicle resting on its side presents a significant hazard and should be stabilized prior to gaining access. Any vehicle, even if it is on its wheels, should be stabilized. It may only be necessary to chock (place a wedge under) the wheels to prevent forward motion. The potential for severe injury to both rescuers and victims from an unstable vehicle is great.

Knowing your personal limitations relative to the rescue scene is very important. The place to try new rescue equipment and technique is the garage, in a structured training program, not in the field, where the lives of the victims and rescuers may be at risk.

STABILIZING THE VEHICLE.   The goal of stabilization is to prevent any unwanted or dangerous movement of the car body on its springs. It is also to ensure that the structural integrity of the car is not going to be compromised by the rescue effort. This includes but is not limited to rolling, tipping, falling, or rocking. Stabilization is accomplished by taking the weight of the vehicle and spreading it out over as great an area as possible. Make as many points of the car as possible come in contact with the ground.

There are many methods of stabilizing a vehicle with hands. The attempt by personnel to lift or stabilize a vehicle is both unsafe and foolhardy. Although several muscular individuals can certainly lift a vehicle, what happens when one of them injures his or her back in the middle of the operation? The use of cribbing material is the safe method of stabilizing a vehicle. With the advent

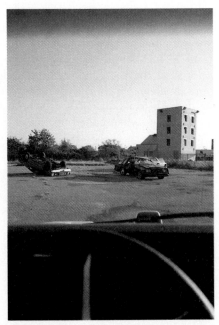

FIGURE 18–18. When approaching the scene, look all around for hazards and indications of activity. Look for hazardous material placards, spillage, and fire. Look for victims who may have been ejected from the vehicle. Initially, look at the scene from a distance for your safety and for the safety of the victims. Decide what initial resources you need and call for them.

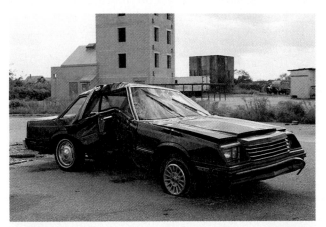

FIGURE 18–19. Look at the car. Is this a high-velocity crash? Is there impact on the passenger area? Are the victims trapped? Some EMS systems take Polaroid pictures of the car so that the physician at the hospital can visualize the damage. Would that be useful here?

of airbags, the ability to quickly stabilize a vehicle has become possible. Use hardwood such as oak for cribbing, and carry several different sizes. It is important that you build a base of large pieces, integrating smaller pieces toward the top. Figure 18–20 illustrates the basic technique for vehicle stabilization using wood cribbing and an airbag. Although air bags and hydraulic jacks are well suited for lifting, they should not be depended upon for total stabilization. They fail to spread the weight evenly, and the potential for slippage exists. These devices should be used in conjunction with cribbing to ensure stabilization. Airbags that are not properly placed by trained personnel have a tendency to slip or shoot out from lift points. The use of airbags requires special training prior to their application in the field.

SUPPORT OPERATIONS.   As the rescue operation proceeds, evaluate the need for support operations such as lighting and establish effective police lines and safety zones.

Gaining Access

Efforts to gain access to the patient should be made in the most expedient manner possible. The route by which you reach the patient is not necessarily the route by which the patient is removed. Your objective at this point is to get into the car and provide lifesaving care and stabilization prior to removal.

Once inside the car, your assessment of the patient's condition may change and, therefore, the priorities of the rescue are altered accordingly. Entering at the points of least resistance is the best approach to gaining access. In general, these are doors, windows, the windshield, the roof, and the floor. When you gain access, take your rescue blanket with you and cover the victim. This serves two purposes: first, it aids in treating the victim for shock by maintaining his or her body temperature; and second, it provides some measure of protection during the rescue.

DOORS

Since the doors of the vehicle are intended for entry, they probably can be used to gain access most expediently. It is always important to keep the rescue operation as simple as possible. For example, if the door is locked and the victim is conscious, ask him or her to unlock the door. It may be all that is needed to gain access. Also, check all the doors, including hatchbacks, before breaking glass.

UNLOCKING THE DOOR.   Frequently, the EMT must unlock the door of a vehicle. Several different techniques exist for doing this. Hook wires consist of a piece of small wire with a hoop. The hook wire is the most efficient tool for entering a locked car when the door lock is equipped with a mushroom-type button (Fig. 18–21). The specific type of wire that is used varies; for example, sometimes the antenna of the car works better than a coat hanger. To be effective with a hook wire, it is important to use a flat-head screwdriver or prying tool to open the window.

SLIM JIM.   The Slim Jim is a device frequently used by car repossession agents and is very effective, causing little or no damage to the vehicle. The drawback with this technique is its basic unreliability. Unless you use the device on a regular basis, your potential for success is limited (Fig. 18–22).

ANTI-THEFT DEVICES.   Anti-theft locks are very common in vehicles manufactured in the 1980s and 1990s. In some vehicles, the anti-theft lock or button comes as a standard option. The device, designed to protect property, prevents a rapid evaluation and evacuation of the patient. The most suitable tool for opening this lock is an 18-inch length of coat hanger wire, with a washer looped at the end. The washer should have a hole of approximately $\frac{1}{2}$ inch; it should then be bent at an angle 45 degrees to its diameter. This tool slips over the door button and, when pulled up, snags the lock.

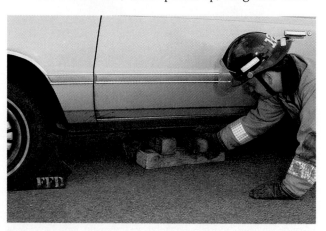

A   B

FIGURE 18–20. (*A*) The airbag and the wheel chock stabilize the car in two directions—forward and backward and up and down. (*B*) The cribbing also provides vehicle stabilization.

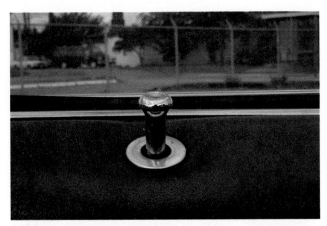

FIGURE 18–21. This is the mushroom-type of door lock.

CUTTING DOOR PANELS.   Cutting door panels is a technique used for gaining access. It is primarily used when opening the door is required to remove a patient. Several devices are quite suitable for this purpose. Screwdriver and hammer combinations, tin snips, panel cutters, axes, and pieces of sharpened leaf springs are all quite capable of doing a quick and efficient job. Figures 18–23 through 18–27 show the proper techniques used to cut door panels.

Taking time to open stuck doors should be done only when the patient's condition or appearance indicates that additional time can be taken. The cutting of door panels is a time-consuming process and sometimes it is quicker to go through the window. The patient's condition must dictate the technique to be used. One other concern is always the chance of compromising the struc-

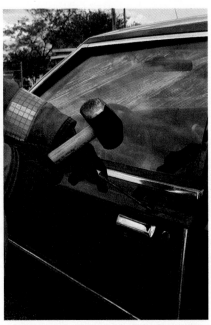

FIGURE 18–23. Cutting the door panel with a screwdriver. Position the edge of the blade against the metal and strike it sharply with a small sledge. Make sure to hold the screwdriver with only the flat edge in the metal.

tural integrity of the vehicle. Remember, for every action that you take during a rescue, some other reaction or reduction of overall structural integrity of the car may occur.

WINDOWS

If the door is locked and the victim is unconscious, the quickest way to gain access is to select the window furthest from the victim and break the glass with the spring-loaded window punch. Since the patient may be in need of immediate lifesaving therapy, breaking glass is a reasonable and necessary response. You may do an

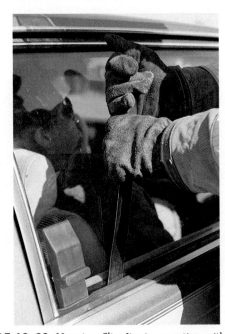

FIGURE 18–22. Here is a Slim Jim in operation with a wedge. The Slim Jim produced commercially is the best type to use. A great deal of practice is required. Instruction manuals in the use of the Slim Jim are available.

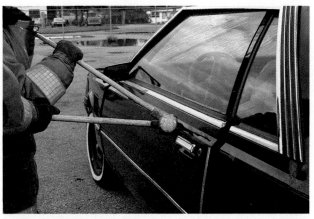

FIGURE 18–24. Cutting the door panel with an ax and sledge. This is a two-person operation. A flat-head ax should be used in this situation. There is a great need for coordination between the two parties involved in the cutting process.

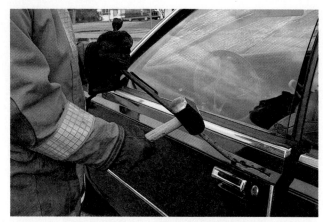

FIGURE 18–25. Cutting the door panel with a tire iron and hammer. A small sledge hammer should be used in this technique. This is very similar to cutting with a screwdriver and, although not the optimal system, can be used in a crisis when other tools are not available.

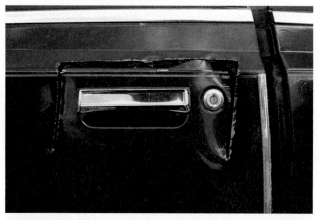

FIGURE 18–26. Once the door panel is completely cut, it should appear as illustrated here. It can then be pulled back and the door opened. Please note that the patient's condition may not allow for this time-consuming method of gaining access. If this is the case, other options should be evaluated.

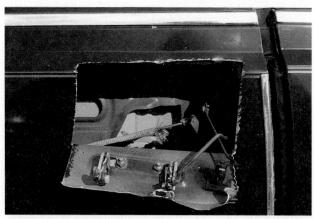

FIGURE 18–27. With the door panel peeled back, the lock mechanism and door latch mechanism are accessible to the rescuer.

initial patient assessment through the window before you are able to enter the car with your whole body.

Spring-loaded window punches are the ideal tools to be used for gaining access and result in the least amount of glass entering the vehicle. If possible, you should practice this technique on a junk car prior to a real situation so that you are familiar with the technique (Figs. 18–28 and 18–29).

Other methods of breaking glass include the use of hammers, axes, Haligan tools, and screwdrivers. All of these methods have drawbacks over the spring-loaded punch. One method of reducing the amount of glass entering the vehicle is to stick contact paper over the window to be broken and then break the glass. A good deal of the glass remains stuck to the paper. One draw-

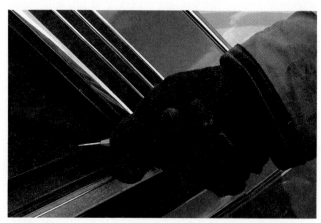

FIGURE 18–28. The spring-loaded center punch is a great tool for breaking window glass in a nonobtrusive way. This device breaks window glass quickly, without showering it throughout the car. It only works on a fully framed and closed window. It is dependent upon complete circumferential pressure to achieve the desired result.

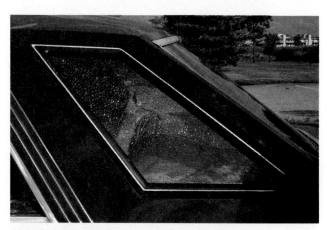

FIGURE 18–29. This is a vehicle side window after the spring-loaded center punch has been used. Note that the center punch does not operate on the windshield because it is laminated glass. It is effective only on side windows because they are made of tempered glass. The breaking quality of the tempered glass is what makes the device work.

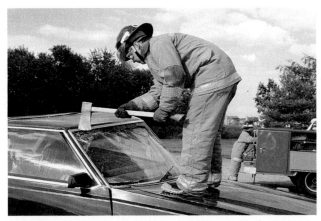

FIGURE 18–30. Cutting the windshield. The use of an ax for cutting the windshield to gain access should be done as a last resort. Full protective clothing is required because in cutting the windshield the glass becomes like particles of sand. Note the position of the EMT as he makes the first downward cuts.

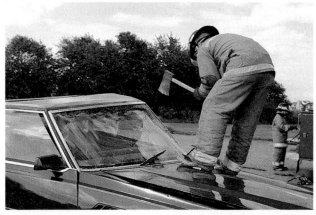

FIGURE 18–31. A flap is cut in a U-shaped pattern and then pulled down.

back to this method is that contact paper does not stick well on wet windows and, therefore, may not always produce the expected result. The word *window* is used here to refer to all the windows on the vehicle, with the exception of the windshield. The windshield is made of laminated glass, which can withstand significant impact and, therefore, cannot be broken with a window punch. Rather, the windshield is cut along the outside with an ax and folded unto the hood (Figs. 18–30 to 18–33A). Being familiar with windshield construction is essential if rescue attempts in which a windshield is involved are to be successful. If you understand how something is put together, you are better able to disassemble it. Windshield mountings have changed in the last 15 years, and it is important that you be familiar with these changes.

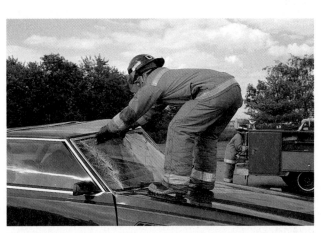

FIGURE 18–32. The EMT grips the windshield and pulls it toward the hood of the vehicle.

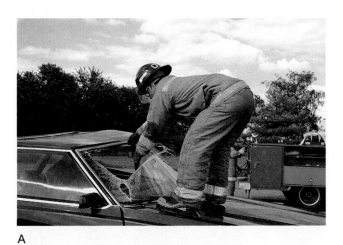

A

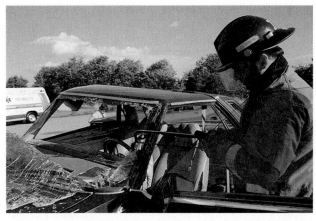

B

FIGURE 18–33. (*A*) As the EMT pulls the windshield back, notice the layer of plastic inside the windshield—this is the lamination. When possible, the windshield should be totally removed from the car in one piece. Although cutting the windshield in a crisis to gain access is an option, preferably the windshield should be removed whole. (*B*) Cutting the door posts for roof removal with a hacksaw is only initiated after all the chrome framing around the windshield has been removed. The cuts are done low and close to the body of the vehicle so that the remaining posts do not further impede the rescue. It is sometimes necessary, when using hand tools, to apply upward pressure on the inside of the roof to allow the saw blade to pass smoothly.

In 1965, windshields were mounted in a rubber channel, making removal significantly easier; it also made the windshield less likely to protect the occupants in the event of a crash. From 1965 to 1969, attempts to use soft adhesives replaced many channel systems. These adhesives sometimes leaked and dried out, and finally, in 1969, mastic compounds were used for the first time. The mastic compounds greatly increased the integrity of windshields but also made their removal more difficult. This is because mastic reseals itself when it is in contact with its original contact point. In newer vehicles, it is paramount to remember that once you separate the windshield from a contact point during removal, any recontacts with that point will seal it again. The use of small wooden wedges or screwdrivers is helpful in preventing that re-contact.

In some trucks, vans, buses, and cars, the U-mount rubber system of windshield placement is still used. The EMT should learn to identify this type of window mount.

CUTTING THE ROOF

If you decide that it is necessary to cut the roof of a vehicle to gain access, you should be aware that there can be potential problems associated with this. There is no question that cutting the roof of a vehicle that has been involved in a crash poses a risk of compromising the total structural integrity of the vehicle. When considering cutting the roof, EMTs should recognize that there are essentially two types of roof cuts—one for gaining access, and one for removing patients. When cutting the roof, remember your initial objective. Are you trying to get in or to get the patient out? In most cars, the roof is primarily constructed of thin sheet metal, supported in several spots by roof posts. When a vehicle is on its wheels, cutting the roof should not affect the structural integrity of the vehicle. In situations where the vehicle is on its side, the structural integrity may be compromised.

Tools that are used to cut door panels may not cut the post of the roof. Tools that do work well are hacksaws and power cutters. Extreme caution should be used when cutting the hatch of a hatchback vehicle. The hydraulic pistons used to make the hatch go up so easily in normal everyday use are fully loaded when the hatch is down. If cut, the attached arm springs out with considerable force and can cause injury to the rescuer.

CUTTING A ROOF FLAP. When cutting a roof flap, the size of the flap is determined by what your purpose is in cutting it and the impact it will have on the structural integrity of the vehicle. Assuming the roof flap is to be cut on a car that is on its side, the first step is to cut the roof posts surrounding the windshield. Next, start at the lowest corner and cut in an upward direction. Save the downward direction for the last cut, because your physical energy may be reduced by this point and gravity can assist you. The cut should be in a U-shaped pattern, with the one intact edge on the bottom. Once the cut has been completed, the metal should be folded down. Then cut the post completely free from the vehicle. All that is remaining is the headliner. Cut it in the same pattern as you cut the roof. Fold the headliner down over the folded metal, which will provide you with some additional protection. You can now treat and remove your patients. One last caution when cutting the roof of a car on its side—be sure that the victims are not being supported by the roof you are cutting. If the victims are leaning against the roof or using it for support, it will be necessary to gain access another way and provide additional, alternative support to the victims during the roof cutting operation.

Another technique for folding the roof is used for the car that is on its wheels. Have a rescuer reach inside the vehicle and lift the roof up slightly. Then take your hacksaw and cut the front posts one-third of the way from the bottom (Fig. 18–33B). Once this has been accomplished, cut the roof on both sides at the point at which you want the fold to occur. For example, if the roof cut is to create more working room in the front of the vehicle, then cut 6 inches behind the back of the front seat (Fig. 18–34). The cuts in the sides of the roof should be approximately 8 inches long, clearing the roof's natural or intended curve. Once you have made all four cuts, crease the roof with an ax and lift the roof from the posts toward the back (Fig. 18–35).

GOING THROUGH THE FLOOR

You should make the decision to go through the floor only when no other method of entrance is possible. For example, you may have to go through the floor if the car has flipped over and the roof is crushed, so that

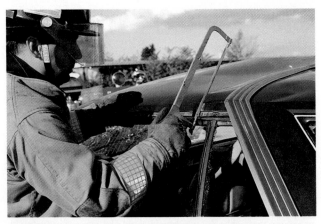

FIGURE 18–34. After the posts are cut, the two cuts are made in the sides of the roof. Make sure that someone is communicating with the victim during this operation—the noise level can be very disconcerting. Victims should understand what is being done to prevent fear and panic from setting in.

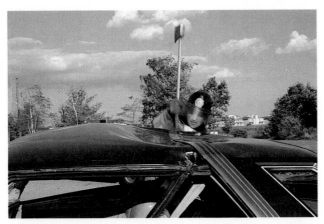

FIGURE 18–35. After all four cuts are made, the ax is used to crease the roof so that it can be peeled back. This and the preceding illustrations show a two-door car. In a four-door car, additional posts might have to be cut. Be extremely careful when cutting a hatch-type roof because of the loaded pistons. It is not recommended that the hatch-type roof be cut because of this danger.

the hood and trunk are touching the ground. It is impossible to open the doors of this vehicle without compromising its structural integrity. In such situations, the door supports the weight of the vehicle. This technique is used to gain access to any potential victims inside the vehicle. To remove the victims, options other than bringing them out through the floor might be available. Floor construction is similar to roof construction, with the exception that there is less spacing between supports. Locate a section of the floor that has a support. An excellent area for entry is the rear foot well. Locate the rubber drain plug in the rear foot well area. Once located, assess the location of the victims by either making a direct visualization or poking out the plug and feeling around. Using the three-side, or U-shaped, fold technique, cut an 18-inch square hole. This will provide you with the access you require to further evaluate your rescue situation and the patient's condition.

Essential Emergency Care

Immediately upon gaining access to the patient, one EMT should assume in-line cervical immobilization; another EMT can then conduct a primary survey. The mechanism of injury should be used to guide you in your assessment (see Chapters 2 and 20). If life-threatening conditions are identified, the rapid extrication procedure should be used if the patient is not trapped in the vehicle. If removal is not possible, every attempt should be made to stabilize the victim in the vehicle; front-seat passengers in need of airway maintenance and ventilation can be managed by lowering the back of the seat (when possible) to facilitate these procedures. As

usual, the principles of management remain the same: airway, breathing, circulation, and so forth.

Disentanglement

Disentanglement represents the most pivotal stage of extrication as it relates to rapid patient removal from the scene. *Your primary focus during the disentanglement stage is removal of the wreckage from the patient, not removal of the patient from the wreckage.* Applying this principle to your operation provides the patient with the most efficient and stabilizing situation. The four steps of the disentanglement process greatly contribute to successful outcomes. *These steps are best described by disassembly, distortion, displacement, and severance.* You should be familiar with all of these operations. All of the tools previously listed are used in these operations.

DOORS. Just as doors are a good place to enter a vehicle, they are also an excellent place through which to rapidly remove patients. However, the door opening may have to be widened. This is best accomplished by distorting the door by having several rescuers pushing and pulling it (Figs. 18–36 and 18–37). Another appropriate tool to be used in this situation is a come along (hand winch). If clear access cannot be gained, then it is appropriate to disassemble the doors from the vehicle. This might also be accomplished by unscrewing or unbolting the hinges.

FREEING THE DRIVER. Freeing the driver is one of the most common extrication problems encountered. The steering wheel, while convenient for driving, pre-

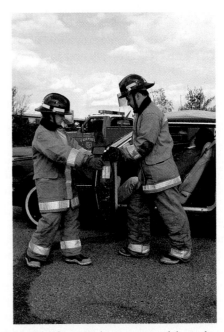

FIGURE 18–36. The EMTs have positioned themselves to further open the door for patient access and removal.

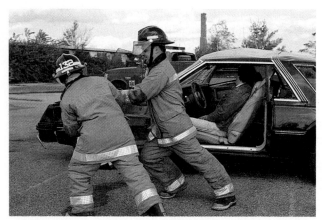

FIGURE 18–37. Pushing and pulling simultaneously is the best method to widen a door opening. The car must, however, be completely stabilized prior to this procedure. This technique can create a rocking type of motion in the nonstabilized vehicle.

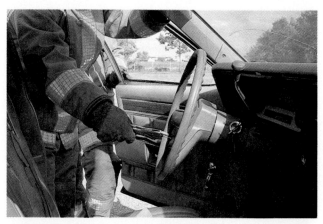

FIGURE 18–38. By using the vise grips you can quickly strip all of the plastic from the steering wheel and expose the metal frame.

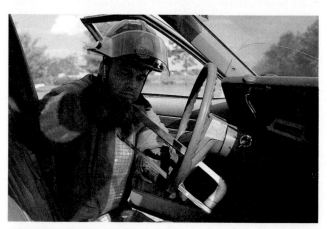

FIGURE 18–39. Once the frame has been exposed, the EMT can cut the frame with a hacksaw. Sometimes this is all that is required to provide enough space to remove a victim.

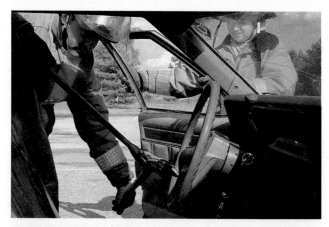

FIGURE 18–40. If a bolt cutter is going to be used to cut the steering wheel frame, have another EMT with proper protective clothing stabilize the wheel to prevent it from hitting the victim when the cut is made. The bolt cutter should have its blades perpendicular to the steering frame, as demonstrated here. It is easier to cut the frame with the plastic or rubber cover removed; however, circumstances may occur that require a cut through the wheel without the plastic removed. This is significantly more difficult, because the plastic or rubber absorbs a great deal of the force being exerted. In any cutting situation, the more material removed from the cutting area, the cleaner and more efficient is the cut.

sents problems during extrication. Sometimes all that is necessary for removal of the driver is a few inches of space. Moving the seat back without unduly jarring the driver is the simplest method. Seats move either manually or electrically, and either method is acceptable if done slowly.

Often, power to the seat is not lost during the accident, but the battery cables may be disconnected during the rescue operation. If it is necessary to disconnect the battery, it is best to disconnect the negative cable. This reduces the likelihood of a spark. Never cut battery cables because you may need them later to move a power seat. If the power to the seat is gone and reconnecting the battery does not work, it may be best to consider trying another procedure for creating extra room. Cutting a portion of the wheel is an appropriate operation. The vise grip and hacksaw are best suited for this purpose. Strip the plastic from the steering wheel with the vise grips (Fig. 18–38) and then cut the metal core with the hacksaw or bolt cutter (Figs. 18–39 and 18–40). You should do this in two locations on parallel sides and then remove the loose portion of the wheel.

PEDALS. The gas and brake pedals present small but annoying obstacles in the disentanglement process. The brake pedal was designed to accept pressure in an up and down motion; therefore, the structural integrity of the pedal from side to side is not great. It is significantly easier to move a brake pedal sideways than it is to move it up and down. For this reason, if you find yourself having to move a brake pedal, do it sideways. This is best accomplished by securing a chain to the pedal and pulling sideways. If the door is still intact, you can wrap the other end of the chain to the door while the door is in the near-closed position and then open the door (Fig. 18–41). Sometimes removal of the victim's shoe can facilitate disentanglement. The EMT should use the simplest and safest method for removing a victim.

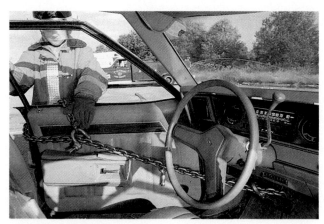

FIGURE 18–41. Moving the brake pedal with a chain is accomplished by using the method illustrated in the photo. When looped shackles are not available, the chain can be wrapped around the door many times and cinched against itself.

POWER SPREADERS AND POWER CUTTERS.

Power spreaders and cutters are useful in operations where human strength is not adequate to accomplish the task. Examples are lifting and pulling of steering columns, stabilizing vehicles, raising dashboards, and pulling seats back. Figure 18–42 illustrates how a hydraulic tool is used to remove a steering wheel from an entrapped patient. Power spreaders and cutters can also be used to cut roof posts for roof removal (Fig.18–43).

Immobilization and Packaging

While the process of disentanglement progresses, the patient can be prepared for removal while cervical immobilization is maintained. A secondary survey can be conducted to identify additional injuries to head, trunk, and extremities. Again, the mechanism of injury should provide the basis for identification of specific types of trauma. For example, a front-end collision would provoke the EMT to carefully examine the patient's anterior head, chest, and abdomen, as well as the knee, femur, and hip region.

When serious injuries are identified, e.g., flail chest, immediate action to stabilize the condition should be taken. More minor injuries can be treated at the end of the survey. If time permits, open wounds should be dressed and bandaged. When possible, fractures should be splinted prior to removal. However, the application of traction splints and long board splints to the lower extremities is sometimes not possible in the confines of an automobile.

The patient should be attached to the short spine board (Fig. 18–44) and removed from the vehicle onto a long spine board (Fig. 18–45). Once again, if life-threatening injuries exist and removal is possible, the rapid extrication procedure should be followed (see Chapter 16).

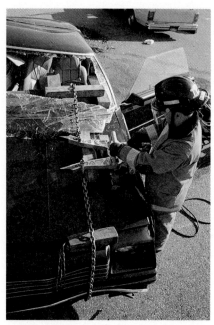

FIGURE 18–42. The hydraulic spreader unit pulling a steering wheel. The use of a power tool of this type requires special training. Power tools have great capability in the hands of a trained professional. In the hands of an untrained individual, they can cause serious injury to both rescuer and victim.

Removal

Once the patient is effectively immobilized, he or she can be removed from the vehicle. Care should be exercised in selection of the exit route. Again, the optimal route follows the path of least resistance. For example, the rear window is a poor choice for removal of the driver or a front-seat passenger. However, the condition and location of wreckage often dictate the options available to the rescuer. Once again, the door adjacent to the occupant is the best choice. A second consideration is personnel. Attempting removal of an adult patient with two EMTs should be avoided. Personnel should be re-

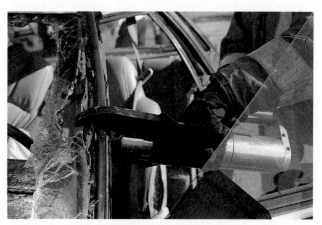

FIGURE 18–43. Hydraulic-powered cutter. Here it is being used to cut a door post for roof removal.

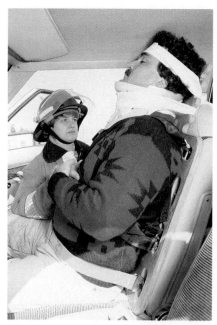

FIGURE 18–44. The victim who is trapped is in need of constant reassurances and support during the rescue operation. When possible, it is appropriate that the person who gained access and made the first patient contact should stay with the victim throughout the rescue. This provides the patient with some sense of stability and an identifiable friend on the scene. Do not become distracted from your patient by the technology. The same rules of patient care apply in rescue as in all emergency care. The victim is depending on you for support and help.

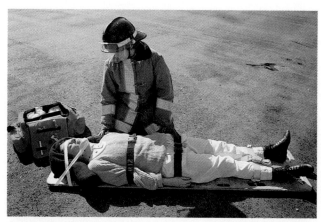

FIGURE 18–45. Once the victim has been removed from the vehicle, it is important to tend to all the injuries that you were unable to treat during the rescue.

Summary

The successful extrication of injured patients from an automobile wreck is a challenge that you are likely to encounter on a regular basis (Fig. 18–45). Your effectiveness depends on your ability to remain calm and to organize the available resources. Safety to yourself, bystanders, and the patient is your first priority. In most cases, rescue personnel concentrate on gaining access and disentanglement. Your role is to assess, treat, immobilize, and safely remove and transport the injured victim (Fig. 18–46). Again, time to definitive care should be a prime consideration. When you are called upon to

cruited based on their experience in handling patients and their individual physical strength. Strong rescuers should be assigned positions that require the greatest effort during movement. The senior EMT should position himself or herself at the patient's head and maintain cervical traction, ensuring the best possible immobilization.

The removal should proceed carefully, without abrupt or jerky movements that could result in loss of in-line immobilization of the spine. The path and steps of removal should be reviewed with the rescuers prior to execution. Each step should be initiated with a verbal cue from the team leader. The patient should be protected during removal. This is particularly important when the windshield or window exit is used. Upon lifting the patient, rescuers should support the patient as one unit. Rescuers should never lift short spinal immobilization devices. As a rule, lift a patient—not a device. In most instances, a wheeled cot stretcher can be positioned adjacent to the exit route to facilitate transfer to the long spine board. The specific technique for the use of short and long spine boards is covered in Chapter 16 on lifts and carries.

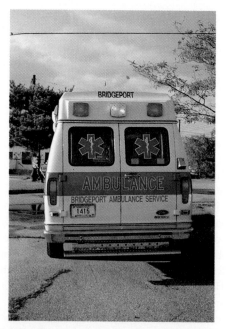

FIGURE 18–46. After all the victims have been removed, the rescue team retrieves all the equipment used and prepares it for the next rescue situation. The EMT on the rescue site should understand the principles of rescue and extrication. The key to successful rescue is cooperation, training, and experience.

effect a rescue you should be prepared to do so with a minimal amount of equipment. Selection of the safest, fastest, and often the simplest method of gaining access and disentanglement should be the guiding principle of the rescue operation. There are many different techniques of extrication. This chapter's purpose is to orient the EMT to extrication. Rescue in and of itself is a skill requiring many hours of training. The EMT should understand some of the rescue options available and the principles on which they are based. The highest priority should be given to the victim and his or her speedy extrication. Several different options in extrication have been presented and discussed in this chapter. However, study of this chapter alone does not qualify the EMT to perform the rescue techniques outlined; only time, experience, and training can achieve that goal.

REVIEW EXERCISES

1. Describe the basic uses of the following devices used in the extrication process:
   Reflectors
   Hacksaw
   Vise grip pliers
   Fire ax
   Bolt cutters
   Tin snips
   Blankets
   Pruning saw
   Bale hooks
   Jacks
   Air chisel
   Wrench—12-inch adjustable crescent
   Screwdrivers
   Hammer
   Wrecking bar and crowbar
   A shovel
   Ropes
   Mastic knife
   Spring-loaded center punch
   Cold chisels
   Storage and maintenance
   Hand winch or come along

2. Describe the basic components of self-protection gear used at a rescue site.

3. Describe the basic methods for gaining access through the following routes:
   Door   Window
   Roof   Floor

4. Describe the techniques for the following extrication techniques:
   Displacing a brake pedal
   Removing a steering wheel

5. List three routes of removal from an automobile.

REFERENCES

American Academy of Orthopaedic Surgeons, Committee on Allied Health: Emergency Care and Transportation of the Sick and Injured, 4th ed. Chicago, American Academy of Orthopedic Surgeons, 1986.

Butman A, Paturas J: Pre-Hospital Trauma Life Support. Akron, OH, Emergency Training, 1986.

Conrad M: Principles of extrication. EMT Journal 3(4): 48–51, 1978.

Essential equipment for ambulances. Bulletin of the American College of Surgeons, May 1970.

Grant H, Murray R: Emergency Care, 4th ed. Bowie, MD, Brady/Prentice-Hall, 1986.

Grant HD: Vehicle Rescue, 2nd ed. Bowie, MD, Robert Brady Co, 1981.

The perilous path from accident to ambulance: Extrication. Emergency Medicine 1(9), 1969.

United States Department of Transportation: EMT—A Patient Handling Manual. Washington, DC, Department of Transportation Traffic Safety Administration, 1976.

United States Department of Transportation: EMT: Crash Vehicle Extrication Manual. Washington, DC, US Government Printing Office, 1979.

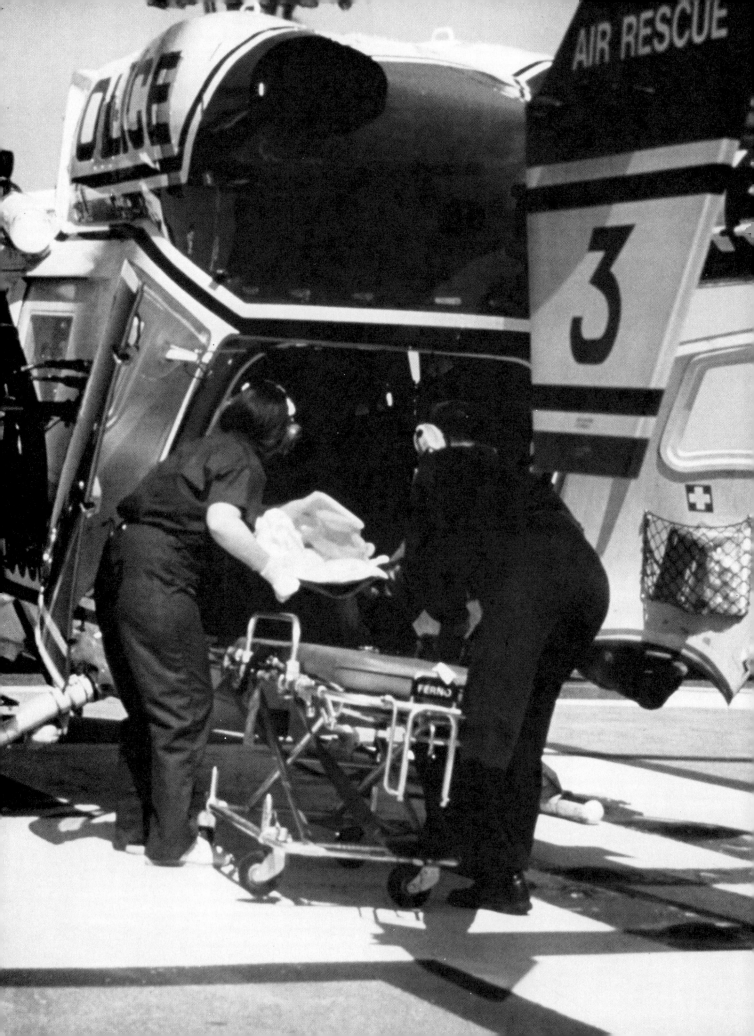

CHAPTER 19

AMBULANCE OPERATIONS

OBJECTIVES

At the conclusion of this chapter the reader will be able to:

1. Describe the privileges given to emergency vehicles for each of the following categories:

Speed	Right-of-way
Warning lights	Parking
Sirens	Turning

2. List four contributing factors to unsafe driving conditions.

3. Describe in narrative the considerations that should be given to:
   Requests for escorts
   Following an escort vehicle
   Intersections

4. List agency contact capabilities of all two-way radio channels in the ambulance.

5. List the correct radio procedures in the following phases of each run:

To the scene	At the facility
At the scene	To the squad station
To the facility	At the squad station

6. List the proper method for beginning and terminating a radio call.

7. Describe what information is required in each area of the trip ticket.

8. Describe where trip report forms should be left and how they are used.

9. Identify the vehicle systems and equipment that require daily inspection.

10. Describe the nonmedical role of the EMT at traffic accidents, crime scenes, and emergency departments.

OPERATING AN EMERGENCY VEHICLE

Overview

In 1976, a fire department ambulance responded to the scene of a cardiac arrest with two EMTs aboard. An off-duty firefighter who lived two blocks away from the scene of the call also responded and initiated CPR with the ambulance crew. The firefighter continued resuscitation efforts while en route to the hospital; the patient's family followed behind. The ambulance was traveling at a speed in excess of 70 mph on local streets, and the patient's family was unable to keep up with it.

At 4:30 AM, the ambulance failed to negotiate a sharp curve, mounted the curb, and struck a tree, killing five people on impact: two firefighters, two EMTs, and the patient.

On impact, the top of the 1973 Chevrolet van was ripped completely off the ambulance, scattering bodies and equipment across the lawn. It was this single accident that prompted the establishment of the Emergency Vehicle Operation Course (EVOC), sponsored by the United States Department of Transportation. Until that time, no standardized curriculum had been developed to train EMTs in the operation of emergency vehicles. While over 100 hours are dedicated to the teaching of acute emergency medicine during the EMT program, and many years of experience may be accumulated, this is all wasted if the EMT never arrives at the scene or fails to deliver the patient to the hospital (Fig. 19–1).

This chapter discusses the concept of low-risk, non-aggressive emergency vehicle operation and gives general guidelines for emergency situations. Ambulance operation differs substantially from police pursuit driving or the handling of fire apparatus. Ambulances are subject to special vehicle and traffic laws, and their operators are charged with the responsibility of preserving human life. While the philosophies and procedures described in this text are a good basic introduction, it is necessary to practice these techniques in a properly supervised EVOC program to gain a full understanding of them. Actual hands-on experience reinforces these ideas, allows the EMT to practice emergency maneuvers in a controlled environment, and gives the EMT a better appreciation of the size and weight of the vehicle.

ARCH OF DRIVER SAFETY

Driving can be thought of as an arch that is constructed of many components, including physical and mental abilities, knowledge of traffic laws, and driver attitude.

The driver of an emergency vehicle must possess many attributes to effectively perform his or her duties. Being physically fit is essential to the driving task, but while driving is considered to be primarily a physical activity, 90% of it is dependent on the driver's attention and concentration on the task. Therefore, mental fitness is an integral component of the arch.

A considerable amount of good judgment is required to select the best alternatives in crisis situations. It is here where the experienced operator, having acquired the proper skills, can anticipate hazards and prepare to take evasive maneuvers.

Some drivers develop good habits, such as using proper turning techniques, using the brake in questionable situations, and using safety restraint devices consistently. Others develop poor habits, including left-foot braking and "palming" the wheel during a turn. Accidents are often avoided because good driving habits have prevailed over bad ones.

Knowledge of how a particular ambulance handles as well as a familiarity with applicable traffic laws is critically important for the emergency vehicle operator. While certain "privileges" are granted to emergency vehicle operators to expedite the delivery of emergency care, EMTs can be held civilly and criminally liable for abuse of any of these exemptions.

The keystone of the arch is attitude. The ambulance operator who assumes that he or she automatically and always has the right-of-way may cause a serious accident. The EMT's paramount concern should be the safe operation of the ambulance, without which he or she cannot possibly perform the job.

Although textbooks can contribute to an individual's bank of knowledge and skills can be quickly developed to perform lifesaving tasks, attitudes cannot be altered so readily. The EMT should carefully assess his or her driving attitude before each tour of duty and examine his or her personal and job-related stresses before accepting the responsibility of operating an ambulance.

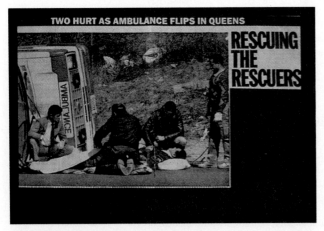

FIGURE 19–1. Newspaper headline from Queens, New York. (From Ambulance Accident Prevention Student Workbook. Albany, New York State Department of Health.)

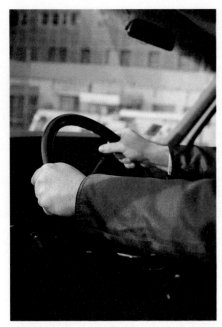

FIGURE 19–2. The 10 o'clock and 2 o'clock positions ensure maximum control and maneuverability.

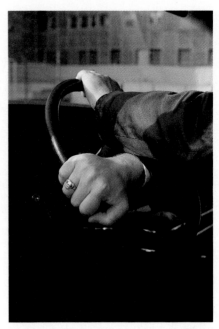

FIGURE 19–3. Hand-over-hand turning.

CONTROL TASKS

Control of a vehicle can be broken into two components: directional control and speed control.

DIRECTIONAL CONTROL. Directional control is dependent upon many factors, including the mechanical condition of the vehicle, road conditions, the physical condition of the driver, and other factors. One of the most important factors, and among the simplest, is the driver's hand position. Emergency vehicle operators should drive with two hands on the wheel whenever possible. Secondary tasks such as radio and siren operation should be delegated to the second EMT, so that the operator can focus full attention on the driving task. The recommended hand positions are 10:00 o'clock and 2:00 o'clock, which allow the optimal position for evasive meneuvers (Fig. 19–2). Turning the steering wheel is accomplished with the hand-over-hand technique, which has proven to be a safe method (Fig. 19–3). Another steering wheel technique is called "shuffling." Shuffling is a method where the hands slide from one position to the next as you turn the steering wheel. Using this technique, your hands never leave the wheel.

Emergency vehicle operators should not vary their driving habits when they enter their own personal cars, as these procedures are applicable to all vehicles and are reinforced by constant practice. It is important to remember, however, that you can drive a Chevy like an ambulance but you cannot drive an ambulance like a Chevy. The ambulance is a light truck that weighs approximately 10,000 pounds and cannot stop as fast as a car (Table 19–1).

SPEED CONTROL. Speed control depends on many of the same factors as directional control, and a loss of control in either case can result in a serious accident (Fig. 19–4). Modern ambulances weigh up to four times more than the standard passenger car and therefore have considerably different handling characteristics (Fig. 19–5). EMTs quickly learn that ambulances have substantially longer stopping distances than their own cars, and the additional weight, combined with improper braking technique, can cause an uncontrollable skid and loss of control. A survey of fully equipped Type III ambulances found that the average vehicle weighs 10,450 pounds without the patient or crew inside. Many EMS services are routinely overloading their ambulances.

TABLE 19–1. Stopping Distances of a Light Axle Truck

Speed (Miles/hour)	Driver Reaction Distance	Vehicle Braking Distance	Total Stopping Distance
10	11	7	18
15	17	17	34
20	22	30	52
25	28	46	74
30	33	67	100
35	39	92	131
40	44	125	169
45	50	165	215
50	55	225	280
55	61	275	336
60	66	360	426

New York State Health Department, EMS Program, Ambulance Accident Prevention Student Workbook. Albany, NY, New York Department of Health, 1989.

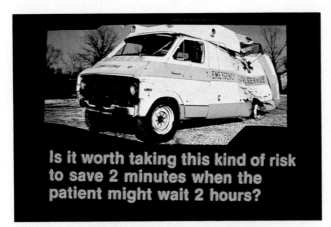

Is it worth taking this kind of risk to save 2 minutes when the patient might wait 2 hours?

FIGURE 19-4. Speed-related accidents. (From Ambulance Accident Prevention Student Workbook. Albany, New York State Department of Health.)

WHAT DOES YOUR AMBULANCE WEIGH?

AMBULANCE	MAX. GROSS VEHICLE WEIGHT	AVG. MFG. CURB WEIGHT
TYPE 1	11,000	8,630
TYPE 2	9,000	7,065
TYPE 3	11,000	8,860

A survey of fully equipped (without crew) TYPE 3 ambulances produced an avg. actual vehicle weight of 10,450 lbs.

FIGURE 19-5. Ambulance weight by type. (From Ambulance Accident Prevention Student Workbook. Albany, New York State Department of Health.)

When the gross vehicle weight is exceeded, the handling and braking of the vehicle are affected.

SEAT BELTS. One of the simplest devices that can help maintain control of any vehicle is an ordinary seat belt. There are no valid excuses for not wearing a seat belt. Not only does a seat belt keep the vehicle operator inside the car in the event of a collision, it keeps him or her in position behind the controls of the vehicle. Most vehicles involved in moving accidents actually have two collisions: the initial impact and a second crash should the driver be unable to control the vehicle following the initial impact. Frequently, the second impact is more severe than the first, because contact is often made with a fixed object such as a parked car or a telephone pole.

The theory that an occupant can be "thrown clear" of the accident has a very low probability. In most circumstances, human beings who are ejected from a moving vehicle, even at low rates of speed, sustain serious injuries. Being thrown from a vehicle increases the chance of death 25 times. Frequently such individuals are struck by other cars and occasionally are even run over by their own vehicle.

The following are a few questions and comments that are often voiced about seat belts: "What happens if I'm in a head-on collision and both my arms are broken and the car's on fire? How can I get out if my seat belt is on?" In all probability, if the collision was severe enough to break both your arms while you were wearing your seat belt, you would have been even more seriously injured or killed had the seat belt not been fastened. Statistically, 1 out of every 200 people involved in collisions while wearing seat belts correctly is injured by them. However, these injuries are much less severe than those sustained by unrestrained occupants. In addition, less than 0.5% of vehicle accidents involve fires.

"If I see an accident about to happen, I can brace myself against the dashboard." A passenger bracing against the dashboard can be compared to a sprinter running at full speed—15 mph. If the sprinter were to run into a wall at that speed with his or her arms extended, he or she would undoubtedly sustain serious injury. If the running speed were accelerated to perhaps 30 mph, the physical insult would be four times as great.

Seat belts should be worn by all vehicle occupants, including patients and those escorting patients in the ambulance. EMTs can be held responsible for any injuries to unrestrained passengers who are in the ambulance while a patient is being transported to the hospital. The seat belt should be worn snugly across the pelvic gridle, not across the lower abdomen, which is highly susceptible to blunt trauma in deceleration accidents (Fig. 19-6). Small children should be restrained in approved child seats, as unrestrained children are frequently ejected from vehicles during a collision. Motor vehicle accidents are the leading cause of death in young children. If you are still not convinced that safety belts save lives, ask any EMT how often he or she has unbuckled a dead person.

Motor Vehicle Laws

The wording of vehicle and traffic laws regarding emergency vehicle operation differs slightly from state to state, but the content is generally consistent. It is recommended that the emergency vehicle operator be familiar with the specific regulations in the community concerning emergency vehicles prior to operating an ambulance. The following examples are paraphrased from the New York State Vehicle and Traffic Law.

DEFINITION OF EMERGENCY OPERATION

Emergency operation is defined as the operation or parking of an emergency vehicle when engaged in trans-

FIGURE 19-6. Proper position of seat belts. (From United States Department of Transportation, National Highway Traffic Safety Administration.)

Wear it right!

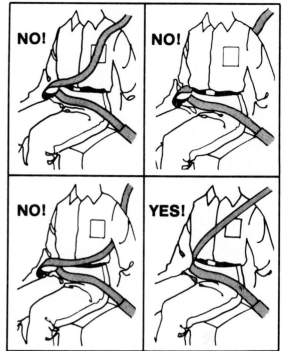

Shoulder belts should be snug. Don't allow more than 1 inch of slack. Never wear the belt behind your back or under your arm. The correct position is over the shoulder, snug across the chest, and low on the lap.

U.S. Department of Transportation
National Highway Traffic Safety Administration

porting a sick or injured person or responding to or working at the scene of an accident, disaster, police call, alarm of fire, or other emergency. Emergency operations shall not include returning from such service.

SPECIFIC EXEMPTIONS

The driver of an authorized emergency vehicle, when involved in an emergency operation, may exercise the following privileges:

The operator may proceed past a steady red signal, a flashing red signal, or a stop sign, but only after slowing down as may be necessary for safe operation.

The operator may exceed the maximum speed limits so long as he or she does not endanger life or property.

The operator may disregard regulations governing the direction of movement or turning in specified directions.

These exemptions shall apply only when the authorized emergency vehicle utilizes an audible warning device and displays appropriate red warning lamps.

The foregoing provisions shall not relieve the driver of an authorized emergency vehicle from the duty to drive with due regard for the safety of all persons, nor shall these provisions protect the driver from the con-

sequences of his or her reckless disregard for the safety of others.

This last paragraph states specifically that while there are certain privileges granted to an emergency vehicle, the operator is responsible for the outcome should an accident occur while exercising any one of these privileges.

Drivers of emergency vehicles are actually held to a higher standard than the average citizen. Take for example, an ambulance en route to a cardiac call with lights and siren on that drives up a narrow one-way street against the flow of traffic. A car pulling out of a parking space strikes the ambulance head-on, causing considerable damage to both vehicles. Despite the fact that the ambulance operator used all warning devices, the fact that he or she was proceeding against traffic on a one-way street makes him or her responsible for the accident.

What does "due regard" mean and how does it affect the driver of an ambulance? Due regard is based on the particular circumstances. In judging due regard, the following criterion is used: Was there "enough" notice of approach to allow other motorists and pedestrians to clear a path and protect themselves? If you do not give notice of the ambulance's approach until a collision is inevitable, you have probably not satisfied the principle of due regard for the safety of others.

In determining whether or not an ambulance was exercising due regard in the use of signaling equipment, for example, the courts consider at least the following points:

Was it reasonably necessary to use the signaling equipment under all of the circumstances?
Was the signaling equipment actually used?
Was the signal given audible and/or visible to the motorists and pedestrians?

An accepted definition of due regard is as follows: A reasonably careful man performing similar duties under the same circumstances would act in the same manner.

Unlike police vehicles and fire apparatus, ambulances are considered emergency vehicles only while engaged in emergency activities. A "true emergency" is defined as any situation in which there is a high probability of death or serious injury to an individual or group of individuals, or a significant loss of property, and the action of an emergency service may reduce the severity of the situation.

Ambulance personnel should respond to all calls in the same manner, keeping in mind that the general public is usually unaware of the fine points of medicine. A typical "seizure" call may in fact be the result of a serious head trauma and the "sick" call may very well be cardiac arrest. Only after you have arrived on the scene and assessed the patient can you determine the severity of the call. How you return to the hospital can be adjusted according to the known condition of the patient. Rapid transportation of serious multitrauma and cardiac patients is frequently contraindicated because a high-speed ambulance ride would worsen their condition or hinder treatment. Speed of transport must be balanced by the need to perform procedures en route (e.g., maintain an airway, positive-pressure ventilation, cardiopulmonary resuscitation).

EMERGENCY LIGHTS

Most state traffic laws mandate the use of emergency lights and a siren when exercising emergency vehicle "privileges." It is important to understand, however, that these warning devices are simply that: warning devices. They do not automatically grant right-of-way; they can only request it. Remember also that use of lights and a siren does not relieve the emergency vehicle operator of liability in the event of an accident.

Emergency warning lights have been shown to be nearly ineffective during periods of low light, such as at dawn and at dusk. A complete spectrum of warning lamps would be required to deal with all light and weather conditions. Each state mandates different colors for various types of emergency vehicles, although red and white warning lamps are the most common. Rear-facing red lamps easily blend in with a field of tail and brake lights, reducing their effectiveness. Some people are color blind to red and are not warned by the lights. Therefore, amber and blue rear-facing warning lamps are preferred. The most effective warning lamps are the ones that are mounted at the eye level of other drivers. These are the vehicle headlights. White lights contain all the colors of the light spectrum, making them most noticeable in all conditions.

As a note of caution, four-way hazard lights should not be used while operating a moving vehicle. They negate the turn signals and the brake lights and therefore create a hazard to other motorists who cannot anticipate the actions of the ambulance. Flashing lights on the rear of an ambulance should flash in tandem rather than one at a time. This helps the on-coming driver to recognize the size of the ambulance, interpret the signal, and react properly.

EMERGENCY SIREN

The emergency vehicle siren is emitted in a cone of sound transmitted ahead of the vehicle. Its effectiveness can also be reduced by a number of factors such as reverberation, absorption, reflection, background noise, and a phenomenon called "vehicle insertion." This means that the ambulance actually projects itself into its own siren cone the faster it goes, thereby limiting its advance warning. At approximately 60 mph (88 feet per second), the siren barely precedes the speeding ambulance, so that vehicles ahead of it cannot respond to its warning. Studies have shown the distance for getting the attention of a motorist traveling at 60 mph to be within 5 feet of the ambulance's bumper.

People respond to a warning sound in a four-step process. First, we *detect* the signal with our personal sensory system. We all are bombarded with so much auditory stimulation that we tend to filter out the noise and only recognize signals that we either are listening for or are unusual and well above the background threshold level.

The next step is *attention* or notice of the signal. Unfortunately, the ambient street noise, closed car windows, and air conditioning and heating fans all cause high sound levels within the automobile. The combination of all this noise can easily mask even the most intense exterior sounds such as a siren.

The next step is to *interpret* the sound by attaching a purposeful meaning to the sound. Unfortunately, EMTs have created part of the problem here, because they sometimes overuse or abuse the use of the siren, which has desensitized the public, so that they frequently do not even turn their heads when they hear a siren. Couple this with all those vehicle theft alarms that go off from time to time, and it becomes evident that people just do not connect the sound of a siren with an emergency.

The last step is a *reaction*, which is an appropriate

action taken by the pedestrians and drivers you expect to warn. Often there are very unpredictable responses by drivers who do not interpret the siren until the last minute. When a person is frightened by the siren, this mini "fight or flight" situation produces a snap reaction that does not always include ample time for logical decision-making.

It is sometimes the case that even the best emergency warning device proves to be inadequate for the task of warning drivers in time for them to take evasive action. A United States Department of Transportation study found that only 26% of the occupants of a closed car with the windows rolled up could tell from which direction the siren sound was coming.

The siren physically affects the ambulance operator and affects his or her abilities as a driver. A normally safe driver feels the effects of the siren as soon as it is switched on. The siren's wail and yelp cause an immediate release of epinephrine in the driver's bloodstream, causing a sympathetic physiologic reaction. As a result, the pulse quickens, the vision narrows, the palms become sweaty, and the muscles tense. The driver's right foot presses down on the accelerator and the ambulance picks up speed, without any conscious effort on the part of the driver. Since the vision is narrowed, the driver is not aware of cross traffic, pedestrians, or other distractions, and can even unconsciously ignore traffic signals in the quest to get to the scene as quickly as possible.

Being aware of this phenomenon is not enough. The ambulance operator must make a conscious effort to overcome the effects of the epinephrine by letting up on the accelerator as soon as the siren is switched on. In addition, the driver must make an effort to check his or her peripheral vision by changing the focus of vision regularly and increasing general awareness of the environment. The driver should alternate checking ahead with checking right, left, the gauges, the grip on the steering wheel.

The siren noise level can also be dangerous to the EMT. The National Institute for Occupational Safety and Health (NIOSH) conducted an investigation of siren noises in ambulances in 1984. NIOSH staff evaluated the effect of siren speaker location on noise levels, monitoring sound levels in the following four locations:

Driver compartment/driver position
Patient compartment/patient position
Ten feet from the siren speakers on an axis to the person minus 45 degrees
One hundred feet on axis to plus or minus 45 degrees from the siren speakers

Exposure to high levels of noise may cause temporary or permanent hearing loss. The extent of damage depends upon the intensity of the noise and the duration of the exposure. There is abundant evidence that protracted noise exposure above 90 decibels (dB) causes hearing loss in a portion of the exposed population.

TABLE 19–2. Standard Permissible Noise Exposure

Exposures (Hours/Day)	Noise Level dBA*
8	90
6	92
4	95
3	97
2	100
1–1$\frac{1}{2}$	102
1	105
$\frac{1}{2}$	110
$\frac{1}{4}$	115

*NIOSH recommends 5 dBA less per level. United States Department of Transportation: Emergency Vehicle Operators Student Manual. Washington, DC, Department of Transportation, 1978.

NIOSH recommend a lower limit standard of 85 dB. Table 19–2 lists the recommended noise limits according to exposure time.

The study found that when siren speakers were located on the roof above the driver, the siren noise within the ambulance had an average intensity of 109 dB in the driver's position (Fig. 19–7) and an average of 91 dB in the patient's position. Siren noise immediately in front of the ambulance created a hazard at 122 dB, exceeding the NIOSH ceiling level of 115 dB. Siren noise 100 feet down range from the ambulance increased from 99 to 105 dB when siren speakers were located in the roof as opposed to on the grill. The study recommends minimizing noise exposure by locating siren speakers in the grill area and keeping the windows in the cab closed. Under these conditions, the noise dB range is certainly much healthier for the ambulance crew and the patients.

The same factors affect the patient being transported. Consider the effects on a cardiac patient of a dose of epinephrine caused by a frantic ambulance ride to the hospital. The increased heart rate would cause a

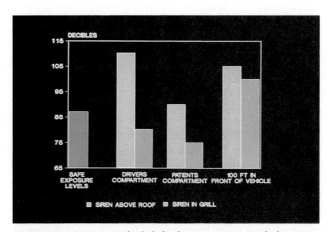

FIGURE 19–7. Siren decibels by location. (From Ambulance Accident Prevention Workbook. Albany, New York State Department of Health.)

compensatory increase in myocardial oxygen demand. With already reduced oxygen levels due to the ischemia, more heart muscle would infarct en route. This would affect the patient in the same way as would jogging to the hospital.

ESCORTS

It is not uncommon for EMTs to use escort vehicles to lead the way to the receiving hospital. Generally, the use of escorts is not a good idea. A driver observing an emergency vehicle crossing an intersection may falsely believe that it is the sole emergency vehicle, causing him or her to proceed through the intersection only to collide into the second vehicle. The only circumstance in which an escort vehicle may be practical is when the ambulance driver is not familiar with the route to the receiving hospital. Extra caution must be taken at all intersections.

Principles of Effective Operation

ROUTE PLANNING

The first order of business once the EMT is dispatched should be to plan the route to the call. The shortest route is not necessarily the quickest one. There are a number of factors that influence response route planning, depending on the environment in which the EMT works. These include traffic congestion during peak "rush hours," construction delays, nonsequential traffic lights, and weather conditions. It is imperative that an area map be carried in the ambulance to plan routes in unfamiliar areas and to select alternate routes when detours are dictated by conditions. Effective preselection of the route allows the EMT to devote full attention to the driving task.

"NATURAL LAWS"

In addition to local and state laws, there are other laws that affect emergency vehicle operation. These are referred to as "natural laws." They affect the two major control tasks of the emergency vehicle operator: speed control and directional control.

GRAVITY. Gravity is most evident when operating the common high-top van ambulance. These vehicles have been modified by their manufacturers to include a heavy fiberglass roof that drastically changes the handling characteristics of the vehicle by raising its center of gravity. In contrast, consider a sports car, with a much lower center of gravity (half the weight of the vehicle above and half the weight below this point). The sports car can turn a sharp corner at 50 mph. If the ambulance

attempted to take the same sharp turn at the same speed, it would flip on its side because its higher center of gravity would pull it over.

During normal operation, the weight of the vehicle is distributed relatively evenly over all the wheels. But during sudden braking, the weight of the vehicle suddenly shifts forward onto the front wheels, making steering more difficult and adding strain on the steering and front braking systems. With little weight on the rear wheels during this maneuver, the rear brakes are considerably less effective in stopping the vehicle and may lock up when increased pedal pressure is applied to stop the ambulance. New antilock braking systems may help considerably, but presently, most ambulances have yet to be equipped with this system.

CENTRIFUGAL FORCE. Centrifugal force is demonstrated by swinging a weight attached to a string over your head. If you let go of the string, the rock flies off in a straight line, not an arc. The force that pulls on a rock is the same as that exerted on a vehicle in a turn. Centrifugal force tends to pull a vehicle out of a curve, on a straight line to the arc. This force increases with the following:

The weight of the vehicle
The sharpness of the curve
The speed of the vehicle
The flatness of the "blank"

Modern road design compensates for centrifugal force by banking the curves in proportion to the sharpness of the curve and by adding "Jersey Walls," preformed concrete barriers that redirect vehicles back onto the road before centrifugal force carries them into the opposite lanes or off the road.

FRICTION. Friction is required to control both the speed and the direction of a vehicle. It is important to distinguish between two types of friction: rolling friction and stopping friction.

Rolling Friction. Contact with the road is essential to steer the vehicle. Furthermore, the front wheels must be rolling to maintain directional control. If rolling friction is lost, for instance, when hitting a patch of ice, directional control is lost and inertia (the property of matter by which it remains at rest or in uniform motion in the same straight line unless acted upon by some external force) and centrifugal force direct the movement of the vehicle. When "peeling rubber" (accelerating quickly from a stop) rolling friction is lost and forward momentum is actually reduced.

Stopping Friction. In the brakes, contact between the pads and the drums (or discs) slows the vehicle down. At the road surface, the tires require friction with the pavement to both stop and steer the vehicle. The shortest stopping distance is achieved when the brakes do not lock up. Locked brakes cause the tires to skid. This sudden increase in friction is converted to heat, which melts the tire rubber. Molten rubber forms beads between the tire and the pavement that actually reduce friction, thereby increasing the stopping distance.

THRESHOLD BRAKING

If the brakes are applied to a point just before they lock (incipient skid), this would be the optimum braking potential. This can be accomplished by depressing the brake pedal to the point where the brakes lock (a squeal is heard on dry pavement) and then letting up slightly to release the lock. The pedal should then be "quivered" at this lock-point for maximum braking potential without loss of friction. This technique is called threshold braking. An added advantage of this technique is that with the front wheels still rolling, directional control is maintained. State-of-the-art antilock braking systems automatically perform this maneuver of alternately locking and unlocking the brakes to maintain steering control.

Each tire has only 20 square inches of contact with the road, about the same as the surface area of your hand. There are a number of factors that can negatively affect friction even further: bad weather; a poor road surface; and items on the road surface such as oil, gravel, and wet leaves. Obviously, a poor tire condition further reduces the operator's ability to maintain control of the vehicle. The tires' tread and air pressure are both critical to vehicle performance and handling, especially for emergency vehicles that are exposed to higher speeds and rougher handling than passenger cars.

OPERATION

One of the major advantages of ambulances is that the driver is positioned high and has a view of the road above other vehicles and well ahead of his or her position in traffic. You can use this advantage to avoid accidents. First, define the safest path well ahead of the ambulance. Certain lanes may be bunched tightly together and therefore may necessitate sudden stops and lane changes. Second, keep a safe distance from the vehicle ahead, allowing time to scan the entire traffic situation, and keep your eyes moving, regularly checking the rear-view and side-view mirrors, the gauges, and your grip on the steering wheel.

Make sure other drivers see you. This is especially important at intersections. By having eye contact with other drivers you ensure that they are aware of you. Make sure that they acknowledge you prior to proceeding into an intersection.

Leave yourself an "out." This is probably the most important concept in accident avoidance. When using the techniques outlined above, you must expect the un-

---

GUIDELINES FOR SAFE DRIVING

- Drive with your headlights on all the time. This is helpful in alerting other drivers to see you and stay away.
- Keep a 4-second following distance whenever driving an ambulance. Remember the stopping distance is much greater than that of a car, which uses the 2-second rule.
- Make gradual changes in acceleration.
- Look far ahead so you can recognize the hazards, understand the defense maneuvers you may have to make, and act correctly in time.
- Apply the brakes smoothly.
- When stopping in traffic, you should always be able to see the rear tire of the vehicle in front of you.
- Maintain adequate cushions of space to the side and rear.
- Make gradual lane changes.
- Always use proper signaling for turns and exits.
- Exercise proper eye movement and use of mirrors.
- Exercise sensible speed control with reduction in
    Reduced visibility/obstructed view
    Reduced road grip
    Sharp changes in direction
- Always be prepared to brake when approaching all intersections and potential hazards.

---

expected and leave yourself an emergency exit route in case of a sudden change in the traffic situation ahead. Do not wait for a crisis to occur before you plan a potential exit. Always leave a space to one side of the vehicle in case the space in front suddenly disappears.

Causes of Ambulance Accidents

DISTANCE

It is the responsibility of any vehicle operator to maintain an assured clear following distance behind the vehicle in front of him. If you fail to do so and collide with the rear of the car in front of you, you are held completely responsible for the accident, regardless of road, vehicle, or weather conditions. If a car cuts in front of the ambulance and stops, the experienced emergency vehicle operator should have a preplanned escape route. In addition, the driver should keep a safe following distance using the 4-second rule. Maintaining a 4-second distance is done by observing the vehicle in front of you passing a stationary object (e.g., light pole, overpass, or even a shadow). If your vehicle passes the same object in 4 seconds or more, you are traveling at a safe distance. If you count less than 4 seconds, you must reduce your speed until that 4-second distance is obtained. This system works at all speeds and in all types of vehicles on a dry road surface. It must be modified in rainy, snowy,

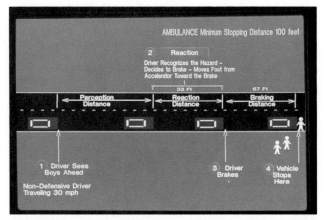

FIGURE 19–8. This illustration demonstrates the distance needed to react and stop a vehicle when faced with a hazard for a nondefensive driver. (From Ambulance Accident Prevention Workbook. Albany, New York State Department of Health.)

or icy conditions. In rainy weather, the time should be doubled to 8 seconds. On icy or snowy roads, the time should be tripled to 12 seconds. Figure 19–8 illustrates braking distances and reaction time.

SPEED

Speed is the greatest contributing factor to accidents. Less than 1% of people involved in crashes at speeds of 70 mph survive. On a 2-mile ambulance run, the difference in arrival time between averaging 30 mph and 60 mph is only 2 minutes. Travelling at 60 mph through most streets, except major interstate highways, is unsafe and imprudent (Fig. 19–9). Operating an ambulance at excessive speeds constitutes irresponsible, dangerous driving. The risks far outweigh the potential benefits. Conditions that should decrease your speed include adverse weather conditions, a poor road surface, high-density urban traffic areas, and school zones.

INTERSECTIONS

Studies have shown that 70% of emergency vehicle accidents occur at intersections, where high-speed vehicles come together at right angles, controlled only by traffic signs or signals. Many EMTs believe that lights and a siren legally grant them the right-of-way. In fact, these warning devices are simply accessories to warn other motorists of your approach. Right-of-way is established on an individual basis, by each driver as he or she reacts to the approaching emergency vehicle. Intersection accidents most often occur when emergency vehicle operators assume that they have the right-of-way or misjudge the speed of their own or other vehicles. Being aware of this statistic is not enough. You must always stop at each intersection when approaching a red light or stop sign and be sure it is safe to proceed before driving on. Be aware that other motorists may try to beat changing traffic signals and that pedestrians frequently try to race across an intersection prior to the arrival of your vehicle.

Even green lights are unsafe for emergency vehicles. Approaching traffic frequently turns left in front of the ambulance, and most motorists take full advantage of right-on-red laws. Impatient drivers may run red lights altogether. Pedestrians are also potential victims. They often seem to be "color blind," crossing regardless of the traffic signals.

What about other emergency vehicles? Depending on the type of call, other agencies (police, fire, rescue, and specialized units) may be responding to your (or a different) call from other directions. Always leave your window open approximately 1 inch to listen for approaching sirens (Fig. 19–10).

Should you be involved in an accident with an emergency vehicle, you may be held personally liable for damages incurred as a result of your actions. Liability may be limited to civil penalties (financial reimbursement

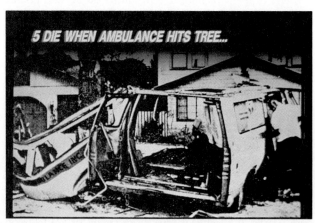

FIGURE 19–9. Speed control is an essential component of safe driving. (From Ambulance Accident Prevention Workbook. Albany, New York State Department of Health.)

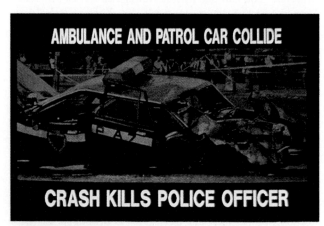

FIGURE 19–10. Emergency vehicles are at increased risk of accident at intersections. The sound of the siren of the other vehicle may be masked by your own. (From Ambulance Accident Prevention Workbook. Albany, New York State Department of Health.)

for damages) or may involve criminal charges (manslaughter, driving while impaired, etc.).

During the trial of an ambulance driver in Binghamton, New York, the judge told the defendant "Everybody keeps calling this a tragic accident; it was tragic but I don't think it was an accident at all." "Somebody propels a 10,000-pound ambulance through an intersection at a high rate of speed against a light, that's not an accident." The defendant was convicted of a misdemeanor assault for running a red light and severely injuring an 18-year-old woman. The woman suffered a broken neck and was in a coma for 5 weeks, and the driver of the ambulance was sentenced to $4\frac{1}{2}$ months in jail and 3 years' probation.

BACKING UP

A certain percentage of ambulance accidents occur when the driver is backing up. Usually fixed objects such as parked cars and emergency room canopies are hit. As these objects do not respond to back-up alarms, it is mandatory that you check behind the ambulance before backing up. Whenever possible, if you are backing and turning, turn from the driver's side and stay close to the driver's side of the vehicle, because you can always see better and have better control of this side of the vehicle. If a police officer, firefighter, or second EMT is available, he or she may assist as a spotter in this maneuver (Fig. 19–11).

The following list summarizes some common elements of accidents that were derived from a 4-year study by New York City Emergency Medical Services.

70% occurred in daylight
70% occurred in an intersection
56% occurred on a clear day
63% occurred on dry roads
53% occurred at traffic signal devices

Summary

Operating an emergency vehicle involves assuming a number of risks not normally taken while driving a passenger car or truck. Accident exposure refers to the risks that a driver takes in responding to an emergency call. This may involve exceeding posted speed limits, traveling the wrong way down one-way streets, or passing red lights. It is incumbent upon you to minimize these risks as much as possible, thereby reducing the possibility of having an accident.

When emergency vehicle exemptions are used, you must show due regard for safety at all times. In the accident described at the beginning of this chapter, the ambulance operator failed to show due regard for safety, and his reckless operation was a major contribution to the deaths of five people.

At all times, it is important to maintain a professional attitude behind the wheel. Even in the busiest EMS systems, you will spend more time driving than performing patient care. Do not let the actions of other drivers affect your abilities as an emergency vehicle operator or an EMT. The results can be disastrous.

RECORD KEEPING

Overview

Record keeping is an essential role of the EMT. The prehospital call report documents all aspects of a given call and represents a valuable part of a patient's record. It is also an important part of a legal defense in the event of a lawsuit. EMTs often view record keeping as a nonessential aspect of their work; however, a call report can be as useful as a well-applied splint to the care of the patient.

Effective record keeping includes the systematic collection of data from the dispatch phase through the transfer of the patient over to the emergency department staff. Times, location, assessment and treatment information, and other information should be carefully documented to ensure that it is readily accessible should the need arise.

Purpose of a Call Report

THE CALL REPORT AS A MEDICAL RECORD

The call report has several distinct purposes. First and foremost, it is a medical record of prehospital care. It provides the physician with a history of the events that surrounded the patient's call for help. During the first critical hours of illness or injury, this information plays an important role in the decision-making process. The mechanism of illness or accident, the vital signs, the chronology of signs and symptoms, and drugs or poisons found on the scene are examples of data that may be lifesaving for a given patient.

LEGAL PROTECTION

A call report is also a critical ingredient for protection from litigation. Should a patient or family member suggest negligence, the best defense is a well-developed record. Since most lawsuits do not occur until weeks or months following an incident, a record may provide the only means of recalling the details of a call. Additionally, the call report serves as evidence of the care given, which reinforces the need to document thoroughly all aspects of assessment and treatment.

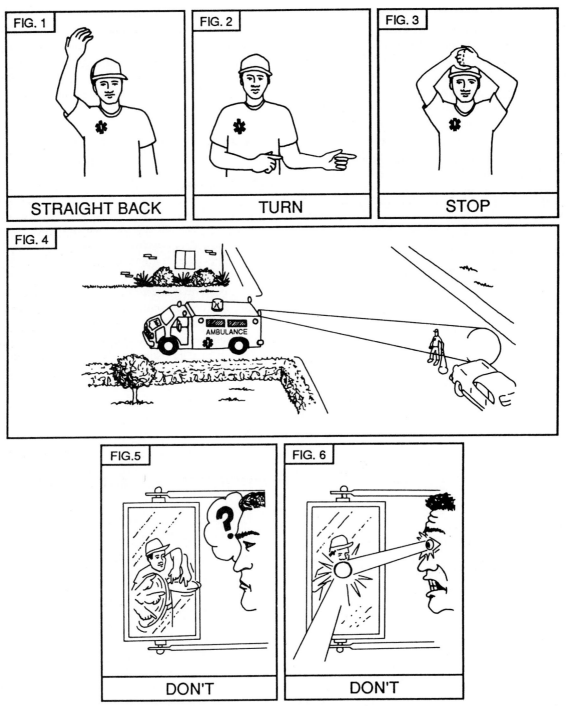

FIGURE 19–11. (*1–3*) Proper hand signals for directing a vehicle. (*4*) The person directing the vehicle should be positioned in lighted view of the driver (the rear spots should be turned on) and should use a flashlight as a wand. (*5*) Never use signals unfamiliar to the driver. (*6*) Never shine the light toward the driver. (From Ambulance Accident Prevention Workbook. Albany, New York State Department of Health.)

QUALITY ASSURANCE

Quality assurance is another use for the prehospital call report. Call reports are often reviewed to evaluate the effectiveness of prehospital care. Audits of records rely upon the validity and reliability of the recorded data to properly evaluate the appropriateness of the care.

Many of the changes that have occurred in EMS systems were based upon this type of review.

CONTINUING EDUCATION

Many EMS systems conduct call review as a primary means of continuing education for EMTs. In these sessions EMTs are asked to present cases to a group of their peers and their physician medical director. The prehospital care is analyzed and critiqued in order to identify areas in need of improvement. This area of continuing education is extremely valuable in that it clarifies specific experiences for field personnel. The success of these sessions largely depends upon the quality of documentation.

ADMINISTRATIVE USES OF THE CALL REPORT

There are several administrative uses for a call report. Planning optimal distribution of ambulances, compiling annual reports, and billing are just a few examples of how call report information is used. You should always approach the record keeping process in such a way as to ensure easy access to these data.

Principles of Record Keeping

The effectiveness of a call report depends on four major factors: accuracy, clarity, proper chronology, and completeness. Many forms used in EMS systems today are structured in such a way as to facilitate adherence to these principles. Boxes that can be checked are often used to save time for the EMT and to allow for computer transfer of essential data. However, no single form can account for all possible categories of information that should be recorded. As an EMT, you must be able to apply individual judgment in determining important entries. For example, if an unconscious patient were to vomit and aspirate while en route to the hospital, a clear notation of this event would be essential to guide follow-up care. A check box system cannot account for all of these variables.

ACCURACY

Every attempt should be made to be accurate and honest about the recorded data. EMTs who forget to record vital signs and create bogus values at a later time are jeopardizing the quality of patient care. Times, diagnostic signs, treatments, and other entries should be as accurate as possible. It may be impossible to be exact about certain data. Times during the call, such as time of arrival at the scene or time of treatments, must often be approximated since they are documented during transport or after arrival at the hospital. In these instances, a review of times should be done from dispatch through arrival at the hospital to develop the best possible approximation of data.

Accuracy is also important when documenting unusual behavior or events. For example, a recorded statement, "The patient was found drunk on the floor of the apartment," is too judgmental, since it concludes that there was alcohol intoxication without definitive evidence. The same event could be recorded "The patient was found disoriented on the apartment floor with an alcohol-like smell on his breath." This statement more accurately reflects the actual observations rather than the conclusions made by the EMT.

CLARITY

Ideally, a call report should be written for the reader. It should be developed clearly and legibly so that the data are easily understood. Any abbreviations or characters used to shorten a statement should be accurate. Care should be used to spell words properly. Many words change meaning when spelled incorrectly. For example, *ileum* refers to a portion of the small intestine, while *ilium* is a section of the pelvic bone. When describing areas of pain or the location of wounds, you should be as exact as possible. "Body diagrams" are useful tools in achieving clarity. The location of wounds, fractures, and other injuries can be drawn on diagrams of the body to identify these locations. Some EMS systems provide diagrams on the ambulance call report (Fig. 19–12).

CHRONOLOGY

The time relationships of response, assessment, treatment, transport, and arrival at the hospital are critical areas of documentation. They provide the physician with

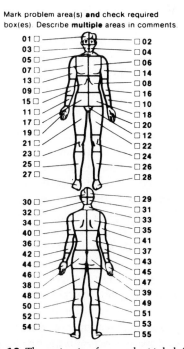

Mark problem area(s) and check required box(es). Describe **multiple** areas in comments.

FIGURE 19–12. The anatomic reference chart is helpful to indicate the location of wounds and pain. It also is useful to describe the burn surface areas. (From New York City Emergency Medical Services: Ambulance Call Report.)

a history of events in the order in which they occurred. For example, if a patient exhibits signs of hypoxia that are abolished following oxygen therapy, the relationship of therapy to this improvement should be clearly noted. Conversely, if a patient's condition deteriorates, the sequence of significant changes should be noted in the order in which they occurred. This allows the physician to more easily identify progressive problems as well as the effectiveness of therapy.

The recordings below illustrate the importance of accurate entries:

Time	Vital Signs	Treatment	Comments
1530	Pulse 140 BP 96/60 Resp. 30	Oxygen nonrebreather Pneumatic antishock garment (PASG)	Patient unresponsive
1534	Pulse 100 BP 110/70 Resp. 24	Transport	Responds to painful stimuli
1540	Pulse 110 BP 90/60 Resp. 30	During transport	Patient unresponsive
1546	Pulse 120 BP 110/70 Resp. 34	Arrival hospital	Patient unresponsive

The above record demonstrates signs consistent with internal bleeding. Oxygen therapy and the application of the PASG resulted in improvement of the patient's status initially, but the patient continued to deteriorate during transport. This example illustrates how the effective documentation of chronology is invaluable to the physician in the emergency department.

COMPLETENESS

Deciding what factors should be included in the report is probably the most difficult task. Needless to say, all assessment, treatments, and reassessment procedures should be recorded in their chronologic order. Events that affected treatment or transport should also be noted. For example, a prolonged extrication time should be recorded to account for delay on the scene. If other EMS providers or first responders participated in the call, their role should be documented. In the case of physicians, their names and addresses should be recorded, especially if definitive care such as drug therapy or defibrillation was administered on the scene. Some EMS systems require treating physicians to accompany the patient following interventions on the scene.

Other unusual occurrences, such as belligerent or

aggressive actions on the part of the patient or the patient's relatives or friends, should be recorded. Avoid being judgmental or attempting to editorialize such events. Simply record the behavior and its implications regarding your treatment of the patient. If a family member rides in the ambulance, it should also be noted on the record.

Occasionally, police or family remove valuables from the patient. A note indicating the person, shield number (in the case of police), and the property removed should be documented.

Components of a Call Record

Although each emergency medical system has its own version of the call report, most records have common components. These include dispatch data, patient data, assessment and treatment data, patient disposition, and special authorization forms (Fig. 19–13).

DISPATCH DATA

The dispatch data usually consist of the call location, the date and time of the call, the crew names or numbers, the type of call, and the sequential times of response, arrival at the scene, removal from the scene, and arrival at the hospital. Most EMS systems use military time to document the respective phases of the call, i.e., 1200 (12 noon), 1530 (3:30 PM), 2400 (midnight), and so on. Some forms may include route information such as cross streets or major thoroughfares. A space may also be provided for a call identification number (Fig. 19–14).

When recording dispatch data, you should confirm the information if it is unclear and repeat the location of a call routinely if radio protocol permits. Most emergency communication systems make every attempt to reduce the time spent on a given dispatch, so that *routine* location confirmation may be inappropriate. However, if there is any doubt, confirmation should occur. Also, if the address seems incorrect based upon your knowledge of the area, you should note this to the dispatcher. The dispatcher frequently has a callback number to confirm questionable information while you respond to the scene.

In many EMS systems, the EMT may receive calls directly from the victim or bystander. Panic and chaos on the scene may make this task difficult. You should firmly direct the interview to ensure the receipt of the call location, the nature of the problem, and the callback number. Some EMS systems also provide for over-the-phone directions, during which you may be able to direct the caller in self-help procedures while he or she awaits

Text continued on page 772

Prehospital Care Report

2 –1128039

Press Down Firmly. You're Making 4 Copies.

M	D	Y

DATE   RUN NO   AGENCY CODE   VEH ID

Name

Address

Ph #

AGE | DOB M | D | Y | SEX M☐ F☐

Physician

Next of Kin

Agency Name

Call Location

CHECK ONE: ☐ Residence ☐ Health Facility ☐ Farm ☐ Indus. Facility
☐ Other Work Loc. ☐ Roadway ☐ Recreational ☐ Other

Call Origin

Dispatch Information

CALL TYPE AS REC'D.	INTERFACILITY TRANSFER
☐ Emergency	☐ Yes
☐ Non-Emergency	TYPE OF TRANSFER
☐ Stand-by	☐ BLS ☐ ALS

MILEAGE
END
BEGIN
TOTAL

HOSPITAL COMMUNICATIONS
☐ Yes ☐ Directly ☐ Thru Dispatch
☐ VHF ☐ UHF ☐ Phone
☐ No ☐ Communications Difficulties

USE MILITARY TIMES
CALL REC'D
ENROUTE
AT SCENE
FROM SCENE
AT DESTIN
IN SERVICE
IN QUARTERS

MECHANISM OF INJURY
☐ MVA (complete seat belt section) ☐ Fall of ____ feet ☐ GSW ☐ Other
☐ Struck by vehicle   ☐ Unarmed assault ☐ Knife _____

☐ Extrication required _____ minutes

Seat belt used?
☐ Yes ☐ No ☐ Unknown

Seat Belt Use Reported By
☐ Crew ☐ Patient
☐ Police ☐ Other

CHIEF COMPLAINT

SUBJECTIVE ASSESSMENT

PRESENTING PROBLEM

☐ Airway Obstruction
☐ Respiratory Arrest
☐ Respiratory Distress
☐ Cardiac Related (Potential)
☐ Cardiac Arrest

☐ Allergic Reaction
☐ Syncope
☐ Stroke/CVA
☐ General Illness/Malaise
☐ Gastro-Intestinal Distress
☐ Diabetic Related (Potential)
☐ Pain _____

☐ Unconscious/Unresp.
☐ Seizure
☐ Behavioral Disorder
☐ Substance Abuse (Potential)
☐ Poisoning (Accidental)

☐ Other _____

☐ Shock
☐ Head Injury
☐ Spinal Injury
☐ Fracture/Dislocation
☐ Amputation

☐ Multiple Trauma
☐ Trauma-Blunt
☐ Trauma-Penetrating
☐ Soft Tissue Injury
☐ Bleeding/Hemorrhage

☐ OB/GYN
☐ Burns
Environmental
☐ Heat
☐ Cold
☐ Hazardous Materials
☐ Obvious Death

PAST MEDICAL HISTORY

☐ Hypertension ☐ Stroke
☐ Seizures ☐ Diabetes
☐ COPD ☐ Cardiac
☐ Allergy ☐ Other (List)
☐ Medication

VITAL SIGNS

TIME	RESP	PULSE	B.P.	LEVEL OF CONSCIOUSNESS	GCS	TS	R PUPILS L	SKIN
	Rate: ☐ Regular ☐ Shallow ☐ Labored	Rate: ☐ Regular ☐ Irregular		☐ Alert ☐ Voice ☐ Pain ☐ Unresp.			☐ Normal ☐ Dilated ☐ Constricted ☐ Sluggish ☐ No-Reaction	☐ Unremarkable ☐ Cool ☐ Pale ☐ Warm ☐ Cyanotic ☐ Moist ☐ Flushed ☐ Dry ☐ Jaundiced
	Rate: ☐ Regular ☐ Shallow ☐ Labored	Rate: ☐ Regular ☐ Irregular		☐ Alert ☐ Voice ☐ Pain ☐ Unresp.			☐ Normal ☐ Dilated ☐ Constricted ☐ Sluggish ☐ No-Reaction	☐ Unremarkable ☐ Cool ☐ Pale ☐ Warm ☐ Cyanotic ☐ Moist ☐ Flushed ☐ Dry ☐ Jaundiced
	Rate: ☐ Regular ☐ Shallow ☐ Labored	Rate: ☐ Regular ☐ Irregular		☐ Alert ☐ Voice ☐ Pain ☐ Unresp.			☐ Normal ☐ Dilated ☐ Constricted ☐ Sluggish ☐ No-Reaction	☐ Unremarkable ☐ Cool ☐ Pale ☐ Warm ☐ Cyanotic ☐ Moist ☐ Flushed ☐ Dry ☐ Jaundiced

OBJECTIVE PHYSICAL ASSESSMENT

COMMENTS

☐ Physical Findings Unremarkable

Head/Neck | Upper Extr. | Chest/Back | Abd/Pelvic | Lower Extr.

1) Pain
2) Wound
3) Fracture/Disloc. Open
4) Fracture/Disloc. Closed
5) Bleeding/Hemorrhage
6) Loss of Motion/Sensation
7) Sprain/Strain
8) Burn ____ Deg ____ %
9) Internal

TREATMENT GIVEN

MEDICAL CONTROL INFORMATION

Insurance Data

☐ Airway Cleared
☐ Oral Airway
☐ Esophageal Obturator Airway/Esophageal Gastric Tube Airway (EOA/EGTA)
☐ EndoTracheal Tube (E/T)
☐ Oxygen Administered @ ____ L.P.M., Method ____
☐ Suction Used
☐ Artificial Ventilation Method ____
☐ C.P.R. in progress on arrival by: ☐ Citizen ☐ Firefighter ☐ Police Officer
☐ C.P.R. Started @ Time ▶ [ ][ ][ ]   Time from Arrest Until C.P.R. ▶ [ ][ ][ ] Minutes
☐ EKG Monitored (Attach Tracing) [Rhythm(s) ____]
☐ Defibrillation/Cardioversion No. Times ____ With ____ Watt/Sec.

☐ Medication Administered (Use Continuation Form)
☐ IV Fluid ____ No. Established ____ No. of Attempts ____
☐ Mast Inflated (Time Inflated: ____)
☐ Bleeding/Hemorrhage Controlled (Method Used: ____)
☐ Spinal Immobilization ☐ Neck ☐ Back
☐ Limb Immobilized by ☐ Fixation ☐ Traction
☐ (Heat) or (Cold) Applied
☐ Vomiting Induced @ Time ____ Method ____
☐ Restraints Applied, Type ____
☐ Baby Delivered @ Time ____ In County ____
   ☐ Alive ☐ Stillborn ☐ Male ☐ Female
☐ Other ____

DISPOSITION (See list)

DISP. CODE

CONTINUATION FORM USED YES ←

CREW

IN CHARGE
☐ EMT
☐ AEMT #

DRIVER'S NAME
☐ EMS-FR
☐ EMT
☐ AEMT #

NAME
☐ EMS-FR
☐ EMT
☐ AEMT #

NAME
☐ EMS-FR
☐ EMT
☐ AEMT #

EMS 100 (11/86) provided by NYS-EMS PROGRAM

AGENCY COPY/**WHITE**   HOSPITAL PATIENT RECORD COPY/**PINK**   RESEARCH COPY/**BLUE**   EXTRA SERVICE COPY/**GREEN**

FIGURE 19–13. A sample call report. (From New York State Department of Health: Prehospital Care Report.)

Call Location

Call Location					
CHECK ONE	☐ Residence	☐ Health Facility	☐ Farm	☐ Indus. Facility	
	☐ Other Work Loc.	☐ Roadway	☐ Recreational	☐ Other	

Place an *X* in the appropriate box indicating the location where the patient was initially found. (Check *ONLY* one box.)

Residence: Private homes, multiple occupancies such as; apartments, dormatories, etc...

(NOTE: May not necessarily be the patient's own residence.)

Health Facility: A place where medical care is routinely provided. (Examples include, hospital, nursing home, doctor's office, health clinic, emergicare clinic, infirmary.)

Farm: National Safety Council Definition: A rural place from which $1000. or more of agricultural products were sold, or normally would have been sold. (Examples: dairy farms, fields where crops are grown, chicken farms, tree farms—includes barns as well as fields.)

Indus. Facility: A place where a product is manufactured or stored. (Examples: warehouses, manufacturing plants, etc.)

Other Work Location: A place of work other than an industrial facility. (Examples: offices.)

Roadway: A place that is designated as a thoroughfare for motor vehicles; to include, passenger vehicles, trucks, and motorcycles. Not a private residence driveway. (Examples: interstates, town or village roads, county roads, streets.)

Recreational: National Safety Council Definition: Recreational places are those organized for recreation or sport but excluding homes and industrial places. (Examples: gymnasium, tennis court, bike or jogging path, basketball courts.)

Other: Any place which has not been defined by any of the other call locations in this section.

Call Origin

Call Origin

Enter the source of the call.
Examples: dispatcher, police, private citizen, walk-in.

Dispatch Information

Dispatch Information

Enter any additional dispatch information provided to your agency or service.
Examples: MVA, unconscious patient; gun shot wound.

Mileage

MILEAGE					
END					
BEGIN					
TOTAL					

Enter the mileage information required by your agency. Indicate the mileage on the responding vehicle's odometer at the beginning of the run and at the end of the run. Subtract the "beginning" reading from the "end" reading and enter the "total" mileage.

Call Type As Rec'd

Both Call Type and Interfacility Transfer Categories must be completed on each PCR.

CALL TYPE AS REC'D
☐ Emergency
☐ Non-Emergency
☐ Stand-by

Place an *X* in the box that indicates how the call was received from the *dispatcher.* Indicate whether the unit responding was dispatched as an emergency, a nonemergency, or a standby.

Emergency: Place an *X* in this box when a call is dispatched as an emergency or a potential emergency even though it may not turn out to be an emergency. This box should also be marked for emergency or critical care Interfacility Transfers (see Interfacility Transfer section).

Nonemergency: Place an *X* in this box for routine calls such as a non-urgent transport from home to hospital, a transport from hospital to home, or a non-urgent call to assist a patient at home. This box should also be marked for non-urgent Interfacility Transfers (see Interfacility Transfer section).

Stand-by: Place an *X* in this box when your unit is dispatched but no patient is treated such as when covering a football game, standing by at a fire, or providing mutual aid at a neighboring station. If an incident occurs during a standby such as an injured football player, a separate PCR should be completed and the appropriate Call Type (emergency, nonemergency) marked.

FIGURE 19–14. Dispatch data form with directions for completion. (From New York State Department of Health: Prehospital Care Report.)
Illustration continued on opposite page

Interfacility Transfer

Both Call Type and Interfacility Transfer Categories must be completed on each PCR.

```
INTERFACILITY TRANSFER
  ☐ Yes
TYPE OF TRANSFER
  ☐ BLS    ☐ ALS
```

YES: Place an *X* in this box when a patient is taken from a hospital or nursing home and is transferred to another hospital or nursing home. This category only applies to *transfers* from one *facility* to another. Transports to or from private residences, doctors' offices, etc. are not considered Interfacility Transfers.

Place an *X* in the appropriate box to indicate the type of treatment (BLS, ALS) the patient received *during* the transfer. This treatment may be given by crew members *or* by nurses, physicians, or other health professionals who accompany the patient *during* the transfer.

BLS: Treatment given that *does not require* the skills of Advanced EMTs.

ALS: Treatment given that *requires* Advanced EMT skills or higher.

If the call being reported on the PCR is *NOT* an interfacility transfer leave this entire section blank.

Hospital Communications

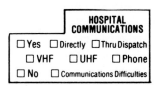

```
         HOSPITAL
      COMMUNICATIONS
☐ Yes  ☐ Directly  ☐ Thru Dispatch
   ☐ VHF    ☐ UHF    ☐ Phone
☐ No   ☐ Communications Difficulties
```

Indicate in this section how you communicated with any hospital. Do not record how you communicated with your dispatch center or other agency.

YES: Place an *X* in the box if you notified a hospital of your ETA (expected time of arrival) or patient information.

Directly: Place an *X* in this box if you communicated with a hospital directly by radio or telephone (not through a dispatch center).

Check all that apply.

VHF: Place an *X* in the box if you communicated *directly* with a hospital using a VHF radio (high band or low band).

UHF: Place an *X* in this box if you communicated *directly* with a hospital using a UHF radio (voice and/or telemetry).

Phone: Place an *X* in this box if you communicated *directly* with a hospital using a telephone.

Thru Dispatch: Place an *X* in this box if your only contact with a hospital was through a dispatch center.

NO: Place an *X* in the box if you did not communicate with a hospital at all.

Check if it applies.

Communications Difficulties: Place an *X* in this box if you encountered difficulties with the communications system or equipment. This category may be checked *in addition to* any of the above.

Call Times

```
              USE MILITARY TIMES
CALL REC'D   [    :    :    ]
ENROUTE      [    :    :    ]
AT SCENE     [    :    :    ]
FROM SCENE   [    :    :    ]
AT DESTIN    [    :    :    ]
IN SERVICE   [    :    :    ]
IN QUARTERS  [    :    :    ]
```

Only enter military times in this section. To calculate military time, see General Instructions.

Call Rec'd

Enter the time the service/agency receives the call. If a unit was reserved ahead of time for a transport, record the time when the vehicle responds. In that case, the call received time and the en route time will be the same.

En route

Enter the time the unit starts toward the incident location.

At Scene

Enter the time the *unit* arrives at the incident location. If the incident is within a structure, the time the emergency vehicle arrives at the structure should be entered.

From Scene

Enter the time of departure from the scene.

FIGURE 19-14. *Continued*

your arrival at the scene. These procedures may include instructing the caller to secure the airway, control bleeding, and even perform cardiopulmonary resuscitation. However, excessive conversations with the caller should be avoided if the person receiving the call is also the responding EMT.

PATIENT DATA

The patient data generally include the name, sex, age, date of birth, and address of the patient. It may also include the patient's religion and the name and telephone number of the next of kin. Some systems include information about health insurance and assistance at the scene (i.e., police, physicians, etc.). Every reasonable attempt at securing this information should be made. Most systems discourage a search of personal property in the absence of police or inhospital personnel. Furthermore, there may not be time to gather this information either at the scene or en route to the hospital if the patient is critically ill and requires your constant attention. In noncritical patients, it should be collected as soon as more important issues have been completed. The prehospital care record often becomes the primary source of basic patient data. For example, a patient who becomes unconscious in your ambulance or upon arrival at the hospital and who has no personal identification on his or her person may encounter delays in needed care. Contacting private physicians, locating patient records, and communicating with relatives are essential activities that may depend upon your accurate collection of the patient data (Fig. 19–15).

ASSESSMENT DATA

During evaluation of the patient, you should attempt to record critical signs and symptoms. Vital signs and Glasgow Coma Scale and trauma scores are examples of values that may be forgotten if not documented early (Figs. 19–16 and 19–17). It may not be possible to make notes during critical care. In these instances, recordings should be made during transport or at the first opportunity after arriving at the hospital.

Some systems carry recording devices (notably in EMT-defibrillation programs) that record voices on the scene and electrocardiograms. This permits more accurate documentation and is invaluable for quality assurance audits by medical directors.

Continuous reassessment of the patient should also be recorded to establish a record of improvement or deterioration during transport. Some systems use a check box format for recording assessment and treatment information. Again, this should not prevent you from making additional notes when necessary to cover contingencies not accounted for in the format. A "com-

ments" section is often provided for this purpose. To establish the chronology of assessment and care, the comments section can also be used to construct a summary of key assessments and treatments. This provides the physician with a concise account of the prehospital care (see Fig. 19–13). Figure 19–18 illustrates a checkbox system for summary assessment data related to the patient's presenting problem.

TREATMENT DATA

Every treatment rendered should be recorded clearly in the call record, and a time relationship should be established. If other providers intervened prior to your arrival, their actions should be noted. If extraordinary factors prevented the timely application of treatment, such as difficulty in gaining access to the patient, weather conditions, or hazards to rescue personnel, they should also be noted. Treatment data also include the transportation method, time of transport, and notification of the hospital. If the patient was taken to a trauma center or other specialty referral hospital, it should be documented. This is of special importance if a closer hospital was bypassed (Fig. 19–19).

PATIENT DISPOSITION INFORMATION

The patient disposition information may include the receiving hospital, special transport modes (such as helicopters), the rationale for facility selection (nearest facility, patient choice, specialty hospital, etc.), the reason for not receiving a patient (i.e., refused medical aid), and the final disposition of the patient at the hospital. There may also be a space provided for the EMT's signature and the signature of the receiving nurse or physician (Fig. 19–20).

AUTHORIZATION FORMS

Ambulance call reports often have authorization or treatment refusal forms on the reverse side of the call report. In cases where patients refuse medical aid or refuse an aspect of care such as oxygen therapy, a signature of this refusal should be obtained. It should be accompanied by the signature of a witness, preferably a relative, friend, or police officer. Obviously, you should first make every effort to convince the patient to accept treatment and/or transport. The refusal signature is of no value if the patient has not been clearly informed of the potential consequences of his or her actions. If standard release forms are not provided, it may be appropriate for you to write one and have it signed by the patient. Occasionally a patient who refuses aid will also refuse to sign. This should be noted and signed by a witness if possible.

Name

Name

Enter the name of the patient. If the name is unknown, write "unknown" and add important identifiers.
Examples: unknown white female, unknown black male.

Address

Address

Enter the mailing address of the patient. Be as complete as possible. If the address is unknown, write "unknown."

Ph #

Ph #

Enter the patient's telephone number.

Age

Enter the age of the patient. The patient's age must be entered even if the date of birth is entered. If the patient's age is unknown, enter the approximate age of the patient. If the patient is less than one year of age, enter either *H* for hours, or *D* for days, or *M* for months.
Examples: 12 hours entered as 12*H*, 5 days entered as 5*D*, 7 months entered as 7*M*.

DOB

Enter the date of the patient's birth. If the date of birth is unknown, leave this section blank. Numbers less than *10* are to be listed as two digits.
Example: January 3, 1905 (01:03:05).

Sex

Place an *X* in the appropriate box to indicate whether the patient is male or female.

Physician

Physician

Enter the name of the patient's personal physician.

Next of Kin

Next of Kin

Enter the name of a relative or guardian and his/her relationship to the patient.

FIGURE 19–15. Patient data form with instructions for completion. (From New York State Department of Health: Prehospital Care Report.)

Patients may also sign to select an institution that is beyond the closest receiving hospital. Some systems have policies that cover these possibilities (Fig. 19–21).

SPECIAL SITUATIONS

Aside from routine documentation, there are certain circumstances that require special notations to prevent medicolegal complications at a later date.

DOCUMENTATION OF DEATH. Some systems permit EMTs to withhold resuscitative methods for victims of cardiac arrest if evidence of irreversible brain damage exists. For example, a patient with complete destruction of the brain or decapitation following an automobile collision may be left on the scene. Instances of obvious death must be recorded clearly. It is not sufficient to record "Dead on Arrival," "DOA," or other general statements. All factors that demonstrate irreversible or biologic death must be noted. These include decomposition of the body, rigor mortis (muscle rigidity following death), or extreme dependent lividity (mottling of the dependent areas of the body due to the gravitational pooling of the blood). Time factors may also be recorded. However, time by itself is never a reason to withhold resuscitation. Following is an example of a well-documented instance of death.

Vital Signs

Enter each set of vital signs in the space provided. If more than three sets are taken, record them in the Comment section.

	TIME	RESP	PULSE	B.P.	LEVEL OF CONSCIOUSNESS	GCS	TS	R	PUPILS	L	SKIN
V I T A L S I G N S	┊ ┊ ┊	Rate: ☐ Regular ☐ Shallow ☐ Labored	Rate: ☐ Regular ☐ Irregular	╱	☐ **A**lert ☐ **V**oice ☐ **P**ain ☐ **U**nresp.			☐ ☐ ☐ ☐ ☐	Normal Dilated Constricted Sluggish No-Reaction	☐ ☐ ☐ ☐ ☐	☐ Unremarkable ☐ Cool ☐ Pale ☐ Warm ☐ Cyanotic ☐ Moist ☐ Flushed ☐ Dry ☐ Jaundiced
	┊ ┊ ┊	Rate: ☐ Regular ☐ Shallow ☐ Labored	Rate: ☐ Regular ☐ Irregular	╱	☐ **A**lert ☐ **V**oice ☐ **P**ain ☐ **U**nresp.			☐ ☐ ☐ ☐ ☐	Normal Dilated Constricted Sluggish No-Reaction	☐ ☐ ☐ ☐ ☐	☐ Unremarkable ☐ Cool ☐ Pale ☐ Warm ☐ Cyanotic ☐ Moist ☐ Flushed ☐ Dry ☐ Jaundiced
	┊ ┊ ┊	Rate: ☐ Regular ☐ Shallow ☐ Labored	Rate: ☐ Regular ☐ Irregular	╱	☐ **A**lert ☐ **V**oice ☐ **P**ain ☐ **U**nresp.			☐ ☐ ☐ ☐ ☐	Normal Dilated Constricted Sluggish No-Reaction	☐ ☐ ☐ ☐ ☐	☐ Unremarkable ☐ Cool ☐ Pale ☐ Warm ☐ Cyanotic ☐ Moist ☐ Flushed ☐ Dry ☐ Jaundiced

Time

Enter the time each set of vitals are taken. *Only enter military time in this section.* To calculate military time, see General Instructions.

Resp.

Record the number of respirations per minute. Also place an *X* in the box that best describes the quality of respiration (regular, shallow, labored).

Pulse

Record the pulse rate per minute. Also place an *X* in the box that best describes the patient's pulse (regular, irregular).

B.P.

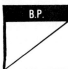

Record the blood pressure (B.P.) as systolic over diastolic pressure. If you are unable to take the patient's blood pressure, explain the reason in the Comment section. If the blood pressure is taken by palpation, record the systolic pressure over *P.* Example: 90/P.

Level of Consciousness

This section denotes level of consciousness by the following acronym (AVPU) which stands for:

A—Alert—Knows his name (person); Knows where he is (place); knows day of week (day).

V—Verbally responds—but not able to respond correctly to all three questions above.

P—Responds to painful stimulus but not oriented to person, place, and/or time.

U—Unresponsive to both painful and verbal stimulus.

Place an *X* in the box that most accurately denotes the patient's level of consciousness at the time this assessment was performed.

FIGURE 19–16. Vital signs section of a call report should record serial vital signs and neurologic signs (i.e., pupils) during the time with the patient. This is helpful to identify evolving problems. Glasgow coma scale and trauma score are explained earlier. (From New York State Department of Health: Prehospital Care Report.) *Illustration continued on opposite page*

Glasgow Coma Scale (GCS)

The Glasgow Coma Scale (GCS), based upon eye opening, verbal, and motor responses, is a practical means of monitoring changes in level of consciousness. If response on the scale is given a number, the responsiveness of the patient can be expressed by summation of the figures. Lowest score is 3; highest is 15. (Refer to GCS guide on back of PCR.)

Record the numeric total of the highest level of responses to the level of consciousness survey.

Example:	**GCS**
Eye Opening — To Pain	2
Verbal Response — Confused	4
Motor Response — Withdraw (Pain)	4
TOTAL GCS SCORE	10

Trauma Score (TS)

The Trauma Score (TS) is a numeric grading system for estimating the severity of injury. The score is composed of the Glasgow Coma Scale (reduced to approximately one-third total value) and measurements of cardiopulmonary function. Each parameter is given a number (high for normal and low for impaired function). Severity of injury is estimated by summing the numbers. The lowest score is 1; and the highest score is 16. (Refer to TS guide on back of PCR.)

Record the numeric estimation of the severity of the injury. The score is composed of one-third the value of the GCS plus the patient's best response to the measurement of cardiopulmonary function.

Example:	*TS*
Glasgow Coma Scale — Points - 10	3
Respiratory Rate — 24-35/min.	3
Respiratory Expansion — Normal	1
Systolic Blood Pressure — 90 mm Hg or greater	4
Capillary Refill — Normal	2
TOTAL TS SCORE	13

Pupils

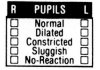

Place an **X** in the box that best describes the eyes' response to light. Record the right pupil under the **R** column and the left under the **L** column. These columns are the patient's right and left sides. Indicate in the Comment section if the pupils are normally uneven or if a patient has an artificial eye.

Skin

SKIN
☐ Unremarkable
☐ Cool ☐ Pale
☐ Warm ☐ Cyanotic
☐ Moist ☐ Flushed
☐ Dry ☐ Jaundiced

Place an **X** only in the boxes that apply. Mark "unremarkable" only if all three assessment categories (temperature, moisture, and color) are within normal limits.

FIGURE 19–16. *Continued*

The patient was found prone, with extreme dependent lividity and rigor mortis present. The patient was pulseless, apneic, and had fixed and dilated pupils. According to family members the patient was last seen two days ago.

This documentation includes both concrete evidence of irreversible death (rigor mortis and dependent lividity) and supporting evidence (pupils, pulse, breathing, and time).

EMOTIONALLY DISTURBED, UNDER-AGE (MINOR), OR UNCONSCIOUS PATIENTS. Whenever possible, minors or unconscious patients should be accompanied by an adult relative or a police officer. This minimizes the chance of later complaints regarding missing property or improper behavior by the EMT. If circumstances prevent accompaniment, delay in transport should not occur. In the case of the emotionally disturbed patient, a police

Text continued on page 780

Glasgow Coma Scale

Eye Opening	Spontaneous	4	
	To Voice	3	
	To Pain	2	
	None	1	
Verbal Response	Oriented	5	
	Confused	4	**Patient's Best Verbal Response**
	Inappropriate Words	3	Arouse patient with voice or painful stimulus.
	Incomprehensible Sounds	2	
	None	1	
Motor Response	Obeys Command	6	
	Localizes Pain	5	**Patient's Best Motor Response**
	Withdraw (pain)	4	Response to command or painful stimulus.
	Flexion (pain)	3	
	Extension (pain)	2	
	None	1	
Total GCS Score		**:3-15**	

Trauma Score*

The Trauma Score is a numerical grading system for estimating the severity of injury[1]. The score is composed of the Glasgow Coma Scale (reduced to approximately one third total value) and measurements of cardiopulmonary function. Each parameter is given a number (high for normal and low for impaired function). Severity of injury is estimated by summing the numbers. The lowest score is 1, and the highest score is 16.

Total Glasgow Coma Scale Points	14-15	5	
	11-13	4	
	8-10	3	
	5-7	2	
	3-4	1	
Respiratory Rate	10-24/min	4	
	24-35/min	3	**Respiratory Rate**
	36/min or greater	2	Number of respirations in 15 seconds: multiply by four.
	1-9/min	1	
	None	0	
Respiratory Expansion	Normal	1	Retractive-use of accessory muscles or intercostal muscle retraction
	Retractive	0	
Systolic Blood Pressure	90 mm Hg or greater	4	**Systolic Blood Pressure**
	70-89 mm Hg	3	
	50-69 mm Hg	2	Systolic cuff pressure; either arm - auscultate or palpate
	0-49 mm Hg	1	No pulse - no carotid pulse
	No Pulse	0	
Capillary Refill	Normal	2	Normal -nail bed, forehead, or lip mucosa color refill in 2 seconds or time taken to mentally repeat "capillary refill"
	Delayed	1	Delayed -more than 2 seconds capillary refill
	None	0	None -no capillary refill
Total Trauma Score		**:1-16**	

*Endorsed by the American Trauma Society

FIGURE 19–17. Glasgow coma scale and trauma score. (From Champion HR, Sacco WJ, Carnazzo AJ, et al: Trauma score. Crit Care Med 9(9): 672–676. Copyright © by Williams & Wilkins, 1981.)

PRESENTING PROBLEM					
	☐ Allergic Reaction	☐ Unconscious/Unresp.	☐ Shock	☐ Multiple Trauma	☐ OB/GYN
	☐ Syncope	☐ Seizure	☐ Head Injury	☐ Trauma-Blunt	☐ Burns
☐ Airway Obstruction	☐ Stroke/CVA	☐ Behavioral Disorder	☐ Spinal Injury	☐ Trauma-Penetrating	Environmental
☐ Respiratory Arrest	☐ General Illness/Malaise	☐ Substance Abuse (Potential)	☐ Fracture/Dislocation	☐ Soft Tissue Injury	☐ Heat
☐ Respiratory Distress	☐ Gastro-Intestinal Distress	☐ Poisoning (Accidental)	☐ Amputation	☐ Bleeding/Hemorrhage	☐ Cold
☐ Cardiac Related (Potential)	☐ Diabetic Related (Potential)				☐ Hazardous Materials
☐ Cardiac Arrest	☐ Pain ________		☐ Other ________		☐ Obvious Death

Allergic Reaction — an abnormal or unexpected reaction to a substance such as a drug, an insect sting or bite, a food, dust, pollen, or chemical.

Syncope — a temporary loss of consciousness; fainting.

Stroke/CVA — a condition characterized by a sudden lessening or a loss of consciousness, sensation and/or voluntary movement. Cerebrovascular accident (CVA) is a medical problem and not a trauma-related problem.

General Illness/Malaise — a vague feeling of physical discomfort or uneasiness often occuring before or during an illness.

Gastro-Intestinal Distress — complaints associated with the stomach and intestines such as nausea, vomiting, diarrhea, stomach pain, indigestion, and passage of blood in the stool.

Diabetic Related (Potential) — signs and symptoms that are consistent with insulin shock or diabetic coma.

Potential Insulin Shock: The patient is hypoglycemic with presenting signs of full, rapid pulse; normal breathing; dizziness; headache; fainting; seizures; disorientation; coma; normal blood pressure.

Potential Diabetic Coma: The patient is hyperglycemic with presenting signs of sweet or fruity smelling breath; rapid, weak pulse; rapid, deep breathing; varying degrees of unresponsiveness up to coma; normal or slightly low blood pressure.

Pain — a sensation in which the patient states he is experiencing distress, discomfort, or suffering. Specify the type and location of pain on the line provided.

Unconscious/Unresponsive — When the patient is comatose and does not react to verbal or painful stimuli.

Seizure — involuntary contraction and relaxation of voluntary muscles (convulsions). These are signs, for example, that may be seen with a grand mal seizure.

Behavioral Disorder — an inappropriate mood or conduct exhibited by the patient.

Select Substance Abuse or Poisoning. Do ***not*** check both categories.

Substance Abuse (Potential) — in injection, ingestion, or inhalation of excessive amounts of any drug including alcohol. Overdose and suicide attempts using drugs and/or alcohol would fall into this category.

Poisoning (Accidental) — the injection, ingestion, exposure, inhalation, or absorption of any substance that will produce a harmful or injurious effect on the body. Substance abuse, overdose, or attempted suicides should ***not*** be recorded under this category.

FIGURE 19–18. Patient assessment data form with instructions for completion. (From New York State Department of Health: Prehospital Care Report.)

TREATMENT GIVEN | **MEDICAL CONTROL INFORMATION**

☐ Airway Cleared
☐ Oral Airway
☐ Esophageal Obturator Airway/Esophageal Gastric Tube Airway (EOA/EGTA)
☐ EndoTracheal Tube (E/T)
☐ Oxygen Administered @ _____ L.P.M., Method _____
☐ Suction Used
☐ Artificial Ventilation Method _____

☐ C.P.R. in progress on arrival by: ☐ Citizen   ☐ Firefighter   ☐ Police Officer

☐ C.P.R. Started @ Time ▶ [   ][   ][   ][   ]   Time from Arrest Until C.P.R. ▶ [   ][   ][   ] Minutes
☐ EKG Monitored (Attach Tracing) (Rhythm(s) _____
☐ Defibrillation/Cardioversion No. Times _____ With _____ Watt/Sec.

☐ Medication Administered (Use Continuation Form)
☐ IV Fluid _____ No. Established _____ No. of Attempts _____
☐ Mast Inflated (Time Inflated _____)
☐ Bleeding/Hemorrhage Controlled (Method Used _____)
☐ Spinal Immobilization   ☐ Neck   ☐ Back
☐ Limb Immobilized by   ☐ Fixation   ☐ Traction
☐ (Heat) or (Cold) Applied
☐ Vomiting Induced @ Time _____ Method _____
☐ Restraints Applied, Type _____
☐ Baby Delivered @ Time _____ In County _____
    ☐ Alive   ☐ Stillborn   ☐ Male   ☐ Female
☐ Other _____

CPR in progress on arrival by:

☐ C.P.R. in progress on arrival by:

Place an *X* in the box if cardiopulmonary resuscitation (CPR) was initiated prior to the arrival of responding emergency personnel.

(NOTE: If the above is checked, check all the following that apply.)

☐ Citizen

Place an *X* in this box if CPR was initiated by an individual who was not part of emergency services personnel, i.e. EMS, fire, or police, who responded in an official capacity.

☐ Firefighter

Place an *X* in box if CPR was initiated by a firefighter who responded to this call in an official capacity.

☐ Police Officer

Place an *X* in box if CPR was initiated by a police officer who responded to this call in an official capacity.

CPR Started

Place an *X* in the box if the patient was given CPR by *anyone* (bystander, first responder, your agency, etc).

@ Time

Enter the time that CPR was first started. Only enter this time if you have a reliable source of information regarding the actual time when CPR was started. Use military time. To calculate military time, see General Instructions.

Time From Arrest Until CPR

Enter the best approximation of the patient's down time prior to CPR being administered by anyone. Only enter this time if you have a reliable source of information regarding the patient's down time. If the time is unknown, leave the boxes blank.

EKG Monitored

Place an *X* in the box if an electrocardiogram (EKG/ECG) was performed and attach sections of the tracing to the agency (white) and hospital (pink) copies of the PCR. Indicate the interpretation of each significant tracing in the space provided.

Defibrillation/ Cardioversion

Place an *X* in the box if the patient was defibrillated or cardioverted. Circle either "defibrillation" or "cardioversion" and record the number of times and the watt/seconds that were used each time.

Medication Administered

Place an *X* in the box if your crew administered any medication(s). List all medications including time, dosage, and route in the Comment section or on an ALS form, if available.

IV

Place an *X* in the box if an intravenous line was established or attempted. Do not mark this section if the IV was started by hospital personnel prior to an Interfacility Transfer (note in Comment section).

Fluid: Indicate the IV fluid (normal saline, D5W, lactated Ringers) administered. List IV medications in the Comment section or on an ALS form, if available.

No. Established: Record the number of intravenous lines that were established.

No. of Attempts: Record the total number of attempts. This is the number of lines that were established *plus* the number that were attempted but were unsuccessful.

Example: IV Fluid *Ringers;* No. Established *1,* No. of Attempts *2.*

FIGURE 19–19. Treatment data form with instructions for completion. (From New York State Department of Health: Prehospital Care Report.)

Disp. Code

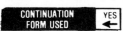

Enter the code number from the list below that corresponds to the disposition entered. Note that each hospital has an individual code number listed on the PCR clipboard. Nontransporting services should only use codes 004 through 010. The disposition list and codes are also printed on the PCR clipboard.

Code	Disposition
001	Nursing Home
002	Other Medical Facility
003	Residence
004	Treated by this Unit and Transported by Another
005	Refused Medical Aid or Transport
006	Call Cancelled En Route
007	Standby Only
008	Gone on Arrival (patient removed prior to arrival)
009	Unfounded (false alarm) (no patient found)
010	Other

ALS Form Used

Place an **X** over the word **YES** if a continuation form was used on this call. This box is to be used if a continuation form is available in your region.

Crew

Enter the names of the crew members. If there are more than four members on the call, list the additional names in the Comment section. The crew member *in charge* of the call should be entered in the *first* box. The *driver's name* must be entered in the *second* box.

When the crew member is an EMT, place an **X** in the box which indicates his/her *highest level* of EMT certification and enter the six-digit NYS certification number in the space provided. If the crew member is not an EMT, only enter the person's name and leave the EMT section blank.

FIGURE 19–20. Patient disposition form with instructions for completion. (From New York State Department of Health: Prehospital Care Report.)

REFUSAL OF TREATMENT/TRANSPORTATION
NEGATIVA A RECIBIR TRATAMIENTO/SER TRASLADADO

RELEASE
EXONERACION DE RESPONSABILIDADES

COMPLETE ON WHITE (AGENCY) COPY ONLY
LLENE UNICAMENTE LA COPIA BLANCA (DE LA AGENCIA)

I hereby refuse (treatment/transport to a hospital) and I acknowledge that such treatment/transportation was advised by the ambulance crew or physician. I hereby release such persons from liability for respecting and following my express wishes.

Mediante la presente declaro que me niego a aceptar el tratamiento/traslado a un hospital y reconozco asimismo que el medico o el personal de la ambulancia recomendaron ese tratamiento/traslado. Consiguientemente, eximo a dichas personas de toda responsabilidad por haber respetado y cumplido mis deseos expresos.

Signed:
Firma: _____

Witness:
Testigo: _____

FIGURE 19–21. Refusal of treatment or authorization forms. (From New York State Department of Health: Prehospital Care Report.)

officer is preferable. Most systems have policies that define these issues clearly.

DYING STATEMENTS. Occasionally, you may find yourself the sole witness to a dying patient's last words. These comments may have a legal or personal significance to family members and should be properly recorded. This is of particular importance in instances of suicide or trauma associated with criminal acts.

HOMICIDE AND SUICIDE. If you are the first person to arrive at the scene of a homicide or suicide, you must carefully document any significant findings. The position of the body, potential mechanisms of injury (such as the presence of an empty bottle of sleeping pills), and other essential facts should be noted. Care should be taken not to unnecessarily disturb the scene of the crime or move the body, since this may be important in the investigation. These and other criminal acts should be reported to the police at the appropriate time.

Confidentiality

All information recorded on an ambulance call report is confidential. Requests by bystanders or reporters should be directed to the police, physician, or administrative staff at the hospital. Certain conditions such as communicable diseases or dog bites may warrant addi-

tional action, such as reporting the event to a specific agency.

COMMUNICATIONS

Introduction

Prehospital care requires the use of many resources to effect the survival of the acutely ill or injured patient. Police, rescue personnel, firefighters, utility companies, and other specialized personnel are examples of resources that cooperate within an EMS system. Communication systems play an essential role in the initial notification of accidents or any emergency requiring medical assistance. Additionally, you may have provisions within your EMS system to communicate with the medical control physician.

A modern communications system literally serves as the central nervous system for emergency medical services personnel. It can document input from a citizen's call for help and can quickly analyze this information for the appropriate ambulance response. Most systems are also capable of coordinating additional activities such as facility selection and notifications. During each of these functions, the communications center must continually monitor the disposition of all assignments and the status of each unit. The diagram in Figure 19–22 demonstrates

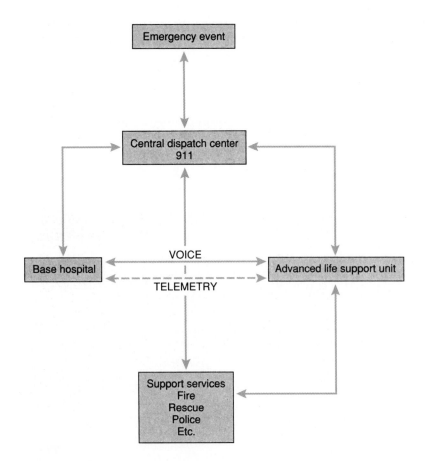

FIGURE 19–22. A centralized 911 dispatch system with telemetry communications to medical control facilities. (From Stapleton E, Best J: Developing a hospital based Ambulance Service. In Pascarelli E (ed): Hospital Based Ambulatory Care. Norwalk, CT, Appleton-Century-Crofts, 1983.)

the basic configuration of a typical EMS communication system.

Aspects of a Communications System

COMMUNICATIONS CENTER

The communications center is responsible for receiving all requests for emergency assistance, triage (sorting calls according to priority), dispatch of available resources, and coordination between other emergency services (e.g., fire, police, hospital, etc.). In small systems, the ambulance base may serve as the communications center. In larger urban systems, a separate center usually exists and may be based at the headquarters of the EMS system. The 911 system has been established in many communities throughout the nation over the last 20 years. This was developed to efficiently use the resources within the EMS system and to provide an easily remembered number for access to emergency assistance. Figure 19–23 shows a dispatcher's work station in a modern-day communications center.

RECEIVING OPERATORS

The individual who receives the call for help is often called the receiving operator. In small systems this role may be assumed by the on-duty EMT or the dispatcher. The receiving operator has the responsibility of obtaining and documenting the call location and other pertinent patient data. In larger urban systems, this person may also be responsible for providing a category status for priority dispatch. This is a tremendous responsibility, since this action establishes which patient receives an emergency medical response first. The most modern systems also have provisions for telephone-directed instructions for self-help. One of these is the Seattle EMS system, which gives structured directions for cardiopulmonary resuscitation when cardiac arrest calls are received. Figure 19–24 shows a receiving operator's work station in a modern communications center.

DISPATCHER

The dispatcher is an individual who communicates with field personnel and other agencies to coordinate the emergency medical response. He or she may also function as the receiving operator in small or medium-sized EMS systems. The dispatcher may also have the responsibility for prioritizing calls and deciding when basic life support versus paramedic units are dispatched. Dispatchers and receiving operators should possess good communication skills and be knowledgeable in emergency care, since they must perform triage. There is a national training program that prepares dispatch personnel for this difficult task. Even with this training, it is also valuable for dispatchers to be trained and experienced EMTs or paramedics. The field experience allows for a more practical understanding of the special circumstances that may arise during a particular response.

HOSPITAL NOTIFICATION AND SELECTION. A very important function of dispatch personnel is to relay information from the field sources to the receiving hospitals or specialty care centers (e.g., trauma, burn, neonate, etc.). It is essential that this type of communication be concise but contain all pertinent information necessary to prepare for the imminent arrival of the patient. A basic description of the patient's status, such as "cardiac arrest," "severe head trauma," or "gunshot wound to the chest," should be given. Pertinent vital signs, including pulse, mental status, respirations, and blood pressure, should be included to clarify the severity of the problem. This kind of information allows the emergency department team to mobilize the appropriate personnel and resources for a specific type of patient.

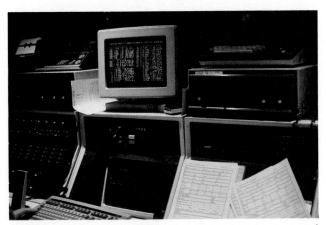

FIGURE 19–23. Dispatcher's work station with computerized dispatch system. (Courtesy of Gustave Pappas.)

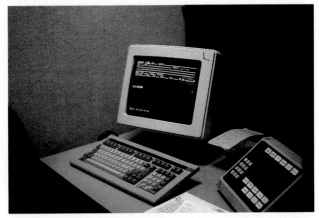

FIGURE 19–24. Receiving operator's work station with computerized dispatch system. (Courtesy of Gustave Pappas.)

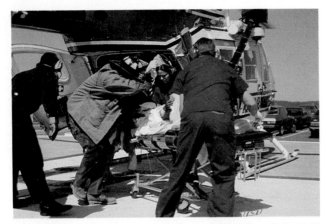

FIGURE 19–25. Helicopters are often mobilized through the EMS dispatch system. The need for resources must be anticipated and communicated to the dispatcher to ensure a timely response.

Dispatchers often have tracking systems in place to determine the status of surrounding hospitals and the basic availability of beds. The communication between the dispatcher and field personnel is essential to determine transport feasibility to specialty care centers and at times to provide air evacuation by helicopter (Fig. 19–25).

RADIO SYSTEMS

Most EMS systems transmit on UHF or VHF frequencies that are designated for this purpose by the federal government. Communications systems may include centralized dispatch centers, mobile radio equipment in vehicles, repeater systems, telephones, and portable hand-held radios. The dispatch console at communications headquarters may consist of a simple two-way radio in small volunteer systems or a computerized system in large metropolitan areas. These larger and highly sophisticated computer systems may recommend available units, prioritize calls based upon the designated

call status as provided by the receiving operator, and keep track of unit availability.

FIELD COMMUNICATION EQUIPMENT. Field personnel may communicate to the dispatch center by telephone, mobile vehicle radios (Fig. 19–26), or portable radios (Fig. 19–27). The range of the radio on the vehicle tends to be greater than that of the portable unit because of the availability of onboard electrical power.

MOBILE DATA TERMINALS. Some systems have computerized dispatch terminals in the ambulance. These terminals allow the dispatcher to communicate with units via a computer screen (Fig. 19–28). This system decreases the amount of voice transmission needed to communicate and clears the airwaves for critical communication. The use of visual data decreases the likelihood of errors in communication that may occur due to verbal misunderstandings. The field personnel can also enter data into the system to communicate with the dispatcher. The dispatcher can maintain a visual status display of each unit to aid in strategically selecting units for calls. Some systems recommend the dispatch of units based on locations and status. Other features of mobile data terminals include the ability to recall the history of a unit during the shift or throughout the response day and to communicate without voice from unit to unit for various purposes, such as exchange of equipment.

REPEATER SYSTEMS. Repeater systems are sometimes used to relay the signals from portable or ambulance radios to the dispatch center or base hospital. Repeaters are strategically based receivers and transmitters that accept the signal from the portable unit or mobile

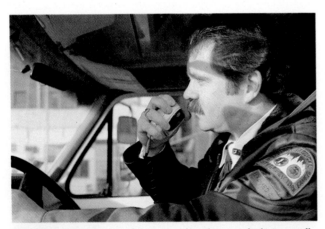

FIGURE 19–26. A radio mounted within a vehicle is usually capable of long-distance transmission because of the increased electrical power.

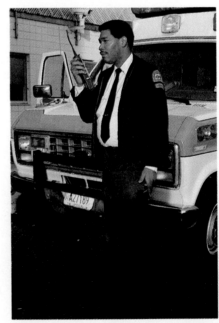

FIGURE 19–27. Portable radios provide the EMT with essential on-the-scene communication capabilities.

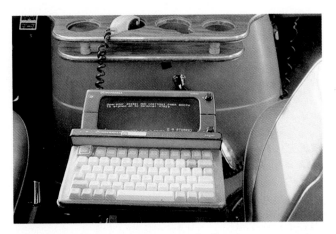

FIGURE 19–28. Mobile data terminals allow for communication to occur without voice transmission.

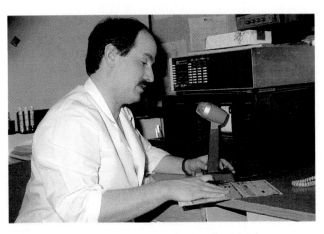

FIGURE 19–29. Physician at a telemetry base station.

radio and relay it with a more powerful signal. They are often located on high ground or in tall buildings. They may also be situated in the emergency vehicle, specifically for boosting and relaying the portable radio signal.

MEDICAL CONTROL

Many EMS systems provide on-line medical control via radio and telephone systems. These systems use base stations, often located at hospitals, and specialized field radio equipment.

TELEMETRY. Telemetry is a method by which biotelemetry data are transferred from one location to another via radio. In EMS systems, telemetry is used to transmit a patient's electrocardiogram (ECG) to a base hospital for interpretation by a physician who then recommends field therapy. ECG information is coded (modulated) into radio waves and decoded (demodulated) at the base hospital into the original form of ECG data. The physician at the medical control facility can then interpret the data and communicate his or her impressions and orders to the field personnel (Fig. 19–29). This is sometimes referred to as on-line medical control. This is done in conjunction with voice communication systems similar to those discussed previously in the dispatch section.

There are several types of biotelemetric systems available throughout the country.

SIMPLEX. Simplex is a push-to-talk (PTT) system similar to a standard radio in which you depress the button to talk and release the button to listen (like an intercom).

DUPLEX. A duplex system permits two-way voice communication similar to a telephone.

MULTIPLEX. This is a combination of simplex and duplex systems that allows for the direct transfer of ECG data at the same time voice communication takes place.

Principles of Communication

Radio communication requires special skills and techniques to ensure the clear and accurate transfer of information. Unlike telephone communications, radio communications must be brief and concise because many units may be competing for time on the same frequency.

When making initial radio contact, you should never interrupt another radio transmission. Most systems use unit codes or designations to identify each caller to the dispatcher. In your initial contact, identify yourself by announcing your code or designation to the dispatcher. Upon acknowledgement by the dispatcher, you can proceed with your brief transmission, using the appropriate codes as explained in the following section. You should speak in a normal voice with the microphone a few inches away from your mouth. You may tend to speak too loudly or quickly while providing patient care in a serious situation, and your message may be garbled. Unlike telephone conversations, only one person may speak at a time on a simplex radio. While you are speaking, you are pushing a button and cannot be interrupted by the person you are speaking to. This is another reason to keep your messages brief. At the end of each exchange between yourself and the dispatcher, give a code to let him or her know that you have finished speaking and ready to listen to a response. This code may be the word "over" or "K." Likewise, wait until the dispatcher gives you this code before pressing the button to speak again. There is also a standardized way to end the call when both parties are finished speaking. These codes differ from one region to another, and you will need to become accustomed to the radio protocols in your particular locality.

The radio should be used to provide the dispatcher with updates on your status. Upon arrival on the scene, you should provide the appropriate signal. At that time you should rapidly access the need for additional units

TABLE 19–3. 10 Codes

Mandatory Codes

10-63	Unit responding on assignment
10-81	Unit at hospital (AH)
10-82	Unit leaving scene with patient(s)
10-88	Unit arrived at scene of incident
10-89	Unit available by radio without Mobile Data Terminal (MDT)
10-97	Unit available by radio and within Center of Rove (COR) area
10-98	Unit available by radio outside COR area
10-99	Unit available by landline at location (specify)

DISPOSITION CODES

10-83	Patient pronounced dead (specify removed/not removed)
10-90	Incident unfounded
10-91	Condition corrected (specify)
10-92	Patient treated and not transported
10-93A	Refused medical aid—release signed (specify by whom)
10-93B	Refused medical aid—release not signed (specify reason)
10-94	Patient treated by (specify) and transported by (specify)
10-95	Triaged out at scene under medical control—patient not transported
10-96	Patient gone on arrival

Message Codes

10-1	Call your station/command by landline
10-2	Return to your station/command
10-3	Call dispatcher by landline
10-4	Acknowledge
10-5	Repeat your last message
10-6	Stand by with your message
10-7	Verify address
10-12	Condition/progress report (specify particulars)
10-13	M.O.S. Requires emergency assistance (specify location/condition)
10-14	Verification of unit status (specify)
10-15	Request for current unit location
10-19	Cancel all responding units except first-due supervisor
10-20	Continue response at reduced speed
10-62	Out of service (specify location/condition)
10-71	Backlog of Priority One calls (specify area)
10-72	Backlog of Priority Two calls (specify area)
10-85	Need additional unit(s) (specify forthwith/no emergency)
10-87	Cancel
10-100	Personal (specify location)

Unusual Situation/Multiple Casualty Incident Codes

10-21	One alarm fire
10-22	Two alarm fire
10-23	Three alarm fire
10-24	Four alarm fire
10-25	Five (or greater) alarm fire (specify)
10-26	Occupied high-rise building incident (automatic 10-86)
10-27	Medical facility incident
10-28	Criminal detention facility incident
10-29	Report of explosive (specify scare, suspected, or device)
10-30	Explosion
10-31	Rapid transit/rail incident (automatic 10-86)
10-32	Ground transport incident
10-33	Structural collapse (building, scaffolding, etc.)
10-34	Construction/demolition incident
10-35	Elevator/escalator incident
10-36	Toxic fumes incident
10-37	Tunnel incident (non-rail)
10-38	Marine/harbor incident
10-39	Aircraft emergency standby response
10-40	Aircraft incident/crash
10-41	Bridge/elevated roadway collapse
10-42	Civil disturbance
10-43	Hostage situation/barricaded person(s)
10-44	Power failure/blackout
10-45	Chemical/fuel pipeline incident
10-46	Bulk oil storage/liquified natural gas facility incident
10-47	Nuclear substance spill/incident
10-48	Hazardous materials solid/incident (specify)
10-49	Environmental incident (earthquake, hurricane, etc.)
10-50	Mutual aid response (specify)
10-58	Planned MCI/standby response
10-59	All other incidents
10-86	Request for 3 ambulances (2 BLS; 1 ALS 2 supervisors (Lieutenant or Captain), one Deputy/Assistant Chief, Field Communications unit, and Technical Services team response.

UNUSUAL SITUATION/MCL CLASSES

Class	Number of victims
Adam	None
Boy	1 to 5
Charlie	6 to 10
David	11 to 25
Eddie	25 to 50
Frank	51 to 75
George	76 to 100
X-Ray	101 to 250
Yankee	251 to 500
Zebra	501 to more

Adapted from New York City Emergency Medical Services: Radio Code Signals—November 1983. New York, Health and Hospitals Corporation, 1983.

or specialized assistance. The dispatcher is again notified when you depart from the scene. When departing, you should notify the hospital if necessary. Remember to be concise!

10 CODES

One method used to condense radio conversations is the use of codes to convert common messages or phrases into short, prearranged numerical sequences. The most common code system is the "10 Codes" (Table 19–3). This system uses the number 10 followed by a series of other numbers, starting with 1, to indicate the status of a unit, relay information, acknowledge communications, or request additional resources.

Summary

Effective communication is an essential skill of the EMT. Whether communicating via radio or providing a history to emergency department personnel, a structured and concise approach is critical to the rapid and accurate exchange of information. The radio and telephone systems represent important tools to prepare hospitals for the imminent arrival of critical patients. The time saved by proper notification can mean the critical difference for the patient.

VEHICLE AND EQUIPMENT MAINTENANCE

Overview

As technology alters and improves the field of EMS, the EMT becomes more and more reliant on the use of equipment to evaluate and treat the patient. Twenty years ago ambulance equipment was minimal and simplistic. Ambulance personnel were faced with very few options for immobilizing, oxygenating, or ventilating an acutely ill or injured patient. In today's EMS systems, a wide range of equipment exists that is more specific to a given patient's needs and, therefore, requires careful consideration by the prehospital provider. For example, a well-equipped ambulance may carry several types of spinal immobilization devices. A Kendrick extrication device is designed primarily for victims of extrication who are sitting upright (Fig. 19–30). A person who is supine is more appropriately treated with a long spine board or a "Miller body splint" (Fig. 19–31). The EMT must assess the situation first and then select the most appropriate option.

Complex variations within each device are another

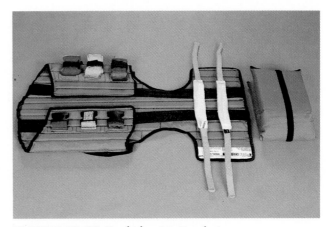

FIGURE 19–30. Kendrick extrication device.

complicating factor facing EMTs today. Twenty years ago, a traction splint consisted of the simple combination of a metal frame combined with bandages. Today, there are several variations of traction devices that use pulley systems, tension meters, and Velcro attachments (Figs. 19–32 through 19–36). This is not to say that they are necessarily more complicated. Most of these splints are easier to apply than their metal and bandage "ancestors," but they represent yet another area where training is necessary for the provider. Since most EMT courses do not have the time to orient students to all the variations of a given device, you need to review the equipment stocked on your own ambulance to ensure familiarity prior to the first call.

The type of equipment stocked on a particular ambulance varies from region to region and system to system. Factors such as cost, types of calls, level of training, and exposure to "state-of-the-art" equipment are likely to account for these differences. The following section discusses the various types of prehospital equipment, as well as some of the variations discussed previously.

The Vehicle

There are three basic types of ambulances used within EMS systems today. Each has advantages and

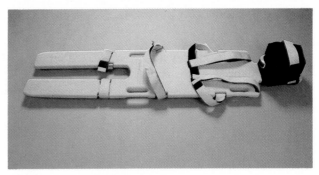

FIGURE 19–31. Miller body splint.

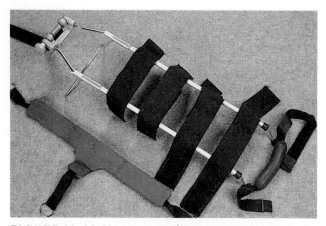

FIGURE 19–32. Hare traction splint.

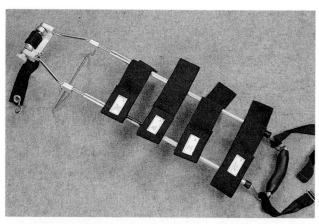

FIGURE 19–33. Ferno traction splint.

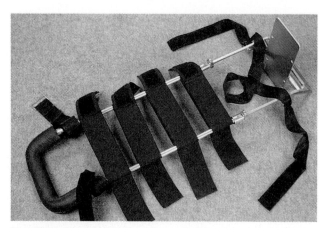

FIGURE 19–34. Kipple traction splint.

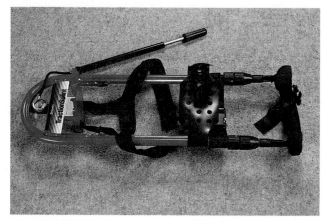

FIGURE 19–35. Donway traction splint.

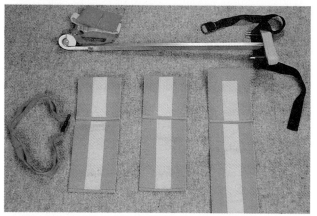

FIGURE 19–36. Sager traction splint.

disadvantages, and they are often selected on the basis of regional needs or the budgetary limitations of a given provider. These vehicles differ in size, weight, turning radius, storage capacity, and interior working space.

THE TYPE I AMBULANCE

The Type I ambulance consists of a box-shaped passenger compartment mounted onto a truck-style chas-

sis (Fig. 19–37). This type of ambulance tends to be more spacious and more powerful than its counterparts. The modular unit allows for some degree of cost efficiency, in that it can be transferred onto a new chassis as the need arises. This type of ambulance generally has a rougher ride and the cab is separated from the passenger compartment. This prevents the driver from going to a partner's aid should the need for assistance arise while en route to the hospital.

THE TYPE II AMBULANCE

The Type II ambulance is a van-style vehicle with a raised roof and an extended rear compartment (Fig. 19–38). Unlike the Type I ambulance, the cab and patient compartments are usually joined to allow easy access by the driver should the need arise. The van also tends to have a smoother ride. However, the space in the patient compartment is smaller and there is generally less storage capacity. The turning radius of a van is better than in the modular type vehicles. This allows for greater mobility and easier parking. The enhanced maneuverability of the van type ambulance is of great value in urban areas with congested traffic and narrow streets.

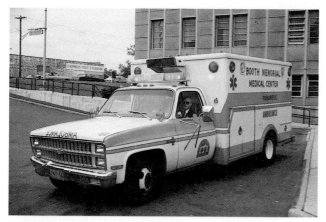

FIGURE 19–37. Type I ambulance.

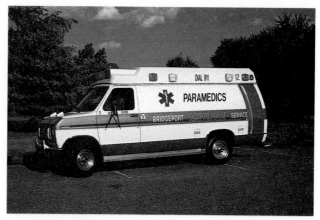

FIGURE 19–38. Type II ambulance.

THE TYPE III AMBULANCE

The Type III ambulance is a modular box, as found in the Type I ambulance, but it is mounted on a van chassis (Fig. 19–39). As in a Type II ambulance, there is usually access to the patient compartment from the cab. The combination of added storage space and better gas mileage than the truck style makes this a popular model in many EMS systems.

Ambulance Equipment

Equipment may vary according to regional requirements and resources, but certain equipment is recommended as standard by regulatory agencies such as the State Department of Health, local EMS administrations, and national agencies. The following chart lists the essential equipment for ambulances.

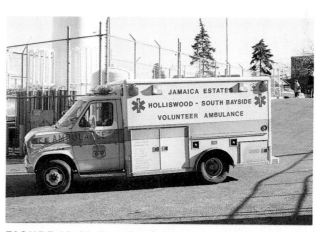

FIGURE 19–39. Type III ambulance.

EQUIPMENT FOR EMS AMBULANCE

Ventilation and Airway Equipment

Suction equipment
  Portable suction apparatus
  Wide-bore tubing, rigid pharyngeal curved suction tip
Oxygen equipment
  Portable and fixed oxygen equipment
  Variable flow regulator, humidifier (on fixed equipment)
  Oxygen administration equipment
    Adequate length tubing
    Masks (adult, child, and infant sizes; non-rebreathing, Venturi, valveless, and nasal prongs)
  Ventilation equipment
    Bag-valve-mask hand-operated, self-reexpanding bag (adult and infant sizes, equal to or greater than 0.85), accumulator (FiO_2, 0.9), clear mask (adult, child, and infant sizes), valve (clear, easily cleanable, operable in cold weather)

Manually triggered demand-valve resuscitator, 40 liter/min flow rate, 40 psi valve
Airway devices
  Nasopharyngeal, oropharyngeal (adult, child, and the infant sizes)

Immobilization Devices (Splints)

Splints
  Traction splints with padded ankle hitch, ischial straps, straps for securing legs to splint
  Lower extremity rigid splints (3-foot and 5-foot appropriate material (cardboard, metal, pneumatic, wood, plastic, etc.)
Backboards
  Long and short
    Head and chin straps
    Handholds for moving patients

Continued

Short (extrication—head to pelvis length)
Long (transport—head to feet)

Bandages, Dressings, and Other Sterile Supplies

Bandages
  Eight triangular bandages, three safety pins each
  Self-adherant roller (2-inch, 3-inch, 4-inch)
  Ace bandages (2-inch, 43-inch, 4-inch)
  Adhesive tape
Dressings and sterile supplies
  Burn sheets
  Sterile dressings, large and small
      Sterile, 2 × 2, 4 × 4, surgical pads, multitrauma
  Vaseline gauze
Obstetric (separate sterile kit)
  Towels
  4 × 4 dressing
  Umbilical tape
  Bulb syringe
  Clamps for cord
  Sterile gloves
  Blanket
  Aluminum foil roll (enough to cover newborn)
Gloves
  Nonsterile latex
  Sterile latex

Other Equipment

Pneumatic antishock garment (PASG)
  Compartmentalized (legs and abdomen separate)
  Control valves (closed/open)
  Inflation pump
  Pediatric and adult sizes
Radio communication equipment
  Two-way communication
  EMT to physician, UHF or VHF
EMT kit
  Sphygmomanometer
  Stethoscope
  Heavy bandage scissors for cutting clothing, belts, boots, etc.
  Mouth gags (commercial or tongue blades covered with gauze)
  Flashlight
Extrication
  Reflectors (triangular) or battery flares
  Wrench (12-inch adjustable crescent)
  Screwdriver (12-inch flat head)
  Screwdriver (8-inch Phillips head)
  Hacksaw (12-inch blade, 18 teeth per inch, oil can with light-grade oil)
  Pliers (12-inch vise grip)
  Hammer (5 lb, 12-inch or 15-inch handle)
  Fire ax (24-inch handle), combination acceptable
  Wrecking bar (24-inch handle)
  Crowbar (51-inch pinchpoint)
  Bolt cutter ($\frac{9}{16}$-inch opening)
  Shovel (49-inch pointed blade or folding heavy-duty entrenching tool)
  Tin snip (double action)
  Ropes (tensile strength 5,400 lb in protective bag)

Hard hat (ANSI Z 89.1), one per occupant
Safety goggles (ANSI Z 37.1), one per occupant
Blanket (large, heavy for patient protection during extrication)
Mastic knife
Bale hooks (2)
Spring-loaded center punch
Gauntlet leather gloves (one pair per occupant)
Pruning saw (heavy duty)

The following additional equipment should be available either on the primary response vehicle or a heavy rescue vehicle with a maximum response time of 10 minutes:

Hydraulic jack/spreader combination (2- to 4-ton minimal)
2 × 4 wood (various lengths for shoring)
Two ropes, 150 feet, $\frac{5}{8}$-inch Kernmantle construction, maximum 2% stretch factor, 11,000-lb minimum tensile strength (must be carried in protective bag)
Swiss seat
Caribiners, locking type, minimum rod stock 10 mm (minimum of 10)
Stokes basket
Come-along (minimum 5 ton with breakaway handle)
Chain (15-inch), grab hook, running hook

Local extrication needs may necessitate additional equipment:

Scuba gear for water rescue
Aerial rescue gear for tall buildings
Mountain rescue equipment, etc.
One air-cutting gun kit, minimum generating pressure, 90 psi, with cylinders and chisels
Hydraulic truck jack, minimum 4 tons
Rappelling harness, one per rescuer

EMT-Intermediate (EMT-I)/EMT-Paramedic (EMT-P)

Should include all EMT-Ambulance (EMT-A) equipment with the additional following supplies:

Intravenous administration equipment (fluid should be in bags, not bottles)
Ringer's lactate (four 1000-ml bags)
Intravenous administration set (three each)
Intravenous catheter with needle ($1\frac{1}{2}$ inches long by 22, 20, 18, 16, 14 gauge, six each)
Venous tourniquet
Antiseptic solution (alcohol wipes preferred)
IV pole or roof hook
Airway
  Esophageal gastric tube airway, mask, 35-ml syringe

EMT-A and EMT-I equipment plus the following should be included:

Airway
  Endotracheal tube (adult, child, and infant sizes)
  10-ml syringes
  Stylettes
  Laryngoscope handle, blades (adult, child, and infant sizes, curved and straight)

Cardiac

    Monitor/defibrillator (with tape write-out)
    Defibrillator pads
    Quick-look paddles
    ECG leads
    Chest attachment pads
    Telemetry radio capability (optional)

Drugs (preloaded when available)

    Drugs used on EMT-P units should be compatible with the standards set by the American Heart Association's Emergency Cardiac Care Committee, as reflected in the Advanced Cardiac Life Support (ACLS) course. The cardiac drugs listed here are based on the 1986 ACLS revision.

    Epinephrine (1 : 1,000), epinephrine (1 : 10,000) sodium bicarbonate, atropine sulfate, dopamine hydrochloride, bretylium tosilate, dobutamine hydrochloride, morphine sulfate (optional), meperidine hydrochloride (Demerol) (optional), nitrous oxide (optional), diazepam (optional), diphenhydramine hydrochloride (Benadryl), propranolol (optional), calcium chloride, isoproterenol, dextrose 50% in water, lidocaine, nitroglycerin, naloxone, xylocaine hydrochloride

Optional equipment

    Mechanical cardiac compression device (EMT-A-I-P) This device provides significant relief from EMT fatigue as well as consistency in rate and depth of cardiac compressions. It should not be used as a substitute for learning and maintaining proficiency in manual CPR skills for the EMT.
    Nitrous oxide administration equipment (EMT-P only)
    Used in England for the past 15 years, this procedure has proved to be effective and safe for the relief of pain during extrication and transport. It does not produce prolonged analgesic effects. This should be used only with a self-administration mask and gas-mixing device that allows a maximum of 50% nitrous oxide partial pressure. Oxygen should never be less than 50% partial pressure.

Care and Maintenance of the Ambulance and Equipment

The finest equipment available is of no value to you or your patient if it is not serviceable or if it presents an infectious threat. Care of your ambulance and equipment starts at the beginning of your working tour, continues after each individual call, and ends with your tour of duty. Embarrassment is the least of your worries if you are transporting an ill or injured patient and your ambulance runs out of gas. A life may be lost if you have two cardiac calls in a row and fail to replace essential resuscitation equipment between calls. The timing of emergency calls is unpredictable, and the best way to safeguard against an ill-prepared unit is to check your equipment and vehicle at definite, regularly specified intervals (Fig. 19–40).

VEHICLE MAINTENANCE

The vehicle should be systematically checked at the beginning of each tour to be sure that it is fueled and in safe, serviceable condition. The easiest and surest way to be certain that all areas of your vehicle are inspected regularly is to use a checklist (Fig. 19–41) that covers all of the following areas.

ENGINE CHECK. Fuel and oil levels should be checked and replaced as needed. The battery should be checked for appropriate fluid level, connections, and signs of corrosion. The cooling system should be checked for fluid levels and hoses should be checked for leaks. Power steering and transmission fluid levels should also be checked and corrected at this time.

OUTSIDE INSPECTION. A complete inspection of the ambulance body should be conducted to establish the condition prior to the first ambulance run. Any dents not noticed previously should be recorded on your check sheet. Tires should be inspected for thread wear, defects, and air pressure. An outer inspection of all light systems

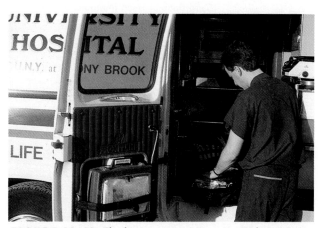

FIGURE 19–40. Checking equipment is an essential preresponse activity for the EMT.

(Name of Ambulance Service)

_____

Technician's Check Sheet

Date _____ Time/Tour _____ Vehicle # _____

VERIFY OPERATION OF ALL EQUIPMENT AND PROVIDE QUANTITY FOR ALL ITEMS—CHECK FOR SHORTAGES AND EXCESS

TRANSPORTATION EQUIPMENT

_____ _____ Cot, Blanket, Linen & Pillow ⟨1⟩
_____ _____ Stair Chair ⟨1⟩
_____ _____ Second Patient Stretcher ⟨1⟩
_____ _____ Cot Fastener ⟨*⟩
_____ _____ Patient Restraints on all Devices

AIRWAY EQUIPMENT

_____ _____ Bag-Valve-Mask ⟨1⟩*
_____ _____ Adult Mask ⟨1⟩*
_____ _____ Child Mask (or Ped BVM) ⟨1⟩*
_____ _____ Lg. Oral Airway ⟨1⟩*
_____ _____ Med. Oral Airway ⟨1⟩*
_____ _____ Sm. Oral Airway ⟨1⟩*
_____ _____ Bite Sticks ⟨2⟩*
_____ _____ Tongue Blades ⟨12⟩
_____ _____ Port o2 & Flow Meter ⟨1; 500#; 15 lpm⟩
_____ _____ Spare Port o2 Cyl. ⟨1; 1000#⟩
_____ _____ Main o2 Cyl. & Flow Meters ⟨2; 500#; 15 lpm⟩
_____ _____ o2 Cylinders secured ⟨*⟩
_____ _____ Cylinders within test date ⟨*⟩
_____ _____ Humidifier (Dry)
_____ _____ Simple o2 Masks*
_____ _____ Non-Rebreather o2 Masks ⟨4⟩*
_____ _____ Nasal Cannula ⟨4⟩*
_____ _____ Oxygen Supply Tubing*
_____ _____ Suction Unit ⟨300 mm/hg⟩*
_____ _____ Portable Suction Unit*
_____ _____ Rigid Suction Catheter ⟨3⟩*
_____ _____ Flex. Suction Catheters ⟨2⟩*
_____ _____ *All Oral Items Clean & Packaged

IMMOBILIZATION EQUIPMENT

_____ _____ Long Spineboard ⟨1⟩
_____ _____ Short Spineboard or equiv. ⟨1⟩
_____ _____ Orthopedic Stretcher
_____ _____ 54" Padded Splints ⟨2⟩
_____ _____ 36" Padded Splints or equiv. ⟨2⟩
_____ _____ 15" Padded Splints or equiv. ⟨2⟩
_____ _____ Sand Bags or Head Immobilizer ⟨1⟩
_____ _____ Lg. Cervical Collar ⟨1⟩
_____ _____ Med. Cervical Collar ⟨1⟩
_____ _____ Sm. Cervical Collars ⟨1⟩
_____ _____ Nine Foot Straps ⟨4⟩
_____ _____ Traction Splints ⟨1⟩

DRESSINGS/BANDAGES

_____ _____ 4 x 4 Dressings ⟨24⟩
_____ _____ 5 x 9 Dressings ⟨6⟩
_____ _____ 10 x 30 Trauma Dressing ⟨2⟩
_____ _____ Conforming Gauze ⟨12, 2 sizes⟩
_____ _____ Triangular Bandages ⟨12⟩
_____ _____ Tape ⟨4, 2 sizes⟩

_____ _____ Sterile Saline ⟨1 L; date⟩
_____ _____ Sterile Water ⟨date⟩
_____ _____ Sterile Burn Sheets ⟨2; date⟩
_____ _____ Aluminum Foil/plastic wrap ⟨1⟩

LINEN

_____ _____ Extra Pillows ⟨1⟩
_____ _____ Extra Blankets
_____ _____ Extra Sheets ⟨2⟩
_____ _____ Extra Pillow Cases ⟨2⟩
_____ _____ Cloth Hand Towels (Apx. 16 x 24) ⟨6⟩
_____ _____ Paper Towels
_____ _____ Facial Tissue ⟨1 box⟩

MISCELLANEOUS EQUIPMENT

_____ _____ Sterile Latex Gloves ⟨2 pr.⟩
_____ _____ Obstetrical Kit ⟨1; pcs. sterile⟩
_____ _____ Safety Pins ⟨12⟩
_____ _____ Emesis Containers ⟨2⟩
_____ _____ Urinal ⟨1⟩
_____ _____ Bed Pan & Toilet Tissue ⟨1⟩
_____ _____ Stocked "First Aid" Kit ⟨1⟩
_____ _____ 12" Screwdriver ⟨1⟩
_____ _____ 24" Wrecking Bar ⟨1⟩
_____ _____ Work Gloves ⟨2 pr.⟩
_____ _____ Hacksaw with spare blade ⟨1⟩
_____ _____ Jumper Cables ⟨1⟩
_____ _____ Flares ⟨6⟩
_____ _____ Fire Extinguisher ⟨1; 10BC⟩
_____ _____ Battery Lantern ⟨1⟩

PERSONAL EQUIPMENT

Stethoscope ⟨1⟩
BP Cuff ⟨1⟩
Flashlight/Penlight ⟨1⟩
Oxygen Wrench

_____

VEHICLE

_____ _____ Vehicle Interior, Exterior & All Equip. Clean and Sanitary ⟨*⟩
_____ _____ Emergency Lights & Siren ⟨*⟩
_____ _____ Headlights, Dir. Signals, Brakes & BU ⟨*⟩
_____ _____ Wipers and Horn ⟨*⟩
_____ _____ DMV Registration ⟨*⟩
_____ _____ DMV Inspection ⟨*⟩
_____ _____ DOH Inspection ⟨*⟩
_____ _____ Tire Condition ⟨*⟩
_____ _____ Heater and AC Operating ⟨*⟩
_____ _____ Exhaust System Condition ⟨*⟩
_____ _____ Vehicle & Glass Condition ⟨*⟩
_____ _____ Fluid Levels-Coolant, PS, Trans.

Tech/EMT _____ Mgr/Supervisor Review _____
Comments:

FIGURE 19–41. Inspection checklist. (Adapted from the New York State Department of Health Ambulance Inspection Sheet.)

should also be done at this time. Doors, windows, and outside compartments should be inspected to ensure that they are operational. The outside of the ambulance should be washed and waxed at regular intervals to prolong the life of the vehicle.

CAB INSPECTION. Brakes can be tested by noting the level to which the brake pedal can be depressed. Turning and stopping signals, all emergency lights, sirens, and the horn should be inspected. Start the ambulance and check all gauges and indicator or warning lights. Windshield wipers, ventilation, and cooling and heating systems should be evaluated. The person who will be driving should adjust the mirrors and seat position if necessary. Mirrors, doors, and storage compartments should be checked to ensure that they are secure and operational. The steering wheel should move freely and soundlessly. Communication equipment should be checked by contacting dispatch and requesting confirmation.

EQUIPMENT MAINTENANCE

A systematic check of the patient compartment and cabinets must be conducted to note missing, dirty, or damaged equipment and to ensure that the compartment itself is clean.

PATIENT COMPARTMENT. The floor and all environmental surfaces should be cleaned at the beginning of each tour and after each call when needed. Local protocols determine specific guidelines for thorough disinfection of the ambulance in special instances such as after transportation of an infectious patient. The stretcher should be wiped with a disinfectant solution after each patient and clean linen should be applied. Dispose of all waste materials in appropriate receptacles. Body fluids, dirty bandages, and needles or syringes require special attention.

VENTILATION, AIRWAY, AND OXYGEN EQUIPMENT. Bag-valve-masks, oxygen-powered resuscitators, other positive-pressure ventilation equipment, and suction devices should be tested to ensure that they are operational (Figs. 19–42 through 19–44). They should be disinfected after each use according to local protocols. Both onboard and portable oxygen tanks should be checked to ensure a sufficient supply. The number of oxygen administration and airway devices should be checked and replaced as needed.

BANDAGES AND STERILE SUPPLIES. Bandages, dressings, burn packs, obstetric kits, and other sterile supplies should be checked to ensure sterility and sufficient quantity. All sterile supplies should be stored in a dust-free, dry location. If they become wet, they should be replaced because sterility can no longer be guaranteed. Expiration dates must be checked periodically and out-

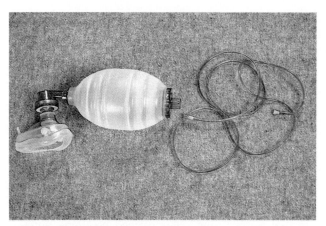

FIGURE 19–42. Bag-valve-mask device.

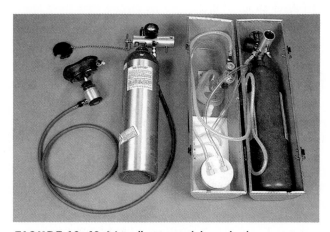

FIGURE 19–43. Manually triggered demand-valve resuscitators.

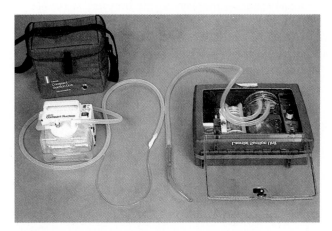

FIGURE 19–44. Battery-operated suction devices.

dated items pulled and discarded. Newly acquired supplies should be placed under the old ones to minimize waste.

STRETCHERS AND IMMOBILIZATION EQUIPMENT. Long spine boards, short spine boards, and stretchers should be stored neatly and be operational. Straps should be examined to ensure that they are in sufficient quantity for each device. Traction and rigid and other types of splinting devices should also be checked. Soiled immobilization equipment should be cleaned after each use.

SAFETY AND EXTRICATION EQUIPMENT. Traffic cones, flares, and other safety devices should be checked. Protective clothing and self-contained breathing apparatus should be carefully inspected to ensure that they are serviceable. Extrication equipment should be tested at regular intervals.

OTHER EQUIPMENT. Diagnostic and specialized equipment such as stethoscopes, sphygmomanometers, and PASG should be checked to ensure that they are present and in working order.

Summary

The EMT relies on various types of equipment to respond, communicate, provide safety, perform patient assessment, and administer patient care.

During the *pre-run* phase of a call, the EMT must check essential equipment to ensure that it is available and operational. This involves daily inspection and replacement and cleaning as needed. In the *dispatch phase*, an EMT must use communication equipment to ascertain the dispatch data. *En route* to the call, the EMT must rely upon the vehicle to provide a safe and reliable ride. This requires careful inspection and maintenance on a daily basis. At *the scene*, the safety of EMTs the patient must be ensured through the use of protective clothing and other equipment.

Finally, during *transport* to the hospital, at *the hospital*, and *en route to the station*, use equipment to provide continued assessment, treatment, and effective communication. Following each call, during the *post-run phase*, it is essential to replace needed supplies.

REVIEW EXERCISES

1. Quote laws relating to the operation of the ambulance and privileges in any of the following categories:
   Speed
   Warning lights
   Sirens
   Right-of-way
   Parking
   Turning
2. Describe the proper use of the siren.
3. Describe the considerations that should be given to:
   Request for escorts
   Following an escort vehicle
   Intersections
4. Describe the effect of the following "natural laws" upon driving an emergency vehicle:
   Gravity   Centrifugal force
   Friction
5. Describe the basic approach to maintaining the proper distances while driving an emergency vehicle.
6. Describe the basic safety procedures for the following situations:
   Approaching intersections
   Backing up
7. List four purposes of a call report.
8. Write a paragraph for each of the following principles of record keeping:
   Accuracy   Clarity
   Chronology   Completeness
9. List four areas of patient data.
10. Give one example of an authorization form and describe its importance.
11. Discuss the importance of confidentiality with record keeping.
12. Describe the roles of the following communications components in an EMS System:
    Receiving operators   Communications center
    Dispatcher   Repeater systems
    Telemetry radios
13. Describe the differences between the simplex, duplex, and multiplex radio systems.
14. Describe the differences between Type I, Type II, and Type III ambulances.
15. Give three examples of vehicle and equipment inspection for the following areas:
    Engine   Outside of vehicle
    Cab inspection   Patient compartment

REFERENCES

American College of Surgeons: Essential equipment for ambulances. American College of Surgeons Bulletin 68:36–638, 1983.

Boyd D: Emergency medical services systems: Hospital based ambulatory care. Norwalk, CT, Appleton-Century-Crofts, 1982.

Cales R, Heilig R: Trauma Care Systems: A Guide to Planning, Implementation, Operation, and Evaluation. Rockville, MD, Aspen, 1986.

Caroline N: Emergency Care in the Streets, 2nd ed. Boston, Little, Brown & Co, 1986.

Grant H, Murray R, Bergeron J: Emergency Care, 5th ed. Englewood Cliffs, NJ, Brady/Prentice-Hall, 1990.

Henry M, Stapleton E: Medical control for EMTs. Journal of Emergency Medical Services, January, 1986.

Montaglione M: Medical record systems for ambulatory care: Hospital based ambulatory care. Norwalk, CT, Appleton-Century-Crofts, 1982.

National Research Council, Committee on EMS, Subcommittee on Medical Control: Medical control in emergency medical services. Washington, DC, National Academy Press, 1981.

New York State Department of Health: Prehospital call report. Albany, Emergency Health Services, 1985.

Stapleton E, Best J: Developing a Hospital Based Ambulance Service: Hospital Based Ambulatory Care. Norwalk, CT, Appleton-Century-Crofts, 1982.

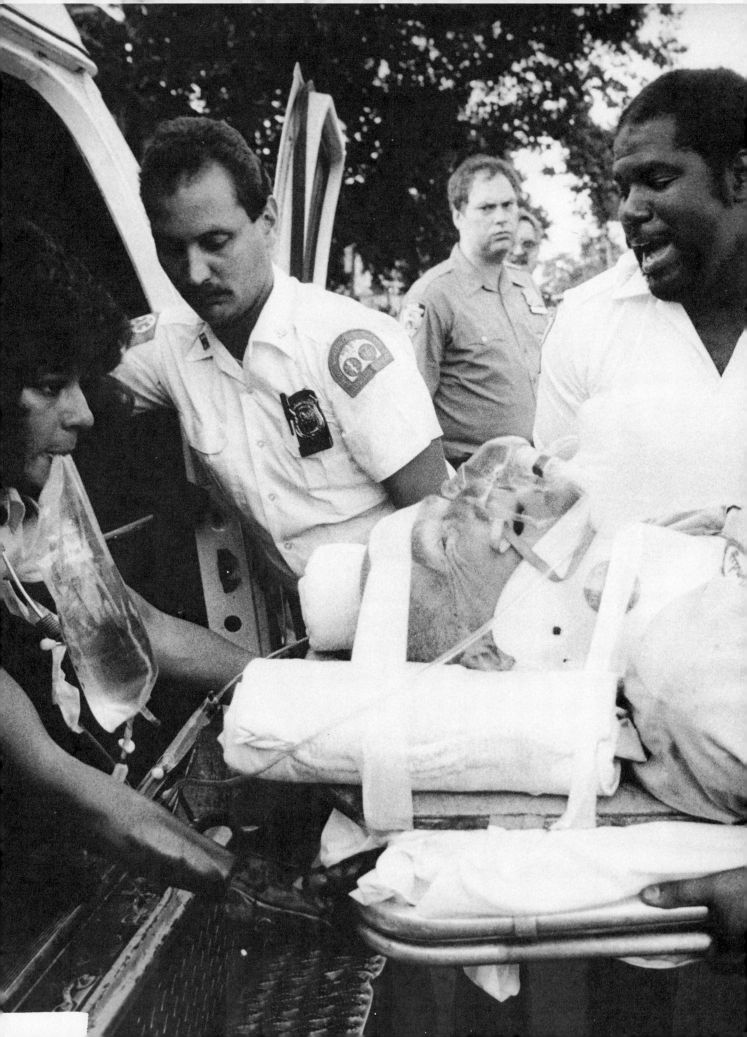

CHAPTER 20

APPROACH TO THE MULTIPLE TRAUMA PATIENT

O B J E C T I V E S

At the conclusion of this chapter the reader will be able to:

---

1. Define *mechanism of injury* and explain why it is such an important element to consider when assessing a patient.

---

2. Explain what is involved in the AMPLE history.

---

3. Demonstrate the approach to the multiple trauma patient.

---

4. Explain the role of the EMT in a trauma system.

INTRODUCTION

Nowhere is the skill of the EMT challenged more than in the care of the patient with multiple trauma. All your assessment and treatment skills are needed with such patients.

The primary objective of prehospital trauma evaluation is the rapid recognition and treatment of the most common, most lethal, and treatable conditions. Prehospital care centers on managing the airway, controlling hemorrhage, initiating treatment for shock, applying spinal immobilization, recognizing life-threatening conditions, and rapidly transporting the patient to appropriate hospitals. Most life-threatening conditions secondary to trauma such as internal bleeding, tension pneumothorax, intracranial hemorrhage, and pericardial tamponade require rapid surgical intervention and cannot be treated definitively in the field. The EMT must be able to identify such conditions early to improve the patient's chances for survival. Decisions regarding the appropriate field treatment and need for rapid transport must be made rapidly and accurately.

Beyond instituting emergency treatment in the field, the EMT plays a crucial role in the care of the trauma patient by initiating a series of decisions that are critical to life and death for the patient. For example, within a trauma system, the EMT is the first trained medical professional to contact the patient. The assessment by the EMT leads to decision-making regarding the extent of field treatment, whether rapid transport is necessary, hospital (trauma center) selection, and mobilization of appropriate hospital staff through advanced notification.

In systems with designated trauma centers, assessment criteria are used in the field to identify patients who should be taken directly to the trauma center. Assessment criteria might be similar to those incorporated in the Trauma Score, which uses measurements such as respiratory function, blood pressure, and capillary refill, and the Glasgow Coma Scale (Table 20–1). The Revised Trauma Score assigns values to findings of respiratory rate, systolic blood pressure, and the Glasgow Coma Scale for use in identifying trauma center candidates (Table 20–2). A system may also have trauma center criteria that incorporate both the mechanism of injury and the anatomy of the injury in addition to physiologic measurements. The American College of Surgeons has published a triage decision scheme (Fig. 20–1) that is a model for local criteria. Study this algorithm and its accompanying notes to better understand your approach to identifying trauma center candidates. Become familiar with the trauma center triage criteria used in your system.

APPROACH TO THE TRAUMA PATIENT

The need for a systematic approach was presented in the patient assessment chapter and reinforced through-

out this text. The assessment of the patient must be done in a systematic and orderly fashion to avoid a delayed response to serious injury or illness.

As discussed previously, the components of assessment include the dispatch review, the scene survey, the primary survey, and the secondary survey. This sequence of evaluation protects the EMT and patient from further injury, allows rapid mobilization of additional resources, ensures priority management for one or more patients, and expedites the comprehensive evaluation and treatment of existing injuries.

The extent of field assessment and treatment varies. Patients who are stable may have a complete primary and secondary survey in the field. However, unstable patients may be transported soon after the primary survey because of the serious nature of their illness or injury.

The Dispatch Review

Upon receipt of a suspected trauma call from the dispatcher, you and your partner must begin to prepare for the worst possible contingencies. EMTs who wait until arrival on the scene to organize their approach are wasting valuable time. When possible, discuss while en route to the scene who will assess the patient, secure the scene, ready equipment, and notify the dispatcher if additional resources are needed.

It is helpful to review the chronologic approach in your mind so that your focus on priorities is maintained.

As always, route selection is another priority. The saving of 1 or 2 minutes by avoiding traffic or construction delays may make the difference in many circumstances.

The Scene Survey

HAZARDS

Once on the scene, the first priority is to ensure the personal safety of EMTs, the patient, and others. Many EMTs and well-intentioned lay people have died on highways because of poor attention to their own safety. The ambulance and traffic-diverting devices should be positioned to provide fair warning to oncoming traffic.

The presence of other hazards should be identified and appropriate precautions taken. For example, when toxic gases might be present the ambulance should be positioned upwind. When explosives are involved, added distance is important.

IDENTIFYING THE NEED FOR ADDITIONAL RESOURCES

The need for additional resources such as fire department and rescue personnel as well as more ambulance

TABLE 20–1. Glasgow Coma Scale and Trauma Score

Glasgow Coma Scale

Eye Opening	Spontaneous	4
	To voice	3
	To pain	2
	None	1
Verbal Response	Oriented	5
	Confused	4
	Inappropriate words	3
	Incomprehensible sounds	2
	None	1
Motor Response	Obeys command	6
	Localizes pain	5
	Withdraw (pain)	4
	Flexion (pain)	3
	Extension (pain)	2
	None	1
Total Score		**3–15**

Trauma Score*

The Trauma Score is a numerical grading system for estimating the severity of injury.[†] The score is composed of the Glasgow Coma Scale (reduced to approximately one-third total value) and measurements of cardiopulmonary function. Each parameter is given a number (high for normal and low for impaired function). Severity of injury is estimated by summing the numbers. The lowest score is 1; and the highest score is 16.

Total Glasgow Coma Scale Points	14–15	5
	11–13	4
	8–10	3
	5–7	2
	3–4	1
Respiratory Rate	10–24/min	4
	25–35/min	3
	36/min or greater	2
	1–9/min	1
	None	0
Respiratory Expansion	Normal	1
	Retractive	0
Systolic Blood Pressure	90 mm Hg or greater	4
	70–89 mm Hg	3
	50–69 mm Hg	2
	0–49 mm Hg	1
	No pulse	0
Capillary Refill	Normal	2
	Delayed	1
	None	0

* *Endorsed by the American Trauma Society.*
[†] *Champion HR. Sacco WJ. Carnazzo AJ, et al: Trauma score. Crit Care Med 9/9:672–676. Copyright © by Williams & Wilkins, 1981.*

units is determined quickly to avoid unnecessary delay. A brief description of the nature of the condition is essential so that the dispatcher and other responding personnel can make informed decisions regarding the number and type of additional resources that are needed. The extent of the fire, the type of entrapment, identification numbers of hazardous materials, or the number of injured victims are examples of pertinent information.

In the event of multiple patients, you must avoid giving all your attention to one patient. Rather, a rapid triage of all patients allows for prioritization in order of need. As additional units arrive on the scene, they can be directed to the most seriously injured in order of triage priority. When the number of personnel permits, the senior or highest trained individual should assume the role of "triage officer" to strategically sort patients and distribute them to the appropriate specialty referral hospital. Review the following categories of injury arranged by order of severity. This categorization is taught in the Advanced Trauma Life Support Course by the American College of Surgeons (see Injuries Grouped by Severity: From Most to Least Severe).

INJURIES GROUPED BY SEVERITY: FROM MOST TO LEAST SEVERE*

Category 1

Combined system injuries; bleeding; open fractures; uncontrolled hemorrhage; severe maxillofacial injuries; severe head, neck, and upper respiratory tract injuries; unstable chest injuries; pelvic fractures; blunt abdominal trauma with hypotension and/or penetrating abdominal wounds; and neurologic injuries producing prolonged loss of consciousness, abnormal posturing, lateralizing signs, or paralysis

Category 2

Patients with open or closed fractures; soft tissue injuries with stabilized bleeding; multiple rib fractures without flail segments; blunt abdominal trauma not producing hypotension; and transient loss of consciousness

Category 3

Patients with uncomplicated fractures, no hypovolemia or hypotension, no neurologic injuries, no abdominal injuries, soft tissue injuries of a moderate degree and chest injuries not producing respiratory distress.

* From Committee on Trauma, American College of Surgeons: Advanced Trauma Life Support Program. Chicago, American College of Surgeons, 1984, p. 183.

MECHANISM OF INJURY

Throughout this text, the importance of the mechanism of injury has been emphasized. It allows you to anticipate and search for injuries associated with a specific type of force. It also may alter your perception of the severity of injury. For example, it would be appropriate to transfer a patient who fell three stories to a trauma center regardless of physical findings. Many patients who have suffered severe head injuries may not develop sig-

nificant neurologic signs for some time after the event. Failure to recognize the mechanism of injury could lead to delayed care in such cases. A sensitive evaluator considers the mechanism of injury in assessing such patients.

Remember that kinetic energy, absorbed by the

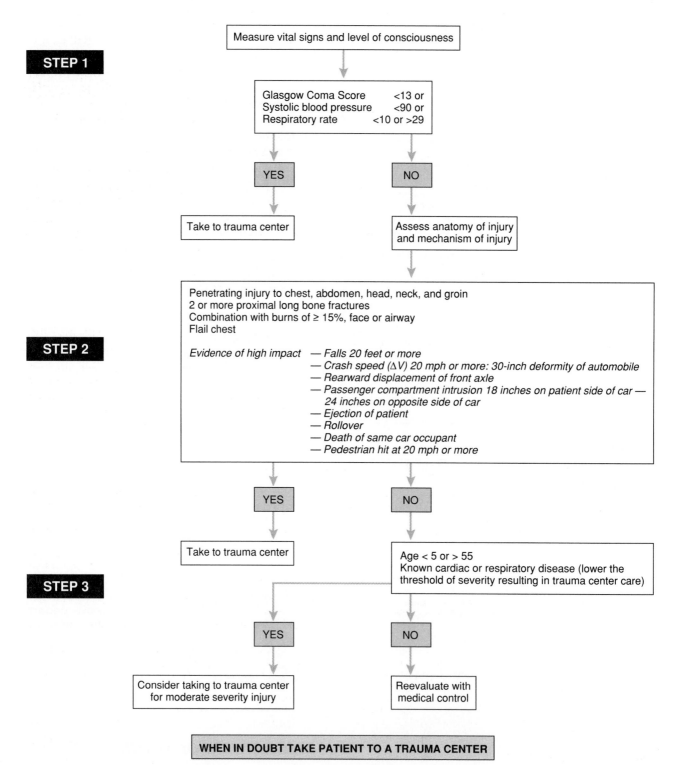

FIGURE 20–1. Triage decision scheme.

Legend continued on following page

TABLE 20–2. Revised Trauma Score

Glasgow Coma Scale	Systolic Blood Pressure	Respiratory Rate	Coded Value
13–15	>89	10–29	4
9–12	76–89	>29	3
6– 8	50–75	6– 9	2
4– 5	1–49	1– 5	1
3	0	0	0

* *With permission from Howard R. Champion.*
When the sum of the coded values is 11 or less, the American College of Surgeons recommends triage to a trauma center (see Fig. 20–1).

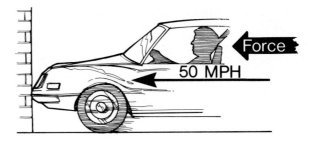

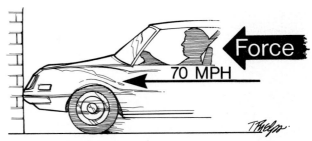

FIGURE 20–2. Kinetic energy increases with speed (velocity squared) of the vehicle. For example, the kinetic energy generated by a 70-mph collision (70 × 70 = 4900) is twice as much as that generated by a 50-mph collision (50 × 50 = 2500). (From Cardona VD, Hurn PD, Mason PJB, et al: Trauma Nursing: From Resuscitation through Rehabilitation. Philadelphia, WB Saunders, 1988, p. 116.)

body in a collision or fall, is greatly increased by the speed at impact. The formula $KE = \frac{1}{2}mv^2$ shows that velocity is squared when computing the kinetic energy. This is illustrated in Figure 20–2. If the kinetic energy is imparted by a bullet, the velocity plays an important factor also. Not only does penetration of the bullet cause damage along its path, but the zone of injury around the path is extended in proportion to the bullet's speed at impact (Fig. 20–3).

Other important aspects to consider with the mechanism of injury are the compression and deceleration forces that damage tissues and organs. Compression forces (Fig. 20–4) and deceleration forces (Fig. 20–5) should be suspected in most cases of blunt trauma. Knowledge of these forces helps EMTs appreciate findings of shock or organ disruption even in the absence of extensive external findings.

Also, when reviewing the mechanism of injury, remember to look for associated injuries. For example, a fall from a height transfers force up the long leg bones to the spine (Fig. 20–6). Associated injuries have been stressed throughout this text. A review is provided in Table 20–3.

FIGURE 20–1

1. Physiologic status thresholds are values of the Glasgow Coma Score, blood pressure, and respiratory rate from which further deviations from normal are associated with less than a 90% probability of survival. Used in this manner, prehospital values can map into the admission trauma score and the quality assessment process.

A variety of physiologic severity scores have been used for prehospital triage and have been found to be accurate, but those contained in the triage guidelines are the simplest to perform and provide an accurate basis for field triage based on physiologic abnormality.

2. Even in the presence of normal physiology, it is important to evaluate the likely presence of injuries that should be treated in a trauma center. A patient who has normal vital signs at the scene of the accident may still have serious or lethal injury. Accurate diagnosis of life-threatening injury at the accident scene is usually unlikely. Thus, it is essential to look for indications that significant forces were applied to the body.

3. Evidence of damage to the automobile can be a helpful guideline to the change in velocity (ΔV). The relationship between ΔV is such that 90% of patients with injury severity scores greater than 15 have been in an accident with ΔV of 20 mph or more. ΔV can be estimated by a rule of thumb that vehicular deformity of 1 inch approximates 1 mph ΔV. However, if contact diameter is less than 1 foot, then $1\frac{1}{2}$ inches deformity approximates 1 mph.

4. Certain other factors that might lower the threshold at which patients should be treated in trauma centers must be considered in field triage. These include: *Age.* Patients over age 55 have an increasing risk of death from even moderately severe injuries. Those of less than 5 years of age have certain characteristics that may merit treatment in a trauma center with special resources for children. *Comorbid factors.* The presence of significant cardiac or respiratory disease are also factors that may merit the triage of patients with moderately severe injury to trauma centers.

5. It is the general intention of these triage guidelines to select patients with an injury severity score* of 15 for trauma center care. Patients with this level of injury severity score have at least a 10% risk of dying from a single severe injury or multiple serious injuries. When there is doubt, the patient is often best evaluated in a trauma center.

(From American College of Surgeons Committee on Trauma: Hospital and Prehospital Resources for Optimal Care of the Injured Patient (Appendices A through J). Chicago, American College of Surgeons, 1987.)

---

* A score used to help evaluate effectiveness of trauma programs.

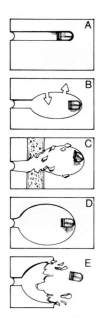

FIGURE 20–3. Effect of bullet wounds. The zone of injury from gunshot wounds increases with the velocity of the weapon. (*A*) Low-velocity wound. (*B*) Higher-velocity with cavitation. (*C*) Same velocity as *B*, plus deformity of bullet and secondary missiles created by fragmented bone. (*D*) Very high velocity with larger cavity. (*E*) Very high velocity with ragged exit wound. (From Cardona VD, Hurn PD, Mason PJB, et al: Trauma Nursing: From Resuscitation through Rehabilitation. Philadelphia, WB Saunders, 1988, p. 118.)

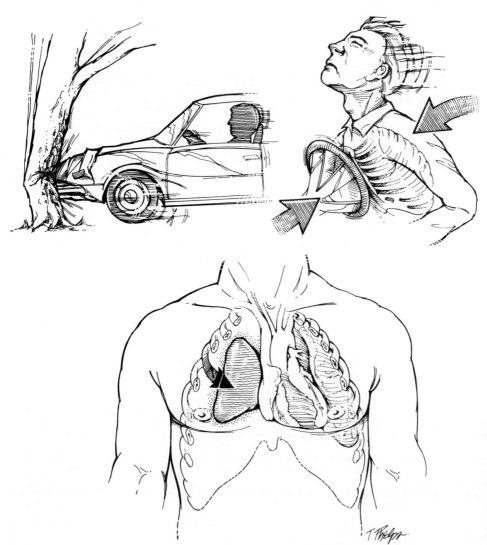

FIGURE 20–4. The compression forces of an automobile collision. As the car suddenly decelerates, the occupant strikes a fixed object (e.g., steering wheel). The posterior thoracic spine continues forward, compressing the internal organs between the sternum and the spine. (From Cardona VD, Hurn PD, Mason PJB, et al: Trauma Nursing: From Resuscitation through Rehabilitation. Philadelphia, WB Saunders, 1988, p. 116.)

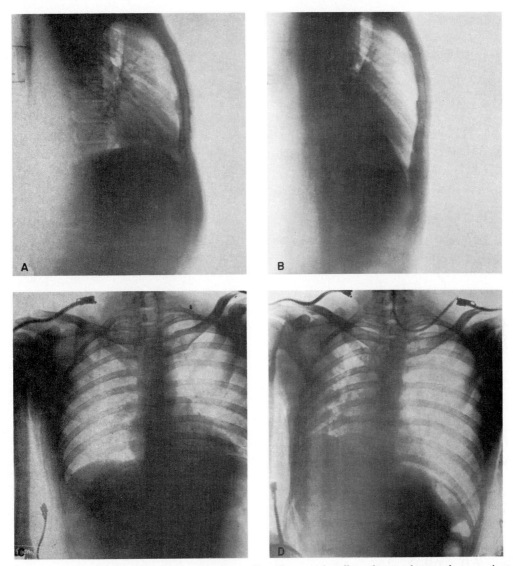

FIGURE 20–5. Acceleration and deceleration forces. These x-ray films illustrate the effect of an accelerating force on the internal organs. (*A*) At rest and (*B*) after a 5-G forward moving force is applied to the body. Note the displacement of the organs toward the posterior thorax. (*C*) At rest and (*D*) after a 5-G lateral moving force is applied to the body. Note the displacement of the organs toward the right lateral thorax. Deceleration forces can tear or otherwise damage internal organs with few external signs of injury. (From Zuidema GD, Rutherford RB, Ballinger WF: The Management of Trauma, 4th ed. Philadelphia, WB Saunders, 1988, p. 393.)

The Primary Survey

As discussed earlier, the primary survey addresses the function of the three critical body systems. Prehospital Trauma Life Support recommends the use of the mnemonic A, B, C, D, E for remembering the critical order of assessment:

A = Airway, for ensuring a patent air passage
B = Breathing, for ensuring adequate ventilation and oxygenation
C = Circulation, for evaluating cardiovascular function and to control bleeding
D = Disability, for evaluating central nervous system function
E = Expose, which acts as a reminder to fully expose and examine the whole patient

AIRWAY

After establishing responsiveness through physical and verbal stimuli, the following evaluation and treatment components are initiated.

As a primary measure, the airway is established. Again, two methods are used for opening the airway:

The head tilt–chin lift is the primary technique for nontraumatic patients and is the most reliable airway maneuver (see Fig. 2–25).
The jaw thrust without head tilt—technique is used in all patients who are suspected to have a spinal injury. This includes all unconscious trauma patients or patients who have a mechanism of injury that may have caused spinal injury such as patients with injuries above the clavicle (see Fig. 2–26).

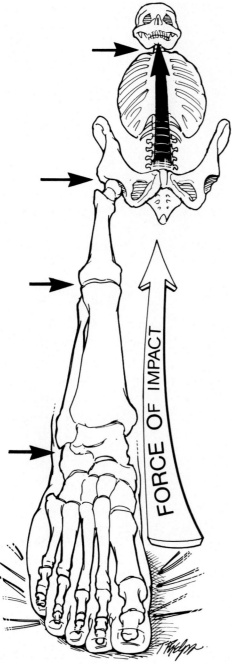

FIGURE 20–6. Forces applied to the foot or heel (as from a fall) would be transmitted along the axis of the leg and spine. Possible injuries might include fractures of the ankle, knee, femur, hip, and spine. (From Cardona VD, Hurn PD, Mason PJB, et al: Trauma Nursing: From Resuscitation through Rehabilitation. Philadelphia, WB Saunders, 1988, p. 118.)

TABLE 20–3. Mechanisms of Injury and Associated Injuries

Mechanism	Common Associated Injuries
Head-on collisions	Head and spinal trauma
	Chest and abdominal trauma
	Flail chest
	Pneumothorax
	Internal hemorrhage
	Lower extremity trauma
	Knee, femur, hip
	Upper extremity trauma
	Protection injury
Side collision	Head and spinal trauma
	Chest and abdominal trauma
	Lateral chest wall injury
	Flail chest
	Pneumothorax
	Internal hemorrhage
	Upper extremity trauma
	Shoulder, clavicle, humerus
	Lower extremity trauma
	Hip/acetabulum
Rear-end collision	Head and spinal trauma
	Contra coup
	Whiplash
Rotational collision force	Varies according to vector; person closest to impact point most injured
Falls	Types of injury depend on impact point
Feet first	Calcaneus (heel)
	Lower extremity
	Spine
Outstretched arm	Wrist, elbow, humerus, shoulder
Penetrating knife injuries	Type of injury depends on size, direction, and location
Missile injuries	Type of injury depends on velocity, location, and range

For ongoing airway maintenance, oropharyngeal, nasopharyngeal, or esophageal airways or endotracheal intubation may be considered, depending on your training level and local protocols.

If manual maneuvers fail to open the airway or secretions impair the ability to ventilate, the airway must be cleared. Suctioning can remove liquid and small particles from the airway. If a complete obstruction with a foreign body is suspected, the airway obstruction sequence described in Chapter 3 should be followed. If relief is not possible by basic life support procedures or if the obstruction is due to crush injuries to the airway, then rapid transport should be considered so that a cricothyrotomy or tracheostomy can be initiated.

BREATHING

The adequacy of breathing is evaluated and ventilation is initiated if necessary. The key signs of adequate ventilation and oxygenation are discussed below.

RESPIRATORY RATE AND DEPTH. Respiratory rates below 12 and above 30 per minute usually require assistance with positive-pressure breathing. Chest excursion is used as the primary determinant of adequate depth of breathing.

SKIN COLOR. Skin that is cyanotic (blue) is indicative of poor oxygenation. If cyanosis is noted, give high-concentration oxygen and, if needed, positive-pressure ventilation.

ACCESSORY MUSCLE USE. Patients in respiratory distress may use their neck and abdominal muscles to assist in breathing. Active use of accessory muscles is a key sign of respiratory problems.

EVIDENCE OF CHEST TRAUMA. Open wounds, bruises, flail chest segments, and signs of fractures should be noted.

TRACHEAL SHIFT AND NECK VEIN DISTENTION. Movement of the trachea from midline is suggestive of a tension pneumothorax. Check if the neck veins are flat (as in hypovolemic shock) or distended (as in obstructive shock).

ABNORMAL RESPIRATORY SOUNDS. Snoring, gurgling, wheezing, and high-pitched sounds (stridor) may suggest inadequate breathing or airway obstruction. Quickly auscultate breath sounds with a stethoscope.

CIRCULATION

The adequacy of circulation is evaluated by checking for pulses and observing other signs of cardiovascular function.

PULSE CHECK. The initial pulse check is performed at the carotid artery in the unresponsive patient to determine the need for cardiac compressions and to recognize impending or existing shock states. Rate, quality, and regularity are noted.

BLOOD PRESSURE. The blood pressure can be estimated by the presence of pulses at the carotid (60 mm Hg), femoral (70 mm Hg), and radial (80 mm Hg) arteries. Although these are not exact figures, they are helpful guides. Auscultate the blood pressure when time permits, at the scene or while en route to the hospital.

SKIN COLOR. Pale, cool, sweaty, or cyanotic skin may suggest poor perfusion and cardiovascular function.

CAPILLARY REFILL. Capillary refill is measured by squeezing nail beds and observing return of color. If this takes longer than 2 seconds or if there is no refill, the test is abnormal and may be an early sign of hypovolemic shock. Note that capillary refill may be delayed "normally" in cold temperatures and in some adult females and elderly patients (Schriger and Baraff, 1988). Also, it may not be delayed when hypovolemia is present. Therefore, use the capillary refill test as one (but not as an absolute) finding when assessing for shock.

BLEEDING. Obvious external hemorrhage is searched for and controlled with direct pressure, elevation, pressure points, and, rarely, a tourniquet.

DISABILITY

The central nervous system function is evaluated by quickly assessing the level of consciousness. The mental status is the most sensitive indicator of central nervous system function. Therefore, the patient's response to verbal and physical stimuli as prescribed in the Glasgow Coma Scale is used. During the primary survey, you do not need to calculate a specific numerical score but rather determine grossly if an altered mental state exists. To do this, use the mnemonic "AVPU." The patient is evaluated according to the following categories:

Alert—The patient communicates clearly without any stimuli.
Verbal—The patient responds to verbal stimuli.
Painful—The patient does not respond to verbal stimuli but does respond to painful stimuli.
Unresponsive—The patient is unresponsive to both verbal and painful stimuli.

If the patient has an altered mental status, and there are no obvious signs of respiratory or cardiovascular problems, you should be highly suspicious of intracranial injury.

EXPOSE

The patient's body should be exposed to identify specific injuries during the primary survey. Special attention should be paid to the head and trunk, since life-threatening conditions arise from these areas. Concern for the patient's privacy should not hamper your evaluation.

MANAGEMENT

If problems are identified during the primary survey, they must be addressed immediately and rapid transport should be considered since surgical intervention may be required. Treatment should be provided as the need is identified during the survey.

CERVICAL IN-LINE IMMOBILIZATION. All patients who have suffered significant blunt trauma should be treated as if they have a spinal injury. Immediate immobilization of the neck and head should be established. A cervical collar is applied for added support. It is important to emphasize that a cervical collar does not constitute adequate immobilization by itself. Until the patient is immobilized to the board, manual immobilization should be maintained.

AIRWAY VIA MANUAL MANEUVERS. Again, the airway should be established and maintained during the survey. If the patient is in a car and has a complete airway obstruction or is in ventilatory arrest or depression, a rapid extrication should be initiated. If an adequate ventilation exists, you may proceed with the survey in the car.

OXYGEN. High-concentration oxygen should be applied on all patients demonstrating signs of respiratory distress or cardiovascular compromise. Ask if there is a history of chronic obstructive pulmonary disease (COPD) and follow local protocols. If the patient is showing signs of ventilatory depression or arrest, he or she should be rapidly extricated in order to institute positive-pressure ventilation.

AIRWAY/VENTILATION VIA MECHANICAL MEANS. If positive-pressure ventilation is indicated, a device should be selected based on the underlying condition. Patients with suspected pneumothorax or flail chest should be ventilated with low pressure devices such as mouth-to-mouth resuscitation, pocket mask, or bag-valve-mask. High-concentration oxygen should be administered as soon as possible. Care should be taken to ventilate smoothly to avoid gastric distention. Cricoid pressure can be maintained during mouth-to-mouth or mask ventilation if enough personnel are available. Chest excursion should be used as a criterion to determine the adequacy of tidal volume during ventilation. If tidal volumes appear inadequate, the airway should be evaluated or an alternate ventilation method should be considered. This is particularly important when using the bag-valve-mask resuscitator, since it commonly produces low tidal volumes. In this instance, pocket mask or mouth-to-mouth ventilation should be considered.

CONTROL HEMORRHAGE AND MANAGE CHEST INJURIES. If the patient exhibits external hemorrhage, bleeding should be controlled with the techniques mentioned previously. Open chest wounds should be sealed with an occlusive dressing.

PASG. If the patient shows signs of circulatory shock, the PASG should be applied promptly according to local protocol. This may call for application and inflation either on the scene or en route.

RAPID TRANSPORT. For patients exhibiting signs of respiratory distress, circulatory shock, or severe central nervous system injury, rapid transport should be initiated. Other essential treatments and continuing assessments can be performed en route.

NOTIFICATION AND FACILITY SELECTION. The hospital should be notified as soon as possible to mobilize necessary personnel and resources. Critical information includes the number of patients, the type of injury, vital signs, mental status, obvious severe injuries, and any other special information such as exposure to toxic chemicals. Facilities should be selected according to local protocol. In some cases, this means the closest hospital; in other cases, direct transportation to a specialty referral center (e.g., trauma or burn center) may be appropriate.

EVALUATION AND CONTINUED MANAGEMENT EN ROUTE. Continue evaluation and observation while en route to avoid undue delay at the scene. Key parameters such as those included in the trauma score should be elicited and recorded at regular intervals. Such information is useful both for making treatment decisions en route as well as identifying a deteriorating condition in critically injured patients or response to prehospital treatment.

The Secondary Survey

Patients who are stable but are suspected of having multiple injuries should be carefully surveyed prior to transport.

The secondary survey includes the history, vital signs, the head-to-toe survey, and the neurologic examination. In some circumstances the secondary survey is deleted due to the presence of severe problems that require immediate transport. When used, it is done systematically to identify "less obvious" problems. The survey described below represents a comprehensive approach to prehospital evaluation. It should be noted that the extent of the secondary survey can be altered, depending upon the mechanism of injury and the circumstances of the environment. For example, a person who has suffered isolated penetrating trauma to a portion of his or her body need not receive an entire head-to-toe survey. In situations where there are multiple casualties, abbreviated examinations may be done to facilitate the timely movement of large numbers of patients.

AMPLE HISTORY

The history is the systematic collection of data from the patient to determine the mechanism of injury or illness and to identify significant medical conditions in the patient's past. The complete approach to collecting a history was described in Chapter 2 of this text. When time permits, a more comprehensive history should be collected on the scene and during transport. However, in the assessment of the trauma patient, the history may be somewhat more condensed to minimize the time spent in the prehospital phase. The American College of Surgeons recommends the collection of an AMPLE history when assessing the trauma patient. AMPLE is the mnemonic used to remember the key historical facts necessary to make a decision in regard to a traumatized patient.

The major aspects of an AMPLE history are Allergies, Medications, Past history, Last meal, Events.

ALLERGIES. Ascertain whether the patient has allergies to avoid complications that may occur inhospital during drug administration. This should be done early in the history, as the patient may become unconscious and therefore unable to relay important information about his or her allergies to you. Drugs commonly used in trauma care to which your patient might be allergic include antibiotics and local anesthetics.

MEDICATIONS. Knowledge of your patient's current medications is essential to management. Medications often point to preexisting disease that may affect the care strategy or alter physical findings.

PAST HISTORY. Significant medical conditions in the patient's past, such as heart disease, diabetes, or COPD, should be made known to the hospital personnel as they are also crucial to patient management.

LAST MEAL. The time of the last oral intake is important because surgical intervention is a common aspect of care in the trauma patient. General anesthesia is dangerous when administered to a patient with a full stomach, since vomiting and aspiration may result.

EVENTS. A description of the events leading up to the injury should be ascertained. Car accidents and other injuries are often precipitated by medical problems. Fainting, hypoglycemia, and cardiac problems are common problems that may result in accidents. Family members or other car passengers may be able to describe the behavior of the victim prior to the accident. The history of physical findings prior to your arrival at the scene is helpful in identifying evolving problems.

VITAL SIGNS

Take the patient's vital signs to identify underlying respiratory or cardiovascular problems that were not identified during the primary survey. Vital signs include respirations, pulse, blood pressure, and temperature.

RESPIRATIONS. Respirations are evaluated according to rate (determined by counting the number of breaths in 30 seconds and multiplying by two), depth (deep, normal, or shallow), and rhythm (abnormal patterns seen in various conditions).

PULSE. The pulse is evaluated on the basis of rate (same as above), quality (bounding, normal, thready), and rhythm (regular or irregular).

BLOOD PRESSURE. When time permits, the blood pressure is auscultated. If auscultation is not possible due to extraneous noises in the environment, the pressure can be palpated. Again, in patients who are unstable, the presence or absence of certain pulses can indicate an approximation of the blood pressure.

TEMPERATURE. The temperature is evaluated by touching the skin and noting the relative temperature (cool, warm, normal), moisture (sweating, dry, normal), and color (pale, blue, flushed, normal).

Head-to-Toe Survey

The head-to-toe survey is performed to identify signs of illness or injury in the various regions of the body. As mentioned in the section on the primary survey, the patient should be exposed to inspect and palpate body regions. Flail segments, contusions, and swelling could be overlooked if the patient is not carefully examined. The sequential approach described below should be followed to ensure a thorough examination. Careful attention should be paid to areas where the patient complains of pain or tenderness.

HEAD

Examine the head for contusions and open wounds. The eyes and the mastoid region should be examined for the presence of Battle's sign or raccoon's eyes, which are suggestive of skull fractures. It is important to note that these findings may not be present in the early stages of injury. Palpate bones for evidence of fractures. Care should be taken during palpation because loose bone fragments may be pushed into underlying brain tissue and cause further damage. Check the pupils for diameter, equality, and reactivity. Look for blood or fluid leaks from the ears and nose (additional signs of skull fracture), as well as for foreign material in the airway. Examine facial bones for underlying fractures.

NECK

Observe the neck region for contusions and open wounds. Use of accessory muscles may indicate the presence of respiratory distress. Distention of the neck veins may indicate tension pneumothorax, pericardial tamponade, or preexisting heart failure. Palpate the cervical spine for deformity, crepitus, and tenderness.

CHEST

Observe the chest for contusions and open wounds (Fig. 20–7). Examine the chest wall for evidence of unstable segments or other signs of fractures. Carefully palpate to determine if there are areas of tenderness or paradoxical breathing. If not done in the primary survey, breath sounds should now be auscultated, taking care to check the various regions of the thorax.

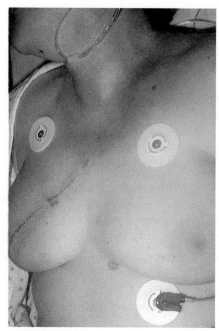

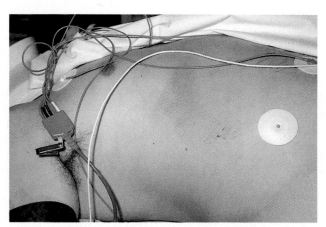

FIGURE 20–7. (*Left*) Abrasion over the right upper ribs suffered when striking the ground after the person was hit by an automobile. Signs of trauma such as this raise the suspicion of internal injuries to the lungs and liver. (*Right*) Abrasion from shoulder belt after 35-mph collision. The patient suffered a fracture of the sterum and was evaluated for myocardial contusion and other internal injuries.

ABDOMEN

Observe the abdomen for contusions and open wounds. Palpate carefully throughout the various quadrants and note tenderness and rigidity. The absence of rigidity or swelling does not rule out the possibility of internal bleeding.

PELVIS

Gently compress the lateral aspects of the pelvis downward and medially to assess for structural integrity. Also palpate the pubic symphysis. Remember that pelvic fractures are often associated with significant blood loss. If pelvic instability is present, a search for signs of internal bleeding or impending hypovolemic shock should be repeated.

EXTREMITIES

Observe the upper and lower extremities for contusions and open wounds. Palpate carefully and note tenderness and deformity. Evaluate distal pulses and sensation to determine if neurovascular compromise has occurred. Capillary refill should be reevaluated to identify the existence of underlying shock states.

THE NEUROLOGIC EXAMINATION

A neurologic examination is performed to assess for brain or spinal cord injury. The mental status and Glasgow Coma Scale can be reevaluated, with a specific score noted.

MOTOR MOVEMENT. Motor function should be evaluated in all extremities to determine whether weakness or paralysis is present.

SENSORY. Sensation in the extremities and at key levels of the trunk is checked to evaluate for any abnormalities.

MANAGEMENT

Upon completion of the secondary survey, wounds and fractures should be sequentially treated according to their priority. If the number of personnel permits, management can occur during the secondary survey. Fractures or minor wounds may be dealt with at the completion of the survey.

The following is a sample protocol for care of the patient with multiple trauma.

P R O T O C O L

MAJOR TRAUMA (INCLUDING TRAUMATIC CARDIAC ARREST)—ADULT

NOTE!

FOR THE PURPOSE OF THIS PROTOCOL, MAJOR TRAUMA IS PRESENT IF THE MECHANISM OF INJURY OR PATIENT'S PHYSICAL FINDINGS MEETS *ANY ONE* OF THE FOLLOWING CRITERIA.

MECHANISM OF INJURY

1. FALL OF TWO OR MORE STORIES (MORE THAN 20 FEET)
2. SURVIVOR OF MOTOR VEHICLE CRASH IN WHICH THERE WAS A DEATH OF A CAR OCCUPANT
3. PATIENT STRUCK BY A VEHICLE MOVING FASTER THAN 20 MPH
4. PATIENT EJECTED FROM THE VEHICLE
5. HIGH-SPEED CRASH WITH RESULTING SEVERE DEFORMITY OF THE VEHICLE
6. ROLLOVER

PHYSICAL FINDINGS

7. PULSE LESS THAN 50/MIN OR GREATER THAN 120/MIN
8. SYSTOLIC BLOOD PRESSURE OF 90 MM HG OR LESS
9. RESPIRATORY RATE LESS THAN 10/MIN OR GREATER THAN 28/MIN
10. GLASGOW COMA SCALE SCORE LESS THAN 13
11. ALL PENETRATING INJURIES OF THE TRUNK, HEAD, NECK, CHEST, ABDOMEN, OR GROIN
12. TWO OR MORE PROXIMAL LONG BONE FRACTURES
13. FLAIL CHEST
14. BURNS THAT INVOLVE 15% OR MORE OF THE BODY SURFACE OR FACIAL/AIRWAY BURNS

A. Establish and maintain airway control while manually stabilizing the cervical spine.

THE FOLLOWING MANAGEMENT MAY BE INSTITUTED BEFORE OR DURING EXTRICATION OR EN ROUTE AS APPROPRIATE. IN NO CASE SHOULD PATIENT TRANSPORT BE DELAYED BECAUSE OF THIS MANAGEMENT!

B. Assess the patient's ventilatory status.

1. IF THE VENTILATORY STATUS IS INADEQUATE:
   a. Insert an oropharyngeal or nasopharyngeal airway if the gag reflex is absent.
   b. Ventilate the patient with an adjunctive device and high-concentration oxygen. MINIMUM RATE OF VENTILATION: 12 TIMES A MINUTE. ENSURE THAT THE CHEST RISES WITH EACH VENTILATION.

AND
EXPOSE THE PATIENT'S CHEST TO LOCATE AND IDENTIFY INJURIES AND TO LISTEN FOR BREATH SOUNDS.
AND
TREAT ANY OPEN CHEST WOUNDS WITH OCCLUSIVE DRESSING, AND STABILIZE IMPALED OBJECTS IN THE CHEST.

2. IF THE VENTILATORY STATUS IS ADEQUATE administer high-concentration oxygen as soon as possible.

3. IF HEAD INJURY IS SUSPECTED, HYPERVENTILATE THE PATIENT WITH HIGH-CONCENTRATION OXYGEN AT A RATE OF ABOUT 20 BREATHS PER MINUTE!

C. Assess the patient's circulatory status.

1. IF THE PULSE IS ABSENT (TRAUMATIC CARDIAC ARREST):
   a. Extricate the patient rapidly.
   b. Initiate transportation IMMEDIATELY.
   c. Perform CPR according to AHA/ARC standards.
   d. Take appropriate steps to control hemorrhage.
   e. (1) Apply and inflate MAST according to the *SHOCK* Protocol (Chapter 5), *OR*
      (2) Elevate the patient's legs 30 degrees if MAST is not available.
   f. Record all patient care information, including all treatment provided, on a prehospital care report.

2. IF THE PULSE IS PRESENT:
   a. Search for any life-threatening hemorrhage and test capillary refill.
   b. Extricate the patient rapidly.
   c. Initiate transportation IMMEDIATELY.
   d. Keep the patient warm en route.
   e. Obtain and record the initial vital signs, including capillary refill, and repeat en route as often as the situation indicates.
   f. Record all patient care information, including all treatment provided, on a prehospital care report.

3. IF LIFE-THREATENING HEMORRHAGE IS PRESENT:
   a. Take appropriate steps to control the hemorrhage.
   b. Extricate the patient rapidly.
   c. Initiate transportation IMMEDIATELY.
   d. Keep the patient warm en route.
   e. Assess for SHOCK en route.
   f. Obtain and record the initial vital signs, including capillary refill, and repeat en route as often as the situation indicates.
   g. Record all patient care information, including all treatment provided, on a prehospital care report.

Continued

4. IF ONE OR MORE SIGNS OF SHOCK ARE PRE-SENT, REFER IMMEDIATELY TO THE *SHOCK PROTOCOL* (Chapter 5).
   a. Extricate the patient rapidly.
   b. Initiate transportation IMMEDIATELY.
   c. (1) Apply and inflate MAST according to the *SHOCK* Protocol (Chapter 5), *OR*
      (2) Elevate the patient's legs 30 degrees if MAST is not available.

d. Keep the patient warm.
e. Obtain and record the initial vital signs, including capillary refill, and repeat en route as often as the situation indicates.
f. Record all patient care information, including all treatment provided, on a prehospital care report.

From Manual for Emergency Medical Technicians. Emergency Medical Services Program. Albany, New York State Department of Health, 1990.

CASE ILLUSTRATIONS

The following case histories are presented to increase your appreciation of the appropriate prehospital approach and the significance of key findings in the primary and secondary surveys. A discussion follows the scenarios to provide rationales for the findings and the therapy given. Additional case presentations are provided in the student study and review guide that accompanies this text.

• CASE HISTORY 1 •

EMTs responded to a "collision." Upon arrival at the scene, the police indicated that there had been a head-on collision at a speed of approximately 40 mph and there were three injured passengers. The scene was already secured by the police. One EMT called for an additional unit, while the other did a triage of the three patients. The first car contained one patient who was alert and complaining of localized shoulder pain but who exhibited no evidence of serious injuries. In the second car, a 25-year-old male was the front seat passenger; the driver was found dead, with massive brain injury. The EMT attended the 25-year-old patient, who was alert and agitated, complaining of shortness of breath and pain in the right hip. The physical assessment revealed:

Respirations: 30 and labored
Pulse: 64 and regular
Blood pressure: 90/palpation
Skin: pale, with profuse sweating
Forehead laceration
Pupils: midpositional, equal and reactive
Paradoxical breathing with subcutaneous emphysema and absent breath sounds in the left chest

The EMTs suspected that the patient had a flail chest, pneumothorax, and possible internal bleeding. They maintained in-line immobilization of the neck, applied high-concentration oxygen via a nonrebreather mask, and rapidly extricated the patient from the car. During extrication it was noted that the right leg was internally rotated and flexed at the hip. Once outside the car, the flail segment was splinted and the PASG were applied. Only one leg of the garment could be attached, due to the position of the leg.

The condition did not change en route and the pulse rate remained at 64.

Questions for Discussion

1. What injuries are likely to be associated with front-end collisions?
2. What are the indications for positive-pressure ventilations with a flail chest?
3. What are the possible causes of a relatively slow pulse (64) in hypovolemic shock?

Discussion of Case History 1

Typical injuries associated with front-end collisions include head and cervical spine injury, injury to the airway, shoulder and clavicle injuries, and blunt trauma to intrathoracic and intra-abdominal organs. Dashboard injuries include tibial and knee fractures, femur fractures, and dislocation of the hip through the acetabulum. The patient described in this scenario manifested many of the classic injuries in front-end collisions.

Caution should be used when providing positive-pressure ventilation in cases of intrathoracic trauma. Injuries to the airway can be complicated by excessive positive pressure. Tension pneumothorax can result by forcing air into the pleural space. The ventilation methods of choice in these patients include bag-valve-mask, mouth-to-mouth, or the pocket mask, since airway pressure can be better controlled.

In the face of internal bleeding, hypovolemic shock, or other causes of tissue hypoxia a compensatory tachycardia is most common. Patients who present with relatively slow pulse rates are likely to have other complicating problems. Increased intracranial pressure may result in a slowing of the pulse associated with an increase in blood pressure. However, the patient described above did not exhibit an increase in blood pressure and there were no other signs of intracerebral bleeding. The pulse may also slow as a result of severe end-stage shock, caused by sustained ischemia to the myocardium. This is an unlikely cause in this patient, since he is still compensated as indicated by his blood pressure and mental status. Drugs that block sympathetic tone may also prevent an increase in pulse. This reinforces the need to obtain a medication history during your assessment. This patient was not on any type of medication.

The cause of the slow heart rate in this patient was related to a cardiac contusion. The contusion resulted in damage to the conduction system, which led to poor conduction "heart block" and the related slowing of the heart rate. The mechanism of injury supported this possible diagnosis, since steering wheel and dashboard injuries are a common mechanism for cardiac contusion (see Fig. 20–4).

• CASE HISTORY 2 •

A 24-year-old woman jumped six stories and landed on a grass surface softened by one week's rainfall. Six-inch depressions in the ground were made by her feet and buttocks. She was alert and oriented, with no history of loss of consciousness, and complained only of pain in the lumbar region.

The physical examination revealed:

Respirations: 20 and normal
Breath sounds: normal
Pulse: 100 and regular
Blood pressure: 100/70
Skin: normal
Pupils: midpositional, equal and reactive
No obvious external evidence of injury
Neurologic examination revealed a Glasgow Coma score
   of 15 and normal motor and sensory function

The EMTs assumed the presence of spinal injury and maintained in-line immobilization of the cervical spine and administered supplemental oxygen via a nasal cannula at 6 liters per minute. The patient was immobilized on a long spine board and transported to the local trauma center.

Questions for Discussion

1. What injuries should be presumed, given the mechanism of injury?
2. What is the likelihood of cervical spine injury without also having head injury?

Discussion of Case History 2

This patient suffered bilateral fractures of the talus (ankle bone), compression fractures of the lumbar spine, and a nondisplaced fracture of the second cervical vertebra (see Fig. 20–6). Because of the mechanism of injury, the EMTs took the appropriate cervical spine precautions. Although there was no internal bleeding, the EMTs maintained a suspicion of internal bleeding and provided a

timely but smooth transport of the patient. The patient had no spinal cord compression, no other severe internal injuries, and went on to good recovery.

This patient made no complaint of pain in the neck or feet. The patient who has suffered severe trauma, let alone one who has jumped six stories, may not give you the most reliable history. This case illustrates the importance of establishing a treatment plan based on knowledge of the mechanism of injury and suspected associated injuries.

• CASE HISTORY 3 •

A 30-year-old man was struck by a van on a local city street. Bystanders reported that he was thrown 15 feet on impact and suffered no loss of consciousness. The EMTs found the patient sitting on the curb about to sign a release, against medical advice, for another unit on the scene. The patient appeared agitated and refused to undergo physical assessment. However, the EMTs convinced the patient to submit to a brief survey.

The patient's skin appeared pale and sweaty, the pupils were midpositional and equal and reactive, and the Glasgow Coma score was 15. The EMTs noted the dent on the van from the impact. An inspection of the patient also revealed a discharge of fluid and blood from the nose and fluid from the right ear.

Although the patient was refusing medical attention, the police and EMTs insisted that the patient accompany them to the hospital. With moderate resistance, they placed the patient on a stretcher and notified the hospital that a potential neurosurgical emergency was en route. Although the patient refused immobilization with a cervical collar and spine board, the EMTs maintained in-line immobilization while en route to the trauma center.

Questions for Discussion

1. What injuries are suggested by the mechanism of injury and the physical findings?
2. What are the medicolegal implications of the attempted treatment and transport of a patient despite his expressed refusal?
3. Can a patient have an epidural hematoma with no initial loss of consciousness?

Discussion of Case History 3

This patient was still agitated upon arrival in the emergency department. The trauma team was present, and one physician asked the EMTs why they had called in the case as a neurosurgical emergency. The EMTs indicated that the mechanism of injury and the physical findings were the basis for their decision.

The patient subsequently lost consciousness; had

focal neurologic deficits; and on computed tomography scan showed an epidural hematoma, which was evacuated.

Classic teachings about epidural hematomas present cases with initial loss of consciousness, clearing of mental status, and subsequent deterioration. This is good for teaching purposes, since it points out that a secondary process (bleeding in the head) is the cause of the coma—not the initial blow (the patient regained consciousness first). However, some patients never lose consciousness until signs of herniation appear, and others remain unconscious from the time of impact.

EMTs should respect a patient's refusal of medical treatment when the patient demonstrates an intact mental status and can understand the consequences of his or her actions. A patient with an injury that may threaten life or well-being should be able to understand both the nature of the injury and the consequences that can develop if no treatment is rendered. It is a judgment made by medical personnel that a patient truly understands the potential ramifications if treatment is declined and is therefore competent to sign a release. The neurologic status of the patient should be carefully documented in such cases.

If the EMTs had not insisted on treating this particular patient, the results may have been disastrous.

Patients often refuse medical attention even when there is good evidence that they have critical injuries or illness. Handling these situation is even more complex when there are associated conditions such as head injury or intoxication from alcohol or other drugs.

As in the emergency department, prehospital personnel must act in the best interest of the patient. If in their judgment the patient is not competent because of the illness, injury, or an altered mental status, they should continue in their attempt to render emergency care. There are no hard rules in situations like this. Recruiting family, friends, or police in your attempt to "protect" the patient is a good practice. A good rule of thumb is to act with the same concern you would want another EMT to show a member of your family. Be familiar with the guidelines and resources available in your system for such cases.

• CASE HISTORY 4 •

A 60-year-old woman was involved in a front-end automobile collision. EMTs arrived on the scene first and found the patient in the car with a weak pulse. After rapid extrication, the pulse was no longer detectable and CPR was begun. Paramedics had also been dispatched and arrived 5 minutes after CPR had been initiated. Cardiac arrest was confirmed, and fixed and dilated pupils and a contusion of the anterior right chest were noted.

CPR was continued, an esophageal airway was inserted, and MAST trousers were applied. An IV was inserted and normal saline was infused. A pulse returned at 130/min, 10 minutes after the paramedics began treatment. Five minutes later the pulse dropped to 40. It was lost en route to the hospital.

Summary of Events

Event	Time	BP	Pulse	Respiration	
Treatment					
Basic life support arrives	00:00	—	(present)		
Extrication	00:05	0	0	0*	CPR begun
Advanced life support arrives	00:10	0	0	0	Airway, MAST, IV fluid
	00:15	0	130	0	
	00:20	0	40	0	Transport
	00:27	0	30	0	Arrives at hospital

* Assisted ventilation only, no spontaneous breathing.

The patient lost all pulses at the hospital and could not be resuscitated.

Question for Discussion

1. How could prehospital care have been altered to potentially improve the outcome for this patient?

Discussion of Case History 4

The essential first step in resuscitation from hypovolemia is restoration of blood volume and control of further bleeding. Delivery of oxygen to the tissues is dependent on both the blood's volume and its hemoglobin content.

Continuous bleeding must be definitively controlled, which in this case meant surgical intervention. Severe hemorrhage ultimately requires replacement with whole blood. IV solutions and MAST trousers address the volume problem and serve as a temporary measure.

In this case, the oxygen, IV, and MAST trousers probably restored enough volume and oxygen to the central circulation to allow a failing heart to generate a pulse. However, without definitive control of internal bleeding, such therapy is limited.

A better judgment in this instance would have been to rapidly transport the patient. The patient was 7 minutes from the hospital. If the EMTs had left immediately after extrication, the patient would have arrived at the hospital 15 minutes earlier. Resuscitation from cardiac arrest due to blunt trauma has an extremely poor outcome. The importance of an early transportation decision in cases involving resuscitation from severe trauma cannot be overemphasized.

A 14-year-old boy was balancing on the railing of a bridge in a public park. He fell 20 feet into 6 inches of water, head first. His friends dragged him 40 feet up a hill to the roadway.

EMTs arrived to find the patient conscious, alert, and oriented, complaining of pain in his neck.

The physical examination revealed the following:

Respirations: 24 and regular
Pulse: 60
Blood pressure: 80/50
Skin: warm and pink
Diaphragmatic breathing with no chest excursion
Breath sounds equal
No sensation below the clavicle and the patient could not move his arms or legs

The patient was immobilized manually and oxygen was provided via a non-rebreather mask. The patient was secured to a long spine board and transported to a trauma center.

Question for Discussion

1. Does the mechanism of injury in this case dictate the need for an early transport decision to rule out intra-abdominal or other occult hemorrhage that may be masked by spinal shock?

Discussion of Case History 5

Studies have shown that internal bleeding is difficult to detect in patients with spinal shock. The pelvis, abdomen, and thorax can contain large quantities of blood that may not be readily apparent on physical examination. Long bone fractures such as the femur can also produce substantial blood loss, which is better appreciated when swelling of the leg is considered as a volume of a cylinder.

This patient, suffering a catastrophic injury to the neck, did not have hypovolemia from other injuries. However, the EMT must remember that such patients cannot complain of pain or tenderness upon abdominal examination despite major injury.

CONCLUSION—EMT: PREHOSPITAL CARE

The skills one learns in caring for the severe trauma patient are transferable to many other cases as well. What is most important is to maintain the proper perspective on the role of the EMT—service to others who are in great need.

We would like to share a story. It is a real story and real names are used. The patient has allowed us to tell his story in the hope that it will help others.

Several years ago, an emergency medical technician team from our hospital responded to a call for "syncope," or fainting. It was a typical type of call—nothing out of the ordinary. Upon arriving at the scene, the EMTs encountered a white-haired gentleman in his sixties who had fainted 10 minutes prior to their arrival and who now complained of abdominal pain and felt very weak. He was pale, very sweaty, and generally looked quite ill. The EMTs proceeded to evaluate the patient. His vital signs were not promising. He had a very rapid pulse and a very low blood pressure. The patient also had a long history of hypertension and cardiovascular disease. Upon physical examination, the EMTs observed signs of poor circulation and oxygenation. When they examined the abdomen, they felt a pulsating mass—an ominous sign of a life-threatening condition—a leaking abdominal aneurysm. The patient was likely to die.

While the EMTs were caring for the patient, the police indicated that someone wanted to speak to the EMTs on the phone. The EMT who answered the phone expected to be talking to the family physician or a family member but instead discovered that he was speaking to Don Jirak, another EMT from the hospital, who happened to be an old friend and long-time associate. At first, Mike, the EMT at the scene, could not figure out why Don was calling him at this patient's home. But assuming that he was arranging for a surgical standby at the hospital, Mike quickly provided a history of the patient's status. At the end of the dialogue, Mike finally asked, "What in the world are you calling me for in the middle of this and, by the way, where did you get this telephone number?"

It turned out that the man Mike was treating was Don Jirak's father. At this point, the perspective on this call underwent a profound change. The patient was now Don Jirak's father. This did not alter the sense of urgency or the quality of care, but it dramatically altered the perspective. Mike told Don to meet them at the hospital and proceeded to complete the treatment and to rapidly transport the patient. Fortunately, one of the best vascular surgeons in the area worked at the hospital. A surgical standby was established, and Mr. Jirak was quickly assessed in the emergency room and transferred to the operating room, where he successfully underwent emergency surgery. Needless to say, the outcome of this particular call was extremely gratifying to everyone involved. This does not imply that other patients who are saved are not special. But to save the family member of a coworker provides a more personal perspective to a sometimes "clinically oriented" profession, and it reminds us of the true nature of emergency care.

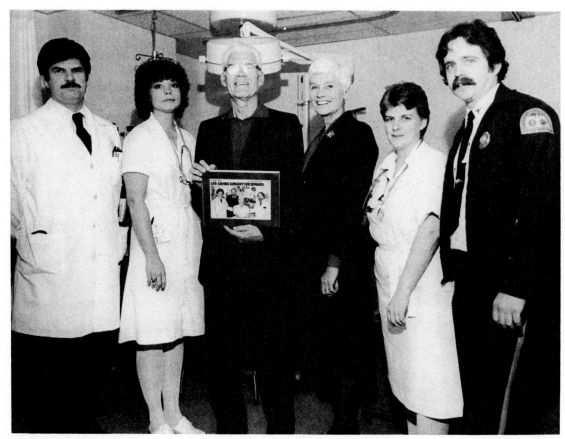

FIGURE 20–8. Mr. Jirak and the emergency medical services system team members who gave him lifesaving care reunite after he recovered.

Our word of advice is that we should all try very hard to maintain the proper perspective. Be dedicated—remembering that this profession is one of service—and maintain a human and humane outlook toward your patients, your coworkers, and yourselves.

Emergency medicine can be very stressful work. Sometimes it is difficult to maintain perspective. But there are many rewards—the birth of a child, a successful resuscitation, and the simple act of helping a mother, father, or other family member through a crisis. Remember that everyone is somebody's Mr. Jirak (Fig. 20–8).

REVIEW EXERCISES

1. List the steps of patient assessment of a trauma patient.

2. List two injuries for each of the following mechanisms:
   Head-on collisions   Fall on feet
   Side-hit collisions   Fall on outstretched arm
   Rear-end hit collisions

3. Define the pneumonic AVPU and describe its components.

4. Define the pneumonic AMPLE and describe its components.

5. List the major components of the trauma score and explain the score's relevance.

6. List the components of the trauma triage algorithm.

REFERENCES

American College of Surgeons Committee on Trauma: Advanced Trauma Life Program. Chicago, American College of Surgeons, 1984 and 1988.

American College of Surgeons Committee on Trauma, Moore EE (ed): Early Care of the injured patient, 4th ed. Philadelphia, BC Decker, 1990.

American College of Surgeons Committee on Trauma, Walt J (ed): Early care of the injured patient, 3rd ed. Philadelphia, WB Saunders, 1982.

Campbell JE: BTLS: Basic Prehospital Trauma Care. Englewood Cliffs, NJ, Brady/Prentice-Hall, 1988.

Campbell JE: Basic Trauma Life Support Advanced Prehospital Care, 2nd ed. Englewood Cliffs, NJ, Brady/Prentice-Hall, 1988.

Hughes S: The basis and practice of traumatology. Rockville, MD, Aspen, 1984.

Nakum A, Melvin J: The biomechanics of trauma. Norwalk, CT, Appleton-Century-Crofts, 1985.

Prehospital Trauma Life Support Committee of the National Association of EMTs: Pre-hospital trauma life support. Akron, OH, Emergency Training, 1986.

Rosen et al (eds): Emergency medicine: concepts and clinical practice. St Louis, CV Mosby, 1983.

Schriger DL, Baraff L: Defining normal capillary refill: Variation with age, sex and temperature. Ann Emerg Med 17(9):113–116, 1988.

Schriger DL, Baraff L: Capillary refill—Is it a useful predictor of hypovolemic states? Ann Emerg Med 20(6):23–27, 1991.

Zuidema GD, Rutherford RB, Ballinger WF: The management of trauma, 4th ed. Philadelphia, WB Saunders, 1985.

GLOSSARY

Abandonment The unilateral severance of a professional provider–patient relationship without giving the patient notice and reasonable time to find substitute treatment.

Abdominal aortic aneurysm Outpouching of the wall of the abdominal aorta that weakens the structure and may potentially leak or burst.

Abduction Movement away from midline.

Abrasion A scrape on the surface of the skin or mucous membrane.

Abruptio placentae Premature separation of the placenta from the uterine wall.

Accessory muscles (of respiration) Muscles used in respiration during strenuous exercise or in instances of respiratory disease or trauma.

Ace bandage Elastic bandage used to support joints.

Acetabulum The socket of the pelvis that articulates with the femur (thigh bone) to form the hip joint.

Acetaminophen (Tylenol) An analgesic (pain reliever) and antipyretic (fever reducer) drug.

Acidosis A state of increased acidity of the blood that may be caused by anaerobic (without oxygen) metabolism such as during cardiac arrest.

Activated charcoal An absorbent material that binds with most toxins and keeps them within the gastrointestinal tract until they are eliminated from the body, thereby preventing absorption.

Active disaster A disaster in which the forces that contributed to or were associated with the disaster are still active, evolving, and ongoing.

Active labor The period of labor during which cervical dilatation progresses from 4 cm to about 8 cm. Contractions during active labor are usually strong and regular.

Acute abdomen Unremitting abdominal pain of recent onset.

Acute urinary retention Retention of urine, usually caused by enlargement of the prostate gland, which obstructs the urethra.

Adduction Movement toward the midline.

Adrenal glands Important pair of glands located above each kidney that are responsible for the production of cortisol, norepinephrine, epinephrine (adrenaline), and other important substances.

AIDS (acquired immunodeficiency syndrome) A condition caused by the human immunodeficiency virus (HIV) that permits the development of opportunistic infections, malignancies, and neurologic disease.

Air chisel A pneumatic chisel used to cut panels of metal, glass, and plastic almost effortlessly.

Air embolism An air bubble introduced into the circulatory system by way of intravenous therapy or an open wound that can result in an obstruction of blood flow.

Air splints Plastic splints that are filled with air to provide circumferential support to an injured extremity.

Airborne transmission Disease transmission by either droplet nuclei (residue of evaporated droplets that may remain suspended in the air for long periods of time) or dust particles in the air containing the infectious agent.

Alkaloids Organic substances (made from plants) that are used as drugs.

Altered mental status Any change in the patient's mental status; can range from mild confusion and abnormal behavior to deep coma, where the patient is totally unresponsive to verbal or painful stimuli.

Alveoli Microscopic air sacs in the lungs in which gas exchange takes place.

Amnesia Memory loss that may be retrograde (amnesia for events before the injury) or antegrade (amnesia for events after the injury).

Amnion The innermost membrane of the sac that encloses the fetus.

Amnionitis Infection of the amniotic fluid with bacteria.

Amniotic fluid Clear, watery liquid that surrounds and cushions the unborn fetus.

Amniotic sac The membranous sac that encloses the fetus.

Amphetamines A group of commonly abused central nervous system stimulant drugs.

Amputation The cutting away from the body of a limb or protruding structure.

Analgesics Drugs used to reduce pain; "pain killers."

Anaphylactoid An anaphylaxis-like reaction.

Anaphylaxis An allergic condition in which an *antibody–antigen* reaction results in a release of substances that can cause shock, bronchoconstriction, and airway obstruction.

Anasarca Severe, generalized body edema.

Anatomy The study of the structure of body parts.

Anemia A reduced amount of hemoglobin or red blood cells per 100 milliliters of blood.

Anemia of pregnancy Refers to the fact that the plasma volume increases during pregnancy, making the blood more dilute. A blood test during pregnancy will reveal a low hematocrit and hemoglobin.

Aneurysm Outpouching of the wall of a blood vessel that weakens the structure and may potentially leak, burst, or dissect (bleeding within and along the layers of a blood vessel).

Angina Temporary ischemic chest pain that is usually caused by exertion or stress and relieved by rest.

Angioedema A condition that results from vasodilation and causes hives and swelling of the face, airway, and other tissues.

Anisocoria Unequal diameter of the pupils.

Anorexia Lack of appetite.

Anterior Toward the front of the body.

Antibiotics Substances that kill or inhibit the growth of microorganisms.

Antibody A protein that combines with an antigen to neutralize toxins that enter the body or to fight infection.

Anticoagulants Substances that interfere with the clotting of blood, e.g., coumadin, heparin.

Antidepressants Drugs used in the treatment of mental depression.

Antidote A substance that neutralizes a poison and its toxic effects.

Antigen A substance that is recognized as foreign to the body and that can cause antibodies or special white cells to form and combine with it.

Antihistamine A substance that can block the effects of histamine.

Antiviral Substances that kill or inhibit the growth of viruses.

Anus Exterior opening of the rectum.

Anxiety A fearful emotional state characterized by increased nervousness, tension, pacing, hand wringing, and trembling.

Aorta The primary artery of the systemic circulation that leaves the left ventricle and delivers blood to arteries in the neck, head, thorax, and abdominal cavity.

Aortic aneurysm Ballooning of the aorta caused by weakness or disease in the aortic wall.

Aortic valve Semilunar valve between the left ventricle and the aorta.

Apgar score A system of quickly evaluating an infant's heart rate, respiratory effort, muscle tone, reflex irritability, and color at birth. The Apgar score is done at 1 minute after birth and repeated 5 minutes after birth.

Apical pulse Pulse felt over the apex of the heart at the 5th intercostal space in the midclavicular line.

Appendicitis Inflammation or infection of the appendix.

Appendicular skeleton The bones of the upper and lower extremities, the shoulder, and the pelvis.

Appendix Wormlike outpocketing of the cecum that has an extremely narrow lumen and no known function.

Aqueous humor Watery fluid that fills the anterior chamber of the eye.

Arc burns Burns that occur as a result of electricity that travels through the air between objects of opposite charge or a highly charged source and the ground.

Arrhythmia Abnormal heart rhythm.

Arterioles Small arteries connecting the larger arteries to the capillaries.

Arteriosclerosis Progressive disease of the arteries that results in narrowing of the lumen, caused by deposits of fat and hardening of the arterial wall.

Arteriosclerotic heart disease Progressive disease of the coronary arteries that results in narrowing of the lumen due to deposits of fat and hardening of the arterial wall.

Artery Muscular blood vessel that carries blood away from the heart.

Articulation The site of connection of bones or cartilage and bone. A joint.

Artifact A disturbance in the electrocardiographic (ECG) tracing caused by many conditions, such as electrical interference, patient or cable movement, dislodging of the cables, muscle tremors, and seizures.

Asphyxiant Anything, often a gas, that will produce asphyxia (absent or extremely impaired exchange of oxygen and carbon dioxide).

Asthma An acute obstructive respiratory disease with narrowing of the airways that is usually precipitated by stress, infection, or an allergic response.

Asystole Cardiac standstill or an absence of any cardiac rhythm; "flat line."

Ataxic breathing A slow and irregular pattern of breathing associated with brainstem injury.

Atelectasis Collapsed alveoli.

Atherosclerosis A buildup of fatty deposits on the lining of arteries that narrows the lumen.

Atoms The smallest units of matter that can bind together chemically to form elements and molecules. The smallest particle of an element.

Atrial fibrillation Abnormal heart rhythm with quivering of the atria and ineffective atrial contraction.

Atrioventricular valves Either of the two valves that separate the atria from the ventricles (mitral or tricuspid valves).

Atrium The relatively thin-walled upper chamber of the heart that receives blood from the body (right side) and lungs (left side).

Auditory canal Curved tube leading inward from the auricle through the temporal bone to the tympanic membrane.

Aura Strange smells, visual or auditory sensations, or motor events in only one part on the body that may herald the onset of a generalized convulsion or seizure.

Auricle External flap of skin and skin-covered cartilage of the ear.

Auscultation Listening for sounds through a stethoscope.

Authorization forms Forms used by EMS personnel to document special requests or refusals by the patient, including refused medical aid forms, request for transport to a particular hospital, refusal of a specific treatment, and so on.

Automatic external defibrillators Defibrillators that interpret the patient's ECG status and automatically initiate or advise defibrillation as needed.

Autonomic nervous system The division of the nervous system consisting of the sympathetic and the parasympathetic nervous systems that controls vital body functions such as heart rate, constriction and dilation of blood vessels, digestion and other involuntary actions.

AV (atrioventricular) node Part of conduction system between the atria and the ventricles that receives impulses from the SA (sinoatrial) node and conducts them to the bundle of His and the bundle branches.

Avulsion (Evulsion) Tearing away of a body part or structure; usually refers to a chunk of skin. The part is often still attached to the body by a small flap or pedicle of skin.

Avulsion fractures Fractures that result from forceful contraction of muscle against resistance, with tearing of a fragment of bone at the site of muscle insertion.

Axial skeleton The bones of the skull and face, the spinal column, and the thoracic cavity.

Bag-valve-mask Mechanical aid used to administer positive-pressure breathing. Usually consists of a bag with an oxygen inlet, a unidirectional valve, and a mask.

Bale hooks A hand-held hook used in pulling and tearing operations of extrication.

Ball-and-socket joint A joint in which the rounded surface of one bone moves within a cup-like indentation in another bone; i.e., the shoulder, hip.

Bandage Material used to secure a dressing in place and to provide pressure over the dressing to aid in the control of bleeding.

Barbiturates A group of drugs that act as central nervous system depressants.

Baroreceptors Receptors that are sensitive to changes in blood pressure; found in the heart, vena cava, aorta, and carotid arteries.

Barotrauma Damage to air-containing structures such as the middle ear or sinuses caused by changes in the environmental pressure (as in flying or under-water diving).

Bartholin's glands   Mucus-secreting glands lying deep in the posterior parts of the labia majora; may become blocked and infected.

Basilar rales   Rales (crackles) heard at the base of the lungs.

Basilar skull fracture   A crack in the *base* or floor of the skull.

Battle's sign   Ecchymosis behind the ears; a sign of basilar skull fracture.

Benzodiazepines   A group of drugs with sedative and hypnotic effects used often to control anxiety.

Bile   Digestive juice produced in the liver and stored in the gallbladder until it is needed for the digestion of fatty foods.

Bilirubin   Pigment that gives bile its color; produced in the liver as a byproduct in the breakdown of red blood cells.

Biologic death   A state of sustained oxygen deprivation after which recovery without brain damage is unlikely.

Biotelemetry   Transmission of biologic data via a radio or other form of communication to a distant location, e.g., hospital.

Blanket drag   A rescue evacuation technique that uses a blanket to drag the patient from a hazardous situation.

Bleb   Blister-like defect in the lung tissue.

Blood pressure   The force exerted by the blood volume on the walls of the vessels. Formula: blood pressure = cardiac output × peripheral vascular resistance (PVR).

Bloody show   Blood-tinged mucus expelled from the vagina as the cervix dilates. May be dark brown, pink, or bright red.

Body language   Messages conveyed through body posture and gestures that we may communicate "unconsciously."

Bolt cutters   A large "scissor-like" device used for cutting large-diameter metal objects, e.g., steering wheel.

Bourdon gauge flowmeter   Type of flowmeter that utilizes gas pressure to monitor flow rates to an oxygen delivery device.

Brachial artery   Artery of the upper arm; it divides into the *radial* and *ulnar* arteries in the forearm.

Bradycardia   Abnormally slow heart rhythm.

Brainstem   The lower part of the brain responsible for a variety of vital functions and regulatory activities including respiratory and circulatory functions.

Breach of duty   A negligent act or omission by a medical provider.

Bridging   The transfer of electricity from one defibrillator paddle to another via the conductive medium, sweat, or other form of moisture on the chest wall.

Bronchi   The branches of the airway from the trachea to the lungs. The trachea divides into right and left main bronchi, which further subdivide many times.

Bronchial   Referring to the bronchi; bronchial sounds are loud and high-pitched breath sounds heard at the top of the sternum and between the scapulas (posteriorly).

Bronchioles   Smallest tubes of the airway, terminating in alveoli.

Bronchoconstriction   Constriction of the bronchioles.

Bronchovesicular sounds   Low-pitched breath sounds heard over the upper/middle sternum and to its left and right are referred to as bronchovesicular; usually have an equal inspiratory and expiratory phase and refer to the bronchial tubes and alveoli in the lungs.

Bundle branch   A branch of the bundle of His carrying impulses to a ventricle.

Bundle of His   Atrioventricular bundle of impulse-conducting fibers in the myocardium.

Capillary   Thin-walled blood vessel where diffusion takes place.

Capillary refill   A diagnostic test in which the nailbed is compressed in order to empty the capillaries and determine the time it takes to refill (return of color is noted).

Carbon dioxide   The waste product gas exhaled by the lungs.

Carbon monoxide   A poisonous gas commonly found in fires, charcoal burners, automobile exhaust fumes, and inadequately ventilated stoves and home heaters.

Carboxyhemoglobin   The combined state of carbon monoxide and hemoglobin that occurs when inhaling carbon monoxide gas.

Cardiac arrest   The cessation of a functional heartbeat.

Cardiac contusion   Bruising of heart tissue.

Cardiac output   The volume of blood pumped by the heart in 1 minute. Calculated by multiplying the number of heartbeats per minute times the amount of blood pumped with each beat (for normal adult at rest = 5 liters/minute).

Cardiogenic shock   Shock secondary to pump failure.

Cardiovascular unresponsiveness   The point in the resuscitation process at which resuscitation of the heart is deemed impossible following the application of basic and advanced life support measures.

Carotid arteries   The primary arteries that supply blood to the brain and that can be palpated in the neck region. They supply 80% of the brain's blood supply.

Carpal bones   The bones forming the wrist.

Carrier (infectious)   A person who shows no signs of the disease yet harbors an infectious organism.

Cartilage   A softer precursor of the bony skeleton, as present in fetal life; sites of bone growth in children. Cartilage persists at the junction of the ribs and sternum and at the surfaces of joints.

Categorization   A system of hospital designation according to the hospital's ability to treat different types of patients. Examples of hospital designations include trauma, cardiac, psychiatric, replantation, and neonatology.

Cathartic   An agent that is given to induce diarrhea. In the treatment of an overdose, cathartics decrease transit time through the gastrointestinal tract and thereby reduce the chance for absorption of drug from the intestine.

Causal connection   A connection between the patient's injury and actions taken or omitted by the health care provider.

Caustic   An agent that has corrosive and burning effects and is destructive to living tissue.

CDC   Centers for Disease Control.

Cecum   The first section of the large intestine.

Cell   The fundamental unit of every living thing.

Central   Located toward the center of the body.

Central nervous system   The controlling and regulating part of the nervous system, which includes the brain, brainstem, and spinal cord.

Central neurogenic hyperventilation   A breathing pattern characterized by regular deep and rapid ventilations.

Centrifugal force   A force that propels objects outward from the center of rotation.

Cephalhematoma   A hematoma between one of the cranial bones and the overlying periosteum.

Cerebellum   An outpocketing of the brain located behind or posterior to the brainstem. It is primarily concerned with coordination of movement and balance.

Cerebral contusion   Bruising or contusion of the brain.

Cerebral hematoma   Bleeding within the brain tissue itself or in the spaces between the meningeal layers that cover the brain.

Cerebrospinal fluid   The fluid between the arachnoid and pia mater that helps protect and cushion the brain and acts like a liquid shock absorber.

Cerebrovascular accident (CVA)   A blockage or disruption of blood flow in an artery feeding the brain.

Cerebrum   The largest and most superior portion of the brain responsible for intellectual functions, motor control, sensory perception, visual stimuli, smell, hearing, and other body functions.

Cerumen   Earwax.

Cervical vertebrae   The first seven vertebrae that form the bones of the neck.

Cervix   The lowermost part or neck of the uterus.

Cesarean section   Surgical abdominal delivery of a baby.

Cheyne-Stokes respiration   A breathing pattern characterized by increasing and then gradual decreasing amplitude and rate of breathing, followed by a period of apnea.

Chickenpox   A communicable viral disease spread by respiratory secretions and contact with the moist vesicles.

Chief complaint   The expression of the patient's main problem in his or her own words.

Cholecystitis   Inflammation or low-grade chronic infection of the gallbladder.

Chronic bronchitis   Inflammation of the bronchi with repeated attacks of coughing and sputum production.

Cirrhosis   Scarring of the liver.

Clavicle   The collar bone.

Cleft palate   A birth defect characterized by a hole or separation in the hard and/or soft palate. May be confined to the inside of the mouth or extend to the upper lip or even involve the nose.

Clinical death   The cessation of pulse and respirations.

Closed disaster A disaster that has physical or geographic boundaries that prevent speedy access to or evacuation of patients.

Closed fractures Fractures of a bone without a break in the skin.

Clothes drag A rescue evacuation technique that uses the patient's clothing to drag the patient along the long axis of the body from a hazardous situation.

Clotting factors Any of several substances in the blood that are required for the complicated mechanism of clotting the blood.

Cocaine A commonly abused stimulant drug that is often snorted through the nose and absorbed by the membranes in the nasopharynx.

Coccyx (coccygeal vertebrae) The lowermost fused vertebrae, commonly called the tail bone.

Cochlea A snail-like tube of the inner ear with nerve receptor cells that transmit auditory messages to the auditory branch of the eighth cranial nerve.

Colon Refers to the large intestine.

Coma A lack of responsiveness to the environment. The patient is unconscious and cannot be aroused by external stimuli.

Comminuted fractures Fractures that have multiple (always more than two) fragments and are caused by severe direct violence.

Comminuted skull fracture A skull fracture that has multiple cracks or segments radiating outward from the point of impact.

Communicable diseases (infectious or contagious) Diseases capable of being spread from one person to another.

Communicable period The time period during which a person can transmit an infectious disease to others.

Communication center The part of the communications system that coordinates receiving calls, triage, dispatch, and other activities of an EMS system.

Compact bone The dense bone that makes up the outer layer of all bones and the central outer portions of long bones.

Compensatory mechanism Dynamic change to compensate for a failing body system. In the circulatory system, a measure to compensate for a diminishing blood volume, e.g., vasoconstriction, increase in the heart rate, redistribution of blood flow.

Competence A condition or quality of being competent, able, or fit to perform a particular task or tasks. A specific legal capability.

Complete abortion Passing all the products of conception.

Compression fractures Fractures resulting from transmitted forces that drive bones together.

Concussion A transient loss of consciousness or of neurologic function as a result of trauma to the brain.

Condyle A rounded projection of bone, usually for articulation with another bone; an *epicondyle* is an eminence above a condyle for the attachment of muscle.

Confidentiality The practice by an EMT of maintaining a patient's right to privacy in each patient encounter.

Congestive heart failure Failure of the heart with resultant backup of blood to the lungs and the systemic circulation, leading to pulmonary and generalized edema.

Conjunctiva Membrane that lines the interior surface of the eyelids and covers the anterior surface of the sclera of the eye.

Conjunctivitis Irritation or infection of the conjunctiva.

Constant flow selector valve Type of flowmeter that uses a flow marking at the adjustment dial to indicate flow rates.

Constipation Difficulty in passing stools, with a feeling of urgency or rectal fullness.

Contact transmission The transmission of an infection from a host to a susceptible person through contact with infectious material.

Contained disaster A situation where the likelihood of further injury is low because the forces responsible for the disaster are exhausted or contained.

Contra coup A mechanism of injury where the injury occurs to the side of the brain opposite to the site of external impact of the blow owing to movement of the brain within the cranial cavity.

Contusion Bruise.

Convergence Convergence is the rapid response of onlookers, rescuers, and press upon the scene of a disaster.

COPD (chronic obstructive pulmonary disease) Long-term lung disease in which air becomes trapped in the alveoli due to bronchospasm, mucus plugs, or collapse of the bronchioles, requiring greater force to exhale.

Cornea Transparent anterior surface covering the pupil and iris through which light can enter the eye.

Coronary arteries Arteries responsible for supplying blood to the heart.

Costal margin Margin of the ribs formed by the costal cartilages, beginning with the 7th to the tips of 12th rib.

Cranium Flat, irregularly shaped bones forming the portion of the head enclosing the brain.

Cravat Triangular bandage folded to form a band around an injured part.

Crepitus A grating or crackling sound heard during auscultation as a result of fluid in the airways or a sensation felt during palpation caused by air beneath the skin or broken bone ends rubbing together

Cribbing Materials or devices, including hardwood and airbags, used to support a large amount of weight during rescue operations.

Cricoid cartilage Band of cartilage below the thyroid cartilage; forms a circle just above the trachea.

Cricothyroid membrane Membrane between the thyroid and cricoid cartilages that is surgically opened to gain access to the airway when facial injuries or obstructions exist above the larynx.

Cricothyroidotomy (cricothyrotomy) Surgical opening of the cricothyroid membrane to provide an airway.

Crowning The presenting part of the fetus is visible and does not recede between contractions.

Cushing's reflex A rising blood pressure with a slow pulse associated with increased intracranial pressure.

Cyanide A poisonous compound (chemical asphyxiant) found in industry, such as electroplating, photography, metallurgy, and metal cleaning in the jewelry industry.

Cyanosis Bluish discoloration of the mucous membranes or skin, resulting from oxygen-depleted hemoglobin.

Debriefing A process used at the end of a disaster to allow EMTs and other rescue personnel to share experiences with professional counselors in order to deal with the psychological and emotional stress.

Decerebrate posturing A posture assumed by a patient in which the arms are extended and internally rotated at the shoulders, with the wrists flexed and the legs extended. Associated with brain injury.

Decomposition The decaying of body tissue that occurs over a prolonged period of time after death.

Decorticate posturing A posture assumed by a patient in which the arms are flexed but the legs are extended. Associated with brain injury.

Deep Away from the surface.

Defibrillation The external application of an electric shock across the heart of sufficient energy to depolarize the heart's cells for the purpose of converting ventricular fibrillation into an organized rhythm.

Defibrillator Device capable of delivering electric shock therapy in order to reverse an otherwise lethal heart rhythm.

Definitive treatment Inhospital treatment needed to stabilize a patient, e.g., surgery, blood transfusion.

Delirium A state of mental confusion, characterized by auditory, visual, tactile, or olfactory hallucinations, that is usually caused by organic causes.

Dependent lividity The discoloration of body tissues in the lower or dependent areas of the body, caused by the collection of coagulated blood.

Depressed skull fracture A fracture where the bone fragments are depressed downward toward the brain.

Depression A condition characterized by loss of pleasure, deep sadness, feelings of hopelessness, difficulty with sleeping, loss of appetite, loss of sex drive, and feelings of guilt.

Dermatome Area of skin innervated by nerve fibers from a particular segment of spinal cord; the mapping of a particular area of innervation.

Dermis Inner layer of skin composed of dense connective tissue that contains the nerves, blood vessels, sweat and sebaceous glands, and hair follicles.

Diabetes Disease that results from failure of the pancreas to produce a sufficient amount of insulin.

Diabetic ketoacidosis A condition resulting from a relatively prolonged insulin deficiency where the blood glucose level rises and fatty acids are produced in the blood.

Diaphragm The primary muscle of respiration that separates the thoracic and abdominal cavities.

Diaphysis The elongated cylindrical portion (shaft) of a long bone.

Diarrhea Frequent watery stools.

Diastole Relaxation phase of the heart cycle.

Diastolic blood pressure The blood pressure measured during the relaxation phase (diastole) of the heart. The pressure at which the sounds heard through a stethoscope disappear or significantly diminish.

Diffusion   A process by which a substance flows from an area of higher concentration to an area of lower concentration.

Digoxin   Heart medication that slows and strengthens the contraction of the heart.

Direct carry   A technique, using two EMTs, to transfer a patient from a bed to a stretcher positioned at a 90-degree angle.

Direct contact transmission   Direct physical transfer of an infectious agent between a susceptible host and an infected or colonized person.

Disaster   An occurrence inflicting widespread destruction and distress, a grave misfortune, a total failure that overwhelms the resources available.

Disentanglement   The part of the extrication process where the rescuers remove materials that are trapping a victim.

Dislocation   The displacement of a bone from its normal anatomic position.

Dispatch communications system   That part of the communications system that receives the call for help and sends the appropriate response vehicles to the scene.

Dispatch data   Information provided to the EMS crew by the dispatcher, including address, type of call, times.

Dispatch review   Phase of patient assessment where information received from the dispatcher is validated and used to plan response.

Disseminated intravascular coagulopathy (DIC)   A severe disruption in the clotting mechanism of the blood, characterized by diffuse clotting and, as the clotting factors are used up, hemorrhage.

Distal   Further away from the trunk.

Diverticulitis   Inflamed or infected diverticulum.

Diverticulum   Abnormal formation of a pouch or pocket in the intestines in which feces may become trapped, leading to infection or inflammation.

Dorsalis pedis   The artery in the foot that is palpable on the dorsal (top) surface of the foot.

Dressing   Any material that covers a wound, prevents introduction of further contamination into the wound, and aids in bleeding control.

Droplet contact transmission   Physical transfer between a susceptible host and an infected or colonized person through contact with the conjunctivae, nose, or mouth or as a result of coughing, sneezing, or talking by an infected person.

Duodenal ulcer   Ulcer or hole in the duodenum, the most proximal portion of the small intestines.

Duodenum   The first section of the small intestines connecting the stomach to the jejunum.

Duty to act   The legal requirement to evaluate and treat a patient. The first necessary ingredient of litigation that can be established by responding in a formal system or by initiating treatment.

Dysphagia   Pain or difficulty in swallowing.

Dyspnea   Difficulty breathing.

Dysuria   Pain or difficulty in urination.

Early labor   The period of labor during which the cervix becomes effaced and dilates to about 4 cm. The contractions of early labor are usually mild and often irregular.

Ecchymosis   Black and blue marks caused by hemorrhage beneath or within the layers of skin.

ECG monitor   The screen, which is a cathode ray tube (CRT), used to display an ECG.

Eclampsia   Seizures between the 20th week of pregnancy and the first week postpartum; associated with hypertension, edema, and protein in the urine.

Ectopic pregnancy   Pregnancy that occurs outside of the uterine cavity.

Edema   Collection of excess fluid within or around the body tissues or cavities.

Effacement   Thinning of the cervix during labor.

Elapid   A group of venomous snakes with grooved fangs; includes the coral snake.

Electrical mechanical dissociation (EMD)   An organized ECG rhythm without a pulse.

Electrocardiogram (ECG)   A tracing from a device that is connected to the body's surface to record the electrical activity of the heart.

Electrodes   A device used with an ECG machine that interfaces with the skin to record the electrical activity of the heart.

Electrolytes   A compound that, when dissolved in water, separates into charged particles capable of conducting an electric current, e.g., sodium, potassium, magnesium.

Emancipated minor   An individual who is under the legal adult age but who is living independent of the parents.

Emboli (singular **embolism**)   Blood clots moving in the bloodstream.

Embryo An unborn baby at the earliest stage of development, usually before the second month of development.

Emergency medical services system (EMSS) The planned configuration of community resources and personnel necessary to provide immediate medical care to patients who have suffered sudden or unexpected illness or injury.

Emergency medical technician-ambulance (EMT-A) Entry-level prehospital emergency care provider. Trained in a program utilizing the structure and guidelines set forth by the Department of Transportation (DOT).

Emergency medical technician-intermediate (EMT-I) An individual who is trained in a number of advanced techniques such as endotracheal intubation or IV therapy. The scope of training varies from system to system.

Emergency medical technician-paramedic (EMT-P) An individual who has completed the standardized national curriculum as prescribed by the DOT. This individual performs advanced techniques such as ECG interpretation, drug therapy, invasive airway techniques, and defibrillation.

Emphysema A disease that is caused by a destruction of alveoli and the loss of elastic recoil within the lung.

Endocardium The smooth inner layer that lines the heart.

Endocrine system A regulatory system that controls certain functions of the body through the secretion of hormones.

Endometriosis The growth of endometrium (tissue from the lining of the uterus) outside the uterine cavity.

Endotracheal intubation The most effective form of airway management; involves the insertion of a tube directly into the trachea.

Endotracheal tube Soft tube with an inflatable cuff that is inserted into the trachea with the aid of a laryngoscope.

Envenomation The process of being poisoned by the bite or sting of an animal.

Epicardium Outer layer of the heart, actually the visceral pericardium.

Epidermis Outermost layer of skin.

Epidural hematoma Hematoma above the dura mater caused by a laceration of an artery traveling along the inner surface of the cranium.

Epigastric region The region located in the center of the upper abdomen just below the breast bone.

Epigastrium Area just below the xiphoid process.

Epiglottis Flap of cartilage that covers the larynx during swallowing to prevent food from entering the lungs.

Epinephrine (adrenaline) A hormone secreted by the adrenal glands that increases sympathetic activity, e.g., increasing heart rate and the force of contraction.

Epiphyseal plates or growth plates The growth plates found at the ends of bones.

Episiotomy A surgical incision made in the perineum from the vagina. An episiotomy is done to facilitate childbirth and to prevent a jagged tear.

Erect The body standing upright.

Erythema A redness of the skin in an area of infection or inflammation.

Esophageal airway A device designed to obstruct the esophagus with a blunt or gastric tube and that permits positive-pressure ventilation through a mask device to the upper airway. The main objective of the device is to prevent air from entering the stomach during mask ventilation and aspiration of vomitus.

Esophageal varices Engorged blood vessels that protrude through the lower esophageal wall where they are subject to erosion by gastric acids.

Esophagus Muscular tube connecting the stomach to the mouth.

Estrogen Female sex hormone.

Ethics The rules or principles that govern right conduct. *Medical ethics* are the values and guidelines that should govern decisions in medicine (Dorland's).

Ethylene glycol A colorless alcohol most commonly found as antifreeze.

Eustachian tube Tube connecting the middle ear to the nasopharynx, allowing for the equalization of air pressure between the middle ear and the outside or atmospheric pressure.

Evisceration Spilling of the abdominal contents through a wound to the abdominal wall.

EVOC Program (Emergency Vehicle Operation Program) A program designed by the Department of Transportation for training emergency personnel in the safe operation of an emergency vehicle.

Exposure   The process of coming in contact with, but not necessarily being infected by, a disease-causing agent.

Extension   Straightening of a joint.

External ear   Includes the auricle and auditory canal, leading to the tympanic membrane.

External intercostals   Muscles of respiration that pull the ribs upward and outward, thereby increasing the anterior-posterior, superior-inferior, and lateral-lateral dimensions of the chest cavity.

External os   The outermost part of the opening between the cervix and the vagina.

Extreme dependent lividity   Mottling of the dependent areas of the body due to the gravitational pooling of the blood following death.

Extremity carry   A rescue evacuation technique where one rescuer supports the victim's legs and the other supports the torso to remove the patient from a hazardous situation.

Extrication   The process by which entrapped patients are rescued from vehicles, buildings, tunnels, or other structures or devices.

Facial artery   Artery of the face that branches off the internal maxillary artery and that can be palpated at the angle of the jaw.

Fallopian tubes   Trumpet-shaped tubes found on both sides of the upper segment of the uterus through which a fertilized egg must travel in order to reach the uterus.

False labor   A condition in which labor pains occur with no dilatation of the cervix. May be identical in appearance to real labor and may last for hours.

Fascia   Tough fibrous membrane, for example, fascia separates the subcutaneous tissue from the skeletal muscles.

Fat embolism   Small particles of fat within the bloodstream that may cause an obstruction of blood flow through a vessel.

Femoral artery   The artery located in the thigh, palpable halfway between the pubic bone and the iliac crest of the pelvis along the inguinal crease.

Femur   The thigh bone; the largest bone in the body.

Fetus   An unborn baby, usually referred to as a fetus after the second month of pregnancy.

Fibula   The bone that forms the posterolateral aspect of the lower leg.

Figure-eight bandage   Dressing used to secure a dressing over a joint while at the same time allowing for mobility.

Firefighter's carry   A rescue evacuation technique where the victim is carried over the shoulder of single rescuer.

Firefighter's drag   A rescue evacuation technique where the rescuer wraps the patient's arms around his or her neck and crawls along the floor from a hazardous situation.

First responders   Police officers, firefighter, or other safety personnel trained in first aid or basic emergency care.

First stage of labor   The period that begins with the first contraction and ends when the cervix has been fully stretched or dilated to a diameter of 10 cm (about 4 inches).

Flaccid muscles   Muscles that are limp and without tone.

Flail chest   Two or more ribs fractured in two or more places, resulting in a disassociation of part of the chest wall structure.

Flexion   Bending of a joint.

Flowmeter   Device that records the quantity of gas leaving a cylinder.

Focal seizures   Seizures affecting only a portion of the body or that manifest as an alteration in consciousness with bizarre behavior.

Fontanelles   Sites in the cranium where the bones do not meet and soft spots are present during infancy.

Foramen   Small opening.

Foramen magnum   An opening in the base of the skull where the lower part of the brain and brainstem exit the skull to connect with the spinal cord.

Frequency   Frequent urination, usually in small amounts; a common symptom of urinary tract infection.

Friction rub   Coarse, grating sound created by inflamed pleura rubbing against the opposite pleural surface.

Frontal bone   The anterior bone of the cranium forming the forehead.

Fundal pressure   Downward pressure applied to the fundus of the uterus to assist in delivery of a baby or placenta.

Fundus   The uppermost part of the uterus.

Vestibule   Part of the inner ear necessary for maintaining position and balance; transmits messages to the brain via the vestibular portion of the eighth cranial nerve.

VHF (very high frequency)   Radio frequency used in EMS systems.

Viscera   The soft organs within the body.

Visceral pain   Visceral or organ pain initiated by ischemia, stretching, or distention of an organ, e.g., intestinal obstruction. Visceral pain is perceived as diffuse and cramping or aching. It is often felt in an area quite removed from the anatomic source.

Visceral peritoneum   Inner layer of peritoneum that covers most of the organs of the abdomen.

Vital capacity   The maximum amount of air that can be exhaled after a maximum inspiration. Average vital capacity for a healthy adult is about 4500 to 5500 ml.

Vital signs   Temperature, respirations, heart rate, and blood pressure.

Vitreous humor   Jelly-like substance that fills the posterior chamber of the eye.

Vocal cords   Two folds of tissue in the larynx that vibrate as air passes between them, allowing speech.

Voluntary nervous system   The division of the nervous system that allows "willful", conscious activities such as walking, speech, and so forth.

Vulva   External female genitalia that includes the folds of skin called the labia majora and labia minora, clitoris, vaginal orifice, and urethral orifice.

Wheeled cot stretcher   The primary transport stretcher used by prehospital personnel that has a wheeled base and comes in multilevel, two-level, and single-level varieties.

Wheezing   High-pitched whistling sounds created by narrowed bronchioles.

White blood cells   Cells whose principle role is to combat and eliminate infecting organisms and foreign materials.

Wire ladder splints   Splints constructed of thin metal rods that are flexible and can be shaped and molded to conform to a fractured extremity.

Wrecking bar   A large device used for prying metal and for leverage in moving objects.

Zygoma   Connects the maxilla and the frontal and temporal bones.

Ulna   The bone forming the medial side of the forearm.

Ulnar artery   The artery located in the medial aspect of the forearm, palpable in the anterior wrist proximal to the little finger.

Umbilical arteries   The two small vessels in the umbilical cord that carry waste products away from the fetus to the placenta.

Umbilical cord   Structure that connects the fetus to the mother, allowing the exchange of nutrients and waste products. Contains three blood vessels surrounded by a clear, gelatinous substance.

Umbilical vein   The largest vessel in the umbilical cord; carries oxygenated and nourishing blood to the fetus.

Umbilicus   Navel.

Universal dressing   See *Multitrauma dressing*.

Universal precautions   Consistent use of appropriate blood and body fluid precautions for all patients, especially in emergency care settings.

Upper airway obstuction   Blockage in the air passages of the larynx, pharynx, or epiglottis.

Urea   End product of protein metabolism excreted in the urine.

Uremia   Buildup of urea in the bloodstream.

Uremic frost   White powdery substance found on the skin of uremic patients as the body attempts to sweat out waste products that the failing kidneys can no longer excrete.

Ureters   Narrow tubes that drain urine from the kidneys into the urinary bladder.

Urethra   Tube leading from the urinary bladder to the external genitalia through which urine is passed.

Urinary bladder   The storage bladder for urine, extending from the ureters to the urethra.

Uterine inversion   A dangerous condition where the uterus actually turns inside out.

Uterus   Hollow, muscular female reproductive organ in which the fetus grows.

Vaccination   Inoculation with a vaccine to establish immunity to a particular disease.

Vagina   The passageway between the cervix and the external female genitalia.

Vaginitis   Infection or inflammation of the vagina.

Vagus nerve   The tenth cranial nerve. Among other actions it carries parasympathetic impulses to the heart, which slow the heart's rate.

Vas deferens   Tube that transports sperm from the testicles to the urethra.

Vasodilation   Widening of the diameter of a blood vessel.

Vasodilatory shock   A state of shock due to loss of vascular tone and vasodilation as found in anaphylaxis and spinal cord injury.

Vectorborne transmission   Transmission of disease from one host to another by a vector, such as an insect.

Vehicle route transmission   Disease transmitted through contaminated items, such as transmission of hepatitis (non-A, non-B) by contaminated blood.

Vein   Blood vessels that return blood to the heart.

Vena cava   One of the major veins that returns blood from the upper and lower body to the heart.

Venom   Poison introduced by the bite or sting of an animal.

Venous return   Refers to the quantity of blood returning to the heart.

Ventilation   The inflow and outflow of air from the atmosphere to the air sacs (alveoli) in the terminal end of the pulmonary tree.

Ventricle   Thick-walled lower chamber of the heart that pumps blood to the lungs (right side) and the body (left side).

Ventricular fibrillation   A chaotic quivering of the heart caused by the firing of multiple ectopic (abnormal location) sites throughout the ventricle that results in cardiac arrest.

Ventricular tachycardia   A rapid dysrhythmia (rate 100 to 200 per minute) that originates within the ventricles and that may or may not be capable of producing a pulse.

Venturi mask   A high-flow mask used to deliver a precise amount of oxygen in a range of 24 to 70%.

Venules   Small veins that connect capillaries to larger veins.

Vernix   A white, creamy substance, much like hand cream, found on the skin of a newborn.

Vertebrae   Thirty-three irregular bones forming the spinal column, including 7 cervical, 12 thoracic, 5 lumbar, 5 sacral (fused), and 4 coccygeal (fused) vertebral bones.

Vesicular sounds   Soft, low-pitched breath sounds heard in most areas of the chest, which have a normally longer inspiratory phase.

Threatened abortion Vaginal bleeding in a pregnant patient with no dilatation of the cervix. There may be suprapubic cramping or pain referred to the lower back similar in nature to either menstrual cramps or labor pains.

Threshold braking The gentle, intermittent application of the brakes to the point just before they lock.

Thrombi (singular **Thrombus**) Blood clots.

Thrombus A blood clot that may or may not obstruct a blood vessel.

Thyroid Endocrine gland located at the base of the neck on both sides of the larynx.

Thyroid cartilage (Adam's apple) Band of cartilage above the cricoid cartilage.

Tibia The major weight-bearing bone of the lower leg; located on the anteromedial side of the lower leg.

Tidal volume Volume of air inspired and expired during one respiratory cycle. Normal tidal volume at rest is approximately 500 cc.

Tin snips A hand-held device used to cut through sheet metal such as roofs or door panels.

Tissue A group of cells working together to serve a given function, e.g., muscle tissue, nerve tissue, connective tissue, and epithelial tissue.

Total lung capacity The total amount of air that the lung can contain after a maximum inspiration. Includes both the *vital capacity* and the *residual volume*. The average total lung capacity for an adult is about 6000 cc.

Tourniquet A constricting band applied over an extremity with enough pressure to completely obliterate blood flow beyond the site of application.

Toxicology The study of poisons.

Trachea Windpipe; part of the airway that connects the larynx to the bronchi.

Tracheal Referring to the trachea; *tracheal sounds* are loud, very high-pitched windy breath sounds heard directly over the trachea that have a relatively equal inspiratory and expiratory phase.

Tracheostomy Surgical opening of the trachea to provide an airway.

Traction splint A device consisting of a metal frame and a pulley system to apply traction to the lower extremity.

Transient ischemic attack (TIA) A temporary loss of brain function secondary to diminished blood supply to part of the brain that completely resolves within 12 hours.

Transition The last phase of the first stage of labor during which the cervix progresses from 8 cm to full dilatation. Contractions are usually strong, long lasting, and close together during this period.

Transverse fractures Fractures at a right angle across the bone; usually produced by a direct force applied perpendicular to a bone.

Traumatic iritis Traumatically induced spasm of the iris muscle; should not be confused with the unilateral fixed and dilated pupil seen with herniation of the brain.

Triage To sort or to choose. The sorting of casualties of war or other disaster to determine the priority of need and proper place of treatment.

Triangular bandage Versatile bandage cut diagonally from a 36- to 42-inch square of cloth, usually muslin. The cloth is folded into a triangle and used for a variety of things, including slings, cravats, and tourniquets.

Tricuspid valve Valve with three flaps located between the right atrium and the right ventricle.

Trimester Any of the three equal periods of time into which the 40 weeks of pregnancy are arbitrarily divided.

Tuberculosis A communicable disease most commonly affecting the respiratory system caused by tubercle bacillus.

Tympanic membrane Eardrum.

Type I ambulance An ambulance designed with a modular box patient compartment mounted on a truck-style chassis.

Type II ambulance Van-style ambulance.

Type III ambulance An ambulance designed with a modular box patient compartment mounted on a van chassis.

Type I diabetics (insulin-dependent diabetics) Patients who have a severe or absolute lack of insulin. Also referred to as *juvenile diabetes*.

Type II diabetics (non–insulin-dependent diabetics) Patients who usually have developed diabetes later in life and may not require insulin injections as part of their treatment. Also referred to as *maturity-onset diabetes*.

Typhoid fever A communicable disease caused by *Salmonella typhi*.

UHF (ultra high frequency) Radio frequency used in EMS systems that is between super high and very high frequency.

Stoma A surgical opening in the neck ("neck breathers"). CPR must be modified to provide mouth-to-stoma breathing directly through the opening.

Stomach A J-shaped hollow, muscular organ of the digestive tract, located in the left upper quadrant of the abdomen between the esophagus and the duodenum.

Stopping friction Friction created by contact of the tire with the road during braking and deceleration.

Strain An injury to a muscle due to stretching beyond normal range.

Stress fractures Fractures that result from overuse or continuous activity.

Stridor A harsh, high-pitched sound created by air flowing through a narrowed upper airway; usually heard on inspiration.

Stroke volume The amount of blood ejected with each contraction of the heart (for normal adult = 70 ml).

Stupor A state of lessened responsiveness. The patient can be aroused, but more stimuli are required than for the lethargic patient.

Subarachnoid hemorrhage Bleeding in the space between the arachnoid and the pia mater.

Subconjunctival hematoma Red blotches on the sclera caused by leakage of small capillaries.

Subcutaneous Beneath the skin; an injection site in the fatty layer of tissues beneath the skin.

Subcutaneous emphysema Entrapment of air beneath the skin as a result of trauma to the airways, lung, esophagus, or skin; characterized by deformity and crepitus of the skin.

Subcutaneous tissue Layer of insulating fat and connective tissue beneath the skin.

Subdural hematomas Hematoma underneath the dura mater, caused by bleeding from the venous network.

Sudden cardiac death Spontaneous, sudden, and unexpected cardiac arrest.

Superficial Toward the surface.

Superior Toward the head.

Supine The position of a body lying on its back.

Supine hypotensive syndrome Sudden hypotension that occurs when a pregnant woman lies supine; caused by compression of the vena cava between the spinal column and the heavy, pregnant uterus.

Suprapubic region The region just above the pubic bone.

Surfactant Substance found in the lungs that increases surface tension and is vital to respiration. Surfactant is diminished or absent in the lungs of a premature infant.

Sympathetic nervous system A division of the autonomic nervous system that modulates an organ's activity; it may cause, for example, the heart rate to increase or the pupils to dilate.

Symphysis pubis The articulation of the pubic bones; a fused joint.

Syncope Transient loss of consciousness.

Systole Contraction phase of the heart.

Systolic blood pressure The blood pressure measured during the contraction phase (systole) of the heart noted by the first sound heard through a stethoscope when taking a blood pressure.

T wave The waveform on an ECG that represents ventricular repolarization. It is the positive deflection following the QRS complex.

Tachypnea Rapid breathing.

Tarsal bones The bones that form the ankle.

Telemetry A method by which biologic data are transferred from one location to another by radio transmissions.

Temporal artery Artery supplying blood to the scalp that is palpable just anterior to the ear.

Temporal bones The bones forming the lateral aspect of the cranium just superior and anterior to the ear.

Tendons Tough connective tissue bands that connect muscle to bone and serve to pull or move bones as muscles contract.

Tension pneumothorax Air trapped in the pleural space due to a one-way valve effect created on the lung wall, which results in increased intrathoracic pressure, respiratory failure, and obstructive shock.

Testicles Male organs of reproduction that contain sperm and semen and produce the male hormone testosterone.

Tetanus ("lockjaw") An infectious disease caused by the bacillus *Clostridium tetani* and its toxins.

Third stage of labor Period that begins when the baby has been born and ends with the delivery of the placenta.

Thoracic vertebrae The twelve vertebrae that are located in the posterior thorax and are the main support for the rib cage.

Sigmoid colon   S-shaped end segment of the large intestines; empties into the rectum.

Simple face mask   A low-flow oxygen device capable of providing oxygen concentrations ranging from 30 to 60% at flow rates of 5 to 12 liters per minute.

Sinoatrial (SA) node   Pacemaker of the heart, located in the right atrium.

Situational reactions   Emotional responses that are a reaction to sudden illness, a death in the family, or some other difficult personal experience.

Skin   The largest organ of the body; provides protective covering and insulation, is a barrier to infection and loss of body fluids, and is important for regulation of body temperature.

Skull   The bones forming the head, consisting of the cranium, the face, and the lower jaw or mandible.

Slim Jim   A device used to open the lock of a car door.

Sling and swathe   An immobilization method using a sling to support an injured extremity with a wrap around the extremity and chest wall.

Small intestine   Small-lumened portion of the digestive tract that contains the duodenum, jejunum, and ileum.

Snoring   A harsh, low-pitched sound usually caused by the tongue partially blocking the upper airway.

Soft tissues   Skin, subcutaneous layer of fat and connective tissue beneath the skin, and the skeletal muscles, tendons, and ligaments.

Source (infectious)   A person, an insect, an object, or another substance that carries or is contaminated by an infectious agent.

Sperm   The male reproductive cell

Spermatic cord   Cord that passes down from the abdomen through the inguinal canal, suspending the testicles in the scrotum.

Spinal column   Thirty-three vertebrae extending from the base of the skull to the tail bone, consisting of 7 cervical, 12 thoracic, 5 lumbar, 5 sacral (fused), and 4 coccygeal (fused) vertebrae.

Spinal cord   The portion of the central nervous system that emerges from the brainstem and is a continuation of nerve tracts from all parts of the brain.

Spinal discs   Soft connective tissue discs that separate vertebra and serve as cushions for shock absorption within the spinal column.

Spinal nerves   Thirty-one pairs of nerves that exit the spinal column. They are grouped as follows: 8 cervical, 12 thoracic, 5 lumbar, 5 sacral, 1 coccygeal.

Spiral fractures   Fractures with long, sharp, pointed bone ends that are produced by twisting or rotatory forces.

Spleen   Organ located under the left diaphragm; contains lymphatic tissue designed to filter the blood and also to produce lymphatic cells.

Spongy bone   Light, lattice-like bone located in flat and irregular bones and in the ends of long bones.

Spontaneous abortion (miscarriage)   Passing of the fetus before 20 weeks of gestation. After 20 weeks of gestation the delivery of a dead fetus would be called a *stillbirth*.

Sprain   An injury to a ligament due to stretching beyond normal range.

Spring-loaded center punch   A spring-operated punch used to break a windshield or window glass to gain access to the passengers in an extrication.

Sputum   Substance expelled from the lungs or throat.

Stair chair   A folding chair used to carry patients who are able to assume the sitting position.

Standardization marker   A control switch on an ECG machine that "standardizes" the voltage of the ECG reading.

Standing orders   The portion of EMS protocols that deals with procedures that may be performed without contacting the medical control physician of a given system.

Starling's law   The force of a contraction is determined by the amount of distention of the fibers of the ventricle during the diastolic filling.

Status epilepticus   A rapid succession of epileptic attacks without an intervening period of consciousness or prolonged continuous seizures.

Sterile field   An area that is established for placement of sterile instruments and that is kept free from contamination.

Sternal retractions   An abnormal sucking in of the sternum of a newborn during respiration; a sign of respiratory distress in a newborn.

Sternum   The breast bone; composed of an upper section (manubrium) middle section (body), and lower section (xiphoid process).

Stimulants   Drugs that result in increased functional activity, such as increased excitability, increased heart rate, or increased gastrointestinal activity.

Stokes basket   A wire mesh stretcher used for specialized and high-angle rescue.

Rigid splints Splints made of a rigid material such as cardboard, wood, metal, or plastic.

Rigor mortis A state of body stiffness that is caused by the depletion of proteins in muscles following death.

Rolling friction Friction created by rolling tires in contact with the road that provides directional control during movement of a vehicle.

Rubella (German measles) A communicable disease spread by respiratory droplets and contact with secretions.

S wave The waveform on an ECG that is the first negative deflection following the R wave.

Sacral vertebrae The portion of the spinal column that is fused with the pelvis to form the pelvic girdle.

Salivary glands Glands that secrete saliva to aid in digestion; located on each side of the face below the ear and within the oral cavity.

Scabies A communicable skin disease caused by a mite.

Scalene muscles Accessory muscles of inspiration in the neck that elevate the upper ribs.

Scapula The shoulder blade.

SCBA Self-contained breathing apparatus.

Scene survey Phase of patient assessment during which the scene is evaluated for safety, numbers of victims, and extent and mechanism of injuries.

Sclera Tough, fibrous, and opaque protective membrane that covers the eye.

Scoop stretcher A specialized device consisting of an aluminum frame and a rectangular tube with shovel-type lateral flaps for sliding under the patient.

Scrotum Pouch of skin that contains the testes and the epididymis.

Sebaceous glands Glands in the dermis that secrete an oily substance called sebum, which helps moisten the skin.

Second stage of labor The period that begins with full dilation of the cervix and ends when the baby is delivered.

Secondary brain injury Later complications that a patient might experience that would cause further brain injury, including increased intracranial pressure, hypoxia, hypoglycemia, hypotension, infection.

Secondary survey Final phase of patient assessment, which includes patient history, vital signs, and head-to-toe survey.

Sedative-hypnotics A group of drugs used to decrease excitability (sedatives) and to help induce sleep (hypnotics).

Seizure A temporary alteration in behavior due to abnormal electrical activity in the brain.

Self-adherent bandage Roll of slightly elastic, gauze-like material that can be wrapped around a dressing on the affected part or extremity. The self-adherent quality makes it easy to work with and allows for its rapid application.

Semiautomatic defibrillators Defibrillators that interpret the patients ECG status and advise the operator of the need or the lack of the need for defibrillation. In the event that defibrillation is needed, the operator proceeds to initiate a defibrillation by pushing a control button.

Semicircular canals Part of the inner ear concerned with position sense.

Semi-coma A condition of unconsciousness or lack of awareness of the environment from which the patient may be aroused.

Semilunar valves Either of two valves separating the ventricles from the outlet arteries.

Sensory nerves Nerves that carry messages back to the brain from sense organs throughout the body.

Septic abortion An abortion with pelvic and/or peritoneal infection.

Septic shock A form of shock resulting from a widely disseminated infection that results in vasodilation and hypovolemia.

Septum A dividing wall such as the wall separating the right and left sides of the heart.

Shock The failure of the circulatory system to adequately perfuse and oxygenate the vital organs of the body.

Short spine board A device used to immobilize and extricate automobile accident victims found in the sitting position.

Shoulder dystocia A condition where the baby's head will deliver spontaneously but the baby's shoulders become wedged in the mother's pelvis.

Shoulder presentation The baby is in the transverse position in the uterus, with the shoulder presenting into the mother's pelvis.

Sickle cell crisis Obstruction of blood flow caused by abnormal sickle-shaped red blood cells; occurs with the hereditary disease *sickle cell anemia* and may present with severe abdominal pain much like that of appendicitis.

Pulse pressure The difference between the systolic pressure and the diastolic pressure; normal pulse pressure is between 30 and 40 mm Hg.

Pump failure Failure of the heart to meet the body's basic oxygen needs. This can be a result of either decreased force of contractions or an abnormal heart rhythm.

Puncture wound Penetrating wound caused by a sharp, pointed object.

Pupil Opening in the front of the eye surrounded by the iris.

Purkinje fibers Impulse-conducting fibers in the myocardium that stimulate contraction.

Pus Liquid product of inflammation; contains white blood cells and a fluid.

Pyelonephritis Inflammation of the kidney, usually caused by infection.

Q wave The waveform on an ECG that is the first downward deflection that occurs before the first positive deflection, or R wave, of the QRS complex.

QRS complex The waveform on an ECG that reflects the depolarization of the ventricles.

Quality assurance Methods for ensuring a high level of patient care.

Raccoon's sign Black and blue areas or ecchymosis around the eyes suggestive of a basilar skull fracture.

Radial artery The artery located in the lateral aspect of the forearm, palpable at the wrist just proximal to the thumb.

Radius The bone forming the lateral side of the forearm.

Rales Crackling sounds heard in the lungs; can result from fluid in the alveoli or airways.

Rapid extrication procedure A specialized rescue removal technique used to quickly extricate a patient from an automobile wreck with minimal flexion, extension, or rotation of the spinal column.

Rectum Most distal section of the digestive tract, where feces is stored until evacuation.

Red blood cells The blood cells that constitute the largest portion of the cellular component; they contain hemoglobin.

Redistribution In hemorrhage, a compensatory response in which there is a reduction of blood flow to the skin, muscles, and digestive system, so that the remaining blood is available to perfuse the vital organs.

Reflectors Traffic-delineation devices, including glass or plastic reflectors, flares, traffic cones, and battery-operated lights.

Reflex activity A type of action mediated through the reflex arc along each segment of the spinal cord, e.g., removal of a hand from a burning object.

Regularly irregular ECG rhythms that have an irregular but distinct pattern that recurs at periodic intervals.

Regulator Device that reduces the very high pressure of gas within a cylinder to a level that will not injure the patient.

Renal colic Severe intermittent pain, usually felt in the back or flank, caused by peristaltic spasms as a kidney stone passes from the kidney through the ureters, causing a partial or total obstruction to the flow of urine.

Repeater systems Strategically based receivers and transmitters that accept the signal from the portable unit or mobile radio and relay it with a more powerful transmitter.

Reservoir (infectious) A source in which infectious agents can live and multiply, such as a sewer.

Residual volume The amount of air that remains in the lungs after a forceful expiration.

Resistance Opposing or counterforce; the inherent ability to resist disease from a microorganism or toxin.

Respiratory arrest Cessation of breathing.

Respiratory failure The state that exists when the respiratory system becomes so ineffective that it can no longer support life.

Respiratory rate Number of breaths taken per minute, normally 12 to 20.

Respiratory shock Shock due to respiratory failure.

Retina Posterior wall of the eye composed of millions of sensory receptors that convert light into nervous impulses that are then transmitted to the brain.

Retroperitoneal space Space behind the peritoneum, bordered anteriorly by the peritoneum and posteriorly by the spine and muscles; contains the kidneys, ureters, adrenal glands, pancreas, portions of the intestinal tract (duodenum), and major vessels, particularly the abdominal aorta and the inferior vena cava.

Rhonchi Low-pitched continuous sounds with a snoring quality created by obstruction in the larger airways.

Polyuria   Passage of abnormally large amounts of urine.

Popliteal artery   An artery beginning in the lower thigh and passing behind the knee, where it may be palpated.

Portal system   A system of veins that receives branches from the esophagus, the stomach, and the small intestine and brings blood to the liver for conversion and storage of nutrients and removal of waste products.

Positive-pressure ventilation   The act of positively forcing air into the lungs.

Posterior   Structures toward the rear of the body.

Posterior tibial artery   The artery passing just behind the ankle bone, where it is palpable between the medial malleolus and the Achilles tendon.

Postmature   Beyond 42 weeks of pregnancy.

Postpartum   Occurring after delivery.

Postpartum hemorrhage   A blood loss of greater than 500 ml that occurs after delivery.

PR interval   The ECG interval that starts with the beginning of the P wave and ends with the QRS complex, between 0.12 and 0.20 second, and reflects atrial depolarization and conduction through the AV node.

Preeclampsia   Hypertension, proteinuria, and edema after the 20th week of pregnancy.

Premature   Before the 38th week of pregnancy.

Presentation   Refers to the part of the baby's body that first enters the pelvis. In *vertex presentation*, the baby is sharply flexed with his chin on his chest, and the occipital or vertex portion of his head is the first portion of his body to enter the pelvis. In *frank breech*, the breech or buttocks are lowermost in the pelvis. In *footling breech*, one or more of the feet enter the pelvis first.

Presenting part   The part of the baby that first enters the pelvis, or the lowermost part.

Pressure-compensated flowmeter   Flowmeter that uses a gravity-regulated ball on a vertical meter to register the flow.

Pressure face   Discoloration of a newborn's face caused by a widespread rupture of tiny surface blood vessels in the baby's face during the birthing process.

Pressure points   Common pulse points where pressure can be applied to collapse an artery and thereby reduce or stop blood flow to a wound.

Priapism   A sustained penile erection.

Primagravida   A pregnant woman who is about to have her first baby.

Primary survey   Phase of patient assessment during which life-threatening conditions are identified and treated.

Progesterone   Hormone produced by the ovaries and the placenta that prepares the body for and permits the continuation of pregnancy.

Prolapsed cord   Slipping of the umbilical cord down past the presenting part.

Prolapsed uterus   A condition where the supporting structures of the uterus fail so that the uterus dips out of the vagina.

Prostate gland   Gland surrounding the neck of the bladder and the upper urethra in males; when enlarged or inflamed (prostatitis), the prostate may cause urinary retention.

Protective custody   The process by which an emotionally disturbed or incompetent patient who is a danger to self or others is moved to a medical facility by police and emergency personnel.

Protocol   Written procedures that guide the EMT in the specific care of a patient; usually established by the physician or physicians who provide local supervision of a given EMS system.

Proximal   Closer to the trunk.

Psychedelic   A group of drugs such as LSD that cause hallucinogenic effects or intensified perception.

Psychogenic shock   Fainting caused by a strong emotional reaction that results in stimulation of the parasympathetic nervous system and vasodilator nerves. The result is dilatation of the blood vessels and a slowing of the heart rate, the combination of which is sufficient to result in fainting.

Psychosis   Disordered thought; the patient has distorted perceptions of reality, with hallucinations and inappropriate responses to the environment.

Pulmonary artery   The artery leaving the right ventricle that returns deoxygenated blood to the lungs.

Pulmonary edema   Fluid in the alveoli, airways, or interstitial space of the lungs.

Pulmonary valve   Semilunar valve between the right ventricle and the pulmonary artery.

Penis   Male organ of reproduction and urination.

Peptic ulcer   Ulcer or hole in the lower end of the esophagus, the stomach, or the duodenum, caused by digestive acids.

Perforation   Tear or hole.

Pericardial tamponade   Accumulation of fluid or air in the pericardial space, leading to compression of the heart's chambers and resulting in the obstruction of venous return to the heart.

Pericarditis   Inflammation or infection of the pericardium.

Pericardium   Double-layered sac surrounding the heart.

Perineum   The pelvic floor.

Periorbital ecchymosis   Bruising around the eyes.

Periosteum   A two layer, hard fibrous membrane that covers bone except at the articular surfaces of joints.

Peripheral   Away from the center of the body.

Peripheral nervous system   The nerves outside the central nervous system, leaving from both the brainstem and the spinal cord.

Peripheral vascular resistance   The sum total of the resistance provided by blood vessels that contributes to the maintenance of blood pressure.

Peristalsis   Wavelike contractions of smooth muscle.

Peritoneal cavity   The space between the visceral and parietal peritoneum.

Peritoneum   The lining of the abdominal cavity and some of it organs.

Peritonitis   Inflammation of the peritoneal cavity.

Periumbilical   The region surrounding the umbilicus.

Permeability   The quality of allowing the passage of fluid and/or substances through a structure, such as a capillary wall or a cell wall.

Pertussis ("whooping cough")   A communicable disease characterized by sudden coughing episodes.

Phalanges   The finger or toe bones.

Pharynx   The passage, extending from the back of the nasal cavity and mouth down to the esophagus and larynx.

Phenols   Also called carbolic acids; used in industry and found in preservatives or disinfectants; can penetrate skin and be absorbed systemically.

Phenothiazines   A class of psychotherapeutic drugs.

Phrenic nerve   Nerve that arises from the spinal cord in the neck and that stimulates the diaphragm to contract.

Physiology   The study of processes and activities of the living organism and its parts.

Pit vipers   A class of poisonous snakes characterized by their elliptical pupils, the pit (heat sensor) between the eyes and nostril, fangs, and a single row of subcaudal plates on the tail.

Placenta   An organ of pregnancy through which nutrients and waste products are exchanged between the mother and the fetus. Also referred to as the "afterbirth," since it is expelled after the baby is born.

Placenta accreta   A condition where the placenta has grown into the uterine wall and will not separate.

Placenta previa   Abnormally low implantation of the placenta so that it covers all or part of the cervical opening.

Plasma   The liquid portion of blood; constitutes 55 to 65% of the blood volume.

Plasma proteins   Proteins floating in plasma (too large to diffuse through the capillary wall) that provide the "pulling force" needed to keep fluid within the vascular space.

Platelets   Disc-shaped bodies in the blood necessary for blood clotting.

Pleura   Serous membranes that line the chest wall (parietal pleura) and cover the lungs (visceral pleura).

Pleuritic chest pain   Pain resulting from or made worse by breathing or coughing.

Pneumonia   An inflammation of alveolar spaces caused by various types of infecting organisms or by aspiration of fluid into the tracheobronchial tree.

Pneumothorax   Air within the pleural space.

Pocket mask   A transparent, semirigid mask used to prevent direct contact with the patient and to give supplemental oxygen during mouth-to-mask ventilations. The mask is sealed by placing the heel of each hand on the border of the mask's edge.

Poison   A substance that, through its chemical action, is harmful and kills, injuries, or impairs an organism.

Polio   An acute communicable disease affecting the central nervous system.

Orthopnea Difficulty breathing when lying down and relieved by sitting up or standing.

Orthostatic change Signs of weakness, an increase in heart rate, or a fall in blood pressure caused by a change from the recumbent to the sitting or standing position.

OSHA Occupational Safety and Health Administration.

Osmosis The process whereby a solvent (water) moves across a membrane (which prevents passage of particles) from an area of lower concentration of particles to an area of higher concentration of particles.

Osteoporosis A decrease in the amount of bone tissue occurring in old age due to more bone breakdown than bone formation, resulting in weaker bones.

Ovaries Female sex glands responsible for housing and maturing the eggs and also for the production of hormones

Overdose Results when a drug is taken in excess or in combination with other agents, to the point where poisoning occurs.

Ovulation Release of a mature egg from one of the ovaries.

Ovum The female reproductive cell.

Oxyhemoglobin Hemoglobin bound to oxygen. Bright red in color, oxyhemoglobin accounts for the pink appearance of the lips and nail beds.

Oxytocin A hormone produced by the pituitary gland that causes the uterus to contract.

P wave The first waveform on an ECG that represents the depolarization of the atria.

Pacemaker SA node; group of cells that initiate the electrical impulses in the heart. Also, a mechanical device implanted to control certain arrhythmias, to provide a backup if the SA node fails, or to serve as the pacemaker.

Packaging The process of immobilizing and securing a victim to a transport device.

Palpation Examination of the patient by touch.

Palpitations Common fluttering sensations in the chest, often described as the heart skipping a beat or a rapid heartbeat.

Pancreas Gland in the upper abdomen behind the stomach responsible for production of insulin and glucagon and many enzymes necessary for digestion.

Pancreatitis Inflammation of the pancreas.

Paradoxical breathing Abnormal breathing as a result of instability of a section of chest wall where the flail segment is moving in the direction opposite that of the intact chest wall.

Paranoia A condition where a patient feels unduly threatened by his or her environment and the person or persons with whom he or she is in contact.

Parasternals Accessory muscles of inspiration that pull up on the cartilaginous portion of the ribs adjacent to the sternum.

Parasympathetic nervous system A division of the autonomic nervous system that modulates an organ's activity, such as slowing of the heart rate or constriction of the pupil.

Paresthesia An abnormal sensation of numbness, tingling, burning, itching, or prickling of the skin.

Parietal bones Bones that form the superior and lateral surfaces of the cranium.

Parietal peritoneum Outer layer of the peritoneum that lines the abdominal cavity.

Paroxysmal nocturnal dyspnea Sudden night-time shortness of breath caused by the gravitational shifting of blood volume and resulting edema in the lungs while sleeping.

PASG Pneumatic anti-shock garment. Air-filled pants that surround the legs and the abdomen; when inflated can be used to treat shock states, immobilize fractures, and control bleeding.

Patella The kneecap.

Pathogenic Causing or producing disease.

Pathologic fractures Fractures that result when diseases have destroyed and weakened bone to the point where minimal stress may lead to fracture.

Patient data Identification information provided by the patient or family of the patient, including the name, sex, age, date of birth, and address of the patient.

PCP (phencyclidine hydrochloride) An anesthetic used in veterinary medicine that is abused for its hallucinogenic effects. Commonly called angel dust.

Pelvic girdle A ring of bones formed by the sacrum and the pelvic bones, including the ileum (2, left and right), the ischium (2), and the pubis (2).

Pelvic inflammatory disease (PID) Ascending infection of the female reproductive tract.

Pelvic inlet Upper part of the pelvic girdle.

Pelvic outlet The lowermost margin of the pelvic cavity through which the fetus must pass to be born.

Myocardial infarction Severe and sustained oxygen deprivation of the myocardium resulting in the death of heart cells; commonly known as *heart attack*.

Myocardial ischemia A state of decreased blood flow to the heart.

Myocardium Muscular middle layer of the heart, which performs the work of contraction.

Naloxone (Narcan) An antidote to narcotics that rapidly reverses the respiratory depression and mental depression caused by narcotics.

Nares The external openings in the nose.

Nasal cannula A low-flow oxygen delivery system, consisting of a thin tube with prongs at the end that slip into the nares, capable of delivering 24 to 40% of oxygen.

Nasal septum A dividing wall between the nostrils, made of cartilage and bone.

Nasopharyngeal airway A soft rubber tube that extends from the nares down into the oropharynx; used to elevate the tongue away from the oropharynx.

Negative pressure Relative vacuum in the pleural space that keeps the lungs expanded.

Neurogenic shock A distributive form of shock that results from injury to the central nervous system causing dilation of blood vessels.

Nitrites A group of drugs that are used as an antidote for cyanide poisoning.

Nitroglycerin Medication usually placed under the tongue for absorption; it reduces the work of the heart by decreasing peripheral vascular resistance while at the same time improving blood flow to the myocardium by dilating the coronary arteries.

Non-rebreather mask A low-flow, high-oxygen concentration device consisting of a reservoir bag beneath a one-way valve that prevents the patient from exhaling into the bag; best used when high concentrations of oxygen are needed, since it can achieve oxygen concentrations up to 90%.

Normal sinus rhythm (NSR) A normal ECG rhythm with a rate of 60 to 100 times a minute.

Nosocomial infections Infectious disease spread by health care workers or within a health care setting.

Oblique fractures Fractures produced by a twisting force with an upward thrust that results in an oblique angle across the bone.

Obstructive shock Shock that results in an obstruction of arterial or venous flow, caused by tension pneumothorax, pericardial tamponade, or embolism.

Occipital bone Posterior bone of the cranium.

Occlusive dressing Airtight dressing usually using sterile plastic wrap, aluminum foil, or petrolatum impregnated gauze.

Omentum Large fold of peritoneum in the anterior abdominal cavity.

Oncotic pressure The "pulling force" created by plasma proteins that retains fluid in the vascular space.

Open disaster A disaster spread over a large open area such as a field where there is easy access to the victims.

Open or compound fracture Fractures that communicate with the external environment because the skin above the fracture site has been broken.

Opioids ("narcotics") A special class of depressants that alter the perception of pain and in overdose may cause a depressed mental status and respiratory arrest.

Optic nerve Cranial nerve that services the eye.

Orbit The outer ridges of the eye socket, made up of the edges of the maxilla, zygoma, and frontal bones.

Orbital muscles Muscles that move the eye.

Organ A structure composed of several types of tissues that work together to serve a given function, e.g., stomach.

Organ system A group of organs working together to perform complex functions, e.g., respiratory system.

Organic brain syndromes A group of disorders associated with brain damage and impaired cerebral function that result in disordered thought, disorientation, confusion, difficulty with attention, or even varying levels of alertness.

Organophosphate A poisonous pesticide.

Orientation A person's awareness of person, place, and time.

Oropharyngeal airway A basic airway device; designed to elevate the tongue away from the oropharynx in unconscious states.

Oropharynx The oral cavity, lying between the soft palate and the epiglottis.

Mediastinum   The space in the center of the chest that contains the heart, great vessels, esophagus and trachea (windpipe), and mainstem bronchi.

Medical control   The active participation of physicians in all phases of the EMS system. Medical control includes protocol development, needs assessment of the system, education, quality assurance, and outcome studies as well as medical direction via telemetry.

Megacolon   Massively dilated segment of the large intestine caused by the collection of fecal material and water in a nonfunctioning colon.

Melanin   Pigment in the epidermis that colors the skin and protects against the sun's radiation.

Melena   Blood in the stool; seen as black, tarry stools with a distinct foul odor.

Meninges   The membranous coverings of the brain and spinal cord consisting of three layers: the *dura* is the tough, leathery outer layer closest to the skull and vertebral column; the *arachnoid* is the middle layer; and the *pia* is the innermost layer, which is adherent to the brain tissue itself.

Meningitis   An inflammation of the coverings of the brain.

Menstruation   Shedding of the lining of the uterus when pregnancy does not occur.

Mental status   Level of consciousness, orientation, verbal behavior, and ability to respond.

Mesentery   Large fold of peritoneum in the posterior abdominal cavity.

Metabolic injuries   Injuries to cells that occur when the energy processes necessary for life are compromised, as by hypoxia or hypoglycemia.

Metacarpal bones   The bones of the hand.

Metaphyses   The ends of the bone shaft.

Methadone   A synthetic narcotic used in the treatment of addiction to opiate-derivative drugs.

Methanol   A poisonous form of alcohol found as "dry gas," windshield washing solution, and fuel for warming food (Sterno).

Microcirculation   The continuous movement of fluids and solutes out of the capillaries and back in from the interstitial fluid.

Microorganisms   Organisms not visible to the naked eye.

Middle ear   Air-filled cavity containing three tiny bones, the *malleus* (hammer), *incus* (anvil), and *stapes* (stirrup), which transmit sound waves from the tympanic membrane of the external ear to the oval window of the inner ear.

Milia   Clogged pores seen as small white spots on a newborn's nose and chin. Milia are harmless and will disappear spontaneously.

Minute volume   Tidal volume × respiratory rate.

Missed abortion   Retention of the fetus for 4 or more weeks after fetal death has occurred.

Mitral valve   Valve with two flaps that is located between the left atrium and the left ventricle.

Molding   Temporary change in shape of the fetal head to allow passage of the head through the pelvis.

Molecules   Small particles made up of more than one atom, which form a chemical substance.

Mononucleosis   Acute infectious disease characterized by swelling of the lymph glands and the spleen.

Morphine   A highly addictive opiate derivative widely used for its analgesic and sedative effects.

Motor and sensory examination   The neurologic examination that tests for the ability to feel and to move body parts.

Motor nerves   Nerves that carry messages to the muscles and various organs to initiate a particular activity.

Mucous membranes   Skin rich in mucus-secreting glands that line the body orifices, such as the linings of the nasopharynx, urethra, bladder, lungs, intestines, and vagina.

Multitrauma dressing (universal dressing)   Large sterile dressing made of thick absorbent material, measuring 9 × 36 inches in size, used to cover large areas of burns or abrasions, as a pressure dressing, or for padding for splints.

Mumps   A communicable viral disease causing inflammation of the parotid glands and other salivary glands.

Muscles   Tissue capable of contraction or shortening. The three types of muscles are *skeletal*, which is striated muscle used for motor functions; *smooth*, which is muscle in structures with autonomic functions, e.g., blood vessels: and *cardiac*, which is the heart muscle.

Mutual aid   A predetermined response system with neighboring communities that ensures a large-scale response of emergency vehicles and personnel, including police, fire department, and ambulances, during a catastrophic incidence.

Lateral recumbent   The position of a body lying on its side.

Lateral rotation   Rotation of an extremity toward the side of the body.

Lay rescuers   A lay person trained in CPR or other first-aid skills.

Lead   A specific arrangement of ECG electrodes, consisting of positive and negative poles, to view the electrical activity of the heart.

LeFort I fracture   A transverse fracture above the roots of the teeth, with instability of the upper teeth and the upper palate.

LeFort II fracture   A fractured triangular segment containing the nasal bones and the frontal process of the maxilla, with instability of the nose as well as the upper teeth.

LeFort III fracture   Fracture line extending through the maxilla, nasal bones, and zygomas, causing instability of the entire midface relative to the base of the skull.

Left atrium   Relatively thin-walled left upper chamber of the heart that receives oxygenated blood from the lungs.

Left ventricle   Thick-walled lower left chamber of the heart that pumps blood to the entire body.

Lethargy   A sleepy, depressed state where the patient may still be arousable with painful and verbal stimuli.

Lice   Small, wingless parasites that can infest the head, body, or pubic area.

Ligaments   Connective tissue that attaches bone to bone.

Linear skull fracture   A skull fracture characterized by a line of non-union or a crack along a bone of the cranium.

Liver   Large, solid organ located in the right upper quadrant of the abdomen; responsible for many valuable tasks, including the filtering of toxins from the bloodstream, the secretion of bile, and the processing of nutrients.

Log roll   A rotation technique used to slide an immobilization device under a patient with minimal flexion, extension, or rotation of the spinal column.

Long spine board   A flat wooden, plastic, or metal device used to maintain spinal immobilization.

Lower airway obstruction   Blockage in the tracheobronchial tree.

LSD (lysergic acid diethylamide)   An abused hallucinatory agent.

Lumbar vertebrae   The five vertebrae that form the lower part of the spinal column extending from the thoracic to the sacral spine.

Lymphatic system   A network of lymph capillaries that drain into larger and larger vessels until they ultimately drain into the right and left subclavian veins.

Main stem bronchi   The first division of the bronchial tree.

Mammalian diving reflex   A reflex mechanism that slows down metabolism, resulting in decreased oxygen consumption and redistribution of blood to more vital organs; occurs upon submersion in cold water and increases the chance for successful resuscitation in cases of cold water drowning.

Mandible   Bone that forms the lower jaw.

Manually triggered demand valve resuscitator   Oxygen-powered, high-pressure apparatus for positive-pressure ventilation; activated by a push button or lever located on the valve or by the negative pressure created by a breathing patient.

Marrow   Substance contained in the center of the shafts of long bones and within the meshwork of spongy bone; responsible for the production of red blood cells.

MAST   Military anti-shock trousers. See *PASG*.

Mastic knife   A razor-sharp, curved device used to remove a windshield and seatbelts.

Mastication   Chewing.

Maxilla   Bone that forms the upper jaw.

McRobert's maneuver   Positioning a pregnant woman flat on her back with her legs spread widely apart and flexed sharply on either side of her abdomen.

Measles   A communicable disease spread by respiratory droplets and contact with nasal secretions.

Meatus   External opening.

Mechanism of injury   The manner in which an injury was incurred; helps in recognizing the type and extent of injury.

Meconium   The substance that makes up the stool of a fetus or newborn.

Medial rotation   Rotation of an extremity toward the midline of the body.

Medial   Toward the midline.

Inner ear   Innermost portion of the ear consisting of the vestibule, three semicircular canals extending at right angles to each other, and the cochlea.

Insecticides   Substances used to kill insects.

Insulin   Hormone produced by the pancreas; necessary for glucose metabolism.

Integumentary system   The skin.

Intercostal nerves   Nerves that arise from the spinal cord in the thorax, travel along the respective ribs, and stimulate the intercostal muscles to contract.

Internal intercostals   Accessory muscles of expiration that pull the ribs down and inward.

Internal os   The innermost part of the opening between the cervix and the vagina.

Interstitial fluid   Fluid surrounding body tissues that is the source for intake of nutrients into the cell and secretion of wastes and other products made within the cell to the outside.

Intestinal infarction   Death of bowel tissue.

Intestine   A tubular organ of the digestive system responsible for the processing and digestion and absorption of food. The *small intestine* is the narrower portion of the tube, over 20 feet long, into which partially digested food is first emptied from the stomach. The *large intestine* is the last, large-lumened portion of the intestine responsible for the absorption of water from intestinal contents and for formation of feces.

Intracerebral hematomas   Bleeding within the substance of the brain.

Intussusception   Telescoping of a portion of the bowel into an adjacent segment of bowel; occurs most often in children under the age of 2 years as a result of peristaltic movement.

Ipecac (syrup of ipecac)   A syrup used to induce vomiting.

Iris   Pigmented circular muscular ring surrounding the pupil that controls the amount of light that enters the eye by constricting or dilating.

Irregularly irregular   ECG rhythms that have no predictable pattern of complexes.

Irritant gases   Gases that cause bronchoconstriction and inflammatory damage to the airway.

Ischemia   Insufficient blood supply to an area.

Ischemic chest pain   Characteristic pain resulting from inadequate blood supply to the myocardium.

Ischium   The portion of the pelvic bone between the ilium and pubic bone.

Jaundice   A yellowing of the skin and/or sclerae of the eyes caused by a buildup of bilirubin in the blood.

Jejunum   The second section of the small intestine which connects the duodenum to the ileum.

Jugular vein   Major vein of the neck, which travels down through the neck just lateral to the carotid arteries.

Kendrick extrication device   A semirigid device used to immobilize and extricate automobile accident victims found in the sitting position.

Keratin   Protein in the epidermis partially responsible for the skin's impermeable barrier.

Ketoacidosis   Metabolic acidosis associated with an excess of ketones in the blood; often associated with diabetes.

Ketoacids   Acids that develop from the breakdown products of fats; include fatty acids.

Kidney stone   Solid particle cystallized out of the urine that may become lodged within the urinary system (kidneys, ureters, bladder, or urethra), causing pain and bleeding.

Kidneys   Pair of organs responsible for filtering liquid waste from the blood and maintaining a proper fluid and electrolyte balance.

Kiesselbach's plexus   Area of the nasal septum within 2 inches of the tip of the nose, where 90% of all nosebleeds occur.

Kussmaul's respirations   A deep and (usually) rapid pattern of respirations used to blow off carbon dioxide as a compensatory response to diabetic ketoacidosis.

Laceration   Tear or cut in the skin or other soft tissues.

Lacrimal glands   Glands responsible for the production and secretion of tears.

Laryngeal edema   Swelling of the larynx and surrounding tissues.

Laryngoscope   A plastic or metal device used to visualize the vocal cords in order to insert an endotracheal tube.

Larynx   Voice box; structure formed by cartilage, bone, and ligaments, which contains the vocal cords.

Lasix (furosemide)   Diuretic (increases the secretion of urine) used to treat congestive heart failure.

Lateral   Toward the side of the body.

Hydraulic jack spreader   A manual pneumatic pump device used for lifting, pulling, and spreading metal during the extrication process.

Hydrocarbons   Molecules made up predominantly of carbon and hydrogen. Materials containing hydrocarbons include gasoline, kerosene, cleaning fluids, and spot removers.

Hydrofluoric acid   An acid used in industry and that is present in grout cleaners.

Hydrogen sulfide   A toxic gas used in industries, such as petroleum and rubber processing.

Hyperbaric chamber   A pressurized chamber used in the treatment of diving-related injuries or inhalation of toxic gases, especially carbon monoxide.

Hypercarbia   Excessive level of carbon dioxide in the bloodstream.

Hypersensitivity   A state of increased sensitivity to stimuli, e.g., allergy to bee stings.

Hypertension   High blood pressure.

Hyperventilation   Increased minute volume due to increased respiratory rate and/or depth.

Hyperventilation syndrome   Common respiratory problem usually precipitated by some emotional event that causes a patient to override the normal stimulus for respiratory rate and volume.

Hypoglycemia   An abnormally low blood sugar level.

Hypothermia (low body temperature)   Abnormally low body temperature, which may be caused by exposure to environmental extremes or physiologic factors that affect heat production or heat loss mechanisms.

Hypoventilation   Decreased minute volume. May be caused by hypoxia, drug overdose, brain injury, stroke, or any other problem that affects brain function.

Hypovolemic shock   Shock resulting from low blood volume caused by hemorrhage, burns, metabolic disorders, or other causes of loss of body fluid.

Hypoxia   Oxygen deficiency.

Hypoxic drive   Condition found in COPD where patients become insensitive to an increase in carbon dioxide in the blood, so that only a decrease in oxygen will stimulate respiration.

Hysterectomy   Surgical removal of the uterus.

Hysteria   An emotional state characterized by excitable responses, including laughing, crying, or screaming, and sometimes by physical symptoms.

Ileocecal junction   Area of connection between the small and large intestines.

Ileum   End segment of the small intestine that connects with the large intestine at the ileocecal junction.

Ilium   The uppermost portion of the pelvic bone that is palpable at the hip region.

Immunity   The state of being immune to or protected from disease.

Immunization   The process of becoming immune to a particular disease.

Impacted fractures   Fractures caused by strong forces that drive bone fragments firmly together.

Implied consent   A type of patient consent in situations where verbal or authorized consent is not possible. This may include unconscious patients, incompetent patients, or severely injured minors whose parents are not immediately available.

Incarcerated hernia   Entrapment of the herniated segment of bowel outside of the peritoneal cavity, leading to loss of blood flow to the area.

Incomplete abortion   Passing some but not all of the products of conception.

Increased intracranial pressure   Increased pressure within the cranium that can lead to herniation (displacement of the brain through the foramen magnum) and brain damage.

Incubation period   The period of time between contact with an infectious agent and occurrence of signs and symptoms of infection.

Indirect contact transmission   Personal contact of the susceptible host with a contaminated intermediate object such as instruments, dressings, or other infective material.

Induced abortion   A voluntary termination of a pregnancy performed by a physician; may also be called an *elective abortion*.

Inevitable abortion   Cramps and vaginal bleeding during pregnancy with dilatation of the cervix.

Infection control   The practice of common-sense actions to block spread of infectious agents.

Inferior   Toward the feet.

Informed consent   A type of patient consent where the patient is made aware of the benefits and consequences of a physician's or health care provider's treatment.

Inguinal hernia   Most common form of hernia; introduction of the intestine into the inguinal canal, sometimes down into the scrotum.

Gaining access   The part of the extrication process where the rescuers gain entry to trapped victims.

Gallbladder   Storage organ in the right upper quadrant beneath the liver that stores and concentrates bile.

Gangrene   Death of tissue due to poor blood supply.

Gastric distention   Distention of the stomach due to accumulation of air.

Gastric lavage   The insertion of a large oral gastric tube into the stomach to remove gastric contents; "pumping the stomach."

Gastritis   Inflammation of the stomach.

Gastroenteritis   Infectious condition that causes both vomiting and diarrhea.

Gauze roller bandage   Cotton and relatively non-elastic roller bandage that comes in various widths. It is most commonly used for extremity and head dressing applications.

Glasgow Coma Scale   A standardized approach to evaluating neurologic function, utilizing eye opening, verbal response, and motor ability.

Glaucoma   Disease of the eye caused by an obstruction to drainage of the aqueous humor, with a resultant buildup of pressure in the eye.

Glucagon   A substance secreted from the pancreas that can cause stored forms of glucose to be released and glucose to be synthesized from other molecules.

Glucose   A sugar molecule (a type of carbohydrate) in a form that is used by the cells for energy.

Glycogen   A stored form of glucose (made of multiple glucose molecules).

Good Samaritan Laws   Specific laws designed to protect the private citizen who is functioning in a nonprofessional capacity and without an expectation of remuneration.

Grand mal seizure   A convulsion that involves three phases: the *tonic* phase, during which there is a sustained contraction of all voluntary muscles; the *clonic* phase, characterized by intermittent contractions and relaxations of the skeletal muscles; and the *postictal* phase, where the patient shows a depressed level of consciousness and confusion.

Greenstick fractures   Incomplete fractures that occur in children where one side of the fractured bone remains intact.

Guarding   Reflex contraction of the musculature overlying an injury or inflammation of the peritoneum.

Gurgling   A sound created by air moving through fluid in the airway.

Hand winch or come along   A hand-operated leverage device used for lifting, pulling, and spreading metal during the extrication process.

Hematemesis   Vomiting blood.

Hematoma   Collection of blood beneath the skin.

Hematuria   Blood in the urine.

Hemoglobin   An oxygen-binding protein found in red blood cells. Responsible for 98% of oxygen transport in the circulatory system.

Hemoptysis   Coughing up blood.

Hemorrhage   Profuse bleeding.

Hemorrhoids   Ballooning of the veins that drain the rectal area.

Hemothorax   Bleeding within the pleural cavity.

Hepatic coma   Coma brought on by a buildup of toxins in the blood secondary to liver failure.

Hepatitis   An infection of the liver caused by one of three different types of viruses: *hepatitis A*—spread by oral–fecal routes and is sometimes called infectious hepatitis; *hepatitis B*—spread by contact with blood and body fluids; *non-A, non-B type*—thought to be spread in a manner similar to hepatitis B.

Hernia   Protrusion of a structure outside of the cavity that usually contains it.

Herniation (brain)   A condition where the substance of the brain is forced through the foramen magnum due to an expanding lesion in the cranium.

Heroin   An opiate derivative drug, commonly abused, that causes central nervous system depression.

Herpes zoster (shingles)   A localized viral infection along a dermatome (nerve) presenting first as pain, then as pustules.

Histamine   A substance normally present in the body that is released during an anaphylactic reaction and that can cause increased cell permeability, edema, increased gastric secretion, dilation of capillaries, and bronchial constriction.

History   Information about the patient, including the chief complaint, history of the present illness, past medical history, medications, and allergies, gathered during a systematic interview with the patient or a significant other.

Homeostasis   The tendency of an organism to maintain a steady internal environment.

Hormones   Chemicals that are secreted by glands and that influence body functions.

Humerus   The bone of the upper arm.

INDEX

NOTE:

Page numbers in italics refer to illustrations;
page numbers followed by "t" refer to tables.